STOELTING'S
ANESTHESIA AND CO-EXISTING DISEASE

STOELTING'S
ANESTHESIA AND CO-EXISTING DISEASE

Roberta L. Hines, MD
Nicholas M. Greene Professor and Chairman
Department of Anesthesiology
Yale University School of Medicine
Chief of Anesthesiology
Yale-New Haven Hospital
New Haven, Connecticut

Katherine E. Marschall, MD, LLD (honoris causa)
Anesthesiologist–retired
New Haven, Connecticut

Seventh Edition

ELSEVIER

ELSEVIER

1600 John F. Kennedy Blvd.
Ste 1800
Philadelphia, PA 19103-2899

STOELTING'S ANESTHESIA AND CO-EXISTING
DISEASE, SEVENTH EDITION

ISBN: 978-0-323-40137-1

Notices

Previous editions copyrighted 2012, 2008, 2002, 1993, 1988, 1983.

Library of Congress Cataloging-in-Publication Data
Names: Hines, Roberta L., editor. | Marschall, Katherine E., editor.
Title: Stoelting's anesthesia and co-existing disease / edited by Roberta L.
 Hines, Katherine E. Marschall.
Other titles: Anesthesia and co-existing disease
Description: Seventh edition. | Philadelphia, PA : Elsevier, [2018] |
 Includes bibliographical references and index.
Identifiers: LCCN 2017000203 | ISBN 9780323401371 (hardcover : alk. paper)
Subjects: | MESH: Anesthesia--adverse effects | Anesthesia--methods |
 Comorbidity | Anesthetics--adverse effects | Intraoperative Complications
Classification: LCC RD82.5 | NLM WO 245 | DDC 617.9/6041--dc23
LC record available at https://lccn.loc.gov/2017000203

Executive Content Strategist: Dolores Meloni
Content Development Manager: Lucia Gunzel
Publishing Services Manager: Catherine Jackson
Senior Project Manager: Daniel Fitzgerald
Designer: Paula Catalano

Printed in China.

Last digit is the print number: 9   8   7   6   5   4   3   2   1

Preface

In 1983 the first edition of *Anesthesia and Co-Existing Disease* by Drs. Robert K. Stoelting and Stephen F. Dierdorf was published with the stated goal "to provide a concise description of the pathophysiology of disease states and their medical management that is relevant to the care of the patient in the perioperative period." Since then, five more editions have been published. The last two editions were published under our editorial leadership.

This seventh edition of *Anesthesia and Co-Existing Disease* continues the tradition of presenting new and updated medical information to the anesthesiology community. New chapters include those on sleep-disordered breathing and critical care medicine. The chapters on geriatric medicine and cancer medicine have major updates, but all chapters contain new information, refer to major medical society guidelines and recommendations that affect the practice of perioperative medicine, and contain many tables, figures, illustrations, and photographs to aid in understanding key concepts. We hope that our readers will continue to find this book relevant to the care of the patient in the perioperative period.

Roberta L. Hines, MD
Katherine E. Marschall, MD

Contributors

Shamsuddin Akhtar, MBBS
Associate Professor of Anesthesiology
Yale University School of Medicine
New Haven, Connecticut
Chapter 5: Ischemic Heart Disease
Chapter 16: Diseases of Aging

Ferne Braveman, MD
Professor of Anesthesiology and of Obstetrics,
Gynecology and Reproductive Sciences
Division Chief
Anesthesiology
Vice Chair Administrative Affairs
Director, Obstetrics & Gynecology Anesthesiology
Yale University School of Medicine
New Haven, Connecticut
Chapter 31: Pregnancy-Associated Diseases

Tricia Brentjens, MD
Associate Professor of Anesthesiology
Columbia University Medical Center
New York, New York
Chapter 17: Diseases of the Liver and Biliary Tract

Jean G. Charchaflieh, MD, MPH, DrPH
Associate Professor of Anesthesiology
Yale University School of Medicine
New Haven, Connecticut
Chapter 1: Sleep-Related Breathing Disorders

Nikhil Chawla, MBBS
Assistant Professor of Anesthesiology
Yale University School of Medicine
New Haven, Connecticut
Chapter 12: Vascular Disease

Ranjit Deshpande, MD, BS
Assistant Professor of Anesthesiology
Yale University School of Medicine
Director, Liver Transplant Anesthesiology
Yale-New Haven Hospital
New Haven, Connecticut
Chapter 3: Restrictive Respiratory
Diseases and Lung Transplantation

Michelle W. Diu, MD
Department of Anesthesiology
Children's Hospital and Medical Center
Assistant Professor of Anesthesiology
University of Nebraska College of Medicine
Omaha, Nebraska
Chapter 30: Pediatric Diseases

Manuel Fontes, MD
Professor of Anesthesiology and Critical Care
Medicine
Yale University School of Medicine
New Haven, Connecticut
Chapter 9: Systemic and Pulmonary
Arterial Hypertension

Loreta Grecu, MD
Associate Professor of Anesthesiology
University of New York at Stony Brook
New York, New York
Chapter 12: Vascular Disease

Paul M. Heerdt, MD, PhD
Professor of Anesthesiology
Yale University School of Medicine
New Haven, Connecticut
Chapter 9: Systemic and Pulmonary
Arterial Hypertension

Antonio Hernandez Conte, MD, MBA
Associate Professor of Anesthesiology
Cedars-Sinai Medical Center
Los Angeles, California
Chapter 26: Infectious Diseases

Adriana Herrera, MD
Assistant Professor of Anesthesiology
Yale University School of Medicine
New Haven, Connecticut
Chapter 6: Valvular Heart Disease

Roberta L. Hines, MD
Nicholas M. Greene Professor and Chairman
Department of Anesthesiology
Yale University School of Medicine
Chief of Anesthesiology
Yale-New Haven Hospital
New Haven, Connecticut
*Chapter 29: Psychiatric Disease,
Substance Abuse, and Drug Overdose*

Natalie F. Holt, MD, MPH
Assistant Professor of Anesthesiology
Yale University School of Medicine
New Haven, Connecticut
Associate Director of Anesthesiology
VA Connecticut Healthcare System
West Haven, Connecticut
Chapter 22: Renal Disease
Chapter 27: Diseases Related to Immune System Dysfunction
Chapter 28: Cancer

Viji Kurup, MBBS
Associate Professor of Anesthesiology
Yale University School of Medicine
New Haven, Connecticut
Chapter 2: Obstructive Respiratory Diseases
*Chapter 3: Restrictive Respiratory Diseases and Lung
Transplantation*

William L. Lanier, Jr., MD
Professor of Anesthesiology
Mayo Clinic
Rochester, Minnesota
Chapter 13: Diseases Affecting the Brain
Chapter 14: Spinal Cord Disorders
*Chapter 15: Diseases of the Autonomic and Peripheral
Nervous Systems*

Linda L. Maerz, MD
Associate Professor of Surgery and Anesthesiology
Yale University School of Medicine
New Haven, Connecticut
Chapter 4: Critical Illness

Adnan Malik, MD
Assistant Professor of Anesthesiology
Yale University School of Medicine
New Haven, Connecticut
Chapter 10: Heart Failure and Cardiomyopathies

Thomas J. Mancuso, MD
Senior Associate in Anesthesiology
Boston Children's Hospital
Associate Professor of Anesthesiology
Harvard Medical School
Boston, Massachusetts
Chapter 30: Pediatric Diseases

Luiz Maracaja, MD
Assistant Professor of Anesthesiology
University of Texas Health Science Center in San Antonio
San Antonio, Texas
Chapter 11: Pericardial Disease and Cardiac Trauma

Katherine E. Marschall, MD, LLD (honoris causa)
Anesthesiologist–retired
New Haven, Connecticut
Chapter 25: Skin and Musculoskeletal Diseases
*Chapter 29: Psychiatric Disease, Substance Abuse, and Drug
Overdose*

Veronica Matei, MD
Assistant Professor of Anesthesiology
Yale University School of Medicine
New Haven, Connecticut
*Chapter 20: Nutritional Diseases:
Obesity and Malnutrition*

Bryan G. Maxwell, MD, MPH
Anesthesiologist
Randall Children's Hospital
Portland, Oregon
Chapter 7: Congenital Heart Disease

Raj K. Modak, MD
Associate Professor
Director of Cardiac Anesthesia
Henry Ford Medical Group
Henry Ford Hospital
Detroit, Michigan
Chapter 11: Pericardial Disease and Cardiac Trauma

Tori Myslajek, MD
Assistant Professor of Anesthesiology
Yale University School of Medicine
New Haven, Connecticut
Chapter 18: Diseases of the Gastrointestinal System

Adriana D. Oprea, MD
Assistant Professor of Anesthesiology
Yale University School of Medicine
New Haven, Connecticut
Chapter 24: Hematologic Disorders

Jeffrey J. Pasternak, MS, MD
Associate Professor of Anesthesiology
Mayo Clinic
Rochester, Minnesota
Chapter 13: Diseases Affecting the Brain
Chapter 14: Spinal Cord Disorders
Chapter 15: Diseases of the Autonomic and Peripheral Nervous Systems

Wanda M. Popescu, MD
Associate Professor of Anesthesiology
Yale University School of Medicine
New Haven, Connecticut
Chapter 10: Heart Failure and Cardiomyopathies
Chapter 20: Nutritional Diseases: Obesity and Malnutrition

Stanley H. Rosenbaum, MA, MD
Professor of Anesthesiology, Internal Medicine & Surgery
Yale University School of Medicine
New Haven, Connecticut
Chapter 4: Critical Illness

Robert B. Schonberger, MD, MA
Assistant Professor of Anesthesiology
Yale University School of Medicine
New Haven, Connecticut
Chapter 21: Fluid, Electrolyte, and Acid-Base Disorders

Denis Snegovskikh, MD
Attending Anesthesiologist
Anesthesia Associates of Willimantic, CT
Willimantic, Connecticut
Chapter 31: Pregnancy-Associated Diseases

Jochen Steppan, MD, DESA
Assistant Professor of Anesthesiology and Critical Care Medicine
Johns Hopkins University School of Medicine
Baltimore, Maryland
Chapter 7: Congenital Heart Disease

Hossam Tantawy, MBChB
Assistant Professor of Anesthesiology and Trauma Surgery
Yale University School of Medicine
New Haven, Connecticut
Chapter 18: Diseases of the Gastrointestinal System
Chapter 19: Inborn Errors of Metabolism

Jing Tao, MD
Assistant Professor of Anesthesiology
Yale University School of Medicine
New Haven, Connecticut
Chapter 2: Obstructive Respiratory Diseases
Chapter 19: Inborn Errors of Metabolism

Russell T. Wall, III, MD
Chair, Department of Anesthesiology and Perioperative Care
MedStar Georgetown University Hospital
Professor of Anesthesiology and Pharmacology
Georgetown University School of Medicine
Washington, DC
Chapter 23: Endocrine Disease

Zachary Walton, MD, PhD
Attending Anesthesiologist
Anesthesia Associates of Willimantic, CT
Willimantic, Connecticut
Chapter 31: Pregnancy-Associated Diseases

Kelley Teed Watson, MD
Anesthesiologist
Anesthesiology of Greenwood, Inc.
Greenwood, South Carolina
Chapter 8: Abnormalities of Cardiac Conduction and Cardiac Rhythm

Christopher A.J. Webb, MD
Assistant Professor of Anesthesiology
Columbia University Medical Center
New York, New York
Chapter 17: Diseases of the Liver and Biliary Tract

Paul David Weyker, MD
Assistant Professor of Anesthesiology
Columbia University Medical Center
New York, New York
Chapter 17: Diseases of the Liver and Biliary Tract

Contents

Sleep-Related Breathing Disorders

JEAN G. CHARCHAFLIEH

Scientific study of sleep in humans dates back only about a century, whereas the development of sleep medicine as a medical discipline dates back only about 50 years. Rapid eye movement (REM) sleep was first described in cats in 1957. The genetic mutation of narcolepsy was first described in dogs in 1999. The *clock gene* mutation was first described in mice in 2005, demonstrating that a mutation in the circadian system clock gene disturbed not only the sleep cycle but also energy balance, resulting in hyperphagia, hyperlipidemia, hyperglycemia, hypoinsulinemia, obesity, metabolic syndrome, and hepatic dysfunction. The term *sleep apnea syndrome* was first

introduced in 1975. Prior to that the term *Pickwickian syndrome* was used. In 1974 one of the first cases of what would be considered *obstructive sleep apnea* (OSA) was described as a case of periodic nocturnal upper airway obstruction in an obese patient with normal control of breathing, a positional increase in upper airway resistance, and associated dysrhythmias (bradycardia and asystole) that resolved with tracheostomy, which was the treatment of choice at that time. In 1981 the treatment of OSA was advanced by the understanding of its pathophysiology and by demonstrating the therapeutic efficacy of continuous positive airway pressure (CPAP) in a patient with severe OSA who was scheduled for tracheostomy but refused the surgery and elected to undergo the "experimental" therapy with CPAP.

PHYSIOLOGY OF SLEEP

Our current understanding of the wake/sleep state maintains that wakefulness is accomplished by a brainstem neuronal pathway known as the *ascending reticular activating system* (ARAS), which involves several neurotransmitters including acetylcholine, dopamine, norepinephrine, histamine, and 5-hydroxytryptamine. Sleep is maintained by inhibition of the ARAS via a hypothalamic nucleus known as the *ventrolateral preoptic* (VLPO) *nucleus.* This involves two neurotransmitters: γ-aminobutyric acid (GABA) and galanin. There is reciprocal inhibition between the ARAS and the VLPO nucleus. The neurotransmitter adenosine promotes sleep by inhibiting cholinergic ARAS neurons and activating VLPO neurons. The timing and duration of sleep are influenced by three factors: (1) sleep homeostasis, which involves buildup of the inhibitory neurotransmitter adenosine during wakefulness, (2) circadian homeostasis, which is regulated by a hypothalamic nucleus that provides GABAergic input to the pineal gland, and (3) environmental *zeitgebers* ("time-givers"), which include light, temperature, eating, body position, and environmental stimulation. Light is the most important zeitgeber. It provides input to the hypothalamus to suppress release of melatonin from the pineal gland, whereas darkness stimulates the release of melatonin, also known as "the hormone of darkness." In normal circadian rhythm, time of onset of release of melatonin under dim light conditions occurs about 2 hours before sleep onset. Temperature is another important zeitgeber. Falling core body temperature promotes falling to sleep, whereas rising body temperature promotes awakening. Caffeine inhibits sleep by blocking the effects of adenosine.

Sleep Stages

Electroencephalography (EEG) is an important method of studying wakefulness and sleep and defining sleep stages. The electrical activity of the brain can be categorized into three states: wakefulness, REM sleep, and non-REM (NREM) sleep. The latter can be further categorized into three stages: N1, N2, and N3, according to the progressive decrease in frequency and increase in amplitude of EEG waveforms. Muscle tone as measured by electromyography (EMG) is normal during wakefulness, decreased during NREM sleep, and abolished during REM sleep. In terms of vegetative functions and energy expenditures, REM sleep matches or exceeds that in awake levels and has been described as a state of an active brain in a paralyzed body.

Sleep occurs in all stages of human life, including in utero, but sleep duration and stage proportions differ according to age. Sleep stages are not equally distributed during the sleep period. Stage N3, also known as *slow wave sleep,* occurs during the first third of the night. REM sleep periods increase in duration and intensity as sleep progresses. REM sleep is defined by three electrical findings: (1) on EEG: low amplitude, mixed frequency waves; (2) on electromyography: low or absent muscle tone (atonia); and (3) on electrooculogram (EOG): rapid eye movements. *Tonic REM sleep* refers to REM sleep–associated muscle atonia. *Phasic REM sleep* refers, in addition to atonia, to phasic bursts of rapid eye movements, muscle twitches, sympathetic activation, and dreaming that is likely to be recalled upon awakening, unlike NREM dreaming, which is less likely to be recalled.

Physiologic Differences Between NREM and REM Sleep

NREM sleep *maintains homeostasis* and autonomic stability at low energy levels—that is, with a low basic metabolic rate and a decreased heart rate, cardiac output, and blood pressure. Hormonal secretion is maintained.

REM is considered a more primitive state of sleep. It *impairs homeostasis* and disrupts autonomic stability. REM-induced autonomic instability manifests as irregularity in heart rate, cardiac output, blood pressure, and tidal volume and suppression of cardiac and respiratory chemoreceptor and baroreceptor reflexes. REM sleep is associated with skeletal muscle *atonia* affecting all skeletal muscles including upper airway dilator muscles and intercostal muscles but with significant sparing of the diaphragm.

Respiratory Control During Wakefulness and Sleep

The brainstem respiratory control center consists of two groups of neurons: a dorsal respiratory group that promotes inspiration and a ventral respiratory group that functions as the respiratory pacing center. The ventral group contains μ-opioid receptors that inhibit respiration when they are activated by endogenous or exogenous opioids. The respiratory control center sends output to the phrenic nerve and the hypoglossal nerve and receives input from three areas of the body: (1) electrical input from the forebrain regarding sleep/wake state, sleep stage, and voluntary control of breathing; (2) chemical input from peripheral and central chemoreceptors regarding pH, $Paco_2$, and Pao_2; and (3) input via the vagus nerve from mechanoreceptors in the lungs and airway. REM sleep decreases all three aspects of breathing control to a greater extent than NREM sleep.

The transition from wakefulness to sleep can be associated with breathing irregularity, including periodic breathing and sleep-onset apnea. After this transition, sleep is usually associated with an increase in airway resistance and $Paco_2$ (2–8 mm Hg) and a decrease in Pao_2 (3–10 mm Hg), chemosensitivity, CO_2 production (10%–15%), tidal volume, and minute ventilation.

Effects of Aging and Disease on Sleep

Aging *decreases* the percentage of sleep in its slow wave portion and in the REM portion and the total time in bed during which one is asleep (also known as *sleep efficiency*). Aging *increases* the time it takes to fall asleep (also known as *sleep latency*) and the incidence of daytime napping.

Disease states can also disrupt sleep quality and quantity and produce vicious cycles in which sleep disruption and the disease state exacerbate each other until the cycle is broken by treating the disease or the sleep disruption or both. Both acute pain (including postoperative pain) and chronic pain disorders (e.g., fibromyalgia, chronic fatigue syndrome) also disrupt the quality and quantity of sleep. Clinically, fibromyalgia and chronic fatigue syndrome manifest with insomnia, nonrefreshing sleep, excessive daytime sleepiness, and fatigue.

Cardiovascular System Physiology During NREM and REM Sleep

NREM sleep increases vagal and baroreceptor control of the cardiovascular system and results in sinus dysrhythmia through the coupling of respiratory activity and cardiorespiratory centers in the brain. REM sleep–induced loss of homeostasis results in irregularity and periodic surges in heart rate, blood pressure, and cardiac output, which can present clinical risk in patients with cardiopulmonary disease or those with underdeveloped cardiorespiratory systems, such as infants (which increases the risk of sudden infant death syndrome). Phasic REM sleep is associated with phasic increases in sympathetic activity, resulting in heart rate and blood pressure surges without a corresponding increase in coronary blood flow. This can result in *nocturnal angina* and nocturnal myocardial infarction. Tonic REM sleep is associated with increased parasympathetic activity, resulting in abrupt decreases in heart rate, including pauses, which in patients with a congenital long QT syndrome or Brugada syndrome can trigger multifocal ventricular tachycardia or even sudden unexplained nocturnal death.

Cerebral Blood Flow, Spinal Cord Blood Flow, and Epileptogenicity During NREM and REM Sleep

NREM sleep is associated with a decrease in cerebral blood flow and spinal cord blood flow, with maintenance of autoregulation. REM sleep is associated with regional increases in cerebral blood flow and impaired autoregulation. Phasic REM sleep periods increase in intensity and duration toward early morning, with resulting early morning surges in blood pressure that can lead to an increased risk of stroke in the early morning hours. OSA is also associated with early morning surges in blood pressure, increased vascular reactivity to Pco_2, and increased intracranial pressure that can result in additional risk of early morning stroke.

NREM sleep is more epileptogenic than both wakefulness and REM sleep because of increased thalamocortical synaptic synchrony and neuronal hyperpolarization, which promote seizure propagation. REM sleep is least epileptogenic because of decreases in thalamocortical synaptic synchrony and interhemispheric neuronal connectivity and the presence of REM-induced muscle atonia.

Effects of Sleep on Energy Balance and Metabolism

Sleep and sleep deprivation are associated with hormonal changes that affect energy metabolism and other endocrine functions. Hormonal release can be regulated by sleep homeostasis, circadian rhythms, or both. There are sleep deprivation–related postprandial increases in both insulin and glucose to levels greater than would occur without sleep deprivation, which indicates insulin resistance. This might explain the association between sleep deprivation and insulin resistance and diabetes mellitus. Sleep deprivation–related thyroid stimulating hormone peak release indicates that sleep deprivation is a hypermetabolic state.

Effects of Drugs on Sleep

Drugs that affect the central nervous system, autonomic nervous system, or immune system may affect sleep architecture and cause sleep disorders. Many drugs are capable of these changes, and some are listed in Table 1.1. Alcohol, barbiturates, benzodiazepines, nonbenzodiazepine GABA receptor agonists such as zolpidem, opioids, acetylcholinesterase inhibitors such as donepezil (which is used to treat Alzheimer's disease), antiepileptic drugs, adrenergic α_1-agonists such as prazosin, adrenergic α_2-agonists such as clonidine, β-blockers such as propranolol, β-agonists such as albuterol, nonsteroidal antiinflammatory drugs, corticosteroids, pseudoephedrine, theophylline, diphenhydramine, tricyclic antidepressants, monoamine oxidase inhibitors, selective serotonin reuptake inhibitors, serotonin and norepinephrine reuptake inhibitors, serotonin antagonist and reuptake inhibitors, dopamine and norepinephrine reuptake inhibitors, antimigraine drugs (triptans), and statins can all cause sleep disruption and sleep disorders.

SPECIFIC SLEEP DISORDERS

Specific sleep disorders are disorders that manifest predominantly but not exclusively with sleep manifestations. They include disorders that manifest primarily as: (1) decreased sleep (insomnia), which is the most common type of sleep disorder, (2) increased sleep (hypersomnias), (3) abnormal sleep behavior (parasomnias), (4) disruptions of circadian rhythm, and (5) sleep-induced exacerbations of certain pathophysiologic problems such as sleep-related movement disorders and sleep-related breathing disorders (SRBDs).

Narcolepsy represents the loss of boundaries between the three distinct states of wakefulness, NREM sleep, and REM sleep. *Parasomnias* represent admixtures of wakefulness with either NREM sleep or REM sleep. The admixture of wakefulness with NREM sleep results in NREM parasomnias that include confusional arousal, sleep terror, and sleep acting

TABLE 1.1	Effects of Drugs on Sleep Architecture and Sleep Disorders		
Drug	Effect on REM Sleep	Effect on Slow Wave Sleep	Effect on Sleep Disorder
Alcohol	↓		↑ Snoring and exacerbation of SRBD
Barbiturates	↓		
Benzodiazepines		↓	
Zolpidem			↑ NREM parasomnia
Opioids	↑ At high doses	↓	↑ Hypoxia with OSA
Prazosin	↑		Resolves nightmares
Clonidine			Induces nightmares
β-Blockers			↑ Daytime sleepiness, Induce nightmares
Corticosteroids			Insomnia
			Bizarre dreams
Caffeine		↓	
Amphetamine	↓	↓	Bruxism
Tricyclic antidepressants	↓		↑ Periodic limb movements, restless legs syndrome (RLS)
MAOIs	↓ To almost zero		
SSRIs	↓		↑ Periodic limb movements, RLS ↑ REM sleep without atonia
SNRIs			↑ Periodic limb movements, RLS REM sleep behavior disorder
Trazodone		↑	
Mirtazapine			↑ Periodic limb movements, RLS
Bupropion	↑		↓ Periodic limb movements
Antipsychotics		↓	↑ Periodic limb movements, RLS
Lithium	↓	↑	Sleep walking
Statins			Insomnia Sleep disruption

MAOIs, Monoamine oxidase inhibitors; *NREM,* non-REM sleep; *OSA,* obstructive sleep apnea; *REM,* rapid eye movement sleep; *SNRIs,* serotonin and norepinephrine reuptake inhibitors; *SRBD,* sleep-related breathing disorder; *SSRIs,* selective serotonin reuptake inhibitors.

(talking, walking, cooking, or eating). REM parasomnias include REM nightmares and REM sleep behavior disorder, which is REM sleep *without* the usual atonia, which allows physical enactment of dreams during REM sleep and can result in injury to self or others.

PATHOGENESIS OF SLEEP-RELATED BREATHING DISORDERS

Pathogenesis of Obstructive Sleep Apnea

The hallmark of OSA is sleep-induced and arousal-relieved upper airway obstruction. The pathogenesis of this airway obstruction is not fully understood. Comorbid conditions that are associated with increased prevalence rates for OSA include hypertension, coronary artery disease, myocardial infarction, congestive heart failure, atrial fibrillation, stroke, type 2 diabetes mellitus, nonalcoholic steatohepatitis (NASH), polycystic ovarian syndrome, Graves disease, hypothyroidism, and acromegaly. *Predisposing factors* include genetic inheritance, non-Caucasian race, upper airway narrowing, obesity, male gender, menopause, use of sedative drugs and alcohol, and cigarette smoking. Direct physiologic mechanisms involved in the pathogenesis of OSA include (1) anatomic and functional upper airway obstruction, (2) a decreased respiratory-related arousal response, and (3) instability of the ventilatory response to chemical stimuli.

Narrowing of the Upper Airway

Airway obstruction can be due to anatomic narrowing or to functional collapse of the airway or to both factors. The most common sites of upper airway obstruction are the retropalatal and retroglossal regions of the oropharynx. Obstruction can be due to bony craniofacial abnormalities or, more commonly, excess soft tissue, such as thick parapharyngeal fat pads or enlarged tonsils. Children have many reasons for anatomic upper airway narrowing, including the very common enlargement of tonsils and adenoids, as well as the much less common congenital airway anomalies. The latter include Pierre-Robin syndrome, Down syndrome, achondroplasia, Prader-Willi syndrome, Klippel-Feil syndrome, Arnold-Chiari malformation type II, maxillary hypoplasia, micrognathia, retrognathia, tracheomalacia, and laryngomalacia.

In adults, acromegaly, thyroid enlargement, and hypothyroidism are additional causes of narrowing of the upper airway. Mallampati developed a clinical classification of oropharyngeal capacity to predict difficult tracheal intubation, and this was later found useful in predicting the risk of OSA as well. For every 1-point increase in the Mallampati score, the odds ratio for OSA is increased by 2.5.

Graves disease can cause OSA by extraluminal compression of the upper airway, and thyroid mass lesions can cause snoring, stridor, or sleep apnea. Toxic goiter may "burn out," leading to hypothyroidism, which increases the risk of OSA by inducing obesity and macroglossia. Acromegaly increases the risk of OSA by maxillofacial skeletal changes, upper airway soft tissue enlargement (including tongue size), and obesity.

Functional collapse of the upper airway occurs when forces that can collapse the upper airway overcome the forces that can dilate the upper airway. *Collapsing forces* consist of intraluminal negative inspiratory pressure and extraluminal positive pressure. *Dilating forces* consist of pharyngeal dilating muscle tone and longitudinal traction on the upper airway by an increased lung volume, so-called tracheal tug. Excessive inspiratory efforts to help overcome upper airway obstruction can lead to even more upper airway collapse by generating excessive negative intraluminal pressure. The supine position enhances airway obstruction by increasing the effect of extraluminal positive pressure against the pharynx, which lacks any bony support. Sleep, particularly REM sleep, decreases muscle tone generally, including that of the upper airway, and decreases lung volume, which decreases the tracheal tug effect. Patients with OSA have a more collapsible upper airway with altered neuromuscular control. Their upper airway muscles have inflammatory infiltrates and denervation changes, which might decrease their ability to dilate the airway during sleep.

The respiratory-related arousal response is stimulated by (1) hypercapnia, (2) hypoxia, (3) upper airway obstruction, and (4) the work of breathing, which is the most reliable stimulator of arousal.

Obesity

Obesity is a risk factor for OSA in all age groups. A *10% increase* in body weight is associated with a 6-fold increase in the odds of having OSA and a *32% increase* in the apnea-hypopnea index. A *10% weight loss* is associated with a 26% *decrease* in the apnea-hypopnea index. Besides affecting the size of subcutaneous cervical fat, obesity could be associated with increased amounts of fat in the tongue and larger parapharyngeal fat pads.

Genetic Factors

Genes can affect the pathogenesis of OSA by influencing the regulation of sleep, breathing, energy metabolism, and craniofacial anatomy; certain alleles have been found to be associated with OSA. Heredity as a factor in OSA development is suggested by familial aggregation of cases of OSA.

Pathogenesis of Central Sleep Apnea

Central sleep apnea (CSA) refers to sleep apnea that is *not* associated with respiratory efforts during the apnea event. This *absence of respiratory effort* could be due to instability of neural control of respiration, weakness of respiratory muscles, or both. Instability of respiratory control may include increased, decreased, or oscillating respiratory drive.

Primary/Idiopathic Central Sleep Apnea

Primary/idiopathic CSA has an unknown cause and manifests as periodic breathing with a cycle length composed of apnea plus the subsequent hyperpnea. There is then an oscillation between hyperventilation and apnea. Increased chemosensitivity to P_{CO_2} predisposing to respiratory control system instability may be the underlying pathogenesis.

Secondary Central Sleep Apnea

The most common form of secondary CSA is narcotic-induced CSA, which is encountered in up to half of patients using opioids chronically. It can manifest either as periodic Biot's breathing or irregular ataxic breathing. The latter is usually associated with significant hypoxia and prolonged apnea.

Central Sleep Apnea With Cheyne-Stokes Breathing

CSA with Cheyne-Stokes breathing was the first form of a sleep-related breathing disorder to be described. In 1818 John Cheyne described the periodic nature of breathing in an obese patient who suffered from a stroke and heart failure. He described the patient as:

A.B., sixty years, of a sanguine temperament, circular chest, and full habit of body, for years had lived a very sedentary life, while he indulged habitually in the luxuries of the table….The patient suddenly developed palpitations and displayed signs of severe congestive heart failure. The only particularity in the last period of his illness, which lasted eight or nine days, was in the state of respiration. For several days his breathing was irregular; it would entirely cease for a quarter of a minute, then it would become perceptible, though very low, then by degrees it became heaving and quick, and then it would gradually cease again. This revolution in the state of his breathing occupied about a minute…this symptom, as occurring in its highest degree, I have only seen during a few weeks previous to the death of the patient.

Congestive heart failure, stroke, and atrial fibrillation are the three most common conditions during which CSA with Cheyne-Stokes breathing is encountered. It is postulated that a significant decrease in ejection fraction and consequent increase in circulation time is at least partially responsible for this condition. The pathophysiology of this form of periodic breathing is described in terms of its four cyclical components: hypopnea, apnea, hypoxia, and hyperventilation (Fig. 1.1).

Pathogenesis of Sleep-Related Hypoventilation Disorders

Sleep-related hypoventilation disorders can be primary or due to a comorbid illness. Primary forms are rare and include the obesity hypoventilation syndrome (OHS/

Pickwickian syndrome) and central alveolar hypoventilation syndrome/Ondine's curse. Comorbid forms are more common, since they are usually associated with (1) common respiratory diseases, such as chronic obstructive pulmonary disease (COPD) or the overlap syndrome (COPD plus OSA); (2) drug-induced respiratory depression; (3) neurologic disorders such as amyotrophic lateral sclerosis, spinal cord injury, or postpolio syndrome; (4) neuromuscular disorders; and (5) restrictive chest wall disorders such as kyphoscoliosis. The clinical features of OHS include: (1) marked obesity, (2) somnolence, (3) twitching, (4) cyanosis, (5) periodic respiration, (6) secondary polycythemia, (7) right ventricular hypertrophy, and (8) right ventricular failure/cor pulmonale. OHS is characterized by hypoventilation during wakefulness, which worsens in the supine position and during sleep.

Pathogenesis of Sleep-Related Hypoxemia Disorder

Sleep-related hypoxemia disorder is due to exacerbation of diurnal hypoxemia due to cardiopulmonary disease.

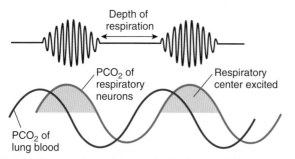

FIG. 1.1 Proposed underlying pathophysiology of Cheyne-Stokes breathing showing changing P_{CO_2} in the pulmonary blood *(red line)* and delayed changes in the P_{CO_2} of the fluids of the respiratory center *(blue line)*. (From Hall JE. Regulation of respiration. In: Hall JE, ed. *Guyton and Hall Textbook of Medical Physiology.* 13th ed. Philadelphia: Elsevier; 2016:539.)

PATHOPHYSIOLOGIC CONSEQUENCES OF SLEEP-RELATED BREATHING DISORDERS

Pathophysiologic Consequences of Obstructive Sleep Apnea

Cardiovascular Consequences (Table 1.2)

The pathophysiology of OSA is the result of three immediate events: apnea episodes, arousals, and increased respiratory effort. Direct and indirect effects of these events can interact and produce significant acute and chronic cardiac, neurologic, and metabolic morbidity and mortality.

Apneic and hypopneic episodes result in hypoxia, which can be prolonged and severe. OSA-induced hypoxia and reoxygenation cycles activate redox-sensitive genes, oxidative stress, inflammatory processes, the sympathetic nervous system, and the coagulation cascade, all of which can contribute to endothelial dysfunction and ultimately to systemic hypertension, pulmonary hypertension, atherosclerosis, right and left ventricular systolic and diastolic dysfunction, coronary artery disease, congestive heart failure, atrial fibrillation, stroke, and sudden cardiac death.

Arousal episodes lead to increased sympathetic system activity and decreased parasympathetic system activity, which results in increases in heart rate, left ventricular afterload, myocardial oxygen consumption, dysrhythmias, myocardial toxicity, and apoptosis. Arousal episodes lead to nonrestorative sleep and chronic sleep deprivation, which are also associated with increased sympathetic activity, inflammation, and a hypermetabolic state.

Increased inspiratory efforts can result in large swings in negative intrathoracic pressure, which are transmitted to the heart, lungs, and great vessels. The increase in transmural pressure in these structures can have multiple detrimental effects.

Swedish national data found that OSA is associated with an increased prevalence of coronary artery disease and that treatment of OSA reduces this risk. Untreated moderate to severe OSA is associated with an increased risk of repeat revascularization after percutaneous coronary intervention, and successful treatment of the OSA reduces this risk. OSA patients having coronary artery bypass surgery have an increased risk

TABLE 1.2	Cardiovascular Consequences of Obstructive Sleep Apnea		
Immediate results	Hypoxemia, hypercarbia	Arousal	Reduced pleural pressure
Intermediate-term clinical consequences	Decreased oxygen delivery Oxidative stress Inflammation Hypercoagulability Pulmonary vascular constriction	Sympathetic activation Parasympathetic inactivation	Increased transmural pressure on heart and great vessels
Long-term clinical consequences	Cardiac dysfunction Endothelial dysfunction Increased right ventricular afterload Right ventricular hypertrophy	Tachycardia Hypertension Increased left ventricular afterload Increased myocardial oxygen consumption Myocardial toxicity Dysrhythmias	Increased right and left ventricular afterload Dysrhythmias, Aortic dilatation Increased lung water

of major adverse perioperative cardiac and cerebrovascular events. They also have a greater risk of significant dysrhythmias and atrial fibrillation in this setting.

Neurologic Consequences

The EEG changes of chronic sleep deprivation include overall slowing of the EEG, a decrease in deeper stages of sleep, and a compensatory increase in lighter stages of sleep. Psychomotor vigilance task testing demonstrates an increase in the number of lapses. OSA-induced disruption of sleep is associated with extensive daytime sleepiness, a decrease in cognition and performance (attention, memory, executive functioning), decreased quality of life, mood disorders, and increased rates of motor vehicle collisions. Caffeine consumption in OSA patients could be a behavioral compensatory mechanism to overcome their daytime sleepiness.

The mortality impact of OSA is evident in moderate to severe OSA. The economic impact is due to increased healthcare utilization, decreased productivity, and years of potential life lost. It is estimated that the yearly incidence of OSA-related motor vehicle accidents alone costs about $16 billion and 1400 lost lives. Treating all drivers with OSA with positive airway therapy (at a cost of ≈ $3 billion a year) would save about $11 billion and about 1000 lives.

Metabolic Consequences

With OSA, multiple mechanisms interact to produce metabolic derangements and disorders that can worsen OSA and produce a vicious cycle that must be broken by treating both of its elements. Pathophysiologic mechanisms of these metabolic derangements include hypoxic injury, systemic inflammation, increased sympathetic activity, alterations in hypothalamic-pituitary-adrenal function, and hormonal changes. The metabolic derangements include insulin resistance, glucose intolerance, and dyslipidemia. Metabolic disorders include type 2 diabetes mellitus, central obesity, and metabolic syndrome. OSA is encountered in 50% of patients with NASH and in 30%–50% of patients with polycystic ovarian syndrome.

Pathophysiologic Consequences of Central Sleep Apnea

Unlike OSA events, CSA respiratory events are *not* associated with increased respiratory effort and may terminate without arousal. Nevertheless, they are associated with hypoxia that can be severe and prolonged and can be associated with severe sleep disruption, including difficulty in establishing or maintaining a refreshing sleep state. The combination of sleep deprivation and hypoxia results in many associated cardiovascular, neurologic, and metabolic derangements.

Pathophysiologic Consequences of Sleep-Related Hypoventilation Disorders

About 90% of patients with OHS also have some degree of OSA, exacerbating their degree of hypoxia and hypercarbia.

The major consequences of hypoxia and hypercarbia include pulmonary hypertension, cor pulmonale, and an increased risk of sudden unexplained nocturnal death. Patients with interstitial lung disease (e.g., interstitial pulmonary fibrosis) usually suffer from even more severe hypoxia and sleep disruption than those with COPD.

PREVALENCE OF SLEEP-RELATED BREATHING DISORDERS

Sleep-related breathing disorders are the second most common category of sleep disorders (after insomnia disorder) and are the most common sleep disorders encountered in sleep medicine clinics. OSA accounts for about 90% of sleep-related breathing disorders. Snoring is more common than OSA and is the most common reason for referral for a sleep study.

Prevalence of Obstructive Sleep Apnea

In 2014 the American Academy of Sleep Medicine (AASM) estimated that OSA affects at least 25 million adults in the United States. The proportion of OSA patients who are *not clinically diagnosed* is estimated to be roughly 80% among men and 90% among women. Patients with hypertension (including drug-resistant hypertension), type 2 diabetes mellitus, coronary artery disease, atrial fibrillation, permanent pacemakers, various forms of heart block, congestive heart failure, a history of stroke, and those coming for bariatric surgery have a much greater prevalence of OSA than the general population, and many of them are undiagnosed.

Prevalence of Central Sleep Apnea

CSA is not common. About 50% of cases of CSA are found in patients with congestive heart failure. Other common comorbidities include chronic renal failure, stroke, multiple sclerosis, neuromuscular disorders, chronic opioid use, and living at higher altitudes.

Prevalence of Obesity Hypoventilation Syndrome

OHS has an estimated prevalence of 0.15%–0.3% in the general population, with higher rates among women than men, probably owing to higher rates of obesity among women than men.

DIAGNOSIS OF SLEEP-RELATED BREATHING DISORDERS

The diagnosis of a sleep-related breathing disorder is based on criteria established by professional organizations, which also provide classifications of sleep disorders. The *International Classification of Diseases,* 10th edition (ICD-10), is developed by the World Health Organization and adopted by many government and billing organizations. The ICD-10 divides

TABLE 1.3	Physiologic Functions Studied During Polysomnography

Electroencephalogram to measure and evaluate sleep stages
Electrooculogram to measure eye movements
Chin electromyogram to measure muscle tone and the presence of REM sleep without atonia
Limb electromyogram to detect periodic limb movements and restless legs syndrome
Electrocardiogram to detect dysrhythmias
Upper airway sound recording to detect snoring
Nasal and oral airflow via a thermal sensor to detect apnea
Nasal airflow via a pressure sensor to detect hypopnea and arousals
Thoracoabdominal inductance plethysmography to detect respiratory efforts
Pulse oximeter to detect oxygen saturation/desaturation
Capnography to detect hypercarbia/hypoventilation
Body position sensor to note body position effects
Video recording or sleep technologist observation to detect parasomnias

TABLE 1.4	Rules for Scoring Respiratory Events During Polysomnography in Adults

Respiratory Event	Scoring Criteria
Obstructive apnea	Apnea for longer than 10 seconds with a ≥ 90% air flow reduction *despite respiratory effort*
Central apnea	Apnea for longer than 10 seconds with a ≥ 90% air flow reduction *without respiratory effort*
Hypopnea	A > 30% reduction in air flow for longer than 10 seconds associated with a ≥ 3% decline in oxygen saturation OR arousal
Hypoventilation	A 10-minute period with a P_{CO_2} > 55 mm Hg or a ≥ 10 mm Hg increase in P_{CO_2} to ≥ 50 mm Hg
Periodic breathing	≥3 consecutive cycles of Cheyne-Stokes breathing with a cycle length ≥ 40 seconds or ≥ 5 episodes of Cheyne-Stokes breathing in 2 hours

sleep disorders into six categories: insomnias, hypersomnias, parasomnias, circadian rhythm sleep disorders, sleep-related movement disorders, and sleep-related breathing disorders. The latter are further divided into four categories: OSA, CSA, sleep-related hypoventilation disorders, and sleep-related hypoxemia disorder.

Polysomnography

Polysomnography (PSG) can be used to differentiate CSA from OSA; assess its severity; detect associated hypoventilation and hypoxia; detect associated EEG, ECG, and limb movement events; and, when indicated, titrate positive airway pressure (PAP) therapy and perform follow-up assessments of any implemented therapy for the sleep-related breathing disorder. Rules for performing and interpreting PSG are published in the *AASM Manual for the Scoring of Sleep and Associated Events*. The manual covers the performance and interpretation of polysomnographic studies and home sleep apnea testing. The impact of these rules extends beyond performing and scoring an individual sleep study. These rules also affect diagnosis rates, which then affect calculations in epidemiologic studies and the implementation of individual and public health therapeutic interventions.

Standard PSG consists of simultaneous recording of multiple (7–12) physiologic parameters during a full night of sleep in a sleep laboratory with a sleep technologist in attendance (Table 1.3). It should contain 6 or more hours of recordings. The recorded PSG study is divided into 30-second periods called *epochs* for scoring purposes. During scoring, each individual epoch must be scored for sleep stage and any respiratory events such as apnea or hypopnea with or without obstruction, cardiac or limb events, and associated arousal. Respiratory events are scored if they last 10 seconds or longer (Table 1.4).

Sleep apnea testing can be done in several ways, each with a decreasing degree of complexity: level 1 testing is PSG; level

2 testing is unattended PSG done at home (rarely done); level 3 testing is home apnea testing in combination with an actigraph (a device that keeps track of movements as an assessment of sleep state); and level 4 testing uses 1–2 channels to monitor pulse oximetry and airflow. Level 4 testing is inadequate for a diagnosis of OSA, since it lacks information about respiratory effort.

Overnight home oximetry is an example of a level 4 home sleep apnea test. Data derived from this monitoring include the hourly frequency of a drop in Sao_2 by 3% or more and the T90, which is the total time spent with an oxygen saturation of less than 90%.

Morphometric Models

The association of anatomic risk factors with sleep apnea has been used to produce morphometric models to predict the likelihood of OSA. One morphometric model uses the triad of BMI, neck circumference, and oral cavity measurements and has a very high sensitivity and specificity. The oral cavity measurements include palatal height, maxillary intermolar distance, mandibular intermolar distance, and overjet (the horizontal distance between the edge of the upper incisors and the labial surface of the lower incisors). Note that overjet is not the same as overbite.

Questionnaires

Multiple tools in the form of questionnaires have been developed for screening populations for OSA. The *Epworth Sleepiness Scale* is used to assess excessive daytime sleepiness. The *Berlin Questionnaire* has three categories assessing snoring, sleepiness, and risk factors. The AASM developed a 10-item questionnaire to detect classic symptoms of OSA, and a 6-item checklist to identify patients who are at high risk for OSA. The American Society of Anesthesiologists (ASA) created an OSA checklist with three categories: predisposing physical characteristics, history of apparent airway obstruction during sleep, and somnolence. Chung et al. used an acronym of some of the clinical features and risk factors of OSA to develop the *STOP-BANG* scoring model. The acronym *STOP* stands for **S**noring, **T**ired (daytime sleepiness), **O**bserved apnea, and high blood **P**ressure; and the acronym *BANG* stands for **B**MI 35 or greater, **A**ge 50 years or older, **N**eck circumference 40 cm (17 inches) or larger, and male **G**ender. Ramachandran et al. developed the *Perioperative Sleep Apnea Prediction* (P-SAP) score based on logistic regression analysis of surgical patient data. It has nine elements: age, male gender, obesity, snoring, diabetes mellitus type 2, hypertension, thick neck, Mallampati class 3 or greater, and reduced thyromental distance. (These questionnaires are available as appendixes to this chapter in Expert Consult online.)

Compared to PSG, most questionnaires demonstrate a trade-off between sensitivity and specificity, with a trend toward decreased specificity as the questionnaire score increases or the severity of OSA increases.

Criteria for the Diagnosis of Obstructive Sleep Apnea in Adults

Elements of the diagnosis of adult OSA include: (1) signs and symptoms such as extreme daytime sleepiness, fatigue, insomnia, snoring, subjective nocturnal respiratory disturbance, and observed apnea; (2) associated medical or psychiatric disorders such as hypertension, coronary artery disease, atrial fibrillation, congestive heart failure, stroke, diabetes mellitus, cognitive dysfunction, and mood disorders; and (3) predominantly obstructive respiratory events recorded during sleep center nocturnal PSG or during out-of-center sleep testing. The sum of apnea and hypopnea events per hour is defined as the *apnea-hypopnea index (AHI)*. The sum of apnea, hypopnea, and arousal events is defined as the *respiratory disturbance index (RDI)*.

Clinical findings of OSA in adults can be divided into three categories: (1) anatomic features; (2) nocturnal and diurnal signs and symptoms of OSA, including loud snoring, gasping, choking, breath-holding, breathing interruption, insomnia, restless sleep, nocturia, bruxism, morning headache, non-refreshing sleep, fatigue, decreased cognitive and executive function, depression and irritability; and (3) commonly associated comorbidities.

Criteria for the Diagnosis of Central Sleep Apnea

Clinical findings of CSA can be divided into two categories: (1) nocturnal and diurnal signs and symptoms, including insomnia, frequent nocturnal awakenings with breath-holding, gasping or choking, mild snoring, breathing interruptions reported by bed partner, nonrestorative sleep, fatigue, and excessive daytime sleepiness; and (2) clinical findings of associated comorbidities, including neuromuscular diseases,

congestive heart failure, stroke, end-stage renal disease, and opioid use. PSG will show apneic periods *without respiratory efforts.*

Criteria for the Diagnosis of Sleep-Related Hypoventilation Disorders

Clinical findings in patients with sleep-related hypoventilation disorders can be divided into three categories: (1) specific signs and symptoms of diseases associated with an increased likelihood of a hypoventilation disorder, including neuromuscular diseases such as amyotrophic lateral sclerosis, postpolio syndrome, and facial muscle weakness in muscular dystrophy; (2) clinical findings due to chronic hypoxia (plethora) and hypercapnia; and (3) clinical findings due to systemic complications of chronic hypoxia and hypercapnia, including polycythemia, right heart failure, liver congestion, and peripheral edema. The BMI is typically over 30 kg/m^2. PSG will demonstrate significant increases in P_{CO_2} during both wakefulness and sleep.

Criterion for the Diagnosis of Sleep-Related Hypoxemia Disorder

The criterion for diagnosis of this disorder is 5 minutes of a sleep-related decrease in oxygen saturation to less than 88% *with or without* hypoventilation.

TREATMENT OF SLEEP-RELATED BREATHING DISORDERS

Treatment of Obstructive Sleep Apnea

Because of its high prevalence rate and a general lack of diagnosis, the first step in management of OSA is detection. In cases of suspected obstructed sleep apnea, objective testing should be performed to confirm the diagnosis and assess its severity using PSG. Testing should be followed by patient education, initiation of treatment, and long-term follow-up to assess the effect of therapy.

Positive Airway Pressure Therapy
The PAP device is an air compressor that delivers air pressurized to specific levels. The device-patient interface can be a facemask, a nasal mask, or nasal pillows. PAP can be continuous (CPAP), bilevel (BiPAP) or autotitrating (APAP). The goal of PAP titration is to select the lowest airway pressure that would eliminate *all* respiratory events, including apneas, hypopneas, arousals, and snoring, so that the respiratory disturbance index decreases to less than 5 per hour, with acceptable oxygenation (Spo$_2$ ≥ 90%) and an acceptable mask leak level. Suggested mechanisms for the efficacy of PAP therapy include (1) increasing the pharyngeal transmural pressure *(pneumatic splint effect),* (2) reducing pharyngeal wall thickness and airway edema, (3) increasing airway tone by mechanoreceptor stimulation, and (4) increasing end-expiratory lung volume and producing a tracheal tug effect.

CPAP consists of a single fixed PAP that is maintained during both inhalation and exhalation. BiPAP consists of two fixed airway pressures: a higher inspiratory pressure and a lower expiratory pressure. The transition from inspiratory to expiratory pressure is based on the machine's detection of expiratory effort. BiPAP mode allows a lower expiratory pressure than what would be required with CPAP. BiPAP is an alternative therapy for OSA in patients requiring high levels of PAP who have difficulty exhaling against a fixed pressure, or who develop gastric distention from swallowing air while on CPAP, or who have co-existing central hypoventilation.

PAP therapy can be titrated either manually or automatically. Manual in-laboratory, PSG-guided, full night titration of fixed PAP is considered the norm. APAP titration consists of a single variable PAP that is maintained during both inhalation and exhalation, with variation from breath to breath according to the presence or absence of apnea, hypopnea, or snoring. APAP is an acceptable alternative for the treatment of uncomplicated moderate to severe OSA that is associated with snoring. APAP mode may improve patient adherence and may minimize the average airway pressure by allowing higher PAP during periods of greater obstruction, such as the supine position and REM sleep, and lower PAP during periods of lesser obstruction.

Expiratory positive airway pressure (EPAP) devices are disposable adhesive valves that direct exhaled airflow into small channels to increase resistance to exhalation and thereby create a degree of expiratory positive airway pressure.

Oral Appliance Therapy

Oral appliance therapy is considered second-tier treatment in the management of OSA. The most common forms of oral appliances for OSA treatment include mandibular advancement devices and tongue retaining devices. Mandibular advancement devices are usually custom-made devices that are fitted to the teeth like a mouth guard and act to advance and stabilize the mandible to increase upper airway capacity (Fig. 1.2). Tongue retaining devices advance and retain the tongue in an anterior position by holding it in a suction cup placed over the front teeth. *(See video at aveotsd.com.)* Mandibular advancement devices are more costly but have greater efficacy and patient

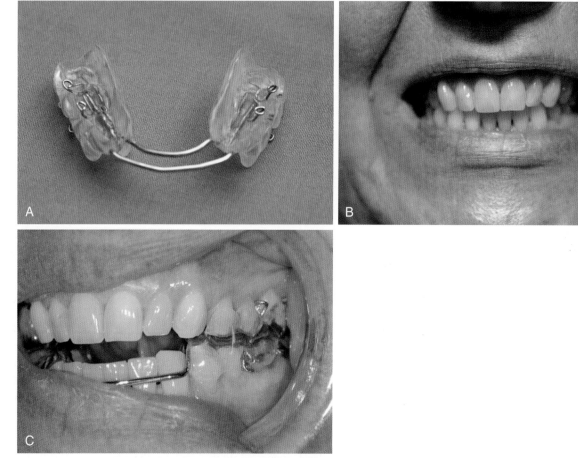

FIG. 1.2 An oral appliance (mandibular advancement device) for use in obstructive sleep apnea. A, Device. B, Natural occlusion of this patient. C, Mandibular advancement device in position. Note the forward movement of the lower teeth/jaw with this device. (From Marcussen L, Henriksen JE, Thygesen T. Do mandibular advancement devices influence patients' snoring and obstructive sleep apnea? A cone-beam computed tomography analysis of the upper airway volume. *J Oral Maxillofacial Surg.* 2015;73:1816-1826.)

compliance. Oral appliance therapy is indicated for the treatment of snoring, mild to moderate OSA, and selected cases of moderate to severe OSA, such as that due predominantly to the supine position or to a disproportionally large tongue relative to oral cavity capacity. This modality has been shown to be effective in reducing sleep interruption, daytime sleepiness, neurocognitive impairment, and cardiovascular complications. Side effects include excessive salivation, temporomandibular joint discomfort, and long-term occlusion changes.

Hypoglossal nerve stimulation uses a nerve stimulator that is implanted in the chest and has electronic sensing leads implanted between the internal and external intercostal muscles in the fourth intercostal space. These sensors detect breathing and signal the device to stimulate the hypoglossal nerve during inhalation, which results in enlargement of upper airway capacity. The system is turned on by the patient before going to sleep and turned off upon awakening.

Surgical Therapy

Surgical treatment of the airway in the form of tracheostomy is the oldest form of therapy for OSA and has a very high rate of efficacy. However, its invasiveness is its major deterrent. In adults, in whom anatomic causes of OSA are relatively uncommon, airway surgery treatment for OSA is considered third-tier therapy. These surgical procedures target soft tissue and bony tissue to enlarge airway capacity at the levels of the nose, palate, and/or tongue base and include maxillomandibular advancement, laser-assisted uvulopalatoplasty, uvulopalato-pharyngoplasty, and palatal implants.

Bariatric surgery aims to restrict caloric intake or absorption or both. Bariatric surgery can be the sole therapy or an adjunctive treatment to PAP therapy in patients with morbid obesity associated with OSA or OHS. *Screening for OSA should be performed in all patients undergoing bariatric surgery.*

Medical Therapy

Adjunctive medical therapy for OSA can be used in combination with any of the other forms of OSA therapy: PAP, oral appliances, or surgery. These adjuncts include diet, exercise, positional therapy, avoidance of alcohol and sedatives before sleep, supplemental oxygen, and pharmacologic therapy, such as with a stimulant drug like modafinil (Provigil). Positional therapy consists of devices that discourage or prevent the patient from sleeping in the supine position.

Comorbid conditions should be treated. Thyroid disorders should be treated surgically, medically, or both as indicated. Acromegaly should be treated surgically, medically, or both as indicated. Bromocriptine and somatostatin therapy can reduce the apnea-hypopnea index in patients with acromegaly by 50%–75%. However, continued PAP therapy is usually required owing to persistent skeletal changes.

Treatment of Central Sleep Apnea

In CSA related to congestive heart failure, first-tier therapy consists of CPAP therapy and nocturnal oxygen supplementation.

This can be augmented with BiPAP or drug therapy with acetazolamide and theophylline after medical optimization of congestive heart failure. Therapies for CSA associated with end-stage renal disease include CPAP, supplemental oxygen, use of bicarbonate during dialysis, and nocturnal dialysis.

Treatment of Sleep-Related Hypoventilation Disorders

Treatment of sleep-related hypoventilation disorders should enhance airway patency and ventilation, which is best achieved using *noninvasive positive pressure ventilation (NIPPV)* in one of three modes: (1) *spontaneous mode,* in which the patient cycles the device from inspiratory PAP to expiratory PAP; (2) *spontaneous timed mode,* in which a backup rate delivers PAP for a set inspiratory time if the patient does not trigger the device within a set period of time; and (3) *timed mode,* in which both the inspiratory time and respiratory rate are fixed. NIPPV is recommended for the treatment of hypoventilation due to *any* sleep-related breathing disorder.

PERIOPERATIVE CONSIDERATIONS IN PATIENTS WITH SLEEP-RELATED BREATHING DISORDERS

Management of sleep-related breathing disorders are a topic of special interest within the specialties of anesthesiology and sleep medicine. In 2011 this combined interest by the two specialties resulted in the establishment of the Society of Anesthesia and Sleep Medicine (SASM), which is an international society with a stated mission "to advance standards of care for clinical problems shared by Anesthesiology and Sleep Medicine, including perioperative management of sleep disordered breathing, and to promote interdisciplinary communication, education and research in matters common to anesthesia and sleep."

The prevalence of OSA among surgical patients is higher than the overall prevalence of 2%–4% in the general population. The perioperative period can exacerbate sleep-related breathing disorders because of (1) sleep deprivation due to anxiety, pain, alterations in circadian rhythms, and nursing interventions; (2) REM sleep rebound, which worsens OSA; and (3) the suppressant effects of anesthetics, sedatives, and analgesics on airway patency, respiratory drive, and arousal. The effect of sleep-disordered breathing on perioperative outcomes has been the subject of many observational studies and systematic reviews, with conflicting findings based on study population, examined outcomes, and study design. The evidence is, however, mostly negative.

PRACTICE GUIDELINES FOR PERIOPERATIVE MANAGEMENT OF PATIENTS WITH OBSTRUCTIVE SLEEP APNEA

The AASM, the ASA, and the Society for Ambulatory Anesthesia (SAMBA) have provided practice parameters for the perioperative management of OSA patients. Algorithms for the perioperative management of OSA patients have also been developed by individual groups.

In 2003 the AASM published a statement for the perioperative management of OSA in which it indicated that the literature is insufficient to develop standards-of-practice recommendations, and that the statement was based on a consensus of clinical experience and published peer-reviewed medical evidence that, unfortunately, was scanty and of limited quality. The statement provided an introduction about OSA and listed the most common factors that contribute to increased perioperative risk in OSA patients, including: (1) increased risk of upper airway obstruction and respiratory depression due to effects of sedative, anesthetic, and narcotic medications; (2) decreased functional residual capacity (FRC) and decreased oxygen reserve due to obesity; and (3) the cardiopulmonary effects of OSA. It described the symptoms and signs of OSA, as well as a description of CPAP therapy, and provided a questionnaire and checklist for preoperative recognition of patients who are at high risk for OSA. The AASM also detailed recommendations for intraoperative and postoperative patient care, including transfer of care.

In 2006 the ASA developed comprehensive practice guidelines for the perioperative management of OSA patients and updated them in 2014. These guidelines provide a checklist for preoperative identification and assessment of OSA and detailed recommendations covering the areas of preoperative evaluation, considerations for inpatient versus outpatient surgery, preoperative preparation, intraoperative management, postoperative management, and criteria for discharge to unmonitored settings.

In 2012, SAMBA produced a consensus statement on preoperative selection of adult patients with OSA scheduled for ambulatory surgery, which concluded that patients *with known OSA* might be considered for ambulatory surgery *if* they were medically optimized and could use their CPAP postoperatively. Patients with *presumed OSA* could be considered for ambulatory surgery *if* they could be managed with *nonopioid analgesia perioperatively.*

The elements of the practice parameters for perioperative care of patients with OSA are noted in Table 1.5.

PERIOPERATIVE OPIOID-INDUCED RESPIRATORY DEPRESSION

The Anesthesia Patient Safety Foundation (APSF) made perioperative opioid-induced respiratory depression a top priority in 2006. In 2011 it held its second conference on this subject and focused on monitoring for this entity. The executive summary of this conference recommended that "all patients receiving postoperative opioid analgesia should have periodic assessment of level of consciousness and continuous monitoring of oxygenation by pulse oximetry," and if supplemental oxygen is provided, "continuous monitoring of ventilation by capnography ($PETCO_2$) or an equivalent method."

In 2009 the ASA provided "Practice Guidelines for the Prevention, Detection, and Management of Respiratory Depression Associated with Neuraxial Opioid Administration." These were updated in 2016. Like the APSF, the ASA recommended that all patients receiving neuraxial opioids be monitored for adequacy of *ventilation, oxygenation, and level of consciousness,* with increased monitoring for patients with high-risk conditions, including unstable medical conditions, obesity, OSA, concomitant administration of opioid analgesics or hypnotics by other routes, and extremes of age. They also recommended administering supplemental oxygen to patients with an altered level of consciousness, respiratory depression, or hypoxemia, and having resuscitative measures available as needed, including narcotic reversal drugs and NIPPV.

KEY POINTS

- Electroencephalography (EEG) is an important method of studying wakefulness and sleep and defining sleep stages. The electrical activity of the brain can be categorized into three states: wakefulness, rapid eye movement (REM) sleep, and non-REM (NREM) sleep. The latter can be further categorized into three stages: N1, N2, and N3, according to the progressive decrease in frequency and increase in amplitude of EEG waveforms. Muscle tone as measured by electromyography is normal during wakefulness, decreased during NREM sleep, and abolished during REM sleep.
- NREM sleep maintains homeostasis and autonomic stability at low energy levels—that is, with a low basic metabolic rate and a decreased heart rate, cardiac output, and blood pressure. Hormonal secretion is maintained.
- REM sleep impairs homeostasis and disrupts autonomic stability. REM-induced autonomic instability manifests as irregularity in the heart rate, cardiac output, blood pressure and tidal volume, and suppression of cardiac and respiratory chemoreceptor and baroreceptor reflexes. REM sleep is associated with skeletal muscle atonia affecting all skeletal muscles, including upper airway dilator muscles and intercostal muscles, but with significant sparing of the diaphragm.
- Specific sleep disorders are disorders that manifest predominantly but not exclusively with sleep manifestations. They include disorders that manifest primarily as: (1) decreased sleep (insomnia), which is the most common type of sleep disorder, (2) increased sleep (hypersomnias), (3) abnormal sleep behavior (parasomnias), (4) disruptions of circadian rhythm, and (5) sleep-induced exacerbations of certain pathophysiologic problems such as sleep-related movement disorders and sleep-related breathing disorders.
- The hallmark of obstructive sleep apnea (OSA) is sleep-induced and arousal-relieved upper airway obstruction.
- Functional collapse of the upper airway occurs when forces that can collapse the upper airway overcome the forces that can dilate the upper airway. Collapsing forces consist of intraluminal negative inspiratory pressure and extraluminal positive pressure. Dilating forces consist of pharyngeal

TABLE 1.5	Perioperative Management of the Patient With Obstructive Sleep Apnea	
Potential Sources of Perioperative Risk	**Perioperative Risk Mitigation**
Lack of institutional protocol for perioperative management of sleep apnea patients	Develop and implement institutional protocol for perioperative management of sleep apnea patients.
Patients with a known diagnosis of obstructive sleep apnea (OSA)	Know sleep study results.
	Know the therapy being used: oral appliance, positive airway pressure (PAP) with settings (mode, pressure level, supplemental oxygen if any).
	Consult sleep medicine specialist as needed.
Patients without a diagnosis of OSA	Use a screening tool to determine the likelihood of OSA: AASM questionnaire, ASA checklist, Berlin questionnaire, or STOP-BANG questionnaire.
Inpatient versus outpatient surgery	Decisions based on institutional protocol containing factors related to: (1) patient, (2) procedure, (3) facility, and (4) postdischarge setting
Preoperative lack of optimization of therapy for OSA	Consult sleep medicine specialist to optimize therapy.
Preoperative sedative-induced airway compromise or respiratory depression	Use preoperative sedation only in a monitored setting.
Intraoperative sedative/opioid/anesthetic-induced upper airway compromise or respiratory depression during monitored anesthesia care (MAC)	Whenever possible, use topical, local, or regional anesthesia with minimal to no sedation.
	Continuous monitoring of ventilation adequacy
	Use of the patient's OSA therapy device during MAC with sedation
	Consider general anesthesia with a secured airway vs. deep sedation with an unsecured airway.
At risk for oxygen desaturation	Elevate head of bed to facilitate spontaneous ventilation/oxygenation.
	Preoxygenate sufficiently.
	Maintain oxygen insufflation by nasal cannula during endotracheal intubation.
Possible difficult mask ventilation or endotracheal intubation	Apply ASA Difficult Airway Algorithm, including the use of laryngeal mask airway, videolaryngoscope, fiberoptic bronchoscope, and transtracheal jet ventilation as indicated.
	Optimize head/neck position for mask ventilation and endotracheal intubation.
Potential difficulty with noninvasive blood pressure monitoring and/or increased risk for cardiovascular complications	Consider intraarterial catheter for blood pressure monitoring and blood sampling for arterial blood gases.
Postextubation airway obstruction in the operating room or postanesthesia care unit with associated risk of negative pressure pulmonary edema	Elevate the head of the bed.
	Extubate only after patient clearly meets objective extubation criteria.
	Maintain readiness for reintubation with the same device used during induction and expect that the difficulty of intubation will be greater than previously.
At risk for postoperative oxygen desaturation	Supplemental oxygen therapy
	Consider nasal airway.
	Consider PAP therapy (this can be initiated de novo in the postoperative setting).
Communication failure during transfer of care	Identify the patient's diagnosis of sleep apnea and its therapy.
	Alert staff about expected problems and their management.
Perioperative opioid-related respiratory depression due to opioids administered by neuraxial route, intravenous route with bolus injection, or via intravenous patient-controlled analgesia (IV-PCA)	Supplemental oxygen as needed
	Continuous electronic monitoring of oxygenation and ventilation
	Maintain patient's OSA therapy whenever possible; use home settings as a guide.
	Avoid background mode with IV-PCA.
	Consider opioid-sparing analgesic techniques (e.g., transcutaneous electrical nerve stimulation), and use nonopioid analgesics (e.g., NSAIDs, acetaminophen, tramadol, ketamine, gabapentin) whenever possible.
Postdischarge opioid-induced respiratory depression and/or exacerbation of OSA	Ensure companionship and a safe home environment for high-risk patients.
	Consult sleep medicine specialist to optimize sleep apnea therapy if needed.

ASA, American Society of Anesthesiologists; *NSAIDs,* Nonsteroidal antiinflammatory drugs.

dilating muscle tone and longitudinal traction on the upper airway by an increased lung volume, so-called tracheal tug.
- *Central sleep apnea* refers to sleep apnea that is not associated with respiratory efforts during the apnea event. This absence of respiratory effort could be due to instability of neural control of respiration, weakness of respiratory muscles, or both. Instability of respiratory control may include increased, decreased, or oscillating respiratory drive.
- Apneic and hypopneic episodes result in hypoxia, which can be prolonged and severe. OSA-induced hypoxia and

reoxygenation cycles activate redox-sensitive genes, oxidative stress, inflammatory processes, the sympathetic nervous system, and the coagulation cascade, all of which can contribute to endothelial dysfunction and ultimately to systemic hypertension, pulmonary hypertension, atherosclerosis, right and left ventricular systolic and diastolic dysfunction, coronary artery disease, congestive heart failure, atrial fibrillation, stroke, and sudden cardiac death.
- Polysomnography can be used to differentiate CSA from OSA, assess its severity, detect associated hypoventilation

and hypoxia, detect associated EEG, ECG, and limb movement events, and, when indicated, titrate positive airway pressure (PAP) therapy and perform follow-up assessment of any implemented therapy for the sleep-related breathing disorder.

- Because of its high prevalence rate and a general lack of diagnosis, the first step in management of OSA is detection.
- Suggested mechanisms for the efficacy of continuous PAP therapy include (1) increasing the pharyngeal transmural pressure (pneumatic splint effect), (2) reducing pharyngeal wall thickness and airway edema, (3) increasing airway tone by mechanoreceptor stimulation, and (4) increasing end-expiratory lung volume and producing a tracheal tug effect.
- The perioperative period can exacerbate sleep-related breathing disorders because of (1) sleep deprivation due to anxiety, pain, alterations in circadian rhythms, and nursing interventions; (2) REM sleep rebound, which worsens OSA; and (3) the suppressant effects of anesthetics, sedatives, and analgesics on airway patency, respiratory drive, and arousal.
- To avoid opioid-induced respiratory depression, all patients receiving opioids, including neuraxial opioids, should be monitored for adequacy of ventilation, oxygenation, and level of consciousness, with increased monitoring for patients with high-risk conditions, including unstable medical conditions, obesity, OSA, concomitant administration of opioid analgesics or hypnotics by other routes, and extremes of age.

RESOURCES

Aurora RN, Casey KR, Kristo D, et al. Practice parameters for the surgical modifications of the upper airway for obstructive sleep apnea in adults. *Sleep.* 2010;33:1408-1413.

Aurora RN, Chowdhuri S, Ramar K, et al. The treatment of central sleep apnea syndromes in adults: practice parameters with an evidence-based literature review and meta-analyses. *Sleep.* 2012;35:17-40.

Biot MC. Contribution a l'ètude de phènomène respiratoire de Cheyne-Stokes. *Lyon Mèd.* 1876;23:517-528, 561-567.

Bradley TD, Logan AG, Kimoff RJ, et al. Continuous positive airway pressure for central sleep apnea and heart failure. *N Engl J Med.* 2005;353: 2025-2033.

Benumof JL. The elephant in the room is bigger than you think: finding obstructive sleep apnea patients dead in bed postoperatively. *Anesth Analg.* 2015;120:491.

Bolden N, Smith CE, Auckley D. Avoiding adverse outcomes in patients with obstructive sleep apnea: development and implementation of a perioperative obstructive sleep apnea protocol. *J Clin Anesth.* 2009;21:286-293.

Chau EH, Lam D, Wong J, et al. Obesity hypoventilation syndrome: a review of epidemiology, pathophysiology, and perioperative considerations. *Anesthesiology.* 2012;117:188-205.

Chung F, Yegneswaran B, Liao P, et al. STOP questionnaire: a tool to screen patients for obstructive sleep apnea. *Anesthesiology.* 2008;108:812-821.

Chung F, Yegneswaran B, Liao P, et al. Validation of the Berlin questionnaire and American Society of Anesthesiologists checklist as screening tools for obstructive sleep apnea in surgical patients. *Anesthesiology.* 2008;108: 822-830.

Chung F, Liao P, Elsaid H, et al. Factors associated with postoperative exacerbation of sleep-disordered breathing. *Anesthesiology.* 2014;120:299-311.

Correa D, Farney RJ, Chung F, et al. Chronic opioid use and central sleep apnea: a review of the prevalence, mechanisms, and perioperative considerations. *Anesth Analg.* 2015;120:1273-1285.

Gay P, Weaver T, Loube D, et al. Positive Airway Pressure Task Force, Standards of Practice Committee, American Academy of Sleep Medicine. Evaluation of positive airway pressure treatment for sleep related breathing disorders in adults. *Sleep.* 2006;29:381-401.

Gross JB, Bachenberg KL, Benumof JL, et al. Practice guidelines for the perioperative management of patients with obstructive sleep apnea: a report by the American Society of Anesthesiologists Task Force on perioperative management of patients with obstructive sleep apnea. *Anesthesiology.* 2006;104:1081-1093.

Johns MW. A new method for measuring daytime sleepiness: the Epworth sleepiness scale. *Sleep.* 1991;14:540-545.

Joshi GP, Ankichetty SP, Gan TJ, et al. Society for Ambulatory Anesthesia consensus statement on preoperative selection of adult patients with obstructive sleep apnea scheduled for ambulatory surgery. *Anesth Analg.* 2012;15:1060-1068.

Kaw R, Pasupuleti V, Walker E, et al. Postoperative complications in patients with obstructive sleep apnea. *Chest.* 2012;141:436-441.

Kaneko Y, Floras JS, Usui K, et al. Cardiovascular effects of continuous positive airway pressure in patients with heart failure and obstructive sleep apnea. *N Engl J Med.* 2003;348:1233-1241.

Lockhart EM, Willingham MD, Abdallah AB, et al. Obstructive sleep apnea screening and postoperative mortality in a large surgical cohort. *Sleep Med.* 2013;14:407-415.

Marin JM, Soriano JB, Carrizo SJ, et al. Outcomes in patients with chronic obstructive pulmonary disease and obstructive sleep apnea: the overlap syndrome. *Am J Respir Crit Care Med.* 2010;182:325-331.

Memtsoudis SG, Stundner O, Rasul R, et al. The impact of sleep apnea on postoperative utilization of resources and adverse outcomes. *Anesth Analg.* 2014;118:407-418.

Meoli AL, Rosen CL, Kristo D, et al. Clinical Practice Review Committee, American Academy of Sleep Medicine. Upper airway management of the adult patient with obstructive sleep apnea in the perioperative period—avoiding complications. *Sleep.* 2003;26:1060-1065.

Mokhlesi B. Obesity hypoventilation syndrome: a state-of-the-art review. *Respir Care.* 2010;55:1347-1365.

Morgenthaler TI, Kapen S, Lee-Chiong T, et al. Standards of Practice Committee, American Academy of Sleep Medicine. Practice parameters for the medical therapy of obstructive sleep apnea. *Sleep.* 2006;29:1031-1035.

Netzer NC, Stoohs RA, Netzer CM, et al. Using the Berlin Questionnaire to identify patients at risk for the sleep apnea syndrome. *Ann Intern Med.* 1999;131:485-491.

Peppard PE, Young T, Palta M, et al. Prospective study of the association between sleep-disordered breathing and hypertension. *N Engl J Med.* 2000;342:1378-1384.

Practice guidelines for the prevention, detection, and management of respiratory depression associated with neuraxial opioid administration: an updated report by the American Society of Anesthesiologists Task Force on Neuraxial Opioids and the American Society of Regional Anesthesia and Pain Medicine. *Anesthesiology.* 2016;124:535-552.

Practice guidelines for the perioperative management of patients with obstructive sleep apnea: an updated report by the American Society of Anesthesiologists Task Force on Perioperative Management of Patients with Obstructive Sleep Apnea. *Anesthesiology.* 2014;120:268-286.

Ramar K, Dort LC, Katz SG, et al. Clinical practice guideline for the treatment of obstructive sleep apnea and snoring with oral appliance therapy: an update for 2015. *J Clin Sleep Med.* 2015;11:773-827.

<http://sasmhq.org/>. Accessed August 15, 2016.

Sateia MJ. International classification of sleep disorders-third edition: highlights and modifications. *Chest.* 2014;146:1387-1394.

Wedewardt J, Bitter T, Prinz C, et al. Cheyne-Stokes respiration in heart failure: cycle length is dependent on left ventricular ejection fraction. *Sleep Med.* 2010;11:137-142.

Obstructive Respiratory Diseases

JING TAO, VIJI KURUP

Anesthesiologists commonly deal with patients with lung diseases and know that such patients are at an increased risk of perioperative pulmonary complications. There is increasing awareness of how these complications contribute to overall morbidity, mortality, and increased hospital length of stay. Perioperative pulmonary complications can also play an important role in determining long-term mortality after surgery. Modification of disease severity and patient optimization prior to surgery can significantly decrease the incidence of these complications.

Obstructive respiratory diseases can be divided into the following groups for discussion of their influence on anesthetic management: (1) acute upper respiratory tract infection (URI), (2) asthma, (3) chronic obstructive pulmonary disease (COPD), and (4) a miscellaneous group of respiratory disorders.

ACUTE UPPER RESPIRATORY TRACT INFECTION

Every year approximately 25 million patients visit their doctors because of a URI. The "common cold" syndrome results in about 20 million days of absence from work and 22 million days of absence from school, so it is likely there will be a population of patients scheduled for elective surgery who have an active URI.

Infectious (viral or bacterial) nasopharyngitis accounts for about 95% of all URIs, with the most common responsible viral pathogens being rhinovirus, coronavirus, influenza virus, parainfluenza virus, and respiratory syncytial virus (RSV). Noninfectious nasopharyngitis can be allergic or vasomotor in origin.

Signs and Symptoms

Most common symptoms of acute URI include nonproductive cough, sneezing, and rhinorrhea. A history of seasonal allergies may indicate an allergic cause of these symptoms rather than an infectious cause. Symptoms caused by bacterial infections will usually present with more serious signs and symptoms such as fever, purulent nasal discharge, productive cough, and malaise. Such patients may be tachypneic, wheezing, or have a toxic appearance.

Diagnosis

Diagnosis is usually based on clinical signs and symptoms. Viral cultures and laboratory tests lack sensitivity, are time and cost consuming, and therefore impractical in a busy clinical setting.

Management of Anesthesia

Most studies regarding the effects of URI on postoperative pulmonary complications have involved pediatric patients.

It is well known that children with a URI are at much higher risk of adverse events such as transient hypoxemia and laryngospasm if they are anesthetized while suffering a URI. However, there are limited data about the adult population in this regard. There is evidence to show an increased incidence of respiratory complications in pediatric patients with a history of copious secretions, prematurity, parental smoking, nasal congestion, reactive airway disease, endotracheal intubation, and in those undergoing airway surgery. Those with clear systemic signs of infection such as fever, purulent rhinitis, productive cough, and rhonchi who are undergoing elective surgery (particularly airway surgery) are at considerable risk of perioperative adverse events. Consultation with the surgeon regarding the urgency of the surgery is necessary. A patient who has had a URI for days or weeks and is in stable or improving condition can be safely managed without postponing surgery. If surgery is to be delayed, patients should not be rescheduled for about 6 weeks, since it may take that long for airway hyperreactivity to resolve. The economic and practical aspects of canceling surgery should also be taken into consideration before a decision is made to postpone surgery.

Viral infections, particularly during the infectious phase, can cause morphologic and functional changes in the respiratory epithelium. The relationship between epithelial damage, viral infection, airway reactivity, and anesthesia remains unclear. Tracheal mucociliary flow and pulmonary bactericidal activity can be decreased by general anesthesia. It is possible that positive pressure ventilation could help spread infection from the upper to the lower respiratory tract. The immune response of the body is altered by surgery and anesthesia. A reduction in B-lymphocyte numbers, T-lymphocyte responsiveness, and antibody production may be associated with anesthesia, but the clinical significance of this remains to be elucidated.

The anesthetic management of a patient with a URI should include adequate hydration, reducing secretions, and limiting manipulation of a potentially sensitive airway. Nebulized or topical local anesthetic applied to the vocal cords may reduce upper airway sensitivity. Use of a laryngeal mask airway (LMA) rather than an endotracheal (ET) tube may also reduce the risk of laryngospasm.

Adverse respiratory events in patients with URIs include bronchospasm, laryngospasm, airway obstruction, postintubation croup, desaturation, and atelectasis. Intraoperative and immediate postoperative hypoxemia are common and amenable to treatment with supplemental oxygen. Long-term complications have not been demonstrated.

ASTHMA

Asthma is one of the most common chronic medical conditions in the world and currently affects approximately 300 million people globally. The prevalence of asthma has been rising in developing countries, and this has been attributed to increased urbanization and atmospheric pollution.

Asthma is a disease of *reversible* airflow obstruction characterized by bronchial hyperreactivity, bronchoconstriction,

TABLE 2.1	Stimuli Provoking Symptoms of Asthma

Allergens
Pharmacologic agents: aspirin, β-antagonists, some nonsteroidal antiinflammatory drugs, sulfiting agents
Infections: respiratory viruses
Exercise: attacks typically follow exertion rather than occurring during it
Emotional stress: endorphins and vagal mediation

and chronic airway inflammation. Development of asthma is multifactorial and includes genetic and environmental causes. It seems likely that various genes contribute to development of asthma and also determine the severity of asthma in an individual. A family history of asthma, maternal smoking during pregnancy, viral infections (especially with rhinovirus and infantile RSV), and limited exposure to highly infectious environments as a child (i.e., farms, daycare centers, and pets) all contribute to the development of asthma. A list of some stimuli that can provoke an episode of asthma are summarized in Table 2.1.

The pathophysiology of asthma is a specific chronic inflammation of the mucosa of the lower airways. Activation of the inflammatory cascade leads to infiltration of the airway mucosa with eosinophils, neutrophils, mast cells, T cells, B cells, and leukotrienes. This results in airway edema, particularly in the bronchi. There is thickening of the basement membrane and the airway wall may be thickened and edematous. The inflammatory mediators implicated in asthma include histamine, prostaglandin D_2 and leukotrienes. Typically there are simultaneous areas of inflammation and repair in the airways.

Signs and Symptoms

Asthma is an episodic disease with acute exacerbations interspersed with symptom-free periods. Most attacks are short lived, lasting minutes to hours, and clinically the person recovers completely after an attack. However, there can be a phase in which a patient experiences some degree of airway obstruction daily. This phase can be mild, with or without superimposed severe episodes, or much more serious, with significant obstruction persisting for days or weeks. *Status asthmaticus* is defined as life-threatening bronchospasm that persists despite treatment. When the history is elicited from someone with asthma, attention should be paid to factors such as previous intubation or admission to the intensive care unit (ICU), two or more hospitalizations for asthma in the past year, and the presence of significant co-existing diseases. Clinical manifestations of asthma include wheezing, productive or nonproductive cough, dyspnea, chest discomfort or tightness that may lead to air hunger, and eosinophilia.

Diagnosis

The diagnosis of asthma depends on both symptoms and signs and objective measurements of airway obstruction. Asthma is diagnosed when a patient reports symptoms of wheezing, chest tightness, or shortness of breath and demonstrates

TABLE 2.2	Most Clinically Useful Spirometric Tests of Lung Function

Forced expiratory volume in 1 sec (FEV$_1$): The volume of air that can be forcefully exhaled in 1 sec. Values between 80% and 120% of the predicted value are considered normal.

Forced vital capacity (FVC): The volume of air that can be exhaled with maximum effort after a deep inhalation. Normal values are $\approx$ 3.7 L in females and $\approx$ 4.8 L in males.

Ratio of FEV$_1$ to FVC: This ratio in healthy adults is 75%–80%.

Forced expiratory flow at 25%–75% of vital capacity (FEF$_{25\%-75\%}$): A measurement of airflow through the midpoint of a forced exhalation.

Maximum voluntary ventilation (MVV): The maximum amount of air that can be inhaled and exhaled within 1 min. For patient comfort, the volume is measured over a 15-sec time period and results are extrapolated to obtain a value for 1 min expressed as liters per minute. Average values for males and females are 140–180 and 80–120 L/min, respectively.

Diffusing capacity (D$_{LCO}$): The volume of a substance (carbon monoxide [CO]) transferred across the alveoli into blood per minute per unit of alveolar partial pressure. CO is rapidly taken up by hemoglobin. Its transfer is therefore limited mainly by diffusion. A single breath of 0.3% CO and 10% helium is held for 20 sec. Expired partial pressure of CO is measured. Normal value is 17–25 mL/min/mm Hg.

airflow obstruction on pulmonary function testing that is at least partially reversible with bronchodilators. Asthma severity depends on the clinical symptoms, the results of pulmonary function testing, and medication usage (Tables 2.2 and 2.3).

Pulmonary Function Testing

Forced expiratory volume in 1 second (FEV$_1$); forced expiratory flow, midexpiratory phase (FEF$_{25\%-75\%}$ [also called *maximum midexpiratory flow rate*]); and peak expiratory flow rate (PEFR) are direct measures of the severity of expiratory airflow obstruction (Fig. 2.1). These measurements provide objective data that can be used to assess the severity and monitor the course of an exacerbation of asthma. The typical asthmatic patient who comes to the hospital for treatment has an FEV$_1$ that is less than 35% of normal. Flow-volume loops show characteristic downward scooping of the expiratory limb of the loop. Flow-volume loops in which the inhaled or exhaled portion of the loop is flat help distinguish wheezing caused by airway obstruction (i.e., due to a foreign body, tracheal stenosis, or mediastinal tumor) from asthma (Figs. 2.2 and 2.3). During moderate or severe asthmatic attacks, the functional residual capacity (FRC) may increase substantially, but total lung capacity (TLC) usually remains within the normal

TABLE 2.3	Classification of Asthma Severity in Youths Older Than 12 Years and in Adults

Components of Severity		Classification of Asthma Severity (Youths $\geq$ 12 years of age and adults)			
		Intermittent	Persistent		
			Mild	Moderate	Severe
Impairment Normal FEV$_1$:FVC: 8–19 yr 85% 20–39 yr 80% 40–59 yr 75% 60–80 yr 70%	Symptoms	$\leq$ 2 days/week	> 2 days/week but not daily	Daily	Throughout the day
	Nighttime awakenings	$\leq$ 2x/month	3–4x/month	> 1x/week but not nightly	Often 7x/week
	Short-acting β_2-agonist use for symptom control (not prevention of EIB)	$\leq$ 2 days/week	>2 days/week but not daily	Daily	Several times per day
	Interference with normal activity	None	Minor limitation	Some limitation	Extremely limited
	Lung function	• Normal FEV$_1$ between exacerbations • FEV$_1$ > 80% predicted • FEV$_1$:FVC normal	• FEV$_1$ < 80% predicted • FEV$_1$:FVC normal	• FEV$_1$ > 60% but < 80% predicted • FEV$_1$:FVC reduced 5%	• FEV$_1$ < 60% predicted • FEV$_1$:FVC reduced > 5%
Risk	Exacerbations (consider frequency and severity)	0–2/year ———— >2/year ——————————————→ ← Frequency and severity may fluctuate over time for patients in any severity category → Relative annual risk of exacerbations may be related to FEV$_1$.			

From National Asthma Education and Prevention Program. *Expert Panel Report 3: Guidelines for the Diagnosis and Management of Asthma (EPR3).* Bethesda, MD: National Heart, Lung, and Blood Institute; 2007.

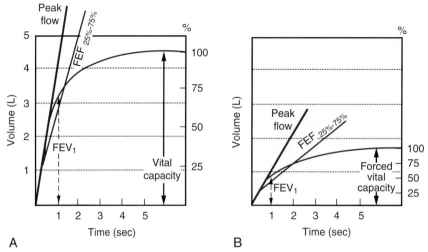

FIG. 2.1   Spirographic changes of a healthy subject (A) and a patient in bronchospasm (B). The forced expiratory volume in 1 second (FEV_1) is typically less than 80% of the vital capacity in the presence of obstructive airway disease. Peak flow and maximum midexpiratory flow rate ($FEF_{25\%-75\%}$) are also decreased in these patients (B). (Adapted from Kingston HGG, Hirshman CA. Perioperative management of the patient with asthma. *Anesth Analg.* 1984;63:844-855.)

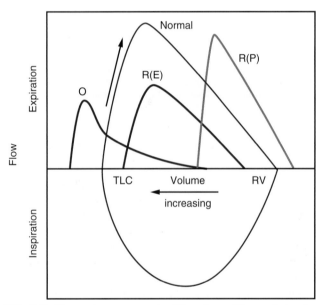

FIG. 2.2   Flow-volume curves in different conditions: obstructive disease, O; extraparenchymal restrictive disease with limitation in inspiration and expiration, R(E); and parenchymal restrictive disease, R(P). Forced expiration is plotted for all conditions; forced inspiration is shown only for the normal curve. By convention, lung volume increases to the left on the abscissa. The arrow alongside the normal curve indicates the direction of expiration from total lung capacity (TLC) to residual volume (RV). (Adapted from Weinberger SE. Disturbances of respiratory function. In: Fauci B, Braunwald E, Isselbacher KJ, et al., eds. *Harrison's Principles of Internal Medicine.* 14th ed. New York: McGraw-Hill; 1998.)

range. Diffusing capacity for carbon monoxide is not changed. Bronchodilator responsiveness provides supporting evidence if asthma is suspected on clinical grounds. In patients with expiratory airflow obstruction, an increase in airflow after inhalation of a bronchodilator suggests asthma. Abnormalities

in pulmonary function test (PFT) results may persist for several days after an acute asthmatic attack despite the absence of symptoms. Since asthma is an episodic illness, its diagnosis may be suspected even if PFT results are normal.

Arterial Blood Gas Analysis

Mild asthma is usually accompanied by a normal PaO_2 and $PaCO_2$. Tachypnea and hyperventilation observed during an acute asthmatic attack do not reflect arterial hypoxemia but rather neural reflexes in the lungs. Hypocarbia and respiratory alkalosis are the most common arterial blood gas findings in the presence of asthma. As the severity of expiratory airflow obstruction increases, the associated ventilation/perfusion mismatching may result in a PaO_2 of less than 60 mm Hg while breathing room air. The $PaCO_2$ is likely to increase when the FEV_1 is less than 25% of the predicted value. Fatigue of the skeletal muscles necessary for breathing may contribute to the development of hypercarbia.

Chest Radiography and Electrocardiography

A chest radiograph in a patient with mild or moderate asthma even during an asthma exacerbation is often normal. Patients with severe asthma may demonstrate hyperinflation and hilar vascular congestion due to mucus plugging and pulmonary hypertension. Chest x-rays can be helpful in determining the cause of an asthma exacerbation and in ruling out other causes of wheezing. The electrocardiogram (ECG) may show evidence of right ventricular strain or ventricular irritability during an asthmatic attack.

The differential diagnosis of asthma includes viral tracheobronchitis, sarcoidosis, rheumatoid arthritis with bronchiolitis, extrinsic compression (thoracic aneurysm, mediastinal neoplasm) or intrinsic compression (epiglottitis, croup) of the upper airway, vocal cord dysfunction, tracheal stenosis, chronic bronchitis, COPD, and foreign body aspiration. Upper airway obstruction produces a characteristic flow-volume loop (see Fig. 2.3A). A history of recent trauma, surgery, or tracheal

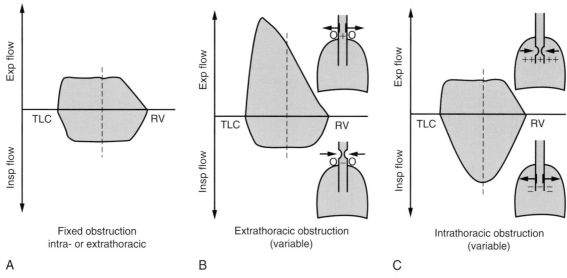

FIG. 2.3   Flow-volume curves in fixed and variable obstruction. A, Fixed obstruction, intrathoracic or extrathoracic. B, Extrathoracic obstruction (variable). C, Intrathoracic obstruction (variable). *Exp,* Expiratory; *Insp,* inspiratory; *RV,* residual volume; *TLC,* total lung capacity. (Adapted from Benumof J, ed. *Anesthesia for Thoracic Surgery.* 2nd ed. Philadelphia: Saunders; 1995.)

TABLE 2.4	Short-Acting Bronchodilators Used for Immediate Relief of Asthma	
Drug	Action	Adverse Effects
Albuterol (Proventil) Levalbuterol (Xopenex) Metaproterenol Pirbuterol (Maxair)	β_2-Agonist: stimulates β_2 receptors in tracheobronchial tree	Tachycardia Tremors Dysrhythmias Hypokalemia

intubation may be present in patients with upper airway obstruction mimicking asthma. Congestive heart failure and pulmonary embolism may also cause dyspnea and wheezing.

Treatment

Historically, treatment of asthma has been directed at preventing and controlling bronchospasm with bronchodilator drugs. However, recognition of the consistent presence of airway inflammation in patients with asthma has resulted in some changes in the pharmacologic therapy of asthma. There is now an emphasis on preventing and controlling bronchial inflammation as well as treating bronchospasm. Asthma treatments can be classified by their role in asthma management and by the timing of their effects (i.e., immediate relief or long-term therapy) (Tables 2.4 and 2.5).

Serial determination of PFTs can be useful for monitoring the response to treatment. When the FEV_1 improves to about 50% of normal, patients usually have minimal or no symptoms.

Status Asthmaticus

Status asthmaticus is defined as bronchospasm that does not resolve despite treatment and is considered life threatening. Emergency treatment of status asthmaticus consists of intermittent or continuous administration of β_2-agonists. β_2-Agonists inhaled via a metered-dose inhaler can be administered every 15–20 minutes for several doses without significant adverse hemodynamic effects, although patients may experience unpleasant sensations resulting from adrenergic overstimulation. Continuous administration of β_2-agonists by nebulizer may be more effective for delivery of these drugs to relieve airway spasm. Intravenous (IV) corticosteroids are administered early in treatment, because it takes several hours for their effect to appear. The corticosteroids most commonly selected are hydrocortisone and methylprednisolone. Supplemental oxygen is administered to help maintain arterial oxygen saturation above 90%. Other drugs used in more intractable cases include magnesium and oral leukotriene inhibitors. Studies on the use of IV magnesium sulfate indicate that it may significantly improve lung function and reduce the rate of hospital admission in children. The National Asthma Education and Prevention Program Expert Panel always has the most recent evidence-based guidelines for treatment of asthma on their website (http://www.nhlbi.nih.gov/about/org/naepp/).

Measurements of lung function can be very helpful in assessing the severity of status asthmaticus and the response to treatment. Patients whose FEV_1 or PEFR is decreased to 25% of normal or less are at risk of developing of hypercarbia and respiratory failure. The presence of hypercarbia (defined as a $Paco_2 > 50$ mm Hg) despite aggressive antiinflammatory and bronchodilator therapy is a sign of respiratory fatigue that requires tracheal intubation and mechanical ventilation. The pattern of mechanical ventilation can be particularly important in the patient with status asthmaticus. The expiratory phase must be prolonged to allow for complete exhalation and

TABLE 2.5	Drugs Used for Long-Term Treatment of Asthma		
Class	Drug	Action	Adverse Effects
Inhaled corticosteroids	Beclomethasone Budesonide (Pulmicort) Ciclesonide Flunisolide Fluticasone (Flovent) Mometasone Triamcinolone	Decrease airway inflammation Reduce airway hyperresponsiveness	Dysphonia Myopathy of laryngeal muscles Oropharyngeal candidiasis
Long-acting bronchodilators	Arformoterol (Brovana) Formoterol Salmeterol	β_2-Agonist: stimulates β_2-receptors in tracheobronchial tree	Therapy with just long-acting bronchodilators can cause airway inflammation and an increased incidence of asthma exacerbations. Should not be used except with an inhaled corticosteroid
Combined inhaled corticosteroids + long-acting bronchodilators	Budesonide + formoterol (Symbicort) Fluticasone + salmeterol (Advair)	Combination of long-acting bronchodilator and inhaled corticosteroid	
Leukotriene modifiers	Montelukast (Singulair) Zafirlukast (Accolate) Zileuton (Zyflo)	Reduce synthesis of leukotrienes by inhibiting 5-lipoxygenase enzyme	Minimal
Anti-IgE monoclonal antibody	Omalizumab (Xolair)	Decreases IgE release by inhibiting binding of IgE to mast cells and basophils	Injection site reaction Arthralgia Sinusitis Pharyngitis Headache
Methylxanthines	Theophylline Aminophylline	Increase cAMP by inhibiting phosphodiesterase, block adenosine receptors, release endogenous catecholamines	Disrupted sleep cycle Nervousness Nausea/vomiting, anorexia Headache Dysrhythmias
Mast cell stabilizer	Cromolyn	Inhibit mediator release from mast cells, membrane stabilization	Cough Throat irritation

cAMP, Cyclic adenosine monophosphate; IgE, immunoglobulin E.

to prevent self-generated or intrinsic positive end-expiratory pressure *(auto-PEEP)*. To prevent barotrauma, some recommend a degree of permissive hypercarbia. When the FEV_1 or PEFR improves to 50% of normal or higher, patients usually have minimal or no symptoms, and at this point the frequency and intensity of bronchodilator therapy can be decreased and weaning from mechanical ventilation can ensue.

When status asthmaticus is resistant to therapy, it is likely that the expiratory airflow obstruction is caused predominantly by airway edema and intraluminal secretions. Indeed, some patients with status asthmaticus are at risk of asphyxia due to mucus plugging of the airways. In rare circumstances when life-threatening status asthmaticus persists despite aggressive pharmacologic therapy, it may be necessary to consider general anesthesia to produce bronchodilation. Isoflurane and sevoflurane are effective bronchodilators in this situation. Treatment of status asthmaticus is summarized in Table 2.6.

Management of Anesthesia

The occurrence of "severe" bronchospasm has been reported in 0.2%–4.2% of all procedures involving general anesthesia performed in asthmatic patients. Factors that are more likely to predict the occurrence of severe bronchospasm include the type of surgery (risk is higher with upper abdominal surgery and oncologic surgery) and the proximity of the most recent asthmatic attack to the date of surgery.

Several mechanisms could explain the contribution of general anesthesia to *increased* airway resistance. Among these are depression of the cough reflex, impairment of mucociliary function, reduction of palatopharyngeal muscle tone, depression of diaphragmatic function, and an increase in the amount of fluid in the airway wall. In addition, airway stimulation by endotracheal intubation, parasympathetic nervous system activation, and/or release of neurotransmitters of pain such as substance P and neurokinins may also play a role.

TABLE 2.6	Treatment of Status Asthmaticus

Supplemental oxygen to maintain $Sao_2 > 90\%$

β_2-Agonists by metered-dose inhaler every 15–20 min or by continuous nebulizer administration

Intravenous corticosteroids (hydrocortisone or methylprednisolone)

Intravenous fluids to maintain euvolemia

Empirical broad-spectrum antibiotics

Anticholinergic (ipratropium) by inhalation

Intravenous magnesium sulfate

Tracheal intubation and mechanical ventilation (when $Paco_2 > 50$ mm Hg)

Sedation and paralysis

Mechanical ventilation parameters:

  High gas flows permit short inspiration times and longer expiration times.

  Expiration time must be prolonged to avoid air trapping and "auto-PEEP."

  Permissive hypercarbia if needed to avoid barotrauma

General anesthesia with a volatile anesthetic to produce bronchodilation

Extracorporeal membrane oxygenation (ECMO) as a last resort

TABLE 2.7	Characteristics of Asthma to Be Evaluated Preoperatively

Age at onset

Triggering events

Hospitalization for asthma

  Frequency of emergency department visits

  Need for intubation and mechanical ventilation

Allergies

Cough

Sputum characteristics

Current medications

Anesthetic history

Preoperative evaluation of patients with asthma requires an assessment of disease severity, the effectiveness of current pharmacologic management, and the potential need for additional therapy before surgery. The goal of preoperative evaluation is to formulate an anesthetic plan that prevents or blunts expiratory airflow obstruction.

Preoperative evaluation begins with a history to elicit the severity and characteristics of the patient's asthma (Table 2.7). On physical examination the general appearance of the patient and any use of accessory muscles of respiration should be noted. Auscultation of the chest to detect wheezing or crepitations is important. Blood eosinophil counts often parallel the degree of airway inflammation, and airway hyperreactivity provides an indirect assessment of the current status of the disease. PFTs (especially FEV_1) performed before and after bronchodilator therapy may be indicated in patients scheduled for major surgery. A reduction in FEV_1 or forced vital capacity (FVC) to less than 70% of predicted, as well as an FEV_1:FVC ratio that is less than 65% of predicted, is usually considered a risk factor for perioperative respiratory complications.

Chest physiotherapy, antibiotic therapy, and bronchodilator therapy during the preoperative period can often improve reversible components of asthma. Measurement of arterial blood gases is indicated if there is any question about the adequacy of ventilation or oxygenation.

Antiinflammatory and bronchodilator therapy should be continued until the time of anesthesia induction. If the patient is currently on or has been treated with high doses of systemic corticosteroids within the past 6 months, supplementation with "stress dose" hydrocortisone or methylprednisolone is indicated. However, hypothalamic-pituitary-adrenal suppression is very unlikely if only *inhaled* corticosteroids are used for asthma treatment. In selected patients a preoperative course of oral corticosteroids may be useful to improve overall lung function. Patients should be free of wheezing and have a PEFR of either greater than 80% of predicted or at the patient's personal best value before surgery.

During induction and maintenance of anesthesia in asthmatic patients, airway reflexes must be suppressed to avoid bronchoconstriction in response to mechanical stimulation of these hyperreactive airways. Stimuli that do not ordinarily evoke airway responses can precipitate life-threatening bronchoconstriction in patients with asthma.

Because it avoids instrumentation of the airway and tracheal intubation, regional anesthesia is an attractive option when the operative site is suitable. Concerns that high sensory levels of anesthesia will lead to sympathetic blockade and consequent bronchospasm are unfounded.

When general anesthesia is selected, induction of anesthesia is most often accomplished with an IV induction drug. Propofol is often used for induction in a *hemodynamically stable* asthmatic patient. It produces smooth muscle relaxation and contributes to decreased airway resistance. Ketamine is a preferred induction drug in a *hemodynamically unstable* patient with asthma.

After general anesthesia is induced, the lungs are often ventilated for a time with a gas mixture containing a volatile anesthetic. The goal is to establish a depth of anesthesia that depresses hyperreactive airway reflexes sufficiently to permit tracheal intubation without precipitating bronchospasm. The lesser pungency of sevoflurane (compared with isoflurane and desflurane) may decrease the likelihood of coughing during this time. An alternative method to suppress airway reflexes before intubation is IV or intratracheal injection of lidocaine (1–1.5 mg/kg) several minutes before endotracheal intubation.

Opioids should also be administered to suppress the cough reflex and to achieve deep anesthesia. However, prolongation of opioid effects can cause postoperative respiratory depression. Remifentanil may be particularly useful because it is an ultra–short-acting opioid and does not accumulate. Most opioids have some histamine-releasing effects, but fentanyl and analogous drugs can be used safely in asthmatic patients. Administration of opioids prior to intubation can help prevent increased airway resistance, but muscle rigidity caused by an opioid could decrease lung compliance and impair ventilation.

Opioid-induced muscle rigidity can be decreased by the combined use of IV anesthetics and neuromuscular blocking drugs.

Insertion of an LMA is less likely to result in bronchoconstriction than insertion of an ET tube. Therefore use of an LMA is often a better method of airway management in asthmatic patients who are *not* at increased risk of reflux or aspiration. During maintenance of general anesthesia, it may be difficult to differentiate light anesthesia from bronchospasm as the cause of a decrease in pulmonary compliance. Administration of a neuromuscular blocker will relieve the ventilatory difficulty resulting from light anesthesia but has no effect on bronchospasm.

Intraoperatively the desired level of arterial oxygenation and carbon dioxide removal is typically provided via mechanical ventilation. In asthmatic patients, sufficient time must be provided for exhalation to prevent air trapping. Humidification and warming of inspired gases may be especially useful in patients with exercise-induced asthma in whom bronchospasm may be due to transmucosal loss of heat. Adequate administration of fluids during the perioperative period is important for maintaining adequate hydration and ensuring that airway secretions are less viscous and can be removed easily. Skeletal muscle relaxation is usually provided with nondepolarizing muscle relaxants. Neuromuscular blockers with limited ability to evoke the release of histamine should be selected.

Theoretically, antagonism of neuromuscular blockade with anticholinesterase drugs could precipitate bronchospasm due to stimulation of postganglionic cholinergic receptors in airway smooth muscle. However, such bronchospasm does not predictably occur after administration of anticholinesterase drugs, probably because of the protective bronchodilating effects provided by the simultaneous administration of anticholinergic drugs.

At the conclusion of surgery, it may be prudent to remove the ET tube while anesthesia is still sufficient to suppress hyperreactive airway reflexes, a technique referred to as *deep extubation*. When it is deemed unwise to extubate the trachea before the patient is fully awake, suppressing airway reflexes and/or the risk of bronchospasm by administration of IV lidocaine or treatment with inhaled bronchodilators should be considered.

During surgery, bronchospasm may be due to light anesthesia rather than asthma itself (Table 2.8). Signs may include high peak airway pressure, upsloping of the end-tidal carbon dioxide ($ETCO_2$) waveform, wheezing, and desaturation. Treatment of intraoperative bronchospasm and wheezing will depend on its cause. Deepening anesthesia with either volatile agents or IV injections of propofol and administration of a rapid-acting β_2-agonist such as albuterol via the ET tube are common first steps. If bronchospasm continues despite these initial therapies, other drugs (e.g., IV corticosteroids, epinephrine, magnesium) may be necessary.

Emergency surgery in the asthmatic patient introduces a conflict between protection of the airway in someone at risk of aspiration and the possibility of triggering significant bronchospasm. In addition, there may not be sufficient time to optimize bronchodilator therapy prior to surgery. Regional anesthesia may be a good option in this situation if the site of surgery is suitable.

CHRONIC OBSTRUCTIVE PULMONARY DISEASE

COPD is a disease of progressive loss of alveolar tissue and progressive airflow obstruction that is *not reversible*. Pulmonary elastic recoil is lost as a result of bronchiolar and alveolar destruction, often from inhaling toxic chemicals such as are contained in cigarette smoke. The World Health Organization (WHO) predicts that by 2030 COPD will be the third leading cause of death worldwide. Risk factors for developing COPD include (1) cigarette smoking, (2) occupational exposure to dust and chemicals, especially in coal mining, gold mining, and the textile industry, (3) indoor and outdoor pollution, (4) recurrent childhood respiratory infections, and (5) low birth weight. α_1-Antitrypsin deficiency is an inherited disorder associated with premature development of COPD. Patients with COPD pose a challenge to the anesthesiologist because intraoperative and postoperative pulmonary complications are more common in this patient population, and the presence of COPD is associated with an increased length of hospital stay and mortality.

COPD causes (1) pathologic deterioration in elasticity or "recoil" within the lung parenchyma, which normally maintains the airways in an open position; (2) pathologic changes that decrease the rigidity of the bronchiolar wall and thus predispose them to collapse during exhalation; (3) an increase in gas flow velocity in narrowed bronchioli, which lowers the pressure inside the bronchioli and further favors airway collapse; (4) active bronchospasm and obstruction resulting from increased pulmonary secretions; and (5) destruction of lung parenchyma, enlargement of air sacs, and development of emphysema.

Signs and Symptoms

Signs and symptoms of COPD vary with disease severity but usually include dyspnea on exertion or at rest, chronic cough, and chronic sputum production. COPD exacerbations are periods of worsening symptoms as a result of an acute worsening in airflow obstruction. As expiratory airflow obstruction

TABLE 2.8	Differential Diagnosis of Intraoperative Bronchospasm and Wheezing

Mechanical obstruction of endotracheal tube
   Kinking
   Secretions
   Overinflation of tracheal tube cuff
Inadequate depth of anesthesia
   Active expiratory efforts
   Decreased functional residual capacity
Endobronchial intubation
Pulmonary aspiration
Pulmonary edema
Pulmonary embolus
Pneumothorax
Acute asthmatic attack

increases in severity, tachypnea and a prolonged expiratory time are evident. Breath sounds are likely to be decreased, and expiratory wheezes are common.

Diagnosis

Patients with COPD will usually report symptoms like dyspnea and chronic cough as well as a history of exposure to risk factors. However, COPD cannot be definitively diagnosed without spirometry.

Pulmonary Function Tests

Results of PFTs in COPD reveal a decrease in the FEV_1:FVC ratio and an even greater decrease in the FEF between 25% and 75% of vital capacity ($FEF_{25\%-75\%}$). An FEV_1:FVC less than 70% of predicted that is not reversible with bronchodilators confirms the diagnosis. Other spirometric findings of

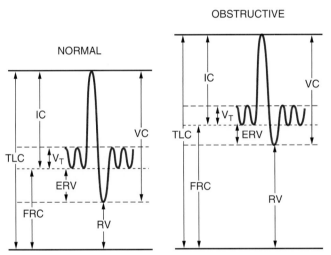

FIG. 2.4 Lung volumes in COPD compared with normal values. In the presence of obstructive lung disease, the vital capacity (VC) is normal to decreased, the residual volume (RV) and functional residual capacity (FRC) are increased, the total lung capacity (TLC) is normal to increased, and the RV:TLC ratio is increased. *ERV,* Expiratory reserve volume; *IC,* inspiratory capacity; *V_T,* tidal volume.

COPD include an increased FRC and TLC (Fig. 2.4). Slowing of expiratory airflow and gas trapping behind prematurely closed airways are responsible for the increase in residual volume (RV). The pathophysiologic "advantage" of an increased RV and FRC in patients with COPD is related to an enlarged airway diameter and increased elastic recoil for exhalation. The cost is the greater work of breathing at the higher lung volumes.

The Global Initiative for Chronic Obstructive Lung Disease (GOLD) works with healthcare professionals and public health officials around the world to raise awareness of COPD and to improve prevention and treatment of this lung disease. GOLD was launched in 1997 in collaboration with the National Heart, Lung, and Blood Institute of the US National Institutes of Health and the WHO. GOLD developed a classification/severity grading system that is now widely used by physicians around the world (Table 2.9).

Chest Radiography

Radiographic abnormalities may be minimal even in the presence of severe COPD. Hyperlucency due to arterial vascular deficiency in the lung periphery and hyperinflation (flattening of the diaphragm with loss of its normal domed appearance and a very vertical cardiac silhouette) suggest the diagnosis of emphysema. If bullae are present, the diagnosis of emphysema is certain. However, only a small percentage of patients with emphysema have bullae.

Computed Tomography

CT is a much more sensitive test compared to simple chest radiography at diagnosing COPD. However, it is not used routinely for this purpose. It is used to screen for lung cancer and to evaluate the lungs prior to lung surgery. Findings indicative of COPD include bronchial wall thickening, alveolar septal destruction, and airspace enlargement.

Arterial Blood Gases

Arterial blood gas measurements often remain relatively normal until COPD is severe. The Pao_2 does not usually decrease

TABLE 2.9	GOLD Spirometric Criteria for COPD Severity (Based on Postbronchodilator FEV_1 Measurement)
Stage	Characteristics
0: At risk	Normal spirometric findings Chronic symptoms (cough, sputum production)
I: Mild COPD	FEV_1:FVC < 70% $FEV_1 \geq 80\%$ predicted, with or without chronic symptoms (cough, sputum production)
II: Moderate COPD	FEV_1:FVC < 70% $50\% \leq FEV_1 < 80\%$ predicted, with or without chronic symptoms (cough, sputum production)
III: Severe COPD	FEV_1:FVC < 70% $30\% \leq FEV_1 < 50\%$ predicted, with or without chronic symptoms (cough, sputum production)
IV: Very severe COPD	FEV_1:FVC < 70% $FEV_1 < 30\%$ predicted or $FEV_1 < 50\%$ predicted plus chronic respiratory failure (i.e., $Pao_2 < 60$ mm Hg and/or $Pco_2 > 50$ mm Hg)

Adapted from Global Initiative for Chronic Obstructive Lung Disease. Global strategy for the diagnosis, management and prevention of COPD: update 2010. http://www.goldcopd.com.

TABLE 2.10	Treatment of Patients With COPD

Smoking cessation
Annual vaccination against influenza
Vaccination against pneumococcus
Inhaled long-acting bronchodilators
Inhaled corticosteroids
Inhaled long-acting anticholinergic drugs
Home oxygen therapy if Pao_2 < 55 mm Hg, hematocrit > 55%, or there is evidence of cor pulmonale
Diuretics if evidence of right heart failure with peripheral edema
Lung volume reduction surgery
Lung transplantation

TABLE 2.11	Treatment of Patients With a COPD Exacerbation

Supplemental oxygen ± noninvasive positive pressure ventilation or mechanical ventilation
Increased dose and frequency of bronchodilator therapy
Systemic corticosteroids
Antibiotics

until the FEV_1 is less than 50% of predicted, and the $Paco_2$ may not increase until the FEV_1 is even lower.

Treatment

Treatment of COPD is designed to relieve symptoms and to slow the progression of the disease.

Smoking cessation and long-term oxygen administration are the two important therapeutic interventions that can alter the natural history of COPD. Smoking cessation should be the first step in treating COPD. This intervention significantly decreases disease progression and lowers mortality by 18%. Smoking cessation causes the symptoms of chronic bronchitis to diminish or entirely disappear, and it eliminates the accelerated loss of lung function observed in those who continue to smoke.

Long-term oxygen administration (home oxygen therapy) is recommended if the Pao_2 is less than 55 mm Hg, the hematocrit is above 55%, or there is evidence of cor pulmonale. The goal of supplemental oxygen administration is to achieve a Pao_2 greater than 60 mm Hg. This goal can usually be accomplished by delivering oxygen through a nasal cannula at 2 L/min. The flow rate of oxygen can be titrated as needed according to arterial blood gas or pulse oximetry measurements. *Relief of arterial hypoxemia with supplemental oxygen administration is more effective than any known drug therapy in decreasing pulmonary vascular resistance and pulmonary hypertension and in preventing erythrocytosis.*

Drug treatment of COPD may include long-acting β_2-agonists, inhaled corticosteroids, and long-acting anticholinergic drugs, often in combination (Table 2.10). This therapy not only improves FEV_1 and dyspnea but also reduces the number of exacerbations of COPD by up to 25%. Other pharmacologic treatments include vaccinations against influenza and pneumococcus, and diuretics in patients with cor pulmonale and right-sided heart failure with peripheral edema. During periods of exacerbation, antibiotics, systemic corticosteroids, and theophylline may become necessary additional treatments (Table 2.11). Exacerbations of COPD may be due to viral or bacterial infection of the upper respiratory tract or may be noninfective, so antibiotic treatment is not always warranted. Diuretic-induced chloride depletion may produce a hypochloremic metabolic alkalosis that depresses the ventilatory drive and may aggravate chronic carbon dioxide retention. Physical training programs can increase the exercise capacity of patients with COPD despite the absence of detectable effects on PFTs. However, prompt deconditioning occurs when the exercise program is discontinued.

Lung Volume Reduction Surgery

In selected patients with severe COPD who are not responding to maximal medical therapy and who have regions of overdistended, poorly functioning lung tissue, lung volume reduction surgery may be considered. Surgical removal of these overdistended areas allows the more normal areas of lung to expand and improves not only lung function but also quality of life. Lung volume reduction surgery is performed via either a median sternotomy or a video-assisted thoracoscopic surgery (VATS) approach. The proposed mechanisms for improvement in lung function after this surgery include (1) an increase in elastic recoil, which increases expiratory airflow; (2) a decrease in the degree of hyperinflation, which results in improved diaphragmatic and chest wall mechanics; and (3) a decrease in the inhomogeneity of regional ventilation and perfusion, which results in improved alveolar gas exchange and increased effectiveness of ventilation. Research is currently underway to examine nonsurgical approaches for achieving benefits similar to those provided by lung volume reduction surgery.

Management of anesthesia for lung volume reduction surgery includes use of a double-lumen endobronchial tube to permit lung separation, avoidance of nitrous oxide, and avoidance of excessive positive airway pressure. Monitoring of central venous pressure as a guide to fluid management is unreliable in this situation.

Management of Anesthesia

A complete history should be taken and geared toward investigating the causes, course, and severity of the COPD. The smoking history, current medications (including any recent use of systemic corticosteroids), exercise tolerance, frequency of exacerbations and the timing of the most recent exacerbation, and the need for hospitalization are all important pieces of information. The requirement for noninvasive positive pressure ventilation (NIPPV) or mechanical ventilation is another key piece of information. Because smoking and COPD are associated with a number of comorbidities, patients should also be questioned regarding the presence and severity of concomitant diseases such as diabetes mellitus, hypertension, peripheral vascular disease, ischemic heart disease, heart failure, cardiac dysrhythmias, and lung cancer. Long-acting bronchodilators, anticholinergics, and inhaled corticosteroids should be continued until the morning of surgery. Patients coming for elective surgery should be optimized prior to surgery to decrease morbidity and mortality after surgery.

The value of routine preoperative pulmonary function testing remains controversial. The results of PFTs and arterial blood gas analysis can be useful for predicting pulmonary function after lung resection, but they do not reliably predict the likelihood of postoperative pulmonary complications after nonthoracic surgery. Clinical findings (smoking, diffuse wheezing, productive cough) are more predictive of pulmonary complications than spirometric test results. Patients with COPD undergoing peripheral surgery do not require preoperative pulmonary function testing. If doubt exists, simple spirometry with measurement of only the FEV_1 can be sufficient to assess the severity of the lung disease.

Even patients defined as high risk by spirometry ($FEV_1 <$ 70% of predicted, FEV_1:FVC ratio < 65%) or arterial blood gas analysis ($Paco_2 > 45$ mm Hg) can undergo surgery, including lung resection, with an acceptable risk of postoperative pulmonary complications. PFTs should be viewed as a management tool to optimize preoperative pulmonary function but not as a means to predict risk. Indications for a preoperative pulmonary evaluation (which may include consultation with a pulmonologist and/or performance of PFTs) typically include (1) hypoxemia on room air or the need for home oxygen therapy without a known cause, (2) a bicarbonate concentration of more than 33 mEq/L or Pco_2 of more than 50 mm Hg in a patient whose pulmonary disease has not been previously evaluated, (3) a history of respiratory failure resulting from a problem that still exists, (4) severe shortness of breath attributed to respiratory disease, (5) planned pneumonectomy, (6) difficulty in assessing pulmonary function by clinical signs, (7) the need to distinguish among potential causes of significant respiratory compromise, (8) the need to determine the response to bronchodilators, and (9) suspected pulmonary hypertension.

Right ventricular function should be carefully assessed by clinical examination and echocardiography in patients with advanced pulmonary disease.

Ventilatory function is quantified under *static conditions* by measuring lung volumes and under *dynamic conditions* by measuring flow rates. With this assessment, expiratory flow rates can be plotted against lung volumes to produce *flow-volume curves*. When flow rates during inspiration are added to these curves, *flow-volume loops* are obtained. The flow rate is zero at TLC before the start of expiration. Once forced expiration begins, the peak flow rate is achieved rapidly, and the flow rate then falls in a linear fashion as the lung volume decreases to RV. During maximal inspiration from RV to TLC, the inspiratory flow is most rapid at the midpoint of inspiration, so that the inspiratory curve is U-shaped.

In patients with COPD there is a decrease in the expiratory flow rate at any given lung volume. The expiratory curve is concave upward due to uniform emptying of the airways. The RV is increased because of air trapping (see Fig. 2.2).

TABLE 2.12	Major Risk Factors for Development of Postoperative Pulmonary Complications

PATIENT RELATED

Age > 60 yr
American Society of Anesthesiologists class higher than II
Congestive heart failure
Preexisting pulmonary disease (chronic obstructive pulmonary disease)
Cigarette smoking

PROCEDURE RELATED

Emergency surgery
Abdominal or thoracic surgery, head and neck surgery, neurosurgery, vascular/aortic aneurysm surgery
Prolonged duration of anesthesia (>2.5 h)
General anesthesia

TEST PREDICTORS

Albumin level of < 3.5 g/dL

Adapted from Smetana GW, Lawrence VA, Cornell JE. Preoperative pulmonary risk stratification for noncardiothoracic surgery. A systematic review for the American College of Physicians. *Ann Intern Med.* 2006;144:581-595.

The major risk factors for the development of postoperative pulmonary complications are shown in Table 2.12. Obesity and mild to moderate asthma have not been shown to be independent risk factors. An algorithm for reducing pulmonary complications in patients undergoing noncardiothoracic surgery is shown in Fig. 2.5.

Risk Reduction Strategies

Strategies to decrease the incidence of postoperative pulmonary complications include preoperative, intraoperative, and postoperative interventions (Table 2.13).

Smoking Cessation

Approximately 20% of American adults smoke, of whom 5%–10% will annually undergo general anesthesia and/or surgery. These times of exposure to general anesthesia and/or surgery offer a window of opportunity for a smoking cessation intervention by a healthcare provider or other individual. This person can be the surgeon, anesthesiologist, nurse, or even a member of an active patient group or community group, who should encourage the patient to stop smoking *at least temporarily* before surgery or preferably permanently. The intervention can be carried out in the surgical clinic or anesthetic preadmission testing clinic, via phone calls by nurses or healthcare workers, or in a letter indicating the risks of postoperative complications caused by smoking. Recent evidence shows that the earlier the intervention before surgery, the more effective it is in reducing postoperative complications and maintaining cigarette abstinence. *Cigarette smoking is the single most important risk factor for the development of COPD and death caused by lung disease.* The effects of smoking on different organ systems are described in Table 2.14. Smoking cessation is strongly encouraged by the US Public Health Service. It recommends systematically identifying all tobacco users who

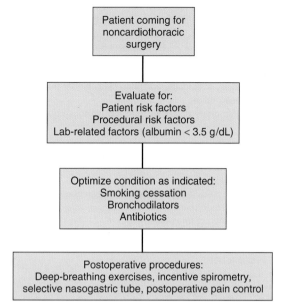

FIG. 2.5 Algorithm for decreasing pulmonary complications in patients undergoing noncardiothoracic surgery. (Adapted from Qaseem A, Snow V, Fitterman N, et al. Risk assessment for and strategies to reduce perioperative pulmonary complications for patients undergoing noncardiothoracic surgery: a guideline from the American College of Physicians. *Ann Intern Med.* 2006;144:575-580.)

TABLE 2.13	Strategies to Decrease Incidence of Postoperative Pulmonary Complications

PREOPERATIVE
Encourage cessation of smoking for at least 6 weeks.
Treat evidence of expiratory airflow obstruction.
Treat respiratory infection with antibiotics.
Initiate patient education regarding lung volume expansion maneuvers.

INTRAOPERATIVE
Use minimally invasive surgery (endoscopic) techniques when possible.
Consider regional anesthesia.
Avoid surgical procedures likely to last longer than 3 hours.

POSTOPERATIVE
Institute lung volume expansion maneuvers (voluntary deep breathing, incentive spirometry, continuous positive airway pressure).
Maximize analgesia (neuraxial opioids, intercostal nerve blocks, patient-controlled analgesia).

Adapted from Smetana GW. Preoperative pulmonary evaluation. *N Engl J Med.* 1999;340:937-944. Copyright 1999 Massachusetts Medical Society.

TABLE 2.14	Effects of Smoking on Different Organ Systems

CARDIAC EFFECTS OF SMOKING
Smoking is a risk factor for development of cardiovascular disease.
Carbon monoxide decreases oxygen delivery and increases myocardial work.
Smoking releases catecholamines and causes coronary vasoconstriction.
Smoking decreases exercise capacity.

RESPIRATORY EFFECTS OF SMOKING
Smoking is the major risk factor for development of chronic pulmonary disease.
Smoking decreases mucociliary activity.
Smoking results in hyperreactive airways.
Smoking decreases pulmonary immune function.

OTHER ORGAN SYSTEM EFFECTS
Smoking impairs wound healing.

come in contact with the healthcare system to urge and help them to quit smoking. The American Society of Anesthesiologists also has a Stop Smoking Initiative and provides resources to help practitioners encourage smoking cessation. The maximum benefit of smoking cessation is not usually seen unless smoking is stopped more than 8 weeks prior to surgery.

Among smokers, predictive factors for the development of pulmonary complications include a lower diffusing capacity than predicted and a smoking history of more than 60 pack-years. Those who have smoked more than 60 pack-years have double the risk of any pulmonary complication and triple the risk of pneumonia compared with those who have smoked less than 60 pack-years. Smoking cessation causes the symptoms of chronic bronchitis to diminish or disappear and eliminates the accelerated loss of lung function observed in those who continue to smoke.

Effects of Smoking Cessation. The adverse effects of carbon monoxide on oxygen-carrying capacity and of nicotine on the cardiovascular system are short lived. The elimination half-life of carbon monoxide is approximately 4–6 hours when breathing room air. Within 12 hours after cessation of smoking, the Pao_2 at which hemoglobin is 50% saturated with oxygen (P_{50}) increases from 22.9 to 26.4 mm Hg, and the plasma levels of carboxyhemoglobin decrease from 6.5% to about 1%. Carbon monoxide may have negative inotropic effects. Despite the favorable effects on plasma carboxyhemoglobin concentration, short-term abstinence from cigarettes has not been proven to decrease the incidence of postoperative pulmonary complications. The sympathomimetic effects of nicotine on the heart are transient, lasting only 20–30 minutes.

Intermediate to Long-Term Effects. Cigarette smoking causes mucus hypersecretion, impairment of mucociliary transport, and narrowing of small airways. In contrast to the rapid favorable effects of short-term abstinence from smoking on carboxyhemoglobin concentrations, improved ciliary and small airway function and decreased sputum production occur slowly *over weeks* after smoking cessation. Cigarette smoking may interfere with normal immune responses and could interfere with the ability of smokers to respond to pulmonary infection following anesthesia and surgery. A decrease in postoperative pulmonary complications resulting from smoking cessation is thought to be related to the physiologic improvement in ciliary action, macrophage activity, and small airway function, as well as a decrease in sputum production. However, these changes take weeks to months to occur. Return of normal immune function requires at least 6 weeks of abstinence from smoking. Some components of cigarette smoke stimulate hepatic enzymes. As with immune responses, it may take 6 weeks or longer for hepatic enzyme activity to return to normal following cessation of smoking.

The optimal timing of smoking cessation before surgery to reduce postoperative pulmonary complications is uncertain, but most data suggest that it is around 6–8 weeks. Smokers scheduled for surgery in less than 4 weeks should be advised to quit and should be offered effective interventions, including behavioral support and pharmacotherapy, to help achieve this goal. Despite the clear advantages of long-term smoking cessation, there can be disadvantages to smoking cessation in the *immediate preoperative period*. These include an increase in sputum production, patient fear of the inability to handle stress, nicotine withdrawal, and symptoms including irritability, restlessness, sleep disturbances, and depression.

Countless methods have been devised to aid in smoking cessation. Most involve some form of counseling and pharmacotherapy. Nicotine replacement therapy, with various delivery systems including patches, inhalers, nasal sprays, lozenges, and gum, is generally well tolerated. The major side effect is local irritation at the site of drug delivery. The atypical antidepressant bupropion in a sustained-release formulation can also aid in smoking cessation. The drug is typically started 1–2 weeks before smoking is stopped.

Nutritional Status

Poor nutritional status with a low serum albumin level (<3.5 mg/dL) is a powerful predictor of postoperative pulmonary complications in COPD patients. Malnutrition can increase the risk of prolonged postoperative air leaks after lung surgery.

Regional Anesthesia

Regional anesthesia is preferred over general anesthesia in patients with COPD; this technique can decrease the risk of laryngospasm, bronchospasm, barotrauma, and hypoxemia associated with positive pressure ventilation and endotracheal intubation. Regional anesthesia is suitable for operations that do not invade the peritoneum and for surgical procedures performed on the extremities. Lower intraabdominal surgery can also be performed using a regional technique. General anesthesia is the usual choice for upper abdominal and intrathoracic surgery. Some studies in patients with COPD suggest that there is a higher incidence of postoperative respiratory failure in patients who undergo general anesthesia, but whether this reflects the nature and complexity of the surgery and/or the operative site, or the selection of anesthetic drugs or technique is unclear.

Regional anesthesia via peripheral nerve blockade carries a low risk of pulmonary complications. However, an interscalene block typically causes ipsilateral phrenic nerve palsy and should be avoided in patients with severe COPD. Regional anesthesia is a useful choice in patients with COPD only if large doses of sedative and anxiolytic drugs will *not* be needed.

It must be appreciated that COPD patients can be extremely sensitive to the ventilatory depressant effects of sedative drugs. Elderly patients may be especially susceptible. Often small doses of a benzodiazepine such as midazolam can be administered without producing undesirable degrees of ventilatory depression. Use of regional anesthetic techniques that produce sensory anesthesia above T6 is not recommended, because such high blocks can impair the ventilatory functions requiring active exhalation; this affects parameters such as expiratory reserve volume, PEFR, and maximum minute ventilation. Clinically this is manifested as an inadequate cough.

General Anesthesia

General anesthesia is often accomplished with volatile anesthetics. Volatile anesthetics are useful because of the ability of these drugs (especially desflurane and sevoflurane) to be rapidly eliminated. Residual ventilatory depression during the early postoperative period is thereby minimized. Volatile anesthetics are also known to cause bronchodilation and have been used to treat bronchospasm in status asthmaticus. Desflurane, however, may cause irritation of the bronchi and increased airway resistance, so there may be an advantage to choosing a less irritating vapor such as sevoflurane for induction and emergence in cases of severe airway reactivity. Emergence from anesthesia with inhalational agents can be prolonged significantly, especially in patients with significant airway obstruction, because air trapping also traps the inhalational drugs as they try to flood out of the various body compartments into the lungs. An alternative is total IV anesthesia with propofol. A short-acting analgesic such as remifentanil can be used to relieve the irritation of the ET tube sufficiently that the required level of propofol can be diminished considerably and the attendant risk of hypotension reduced.

Nitrous oxide should be used with great caution owing to the possibility of enlargement or rupture of bullae, resulting in development of a tension pneumothorax. Another potential disadvantage of nitrous oxide is the limitation on inspired oxygen concentration it imposes. It is important to remember that inhaled anesthetics may attenuate regional hypoxic pulmonary vasoconstriction and produce more intrapulmonary shunting. Increasing the fraction of inspired oxygen (FIO_2) may be necessary to offset this loss of hypoxic pulmonary vasoconstriction.

Opioids may be less useful than inhaled anesthetics for maintenance of anesthesia in patients with COPD, because they can be associated with prolonged ventilatory depression as a result of their slow rate of metabolism or elimination. Even the duration of ventilatory depression produced by drugs such as thiopental and midazolam may be prolonged in patients with COPD compared to healthy individuals.

An ET tube bypasses most of the natural airway humidification system, so humidification of inspired gases and use of low gas flows are needed to keep airway secretions moist.

Patients with COPD are at increased risk of lung injury during mechanical ventilation in the perioperative period. The goals of mechanical ventilation must be to avoid dynamic hyperinflation of the lungs and prevent development of auto-PEEP. Most studies show low tidal volumes (6–8 mL/kg), peak airway pressures less than 30 cm H_2O, and FIO_2 titrated to keep SpO_2 greater than 90% result in lower levels of inflammatory markers in bronchoalveolar lavage fluid of mechanically ventilated patients. Patients with moderate to severe COPD can have cystic air spaces in the lungs that carry a risk of rupture once positive pressure ventilation is instituted. *In patients with COPD who become hemodynamically unstable during mechanical ventilation, the differential diagnosis must include tension pneumothorax and bronchopleural fistula.*

The phenomenon of *air trapping*, also called *auto PEEP, intrinsic PEEP,* or *dynamic hyperinflation,* occurs when positive pressure ventilation is applied and insufficient expiratory time is allowed. This contributes to increased intrathoracic pressure, impedes venous return, and transmits the elevated intrathoracic pressure to the pulmonary artery. An increase in pulmonary vascular resistance can lead to right ventricular strain. Hyperinflated lungs may exert direct pressure on the heart, limiting its ability to expand fully during diastole even with adequate preload. Shift of the ventricular septum and ventricular interdependence due to the shared pericardium may cause a distended right ventricle to impinge on filling of the left ventricle.

Air trapping can be detected during mechanical ventilation intraoperatively by the following methods:

1. Capnography shows that the carbon dioxide concentration does not plateau but is still upsloping at the time of the next breath. This indicates that there is still admixture of air from dead space reducing the $ETCO_2$.
2. Direct measurement of flow may be displayed graphically by the ventilator, showing that the expiratory flow has not reached baseline (zero) before initiation of the next breath.
3. Direct measurement of the resulting PEEP can be performed using more advanced ventilators that are capable of an expiratory hold.

Air trapping can cause serious hemodynamic instability by increasing intrathoracic pressure and decreasing preload. Treatment includes decreasing respiratory rate and increasing expiratory time and, if immediate intervention is needed, disconnecting the patient from the ventilator to allow for complete exhalation.

Much like patients with asthma, patients with COPD are prone to bronchospasm. Bronchospasm is often due to airway manipulation during induction and/or to light anesthesia during maintenance. Treatments include deepening anesthesia with either a volatile anesthetic or propofol, delivering a short-acting bronchodilator through the ET tube, suctioning secretions, and administration of IV corticosteroids and/or epinephrine if initial management options fail.

Although traditionally most anesthesiologists have used high inspired oxygen concentrations in the perioperative setting, a number of studies have questioned this practice. Oxygen can be split in tissues to produce reactive oxygen species (ROS), which can have a deleterious effect on nuclear and cell membranes. Surgery, anesthesia, and patient positioning predispose to airway closure and atelectasis. The time from airway occlusion to atelectasis is dependent on the composition of the alveolar gas and is faster in lung units containing 100% oxygen compared to those containing air.

The hazard of pulmonary barotrauma in the presence of bullae should be appreciated, particularly when high positive airway pressures are required to provide adequate ventilation. If spontaneous breathing is permitted during anesthesia in patients with COPD, it should be appreciated that the ventilatory depression produced by volatile anesthetics may be greater in these patients than in individuals without COPD.

Postoperative
Prevention of postoperative pulmonary complications is based on maintaining adequate lung volumes, especially FRC, and facilitating an effective cough. Identification of the FRC as the most important lung volume during the postoperative period provides a specific goal for therapy.

Lung Expansion Maneuvers
Lung expansion maneuvers (deep breathing exercises, incentive spirometry, chest physiotherapy, positive pressure breathing techniques) are of proven benefit in preventing postoperative pulmonary complications in patients at high risk. These techniques decrease the risk of atelectasis by increasing lung volumes. All regimens seem to be efficacious in decreasing the frequency of postoperative pulmonary complications compared with no therapy. Incentive spirometry is simple and inexpensive and provides objective goals for and monitoring of patient performance. Patients are given a particular inspired volume as a goal to achieve and hold. This provides sustained lung inflation, which is important for reexpanding collapsed alveoli. The major disadvantage of incentive spirometry is the need for patient cooperation to accomplish the treatment. Providing education in lung expansion maneuvers *before* surgery decreases the incidence of pulmonary complications to a greater degree than beginning education *after* surgery.

Continuous positive airway pressure (CPAP) is reserved for the prevention of postoperative pulmonary complications in patients who are not able to perform deep-breathing exercises or incentive spirometry. Nasal positive airway pressure can also minimize the expected decrease in lung volumes after surgery.

Postoperative neuraxial analgesia with opioids may permit early tracheal extubation. The sympathetic blockade, muscle weakness, and loss of proprioception that are produced by local anesthetics are not produced by neuraxial opioids. Therefore early ambulation is possible. Ambulation serves to increase FRC and improve oxygenation, presumably by improving ventilation/perfusion matching. Neuraxial opioids may be especially useful after intrathoracic and upper abdominal surgery. Breakthrough pain may require treatment with systemic opioids. Sedation may accompany neuraxial opioid administration, and delayed respiratory depression can be seen especially when poorly lipid-soluble opioids such as morphine are used.

Neuraxial analgesia has been proven to decrease the incidence of postoperative pneumonia when compared to parenteral opioids. Postoperative neuraxial analgesia is recommended after high-risk thoracic, abdominal, and major vascular surgery. Intermittent or continuous intercostal nerve or paravertebral nerve blocks may be alternatives if neuraxial analgesia is contraindicated or technically difficult.

Continued mechanical ventilation during the immediate postoperative period may be necessary in patients with severe COPD who have undergone major abdominal or intrathoracic surgery. Patients with preoperative FEV_1:FVC ratios of less than 0.5 or with a preoperative $Paco_2$ of more than 50 mm Hg are likely to need a period of postoperative mechanical ventilation. If the $Paco_2$ has been increased for a long period, it is important not to correct the hypercarbia too quickly because this will result in a significant metabolic alkalosis that can be associated with cardiac dysrhythmias and central nervous system irritability and even seizures.

When continued mechanical ventilation is necessary, Fio_2 and ventilator settings should be adjusted to keep the Spo_2 around 90% and the $Paco_2$ in a range that maintains the arterial pH at 7.35–7.45. Reduction of the respiratory rate or the I:E ratio allows more time for exhalation and thus reduces the likelihood of air trapping. However, this may also lower the tidal volume and minute ventilation and exacerbate hypercapnia, hypoxia, and acidosis. Pulmonary vascular resistance may then increase and can lead to right ventricular strain. Electrolyte shifts resulting from acidemia can cause cardiac dysrhythmias in patients with COPD or asthma. Extubation of the high-risk patient to CPAP or bilevel positive airway pressure (BiPAP) may reduce the air trapping and work of breathing. However, use of positive airway pressure in the setting of an unprotected airway raises concern about insufflation of the stomach and the risk of vomiting and aspiration. Treatment with sympathomimetic bronchodilators such as albuterol and inhaled anticholinergics such as ipratropium may improve airflow if a reactive component of air trapping is present.

Patients with severe COPD and a tenuous postextubation respiratory status may respond to a trial of BiPAP, which can lower the respiratory rate, decrease the work of breathing, and decrease the need for reintubation.

Early mobilization postoperatively can decrease pulmonary complications by promoting deeper breathing, lung expansion, and cough.

LESS COMMON CAUSES OF EXPIRATORY AIRFLOW OBSTRUCTION

Bronchiectasis

Bronchiectasis is associated with irreversible airway dilation in patients with either focal or diffuse lung involvement by this disease. Despite the availability of antibiotics, bronchiectasis is an important cause of chronic productive cough with purulent sputum and accounts for a significant number of cases of massive hemoptysis.

Pathophysiology

Bronchiectasis is characterized by localized irreversible dilatation of bronchi caused by destructive inflammatory processes involving the bronchial wall. For example, bacterial or mycobacterial infections can cause inflammation and destruction of medium-sized airways that can eventually lead to airway collapse, airflow obstruction, and an inability to clear secretions. The most important consequence of bronchiectatic destruction of airways is an increased susceptibility to recurrent or persistent bacterial infection, which reflects impaired mucociliary activity and pooling of mucus in dilated airways. Once bacterial superinfection is established, it is nearly impossible to eradicate, and daily expectoration of purulent sputum persists.

Diagnosis

The history of a chronic cough productive of purulent sputum is highly suggestive of bronchiectasis. Patients may also complain of hemoptysis, dyspnea, wheezing, and pleuritic chest pain. Clubbing of the fingers occurs in most patients with significant bronchiectasis and is a valuable diagnostic clue, especially since this change is not characteristic of COPD. Pulmonary function changes vary considerably and range from no change to alterations characteristic of COPD or restrictive lung disease. CT provides excellent images of bronchiectatic airways and can be used to confirm the presence and extent of the disease. It will usually show dilated bronchi much larger in diameter than their adjacent blood vessels.

Treatment

Bronchiectasis is treated with antibiotics and chest physiotherapy. Other treatments include yearly immunization against influenza, bronchodilators, systemic corticosteroids, and oxygen therapy. Results of periodic sputum cultures guide antibiotic selection. *Pseudomonas* is the most common organism cultured. *Massive hemoptysis,* defined as hemoptysis of more than 200 mL over a 24-hour period, may require surgical resection of the involved lung segment or selective bronchial arterial embolization. Chest physiotherapy with chest percussion and vibration can aid bronchopulmonary drainage. Surgical resection has played a declining role in the management of bronchiectasis in the modern antibiotic era and is considered only in the rare instance in which severe symptoms persist or recurrent complications occur.

Management of Anesthesia

Much like patients with other types of obstructive airway disease, a detailed history should be elicited from the patient, including severity of disease, frequency of exacerbations, and the date of the most recent exacerbation. Home medications should be continued until the morning of surgery. Elective procedures should be delayed if there are signs of active pulmonary infection with respiratory compromise or systemic involvement. During general anesthesia, the patient may need to be suctioned frequently through the ET tube to manage secretions. If the patient is undergoing surgery for management of an empyema or hemoptysis, a double-lumen endobronchial tube must be used to prevent spillage of purulent sputum into normal areas of the lungs. Nasal endotracheal intubation should be avoided because of the high rate of concurrent chronic sinusitis in these patients.

Cystic Fibrosis

Cystic fibrosis (CF) is an autosomal recessive disorder. It affects an estimated 30,000 persons in the United States.

Pathophysiology

The cause of CF is a mutation in a single gene on chromosome 7 that encodes the cystic fibrosis transmembrane conductance regulator *(CFTR)*. This regulator should produce a protein that helps salt and water move in and out of cells. The dysfunctional regulator blocks this movement and results in the production of an abnormally thick mucus outside of epithelial cells. Decreased chloride transport is accompanied by decreased transport of sodium and water, which results in dehydrated viscous secretions that are associated with luminal obstruction, as well as destruction and scarring of various glands and tissues. This causes damage to the lungs (bronchiectasis, COPD, sinusitis), pancreas (diabetes mellitus), liver (cirrhosis), gastrointestinal tract (meconium ileus), and reproductive organs (azoospermia). The primary cause of morbidity and mortality in patients with CF is chronic pulmonary infection.

Diagnosis

The presence of a sweat chloride concentration greater than 70 mEq/L plus the characteristic clinical manifestations (cough, chronic purulent sputum production, exertional dyspnea) or family history of the disease confirms the diagnosis of CF. DNA analysis can identify the more than 90% of patients having the *CFTR* mutation. Chronic pansinusitis is almost universal. The presence of normal sinuses on radiographic examination is strong evidence that CF is *not* present. Malabsorption with a response to pancreatic enzyme treatment is evidence of the exocrine insufficiency associated with CF. Obstructive azoospermia confirmed by testicular biopsy is also strong evidence of CF. Bronchoalveolar lavage typically shows a high percentage of neutrophils, which is a sign of airway inflammation. COPD is present in virtually all adult patients with CF and follows a relentless downhill course.

Treatment

Treatment of CF is similar to that for bronchiectasis and is directed toward alleviation of symptoms (mobilization and clearance of lower airway secretions and treatment of pulmonary infection), correction of organ dysfunction (pancreatic enzyme replacement), nutrition, and prevention of intestinal obstruction. Gene therapy is currently being investigated as a treatment for CF. This involves insertion of a normal *CFTR* gene into lung cells of CF patients.

Clearance of Airway Secretions

The abnormal viscoelastic properties of the sputum in patients with CF lead to sputum retention resulting in airway obstruction. The principal nonpharmacologic approach to enhancing clearance of pulmonary secretions is chest physiotherapy with postural drainage. High-frequency chest compression with an inflatable vest and airway oscillation with a flutter valve are alternative methods of physiotherapy that are less time consuming and do not require trained personnel.

Bronchodilator Therapy

Bronchial reactivity to histamine and other provocative stimuli is greater in patients with CF than in individuals without the disease. Bronchodilator therapy can be considered if patients are known to have a response to inhaled bronchodilators. A response is defined as an increase of 10% or more in FEV_1 after bronchodilator administration.

Reduction in Viscoelasticity of Sputum

The abnormal viscosity of airway secretions is due primarily to the presence of neutrophils and their degradation products. DNA released from neutrophils forms long fibrils that contribute to the viscosity of the sputum. Recombinant human deoxyribonuclease I (dornase alfa [Pulmozyme]) can cleave this DNA and increase the clearance of sputum.

Antibiotic Therapy

Patients with CF have periodic exacerbations of pulmonary infection that are recognized primarily by an increase in symptoms and in sputum production. Antibiotic therapy is based on identification and susceptibility testing of bacteria isolated from the sputum. In patients in whom cultures yield no pathogens, bronchoscopy to remove lower airway secretions may be indicated. Many patients with CF are given long-term maintenance antibiotic therapy in the hope of suppressing chronic infection and development of bronchiectasis.

Management of Anesthesia

Management of anesthesia in patients with CF follows the same principles as outlined for patients with COPD and bronchiectasis. Elective surgical procedures should be delayed until optimal pulmonary function can be ensured by controlling bronchial infection and facilitating removal of airway secretions. Vitamin K treatment may be necessary if hepatic function is poor or if absorption of fat-soluble vitamins from the gastrointestinal tract is impaired. Maintenance of anesthesia with volatile anesthetics permits the use of high inspired concentrations of oxygen, decreases airway resistance by decreasing bronchial smooth muscle tone, and decreases the responsiveness of hyperreactive airways. Humidification of inspired gases, hydration, and avoidance of anticholinergic drugs are important to maintain secretions in a less viscous state. Frequent tracheal suctioning may be necessary. Patients should regain their full airway reflexes and ventilatory abilities before extubation to decrease risk of aspiration. Postoperative pain control is extremely important to allow for deep breathing, coughing, and early ambulation so that pulmonary complications such as pneumonia, hypoxia, and atelectasis can be prevented.

Primary Ciliary Dyskinesia

Primary ciliary dyskinesia is characterized by congenital impairment of ciliary activity in respiratory tract epithelial cells and sperm tails (spermatozoa are alive but immobile). As a result of impaired ciliary activity in the respiratory tract, chronic sinusitis, recurrent respiratory infections, and bronchiectasis develop. Not only is there infertility in males, but fertility is decreased in females, since oviducts also have ciliated epithelium. The triad of chronic sinusitis, bronchiectasis, and situs inversus is known as *Kartagener's syndrome.* It is speculated that the normal asymmetrical positioning of body organs is dependent on normal ciliary function of the embryonic epithelium. In the absence of normal ciliary function, placement of organs to the left or the right is random. As expected, approximately half of patients with congenitally nonfunctioning cilia manifest situs inversus. However, isolated dextrocardia is almost always associated with congenital heart disease.

Preoperative preparation is directed at treating active pulmonary infection and determining whether any significant organ inversion is present. Regional anesthesia is preferable to general anesthesia in these patients to help decrease postoperative pulmonary complications. In the presence of dextrocardia, it is necessary to reverse the position of the ECG leads to permit their accurate interpretation. Inversion of the great vessels is a reason to select the left internal jugular vein for central venous cannulation. Uterine displacement in parturient women is logically to the right in these patients. Should a double-lumen endobronchial tube be considered, it is necessary to appreciate the altered anatomy introduced by pulmonary inversion. In view of the high incidence of sinusitis, nasopharyngeal airways should be avoided.

Bronchiolitis Obliterans

Bronchiolitis obliterans is a disease of the small airways and alveoli occurring in childhood as a result of infection with RSV. It is a rare cause of COPD in adults. However, this process may accompany viral pneumonia, collagen vascular disease (especially rheumatoid arthritis), and inhalation of nitrogen dioxide (silo filler's disease), or it may be a sequela of graft-versus-host disease after bone marrow transplantation or lung transplantation. It causes airway and alveolar destruction, resulting in airflow obstruction. *Bronchiolitis obliterans with organizing pneumonia (BOOP)* is a clinical entity that shares certain features of interstitial lung disease and bronchiolitis obliterans. *Treatment of bronchiolitis obliterans is usually ineffective,* although corticosteroids may be administered in an attempt to suppress inflammation involving the bronchioles. BOOP, however, *does respond* well to corticosteroid therapy. Symptomatic improvement may also accompany the use of bronchodilators.

Tracheal Stenosis

Tracheal stenosis typically develops after prolonged intubation of the trachea either with an ET tube or a tracheostomy tube. Tracheal mucosal ischemia that may progress to destruction of cartilaginous rings and subsequent circumferential constricting scar formation is minimized by the use of high-volume, low-pressure cuffs on tracheal tubes. Infection and hypotension may also contribute to events that culminate in tracheal stenosis.

Diagnosis
Tracheal stenosis becomes symptomatic when the lumen of the adult trachea is decreased to less than 5 mm in diameter. Symptoms may not develop until several weeks after tracheal extubation. Dyspnea is prominent even at rest. These patients must use accessory muscles of respiration during all phases of the breathing cycle and must breathe slowly. PEFRs are decreased. Stridor is usually audible. Flow-volume loops typically display flattened inspiratory and expiratory curves characteristic of a fixed airway obstruction. (see Fig. 2.3A). CT of the trachea will demonstrate tracheal narrowing.

Management of Anesthesia
Tracheal dilation can be used as a temporizing measure to treat tracheal stenosis in some patients. This can be done bronchoscopically using balloon dilators or surgical dilators or laser resection of the tissue at the stenotic site. A tracheobronchial stent could also be inserted as either a temporary or longer-term solution to this problem. The most successful treatment is surgical tracheal resection and reconstruction with primary reanastomosis. This produces excellent long-term results. For this procedure, translaryngeal endotracheal intubation is accomplished. After surgical exposure, the distal normal trachea is opened and a sterile cuffed tube is inserted and attached to the anesthetic circuit. Maintenance of anesthesia with volatile anesthetics is useful for ensuring a maximum inspired concentration of oxygen. High-frequency ventilation can be helpful in selected patients. Anesthesia for tracheal resection may be facilitated by the addition of helium to the inspired gases. This decreases the density of the gas mixture and may improve flow through the area of tracheal narrowing.

KEY POINTS

- Surgical patients with preexisting respiratory disease are at increased risk of respiratory complications both during and after surgery.
- The anesthetic management of a patient with a recent upper respiratory tract infection (URI) should focus on reducing secretions and limiting manipulation of a potentially hyperresponsive airway.
- If a patient with a URI appears toxic, elective surgery should be delayed.
- Asthma treatment is classified into immediate and long-term therapy. Immediate therapy for bronchospasm

consists mainly of short-acting β-adrenergic agonists, whereas long-term relief includes long-acting β-agonists, inhaled corticosteroids, leukotriene modifiers, and/or monoclonal antibodies.

- In asthmatic patients the goal during induction and maintenance of anesthesia is to depress airway reflexes sufficiently to avoid bronchoconstriction in response to mechanical stimulation of the airway.
- In COPD, smoking cessation and long-term oxygen therapy are the only two interventions that may decrease disease progression and mortality. Drug therapies including inhaled β-adrenergic agonists, inhaled corticosteroids, and anticholinergic drugs are managed with a goal of decreasing exacerbation frequency.
- Pulmonary function tests (PFTs) have limited value in predicting the likelihood of postoperative pulmonary complications, and the results of PFTs in isolation should not be used to deny a patient access to surgery/anesthesia.
- Regional anesthesia, if indicated, is preferred over general anesthesia in patients with COPD, because this technique may decrease complications such as bronchospasm, barotrauma, and the need for positive pressure ventilation.
- COPD patients receiving general anesthesia should be ventilated at slow respiratory rates to allow sufficient time for full exhalation to occur. This minimizes the risk of air trapping and auto-PEEP.

- Prophylaxis against the development of postoperative pulmonary complications is based on restoring diminished lung volumes, especially functional residual capacity, and facilitating production of an effective cough to remove airway secretions.
- Intraoperative bronchospasm due to obstructive lung disease should be treated by deepening the anesthetic, administering bronchodilators (including β-adrenergic agonists, corticosteroids, and epinephrine), and suctioning secretions as needed.

RESOURCES

American Society of Anesthesiologists Stop Smoking Initiative. https://www.asahq.org/resources/clinical-information/asa-stop-smoking-initiative.

Applegate R, Lauer R, Lenart J, et al. The perioperative management of asthma. J Aller Ther. 2013:S11:007.

Barrera R, Shi W, Amar D, et al. Smoking and timing of cessation: impact on pulmonary complications after thoracotomy. Chest. 2005;127:1977-1983.

Burns KE, Adhikari NK, Keenan SP, et al. Use of non-invasive ventilation to wean critically ill adults off invasive ventilation: meta-analysis and systematic review. BMJ. 2009;338:b1574.

Fanta C. Asthma. N Engl J Med. 2009;360:1002-1014.

Lazarus SC. Emergency treatment of asthma. N Engl J Med. 2010;363:755-764.

Licker M, Schweizer A, Ellenberger C, et al. Perioperative medical management of patients with COPD. Int J Chron Obstruct Pulmon Dis. 2007;2:493-515.

Lumb A, Biercamp C. Chronic obstructive pulmonary disease and anaesthesia. Contin Educ Anaesth Crit Care Pain. 2014;14:1-5.

CHAPTER 3

Restrictive Respiratory Diseases and Lung Transplantation

RANJIT DESHPANDE, VIJI KURUP

Patients with restrictive lung disease present unique challenges in intraoperative management and postoperative care. Certain types of surgery, such as cardiac, thoracic, vascular, and trauma surgery, have a significant incidence of perioperative respiratory compromise in this patient population. Restrictive lung disease is associated with high perioperative morbidity and mortality. Although a number of conditions can cause restrictive lung disease, all share some common characteristics, and they differ from obstructive lung disease in several key features. Restrictive lung diseases are characterized by a *decrease in all lung volumes, especially total lung capacity (TLC),* a decrease in lung compliance, and preservation of expiratory flow rates (Fig. 3.1).

Restrictive lung diseases affect both lung expansion and lung compliance ($\Delta V/\Delta P$). The hallmark of restrictive lung disease is an inability to increase lung volume in proportion to an increase in pressure in the alveoli. These disorders can result from connective tissue diseases, environmental factors and other conditions that lead to pulmonary fibrosis, any conditions that increase alveolar or interstitial fluid, and any conditions that limit appropriate excursion of the chest/diaphragm during breathing. These conditions lead to a reduction in available surface area for gas diffusion, leading to ventilation/perfusion mismatching and hypoxia. Intrinsic or extrinsic pathologies can affect the ability of the lung to expand. As the elasticity of the lungs worsens, patients become symptomatic owing to hypoxia, inability to clear lung secretions, and hypoventilation. This leads to restrictive lung disease manifested by a reduced forced expiratory volume in the first second (FEV$_1$) and forced vital capacity (FVC), with a normal or increased FEV$_1$/FVC ratio and a reduced diffusing capacity for carbon monoxide (D$_{LCO}$). However, the principal feature of these diseases is a decrease in TLC (Fig. 3.2).

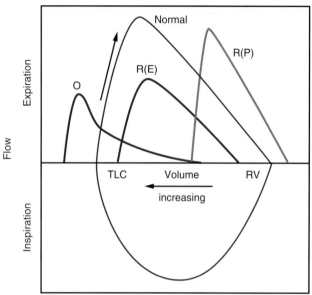

FIG. 3.1 Flow-volume curves in different conditions: obstructive disease, O; extraparenchymal restrictive disease with limitation in inspiration and expiration, R(E); and parenchymal restrictive disease, R(P). Forced expiration is plotted for all conditions; forced inspiration is shown only for the normal curve. By convention, lung volume increases to the left on the abscissa. The arrow alongside the normal curve indicates the direction of expiration from total lung capacity (TLC) to residual volume (RV). (Adapted from Weinberger SE. Disturbances of respiratory function. In: Fauci B, Braunwald E, Isselbacher KJ, et al., eds. *Harrison's Principles of Internal Medicine.* 14th ed. New York: McGraw-Hill; 1998.)

TLC is used to classify restrictive lung disease as mild, moderate, or severe. *Mild* disease is indicated by a TLC that is 65%–80% of the predicted value, *moderate* by a TLC that is 50%–65% of the predicted value, and severe by a TLC that is less than 50% of the predicted value. Restrictive lung disease can be further classified according to its causes as indicated in Table 3.1.

ACUTE INTRINSIC RESTRICTIVE LUNG DISEASE (ALVEOLAR AND INTERSTITIAL PULMONARY EDEMA)

Pulmonary Edema

Pulmonary edema is due to leakage of intravascular fluid into the interstitium of the lungs and eventually into the alveoli. Acute pulmonary edema can be caused by *increased capillary pressure* (hydrostatic or cardiogenic pulmonary edema) or by *increased capillary permeability.* Pulmonary edema typically appears as bilateral symmetrical perihilar opacities on chest radiography. This "butterfly" fluid pattern is more commonly seen with increased *capillary pressure* than with increased *capillary permeability.* The presence of air bronchograms suggests increased-permeability pulmonary edema. Cardiogenic pulmonary edema is characterized by marked dyspnea, tachypnea, and signs of sympathetic nervous system activation (hypertension, tachycardia, diaphoresis) that is often more pronounced than that seen in patients with increased-permeability pulmonary edema. Pulmonary edema caused by increased capillary permeability is characterized by a high concentration of protein and secretory products in the edema fluid. Diffuse alveolar damage is typically present with the increased-permeability pulmonary edema associated with acute respiratory distress syndrome (ARDS).

Aspiration

Aspirated acidic gastric fluid is rapidly distributed throughout the lungs and produces destruction of surfactant-producing

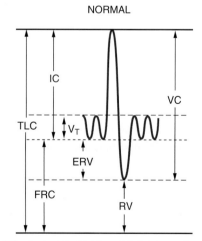

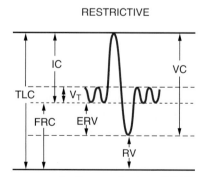

FIG. 3.2 Lung volumes in restrictive lung disease compared with normal values. *ERV,* Expiratory reserve volume; *FRC,* functional residual capacity; *IC,* inspiratory capacity; *RV,* residual volume; *TLC,* total lung capacity; *VC,* vital capacity; *VT,* tidal volume.

TABLE 3.1	Causes of Restrictive Lung Disease

ACUTE INTRINSIC RESTRICTIVE LUNG DISEASE (PULMONARY EDEMA)
Acute respiratory distress syndrome
Aspiration
Neurogenic problems
Opioid overdose
High altitude
Reexpansion of collapsed lung
Upper airway obstruction (negative pressure)
Congestive heart failure

CHRONIC INTRINSIC RESTRICTIVE LUNG DISEASE (INTERSTITIAL LUNG DISEASE)
Sarcoidosis
Hypersensitivity pneumonitis
Eosinophilic granuloma
Alveolar proteinosis
Lymphangioleiomyomatosis
Drug-induced pulmonary fibrosis

DISORDERS OF THE CHEST WALL, PLEURA, AND MEDIASTINUM
Deformities of the costovertebral skeletal structures
    Kyphoscoliosis
    Ankylosing spondylitis
Deformities of the sternum
Flail chest
Pleural effusion
Pneumothorax
Mediastinal mass
Pneumomediastinum
Neuromuscular disorders
    Spinal cord transection
    Guillain-Barré syndrome
    Disorders of neuromuscular transmission
    Muscular dystrophies

OTHER
Obesity
Ascites
Pregnancy

cells and damage to the pulmonary capillary endothelium. As a result, there is atelectasis and leakage of intravascular fluid into the lungs, producing capillary permeability pulmonary edema. The clinical picture is similar to that of ARDS. Arterial hypoxemia is present. There may also be tachypnea, bronchospasm, and acute pulmonary hypertension. Chest radiography may not demonstrate evidence of aspiration pneumonitis for 6–12 hours after the event. Evidence of aspiration, when it does appear, is most likely to be in the superior segment of the right lower lobe if the patient aspirated while in the supine position.

Measurement of *gastric fluid pH* is useful, since it reflects the pH of the aspirated fluid. Measurement of *tracheal aspirate pH* is of *no value* because the aspirated gastric fluid is rapidly diluted by airway secretions. The aspirated gastric fluid is also rapidly redistributed to peripheral lung regions, so lung lavage is *not* useful unless there has been aspiration of particulate material.

Aspiration pneumonitis is best treated by delivery of supplemental oxygen and positive end-expiratory pressure (PEEP). Bronchodilation may be needed to relieve bronchospasm. There is *no evidence* that prophylactic antibiotics decrease the incidence of pulmonary infection or alter outcome. Corticosteroid treatment of aspiration pneumonitis remains controversial.

Neurogenic Pulmonary Edema

Neurogenic pulmonary edema develops in a small proportion of patients experiencing acute brain injury. Typically this form of pulmonary edema occurs minutes to hours after central nervous system (CNS) injury and may manifest during the perioperative period. There is a massive outpouring of sympathetic impulses from the injured CNS that results in generalized vasoconstriction and a shift of blood volume into the pulmonary circulation. Presumably the increased pulmonary capillary pressure from this acute translocation of blood volume leads to transudation of fluid into the interstitium and alveoli. Pulmonary hypertension and hypervolemia can also injure blood vessels in the lungs.

The association of pulmonary edema with a recent CNS injury should suggest the diagnosis of neurogenic pulmonary edema. The principal entity in the differential diagnosis is aspiration pneumonitis. Unlike neurogenic pulmonary edema, chemical pneumonitis resulting from aspiration frequently persists longer and is often complicated by bacterial infection.

Drug-Induced Pulmonary Edema

Acute noncardiogenic pulmonary edema can occur after administration of a number of drugs, but especially opioids (heroin) and cocaine. High-permeability pulmonary edema is suggested by the high protein concentration in the pulmonary edema fluid in this situation. Cocaine can also cause pulmonary vasoconstriction, acute myocardial ischemia, and myocardial infarction. There is no evidence that administration of naloxone speeds resolution of opioid-induced pulmonary edema. Treatment of patients who develop drug-induced pulmonary edema is supportive and may include tracheal intubation for airway protection and mechanical ventilation.

High-Altitude Pulmonary Edema

High-altitude pulmonary edema may occur at heights ranging from 2500–5000 meters and is influenced by the rate of ascent to that altitude. The onset of symptoms is often gradual but typically occurs within 48–72 hours at high altitude. Fulminant pulmonary edema may be preceded by the less severe symptoms of *acute mountain sickness*. The cause of this high-permeability pulmonary edema is presumed to be hypoxic pulmonary vasoconstriction, which increases pulmonary vascular pressure. Treatment includes administration of oxygen and prompt descent from the high altitude. Inhalation of nitric oxide may improve oxygenation.

Reexpansion Pulmonary Edema

Rapid expansion of a collapsed lung may lead to pulmonary edema in that lung. The risk of reexpansion pulmonary edema after relief of a pneumothorax or pleural effusion is related to the amount of air or liquid that was present in the pleural space (>1 liter increases the risk), the duration of collapse (>24 hours increases the risk), and the rapidity of reexpansion. The high protein concentration in this edema fluid suggests that enhanced capillary membrane permeability is important in the development of this form of pulmonary edema. Treatment of reexpansion pulmonary edema is supportive.

Negative Pressure Pulmonary Edema

Negative pressure pulmonary edema follows relief of acute upper airway obstruction. It is also called *postobstructive pulmonary edema*. It can be caused by postextubation laryngospasm, epiglottitis, tumors, obesity, hiccups, or obstructive sleep apnea in *spontaneously breathing* patients. Spontaneous ventilation is necessary to create the marked negative pressure that causes this problem. The time to onset of pulmonary edema after relief of airway obstruction ranges from a few minutes to as long as 2–3 hours. Tachypnea, cough, and failure to maintain oxygen saturation above 95% are common presenting signs and may be confused with pulmonary aspiration or pulmonary embolism. It is possible that many cases of postoperative oxygen desaturation are due to some degree of unrecognized negative pressure pulmonary edema.

The pathogenesis of negative pressure pulmonary edema is related to the development of high negative intrapleural pressure by vigorous inspiratory efforts against an obstructed upper airway. This high negative intrapleural pressure decreases the interstitial hydrostatic pressure, increases venous return, and increases left ventricular afterload. In addition, such negative pressure leads to intense sympathetic nervous system activation, hypertension, and central displacement of blood volume. Together these factors produce acute pulmonary edema by increasing the transcapillary pressure gradient.

Maintenance of a patent upper airway and administration of supplemental oxygen are usually sufficient treatment, since this form of pulmonary edema is typically self-limited. Mechanical ventilation may occasionally be needed for a brief period. Hemodynamic monitoring reveals normal right and left ventricular function. Central venous pressure and pulmonary artery occlusion pressure are also normal. Radiographic evidence of this form of pulmonary edema resolves within 12–24 hours.

Management of Anesthesia in Patients With Pulmonary Edema

Elective surgery should be delayed in patients with pulmonary edema, and every effort must be made to optimize cardiorespiratory function prior to surgery. Large pleural effusions may need to be drained. Persistent hypoxemia may require mechanical ventilation and PEEP. Hemodynamic monitoring may be useful in both the assessment and treatment of pulmonary edema.

Patients with pulmonary edema are critically ill. Intraoperative management should be a continuation of critical care management and include a plan for intraoperative ventilator management. The best way to ventilate patients with acute respiratory failure due to acute pulmonary edema has not been determined. However, because the pathophysiology is similar to that of acute lung injury and because there is the risk of hemodynamic compromise and barotrauma with the use of large tidal volumes and high airway pressures, it is reasonable to ventilate with low tidal volumes (e.g., 6 mL/kg) with a ventilatory rate of 14–18 breaths per minute while attempting to keep the end-inspiratory plateau pressure at less than 30 cm H_2O. Typical anesthesia ventilators may not be adequate for patients with severe pulmonary edema, and more sophisticated intensive care unit (ICU) ventilators may be needed. Patients with restrictive lung disease typically have rapid, shallow breathing. Tachypnea is likely during the weaning process and should not be used as the sole criterion for delaying extubation if gas exchange and results of other assessments are satisfactory.

ACUTE RESPIRATORY FAILURE

Overview

Respiratory failure is the inability to provide adequate arterial oxygenation and/or elimination of carbon dioxide. It has a myriad of causes. Acute respiratory failure is considered to be present when the PaO_2 is below 60 mm Hg despite oxygen supplementation and in the absence of a right-to-left intracardiac shunt. In the presence of acute respiratory failure, $PaCO_2$ can be increased, unchanged, or decreased depending on the relationship of alveolar ventilation to metabolic production of carbon dioxide. A $PaCO_2$ above 50 mm Hg in the absence of respiratory compensation for metabolic alkalosis is consistent with the diagnosis of acute respiratory failure.

Acute respiratory failure is distinguished from *chronic respiratory failure* based on the relationship of $PaCO_2$ to arterial pH (pHa). Acute respiratory failure is typically accompanied by abrupt increases in $PaCO_2$ and corresponding decreases in pHa. With chronic respiratory failure, the pHa is usually between 7.35 and 7.45 despite an increased $PaCO_2$. This normal pHa reflects renal compensation for chronic respiratory acidosis via renal tubular reabsorption of bicarbonate.

Respiratory failure is often accompanied by a decrease in functional residual capacity (FRC) and lung compliance. Increased pulmonary vascular resistance and pulmonary hypertension are likely to develop if respiratory failure persists. ARDS is a condition that falls within the spectrum of acute respiratory failure.

Treatment of acute respiratory failure is directed at initiating specific therapies that support oxygenation and ventilation. The three principal goals in the management of acute respiratory failure are: (1) a patent upper airway, (2) correction of hypoxemia, and (3) removal of excess carbon dioxide.

Mechanical Support of Ventilation

Supplemental oxygen can be provided to spontaneously breathing patients via nasal cannula, Venturi mask, nonrebreathing mask, or T-piece. These devices seldom provide inspired oxygen concentrations higher than 50% and therefore are of value only in correcting hypoxemia resulting from mild to moderate ventilation/perfusion mismatching. When these methods of oxygen delivery fail to maintain the Pa_{O_2} above 60 mm Hg, continuous positive airway pressure (CPAP) by face mask can be initiated. CPAP may increase lung volumes by opening collapsed alveoli and decreasing right-to-left intrapulmonary shunting. A disadvantage of CPAP by face mask is that the tight mask fit required may increase the risk of pulmonary aspiration should the patient vomit. Maintenance of the Pa_{O_2} above 60 mm Hg is adequate because hemoglobin saturation with oxygen is over 90% at this level. In some patients it may be necessary to perform tracheal intubation and institute mechanical ventilation to maintain acceptable oxygenation and ventilation. Typical devices that provide positive pressure ventilation include volume-cycled and pressure-cycled ventilators.

Volume-Cycled Ventilation

Volume-cycled ventilation provides a fixed tidal volume, and inflation pressure is the dependent variable. A pressure limit can be set, and when inflation pressure exceeds this value, a pressure relief valve prevents further gas flow. This valve prevents the development of dangerously high peak airway and alveolar pressures and warns that a change in pulmonary compliance has occurred. Large increases in peak airway pressure may reflect worsening pulmonary edema, development of a pneumothorax, kinking of the tracheal tube, or the presence of mucus plugs in the tracheal tube or large airways. Tidal volume is maintained despite small changes in peak airway pressure. A disadvantage of volume-cycled ventilation is the inability to compensate for leaks in the delivery system. The primary modalities of ventilation using volume-cycled ventilation are *assist-control ventilation* (AC) and *synchronized intermittent mandatory ventilation* (SIMV) (Fig. 3.3).

Assist-Control Ventilation

In the control mode, a preset respiratory rate ensures that a patient receives a predetermined number of mechanically delivered breaths even if there are no inspiratory efforts. In the assist mode, however, if the patient can create some negative airway pressure, a breath at the preset tidal volume will be delivered.

Synchronized Intermittent Mandatory Ventilation

The SIMV technique allows patients to breathe spontaneously at any rate and tidal volume while a defined minute ventilation

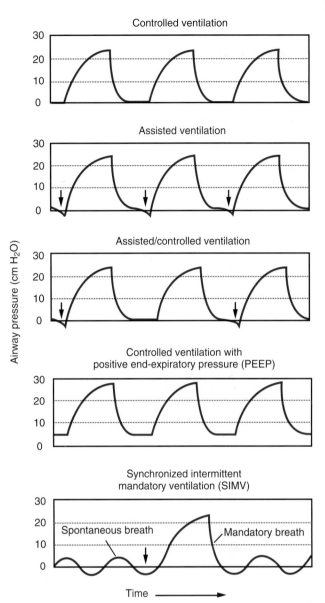

FIG. 3.3 Tidal volume and airway pressures produced by various modes of ventilation delivered through an endotracheal tube. Arrows indicate initiation of a spontaneous breath by the patient, who triggers the ventilator to deliver a mechanically assisted breath.

is provided by the ventilator. The gas delivery circuit is modified to provide sufficient gas flow for spontaneous breathing and permit periodic mandatory breaths that are synchronous with the patient's inspiratory efforts. Theoretical advantages of SIMV compared to assist-control ventilation include continued use of respiratory muscles, lower mean airway and mean intrathoracic pressure, prevention of respiratory alkalosis, and improved patient-ventilator coordination.

Pressure-Cycled Ventilation

Pressure-cycled ventilation (PCV) provides gas flow to the lungs until a preset airway pressure is reached. Tidal volume is the dependent variable and varies with changes in lung compliance and airway resistance.

Management of Patients Receiving Mechanical Support of Ventilation

Critically ill patients who require mechanical ventilation may benefit from continuous infusion of sedative drugs to treat anxiety and agitation and to facilitate coordination with ventilator-delivered breaths. Inadequate sedation or agitation can lead to life-threatening problems such as self-extubation, acute deterioration in gas exchange, and barotrauma. The need for neuromuscular blockade can be reduced by the optimum use of sedation. However, when acceptable sedation without hemodynamic compromise cannot be achieved, it may be necessary to produce skeletal muscle paralysis to ensure appropriate ventilation and oxygenation.

Sedation

Benzodiazepines, propofol, and opioids are the drugs most commonly administered to decrease anxiety, produce amnesia, increase patient comfort, and provide analgesia during mechanical ventilation. *Continuous infusion of drugs rather than intermittent injection* provides a more constant and desirable level of sedation. Daily interruption of sedative infusions to allow the patient to "awaken" may facilitate evaluation of mental status and ultimately shorten the period of mechanical ventilation. Continuous infusion of propofol is uniquely attractive for this purpose because the brief context-sensitive half-time of this drug is not influenced by the duration of the infusion, and rapid awakening is predictable. Prompt recovery from the effects of a remifentanil infusion is also not affected by the duration of the drug infusion.

Muscle Relaxants

When sedation is inadequate or hypotension accompanies the administration of drugs used for sedation, the use of nondepolarizing neuromuscular blocking drugs to produce skeletal muscle relaxation may be necessary to permit optimal mechanical ventilation. The dependence of certain of these drugs on renal clearance should be considered. It is better to use intermittent rather than continuous skeletal muscle paralysis to allow periodic assessment of the adequacy of sedation and the need for ongoing paralysis. Monitoring of neuromuscular blockade and titration of muscle relaxant doses so that two twitch responses remain in the train-of-four is prudent. *Acute quadriplegic myopathy,* also known as the *acute myopathy of intensive care,* is associated with prolonged drug-induced skeletal muscle paralysis in mechanically ventilated patients.

Complications of Mechanical Ventilation
Infection

In mechanically ventilated patients with acute respiratory failure, tracheal intubation is the single most important predisposing factor for development of nosocomial pneumonia *(ventilator-associated pneumonia).* The major pathogenic mechanism is microaspiration of contaminated secretions around the tracheal tube cuff. Diagnosis of pneumonia in the presence of acute respiratory failure may be difficult, since fever and pulmonary infiltrates may already be present in association with the cause of the acute respiratory failure.

Nosocomial sinusitis is strongly related to the presence of a nasotracheal tube. Treatment of nosocomial sinusitis includes administration of antibiotics, replacement of nasal tubes with oral tubes, and use of decongestants and head elevation to facilitate sinus drainage.

Barotrauma

Barotrauma may present as subcutaneous emphysema, pneumomediastinum, pulmonary interstitial emphysema, pneumoperitoneum, pneumopericardium, arterial gas embolism, or tension pneumothorax. These examples of *extraalveolar air* almost always reflect dissection or passage of air from overdistended and ruptured alveoli. Infection increases the risk of barotrauma, presumably by weakening pulmonary tissue. Tension pneumothorax is the most common life-threatening manifestation of ventilator-induced barotrauma. Hypotension, worsening hypoxemia, and increased airway pressure suggest the presence of a tension pneumothorax.

Atelectasis

Atelectasis is a common cause of hypoxemia that develops during mechanical ventilation. Migration of the tracheal tube into the left or right main bronchus or development of mucus plugs should be considered when abrupt worsening of oxygenation occurs in the absence of hypotension. *Arterial hypoxemia resulting from atelectasis is not responsive to an increase in F_{IO_2}.* Other causes of sudden hypoxemia in mechanically ventilated patients include tension pneumothorax and pulmonary embolism, but in contrast to atelectasis, these are usually accompanied by hypotension. Bronchoscopy may be necessary to remove mucus plugs responsible for persistent atelectasis.

Monitoring of Treatment

Monitoring the progress of treatment of acute respiratory failure includes evaluation of pulmonary gas exchange (arterial and venous blood gases, pHa) and cardiac function (cardiac output, cardiac filling pressures, intrapulmonary shunt).

Adequacy of oxygen exchange across alveolar-capillary membranes is reflected by the Pa_{O_2}. The efficacy of this exchange is paralleled by the difference between the calculated alveolar P_{O_2} (PA_{O_2}) and the measured Pa_{O_2}. Calculation of $PA_{O_2} - Pa_{O_2}$ is useful for evaluating the gas-exchange function of the lungs and for distinguishing among the various causes of arterial hypoxemia (Table 3.2).

Significant desaturation of arterial blood occurs only when the Pa_{O_2} is less than 60 mm Hg. Ventilation/perfusion mismatching, right-to-left intrapulmonary shunting, and hypoventilation are the principal causes of arterial hypoxemia. Increasing the inspired oxygen concentration is likely to improve Pa_{O_2} in all of these conditions, with the exception of a significant right-to-left intrapulmonary shunt.

Compensatory responses to arterial hypoxemia vary. As a general rule these responses are stimulated by an acute decrease

TABLE 3.2	Mechanisms of Arterial Hypoxemia				
Mechanism		Pa_{O_2}	Pa_{CO_2}	$PA_{O_2} - Pa_{O_2}$	Response to Supplemental Oxygen
Low inspired oxygen concentration (altitude)		Decreased	Normal to decreased	Normal	Improved
Hypoventilation (drug overdose)		Decreased	Increased	Normal	Improved
Ventilation/perfusion mismatching (COPD, pneumonia)		Decreased	Normal to decreased	Increased	Improved
Right-to-left intrapulmonary shunt (pulmonary edema)		Decreased	Normal to decreased	Increased	Poor to none
Diffusion impairment (pulmonary fibrosis)		Decreased	Normal to decreased	Increased	Improved

TABLE 3.3	Mechanisms of Hypercarbia			
Mechanism		Pa_{CO_2}	V_D/V_T	$PA_{O_2} - Pa_{O_2}$
Drug overdose		Increased	Normal	Normal
Restrictive lung disease (kyphoscoliosis)		Increased	Normal to increased	Normal to increased
Chronic obstructive pulmonary disease		Increased	Increased	Increased
Neuromuscular disease		Increased	Normal to increased	Normal to increased

in Pa_{O_2} below 60 mm Hg. Compensatory responses are also present in chronic hypoxemia when the Pa_{O_2} is less than 50 mm Hg. These responses to arterial hypoxemia include (1) carotid body–induced increase in alveolar ventilation, (2) regional pulmonary artery vasoconstriction (hypoxic pulmonary vasoconstriction) to divert pulmonary blood flow away from hypoxic alveoli, and (3) increased sympathetic nervous system activity to enhance tissue oxygen delivery by increasing cardiac output. With chronic hypoxemia there is also an increase in red blood cell mass to improve the oxygen-carrying capacity of the blood.

The adequacy of alveolar ventilation relative to the metabolic production of carbon dioxide is reflected by the Pa_{CO_2} (Table 3.3). The efficacy of carbon dioxide transfer across alveolar capillary membranes is reflected by the *dead space–to–tidal volume ratio:* V_D/V_T. This ratio indicates areas in the lungs that receive adequate ventilation but inadequate or no pulmonary blood flow. Ventilation to these alveoli is described as "wasted ventilation" or *dead-space ventilation.* Normally the V_D/V_T is less than 0.3, but it may increase to 0.6 or more when there is an increase in dead-space ventilation. An increased V_D/V_T occurs in the presence of acute respiratory failure, a decrease in cardiac output, and pulmonary embolism.

Hypercarbia is defined as a Pa_{CO_2} above 45 mm Hg. *Permissive hypercapnia* is the strategy of allowing Pa_{CO_2} to increase to up to 55 mm Hg or more in spontaneously breathing patients to avoid or delay the need for tracheal intubation and mechanical ventilation. Symptoms and signs of hypercarbia depend on the rate of increase and the ultimate level of Pa_{CO_2}. Acute increases in Pa_{CO_2} are associated with increased cerebral blood flow and increased intracranial pressure. Extreme increases in Pa_{CO_2} to over 80 mm Hg result in CNS depression.

Mixed Venous Partial Pressure of Oxygen

The mixed venous partial pressure of oxygen (Pv_{O_2}) and the arterial-venous oxygen content difference ($Ca_{O_2} - Cv_{O_2}$) reflect the overall adequacy of the oxygen transport system (cardiac output) relative to tissue oxygen extraction. For example, a decrease in cardiac output that occurs in the presence of unchanged tissue oxygen consumption causes Pv_{O_2} to decrease and $Ca_{O_2} - Cv_{O_2}$ to increase. These changes reflect the continued extraction of the same amount of oxygen by the tissues during a time of decreased tissue blood flow. A Pv_{O_2} below 30 mm Hg or a $Ca_{O_2} - Cv_{O_2}$ above 6 mL/dL indicates the need to increase cardiac output to facilitate tissue oxygenation. A pulmonary artery catheter permits sampling of mixed venous blood, measurement of Pv_{O_2}, and calculation of Cv_{O_2}.

Arterial pH

Measurement of pHa is necessary to detect acidemia or alkalemia. Metabolic acidosis predictably accompanies arterial hypoxemia and inadequate delivery of oxygen to tissues. Acidemia caused by respiratory or metabolic derangements is associated with dysrhythmias and pulmonary hypertension.

Alkalemia is often associated with mechanical hyperventilation and diuretic use, which lead to loss of chloride and potassium ions. The incidence of dysrhythmias may be increased by respiratory alkalosis. The presence of alkalemia in patients recovering from acute respiratory failure can delay or prevent successful weaning from mechanical ventilation because of the compensatory hypoventilation that will occur in an effort to correct the pH disturbance.

Intrapulmonary Shunt

Right-to-left intrapulmonary shunting occurs when there is perfusion of alveoli that are not ventilated. The net effect is a decrease in Pa_{O_2}, reflecting dilution of oxygen in blood exposed to ventilated alveoli with blood containing little oxygen coming from unventilated alveoli. Calculation of the shunt fraction provides a reliable assessment of ventilation/perfusion matching and serves as a useful estimate of the response to various therapeutic interventions during treatment of acute respiratory failure.

A physiologic shunt normally comprises 2%–5% of cardiac output. This degree of right-to-left intrapulmonary shunting reflects the passage of pulmonary arterial blood directly to the left side of the circulation through the bronchial and thebesian veins. It should be appreciated that determination of the shunt fraction in a patient breathing less than 100% oxygen reflects the contribution of ventilation/perfusion mismatching as well as right-to-left intrapulmonary shunting. Calculation of the shunt fraction from measurements obtained when the patient breathes 100% oxygen eliminates the contribution of ventilation/perfusion mismatching.

Weaning From the Ventilator

Mechanical ventilatory support is withdrawn when a patient can maintain oxygenation and carbon dioxide elimination without assistance. When determining whether the patient can be safely weaned from mechanical ventilation and will tolerate extubation, important considerations include that the patient is alert and cooperative and is able to tolerate a trial of spontaneous ventilation without excessive tachypnea, tachycardia, or respiratory distress. Some of the guidelines that have been proposed for indicating the feasibility of discontinuing mechanical ventilation include (1) vital capacity of more than 15 mL/kg, (2) alveolar-arterial oxygen difference of less than 350 cm H_2O while breathing 100% oxygen, (3) Pao_2 of more than 60 mm Hg with an Fio_2 of less than 0.5, (4) negative inspiratory pressure of more than −20 cm H_2O, (5) normal pHa, (6) respiratory rate lower than 20 breaths per minute, and (7) V_D/V_T of less than 0.6. Breathing at rapid rates with low tidal volumes usually signifies an inability to tolerate extubation. Ultimately the decision to attempt withdrawal of mechanical ventilation is individualized and considers not only pulmonary function but also the presence of co-existing medical problems.

When a patient is ready for a trial of withdrawal from mechanical support of ventilation, three options may be considered: (1) synchronized intermittent mandatory ventilation, which allows spontaneous breathing amid progressively fewer mandatory breaths per minute until the patient is breathing unassisted; (2) intermittent trials of total removal of mechanical support and breathing through a T-piece; and (3) use of decreasing levels of pressure-support ventilation. Overall, correcting the underlying condition responsible for the need for mechanical ventilation is more important for successful extubation than the particular weaning method. Deterioration in oxygenation after withdrawal of mechanical ventilation may reflect progressive alveolar collapse, which can be responsive to treatment with CPAP or noninvasive positive pressure ventilation (NIPPV) rather than reinstitution of mechanical ventilation.

Several things may interfere with successful withdrawal from mechanical ventilation and extubation. Excessive workload on the respiratory muscles imposed by hyperinflation, copious secretions, bronchospasm, increased lung water, or increased carbon dioxide production from fever or parenteral nutrition greatly decreases the likelihood of successful tracheal extubation. Use of noninvasive ventilation (NIV) as a bridge to discontinuation of mechanical ventilation may be considered. This involves early extubation with immediate application of a form of NIV. This method of weaning may be associated with a decreased incidence of nosocomial pneumonia, a shorter ICU stay, and a reduction in mortality. However, NIV may impair the ability to clear airway secretions if the patient does not have a good cough, and there may be inadequate minute ventilation. Careful patient selection is required if this modality is being considered.

Tracheal Extubation

Tracheal extubation should be considered when patients tolerate 30 minutes of spontaneous breathing with CPAP of 5 cm H_2O without deterioration in arterial blood gas concentrations, mental status, or cardiac function. The Pao_2 should remain above 60 mm Hg with an Fio_2 less than 0.5. Likewise the $Paco_2$ should remain below 50 mm Hg, and the pHa should remain above 7.30. Additional criteria for tracheal extubation include the need for less than 5 cm H_2O PEEP, spontaneous breathing rates lower than 20 breaths per minute, and a vital capacity above 15 mL/kg. Patients should be alert, with active laryngeal reflexes and the ability to generate an effective cough and clear secretions. Protective glottic closure function may be impaired following tracheal extubation, which results in an increased risk of aspiration.

Oxygen Supplementation

Oxygen supplementation is often needed after tracheal extubation. This need reflects the persistence of ventilation/perfusion mismatching. Weaning from supplemental oxygen is accomplished by gradually decreasing the inspired concentration of oxygen, as guided by measurements of Pao_2 and/or monitoring of oxygen saturation by pulse oximetry.

ACUTE RESPIRATORY DISTRESS SYNDROME

Adult ARDS is caused by inflammatory injury to the lung and is manifested clinically as acute hypoxemic respiratory failure. Events that can cause direct or indirect lung injury and lead to ARDS are listed in Table 3.4. Sepsis is associated with the highest risk of progression to ARDS. Rapid-onset respiratory failure accompanied by refractory arterial hypoxemia, with radiographic findings indistinguishable from cardiogenic pulmonary edema, are the hallmarks of ARDS. Proinflammatory cytokines lead to the increased alveolar capillary membrane permeability and alveolar edema seen in this condition. The acute phase of ARDS usually resolves completely but in some patients may progress to fibrosing alveolitis with persistent arterial hypoxemia and decreased pulmonary compliance.

Diagnosis

The previous definition of ARDS came from the American-European Consensus Conference of 1994, but this has now

TABLE 3.4	Clinical Disorders Associated With Acute Respiratory Distress Syndrome

DIRECT LUNG INJURY
Pneumonia
Aspiration of gastric contents
Pulmonary contusion
Fat emboli
Near drowning
Inhalational injury
Reperfusion injury

INDIRECT LUNG INJURY
Sepsis
Trauma associated with shock
Multiple blood transfusions
Cardiopulmonary bypass
Drug overdose
Acute pancreatitis

TABLE 3.5	The Berlin Definition of Acute Respiratory Distress Syndrome

Lung injury of acute onset with 1 week of an apparent clinical insult and with progression of pulmonary symptoms
Bilateral opacities on lung imaging not explainable by other lung pathology
Respiratory failure not explained by heart failure or volume overload
Decreased arterial Pao_2/Fio_2 ratio:
    Mild ARDS: ratio is 201–300
    Moderate ARDS: ratio is 101–200
    Severe ARDS: ratio is <101

From the ARDS Definition Task Force. Acute respiratory distress syndrome: the Berlin definition. *JAMA*. 2012;307:2526-2533.

been supplanted by the Berlin definition of ARDS, which is the result of the work of a task force empowered by critical care societies from several countries (Table 3.5). The focus of the new definition is on oxygenation, timing of disease onset, and imaging results. The term *acute lung injury* is no longer used. Instead, ARDS is now classified as *mild* (200 mm Hg < Pao_2/Fio_2 ≤ 300 mm Hg), *moderate* (100 mm Hg < Pao_2/Fio_2 ≤ 200 mm Hg) or *severe* (Pao_2/Fio_2 ≤ 100 mm Hg). The calculation of the Pao_2/Fio_2 ratio must now be calculated with CPAP or PEEP of at least 5 cm H_2O.

Pulmonary artery occlusion pressure is no longer a part of the definition of ARDS. Bilateral findings on chest radiography in at least three lung quadrants not explained by pleural effusion or atelectasis are seen. Echocardiography helps rule out a cardiogenic cause of pulmonary edema.

Pulmonary hypertension can be due to pulmonary artery vasoconstriction and obliteration of portions of the pulmonary capillary bed and when severe can cause acute right-sided heart failure. Death from ARDS is most often a result of sepsis or multiple organ failure rather than respiratory failure, although some deaths are directly related to lung injury.

TABLE 3.6	Treatment of Acute Respiratory Distress Syndrome

Oxygen supplementation
Tracheal intubation
Mechanical ventilation
Positive end-expiratory pressure
Optimization of intravascular fluid volume
Diuretic therapy
Inotropic support
Glucocorticoid therapy (?)
Removal of secretions
Control of infection
Nutritional support
Administration of inhaled β_2-adrenergic agonists

Clinical Management

Management of a patient with ARDS is mainly supportive. Supportive care consists of mechanical ventilation, antibiotics, stress ulcer prophylaxis, venous thromboembolism prophylaxis, and early enteral feeding (Table 3.6).

The best form of mechanical ventilation in patients with ARDS has been a topic of great debate. Two schools of thought exist: one believes in *protective ventilation* and the other believes in *open lung ventilation*. In addition to lung overdistention, cyclic opening and closing of small airways and alveolar units during tidal mechanical ventilation can lead to a form of lung injury called *atelectrauma*. Several trials have examined the effects of open lung ventilation and protective lung ventilation in limiting atelectrauma.

Overinflation of the lungs is deleterious because it appears to be the main mechanism of *ventilator-induced lung injury*. Limiting end-inspiratory lung stretch to minimize mortality in ARDS patients has been evaluated, and a mortality benefit of 22% was noted in patients ventilated with "low" (6 mL/kg) tidal volumes compared to higher lung volumes. This mortality benefit did not appear to have any relationship to baseline lung compliance or to the underlying factor responsible for the development of ARDS. It was noted that inflammatory mediator concentrations, especially those of interleukin (IL)-6, were lower in the survival group.

Other studies addressed the potential superiority of an open lung ventilation approach in which PEEP was titrated to the highest value possible while keeping plateau pressure below 28–30 cm H_2O. Patients treated according to the open lung approach had significantly more ventilator-free days and organ failure–free days, but in-hospital mortality, 28-day mortality, and 60-day mortality were not improved.

Prone positioning and extracorporeal membrane oxygenation (ECMO) have been proposed as therapies for the life-threatening refractory hypoxemia in patients with severe ARDS. Both of these strategies have demonstrated improvement in oxygenation.

Prone positioning exploits gravity and repositioning of the heart in the thorax to recruit lung units and improve ventilation/perfusion matching. It appears that prone position ventilation is beneficial in selected patients with severe ARDS, as indicated by an improvement in oxygenation as well as a mortality benefit.

Extracorporeal lung support (ECLS) techniques like ECMO can be considered in patients with severe hypoxemic and/or hypercapnic respiratory failure as a possible rescue therapy. The aim of this strategy is to rest the lungs until the severe hypoxemia and respiratory acidosis have resolved. The benefits and timing of venovenous ECMO in ARDS remains controversial.

Additional supportive therapies are crucial in the management of ARDS. Optimal fluid management, neuromuscular blockade, inhaled nitric oxide, prostacyclin (PGI_2) administration, recruitment maneuvers, surfactant replacement therapy, glucocorticoids, and ketoconazole have all been implicated in improved outcomes in ARDS.

A positive fluid balance is an independent risk factor for mortality in critically ill patients. Conservative fluid therapy is essential in managing pulmonary issues. Hypervolemia can lead to increased vascular permeability in already damaged lung tissue. Fluid-restrictive therapy has been associated with more mechanical ventilation–free days and a shorter ICU length of stay but no difference in 60-day mortality.

Use of neuromuscular blockers has been associated with less barotrauma and less secretion of both pulmonary and systemic proinflammatory mediators. However, given the potential adverse effect of these medications in terms of causing ICU-acquired myopathy, their use should be limited to severely hypoxemic patients for as brief a period as possible.

Inhaled nitric oxide (NO) has been proposed to treat refractory hypoxemia, owing to its vasodilatory effects on vascular smooth muscle. It can help improve ventilation/perfusion matching and decrease pulmonary vascular resistance and pulmonary artery pressure. Several studies have noted a transient improvement in oxygenation but no reduction in mortality.

CHRONIC INTRINSIC RESTRICTIVE LUNG DISEASE (INTERSTITIAL LUNG DISEASE)

Pulmonary Fibrosis

Interstitial lung disease is characterized by changes in the intrinsic properties of the lungs and is most often caused by *pulmonary fibrosis*. This produces a chronic restrictive form of lung disease. Pulmonary hypertension and cor pulmonale develop as progressive pulmonary fibrosis results in the loss of pulmonary vasculature. Dyspnea is prominent, and breathing is rapid and shallow.

Sarcoidosis

Sarcoidosis is a systemic granulomatous disorder that involves many tissues but has a predilection for intrathoracic lymph nodes and the lungs. Many patients have no symptoms at the time of presentation, and the disease is often identified only because of abnormal findings on chest radiography. Some patients may have respiratory symptoms such as dyspnea and cough. Ocular sarcoidosis may produce uveitis; myocardial sarcoidosis may produce conduction defects and dysrhythmias. The most common form of neurologic involvement in sarcoidosis is unilateral facial nerve palsy. Endobronchial sarcoid is common. Laryngeal sarcoidosis occurs in up to 5% of patients and may interfere with the passage of adult-size tracheal tubes. Cor pulmonale may develop. Hypercalcemia occurs in fewer than 10% of patients but is a classic manifestation of sarcoidosis.

Mediastinoscopy may be necessary to provide lymph node tissue for the diagnosis of sarcoidosis. Angiotensin-converting enzyme activity is increased in patients with sarcoidosis and is presumably due to production of this enzyme by cells within the granuloma. However, this increase in angiotensin-converting enzyme activity *does not* have useful diagnostic or prognostic significance. Corticosteroids are administered to suppress the manifestations of sarcoidosis and to treat the hypercalcemia.

Hypersensitivity Pneumonitis

Hypersensitivity pneumonitis is characterized by diffuse interstitial granulomatous reactions in the lungs after inhalation of dust containing fungi, spores, and animal or plant material. Signs and symptoms of hypersensitivity pneumonitis include the onset of dyspnea and cough 4–6 hours after inhalation of the antigens. This is followed by leukocytosis, eosinophilia, and often arterial hypoxemia. Chest radiography shows multiple pulmonary infiltrates. Repeated episodes of hypersensitivity pneumonitis may lead to pulmonary fibrosis.

Eosinophilic Granuloma

Pulmonary fibrosis accompanies the disease process known as *eosinophilic granuloma* (histiocytosis X). No treatment has been shown to be beneficial for this disease.

Alveolar Proteinosis

Pulmonary alveolar proteinosis is a disease of unknown etiology characterized by deposition of lipid-rich proteinaceous material in the alveoli. Dyspnea and arterial hypoxemia are the clinical manifestations. This process may occur independently or in association with chemotherapy, AIDS, or inhalation of mineral dusts. Although spontaneous remission may occur, treatment of severe cases requires whole-lung lavage to remove the alveolar material and improve macrophage function. Lung lavage in patients with hypoxemia may temporarily decrease the level of oxygenation further. Airway management during anesthesia for lung lavage includes placement of a double-lumen endobronchial tube to facilitate lavage of each lung separately and optimize oxygenation during the procedure.

Lymphangioleiomyomatosis

Lymphangioleiomyomatosis is proliferation of smooth muscle in airways, lymphatics, and blood vessels that occurs in women of reproductive age. Pulmonary function tests show restrictive and obstructive lung disease with a decrease in diffusing capacity. Lymphangioleiomyomatosis presents clinically as progressive dyspnea, hemoptysis, recurrent pneumothorax, and pleural effusions. Nearly all lymphangioleiomyomatosis cells express progesterone receptors. Progesterone or tamoxifen can be used for treatment, but there is still progressive deterioration in pulmonary function, and most patients die within 10 years of the onset of symptoms.

Management of Anesthesia in Patients With Chronic Interstitial Lung Disease

Patients usually have dyspnea and nonproductive cough. Cor pulmonale may be present. Coarse breath sounds with crepitations can be heard. A chest radiograph may show a ground glass or nodular pattern. Arterial blood gas analysis reveals hypoxemia with normocarbia. Pulmonary function tests show restrictive ventilatory defects, and the diffusing capacity is decreased. A vital capacity of less than 15 mL/kg indicates severe pulmonary dysfunction. Infection should be treated, secretions cleared, and smoking stopped preoperatively.

Patients with interstitial lung disease tolerate apneic periods very poorly because of their small FRC and low oxygen stores. General anesthesia, the supine position, and controlled ventilation all contribute to further decreases in FRC. Alterations in FRC and the risk of hypoxia continue into the postoperative period. Uptake of inhaled anesthetics is faster in these patients because of the small FRC. Peak airway pressures should be kept as low as possible to minimize the risk of barotrauma.

CHRONIC EXTRINSIC RESTRICTIVE LUNG DISEASE

Thoracic Extrapulmonary Causes

Chronic extrinsic restrictive lung disease is often due to disorders of the thoracic cage (chest wall) that interfere with lung expansion. Deformities of the sternum, ribs, vertebrae, and costovertebral structures include conditions such as ankylosing spondylitis, flail chest, scoliosis, and kyphosis. The lungs are compressed and lung volumes are reduced. The work of breathing is increased because of the abnormal mechanical properties of the chest and the increased airway resistance that results from decreased lung volumes. Any thoracic deformity may cause compression of the pulmonary vasculature and lead to right ventricular dysfunction. Recurrent pulmonary infection resulting from a poor cough is common.

The two basic types of costovertebral skeletal deformity are *scoliosis* (lateral curvature with rotation of the vertebral column) and *kyphosis* (anterior flexion of the vertebral column). They may present in combination as *kyphoscoliosis,* which leads to severe restrictive impairment of lung function.

Kyphoscoliosis may be idiopathic, due to a neuromuscular disorder, or associated with congenital vertebral malformations.

Idiopathic kyphoscoliosis accounts for 80% of cases. This commonly begins during late childhood or early adolescence and may progress in severity during the years of rapid skeletal growth. Patients with neuromuscular disorders producing kyphoscoliosis have more respiratory compromise than those with idiopathic kyphoscoliosis. This deformity of the spine results in a decrease in ventilatory capacity of the lung and an increase in the work of breathing. The deformity also leads to a raised hemidiaphragm on the side of the concavity. The severity of this disorder is usually measured by the degree of spinal curvature (Cobb angle). The greater the Cobb angle, the greater the respiratory compromise. Mild to moderate kyphoscoliosis (scoliotic angle < 60 degrees) is associated with minimal to mild restrictive ventilatory defects. A Cobb angle of more than 70 degrees puts the patient at increased risk of respiratory dysfunction. Dyspnea may occur during exercise, but as the skeletal deformity worsens the vital capacity declines and dyspnea becomes a common complaint even with moderate exertion. Severe deformities (scoliotic angle > 100 degrees) can lead to chronic alveolar hypoventilation, hypoxemia, secondary erythrocytosis, pulmonary hypertension, and cor pulmonale. Respiratory failure is most likely in patients with kyphoscoliosis associated with a vital capacity of less than 45% of the predicted value and a scoliotic angle of more than 100 degrees.

Compression of underlying lung tissue results in an increased alveolar-arterial oxygen difference. It is important to note that during the nonphasic period of REM sleep, these patients are at increased risk of hypoventilation. Nocturnal hypoventilation may sometimes be the presenting feature of this condition. NIV strategies can be used to help manage this problem. Indications for NIV in these patients include symptoms suggestive of nocturnal hypoventilation, signs of cor pulmonale, nocturnal oxygen desaturation, or an elevated daytime $Paco_2$. Perioperatively, patients with severe kyphoscoliosis are at increased risk of developing pneumonia and hypoventilation when exposed to CNS depressant drugs. Supplemental oxygen therapy augmented by nocturnal ventilatory support may be needed.

Pectus excavatum, also called *funnel chest* or *concave chest,* is a chest wall deformity in which the body of the sternum, mostly the lower end, is curved inward. This deformity can restrict chest expansion and reduce vital capacity. In most patients with pectus excavatum, there are no significant functional limitations. Lung volumes and cardiovascular function are preserved. Surgical correction is indicated when the sternal deformity is accompanied by evidence of pulmonary restriction or cardiovascular dysfunction.

Pectus carinatum, also called *pigeon chest,* is a deformity of the sternum characterized by outward protuberance of the sternum and ribs. The etiology is unknown, though it does run in families. This is usually a condition of cosmetic concern, but some children do have respiratory symptoms or asthma.

Multiple rib fractures, especially when they occur in a parallel vertical orientation, can produce a *flail chest* characterized by paradoxical inward movement of the unstable portion of the thoracic cage while the remainder of the thoracic cage moves outward during inspiration. At least three or more anteriorly or posteriorly fractured ribs must be present to have a flail chest. The flail portion of the chest moves outward during exhalation. A flail chest results in pain, increased work of breathing, inability to cough and clear secretions, and splinting of the injured hemithorax, with resulting atelectasis and delayed healing. There is also underlying lung contusion that results in low compliance and FRC. Flail chest can also result from dehiscence of a median sternotomy. Tidal volumes are diminished because the region of the lung associated with the chest wall abnormality paradoxically increases its volume during exhalation and deflates during inspiration. The result is progressive hypoxemia and alveolar hypoventilation and increased work of breathing. Treatment of a flail chest includes positive pressure ventilation until a definitive stabilization procedure can be carried out.

Pleural disorders include conditions such as trapped lung syndrome, pleural effusion, empyema, and pneumothorax. The pleura is a thin membrane that covers the entire surface of the lung, inner rib cage, diaphragm, and mediastinum. There are two pleural membranes: the *visceral pleura,* which covers the lungs, and the *parietal pleura,* which underlies the rib cage, diaphragm, and mediastinum.

Pleural effusion refers to accumulation of fluid in the pleural space. Diagnosis can be made with chest radiography, computed tomography (CT) scan of the chest, or bedside ultrasonography. Chest radiography will reveal blunting of the costophrenic angle and a characteristic homogeneous opacity that forms a concave meniscus with the chest wall. Apparent elevation or changes in the contour of the diaphragm may signify a subpulmonic effusion. However, chest radiography is not a very sensitive tool for diagnosis of pleural effusion, since there must be at least 250 mL of effusion before it can be detected by this method. The sensitivity and specificity of ultrasound for diagnosing pleural effusion is much better and approaches 100% in experienced hands. This methodology can also reveal septae within the effusion and can distinguish between transudates and exudates.

Various types of fluid may accumulate in the pleural space, including blood (hemothorax), pus (empyema), lipids (chylothorax), and serous liquid (hydrothorax). Diagnosis of the cause of pleural effusion is possible by analysis of pleural fluid after a thoracentesis. The distinction between transudate and exudate points to potential diagnoses and the need for further evaluation. Bloody pleural effusion is common in patients with malignant disease, trauma, or pulmonary infarction. Surgical treatment is usually required for an effusion that cannot be drained by needle/small catheter thoracentesis. Pleurodesis, decortication, pleuroperitoneal shunts, and closure of diaphragmatic defects are some of the surgical options for treating recurrent effusions.

Pneumothorax is the presence of gas in the pleural space caused by disruption of either the parietal pleura (from an external penetrating injury) or visceral pleura (from a tear or rupture in the lung parenchyma). The visceral pleura usually separates from the parietal pleura, and the air can be seen between the visceral pleural lining and the rib cage. When the gas originates from the lung itself, the rupture may occur in the absence of known lung disease (spontaneous pneumothorax) or as a result of some known parenchymal lung pathology (secondary pneumothorax).

Idiopathic *spontaneous pneumothorax* occurs most often in tall, thin men aged 20–40 years and is due to rupture of apical subpleural blebs. Smoking cigarettes increases the risk of spontaneous pneumothorax 20-fold. Most episodes of spontaneous pneumothorax occur while patients are at rest. Exercise or airline travel does not increase the likelihood of spontaneous pneumothorax. Women with subpleural and diaphragmatic endometriosis can have rupture of these nodules at the time of menstruation, causing a pneumothorax. This particular kind of pneumothorax is termed *catamenial pneumothorax.*

Underlying lung diseases associated with *secondary pneumothorax* include emphysema, cystic fibrosis, and lung abscess. As the air that is trapped in the thoracic cavity continues to expand, it leads to an increase in intrathoracic pressure and can cause compromise of cardiac function (i.e., tension pneumothorax).

Tension pneumothorax is a medical emergency and develops when gas enters the pleural space during inspiration and is prevented from escaping during exhalation. The result is a progressive increase in the amount and pressure/tension in the trapped air (Fig. 3.4). Patients are usually in respiratory distress, with an increased respiratory rate, shortness of breath, hypoxia, and pleuritic chest pain. The trachea may be deviated to the side *away from* the pneumothorax. Auscultation reveals decreased/absent breath sounds on the side of the pneumothorax, with hyperresonance on percussion. Vital signs show tachycardia and hypotension. If the patient is being mechanically ventilated, increased airway pressures and decreased tidal volumes can be observed. Tension pneumothorax occurs in fewer than 2% of patients experiencing idiopathic spontaneous pneumothorax but can occur with rib fractures, insertion of central lines, and barotrauma in patients undergoing mechanical ventilation. More than 30% of the pneumothoraces that develop in patients on mechanical ventilation are tension pneumothoraces. Dyspnea, hypoxemia, and hypotension may be severe. Immediate evacuation of gas through a needle or a small-bore catheter placed into the second anterior intercostal space can be life saving.

Treatment of a symptomatic pneumothorax requires evacuation of air from the pleural space by aspiration through a needle or small-bore catheter or placement of a chest tube. Aspiration of a pneumothorax followed by catheter removal is successful in most patients with a small to moderate-sized primary spontaneous pneumothorax. When the pneumothorax is small (<15% of the volume of the hemithorax) and symptoms are absent, observation may suffice.

When a pneumothorax occurs during anesthesia, immediate discontinuation of nitrous oxide and administration of 100% oxygen must commence. If the patient has a tension

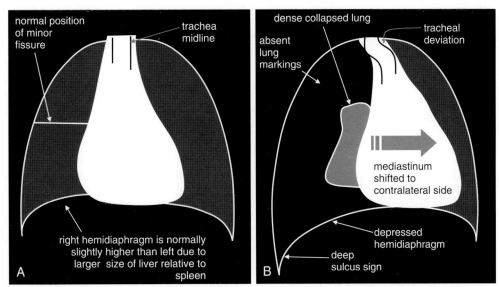

FIG. 3.4   Changes in pressure and volume on chest x-ray. A, Lungs and mediastinum under normal conditions of pressure and volume. The heart and airway are near the midline. The minor fissure is in normal position. The right diaphragm is usually slightly higher than the left because of the larger size of the liver relative to the spleen. B, Increased pressure results in mediastinal shift and tracheal deviation to the opposite side. In the case of a right-sided tension pneumothorax, the right hemidiaphragm may be displaced in a caudad direction and may be lower than the left hemidiaphragm—the reverse of their normal positions. In addition, in any tension pneumothorax the costophrenic angle may be extremely deep on the abnormal side owing to a hyperinflated pleural space—the "deep sulcus sign." (From Broder JS. *Diagnostic Imaging for the Emergency Physician.* Philadelphia: Saunders; 2011.)

pneumothorax, needle/catheter decompression must be performed, followed by chest tube placement. Oxygen supplementation accelerates reabsorption of air from the pleural space.

Pneumomediastinum may follow a tear in the esophagus or tracheobronchial tree or alveolar rupture, although it most often occurs without a known cause. Spontaneous pneumomediastinum has been observed after recreational cocaine use. Symptoms of retrosternal chest pain and dyspnea are typically abrupt in onset and usually follow an exaggerated breathing effort, such as a cough, emesis, or Valsalva maneuver. Subcutaneous emphysema may be extensive in the neck, arms, abdomen, and scrotum. Gas in the mediastinum may decompress into the pleural space, leading to pneumothorax. The diagnosis of pneumomediastinum is established by chest radiography. Spontaneous pneumomediastinum resolves without specific therapy. When pneumomediastinum is a result of organ rupture, surgical drainage and repair may be necessary.

Pleural fibrosis may follow hemothorax, empyema, or surgical pleurodesis for the treatment of recurrent pneumothorax. Despite obliteration of the pleural space, functional restrictive lung abnormalities remain but are usually minor. Surgical decortication to remove thick fibrous pleura is considered only if the restrictive lung disease is very symptomatic.

Acute mediastinitis usually results from bacterial contamination after esophageal perforation. Symptoms include chest pain and fever. It is treated with broad-spectrum antibiotics and surgical drainage.

The *anterior mediastinal compartment* is anterior to the pericardium and includes lymphatic tissue, the thymus, and potentially the thyroid (Fig. 3.5). *Mediastinal masses* most commonly found in the anterior mediastinum are thymomas, germ cell tumors, lymphomas, intrathoracic thyroid tissue, and parathyroid lesions. Thymomas comprise 20% of mediastinal neoplasms in adults and are the most common primary anterior mediastinal neoplasms in this patient population. Symptoms due to myasthenia gravis affect one third of patients with thymomas. Middle mediastinal lesions include tracheal masses, bronchogenic and pericardial cysts, enlarged lymph nodes, and proximal aortic disease (i.e., aneurysm or dissection). Posterior mediastinal masses include neurogenic tumors and cysts, meningocele, lymphoma, descending aortic aneurysm, and esophageal disorders such as diverticula and neoplasms.

Patients with systemic lymphoma often have involvement of the mediastinum, and 5%–10% of patients with lymphoma have primary mediastinal lesions at clinical presentation. Mediastinal cysts can arise in the pericardium, bronchi, esophagus, stomach, thymus, and thoracic duct, and although benign, they can produce compressive symptoms. Lung cancer can manifest with mediastinal adenopathy, a sign of advanced-stage disease. In the evaluation of mediastinal widening, contrast-enhanced CT can distinguish between vascular structures, soft tissues, and calcifications. Large mediastinal tumors may be associated with progressive airway obstruction, loss of lung volumes, pulmonary artery and/or cardiac compression, and superior vena cava obstruction.

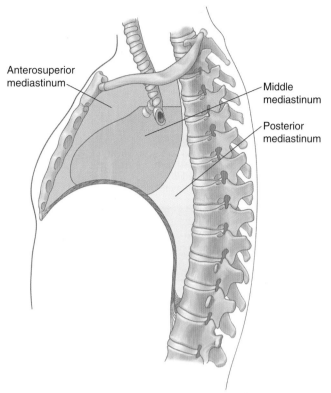

FIG. 3.5 Anatomic location of the mediastinal compartments in the three-compartment model. (This model has no specific superior compartment.) (From Liu W, Deslauriers J. Mediastinal divisions and compartments. *Thorac Surg Clin.* 2011;21:183-190.)

Treatment of a mediastinal mass depends on the underlying pathology. Many require surgical resection, radiation, chemotherapy, or careful surveillance over time.

Anesthetic management of patients with mediastinal masses can present significant challenges. Preoperative evaluation of such patients includes measurement of a flow-volume loop, chest imaging studies, and clinical evaluation for evidence of tracheobronchial compression. The size of the mediastinal mass and the degree of tracheal compression can be established by CT scan, and this study is also a useful predictor of whether airway difficulties during anesthesia are likely. Flexible fiberoptic bronchoscopy *under topical anesthesia* can be a useful tool for evaluating the degree of airway obstruction. Unfortunately the severity of preoperative pulmonary symptoms *has no relationship* to the degree of respiratory compromise that can be encountered during anesthesia. Indeed, a number of *asymptomatic* patients have developed severe airway obstruction during anesthesia. Preoperative radiation of a malignant mediastinal mass to decrease its size should be considered whenever possible. A local anesthetic technique is best for *symptomatic* patients requiring a diagnostic tissue biopsy. During anesthesia, the tumor may increase in size because of venous engorgement, and its position may shift somewhat. As a result, it can compress the airway, vena cava, pulmonary artery, or atria and create life-threatening hypoxemia, hypotension, or even cardiac arrest.

The method of induction of anesthesia and tracheal intubation in the presence of mediastinal tumors depends on the preoperative assessment of the airway. Visible external edema associated with superior vena cava syndrome is likely to be accompanied by similar edema inside the mouth and hypopharynx. If edema resulting from caval obstruction is severe, it may be necessary to establish intravenous access in the legs rather than in the arms. Invasive blood pressure monitoring should be established. Symptomatic patients may need to be in the sitting position to breathe adequately. If so, anesthetic induction should proceed in the sitting position until the airway has been secured. Topical anesthesia of the airway, with or without light sedation, can be used to facilitate fiberoptic laryngoscopy. If severe airway obstruction occurs, it can be alleviated by placing the patient in the lateral or prone position. Spontaneous ventilation throughout surgery is recommended whenever possible. Worsening of superior vena cava syndrome may occur as a result of excessive fluid administration. Diuretics may decrease the tumor volume, but the reduction in preload in these patients with already compromised venous return can result in significant hypotension. Surgical bleeding is often more than expected because of the increased central venous pressure. Postoperatively, tumor swelling as a result of partial resection or biopsy may increase symptoms of airway obstruction and require reintubation of the trachea.

Bronchogenic cysts are fluid- or air-filled cysts arising from the primitive foregut that are lined with respiratory epithelium. They are typically located in the mediastinum or lung parenchyma. These cysts may be asymptomatic, the focus of recurrent pulmonary infection, or the cause of life-threatening airway obstruction. Cysts located in the mediastinum are more likely to be filled with fluid than air and are usually not in direct communication with the airways. These masses cause symptoms of airway compression as they grow. Surgical excision may be necessary.

Theoretical concerns in patients with bronchogenic cysts include hazards related to nitrous oxide administration and the use of positive pressure ventilation. Nitrous oxide can diffuse into air-filled bronchogenic cysts and cause their expansion, with associated life-threatening respiratory or cardiovascular compromise. Institution of positive pressure ventilation in patients with cysts that extrinsically compress the tracheobronchial tree may have a ball-valve effect resulting in air trapping. Despite these concerns, clinical experience confirms that nitrous oxide and positive pressure ventilation are often safely used in patients with bronchogenic cysts.

Extrathoracic Causes

Neuromuscular disorders that interfere with the transfer of CNS input to the skeletal muscles necessary for inspiration and exhalation can result in restrictive lung disease. These abnormalities of the spinal cord, peripheral nerves, neuromuscular junction, or skeletal muscles may result in restrictive pulmonary defects characterized by an inability to generate normal inspiratory and expiratory respiratory pressures. In contrast to *mechanical disorders* of the thoracic cage, in which an effective cough is typically preserved, the *expiratory muscle weakness* characteristic of neuromuscular disorders *prevents generation of a sufficient expiratory airflow velocity to provide a forceful cough.* Acute respiratory failure is likely when pneumonia occurs (caused by retained secretions resulting from this ineffective cough) or central or respiratory depressant drugs are administered. Patients with neuromuscular disorders are dependent to some degree on their state of wakefulness to maintain adequate ventilation. During sleep, hypoxemia and hypercapnia may develop and contribute to the development of cor pulmonale. Vital capacity is an important indicator of the total impact of a neuromuscular disease on ventilation.

Breathing is maintained solely or predominantly by the diaphragm in quadriplegic patients with *spinal cord injury* at or below C4. Higher levels of injury result in diaphragmatic paralysis. Because the diaphragm is active only during inspiration, coughing, which requires activity by the muscles involved in exhalation including those of the abdominal wall, is almost totally absent. Normally, intercostal muscles are required to stabilize the upper rib cage against inward collapse when negative intrathoracic pressure is produced by descent of the diaphragm. With *diaphragmatic breathing* there is a paradoxical *inward motion* of the upper thorax during inspiration. This results in a diminished tidal volume. When quadriplegic patients are in the upright position, the weight of the abdominal contents pulls on the diaphragm and the absence of abdominal muscle tone results in less efficient function of the diaphragm. Abdominal binders can serve to replace lost abdominal muscle tone and may be useful whenever tidal volume decreases significantly in the upright position. Quadriplegic patients have mild degrees of bronchial constriction caused by parasympathetic tone that is unopposed by sympathetic activity from the spinal cord. Use of anticholinergic bronchodilating drugs can reverse this abnormality. Respiratory failure rarely occurs in quadriplegic patients in the absence of complications such as pneumonia.

Respiratory insufficiency that requires mechanical ventilation occurs in 20%–25% of patients with *Guillain-Barré syndrome.* Ventilatory support is needed on average for 2 months. A small number of patients have persistent skeletal muscle weakness and are susceptible to recurring episodes of respiratory failure in association with pulmonary infection.

Myasthenia gravis is the most common disease affecting neuromuscular transmission that may result in respiratory failure. Patients with myasthenia gravis are resistant to succinylcholine and sensitive to nondepolarizing muscle relaxants. Myasthenic syndrome (Eaton-Lambert syndrome) may be confused with myasthenia gravis. Prolonged skeletal muscle paralysis or weakness may occur following administration of nondepolarizing neuromuscular blocking drugs.

Patients with *Duchenne muscular dystrophy, myotonic dystrophy,* and other forms of muscular dystrophy are predisposed to pulmonary complications and respiratory failure. Chronic alveolar hypoventilation caused by *inspiratory muscle*

weakness may develop. *Expiratory muscle weakness* impairs cough. Weakness of the swallowing muscles may lead to pulmonary aspiration of gastric contents. As with all neuromuscular syndromes, CNS depressant drugs should be avoided or administered in minimal dosages. Nocturnal ventilation with noninvasive techniques such as nasal intermittent positive pressure or external negative pressure ventilation may be useful.

In the absence of complications, neuromuscular disorders rarely progress to the point of hypercapnic respiratory failure unless *diaphragmatic weakness or paralysis* is present. Thus quadriplegic patients who have preserved phrenic nerve function are unlikely to develop respiratory failure in the absence of pneumonia or administration of CNS depressants. In the supine position, patients with diaphragmatic paralysis may develop a ventilatory pattern similar to that seen with a flail chest. In the upright posture, these patients experience a significant increase in vital capacity and improved oxygenation and ventilation. Most cases of unilateral diaphragmatic paralysis are a result of neoplastic invasion of the phrenic nerve. In the absence of associated pleuropulmonary disease, most adult patients with *unilateral diaphragmatic paralysis* remain asymptomatic, and this defect is detected as an incidental finding on chest radiography. In contrast, infants are more dependent on bilateral diaphragmatic function for adequate respiratory function. In symptomatic infants and adults, plication of the hemidiaphragm may be necessary to prevent flail motion of the thoracic cage.

Transient diaphragmatic dysfunction may occur after abdominal surgery. Lung volumes are decreased, the alveolar-arterial oxygen difference increases, and the respiratory rate increases. These changes may be a result of irritation of the diaphragm, which causes reflex inhibition of phrenic nerve activity. As a result of this postoperative diaphragmatic dysfunction, atelectasis and arterial hypoxemia may occur. Incentive spirometry may alleviate these abnormalities.

Obesity is an increase in body mass index (BMI) and is associated with decreases in FEV_1, FVC, FRC, and expiratory reserve volume (ERV). With a BMI over 40 kg/m^2 there is also a decrease in residual volume (RV) and TLC. With extreme clinical obesity, FRC may exceed closing volume and approach RV. Central obesity is associated with worse lung function and respiratory symptoms. An increased waist-to-hip ratio and/or abdominal girth has a good correlation with impaired lung function. Buildup of adipose tissue in the anterior abdominal wall and viscera hinders diaphragmatic movement, diminishes basal lung expansion during inspiration, and causes closure of peripheral lung units. This leads to ventilation/perfusion abnormalities and arterial hypoxemia, which results in respiratory compromise, especially during sleep and in the perioperative period. Adipose cells release adipocytokines that play a part in the systemic inflammation triggered by obesity-related hypoxemia and obesity-related respiratory disorders such as obstructive sleep apnea, obesity hypoventilation syndrome, and chronic obstructive pulmonary disease.

Changes associated with *pregnancy* can lead to restrictive lung physiology in several ways. The thorax undergoes structural changes, with the subcostal angle of the rib cage and the circumference of the lower chest wall increasing and the diaphragm moving cranially. Increased levels of the hormone relaxin cause stretching of the lower rib cage ligaments. The subcostal angle widens from 68 to 103 degrees (Fig. 3.6). The anteroposterior diameter and transverse diameter of the chest wall increases by approximately 2 cm, leading to an increase in the circumference of the rib cage. These changes peak at the 37th week of pregnancy. Chest wall configuration normalizes about 6 months postpartum, except for the subcostal angle, which remains wider by about 20%. The enlarging uterus pushes the diaphragm up by about 4 cm.

Static lung function stays the same in pregnancy, except for a decrease in FRC and its components ERV and RV. This reduction in FRC is expected secondary to the elevation of the diaphragm, downward pull of the abdomen, and the changes in chest wall compliance. FRC typically decreases by 15%–20% or 200–300 mL. Intrinsic lung compliance is unaffected

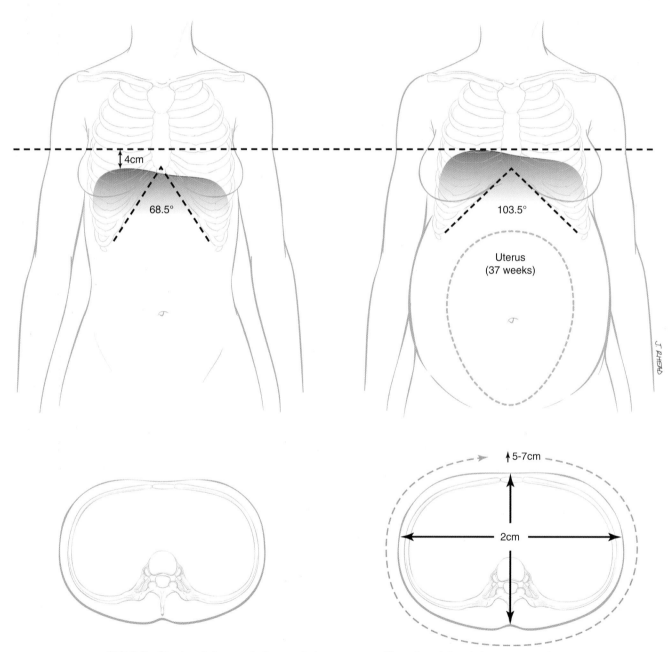

FIG. 3.6 Chest wall changes that occur during pregnancy. The subcostal angle increases, as does the anterior-posterior and transverse diameter of the chest wall and the chest wall circumference. These changes compensate for the 4-cm elevation of the diaphragm so that total lung capacity is not severely reduced. (From Hegewald MJ, Crapo RO. Respiratory physiology in pregnancy. *Clin Chest Med.* 2011;32:1-13.)

by pregnancy. At term, FRC decreases by another 25% in the supine compared to the sitting position. Although the FRC is decreased in both obesity and pregnancy, the RV is *increased* in obesity but *decreased* in pregnancy.

Laparoscopic surgery is one of the most common surgical techniques and has several advantages over traditional surgery, including decreased postoperative pain, a shorter length of stay in the hospital, and cosmetic appeal. However, it requires a *pneumoperitoneum* to allow for visualization of intraabdominal structures. Carbon dioxide is the most commonly used gas for insufflation because it is extremely soluble and diffuses easily through biological membranes. This property of CO_2 helps it equilibrate but can also lead to hypercarbia and respiratory acidosis. Intraabdominal pressure (IAP) is raised from less than 5 mm Hg to approximately 15 mm Hg. Insufflation above 15 mm Hg pressure has significant effects on lung and chest wall compliance. Decreases in lung volume and the ventilation/perfusion mismatch can be offset to some degree by application of PEEP. Pneumothorax, pneumomediastinum, and pneumopericardium can be seen in a few patients. Diagnosis can be confirmed by auscultation or ultrasound. The addition of Trendelenburg positioning worsens the effects of pneumoperitoneum.

ANESTHETIC MANAGEMENT OF PATIENTS WITH RESTRICTIVE LUNG DISEASE

Restrictive lung disease does not influence the choice of drugs used for induction or maintenance of anesthesia. Drugs with prolonged respiratory depressant effects that may persist into the postoperative period should be avoided. Vigilance for development of a pneumothorax and the need to avoid or discontinue nitrous oxide must be maintained. Regional anesthesia can be considered for peripheral operations, but involvement of sensory/motor levels above T10 can be associated with impairment of the respiratory muscle activity needed by these patients to maintain acceptable ventilation. Mechanical ventilation during the intraoperative period facilitates optimal oxygenation and ventilation. Since the lungs are poorly compliant, increased inspiratory pressures may be necessary. Postoperative mechanical ventilation is often required in patients with significantly impaired pulmonary function. Restrictive lung disease does contribute to the risk of perioperative pulmonary complications.

DIAGNOSTIC PROCEDURES IN PATIENTS WITH LUNG DISEASE

Fiberoptic bronchoscopy has generally replaced rigid bronchoscopy for visualizing the airways and obtaining samples for culture, cytologic examination, and biopsy. Pneumothorax occurs in 5%–10% of patients after transbronchial lung biopsy and in 10%–20% after percutaneous needle biopsy of peripheral lung lesions. The principal contraindication to pleural biopsy is a coagulopathy.

Mediastinoscopy is performed under general anesthesia through a small transverse incision just above the suprasternal notch. Blunt dissection along the pretracheal fascia is performed, which permits biopsy of paratracheal lymph nodes down to the level of the carina. Potential complications include pneumothorax, mediastinal hemorrhage, venous air embolism, and injury to the recurrent laryngeal nerve, leading to hoarseness and vocal cord paralysis. The mediastinoscope can also exert pressure on the right innominate artery, causing loss of pulses in the right arm and compromise of right carotid artery blood flow.

LUNG TRANSPLANTATION

Overview

The four principal approaches to lung transplantation are (1) single-lung transplantation, (2) bilateral sequential lung transplantation, (3) heart-lung transplantation, and (4) transplantation of lobes from living donors. Table 3.7 lists the typical indications for lung transplantation.

Fibrotic lung disease responds well to single-lung transplantation because both ventilation and perfusion are distributed preferentially to the transplanted lung. Bilateral sequential lung transplantation involves sequential performance of two single-lung transplants at one surgery. In the absence of severe pulmonary hypertension, cardiopulmonary bypass can usually be avoided by ventilating the contralateral lung during each implantation. The primary indications for double-lung transplantation are cystic fibrosis and other forms of bronchiectasis. The presence of cor pulmonale is not an indication for heart-lung transplantation, because recovery of right ventricular function is typically rapid and complete after lung transplantation alone. In patients with pulmonary hypertension, high pulmonary vascular resistance in the remaining native lung requires the allograft to handle nearly the entire cardiac output. This could result in reperfusion pulmonary edema and poor allograft function in the period immediately after surgery. Immunosuppression is initiated intraoperatively and continued for life.

Management of Anesthesia for Primary Lung Transplantation Surgery

Management of anesthesia for lung transplantation follows the same principles used when pneumonectomy is performed.

TABLE 3.7	Indications for Lung Transplantation

Chronic obstructive pulmonary disease
Cystic fibrosis
Idiopathic pulmonary fibrosis
Primary pulmonary hypertension
Bronchiectasis
Eisenmenger syndrome

Adapted from Singh H, Bossard RF. Perioperative anaesthetic considerations for patients undergoing lung transplantation. *Can J Anaesth*. 1997;44:284-299.

Patients selected for lung transplantation most often have restrictive lung disease and a large $PaO_2 - PaO_2$. They generally have progressive and/or irreversible pulmonary disease. Cancer is regarded as a contraindication to transplantation because of the risk of cancer recurrence with immunosuppression. Mild to moderate degrees of pulmonary hypertension and some degree of right-sided heart failure are often present. Smokers should have quit smoking at least 6–12 months before transplantation. The ability of the right ventricle to maintain an adequate stroke volume in the presence of the acute increase in pulmonary vascular resistance produced by clamping the pulmonary artery before the native lung is removed needs to be assessed. Evaluation of oxygen dependence and steroid use, hematologic and biochemical analyses, and tests of lung and other major organ system function are also required prior to surgery.

Posterolateral thoracotomy is performed for single-lung transplantation, and a clam-shell thoracotomy for bilateral or sequential lung transplantation. Cardiopulmonary bypass may be needed if cardiac or respiratory instability develops during the procedure. The lung with *worse perfusion* is removed in single-lung transplantation. Monitoring includes placement of intraarterial and pulmonary artery catheters. Pulmonary artery pressure monitoring is especially important. During the surgery, the pulmonary artery catheter may need to be withdrawn from the native pulmonary artery to be stapled and refloated into the pulmonary artery of the nonoperative lung. Transesophageal echocardiographic monitoring can be used to evaluate right and left ventricular function and fluid balance. There are no specific recommendations regarding drugs for induction and maintenance of anesthesia and skeletal muscle paralysis for lung transplantation. Drug-induced histamine release is undesirable. Drug-induced bronchodilation is useful.

The trachea is intubated with a double-lumen endobronchial tube, and its proper placement is verified by fiberoptic bronchoscopy. Potential intraoperative problems include hypoxia, especially during one-lung ventilation. CPAP to the nondependent lung, PEEP to the dependent lung, or some form of differential lung ventilation may be needed to minimize intrapulmonary shunting and hypoxia. Severe pulmonary hypertension and right ventricular failure can occur when the pulmonary artery is clamped. Infusion of a pulmonary vasodilator (e.g., prostacyclin) or inhalation of nitric oxide may be helpful in controlling pulmonary hypertension in this situation. If hypoxia cannot be controlled despite all of these maneuvers, support with partial cardiopulmonary bypass is required. Connection of the donor lung to the recipient is usually performed in the sequence of pulmonary veins to the left atrium, then anastomosis of the pulmonary artery, and finally anastomosis of the bronchus.

Postoperative mechanical ventilation is continued as needed. The principal causes of mortality with lung transplantation are bronchial dehiscence and respiratory failure due to sepsis or rejection. The denervation of the donor lung deprives patients of normal cough reflexes from the lower airways and predisposes to the development of pneumonia. In the absence of rejection, pulmonary function test results can be normal.

Management of Anesthesia for Patients With Prior Lung Transplantation

Anesthetic management of patients with a prior lung transplant should focus on (1) the function of the transplanted lung, (2) the possibility of rejection or infection in the transplanted lung, (3) the effect of immunosuppressive therapy on other organ systems and the effect of other organ system dysfunction on the transplanted lung, (4) the disease in the native lung, and (5) the planned surgical procedure and its likely effects on the lungs.

Evaluation before surgery includes obtaining a history suggestive of rejection or infection, auscultation of the lungs, and evaluation of the results of pulmonary function tests, arterial blood gas analyses, and chest radiographs. If rejection or infection is suspected, elective surgery should be postponed. The side effects of immunosuppressive drugs should be noted. Hypertension and renal dysfunction related to cyclosporine therapy are present in many patients.

Because transplanted lungs may have ongoing rejection that can adversely affect pulmonary function, it is recommended that spirometry be performed preoperatively. However, it may be difficult to differentiate between chronic rejection and infection. With chronic rejection the FEV_1, vital capacity, and TLC decrease and arterial blood gas values show an increased alveolar-arterial oxygen gradient, but carbon dioxide retention is rare. *Bronchiolitis obliterans,* the lung disease caused by chronic rejection, usually presents as a nonproductive cough developing later than the third month following transplantation. Symptoms can mimic those of an upper respiratory tract infection and include fever and fatigue. Dyspnea occurs within months and is followed by a clinical course similar to that of COPD. Chest radiographs show peribronchial and interstitial infiltrates.

Premedication is acceptable if pulmonary function is adequate. Antisialagogues can be particularly useful, since secretions can be excessive. Supplemental corticosteroids may be needed. A major cause of morbidity and mortality in transplant recipients is infection. Prophylactic antibiotics are indicated, and strict aseptic technique is required for placement of intravascular catheters. Lung denervation has limited effects on the pattern of breathing, but bronchial hyperreactivity and bronchoconstriction are common. Denervation ablates afferent sensation *in the lung below the level of the tracheal anastomosis.* Patients lose the cough reflex and are prone to retention of secretions and silent aspiration. The response to carbon dioxide rebreathing is normal.

Because lung transplant recipients lack a cough reflex, they do not clear secretions unless they are awake. Because of the diminished cough reflex, the potential for bronchoconstriction, and the increased risk of pulmonary infection, it is recommended that regional anesthesia be selected whenever possible. Epidural and spinal anesthesia are acceptable.

However, paralysis of intercostal muscle function may have special implications in these patients. In addition, any nerve blockade procedure carries the risk of infection. The importance of using sterile technique in this high-risk population cannot be overemphasized. Fluid preloading before spinal or epidural anesthesia may be risky because disruption of the lymphatic drainage in the transplanted lung causes interstitial fluid accumulation. This is particularly problematic during the early posttransplantation period.

In heart-lung transplant recipients, fluid management may be particularly challenging because the heart requires adequate preload to maintain cardiac output, but the lungs have a lower-than-normal threshold for developing pulmonary edema. In this situation, invasive hemodynamic monitoring may be very useful, but the benefits must be balanced against the risk of infection. Transesophageal echocardiography can be useful for monitoring volume status and cardiac function. If a central venous catheter is inserted via the internal jugular vein, it is prudent to *select the internal jugular vein on the side of the native lung.* Cardiac denervation is another consideration in patients who have undergone heart-lung transplantation. These patients may develop intraoperative bradycardia that does not respond to administration of atropine. Epinephrine and/or isoproterenol may be required to increase the heart rate.

An important goal of anesthetic management is prompt recovery of adequate respiratory function and early tracheal extubation. Volatile anesthetics are well tolerated, and use of nitrous oxide is acceptable in the absence of bullous lung disease. Immunosuppressive drugs may interact with neuromuscular blocking drugs, and the impaired renal function caused by immunosuppressive drugs may prolong the effects of certain muscle relaxants. The effects of nondepolarizing neuromuscular blockers are routinely antagonized pharmacologically at the conclusion of surgery because even minimal residual muscle weakness can compromise ventilation in these patients.

When an endotracheal tube is positioned, it is best to place the cuff just below the vocal cords to minimize the risk of traumatizing the tracheal anastomosis. Inadvertent endobronchial intubation of the native or transplanted lung must be avoided. If the surgical procedure requires use of a double-lumen endobronchial tube, it is preferable to place the endobronchial portion of the tube in the native bronchus so as to avoid contact with the tracheal anastomosis. In patients with a single lung transplant, positive pressure ventilation may be complicated by differences in lung compliance between the native and transplanted lung.

Physiologic Effects of Lung Transplantation

Single or bilateral lung transplantation in patients with end-stage lung disease can dramatically improve lung function. Peak improvement is usually achieved within 3–6 months. Arterial oxygenation rapidly returns to normal, and supplemental oxygen is no longer needed. In patients with pulmonary vascular disease, both single and bilateral lung transplantation result in immediate and sustained normalization of pulmonary vascular resistance and pulmonary artery pressure. This is accompanied by a prompt increase in cardiac output and a gradual remodeling of the right ventricle, with a decrease in right ventricular wall thickness. Exercise capacity improves sufficiently to permit most lung transplant recipients to resume an active lifestyle.

The innervation of the lung, the lymphatic drainage of the lung, and the bronchial circulation are disrupted when the donor pneumonectomy is performed. The principal effect of lung denervation is loss of the cough reflex, which places patients at risk of aspiration and pulmonary infection. Mucociliary clearance is impaired during the early postoperative period. Lymphatic drainage disrupted by transection of the trachea and bronchi may be reestablished during the first few weeks postoperatively. Often a blunted ventilatory response to carbon dioxide persists even though pulmonary function improves.

Mild transient pulmonary edema is common in a newly transplanted lung. In some patients, however, pulmonary edema is sufficiently severe to cause a form of acute respiratory failure termed *primary graft failure.* This diagnosis is confirmed by the appearance of infiltrates on chest radiographs and severe hypoxemia during the first 72 hours postoperatively. Treatment is supportive and includes mechanical ventilation. Mortality is high.

Dehiscence of the bronchial anastomosis mandates *immediate* surgical correction or retransplantation. Stenosis of the bronchial anastomosis is the most common airway complication and typically occurs several weeks after transplantation. Evidence of clinically significant airway stenosis includes focal wheezing, recurrent lower respiratory tract infection, and suboptimal pulmonary function.

The rate of infection in lung transplant recipients is several times higher than that in recipients of other transplanted organs and is most likely related to exposure of the allograft to the external environment. Bacterial infection of the lower respiratory tract is the most common manifestation of pulmonary infection. A ubiquitous organism acquired by inhalation is *Aspergillus,* which frequently colonizes the airways of lung transplant recipients. However, clinical infection with *Aspergillus* develops in only a small number of patients.

Acute rejection of a lung allograft is a common event and is usually seen during the first 100 days following transplantation. Clinical manifestations are nonspecific and include malaise, low-grade fever, dyspnea, impaired oxygenation, and leukocytosis. Transbronchial lung biopsy is needed for a definitive diagnosis. Treatment of acute rejection consists of intravenous methylprednisolone. Most patients have a prompt clinical response, although histologic evidence of rejection may persist even in the absence of clinical symptoms and signs.

Chronic rejection is manifested as bronchiolitis obliterans, a fibroproliferative process that targets the small airways and leads to submucosal fibrosis and luminal obliteration. Bronchiolitis obliterans is uncommon during the first 6 months following transplantation, but its incidence exceeds 60% in patients who survive at least 5 years. The onset of this syndrome is insidious and is characterized by dyspnea, cough, and colonization of the airways with *Pseudomonas aeruginosa,* which produces recurrent bouts of purulent tracheobronchitis. The overall prognosis is poor. Retransplantation is the only definitive treatment for severe bronchiolitis obliterans.

KEY POINTS

- Surgical patients with restrictive lung disease are at increased risk of perioperative pulmonary complications.
- Increases in both interstitial and alveolar fluid can cause acute intrinsic restrictive lung disease. Cardiogenic and noncardiogenic pulmonary edema, pulmonary edema associated with acute neurologic injury, high-altitude pulmonary edema, pulmonary aspiration, reexpansion pulmonary edema, and negative pressure pulmonary edema can all be causes of this form of lung disease.
- Thoracic abnormalities such as those of the chest wall, pleura, and spine (e.g., pectus excavatum, kyphoscoliosis, pleural effusion, flail chest, bronchogenic cysts, pneumothorax, mediastinal tumors) can all cause extrinsic restrictive lung disease.
- Extrathoracic causes of restrictive lung disease include (1) neuromuscular disorders associated with limited or absent function of the respiratory muscles, including the diaphragm, (2) obesity, and (3) pneumoperitoneum during laparoscopic surgery.
- The most effective treatment for aspiration pneumonitis is delivery of supplemental oxygen and initiation of therapy with positive end-expiratory pressure (PEEP).
- Adult acute respiratory distress syndrome (ARDS) is a syndrome with many risk factors that trigger acute onset of respiratory insufficiency. Despite the diverse pathologic entities that can cause this syndrome, they all have

in common the following features: significant hypoxemia, increased pulmonary capillary permeability causing alveolar edema, and neutrophil infiltration into the alveoli. The Berlin definition and criteria classify ARDS as mild, moderate, and severe based on the value of the Pao_2/Fio_2 ratio as measured with CPAP or PEEP of at least 5 cm H_2O.
- The principal effect of lung denervation from lung transplantation is loss of the cough reflex, which places patients at risk of aspiration and pulmonary infection. Only while awake will patients clear pulmonary secretions.
- In heart-lung transplant recipients, fluid management is a challenge because the heart requires adequate preload to maintain cardiac output, but the lungs have a low threshold for developing pulmonary edema.

RESOURCES

Arcasoy SM, Kotloff RM. Lung transplantation. *N Engl J Med.* 1999;340:1081-1091.

Hayden P, Cowman S. Anesthesia for laparoscopic surgery. *Contin Educ Anaesth Crit Care Pain.* 2011;11:177-180.

The ARDS Definition Task Force: acute respiratory distress syndrome: the Berlin definition. *JAMA.* 2012;307:2526-2533.

Burns KE, Adhikari NK, Keenan SP, et al. Use of non-invasive ventilation to wean critically ill adults off invasive ventilation: meta-analysis and systematic review. *BMJ.* 2009;338:b1574.

Janz DR, Ware LB. Approach to the patient with the acute respiratory distress syndrome. *Clin Chest Med.* 2014;35:685-696.

Kostopanagiotou GMDP, Smyrniotis VMDP, Arkadopoulos NMD, et al. Anesthetic and perioperative management of adult transplant recipients in nontransplant surgery. *Anesth Analg.* 1999;89:613-622.

Qaseem A, Snow V, Fitterman N, et al. Risk assessment for and strategies to reduce perioperative pulmonary complications for patients undergoing noncardiothoracic surgery: a guideline from the American College of Physicians. *Ann Intern Med.* 2006;144:575-580.

Smetana GW, Lawrence VA, Cornell JE. Preoperative pulmonary risk stratification for noncardiothoracic surgery: a systematic review for the American College of Physicians. *Ann Intern Med.* 2006;144:581-595.

Ware LB, Matthay MA. Acute pulmonary edema. *N Engl J Med.* 2005;353:2788-2796.

Critical Illness

LINDA L. MAERZ, STANLEY H. ROSENBAUM

Critical illness has been documented since the beginning of recorded history, an inherent component of the human experience. However, *critical care* is a recent development made possible by the technical and scientific advances of the 20th century. If the whole of critical illness could be reduced to a single common element, that element would be disordered perfusion. Simply stated, our effort to correct this imbalance is critical care.

Patients who would have succumbed to their critical illness a century ago now have a chance to return to a state of health that allows them to enjoy additional years of productive and fulfilling life. Perhaps more than any other segment of society, the rapidly growing geriatric population will continue to produce an ever greater demand for critical care services. As the critically ill patient population grows, emphasis on patient safety, harm prevention, and improved outcomes must also grow. Over the course of recent decades, critical care has evolved into much more than a conglomeration of technology, pharmaceuticals, and policies. Rather, the subspecialty has become a multidisciplinary and interprofessional endeavor focused on the integration of clinicians with complementary fields of expertise working together to deliver the highest quality of care to our sickest patients. To provide maximum benefit with the least potential for harm, diverse expertise requires excellent communication among the practitioners rendering care. Just as disordered perfusion is the essence of critical illness, communication is the cornerstone of critical care.

Although crucial in every critical care environment, teamwork is of paramount importance in the surgical intensive care unit (SICU) and operating rooms (ORs). Critically ill individuals who require operative intervention comprise a unique patient population. Anesthesiologists and surgeons bring singular viewpoints and expertise to the shared management of these patients. This chapter will provide a unique perspective on the underlying pathophysiology of this patient population. In turn, this perspective will provide a framework for an enhanced understanding of the general management and special scenarios encountered in the care of critically ill surgical patients.

PATHOPHYSIOLOGY OF THE CRITICALLY ILL PATIENT UNDERGOING SURGERY

Shock: Disordered Perfusion

Shock is an abnormality of the circulatory system that causes inadequate organ perfusion and tissue oxygenation. No single parameter can diagnose shock. Rather, the initial diagnosis is based on clinically apparent inadequacy of tissue perfusion and oxygenation. Over 4 decades ago, Hinshaw and Cox proposed a classification of shock involving four subsets: hypovolemic, cardiogenic, obstructive, and distributive. These descriptors are further grouped into two categories based on hemodynamic profiles: hypodynamic shock and hyperdynamic shock. These classifications provide a basis for developing differential diagnoses and management plans. However, the individual patient's clinical status may be much more complex, with overlapping types of shock physiology. For example, early in septic shock, a primarily distributive state, hypovolemia may be the primary clinical manifestation prior to the initiation of volume resuscitation.

Hypodynamic Shock

Hypodynamic shock is characterized by a low cardiac index and vasoconstriction. Decreased cardiac output results in increased oxygen extraction and lactic acidosis. Organ dysfunction is directly related to inadequate blood flow.

Hypovolemic Shock

Common causes of hypovolemic shock include hemorrhage, dehydration, and massive capillary leak. Decreased cardiac filling pressures are the hallmark of these conditions.

Cardiogenic Shock

The most common cause of cardiogenic shock is acute myocardial infarction (MI) involving 40% or more of the left ventricular mass. Cardiomyopathies and valvular lesions are other etiologies. In contrast to hypovolemic shock, cardiac filling pressures are increased in cardiogenic shock.

Obstructive Shock

The most common causes of obstructive shock include pericardial tamponade, acute pulmonary embolism, and tension pneumothorax. Cardiac filling pressures are usually increased owing to outflow obstruction, impaired ventricular filling, or decreased ventricular compliance. Therefore the clinical manifestations of cardiogenic and obstructive shock may be similar.

Hyperdynamic Shock

Hyperdynamic shock is *distributive shock* characterized by a high cardiac index and vasodilation. Unlike hypodynamic shock, oxygen extraction may be normal or decreased despite clinically significant hypoperfusion. Filling pressures can be increased or normal, depending on volume status and myocardial performance. *Maldistribution of blood flow,* rather than inadequate blood flow, is the etiology of organ dysfunction. Common causes of hyperdynamic shock are sepsis, severe trauma, anaphylaxis, specific drug intoxications, neurogenic shock, adrenal insufficiency, and severe pancreatitis.

Septic Shock

Sepsis is the most common etiology of hyperdynamic distributive shock. Direct mediators of the inflammatory response and tissue hypoperfusion result in cellular injury and organ dysfunction in septic patients.

Traumatic Shock

Severe trauma may result in traumatic shock through an inflammatory mechanism that is similar to the genesis of septic shock on a molecular, cellular, and phenotypic level. Shock in trauma patients is especially likely to be multifactorial, including a distributive immunologically mediated response to injury as well as shock resulting from hemorrhage.

Inflammation: Sepsis and the Systemic Response to Trauma

Commonalities of Systemic Inflammation

Sepsis and severe trauma are two of the most common clinical diagnoses encountered in the SICU. *Sepsis,* defined as a systemic inflammatory response to infection, has an incidence of over 900,000 cases per year in the United States. Trauma is the leading cause of morbidity and mortality for individuals younger than age 45. Systemic inflammation is the common denominator in both sepsis and severe trauma. This inflammatory response results from local or systemic release of infection-associated or injury-associated molecules, which use similar signaling pathways to marshal the soluble and cellular effectors necessary to restore homeostasis. Minor infections and minimal traumatic insults cause a *localized* inflammatory response that is transient and usually beneficial. However, severe sepsis and major trauma may result in dysregulated amplified reactions, leading to *systemic* inflammation and multiple organ failure in a significant percentage of these patients. This detrimental amplification of inflammation occurs in up to one-third of severely injured patients. Damage-associated molecular patterns are molecules that result from tissue and cellular injury. They interact with various receptors to initiate a *sterile* systemic inflammatory response following severe traumatic injury. These receptors are the same receptors that sense invading microorganisms. Hence a similar form of systemic inflammation occurs whether the patient is septic or severely injured.

Primary Goals: Surviving Sepsis

Autodysregulation in the septic patient can lead to severe sepsis or septic shock. Severe sepsis is acute organ dysfunction or tissue hypoperfusion due to documented or suspected infection. *Sepsis-induced tissue hypoperfusion* is defined as infection-associated hypotension, an elevated lactate level, and/or oliguria. *Septic shock* is severe sepsis *plus* hypotension refractory to fluid resuscitation. When severe sepsis or septic shock are encountered in the perioperative period, or if an infection potentially amenable to surgical therapy is suspected, affected patients are admitted to the SICU for intensive management.

The Surviving Sepsis Campaign (SSC) was established in 2002 to facilitate a worldwide reduction in sepsis mortality. Initial priorities included (1) building awareness of sepsis, (2) improving the diagnosis, (3) increasing the use of appropriate treatments, (4) educating healthcare professionals, (5) improving post-ICU care, (6) developing guidelines of care, and (7) implementing performance improvement programs. The original SSC guidelines were published in 2004 and revised in 2008. The most current iteration was published in 2013 and is specifically directed toward the management of patients with severe sepsis and septic shock.

These guidelines are broadly classified into (1) recommendations directly targeting severe sepsis and septic shock and (2) those targeting the general care of the critically ill patient. These recommendations are not perfect with respect to scientific rigor, but the evidence-based recommendations regarding acute management of severe sepsis and septic shock provide the foundation for improved outcomes in this large subset of critically ill patients.

General Resuscitative Measures
The SSC guidelines recommend protocols to deal with quantitative resuscitation of patients with sepsis-induced hypoperfusion during the first 6 hours of management. The guidelines recommend the following end points of resuscitation: (1) central venous pressure (CVP) 8–12 mm Hg, (2) mean arterial pressure (MAP) 65 mm Hg or greater, (3) urine output 0.5 mL/kg/h or greater, and (4) a superior vena cava oxygen saturation (central venous oxygen saturation [$Scvo_2$]) of 70% or a mixed venous oxygen saturation (Svo_2) of 65%. An additional end point is normalization of lactate in those patients who present with elevated lactate levels as markers of tissue hypoperfusion. These end points are not absolute indicators of the adequacy of resuscitation. Resuscitative end points must be individualized. This is particularly true concerning reliance on CVP for assessing volume responsiveness during resuscitation. The inaccuracy of this measurement in many patient populations has been well documented.

Diagnosis of Septic Source
Blood cultures should be obtained prior to initiation of antibiotic therapy. If indicated, imaging studies should be performed to confirm potential sources of infection.

Empirical Antibiotic Therapy and Infection Source Control
Administration of broad-spectrum antimicrobials should occur within 1 hour of recognition of septic shock or severe sepsis. When appropriate, the choice of antimicrobial drugs should be reassessed daily for the potential to deescalate from broad-spectrum antibiotics to more specifically tailored antibiotics. Infection source control should occur within 12 hours of diagnosis if the source can be identified.

Fluid Resuscitation
Initial fluid resuscitation should be undertaken with crystalloid. The recommended initial fluid challenge is 30 mL/kg. Volume resuscitation should continue as long as the patient demonstrates volume responsiveness based on either dynamic or static variables. The addition of albumin to the resuscitation fluid can be considered in patients who continue to require substantial quantities of crystalloid to maintain an adequate MAP. *Hetastarch should be avoided.*

Vasopressor and Inotropic Medications
Once intravascular volume is deemed to be optimal, vasopressors may be necessary to achieve adequate perfusion pressures, typically targeted to a MAP of 65 mm Hg or greater. However,

if the degree of shock is profound, volume resuscitation may occur simultaneously with the initiation of vasopressor support, particularly if diastolic hypotension is severe. Norepinephrine is the first-line vasopressor for management of septic shock. Epinephrine can be added when an additional drug is required to maintain an adequate MAP. Low-dose vasopressin can also be added at the nontitratable "sepsis dose" (typically 0.03–0.04 U/min) but should not be used as the initial vasopressor. Dopamine is not recommended as an alternative to norepinephrine except in selected patients such as those with a low risk of tachydysrhythmias and absolute or relative bradycardia. Dobutamine can be added to vasopressor support in the presence of myocardial dysfunction or when hypoperfusion persists despite adequacy of intravascular volume and MAP.

Steroid Management
Empirical intravenous (IV) corticosteroids should be avoided if adequate volume resuscitation and vasopressor therapy restore hemodynamic stability.

Hemoglobin Target
A hemoglobin of 7–9 g/dL is the usual target in the absence of persistent tissue hypoperfusion, coronary artery disease, or acute hemorrhage. The transfusion trigger is generally 7 g/dL.

Ventilator Measures for Sepsis-Induced Acute Respiratory Distress Syndrome
First and foremost, a low tidal volume and limitation of inspiratory plateau pressure are recommended for ventilator management of sepsis-induced acute respiratory distress syndrome (ARDS). Application of at least a minimal amount of positive end-expiratory pressure (PEEP) is also advised; higher levels of PEEP are used for moderate or severe ARDS. Recruitment maneuvers can be used in patients with severe refractory hypoxemia. Prone positioning may be used in patients with a Pao_2/Fio_2 ratio of 100 mm Hg or less in critical care units familiar with this mode of hypoxemic rescue. A short course of neuromuscular blockade (≤48 hours) for adjunctive management of early ARDS and a Pao_2/Fio_2 less than 150 mm Hg can be undertaken. However, neuromuscular blockade should be avoided in septic patients who do not have ARDS. The head of the bed should be elevated in all mechanically ventilated patients unless contraindicated. In patients with established ARDS who are adequately volume resuscitated, a conservative fluid strategy should be employed. Finally, protocols for weaning and minimizing of sedation should be used.

General Critical Care Management
Protocols for blood glucose management are recommended, targeting a blood glucose level of 180 mg/dL or less. Continuous venovenous hemofiltration (CVVH) and intermittent hemodialysis are considered equivalent in patients with severe sepsis and acute renal failure, because they achieve similar short-term survival rates. However, CVVH is much better tolerated in hemodynamically unstable patients with septic

shock. Additional recommendations call for venous thromboembolism prophylaxis, stress ulcer prophylaxis, and enteral feeding initiation within 48 hours. Finally, the goals of care, including treatment plans and end-of-life discussions if appropriate, should occur as soon as possible but within 72 hours of ICU admission.

A Genomic and Molecular Perspective
Systemic Inflammatory Response Syndrome

The similarity between the pathophysiologic response to sepsis and to traumatic injury is immunologically mediated and, by extrapolation, is a genomic and molecular phenomenon. Traumatic injury activates the innate immune system, which results in a *systemic inflammatory response* that ideally limits damage and restores homeostasis. The physiologic manifestations of this *systemic inflammatory response syndrome* (SIRS) are noted in the SIRS criteria: (1) temperature 38°C or higher or 36°C or lower, (2) heart rate 90 beats per minute or higher, (3) respiratory rate 20 breaths per minute or higher, $Paco_2$ 32 mm Hg or lower, or the need for mechanical ventilation, and (4) white blood cell count 12,000/mm^3 or higher, 4000/mm^3 or lower, or 10% or more band forms. Sepsis requires both an identifiable source of infection *plus* the SIRS criteria. Conversely it is widely accepted that systemic inflammation following trauma is sterile.

The two general components of SIRS include: (1) an acute *proinflammatory response* mediated by an increase in the expression of innate immunity genes and (2) an *antiinflammatory response* that modulates the proinflammatory phase to affect the restoration of homeostasis. It is likely that both components of the response occur simultaneously rather than sequentially following severe traumatic injury. The degree of SIRS following trauma is proportional to the severity of the injury and is an independent predictor of organ dysfunction and mortality.

Compensatory Antiinflammatory Response Syndrome

The compensatory antiinflammatory response syndrome (CARS) is associated with the antiinflammatory component of SIRS. It is a *suppression of adaptive immunity* mediated by suppression of associated genes. A major consequence of CARS is the enhanced susceptibility of critically ill patients to nosocomial infections. This has been demonstrated in animal "two-hit" models, manifested as an increased susceptibility to infection after a first insult.

Persistent Inflammation, Immunosuppression, and Catabolism Syndrome

Chronic critical illness describes patients who survive their initial episode of critical illness but remain dependent on ICU care and never fully recover. Persistent inflammation, immunosuppression, and catabolism syndrome (PICS) describes this form of chronic critical illness. Severely injured trauma patients with complicated outcomes are older and sicker and require more ventilator days compared to their "uncomplicated" counterparts. They have persistent leukocytosis and low lymphocyte and albumin levels. Genomic analysis of these complicated patients demonstrates persistent expression of changes consistent with defects in the adaptive immune response and increased inflammation. Clinically this manifests as persistent inflammation, including a prolonged acute phase response, immunosuppression, protein catabolism, malnutrition, and reduced functional and cognitive abilities. The unifying pathology is low-level inflammation inducing immune suppression and progressive protein catabolism. These patients typically have a long and complicated course culminating in transfer to a long-term acute care facility where they experience a further protracted decline and death.

Hemorrhage: The Exsanguinating Patient

Acute blood loss and its sequelae are the leading causes of early preventable death in surgical patients. Massive hemorrhage is typically associated with the severely injured trauma patient, but any operation can be complicated by intraoperative or postoperative hemorrhage. Additional clinical scenarios associated with life-threatening blood loss include gastrointestinal hemorrhage and obstetrical hemorrhage. Management of these patients includes definitive control of the bleeding source in the OR or angiography suite and perioperative management in the SICU. Resuscitative strategies are employed to keep the bleeding patient alive long enough to undergo hemorrhage control. Management of the exsanguinating patient is a prototype of multidisciplinary teamwork: surgeons, anesthesiologists, and intensivists work together to effect a life-saving intervention.

Classification of Hemorrhage

Hemorrhage is classified into four categories based on the initial clinical presentation. This allows estimation of the percentage of acute blood loss. ***Class I hemorrhage*** describes blood loss of up to 15% of blood volume or up to about 750 mL in a 70-kg male. Clinical symptoms may be minimal with no significant change in vital signs. Blood transfusion is typically not required in this circumstance. ***Class II hemorrhage*** describes blood loss of 15%–30% of blood volume or approximately 750–1500 mL. Tachycardia, tachypnea, and a decreased pulse pressure occur. The decreased pulse pressure is due to a rise in diastolic pressure due to an increase in circulating catecholamines. Notably there is not a significant decrease in systolic blood pressure. Subtle central nervous system changes such as anxiety may be apparent. Urine output is only minimally decreased. Some of these patients may require blood transfusion. ***Class III hemorrhage*** describes blood loss of 30%–40% of blood volume or about 1500–2000 mL. These patients present with classic signs including marked tachycardia, tachypnea, systolic hypotension, significant changes in mental status, and oliguria. In an otherwise uncomplicated patient, this is the least amount of blood loss that causes a decrease in systolic blood pressure. These patients almost always require transfusion of blood products. ***Class IV hemorrhage*** describes blood loss of over 40% of blood volume or over 2000 mL. This degree of blood loss is immediately life threatening. Marked tachycardia, significant and sustained hypotension, a very narrow pulse pressure, negligible urine output, markedly depressed mental status, and cold pale skin are characteristic. These patients require transfusion of blood products and immediate control of the bleeding source. Loss of more than half of the blood volume results in loss of consciousness and bradycardia.

Coagulopathy Associated With Massive Hemorrhage and Injury

Excessive blood loss of any etiology, prolonged shock, severe injuries, and traumatic brain injury with disruption of the blood-brain barrier have all been demonstrated to disrupt normal coagulation and result in a coagulopathy. This perturbation is manifested as abnormal clot formation or fibrinolysis or both. The coagulopathy leads to further bleeding, resulting in *the "lethal triad" of hypothermia, acidosis and coagulopathy. Depletion coagulopathy* causes abnormalities in traditionally measured coagulation parameters such as the international normalized ratio (INR) and the activated partial thromboplastin time (aPTT) and is a predictor of mortality. *Fibrinolytic coagulopathy* does not cause abnormalities of INR and PTT and predicts infection, organ failure, and mortality.

Damage Control Resuscitation
Overview and General Principles

Damage control resuscitation or *hemostatic resuscitation* is a useful adjunct in the prevention and reversal of the aforementioned coagulopathy associated with massive hemorrhage and injury. General principles include early hemorrhage control, permissive hypotension until hemorrhage is controlled, avoidance of crystalloids, and early use of blood components facilitated by implementation of institutionally based massive transfusion protocols. Correction of hypothermia, acidosis, and hypocalcemia are important adjuncts.

Limitation of Crystalloid Use. Rapid and large-volume crystalloid infusion in exsanguinating patients can worsen bleeding by clot disruption, dilutional coagulopathy, thrombocytopenia, anemia, and acidosis. Crystalloid resuscitation in massively bleeding trauma patients has been associated with substantial increases in morbidity and ICU and hospital length of stay. Additionally, *albumin and starch-based fluids should not be used as resuscitative adjuncts in actively bleeding patients.*

Optimal Transfusion Practice. Patients who require *massive transfusion,* defined as transfusion of 10 units of packed red blood cells (PRBCs) in 24 hours, benefit from early delivery of component therapy using standardized protocols. Massive transfusion protocols (MTPs) have been demonstrated to optimize this process and improve outcomes. Reduction in 24-hour and 30-day mortality, decreased intraoperative crystalloid administration, and reduced postoperative blood product use have been demonstrated when MTPs are implemented.

Determination of the optimal ratio of blood component delivery has been the subject of numerous investigations. It appears that *high-ratio protocols* are optimal, with recent data indicating that a *1:1:1 ratio of units of plasma:platelets:PRBCs* is associated with improved hemostasis and a decreased mortality due to exsanguination at 24 hours. These high-ratio protocols apply only to patients who require massive transfusion. They do not improve survival in patients who are not massively bleeding, and, in fact, may worsen outcomes in those patients.

Role of Procoagulants in the Exsanguinating Patient
Clotting Factors

Fresh frozen plasma (FFP) contains all of the clotting factors. Individual recombinant clotting factors are also available for the management of a coagulopathy due to inadequate amounts of one or a few clotting factors. The most widely studied and utilized recombinant clotting factor in the past 2 decades has been recombinant human coagulation factor VIIa (rFVIIa), approved in 1999 for the treatment of bleeding in patients with hemophilia and in patients who have inhibitors to factor VIII or factor IX. The clotting mechanism is initiated by activation of factors IX and X in the presence of tissue factor. Activated factor X, in conjunction with factor V, calcium, and phospholipids, converts prothrombin to thrombin, which converts fibrinogen to fibrin. Thrombin generation on the surface of activated platelets is also promoted. This process results in formation of a fibrin-platelet plug at the site of vascular injury.

Bleeding surgical and trauma patients are obviously different than those with hemophilia, since massive blood loss results in *deficiency of all clotting factors,* platelets, and RBCs. The use of rFVIIa was never approved for use in trauma patients, but its off-label use in this population was initially widespread. It was also used by the US military during the Iraq and Afghanistan conflicts. As rFVIIa was subjected to further investigation, it became apparent that this intervention *failed* to improve outcomes in trauma patients, and concern developed regarding the risk of thrombotic complications. At present the consensus is that there are no proven clinically significant benefits of rFVIIa as a general hemostatic agent in patients who do not have hemophilia. *Especially given its potential thrombotic risks, the use of rFVIIa as a general hemostatic agent in patients without hemophilia is not recommended.* When damage control resuscitation using high-ratio blood component replacement is employed, *all of the clotting factors,* platelets, and RBCs required for clot generation are administered, making use of individual recombinant factors unnecessary.

One special scenario in which low-volume rapid reversal of coagulopathy is essential is the management of elderly trauma patients who are anticoagulated with warfarin, particularly in the setting of traumatic brain injury. Rapid infusion of large volumes of FFP is often impossible owing to comorbidities predisposing to volume overload (e.g., congestive heart failure, renal failure). Prothrombin complex concentrates (PCCs) provide rapid and low-volume delivery of vitamin K–dependent clotting factors. These products contain factors II, IX, and X, with variable quantities of factor VII and the anticoagulant proteins C and S. The prothrombin complex concentrate that includes factor VII is 4-factor PCC. In addition to use in traumatic brain injury, studies have demonstrated prothrombin complex concentrates can be effective in rapidly reversing coagulopathy to allow for surgery or to control postoperative bleeding in patients who have been taking warfarin. There are no data to support use of prothrombin complex concentrates in the absence of warfarin use, but these products are often used as salvage therapy for reversal of persistent coagulopathy that occurs despite appropriate use of blood component therapy.

Antifibrinolytic Agents

Under normal circumstances, plasmin initiates clot resolution by degradation of fibrin. Trauma-associated coagulopathy is characterized by poor clot formation and rapid lysis of clots. Tranexamic acid is an antifibrinolytic drug that binds with plasminogen to prevent its activation to plasmin, thereby interfering with the process of clot lysis and slowing bleeding. Experts in trauma resuscitation have developed evidence-based guidelines for the use of tranexamic acid in adult trauma patients. Administration should be limited to patients with severe hemorrhagic shock (systolic blood pressure < 75 mm Hg) with known predictors for fibrinolysis or with documented fibrinolysis on thromboelastography. It should be administered *only if* the time since injury is less than 3 hours. The recommended dose is 1 gram IV over 10 minutes followed by 1 gram by infusion over 8 hours.

The Anticoagulated Patient

A special subset of patients develop life-threatening hemorrhage while being anticoagulated for management of comorbid conditions. Patients taking antiplatelet drugs can also be included in this group. The fundamental principle of anticoagulation is inhibition of thrombin and/or platelet activation. Thrombin generates fibrin from fibrinogen and activates factor V, factor VII, and platelets. Activated platelets adhere to injured endothelium, express glycoprotein IIb/IIIa receptors, aggregate, and increase thrombin generation from prothrombin. Reversal of the effects of anticoagulants and antiplatelet drugs are adjunctive measures in the management of acute hemorrhage. The decision to reverse the therapeutic effects of these drugs in an individual patient is based on a risk-benefit analysis, weighing the risk of ongoing hemorrhage versus the risk of thrombosis.

For a detailed discussion of the currently available anticoagulant and antiplatelet medications, their mechanisms of action, and the availability of antidotes for their activity, see Chapter 24, "Hematologic Disorders."

Platelet Dysfunction and Thrombocytopenia

Inhibition of platelet activation is crucial for the management of patients who have ischemic cardiovascular disease and atherosclerosis. Platelet inhibitors and antiplatelet drugs increase the risk of bleeding.

Aspirin is an irreversible platelet cyclooxygenase and thromboxane A_2 inhibitor and is also a relatively weak antiplatelet agent. More potent antiplatelet drugs include the glycoprotein IIb/IIIa receptor antagonists (abciximab, tirofiban, and eptifibatide). Additional potent antiplatelet drugs include clopidogrel, prasugrel, and ticagrelor, which selectively and irreversibly bind to the P2Y12 receptor to inhibit the adenosine diphosphate–dependent mechanism of glycoprotein IIb/IIIa receptor expression and platelet activation.

Clopidogrel is the major antiplatelet drug in current use. Dual antiplatelet therapy (i.e., *aspirin and clopidogrel*) is standard treatment following revascularization by percutaneous coronary intervention (PCI) with stent placement. Dual therapy is recommended for up to 4 weeks after placement of bare-metal stents and for 6–12 months after placement of drug-eluting stents. *Methods for monitoring the effects of clopidogrel have not been established, and specific therapy in the event of associated bleeding is not available.* In patients who have coronary artery stents and require surgery, the operation should be deferred for more than 6 weeks after bare-metal stent placement and more than 6 months after drug-eluting stent placement if possible. In patients who require surgery within 6 weeks of bare-metal stent placement or within 6 months of drug-eluting stent placement, antiplatelet therapy should be continued perioperatively. The actively bleeding patient with recent placement of coronary stents comprises a third category. In these patients the risks and benefits of stopping clopidogrel must be weighed against the risk of stent thrombosis and against the need for surgical intervention.

Platelet dysfunction without thrombocytopenia may occur in many clinical circumstances, including inherited and acquired coagulopathies. Desmopressin (DDAVP) is a synthetic analogue of the natural hormone arginine vasopressin. DDAVP injection has been approved for and is indicated in patients with hemophilia A with factor VIII coagulant activity levels above 5% and for patients with mild to moderate classic von Willebrand disease (type I) with factor VIII levels above 5%. In these patients the bleeding time is shortened or corrected by release of endogenous factor VIII from storage pools. DDAVP has also been demonstrated to shorten or correct the bleeding time in uremia, but the mechanism of this action is unknown. The use of DDAVP in the actively hemorrhaging patient with platelet dysfunction is not well established.

Thrombocytopenia is the most common coagulation disorder in the ICU and is defined as a platelet count below 150,000/mm^3. The two most important etiologies of thrombocytopenia in this setting are sepsis and heparin-induced thrombocytopenia (HIT). However, other potential causes are many and are generally classified according to whether platelets are consumed, sequestered, or underproduced. HIT is a special circumstance, and platelet transfusion should be avoided in these patients because of the risk of exacerbation of the prothrombotic state. Likewise, platelets are not usually transfused if the thrombocytopenia is due to immune-mediated destruction, thrombotic thrombocytopenic purpura, hemolytic uremic syndrome, or uncomplicated cardiac bypass surgery.

The threshold for prophylactic transfusion of thrombocytopenic ICU patients is not clear. However, we do know that thrombocytopenia is associated with an increased risk of bleeding with surgery or invasive procedures only when the platelet count is below 50,000/mm³. Spontaneous bleeding, especially intracerebral bleeding, usually does not occur until the platelet count is below 10,000/mm³. Therefore in the absence of active bleeding or the need for an invasive procedure, most patients with very low platelet counts and no associated risk factors for bleeding are transfused when the platelet count is below 10,000/mm³. If they have additional risk factors for bleeding, the trigger is typically less than 20,000/mm³. In the presence of an associated coagulopathy, active bleeding, or platelet dysfunction, a more liberal transfusion strategy is undertaken, but guidelines for platelet transfusion triggers are not well established.

In the massively hemorrhaging patient, platelet transfusions in conjunction with correction of plasma coagulation factor deficits are indicated when the platelet count is below 50,000/mm³ or below 100,000/mm³ in the presence of diffuse microvascular bleeding. If the patient meets criteria for activation of a massive transfusion protocol, a 1:1:1 ratio of units of plasma:platelets:PRBCs should be administered.

Acute Cardiopulmonary Instability

Acute cardiovascular or pulmonary decompensation in the immediate perioperative period is a significant cause of morbidity and mortality in the critically ill surgical patient. Rapid assessment, diagnosis, and treatment are key to limiting morbidity and preventing mortality. Pattern recognition and attention to detail allow precision in the management of these conditions.

Hemodynamic Compromise and Circulatory Collapse
Cardiac Etiologies

Circulatory collapse attributable to cardiac dysfunction can involve the myocardium, the pericardium, the cardiac valves, and the outflow tract of the heart. Disease processes involving these components of the heart are reviewed in detail elsewhere in this textbook. However, principles pertaining to the acute deterioration typical of critically ill surgical patients are highlighted here.

Acute deterioration attributable to myocardial dysfunction is most often associated with an acute coronary syndrome (ACS), which includes a continuum of associated disorders including ST-segment elevation myocardial infarction (STEMI), non–ST-segment elevation myocardial infarction (NSTEMI), and unstable angina pectoris (UA). The pathophysiology shared by these disorders is rupture of a previously quiescent atherosclerotic plaque, which triggers the release of vasoactive substances and activation of platelets and the coagulation cascade. All patients suspected of ACS should be treated with supplemental oxygen, sublingual nitroglycerine (unless systolic pressure is < 90 mm Hg), and aspirin. Despite the common etiology of the subtypes of ACS, rapid recognition of the STEMI variant is crucial, since these patients benefit from immediate reperfusion and should be treated with

fibrinolytic therapy or urgent revascularization. Conversely, fibrinolytics have demonstrated *no benefit* and an *increased risk of adverse events* when used in patients with NSTEMI or unstable angina. Multiple clinical trials have demonstrated that the early administration of fibrinolytic agents in STEMI reduces infarct size, preserves left ventricular function, and reduces short- and long-term mortality. Tissue plasminogen activator (tPA) is the fibrinolytic drug most commonly used. However, systemic fibrinolysis poses a special problem in the trauma and surgical patient population because trauma or major surgery within 2 weeks of fibrinolysis that could be a source of rebleeding is an *absolute contraindication* to fibrinolytic therapy in STEMI. In the surgical patient, the risk of thrombolysis may be prohibitive, and emergency coronary angiography with a PCI may be preferable. However, PCI mandates use of antiplatelet drugs and immediate adjunctive therapeutic anticoagulation, which can also be problematic in the trauma or surgical patient. A risk-benefit analysis of reperfusion by each method is imperative for each patient. If a patient is deemed to be a candidate for reperfusion, the time to revascularization is crucial. A medical contact-to-needle time for initiation of fibrinolytic therapy of under 30 minutes or a medical contact-to-balloon time for PCI of under 90 minutes are the currently accepted goals. In patients with diffuse and complex coronary lesions, coronary artery bypass grafting (CABG) may be preferred. The invasive nature of CABG must be weighed against the likelihood of a requirement for repeated interventions after initial PCI. PCI may be a reasonable alternative in patients with complex coronary lesions and severe co-existing diseases that substantially increase the risk of coronary bypass surgery.

Cardiogenic shock, resulting from either left ventricular pump failure or mechanical complications, is the next leading cause of in-hospital death after MI. *Systolic dysfunction* results in decreased cardiac output and decreased stroke volume. Systemic perfusion is decreased, which results in compensatory vasoconstriction and fluid retention, which can contribute to further myocardial dysfunction. Hypotension causes a decrease in coronary perfusion pressure and worsens myocardial ischemia. *Diastolic dysfunction* can also cause an increase in left ventricular end-diastolic pressure, pulmonary congestion, and hypoxemia, which can also worsen myocardial ischemia. Interruption of this cycle of ischemia and myocardial dysfunction is the basis for treatment of cardiogenic shock. Adequate oxygenation and ventilation are maintained with endotracheal intubation and mechanical ventilation if necessary. Electrolyte abnormalities are corrected, narcotics are administered, and dysrhythmias and heart block are corrected with antidysrhythmic drugs, cardioversion, or pacing. Preload should be optimized and is especially important in patients who have right ventricular infarction. If hypotension persists despite adequate volume resuscitation, vasopressors may be needed to maintain coronary perfusion pressure. Norepinephrine is superior to dopamine for management of hypotension in cardiogenic shock. Phenylephrine may be added if tachydysrhythmias are problematic. If tissue perfusion is inadequate despite achieving an adequate blood pressure, inotropic support and/or intraaortic balloon pump (IABP) counterpulsation are initiated. Dobutamine, a selective β_1-adrenergic receptor agonist, is the initial drug of choice in patients with systolic pressures above 80 mm Hg. Phosphodiesterase inhibitors (e.g., milrinone) are less dysrhythmogenic than catecholamines but may cause hypotension. Intraaortic balloon counterpulsation reduces systolic afterload, augments diastolic perfusion pressure, increases cardiac output, and improves coronary blood flow, all without increasing oxygen demand. However, IABP counterpulsation does not improve blood flow distal to a critical coronary stenosis and has not been demonstrated to improve mortality when used without reperfusion therapy or revascularization. Rather, use of an IABP can serve as a bridge to help stabilize patients prior to definitive therapeutic measures. Ventricular assist devices may also be used in appropriate clinical settings. Randomized trials have demonstrated that cardiogenic shock in the setting of acute MI is a class I indication for emergency revascularization, either by PCI or CABG. Systemic fibrinolysis is *not* a preferred option in this circumstance.

Additional complications of acute MI include postinfarction angina, ventricular free wall rupture, ventricular septal rupture, acute mitral regurgitation, and right ventricular infarction. A high index of suspicion and familiarity with the presentation of these entities allows for their prompt diagnosis and treatment.

Postinfarction angina is a syndrome of chest pain that may occur at rest or with minimal activity that occurs 24 hours or later after an acute MI. It may result from ischemia around the fresh infarction or at a distance and is generally associated with a poor long-term prognosis. It can be diagnosed clinically and evaluated by coronary angiography and is an indication for revascularization. PCI is useful for anatomically appropriate lesions. CABG is considered in patients with left main coronary artery disease, three-vessel coronary artery disease, and for lesions unsuitable for percutaneous interventions. IABP counterpulsation is often required as a bridge to revascularization if the angina cannot be controlled medically or if the patient is hemodynamically unstable.

Ventricular free wall rupture may occur during the first week after infarction. The typical patient is elderly, female, and hypertensive. Left ventricular pseudoaneurysm formation with leakage may be a sentinel event, presenting as chest pain, nausea, and anxiety, but frank rupture is catastrophic and presents with shock and electromechanical dissociation. Echocardiography will demonstrate a pericardial effusion. Postinfarction pericardial effusions larger than 10 mm in width on echo images taken in diastole are frequently associated with cardiac rupture. Pericardiocentesis may be required to relieve acute tamponade but is best performed in the OR immediately prior to thoracotomy and ventricular repair.

Ventricular septal rupture presents with severe heart failure or cardiogenic shock. Auscultation demonstrates a pansystolic murmur and a parasternal thrill. The hallmark on echocardiography is a left-to-right intracardiac shunt. Rapid

institution of IABP counterpulsation and supportive pharmacologic therapy must be undertaken. Operative repair should occur within 48 hours of the rupture.

Acute mitral regurgitation is usually associated with an inferior wall MI and ischemia or infarction of the posterior papillary muscle, but anterior papillary muscle rupture is also possible. Papillary muscle rupture occurs in a bimodal distribution: either within 24 hours or as late as 3–7 days after an acute MI. The presentation is catastrophic, with pulmonary edema, hypotension, and cardiogenic shock. The murmur may be limited to early systole, soft or even inaudible. Echocardiography is essential for diagnosis. Management may include afterload reduction, IABP counterpulsation, inotropic support, and vasopressor therapy as a bridge to surgical valve repair or replacement, which should occur as soon as possible.

Right ventricular infarction occurs in up to one-third of patients with inferior wall MI. The classic presentation is a clear chest x-ray and jugular venous distention in a patient with a known inferior wall MI. ST-segment elevation is present in the right precordial leads. Right atrial and right ventricular end-diastolic pressures are elevated, pulmonary artery occlusion pressure is normal to low, and cardiac output is low. Echocardiography demonstrates decreased right ventricular contractility. Right ventricular preload should be maintained with volume resuscitation. Some patients may require inotropic support or IABP counterpulsation. Reperfusion of the occluded coronary artery is also imperative.

Acute deterioration associated with pericardial pathology is usually caused by pericardial effusion and/or cardiac tamponade. A pericardial effusion may be characterized as a transudate, an exudate, a pyopericardium, or a hemopericardium. Large effusions are common with cancer. Loculated effusions tend to occur in the postsurgical patient, the trauma patient, and those with purulent pericarditis. Heart sounds are distant. Symptoms include orthopnea, cough, and dysphagia. Pericarditis is associated with typical chest pain, a pericardial friction rub, fever, and diffuse ST-segment elevation. Large effusions look like globular cardiomegaly on chest x-ray. (See Chapter 11, "Pericardial Disease and Cardiac Trauma," for details about pericardial diseases). The size of an effusion can be graded by echocardiography, which can also detect signs of cardiac tamponade. One-third of patients with asymptomatic large pericardial effusions will go on to develop cardiac tamponade. Triggers for the development of tamponade include hypovolemia, tachydysrhythmias, and acute pericarditis. Pericardiocentesis is indicated for immediate management of tamponade. Patients with very large effusions, electrical alternans, or pulsus paradoxus should also undergo pericardiocentesis. Patients with penetrating cardiac wounds, postinfarction myocardial rupture, or dissecting aortic hematomas presenting as tamponade require emergency cardiac surgery.

Valvular heart disease can present in two ways in the critically ill patient: (1) acute valve dysfunction resulting in acute heart failure and (2) decompensation of chronic valve disease. Regurgitation is the most common type of acute valve dysfunction. Although stenosis is typically chronic and slowly progressive, acute decompensation may occur if there is a significant superimposed hemodynamic demand. For instance, previously asymptomatic mitral stenosis may present with pulmonary edema in the setting of systemic infection, and asymptomatic aortic stenosis may present with cardiogenic shock in the setting of acute gastrointestinal hemorrhage. Echocardiography is essential in the diagnosis of all of these entities.

In addition to acute MI, common etiologies of acute mitral regurgitation include endocarditis and mitral valve prolapse. These patients can present with pulmonary edema, and the characteristic murmur may be soft or absent. Surgical repair should occur as soon as possible.

Causes of acute aortic regurgitation include endocarditis and aortic dissection. The diastolic murmur may be indistinct. Treatment is emergency surgery.

Rheumatic mitral stenosis usually occurs in young women and may present during pregnancy. Acute decompensation can often be treated conservatively. Percutaneous balloon mitral valvulotomy is the preferred intervention in this situation.

Aortic stenosis is common in the elderly patient population. Decompensation occurs with an increased hemodynamic demand. A systolic murmur is auscultated. Conservative management for decompensation is appropriate. Aortic valve replacement is performed for severe symptomatic disease.

Mechanical valves are subject to valve thrombosis, and management of this problem is controversial. Options include therapeutic anticoagulation, surgical intervention with valve replacement, and systemic thrombolytic therapy. Tissue valves degenerate within 10–15 years after implantation. Acute regurgitation associated with tissue valves is similar to native valve regurgitation and requires valve replacement.

Obstruction to cardiac outflow is most commonly encountered in patients with a *pulmonary embolism, which is the most common preventable cause of hospital death*. Acute pulmonary embolism can be divided into several overlapping syndromes: (1) transient dyspnea and tachypnea, (2) pulmonary infarction or congestive atelectasis manifested by pleuritic chest pain, cough, hemoptysis, pleural effusion or pulmonary infiltrates, (3) right ventricular failure associated with severe dyspnea and tachypnea, (4) cardiovascular collapse with hypotension, syncope, and coma (massive pulmonary embolism), and (5) nonspecific symptoms including confusion, coma, pyrexia, wheezing, recalcitrant heart failure, and dysrhythmias. Thrombolytic therapy is indicated for patients with cardiovascular collapse and for some who have clinical evidence of right ventricular failure or right ventricular hypokinesis on echocardiography. Thrombolytic therapy provides rapid lysis of a pulmonary embolism and rapid restoration of right ventricular function. However, many trauma and surgical patients are *not* candidates for systemic thrombolysis, but some may be candidates for catheter-directed thrombolytic therapy. Thoracotomy and surgical pulmonary embolectomy remains an option for life-threatening hemodynamic collapse due to a pulmonary embolism when thrombolysis and catheter-directed therapy are not feasible.

Peripheral Etiologies

Peripheral etiologies of cardiovascular collapse in the critically ill patient include loss of vascular tone and massive hemorrhage. An understanding of the differential diagnosis and presentation of these entities leads to rapid identification of the culprit and targeted management.

Loss of vascular tone leading to cardiovascular collapse is most common in distributive shock. Etiologies include sepsis, severe trauma, anaphylaxis, specific drug intoxications, neurogenic shock, adrenal insufficiency, and severe pancreatitis. A special circumstance is intraoperative vasodilation associated with the use of volatile anesthetics. The systemic hemodynamic effects of volatile anesthetics are determined by myocardial depression, direct arterial and venous vasodilation, and autonomic nervous system activity. All volatile anesthetics can cause a concentration-dependent decrease in arterial blood pressure that can be mitigated by surgical stimulation or by judicious administration of a vasoconstrictor such as phenylephrine.

Massive hemorrhage may occur in a number of different clinical circumstances. Etiologies of hemorrhage that are *visible* include penetrating trauma with blood loss emanating from the wounds, hemorrhage occurring intraoperatively, upper and lower gastrointestinal blood loss, and obstetric or gynecologic uterine hemorrhage. Etiologies of hemorrhage that *are not readily apparent by direct observation* include hemorrhage into the thoracic cavity, abdomen, or pelvis as a result of blunt or penetrating trauma; hemorrhage into the extremities as a result of long-bone fractures; spontaneous hemorrhage of solid organs or major blood vessels (e.g., ruptured or leaking aneurysms); and postoperative hemorrhage. A particularly high index of suspicion and clinical acumen is required to rapidly diagnose and treat clinically significant occult hemorrhage.

Acute Exacerbation of Respiratory Failure
Anatomic Mechanical Etiologies

The most common causes of pneumothorax in the ICU include invasive procedures (most often placement of subclavian and internal jugular central venous catheters) and barotrauma. Pneumothorax can also occur in any trauma patient as a result of either blunt or penetrating injury to the chest. Tension pneumothorax is perhaps the most dramatic example of acute life-threatening respiratory failure originating from an anatomic mechanical etiology. Tension physiology occurs when a "one-way" valve air leak tracks from a defect in the lung or through a defect in the chest wall into the pleural space. Air accumulates and is trapped in the ipsilateral thoracic cavity, eventually completely collapsing the affected lung. The mediastinum is displaced contralaterally, decreasing venous return and compressing the opposite lung. Malperfusion results from the lack of venous inflow, with a resultant decline in cardiac output. Obstructive shock ensues. This typically begins as respiratory distress and, if left untreated, progresses to hemodynamic collapse. Nonspecific signs and symptoms include chest pain, air hunger, respiratory distress, tachycardia, hypotension, neck vein distention, and cyanosis. Specific signs signifying this diagnosis include tracheal deviation away from the affected side, unilateral absence of breath sounds, and a distended hemithorax without respiratory movement. In the mechanically ventilated patient, increasing peak and plateau airway pressures, decreasing compliance, and auto-PEEP may be noted. Additionally, the patient may be difficult to bag ventilate, and difficulty delivering the prescribed mechanical tidal volume may occur.

Tension pneumothorax is diagnosed clinically, and treatment should not be delayed to wait for radiologic confirmation. Immediate decompression is required and may be initially managed by inserting a large-caliber needle into the second intercostal space in the midclavicular line of the affected hemithorax. This temporizes the situation to allow definitive treatment, which consists of insertion of a chest tube into the fifth intercostal space just anterior to the midaxillary line. Successful decompression results in rapid restoration of hemodynamics.

Laparoscopic operations are widely performed, even in critically ill patients. Carbon dioxide (CO_2) is insufflated into the peritoneal cavity. Particularly in a patient with already perturbed hemodynamics, this may interfere with cardiac, circulatory, and respiratory function. A carbon dioxide pneumoperitoneum may result in hypercapnia and acidosis, which in turn can lead to decreased cardiac contractility, a propensity for dysrhythmias, and vasodilation. From a respiratory standpoint, adverse effects include a decreased functional residual capacity, vital capacity, and compliance, as well as increased atelectasis and peak airway pressures. These effects may persist into the postoperative period, further complicating perioperative cardiopulmonary management.

Airway Circuit Mechanical Etiologies

Capnometry is the measurement of expired CO_2 and is a useful diagnostic tool. Changes in the shape of the expired CO_2 waveform in an intubated patient can alert the intensivist or anesthesiologist to developing problems. The end-expiratory (end-tidal) CO_2 pressure ($PETCO_2$) underestimates $PaCO_2$ by 1–5 mm Hg under physiologic conditions because of normally occurring alveolar dead space. Monitoring of $PETCO_2$ during mechanical ventilation can be used to assess cardiovascular status, $PaCO_2$ trends, and adequacy of ventilation. Factors that increase alveolar dead space widen the $PETCO_2$-$PaCO_2$ gradient. Pulmonary embolism acutely increases alveolar dead space. Therefore an abrupt decrease in $PETCO_2$ indicates a sudden decrease in cardiac output or pulmonary embolism. Disappearance of the capnograph waveform may indicate cardiovascular collapse or massive airway obstruction, but it is usually due to disconnection from the ventilator circuit. Capnometry is the confirmation method of choice to confirm proper placement of an endotracheal tube and has been used to assess efficacy of chest compression during cardiopulmonary resuscitation.

Primary Pulmonary Etiologies

Pulmonary pathology common in critically ill patients can pose special challenges in perioperative management. Asthma, emphysema, and bronchitis may complicate management in the intraoperative, immediately postoperative, and extended postoperative periods.

Bronchospasm is a potentially serious problem encountered in the intraoperative management of patients undergoing general anesthesia. Although volatile anesthetics are bronchodilators, bronchospasm can still occur and may have grave consequences. Transient increases in airway resistance frequently occur after endotracheal intubation and may be caused by an increase in bronchiolar smooth muscle tone. Even otherwise healthy patients undergoing stimulation of the pulmonary parenchyma or airways are at risk for bronchospasm. This occurrence can be reduced by the administration of bronchodilator therapy directly into the airway. Patients with either quiescent or active asthma are at even greater risk. Patients without recent symptoms of asthma have a low frequency of perioperative respiratory complications, but perioperative bronchospasm develops in over 5% of patients who carry a diagnosis of asthma. In asthmatics, prophylactic steroids and bronchodilators can reduce the bronchoconstriction associated with tracheal intubation, as does the use of topical lidocaine with flexible fiberoptic intubation. A number of patients who incur bronchospasm intraoperatively will have an intractable course and suffer brain damage or death, and only half of these seriously affected patients will have a history of asthma or chronic obstructive pulmonary disease (COPD).

COPD comprises three disorders: emphysema, peripheral airway disease, and chronic bronchitis. Any individual patient may have one or any combination of these components. The predominant clinical feature of COPD is impairment of expiratory airflow. Flow limitation is especially prominent in emphysema. The primary problem here is loss of lung elastic recoil, which results in marked dyspnea on exertion. Mechanical compression of airways by overinflated alveoli is a primary cause of airflow obstruction in emphysema. Patients with severe airflow limitation are at risk of hemodynamic collapse with the institution of positive pressure ventilation, owing to dynamic pulmonary hyperinflation. In addition to flow limitation, baseline hypercarbia, hypoxemia, and right ventricular dysfunction may make weaning from mechanical ventilation in the immediate postoperative period challenging in patients with COPD. Finally, severe life-threatening COPD exacerbations can be encountered in SICU patients and are characterized by a pH less than 7.30 and a PaO_2 less than 60 mm Hg; these episodes require oxygen supplementation and pharmacologic and ventilatory treatment. Administering noninvasive pressure support ventilation (PSV) and CPAP during COPD exacerbations may reduce intubation rates, complications, inhospital mortality, and hospital length of stay. If mechanical ventilation is used, minute ventilation should be targeted to the predecompensation CO_2 level to minimize alveolar hyperinflation and avoid rebound respiratory acidosis when extubation occurs.

Inhaled anesthetics decrease the rate of mucus clearance by decreasing ciliary beat frequency, disrupting metachronism or altering the characteristics of mucus. Pulmonary surfactant decreases the work of breathing by reducing alveolar surface tension. Volatile anesthetics cause reductions in phosphatidylcholine, the main lipid component of surfactant. Altered mucociliary function in mechanically ventilated patients can contribute to postoperative hypoxemia and atelectasis. Patients at greatest risk have excessive or abnormal mucus or surfactant production or acute lung injury. Examples of high-risk patients include those with chronic bronchitis, cystic fibrosis, and those receiving chronic mechanical ventilation. Difficulty with retained secretions in patients with chronic bronchitis can be very challenging postoperatively.

Metabolic Derangements

An extensive discussion of disease-based metabolic derangements is covered elsewhere in this textbook. In this section, conditions of particular relevance to the management of the critically ill perioperative patient are reviewed.

Malnutrition

Optimization of nutrition therapy and mitigation of malnutrition are primary therapeutic goals and improve outcomes. Basal energy expenditure (BEE) in hospitalized patients is estimated using the Harris-Benedict equations:

$$BEE \ (men) = 66.47 + 13.75 \ (weight \ in \ kg) + 5.0 \ (height \ in \ cm) - 6.78 \ (age \ in \ years)$$

$$BEE \ (women) = 655 + 9.56 \ (weight \ in \ kg) + 1.85 \ (height \ in \ cm) - 4.68 \ (age \ in \ years)$$

Minimally stressed patients require 25 kcal/kg/day, which is about 1.1 times greater than the calculated resting energy expenditure. The provision of 30 kcal/kg/day is required for most postsurgical patients. Trauma and sepsis increase energy substrate demands even further, such that severely stressed patients require 30–35 kcal/kg/day, and burn patients require 35–40 kcal/kg/day, which is 2 times greater than the calculated resting energy expenditure. Substrate requirements for protein synthesis must also be met. Higher protein intake may benefit healing in selected hypermetabolic or critically ill patients. Provision of 1 gram of protein/kg/day is appropriate in minimally stressed patients. Provision of 2 g/kg/day in severely stressed patients and 2.5 g/kg/day in burn patients helps limit the use of their protein stores as an energy source.

Oral intake is not possible for many critically ill patients. Therefore nutrition therapy is necessary. In addition to meeting the aforementioned goals for caloric and protein intake, nutrition therapy modulates and restores physiologic immune responses to critical illness. When provided enterally, nutrition therapy also maintains the functional and anatomic integrity of the gut.

In general, *enteral nutrition* is preferred over parenteral nutrition and should be initiated early, within 24–48 hours of ICU admission. Management strategies to optimize the success of enteral feeding include feeding *distal* to the stomach, directly into the small bowel (facilitated by placement of nasojejunal tubes); elevating the head of the bed to 30–45 degrees; and using directed feeding protocols. Small-volume ("trophic" or "trickle") feeding may not be sufficient to maintain gut integrity and normal mucosal permeability. Rather, 50%–60% of caloric requirements are needed to achieve these therapeutic end points. In patients who do not tolerate enteral nutrition at goal rates, individualized energy supplementation with *supplemental parenteral nutrition* has been demonstrated to reduce nosocomial infections. Full *parenteral nutrition* should be started early in severely malnourished patients and in patients with a nonfunctional gastrointestinal tract.

Overfeeding

Overfeeding usually occurs when caloric needs are overestimated. This can happen when actual body weight is used to calculate the basal energy expenditure in critically ill patients with significant fluid overload and/or significant obesity. Estimated dry weight or adjusted lean body weight should be used to calculate the BEE in these circumstances. Overfeeding can lead to increased oxygen consumption, increased CO_2 production, prolonged ventilatory requirements, fatty liver, suppression of leukocyte function, hyperglycemia, and increased susceptibility to infection.

Refeeding Syndrome

Refeeding syndrome can occur with rapid and excessive initiation of enteral or parenteral feeding in patients who have severe malnutrition due to starvation, alcoholism, delayed nutritional support, anorexia nervosa, or massive weight loss. When feeding is initiated in these patients, a shift from fat to carbohydrate metabolism triggers insulin release, which causes cellular uptake of electrolytes, especially phosphorous, magnesium, potassium, and calcium. Adverse clinical consequences of these electrolyte abnormalities include cardiac dysrhythmias, confusion, respiratory failure, and even death. Prevention of refeeding syndrome includes (1) correction of underlying electrolyte and volume deficits, (2) administration of thiamine prior to the initiation of feeding, and (3) slow initiation of feeding with a gradual increase in nutritional support over the course of the first week.

Hyperglycemia

Blood glucose levels are normally tightly regulated within a narrow range of 60–140 mg/dL in both the fed and fasted states. *Diabetic hyperglycemia* is defined as a fasting blood glucose concentration of 126 mg/dL or higher and a fed blood glucose concentration of over 200 mg/dL. There are no clear guidelines for defining hyperglycemia in the critically ill patient.

Stress-induced hyperglycemia occurs in critically ill patients and results from the effects of complicated hormonal, cytokine, and nervous system signals on glucose metabolic pathways. This hyperglycemia is due to insulin resistance in the liver and skeletal muscle. Hepatic insulin resistance causes increased hepatic gluconeogenesis and glucose production. Decreased glycogen synthesis and a shift from insulin-dependent to non–insulin-dependent glucose uptake occurs in skeletal muscle. Additionally, increased levels of stress mediators such as glucagon, cortisol, and growth hormone increase hepatic gluconeogenesis, while increased levels of epinephrine and norepinephrine increase hepatic glycogenolysis. Interleukins (IL-1 and IL-6) and tumor necrosis factor (TNF) may enhance both of these hyperglycemic mechanisms. Finally, exercise-stimulated glucose uptake into skeletal muscle is eliminated when critically ill patients are immobilized.

Paradigm Shifts. Until the beginning of this millennium, blood glucose levels of up to 220 mg/dL were routinely tolerated in critically ill patients. It was suggested that this stress response was beneficial for organs that rely solely on glucose for their energy supply, such as the brain and RBCs. Subsequently, stress hyperglycemia has been shown to be associated with adverse outcomes in critically ill patients. *In patients without diabetes mellitus,* hyperglycemia has an almost linear relationship with mortality risk. *In patients with established diabetes* the relationship between hyperglycemia and mortality is significantly blunted. It has been difficult to establish how tightly blood glucose levels should be controlled in ICU patients.

Van den Berghe's landmark study in 2001 supported the use of *intensive insulin therapy* to target tight glycemic control in critically ill patients, with a goal of a blood glucose of 80–110 mg/dL. In 2009 the NICE-SUGAR trial demonstrated an increase in mortality and an increase in the incidence of hypoglycemia in critically ill patients managed with this intensive insulin regimen. This and similar studies have resulted in widespread adoption of higher blood glucose targets in the critically ill population. Many of the studies support a blood glucose range of 140–180 mg/dL. Recent literature has also indicated that glucose variability over time may be an even more important determinant of mortality than the absolute blood glucose level at any given time.

Sick Euthyroid Syndrome

Critical illness can cause many nonspecific alterations in thyroid hormone concentrations in patients who do not have intrinsic thyroid dysfunction. These alterations relate to the severity of the critical illness and are termed the *sick euthyroid syndrome.*

The alterations in thyroid hormone concentrations in the critically ill represent a continuum of changes that depends on the severity of the illness and can be categorized into distinct stages. The stages reflect the severity of critical illness and are designated *mild, moderate, severe,* and *recovery.* The alterations in thyroid function are usually associated with alterations in other endocrine systems, such as decreases in serum gonadotropin and sex hormone concentrations and increases in adrenocorticotropic hormone (ACTH, or corticotropin) and cortisol levels. Sick euthyroid syndrome is then functionally part of a systemic reaction to illness involving the immune and endocrine systems.

Low T_3 State

A substantial depression of serum triiodothyronine (T_3) levels is seen *throughout all stages* of the sick euthyroid syndrome and can occur as early as 24 hours after onset of illness. This is accompanied by a reciprocal increase in reverse T_3.

Low T_4 State

As the severity and duration of the illness increases, serum *total thyroxine (T_4) levels* become abnormal. Their decline correlates with prognosis in the critically ill patient. Mortality increases as serum total T_4 levels decrease below 4 µg/dL and approaches 80% for levels below 2 µg/dL. Of note, *free T_4 hormone levels* are normal even when total T_4 levels are decreased. This may be why these patients appear clinically euthyroid. This low T_4 state is unlikely to result from hormone deficiency, but rather is a marker of multisystem failure in critically ill patients.

Recovery State

As acute illness resolves, so do the altered thyroid hormone concentrations. This stage is characterized by modest increases in serum thyroid stimulating hormone (TSH) levels. The recovery stage may be prolonged, and it may take weeks to months following hospital discharge for thyroid hormone levels to return to normal.

Treatment

Thyroid hormone replacement therapy is *not* of benefit in the vast majority of sick euthyroid patients. In the absence of *clinical evidence of hypothyroidism,* there is no good evidence for thyroid hormone replacement in patients who have decreased thyroid hormone concentrations due to the sick euthyroid syndrome.

Utility of Thyroid Function Tests in the Critically Ill Patient

Because of the high prevalence of abnormal thyroid function tests and the low prevalence of actual thyroid dysfunction, routine screening of critically ill patients for thyroid dysfunction is not recommended. Thyroid function tests should only be obtained if there is a high clinical suspicion for intrinsic thyroid dysfunction. The best tests to order are free T_4 and TSH. Interpretation of results must occur in the context of the duration, severity, and stage of the critical illness.

A mildly elevated TSH and low free T_4 may be indicative of primary hypothyroidism early in an acute illness but not in the recovery stage. The clinical context is very relevant. A history of thyroid disease or use of medications that may affect thyroid function should be sought. An increased TSH and low free T_4 are more likely to be indicative of true hypothyroidism in a hypothermic, bradycardic patient but not in a normothermic patient with normal vital signs. If both TSH and free T_4 are normal, intrinsic thyroid dysfunction is not present.

Relative Adrenal Insufficiency

Adrenal insufficiency is the inability of the adrenal gland to produce enough adrenocortical steroid hormones to satisfy bodily needs. *Primary adrenal insufficiency* is usually caused by an autoimmune disorder that destroys more than 90% of the adrenal cortex. *Secondary adrenal insufficiency* is caused by low ACTH levels. *Tertiary adrenal insufficiency* is caused by long-term treatment with steroid hormones, which induces feedback inhibition of the hypothalamic-pituitary-adrenal axis.

Relative adrenal insufficiency in critically ill patients occurs when the baseline plasma cortisol level is less than 18–25 μg/mL. This insufficiency may be due to sepsis, impaired pituitary ACTH release, decreased adrenal responsiveness to ACTH, a reduction in cortisol synthesis, impaired cortisol transport, or an impaired response to cortisol at the tissue level. Septic shock is the most common cause of relative adrenal insufficiency. *Septic shock refractory to volume resuscitation and vasopressor therapy is an indication for steroid replacement.* The steroids can be tapered when vasopressors are no longer required. Steroid therapy in septic patients *without* refractory shock is not recommended.

Acute Renal Dysfunction

Acute renal dysfunction, also called *acute kidney injury* (AKI) or *acute renal failure* (ARF) is common and occurs in up to one-third of ICU patients. In the majority of critically ill patients, its etiology is multifactorial and attributable to hypotension, sepsis, and nephrotoxic medications. The associated mortality can be as high as 50% and generally is part of multiple organ failure. The mortality of acute renal dysfunction increases as the number of organs that fail increases. Mortality is 53% with two organ failures, 80% with three organ failures, and 100% with five organ failures. However, acute renal dysfunction even by itself is associated with increased morbidity and mortality. The risk of developing acute renal dysfunction increases with age, baseline chronic kidney disease, oliguria, and sepsis.

Acute renal failure has traditionally been defined as an abrupt decrease in glomerular filtration rate (GFR) with a resultant retention of urea and other nitrogenous waste products along with dysregulation of body fluids and electrolytes. However, this definition is *qualitative*, not quantitative, and is of limited clinical utility. Until 2004 there was no quantitative definition or characterization of ARF. With the establishment of standardized criteria, the ability to effectively characterize ARF has enhanced precise communication from a clinical standpoint and has improved the rigor of research initiatives.

RIFLE Criteria

In 2004 the Acute Dialysis Quality Initiative (ADQI) group established the RIFLE criteria to define ARF in critically ill patients: **R** = risk, **I** = injury, **F** = failure, **L** = loss, **E** = end-stage. The first three stages (**R, I, F**) reflect progressively severe increases in serum creatinine, decreases in GFR, and the severity of oliguria within a *7-day period.* The last two stages (L, E) reflect longer-term renal function outcomes; **L** describes complete loss of kidney function requiring renal replacement therapy for longer than 4 weeks, and **E** describes end-stage kidney disease requiring dialysis for longer than 3 months.

AKIN Criteria

In 2007 the Acute Kidney Injury Network (AKIN) proposed the term *AKI* to represent the entire spectrum of ARF. The AKIN criteria are based on the acute changes in serum creatinine or urine output comprising stages 1, 2, or 3 AKI. These criteria simplify the RIFLE definitions by describing only 3 stages evaluated over a *48-hour period.* Measurement of GFR was eliminated, and an increase in serum creatinine of as little as 0.3 mg/dL was incorporated into stage 1 AKI.

KDIGO Criteria

In 2013 the AKIN criteria were further modified by the Kidney Disease: Improving Global Outcomes (KDIGO) group. This work represented the first ever international multidisciplinary clinical practice guidelines for AKI and focused on definitions, risk assessment, evaluation, and treatment. *AKI is defined as any* of the following (with 3 stages of severity, 1, 2, and 3):

- an increase in serum creatinine by 0.3 mg/dL or more within 48 hours, *or*
- an increase in serum creatinine by 1.5 or more times baseline within the prior 7 days, *or*
- urine output less than 0.5 mL/kg/h for 6 hours

Cirrhosis

Cirrhosis is characterized by fibrous infiltration throughout the liver, a consequence of sustained wound healing in response to chronic liver injury. It leads to end-stage liver disease (ESLD). Complications of ESLD include hyperbilirubinemia, malnutrition, decreased hepatic synthetic function, coagulopathy, portal hypertension, hepatic encephalopathy, and extreme fatigue. Patients with these complications are frequently managed in the ICU because of the critical nature of these issues. The Child-Pugh score is useful in predicting the surgical risk of intraabdominal surgery in cirrhotic patients. Variables used to calculate this score include the bilirubin level, albumin level, INR, and the presence of encephalopathy and/or ascites. Class A cirrhosis carries an overall surgical mortality of 10%; class B, 30%; and class C, 75%–80%. Perioperative mortality and morbidity correlates well with the Child-Pugh score. The Model for End-Stage Liver Disease (MELD) score is a linear regression model based on the INR, bilirubin level, and creatinine level. The MELD score has been the sole method of liver transplant allocation in the United States since 2002. A minimum MELD score of 18 is necessary to have a survival benefit with liver transplantation. MELD is also useful for predicting mortality in patients undergoing nontransplant surgical procedures. Patients with a MELD below 10 can safely undergo elective surgery; those with a MELD 10–15 may undergo surgery with caution; those with a MELD above 15 should not undergo elective surgery. Familiarity with the Child-Pugh and MELD classifications is important for the surgical intensivist, since patients with ESLD are likely to be managed in the SICU following nontransplant surgical procedures and after liver transplantation.

Fulminant Hepatic Failure

Fulminant hepatic failure (FHF), otherwise known as *acute liver failure,* is uncommon. It is defined as the presence of hepatic encephalopathy and coagulopathy (INR > 5.0) within 26 weeks of the first appearance of symptoms in patients with no history of underlying liver disease. Loss of hepatocyte function initiates multisystem organ dysfunction and terminates in death. Complications include worsening encephalopathy, cerebral edema, sepsis, ARDS, hypoglycemia, coagulopathy, gastrointestinal hemorrhage, pancreatitis, and ARF. Acetaminophen toxicity, idiosyncratic drug reactions, and hepatotropic viruses are the most common causes of acute hepatic failure in the United States. Acute hepatic failure accounts for 5%–6% of liver transplantations. A liver transplant is the only definitive treatment option for these patients, who are unlikely to recover spontaneously. Without liver transplantation the mortality rate for fulminant hepatic failure is 50%–80%. Grade III or IV hepatic encephalopathy is an indication for endotracheal intubation and diagnostic and therapeutic modalities to treat intracranial hypertension, which is the major cause for early mortality in acute hepatic failure. This intracranial hypertension is due to cerebral hyperemia, osmotic factors, and derangements of the blood-brain barrier. Continuous monitoring of intracranial pressure (ICP) is initiated when grade III encephalopathy occurs. Elevated ICP is managed with hyperventilation, mannitol, mild hypothermia, and therapeutic sedation. CVVH is the preferred method if renal replacement therapy is required. It avoids the hemodynamic fluctuations that may be particularly problematic in this situation.

Neurologic Disorders

The purpose of this section is to highlight those neurologic entities of particular importance in the management of the critically ill perioperative patient.

Pain, Agitation, and Delirium

Pain, agitation, and delirium are pervasive conditions in the critically ill patient population and have the potential to adversely affect outcomes if not managed properly. The principles outlined here pertain to *adult* ICU patients.

Pain and Analgesia

The International Association for the Study of Pain defines *pain* as an "unpleasant sensory and emotional experience associated with actual or potential tissue damage or described in terms of such damage." The ability to reliably assess pain is key to optimal management of pain. Critically ill patients may be unable to communicate effectively. Therefore it is necessary to use alternative assessment methods to detect, quantify, and manage their pain. These patients may experience pain at rest; pain as a sequela of surgery, trauma, burns, or cancer; and pain related to ICU procedures. Unrelieved pain has significant and long-lasting psychological consequences, including chronic pain, posttraumatic stress disorder (PTSD), and low health-related quality of life. The physiologic consequences of pain include increased levels of catecholamines, which cause arteriolar vasoconstriction and impaired tissue perfusion and oxygen delivery. Catabolic hypermetabolism causes hyperglycemia, lipolysis, and muscle wasting. Wound healing is also impaired, increasing the risk of wound infection.

The Behavioral Pain Scale (BPS) and the Critical Care Pain Observation Tool (CPOT) are the most reliable behavioral pain scales available for use in medical, postoperative, and trauma patients (adult ICU patients) who are unable to self-report pain and in whom motor function is intact. *Vital signs should not be used as a sole determinant of pain assessment.*

IV opioids are the first-line drugs to treat nonneuropathic pain in critically ill patients. Nonopioid analgesics should be considered only to decrease the dose of opioids used and to decrease opioid-related side effects. Gabapentin or carbamazepine should be added to IV opioids for management of neuropathic pain. Thoracic epidural anesthesia/analgesia should be considered for postoperative analgesia in patients undergoing abdominal aortic aneurysm surgery and for management of pain associated with rib fractures.

Agitation and Sedation

Agitation and anxiety are common in critically ill patients and lead to adverse clinical outcomes. The first step in management is identification and treatment of the underlying causes of agitation, including pain, delirium, hypoxemia, hypoglycemia, hypotension, and withdrawal syndromes. Maintenance of patient comfort, pain control, reorientation, and environmental hygiene to maintain normal sleep patterns should be optimized before sedatives are prescribed.

Prolonged deep sedation has negative consequences. Therefore sedative medications should be titrated to maintain light rather than deep sedation in ICU patients. Sedation scales, sedation protocols designed to minimize sedative use, and use of nonbenzodiazepine medications are associated with improved outcomes, including fewer days of mechanical ventilation, fewer days in the ICU and fewer days in the hospital, less delirium, and less long-term cognitive dysfunction.

The Richmond Agitation-Sedation Scale (RASS) and the Sedation-Agitation Scale (SAS) are the most reliable sedation assessment tools for adult ICU patients. However, these are subjective tests. Objective measures of brain function include auditory evoked potentials, Bispectral Index, Narcotrend Index, Patient State Index, and state entropy. These parameters can be used as adjuncts to subjective sedation assessments in patients receiving neuromuscular blockade. Electroencephalogram (EEG) monitoring should be used to monitor brain electrical activity in patients who have known or suspected seizures or to titrate electrosuppressive medications to achieve burst suppression in patients who have intracranial hypertension.

When a sedative is required, dexmedetomidine or propofol are generally preferred. Dexmedetomidine has no active metabolites, and side effects include bradycardia, hypotension, hypertension with the loading dose, and loss of airway reflexes. Propofol also has no active metabolites, and side effects include hypotension, respiratory depression, hyper-triglyceridemia, pancreatitis, and *propofol infusion syndrome.* The latter is rare but lethal and is associated with infusion of propofol at 4 mg/kg/h or greater for 48 hours or longer. The syndrome is characterized by acute refractory bradycardia that may lead to asystole. Metabolic acidosis, rhabdomyolysis, hyperlipidemia, and an enlarged or fatty liver may also be present. Hyperkalemia and a cardiomyopathy with acute cardiac failure may also occur. In addition to the high propofol dosage, risk factors for propofol infusion syndrome include poor oxygen delivery, sepsis, and severe cerebral injury.

Delirium

Delirium is characterized by acute onset of cerebral dysfunction resulting in (1) an altered level of consciousness (reduced awareness of the environment) with a reduced ability to focus, sustain, or shift attention and (2) either a change in cognition (i.e., memory deficits, disorientation, or language disturbance) or the development of a perceptual disturbance (i.e., hallucinations or delusions). The underlying pathophysiology is poorly understood.

Patients can be agitated (hyperactive delirium), calm, or lethargic (hypoactive delirium). Hyperactive delirium is more easily diagnosed and is associated with hallucinations and delusions. Hypoactive delirium is associated with confusion and sedation and is frequently misdiagnosed or even entirely overlooked. Delirium may be a disease-induced syndrome (e.g., a manifestation of organ dysfunction in severe sepsis), iatrogenic (e.g., from exposure to sedative or opioid medications), or environmentally induced (e.g., from prolonged use of physical restraints or immobilization).

Several risk factors are associated with the development of delirium in the ICU: preexisting dementia, history of hypertension, history of alcoholism, and a high severity of illness at the time of ICU admission. Coma is an independent risk factor. Opioids and benzodiazepines may be associated with the development of delirium in adult ICU patients.

Delirium is very common; 80% of mechanically ventilated patients may be affected. It is also an independent predictor of negative outcomes in ICU patients, including increased mortality, hospital length of stay, cost, and long-term cognitive impairment.

Routine monitoring for delirium should be undertaken in all ICU patients. The Confusion Assessment Method for the ICU (CAM-ICU) and the Intensive Care Delirium Screening Checklist (ICDSC) are the most reliable delirium monitoring tools for adult ICU patients.

In mechanically ventilated patients who require sedation, dexmedetomidine infusion may be associated with a lower prevalence of delirium compared to a benzodiazepine infusion. Early mobilization may reduce the incidence and duration of delirium. There are no drugs that can prevent delirium. There is also no evidence that haloperidol reduces the overall duration of delirium in ICU patients. Nonetheless, use of haloperidol is widespread for episodic acute management of the potentially dangerous behaviors associated with agitated delirium. Given the lack of definitive drug treatment options, the key to management of delirium is mitigation of risk factors and prevention.

Global strategies to manage pain, agitation, and delirium in all ICU patients should include: (1) daily sedation interruption or a "light" level of sedation in mechanically ventilated patients, (2) analgesia-first sedation in mechanically ventilated patients, (3) promoting normal sleep cycles by optimizing the environment, and (4) an interdisciplinary team approach incorporating provider education, protocols, order sets, and checklists to facilitate optimal management of pain, agitation, and delirium.

Metabolic Encephalopathy

Coma is uninterrupted loss of the capacity for arousal, which is due to an acute or subacute brain insult causing either diffuse or bilateral cerebral dysfunction, failure of the brainstem-thalamic ascending reticular activating system or both. The eyes are closed, sleep/wake cycles are absent, and stimulation elicits only reflex responses at best. Nonstructural disorders such as metabolic or toxic pathology induce coma by depressing the brainstem and cerebral arousal mechanisms and are common in critically ill patients. The anatomic target of metabolic brain disease has not been precisely defined. Onset of coma can be abrupt or may evolve more slowly after a period of inattention or confusion.

The primary abnormalities in metabolic encephalopathy are altered arousal and cognitive function. Additional symptoms revolve around abnormalities of the sleep/wake cycle, autonomic dysfunction and abnormal breathing patterns. A primary distinguishing feature of diffuse metabolic encephalopathy is preservation of the pupillary light response. Exceptions to this rule include an overdose of anticholinergic drugs, near-fatal anoxia, and malingering. Elderly patients with serious systemic illnesses or who have undergone complicated surgery are particularly prone to metabolic encephalopathy.

Metabolic encephalopathy manifests as multilevel central nervous system dysfunction. Misperception, disorientation, hallucinations, concentration and memory deficits, and hypervigilance may progress to coma. Motor abnormalities are typically bilateral and symmetrical. Examples include tremor, asterixis, and multifocal myoclonus. Hypoactivity or hyperactivity may be present, depending on the etiology of the encephalopathy. Seizures may occur after substance withdrawal and with hypoglycemia, hepatic failure, uremia, abnormal calcium levels, or toxin ingestion. Hypothermia or hyperthermia may occur as a result of autonomic dysfunction.

Etiologies of metabolic encephalopathy include toxin ingestion, substance withdrawal, hypoglycemia, hypoxemia, hepatic dysfunction, uremia, electrolyte imbalances, pancreatic inflammation, and infection. Initial therapy of all patients with metabolic encephalopathy includes maintenance of adequate oxygenation and ventilation, maintenance of circulation and perfusion, empirical administration of glucose and thiamine, seizure control if indicated, careful and mild sedation if indicated in agitated patients, specific antidotes for reversal of the effects of ingested substances, and maintenance of normothermia. Once these supportive measures are established, efforts can be focused on a search for and treatment of the specific underlying etiology.

Critical Illness Polyneuropathy

Critical illness polyneuropathy is a diffuse sensorimotor peripheral neuropathy that develops in the setting of multiple organ failure and sepsis. This entity is probably *the most common neuromuscular cause of prolonged ventilator dependency in patients without prior neuromuscular disease.* Symptoms include extremity muscle weakness and wasting, distal sensory loss, and paresthesias. Deep tendon reflexes are usually diminished. Electrodiagnostic studies are important to establish a definitive diagnosis because the clinical findings may not be readily discernible in the critically ill patient. The pathophysiology is unknown. However, it has been suggested that increased microvascular permeability may result in endoneural edema and axonal hypoxia and degeneration. It is important to distinguish this disease entity from Guillain-Barré syndrome.

The severity of critical illness neuropathy is correlated with ICU length of stay, the number of invasive procedures, hyperglycemia, hypoalbuminemia, and the severity of multiple organ failure. Overall prognosis is dependent on recovery from the underlying critical illness. Most survivors recover from the neuropathy in several months. Even though ventilator dependence may be prolonged, critical illness polyneuropathy does *not* worsen long-term prognosis. However, the prognosis can be adversely effected when compression neuropathies complicate this disorder.

Acute Quadriplegic Myopathy

Acute quadriplegic myopathy, otherwise known as *acute myopathy of intensive care,* develops in critically ill patients *without* preexisting neuromuscular disease. It usually occurs in the setting of severe pulmonary disease for which neuromuscular blockade has been used to facilitate mechanical ventilation, and high-dose corticosteroids have been administered at the same time. Typically it occurs in those in whom nondepolarizing neuromuscular blockade was used for more than 2 days. This disorder is characterized by an acute necrotizing myopathy. Diffuse flaccid quadriparesis with involvement of respiratory muscles and muscle wasting occurs after several days of induced paralysis. Sensation is intact, but deep tendon reflexes are diminished. Creatine kinase levels are usually elevated. The paralysis is severe and may prolong the period of mechanical ventilation, but the prognosis for recovery from the myopathy is good. Functional recovery occurs over weeks to months. In general, high-dose corticosteroids should be avoided when neuromuscular blockade is required.

Prolonged Effects of Neuromuscular Blockade

Prolonged neuromuscular blockade may occur with most depolarizing or nondepolarizing neuromuscular blockers, especially in the setting of hepatic or renal insufficiency.

Acidosis and hypermagnesemia are also predisposing factors. This phenomenon occurs with vecuronium, which is metabolized by the liver. Atracurium and cisatracurium rarely cause this problem because they do not require organ metabolism for their clearance. If a peripheral nerve stimulator is used to monitor muscle twitch responses to a train-of-four stimulus during neuromuscular blockade, drug dosing can be titrated to preserve one or two twitches. This will reduce the overall amount of neuromuscular blocker used and thus prevent overdosing and this prolonged paralytic effect.

GENERAL PRINCIPLES OF PERIOPERATIVE MANAGEMENT IN THE CRITICALLY ILL PATIENT

Although intensive care is complex and multifaceted, several general principles apply to perioperative management of the critically ill surgical patient. Implementation of these principles is important when care of the patient is transitioned from the SICU to the OR and back again. A shared understanding of these concepts is key to the communication between the surgeons and anesthesiologists caring for this patient population.

Intravenous Fluid Management

Parenteral Solutions

IV fluids are used for resuscitation and maintenance of critically ill patients. Maintenance fluid therapy replaces fluids normally lost over the course of a day. Resuscitative fluid therapy replaces preexisting deficits and ongoing fluid losses. Maintenance and resuscitative fluid therapy can occur simultaneously, but different fluids may be used for these two needs. Parenteral solutions are either crystalloids or colloids. Fluid selection is based on maintenance requirements, fluid deficits, ongoing fluid losses, and clinical context.

Lactated Ringer (LR) solution is a crystalloid that has a composition similar to plasma. It is usually used as a resuscitative fluid to replace loss of fluid that has a similar composition to plasma. LR has a relatively low sodium content (130 mEq/L) and is therefore mildly hypotonic. Hyponatremia can occur with excessive or prolonged use. This is problematic in patients who have traumatic brain injury, since they require a higher plasma osmolality. The lactate in LR solution is sodium lactate, which dissociates when infused. The lactate anions are metabolized to bicarbonate and *do not contribute to acidosis.*

Normal saline solution is another resuscitative crystalloid and contains 154 mEq/L of both sodium and chloride. Normal saline is excellent for the treatment of hyponatremic hypochloremic metabolic alkalosis. However, in other clinical circumstances the excessive chloride load can lead to hyperchloremic metabolic acidosis, which can worsen a preexisting acidosis.

Hypertonic saline solutions are administered to replace sodium deficits in *symptomatic* hyponatremia. The most widely used formulations are 3% NaCl and 1.5% NaCl. The former is infused through a central venous catheter, but the latter may be administered peripherally. Hypertonic saline solutions have also been used in the resuscitation of hypovolemia in trauma and burn patients. Intravascular volume is increased more quickly, and the total resuscitation volume may be decreased compared to standard crystalloids. However, significant acid-base and electrolyte abnormalities often occur.

Naturally occurring colloids include albumin (5% and 25% are available in the United States) and FFP. Albumin solutions are typically prepared in normal saline; therefore large-volume resuscitation might cause hyperchloremic metabolic acidosis. In 2004 the SAFE (Saline versus Albumin Fluid Evaluation) trial demonstrated that albumin is as safe as saline in the vast majority of patients.

Hydroxyethyl starch preparations are the most common *synthetic colloids.* They are categorized by their average molecular weight, degree of substitution (i.e., number of hydroxyethyl groups per 100 glucose groups), and concentration. Starches include hetastarch, pentastarch, and tetrastarch; 6% solutions have been the most commonly used formulations in the United States. The vehicles for the starches differ. Hespan is a 6% solution of hetastarch in normal saline, and Hextend is a 6% solution of hetastarch in a solution similar to LR solution. Starch solutions provide little free water. Therefore starch administration must occur in conjunction with maintenance fluids so as to minimize the likelihood of hyperoncotic renal injury. Some interventional trials have noted an association between starch administration and AKI. Starches were used much more frequently in the past, but now their use has fallen out of favor.

Maintenance Fluid Therapy

Weight-based formulas are used to calculate *maintenance fluid requirements* and *take into account both sensible and insensible losses.* A commonly used formula is the "4-2-1 Rule":

- first 10 kg of body weight: 4 mL/kg/h
- second 10 kg of body weight: 2 mL/kg/h
- each additional 10 kg of body weight: 1 mL/kg/h

For example, the hourly maintenance fluid requirement for a 70-kg patient using this formula is 110 mL/h. For patients who have clinically severe obesity, the adjusted body weight rather than the actual body weight is used to calculate the maintenance fluid rate:

$$\text{Adjusted body weight} = \text{ideal body weight (IBW)} + 1/3 (\text{actual body weight} - \text{IBW})$$

Maintenance fluids are hypotonic and usually contain 5% dextrose. The prototypical maintenance fluid for adults is D_5-1/2 normal saline + 20 mEq KCl/L. Dextrose is an aid in gluconeogenesis, and sodium and potassium are provided in a quantity based on daily requirements. However, potassium should be excluded from solutions provided to patients who have renal impairment or anuria.

Resuscitative Fluid Therapy: Crystalloid Versus Colloid

Resuscitative fluid therapy replaces preexisting deficits and ongoing fluid losses. Crystalloid solutions are used most commonly.

In particular a dextrose-free isotonic (or nearly isotonic) salt solution, such as LR solution, is used in surgical patients.

The capillary endothelium is permeable to isotonic and hypotonic salt solutions, and crystalloid distributes between the intravascular and interstitial spaces in proportion to the relative volumes of these spaces. The intravascular space comprises 25% of the extracellular fluid, and the interstitial space comprises 75% of the extracellular fluid (a 1:3 ratio). Therefore for each liter of crystalloid infused intravenously, 250 mL remains in the intravascular space and 750 mL diffuses into the interstitial space.

Another disadvantage of crystalloid solutions is their proinflammatory effect. From a historical perspective, these disadvantages of crystalloid therapy have been the basis of the crystalloid-versus-colloid debate.

Under normal physiologic conditions the average leakage rate of infused albumin and other isooncotic solutions into the interstitial space is approximately 25%–35%. For each liter of 5% albumin infused intravenously, roughly 750 mL remains in the intravascular space and 250 mL diffuses into the interstitial space. This relationship is *opposite to* that of crystalloid isotonic salt solutions. At least in theory the ratio of intravascular filling between colloid and crystalloid solutions is 3:1. However, this effect of albumin has been overly simplified. Even under physiologic conditions, leakage of albumin is highly variable and dependent on the unique characteristics of various capillary beds. Furthermore, surgical patients, particularly those who are critically ill, have significant perturbations of microvascular permeability. In a severely inflamed capillary bed, up to half of infused albumin may diffuse into the interstitial space. Albumin appears to be safe in most patient populations but may not provide a survival advantage over isotonic salt solutions. The major exception is patients with traumatic brain injury who have an increased risk of death after administration of albumin.

The synthetic plasma expanders, including hydroxyethyl starch preparations, are alternatives to albumin. In 2012, several papers were published that compared hydroxyethyl starch to crystalloid in subsets of critically ill patients. These studies indicated that patients with severe sepsis may have a higher risk of death and a higher likelihood of requiring renal replacement therapy if treated with hydroxyethyl starch as opposed to crystalloid resuscitation fluids. In addition, at least one of the papers demonstrated that use of synthetic colloids to reverse shock resulted in only a marginally lower total volume of resuscitation fluid.

The most recent Cochrane review of the colloid-versus-crystalloid debate was published in 2013 and demonstrated that *there is no evidence to indicate that resuscitation with colloids, compared to resuscitation with crystalloids, reduces the risk of death in patients with trauma, burns, or following surgery.* The use of hydroxyethyl starch might actually increase mortality. Since colloids are not associated with improved survival and are more expensive than crystalloids, continued use of colloids in clinical practice may not be justified.

Interruption of Enteral Nutrition Preoperatively

The primary objective of preoperative fasting is to reduce the risk of pulmonary aspiration. In 2011 the American Society of Anesthesiology published practice guidelines pertaining to preoperative fasting in healthy patients undergoing elective procedures. Fasting for 2 hours after ingestion of clear liquids was recommended, as was fasting for 6 hours after a light meal and 8 hours after a fatty meal.

Critically ill patients frequently undergo surgery or interventions that traditionally mandate nil per os (NPO) status. However, it is not clear what this means in those patients whose enteric intake bypasses the stomach (e.g., patients fed via a nasojejunal tube or a feeding jejunostomy). Given the very significant degree of malnutrition present in critically ill surgical patients, stopping nutritional support prior to surgery or procedures is not inconsequential. In addition, many of these procedures are scheduled on an "add-on" basis without a specific start time. If tube feedings are discontinued at midnight prior to the planned operation and the case does not start until evening, nutritional support will have been interrupted in excess of 18 hours prior to the beginning of surgery.

At present there are no widely accepted guidelines pertaining to discontinuation of tube feedings in the critically ill patient population. Some institutions have developed internal guidelines, whereas other hospitals leave the decision of when to stop tube feeding preoperatively to the anesthesiologist managing the patient in the OR.

In this patient population the risk for aspiration can be assessed by evaluating the following clinical parameters:
- surgery: intraabdominal versus extraabdominal
- preoperative airway status: intubated versus not intubated
- tube feeding route: gastric versus postpyloric
- if feeding by a postpyloric route: gastric drainage versus no gastric drainage

Using this assessment, a patient considered at high risk of aspiration will be one about to undergo an intraabdominal operation who is not yet intubated and who is receiving intragastric feedings. Conversely a patient at low risk will be one about to undergo an extraabdominal operation who is already intubated and is receiving jejunal feedings with concomitant nasogastric tube suction drainage. Additional clinical considerations may include the potential for a difficult airway in a patient who is not already intubated and patient factors that increase the risk for aspiration, such as gastrointestinal motility disorders and diabetes mellitus.

A risk-benefit analysis should be undertaken with respect to the timing of preoperative cessation of tube feedings. The risk of aspiration versus the impact of withholding nutritional support for a period of time must be considered.

Administration of Blood Products

Transfusion of blood products is an integral component of the management of severely injured or hemorrhaging patients. The process whereby blood products are obtained varies depending on the clinical urgency of the situation.

Process for Availability of Blood Products Intraoperatively

Routine preoperative crossmatching of blood for surgical cases means that the crossmatched units of blood are unavailable to other patients for 24–48 hours. Additionally, for certain elective surgical procedures the number of crossmatched units ordered frequently exceeds the number of units transfused. High crossmatch-to-transfusion ratios (CTRs) result in inefficiency and wastage of blood products. For surgery in which the average number of units transfused per case is less than 0.5, the ABO-Rh type and a screen for unexpected antibodies (i.e., type and screen) can be determined instead of a complete type and crossmatch. In general, blood banks try to maintain CTRs of 2.1–2.7.

Another approach incorporates the maximal surgical blood order schedule (MSBOS). This is a list of surgical procedures and the maximal number of units of blood that a particular blood bank will crossmatch for each procedure. This schedule is hospital specific and based on the blood transfusion experience for surgical cases in that hospital. The MSBOS is developed by the suppliers and users of blood products in the hospital, including blood bank personnel, anesthesiologists, and surgeons. In recent years, many blood banks have implemented information technology systems to facilitate this process by interfacing scheduled OR cases with the MSBOS.

Emergency Transfusion

In many situations the need for blood products is urgent, before completion of compatibility testing can occur. Anesthesiologists and surgeons who work in high-volume trauma centers and high-acuity SICUs must make decisions regarding how much and exactly how the crossmatch process can be attenuated in emergencies. If time permits, the best option when using uncrossmatched blood is to obtain an ABO-Rh typing and an immediate-phase crossmatch. This will provide type-specific partially crossmatched blood and takes 1–5 minutes. Serious hemolytic reactions that result from errors in ABO typing are eliminated. The next best option is type-specific uncrossmatched blood; the ABO-Rh type is determined. For patients who have never been exposed to foreign RBCs, most ABO type-specific transfusions occur without significant issues. Approximately 1 in 1000 patients has an unexpected antibody detected on the crossmatch. Complications resulting from incompatibility are more likely to occur in patients who have been previously transfused or who have been pregnant. For these previously exposed patients the incidence of unexpected antibody detection is 1 in 100.

Type O Rh-negative PRBCs are designated as *universal donor blood*. Type O blood lacks the A and B antigens and is not hemolyzed by anti-A or anti-B antibodies in recipient blood. This blood is used in emergency situations when typing and crossmatching are not available in the timeframe required for life-saving intervention. Type O Rh-negative blood is generally available. In hospitals that have a massive transfusion protocol, type O Rh-negative red cells are used in addition to thawed plasma and platelet concentrates.

Reconstitution of PRBCs

PRBCs are transfused in many clinical situations with varying degrees of urgency. Administration is facilitated by reconstituting the PRBCs with crystalloid or colloid. However, crystalloids containing calcium, such as LR solution, should *not* be used because clotting may occur. This is important to note, since LR solution is frequently being used in the management of surgical and trauma patients. In addition, administration of very hypotonic fluids may cause hemolysis of the transfused PRBCs. Solutions recommended for the reconstitution of PRBCs include D_5-1/2 normal saline, D_5-normal saline, normal saline, and Normosol-R.

Mitigation of Surgical Site Infections

Surgical site infections (SSIs) are infections of the tissues, organs, and spaces exposed by surgeons during an operation. Classification includes superficial incisional (skin and subcutaneous tissues), deep incisional, and organ/organ space infections. Surgical wounds are further classified based on the magnitude of the bacterial load present at surgery: class I (clean), class ID (clean with device implantation), class II (clean/contaminated), class III (contaminated), and class IV (dirty). Hospitals in the United States are required to conduct surveillance for development of SSIs for a period of 30 days after surgery. Adherence to preventive measures has become a surrogate measure of quality. SSIs are clearly associated with morbidity, mortality, substantial healthcare costs, and patient inconvenience and dissatisfaction.

Risk Factors

The development of SSIs is primarily related to (1) host factors, (2) duration of the procedure, and (3) degree of contamination. Patient risk factors include advanced age, immunosuppression, obesity, diabetes mellitus, chronic inflammation, malnutrition, smoking, renal failure, peripheral vascular disease, anemia, radiation, chronic skin disease, microbial carrier status, and recent surgery. This list indicates that critically ill patients are at especially high risk for development of SSIs. In addition to prolonged procedures, risk factors related to the surgery itself include open compared to laparoscopic surgery, poor skin preparation, contaminated instruments, inadequate antibiotic prophylaxis, local tissue necrosis, blood transfusion, hypoxemia, and hypothermia. Finally, in addition to the bacterial burden, specific microbial risk factors include prolonged hospitalization resulting in colonization with nosocomial organisms, toxin secretion, and resistance to clearance.

Preventive Measures

The incidence of SSIs can be reduced if preventive measures are implemented. These measures require a collaborative approach including the anesthesiologist, the surgeon, and the OR nursing team. Appropriate patient preparation includes hair removal at the operative site, using clippers rather than razors. Skin preparation of the operative site with an appropriate antiseptic must be performed. Maintenance of perioperative normoglycemia and normothermia and avoidance of hypoxemia are also important. For class III and IV wounds the skin should not be closed. Rather the superficial aspects of the wound should be packed open and allowed to heal by secondary intention. Appropriate perioperative antibiotic administration must also be undertaken.

General Principles of Prophylactic Perioperative Antibiotic Administration

Revised clinical practice guidelines for antimicrobial prophylaxis in surgery were published in 2013. Effective implementation in the OR requires clear communication between all members of the anesthesiology, surgery, and nursing teams. An ideal antimicrobial agent for surgical prophylaxis should: (1) prevent an SSI, (2) prevent SSI-related morbidity and mortality, (3) reduce the duration and cost of health care, (4) produce no adverse effects, and (5) have no adverse consequences for the normal microbial flora of the patient or hospital. Therefore the ideal antibiotic should be: (1) active against the pathogens most likely to contaminate the surgical site, (2) dosed to ensure adequate serum and tissue concentrations during the period of potential contamination, (3) safe, and (4) administered for the shortest effective period to minimize adverse effects, resistance, and cost.

Surgical wounds of class ID, II, III, and IV require antibiotic prophylaxis. Specific drugs are selected based on their activity against microbes likely to be present at the surgical site. It appears that the optimal timing for administration of preoperative doses of prophylactic antibiotics is within the 60 minutes prior to surgical incision. Weight-based dosing in obese patients is advised. Intraoperative redosing to ensure continued adequate serum and tissue concentrations of the antibiotic is advised if the duration of the operation exceeds two half-lives of the drug or if there is excessive blood loss. The redosing interval should be measured from the time of administration of the preoperative dose, *not* from the time of skin incision. Redosing may not be necessary if patient factors result in prolongation of the drug's half-life (e.g., renal insufficiency). In general, recommendations for the duration of prophylactic antibiotic therapy include one preoperative dose, appropriate intraoperative redosing if indicated, and continuation for no longer than 24 hours postoperatively. Continuing antibiotics is not indicated based on the presence of indwelling drains or intravascular catheters.

Ongoing Antimicrobial Management of Established Infections in the OR

Critically ill surgical patients already in the SICU but proceeding to the OR for various indications are frequently under treatment for established infections. Scheduled dosing of prescribed antimicrobial therapy should continue intraoperatively.

Venous Thromboembolism Prophylaxis

The American College of Chest Physicians published its latest Guidelines for Antithrombotic Therapy and Prevention of Thrombosis in 2012. In 2016 they published additional Guidelines for Antithrombotic Therapy for Venous Thromboembolic Disease. These guidelines provide evidence-based recommendations for management of anticoagulant therapy, including anticoagulation for venous thromboembolism (VTE) prophylaxis in critically ill patients, a subset of patients at significant risk for the development of VTE.

Critically Ill Nonsurgical Patients

General recommendations for venous thromboembolism prophylaxis in critically ill nonsurgical patients include drug administration with low-molecular-weight heparin (LMWH) or low-dose unfractionated heparin. If these patients are actively bleeding or at high risk for significant bleeding, *mechanical* prophylaxis with intermittent pneumatic compression is recommended until the bleeding risk is decreased, at which time anticoagulant drug therapy can be added to the mechanical thromboprophylaxis.

Critically Ill Surgical Patients

Critically ill surgical patients are at high risk for venous thromboembolism. Various risk assessment models can place patients into risk categories based on the type of surgery performed and particular patient characteristics. Many SICU patients fall into the high-risk and very-high-risk categories. These high risk patients can be further subdivided into nonorthopedic surgical patients and orthopedic surgical patients.

Nonorthopedic Surgical Patients

Nonorthopedic surgical patients include those undergoing general and abdominal-pelvic operations, such as gastrointestinal, urologic, gynecologic, bariatric, vascular, plastic, or reconstructive procedures. For patients at high risk for VTE but not at high risk for major bleeding complications, LMWH or low-dose unfractionated heparin and mechanical prophylaxis are recommended. Patients having cancer surgery should have *extended-duration* prophylaxis (4 weeks) with LMWH. For patients at high risk for bleeding complications or those in whom the consequences of bleeding are particularly dangerous, mechanical prophylaxis is recommended. When the risk of bleeding diminishes, pharmacologic prophylaxis should be initiated. If LMWH and low-dose unfractionated heparin are contraindicated, low-dose aspirin, fondaparinux, or mechanical prophylaxis are recommended.

Cardiac surgery patients with an uncomplicated postoperative course should receive only mechanical prophylaxis. If the hospital course is prolonged by nonhemorrhagic surgical complications, pharmacologic thromboprophylaxis with low-dose unfractionated heparin or LMWH can be added.

For thoracic surgery patients at high risk for venous thromboembolism who are not at high risk of bleeding, low-dose heparin or LMWH plus mechanical prophylaxis are recommended. If these patients are at high risk of bleeding,

mechanical prophylaxis is recommended until the risk of bleeding diminishes and pharmacologic prophylaxis can be initiated.

For patients undergoing craniotomy, only mechanical prophylaxis is recommended. However, patients at very high risk for VTE (e.g., those undergoing craniotomy for malignancy) can have pharmacologic prophylaxis added once hemostasis is established and the risk of bleeding has decreased.

For patients undergoing spinal surgery, mechanical prophylaxis is recommended. For those at high risk for VTE (e.g., those with malignancy or those undergoing a combined anterior-posterior approach) the addition of pharmacologic prophylaxis is recommended once adequate hemostasis has been achieved and the risk of bleeding has decreased.

For major trauma patients at high risk for VTE (including those with acute spinal cord injury and traumatic brain injury), mechanical prophylaxis can be added to pharmacologic prophylaxis if not contraindicated by lower extremity trauma. If LMWH or low-dose unfractionated heparin are contraindicated, mechanical prophylaxis can be used if not contraindicated by lower extremity injury. Pharmacologic prophylaxis can be added when the risk of bleeding diminishes or the contraindication to heparin resolves.

In many instances the decision-making process for initiation of pharmacologic venous thromboembolism prophylaxis in critically ill surgical patients is complex and requires specific collaboration and communication between the operative surgeon and the surgical intensivist. A particularly complex subset is the multiply injured trauma patient. Ongoing collaboration must involve the surgical intensivist, the trauma surgeon, and consulting surgeons. For example, in traumatic brain injury the decision to initiate pharmacologic VTE prophylaxis occurs when all agree that the risk of neurologic compromise due to further intracranial hemorrhage has been minimized. Typically this occurs when sequential computed tomography (CT) imaging of the head is stable, usually in the timeframe of 24–72 hours after injury; low-dose unfractionated heparin is preferred over LMWH in this situation. Of course, this decision is further complicated if there are other sources of hemorrhage in the multisystem trauma patient that remain an issue.

Orthopedic Surgical Patients

Patients undergoing major orthopedic surgery including total hip arthroplasty, total knee arthroplasty, and hip fracture surgery are sometimes managed in the SICU postoperatively because of their complex comorbidities and adverse intraoperative events. Therefore it is important for the surgical intensivist to understand VTE prophylaxis paradigms in this patient population.

For patients undergoing total hip or total knee arthroplasty, one of the following is recommended for a *minimum* of 10–14 days: LMWH, low-dose unfractionated heparin, fondaparinux, apixaban, dabigatran, rivaroxaban, warfarin, aspirin, or mechanical prophylaxis. In patients undergoing hip fracture surgery, the newer "novel" oral anticoagulant drugs such as apixaban, dabigatran, and rivaroxaban are *not used*. For all of these patients, LMWH prophylaxis should begin 12 or more hours preoperatively or 12 or more hours postoperatively.

It is also important to note that thromboprophylaxis must be extended well into the posthospital phase of recovery—for up to 35 days from the day of surgery. Dual mechanical and drug prophylaxis is recommended throughout the duration of hospitalization. For patients who decline or are uncooperative with injections or use of pneumatic devices, apixaban or dabigatran are recommended. Patients undergoing these major orthopedic operations who have an increased risk of bleeding should receive mechanical prophylaxis.

In none of the above categories of patients is *routine* deep vein thrombosis ultrasound surveillance recommended, nor is the use of inferior vena cava filters recommended for primary VTE prevention.

Glycemic Management

Perioperative Impact of Diabetes Mellitus

Diabetes mellitus afflicts many critically ill patients. Because this disease affects multiple organ systems, its perioperative impact can be significant. Diabetes affects oxygen transport because glucose binds covalently to hemoglobin, thereby altering the allosteric interactions between β chains. This may decrease oxygen saturation and RBC oxygen transport. Autonomic dysfunction is mediated by lack of appropriate vasoconstriction, which predisposes to hypothermia and orthostatic hypotension. Additionally, the changes in heart rate that occur with administration of atropine and β-blockers are blunted in patients who have autonomic dysfunction. Diabetics are at increased risk of coronary artery disease and are more likely to have silent myocardial ischemia than their nondiabetic counterparts. Life-saving surgery may be mandated before the various risk factors of diabetes mellitus have been optimized. Because diabetes adversely affects gastrointestinal motility, including gastric emptying, diabetics should be managed as if they have a full stomach. Preoperative treatment with drugs that inhibit gastric acid secretion and neutralize gastric acid is needed as is a rapid-sequence induction.

Perioperative and Intraoperative Glycemic Control Regimens

Several factors impact perioperative and intraoperative glycemic management. The differentiation between type 1 and type 2 diabetes is especially important because type 1 patients are at risk for ketonemia if insulin is withheld. This risk is increased with surgical stress and with critical illness. Preexisting long-term glucose control also affects management and is best assessed by measurement of glycosylated hemoglobin (hemoglobin A_{1c}), which is a measure of glucose control over the prior 2–3 months. An elevated hemoglobin A_{1c} correlates with complication rates in diabetics, and the quantity of insulin normally required by a diabetic is important in the determination of how blood glucose should be managed intraoperatively.

There are many different protocols for preoperative and intraoperative insulin management, but there is a paucity of prospective studies comparing regimens. This is particularly true for management of critically ill patients, for which there is no consensus about the method of insulin therapy or the exact range of blood glucose that is considered optimal. However, several general concepts are useful. First, effective perioperative glucose management incorporates careful monitoring. The blood glucose monitoring equipment must be readily available, accurate, and efficient. Continuous glucose monitoring devices and other advances for use in the acute care setting are under development. Second, protocols and standards for utilization must be individualized and validated for use in the ICU and OR in which the protocols will be used. What works in one hospital may not work in another because of variability in equipment, training of providers, and the level of expertise and experience in those rendering care.

Steroid Management

Indications for Administration of Stress Steroid Dosing

Perioperative stress is related to the extent of the operation and the depth of anesthesia. One can postulate that the presence of critical illness also impacts the degree of physiologic stress. Additionally, deep general anesthesia or regional anesthesia delay the glucocorticoid surge in response to stress. Some patients who have suppressed adrenal function due to administration of exogenous steroids will have perioperative cardiovascular issues if they do not receive perioperative supplemental steroids. This is because glucocorticoids mediate catecholamine-induced increases in cardiac contractility and maintenance of vascular tone. However, it must be kept in mind that when these patients develop hypotension perioperatively, glucocorticoid or mineralocorticoid deficiency *is not* usually the etiology. Alternative explanations should be sought, especially in the critically ill patient, in whom other etiologies of hypotension are *much more common*. Nonetheless, when acute adrenal insufficiency occurs, it is life threatening.

It is not unusual to lack laboratory data defining the adequacy of the pituitary-adrenal axis available preoperatively, especially in patients undergoing emergency surgery. *Steroid supplementation for any patient who has received steroids within the past year should be considered.* This includes topical steroids but not inhaled steroids. Many different dosages and tapering regimens are employed. Often a patient is administered the estimated maximum quantity of glucocorticoid the body usually manufactures in response to maximal stress. Depending on the overall condition of the patient and the burden of critical illness, the dose can be decreased gradually until the usual maintenance dose of glucocorticoids is achieved or the steroids have been completely stopped.

Risks Associated With Stress Steroid Dosing

Rare complications associated with perioperative glucocorticoid supplementation include aggravation of hypertension, fluid retention, stress ulcers, and psychosis. *More common* complications include abnormal wound healing and an increased rate of infection. The effect on wound healing specifically attributed to short-term perioperative supplementation is probably very small. The increased risk of infection in patients taking long-term steroids is documented, but it is unclear whether or not perioperative steroid supplementation increases this risk.

Thermal Regulation

Body temperature is controlled by a negative feedback system in the hypothalamus. Eighty percent of the thermal input is derived from core body temperature, which is measured using distal esophageal, nasopharyngeal, or tympanic membrane thermometers. The hypothalamus coordinates increases in heat production (nonshivering thermogenesis and shivering), increases in heat loss (sweating), and decreases in heat loss (vasoconstriction) to maintain normothermia.

Hypothermia

Mild hypothermia is common during surgery and anesthesia, including both general and neuraxial anesthesia. General anesthetics decrease the threshold for vasoconstriction and shivering by 2°–3°C. The major initial cause of hypothermia in the OR is core-to-peripheral redistribution of body heat. Neuraxial anesthesia impairs both central and peripheral thermoregulation. Cool OR environments also contribute to hypothermia. Large randomized trials have proven that even mild hypothermia (35°–35.5°C) causes an increase in adverse outcomes, including cardiac complications, wound infections, coagulopathy, need for transfusion, prolonged recovery times, and increased hospital length of stay. Hypothermia may decrease the triggering of malignant hyperthermia and reduce its severity.

The effects of hypothermia are especially pronounced in critically ill surgical patients who are undergoing emergent surgery for control of massive hemorrhage. Hypothermia is one component of the *lethal triad* of *hypothermia, coagulopathy, and acidosis* that if left untreated leads to death. Core temperature should be monitored in any critically ill patient undergoing surgery, with a goal temperature of 36°–37°C. Active cutaneous warming is key, and forced-air warming offers the best combination of efficacy, safety, and price. Infused fluids and blood products should be warmed in patients undergoing large-volume resuscitation. Additional measures ensure that irrigation of the Foley catheter, nasogastric tube, or any body cavity is performed with warmed fluid. Active airway heating and humidification can also be performed via the endotracheal tube.

Hyperthermia

Etiologies of increased core temperature result from augmented thermogenesis (i.e., malignant hyperthermia), excessive heating (i.e., passive hyperthermia), or an increase in the thermoregulatory target (i.e., fever). The particular cause should be sought and treated.

Malignant Hyperthermia

Malignant hyperthermia (MH) is an anesthetic-related disorder of increased skeletal muscle metabolism. Anesthetic drugs known to trigger MH include ether, halothane, enflurane, isoflurane, desflurane, sevoflurane, and depolarizing muscle relaxants (succinylcholine). Malignant hyperthermia is inherited in an autosomal dominant pattern. The abnormal function of the skeletal muscle ryanodine receptor is associated with abnormal intracellular calcium metabolism. Tachycardia, an increased $PETCO_2$, muscle rigidity, and an increased body temperature above 38.8°C (with no other apparent cause) are associated with this increased metabolism. Central thermoregulation remains intact during an MH crisis, but efferent heat loss mechanisms are compromised by the increased peripheral vasoconstriction resulting from the extremely high catecholamine concentrations. Dantrolene normalizes myoplasmic calcium concentrations, restores normal muscle metabolism, and reverses the signs of metabolic stimulation. Affected patients are typically managed in the SICU postoperatively.

SPECIAL SCENARIOS IN THE MANAGEMENT OF THE CRITICALLY ILL SURGICAL PATIENT

Transporting the Critically Ill Patient to and From the Operating Room

Transport of critically ill and mechanically ventilated patients from the ICU to other locations in the hospital is a common phenomenon. Typical destinations include diagnostic radiology, interventional radiology, and the OR. Critically ill patients who require transport out of the ICU for diagnostics or therapeutics have higher severity-of-illness scores on admission than do those who do not require transport. Children and trauma patients require more frequent trips for diagnostics than other patients.

These trips can be life threatening. Physiologic stress is common, and almost all transported patients experience temporary changes in vital signs that may require intervention. Unplanned events are common, and all are potentially life threatening. Included is equipment failure. Complex and numerous pieces of equipment must accompany the patient. Common equipment-related adverse events include ECG lead disconnection and monitor power failure. More serious events directly related to the patient include changes in cardiorespiratory physiology, such as gas exchange deterioration, need for intubation or reintubation, heart rate, and blood pressure variability (hypotension and dysrhythmias); elevated intracranial pressure; anoxic brain injury; and death.

General Principles

Specific guidelines for in-hospital transport have been published by the American Society for Critical Care Medicine. *The first rule of transport is that the patient must be stabilized prior to transport.* A requirement for sedation during the trip must be anticipated. Equipment and medication checklists must be confirmed prior to the trip. The receiving location must confirm that they have the equipment and staff needed to appropriately care for the patient on arrival. Adequate medical supervision for the trip must be immediately available. The frequency of unplanned events is decreased if the accompanying physician has a high level of experience. Equipment for the trip includes a portable resuscitation kit that contains everything on a crash cart, including emergency cardiovascular drugs. The airway compartment includes everything required for intubation or reintubation. An oxygen cylinder with low-pressure alarms, a flowmeter, and oxygen tubing are essential. *The critically ill patient in transit should be monitored just as closely as was necessary in the ICU immediately prior to transport.*

Maintenance of Therapies

Whatever specific therapies the patient is being treated with must continue en route and at the destination. The most important example is mechanical ventilation. A mechanical ventilator rather than manual ventilation devices is preferred for transport. The manual devices are associated with more variability in CO_2 and pH, often caused by unintentional hyperventilation. These devices are also associated with more deterioration in Pao_2.

In patients whose hemodynamics are dependent on ventricular assist devices and IABP counterpulsation, personnel experienced in the operation of these devices must be present during the transport and at the destination. Medication infusions are maintained during transport and continued at the destination. If possible, blood product transfusions are completed prior to transport; however, if a patient must be moved to a location such as the OR or interventional radiology for definitive therapy, transfusion may be ongoing during transport.

In addition to intravascular catheters, great care should be taken to maintain the integrity and functionality of other indwelling devices. These include chest tubes, gastric decompression tubes, feeding tubes, surgical drains, and Foley and other types of urinary drainage catheters.

Contraindications to Transport

Transport out of the ICU is contraindicated when there is an inability to provide adequate oxygenation and ventilation during transport or at the receiving location. It is also contraindicated when there is an inability to adequately monitor cardiovascular hemodynamics during transport or at the destination. Transport out of the ICU is also contraindicated if the patient is hemodynamically unstable, unless the destination will provide the means to achieve restoration of hemodynamic integrity.

A risk-benefit analysis of all transports should be undertaken prior to embarking on movement of a critically ill patient to an alternate location. In recent years, fortunately, bedside alternatives for many diagnostic and therapeutic procedures have been developed.

Specific Operations in Critically Ill Patients

Patients come to the SICU after surgery. Some elective surgery mandates intensive monitoring even in a stable patient. However, many emergent operations result in an unstable patient whose physiology must be repaired. Although circumstances requiring intensive care can occur after any operation, two surgical scenarios of particular interest to the surgical intensivist deserve specific review: abdominal compartment syndrome and damage control in the critically injured trauma patient. Common operative procedures that facilitate management of the critically ill patient will also be discussed: tracheostomy and enteral feeding access.

Abdominal Compartment Syndrome
Definitions

Abdominal compartment syndrome is a recently recognized pathologic entity, physiologically characterized in the laboratory in 1985 and clinically defined in 1989. Abdominal compartment syndrome is distinct from intraabdominal hypertension. *Intraabdominal pressure* (IAP) can be measured by determining bladder pressure as transmitted through a Foley catheter. Normal intraabdominal pressure is 2–5 mm Hg, but it can be as high as 12 mm Hg in obese or pregnant adults. Intraabdominal pressure is higher in critically ill patients, typically 5–7 mm Hg.

Intraabdominal hypertension is defined as an intraabdominal pressure of 12 mm Hg or higher and can be graded: grade I is 12–15 mm Hg, grade II is 16–20 mm Hg, grade III is 21–25 mm Hg, and grade IV is over 25 mm Hg. *Abdominal compartment syndrome is defined as a sustained intraabdominal pressure above 20 mm Hg associated with new onset of organ dysfunction or failure.* Abdominal perfusion pressure is measured as the difference between MAP and intraabdominal pressure. An abdominal perfusion pressure of at least 60 mm Hg is required to maintain adequate perfusion to the viscera contained in the abdomen. End-organ dysfunction occurs if the perfusion pressure goes below this critical level.

Abdominal compartment syndrome can be further characterized as primary, secondary, and tertiary. Primary abdominal compartment syndrome is caused by abdominopelvic pathology that creates a space-occupying or expanding lesion, such as a ruptured abdominal aortic aneurysm, abdominal trauma or retroperitoneal hemorrhage. Secondary abdominal compartment syndrome (extraabdominal compartment syndrome) is caused by massive bowel edema due to extraabdominal conditions requiring massive fluid resuscitation in the presence of capillary leak, such as sepsis and burns. Tertiary abdominal compartment syndrome (recurrent abdominal compartment syndrome) occurs after resolution of an earlier episode of primary or secondary abdominal compartment syndrome.

Significance: Progressive Organ Failure

The common characteristic of all types of abdominal compartment syndrome is progressive organ failure, including failure of the kidneys, splanchnic bed, lungs, heart, and brain. If abdominal compartment syndrome is not recognized and treated expeditiously, hemodynamic collapse and death ensue.

Treatment

Nonoperative management of abdominal compartment syndrome includes sedation and paralysis to relax the abdominal wall, evacuation of intraluminal gastrointestinal contents, evacuation of large abdominal fluid collections, optimization of abdominal perfusion pressure with vasopressor support if necessary, and correction of a positive fluid balance. If these maneuvers are unsuccessful in correcting organ dysfunction, definitive management includes a decompressive laparotomy and temporary abdominal closure until the underlying disease process is reversed.

Damage Control in the Trauma Patient

Damage control surgery is applied to trauma patients who have devastating cervical, truncal, or extremity injuries and intraoperative physiologic compromise termed the *lethal triad:* hypothermia, coagulopathy, and acidosis. Definitive repair of all injuries and closure of the incision is impossible in some patients, too time consuming in others, and may cause a postoperative compartment syndrome (e.g., abdominal compartment syndrome) following trauma laparotomy. Surgical management of these severely injured patients is staged.

The Initial Operation: A Band-Aid for Anatomy to Facilitate Repair of Physiology

The initial operation is limited to control of hemorrhage and gross contamination. Hemorrhage is controlled via rapid repair, ligation or shunting of major vascular injuries, and packing of organs or compartments. Major injuries to the gastrointestinal tract are resected and left in discontinuity, without anastomosis. A quick temporary closure is employed to cover the surgical incision. The anesthesiology team provides ongoing resuscitation following a massive transfusion protocol while the surgeons are operating. Ideally this operation is completed within 2 hours, and the patient is then transported to the ICU.

The SICU Resuscitation: Abrogation of the Lethal Triad

On arrival to the SICU the patient is aggressively rewarmed and resuscitation is ongoing, with infusion of blood, blood products, vasopressors, and inotropes if indicated to manage hemorrhagic and traumatic shock. As coagulopathy is corrected and nonsurgical bleeding ceases, perfusion is restored and acid-base balance normalizes. Supportive management can limit some organ failure, such as acute lung injury and AKI. This SICU phase is variable in length but may require 48–72 hours.

The Definitive Operation: Restoration of Anatomy

Ideally the patient is taken back to the OR when hypotension, coagulopathy, acidosis, and hypothermia have resolved, and when the postresuscitation diuretic phase has begun. Definitive repairs are performed, missed injuries are sought and managed, gastrointestinal continuity is restored (either with anastomoses or ostomies), and formal closure of the incision is undertaken if possible.

After Damage Control: Subsequent Operative Interventions

Saving a life comes at a price. Some of the patients who survive injury and the damage control required to repair it must undergo multiple subsequent interventions and operations. Particularly after damage control for abdominal trauma, definitive closure of the surgical incision is not always feasible at the time of the first repeat laparotomy. This results in an open abdomen, which mandates subsequent repeat laparotomies. If primary closure of the abdominal wall is not ultimately possible, common management includes insertion of absorbable mesh and eventual application of a skin graft. This will result in loss of abdominal domain and a large ventral incisional hernia.

After the patient has sufficiently recovered from the acute illness, a major definitive restorative operation can be undertaken, including repair of fistulas, closure of ostomies, and the hernia repair, typically with abdominal wall reconstruction. Because of the magnitude of these operations, some patients require monitoring in the SICU in the immediate postoperative period. The time frame from initial injury to these operations is typically 6–12 months.

Common Operations to Facilitate Management of the Critically Ill Patient

Tracheostomy

Tracheostomy is indicated in critically ill patients who require prolonged intubation, typically longer than 2 weeks. Additional indications include access for frequent pulmonary suctioning, the presence of neurologic deficits that compromise protective airway reflexes, and facial trauma or operations that anatomically compromise the upper airway. The procedure can be performed either via a percutaneous or open technique. When the indication for tracheostomy has resolved, decannulation is undertaken, and the opening spontaneously closes, usually over a 2-week period.

Enteral Feeding Access

If nasoenteric feeding is anticipated for longer than 30 days, long-term percutaneous or surgical feeding access should be considered. The most common indications for prolonged enteral feeding in the critically ill patient are prolonged mechanical ventilation, impaired swallowing, oropharyngeal or esophageal obstruction, and major facial trauma.

Long-term gastric feeding access can be obtained via a percutaneous, laparoscopic, or open surgical technique. The percutaneous endoscopic gastrostomy (PEG) is one of the most frequently employed methods to achieve durable feeding access. Long-term jejunal feeding access is usually obtained via a laparoscopic or open surgical approach. However, direct percutaneous endoscopic jejunostomy (DPEJ) is available in some institutions. This is more technically challenging than PEG placement. A PEG can also be converted to jejunal access (PEG-jejunal tube) via a two-stage procedure in which a PEG is placed first. This is followed by passing the jejunal feeding tube through the PEG under fluoroscopic guidance. Jejunal access is desired in patients who are at high risk of aspiration or are otherwise intolerant of gastric feeding.

KEY POINTS

- Communication and teamwork between anesthesiologists and surgeons are the basis of optimal care delivery to critically ill patients who require surgical intervention.
- Shock is an abnormality of the circulatory system that causes inadequate organ perfusion and tissue oxygenation. Subsets of shock based on differential hemodynamic profiles include hypovolemic, cardiogenic, obstructive, and distributive.
- Sepsis and severe trauma are two of the most common diagnoses encountered in the SICU. Systemic inflammation is a common denominator in these two conditions. Septic shock and traumatic shock result when the immune response to either of these insults is dysregulated, resulting in an amplified systemic inflammatory response and multiple organ failure.
- The Surviving Sepsis Campaign guidelines provide evidence-based recommendations for the management of patients with severe sepsis and septic shock. These recommendations include low-tidal-volume mechanical ventilation for management of sepsis-induced acute respiratory distress syndrome, implementation of ventilator weaning protocols, and protocols for management of blood glucose, targeting a goal of 180 mg/dL or lower.
- *Systemic inflammatory response syndrome* (SIRS), *compensatory antiinflammatory response syndrome* (CARS), and *persistent inflammation, immunosuppression, and catabolism syndrome* (PICS) represent a continuum of immunologically and genomically mediated consequences of the pathophysiologic response to sepsis and severe injury.
- Ideal management of massive hemorrhage includes prompt control of the bleeding source and damage control resuscitation, including implementation of an institutionally specific massive transfusion protocol. Class III hemorrhage—loss of 30%–40% of total blood volume—results in hemorrhagic shock and is the least amount of blood loss that consistently causes a decrease in systolic blood pressure. *In the exsanguinating patient,* administration of crystalloid should be minimized, and blood component therapy in a 1:1:1 ratio of units of fresh frozen plasma, platelets, and packed red blood cells (PRBCs) has been demonstrated to improve hemostasis and decrease mortality due to exsanguination at 24 hours.
- Prothrombin complex concentrates provide for rapid low-volume reversal of warfarin-induced coagulopathy in elderly patients who have traumatic brain injury.
- Tranexamic acid in the management of hemorrhagic shock is of most benefit in patients who present with severe shock (systolic blood pressure < 75 mm Hg) within 3 hours of the time of injury.
- The use of 4-factor prothrombin complex concentrate as an adjunct to reversal of the new "novel" oral anticoagulants is not specific or targeted, nor has its use for this indication been validated in clinical trials.
- The trigger for platelet transfusion in patients undergoing surgery or invasive procedures is below 50,000/mm³. The

trigger for empirical platelet transfusion in patients without additional risk factors for bleeding is below 10,000/mm³, and for patients with additional risk factors for bleeding it is below 20,000/mm³.
- In the massively hemorrhaging patient, platelet transfusions in conjunction with correcting plasma coagulation factor deficits are indicated when the platelet count is below 50,000/mm³ or below 100,000/mm³ in the presence of diffuse microvascular bleeding.
- Circulatory collapse attributable to cardiac dysfunction can involve the myocardium, the pericardium, the cardiac valves, and the outflow tract of the heart.
- Rapid recognition of an ST-segment elevation myocardial infarction is crucial, since these patients benefit from immediate reperfusion and, in the appropriate clinical circumstances, should be treated with fibrinolytic therapy or urgent revascularization either by percutaneous coronary intervention or coronary artery bypass surgery.
- Massive pulmonary embolism in the critically ill patient can be managed with systemic thrombolysis, catheter-directed thrombolysis, or surgical pulmonary embolectomy.
- Tension pneumothorax is a clinical, not radiographic, diagnosis and must be treated with immediate decompression of the involved hemithorax.
- A sudden decrease in PETCO₂ is usually a result of a circuit disconnection, airway obstruction, an abrupt decrease in cardiac output, or pulmonary embolism.
- The optimal target for glycemic management in the critically ill patient population remains elusive and has undergone a significant paradigm shift in the past 2 decades. At present the literature supports a target blood glucose range of 140–180 mg/dL.
- In the absence of clinical evidence of hypothyroidism, thyroid hormone replacement in patients who have low measured thyroid hormone concentrations due to the sick euthyroid syndrome is not indicated.
- If intrinsic thyroid dysfunction is suspected in the critically ill patient, the best tests to obtain are a free T₄ and TSH.
- In the setting of relative adrenal insufficiency, septic shock refractory to volume resuscitation and vasopressor therapy is an indication for steroid replacement. A typical regimen is hydrocortisone 50 mg IV every 6 hours. Steroid therapy for sepsis in the absence of refractory shock is not recommended.
- Acute kidney injury (AKI) is a significant cause of morbidity and mortality in the critically ill patient population. The Kidney Disease: Improving Global Outcomes group developed criteria that categorize patients according to the degree of AKI based on the absolute change in serum creatinine during a particular time interval and the reduction in urine volume.
- Child-Pugh and MELD scores are used to predict surgical mortality in patients with cirrhosis and end-stage liver disease undergoing nontransplant surgical procedures.
- Delirium is a poorly understood form of cerebral dysfunction that afflicts many ICU patients and is an independent

predictor of negative outcomes. Features include inattention, reduced awareness of the environment, and either a change in cognition or the development of perceptual disturbances. The key to management of delirium is mitigation of its risk factors and prevention.

- Global strategies to manage pain, agitation, and delirium in the ICU include minimizing sedation and optimizing normal sleep/wake cycles.
- Critical illness polyneuropathy develops in patients who have multiple organ failure, and sepsis and is likely the most common neuromuscular cause of prolonged ventilator dependency in patients without prior neuromuscular disease.
- Acute quadriplegic myopathy (acute myopathy of intensive care) most frequently occurs in the setting of severe pulmonary disease in which neuromuscular blockade is used to facilitate mechanical ventilation and high-dose corticosteroids are administered at the same time.
- There is no evidence to indicate that resuscitation with colloids, compared to resuscitation with crystalloids, reduces the risk of death in patients with trauma, burns, or following surgery.
- Lactated Ringer solution and significantly hypotonic crystalloid solutions should not be used to reconstitute PRBCs.
- Appropriate perioperative antibiotic prophylaxis should be administered within 60 minutes of incision time, should be dose-adjusted in obese patients, should be redosed intraoperatively during long procedures or if the blood loss exceeds 1500 mL, and should not be continued longer than 24 hours postoperatively.
- Perioperative stress-dose steroid supplementation should be considered for any patient who has received corticosteroids within the past year.
- Hypothermia in the critically ill perioperative patient is associated with adverse outcomes and should be corrected.
- Malignant hyperthermia is inherited in an autosomal dominant pattern and is treated with dantrolene. Clinical manifestations in the anesthetized patient include tachycardia, an increased $PETCO_2$, muscle rigidity, and a body temperature above 38.8°C (without another explanation).
- *Abdominal compartment syndrome* defines a sustained intraabdominal pressure above 20 mm Hg and is associated with new onset of organ dysfunction or failure. If medical management is unsuccessful, decompressive laparotomy with a temporary abdominal closure provides definitive management.
- Damage control surgery is applied to trauma patients who have devastating cervical, truncal, or extremity injuries and intraoperative physiologic compromise termed the *lethal triad*: hypothermia, acidosis, and coagulopathy.
- Tracheostomy and enteral feeding access are elective operative procedures performed in critically ill patients that facilitate optimal management.

RESOURCES

American College of Surgeons Committee on Trauma. *Advanced Trauma Life Support Student Course Manual.* 9th ed. Chicago: American College of Surgeons; 2012.

Barr J, Puntillo K, Ely EW, et al. Clinical practice guidelines for the management of pain, agitation, and delirium in adult patients in the intensive care unit. *Crit Care Med.* 2013;41:263-306.

Bratzler DW, Dellinger EP, Olsen KM. Clinical practice guidelines for antimicrobial prophylaxis in surgery. *Surg Infect.* 2013;14:73-156.

Carr JA. Abdominal compartment syndrome: a decade of progress. *J Am Coll Surg.* 2013;216:135-146.

Crowther M, Crowther MA. Antidotes for novel oral anticoagulants: current status and future potential. *Arterioscler Thromb Vasc Biol.* 2015;35:1736-1745.

Dellinger RP, Levy MM, Rhodes A, et al. Surviving Sepsis Campaign: international guidelines for management of severe sepsis and septic shock: 2012. *Crit Care Med.* 2013;41:580-637.

Guyatt GH, Akl EA, Crowther M, et al. Executive summary: antithrombotic therapy and prevention of thrombosis. 9th ed. American College of Chest Physicians evidence-based clinical practice guidelines. *Chest.* 2012;141(suppl):7S-47S.

Holcomb JB, Tilley BC, Baraniuk S, et al. Transfusion of plasma, platelets, and red blood cells in a 1:1:1 vs a 1:1:2 ratio and mortality in patients with severe trauma: the PROPPR randomized clinical trial. *JAMA.* 2015;313:471-482.

Kellum JA. Lameire N for the KDIGO AKI Guideline Work Group. Diagnosis, evaluation, and management of acute kidney injury: a KDIGO summary (Part 1). *Crit Care.* 2013;17:204.

Kirkpatrick AW, Roberts DJ, De Wade J. Intra-abdominal hypertension and the abdominal compartment syndrome: updated consensus definitions and clinical practice guidelines from the World Society of the Abdominal Compartment Syndrome. *Intensive Care Med.* 2013;39:1190-1206.

Levy JH, Key NS, Azran MS. Novel oral anticoagulants: implications in the perioperative setting. *Anesthesiology.* 2010;113:726-745.

Napolitano LM, Cohen MJ, Cotton BA, et al. Tranexamic acid in trauma: how should we use it? *J Trauma Acute Care Surg.* 2013;74:1575-1586.

Perel P, Roberts I, Ker K. Colloids versus crystalloids for fluid resuscitation in critically ill patients. *Cochrane Database Syst Rev.* 2013. CD000567.

Wyrzykowski AD, Feliciano DV. Trauma damage control. In: Mattox KL, Moore EE, Feliciano DV, eds. *Trauma.* 7th ed. New York: McGraw-Hill Medical; 2013:725-746.

Ischemic Heart Disease

SHAMSUDDIN AKHTAR

The prevalence of ischemic heart disease and atherosclerotic vascular disease in the United States increases significantly with age (Fig. 5.1). By some estimates, 30% of patients who undergo surgery annually in the United States have ischemic heart disease. Angina pectoris, acute myocardial infarction (AMI), and sudden death are often the first manifestations of ischemic heart disease, and cardiac dysrhythmias are probably the major cause of sudden death in these patients. The two most important risk factors for the development of atherosclerosis involving the coronary arteries are male gender and increasing age (Table 5.1). Additional risk factors include hypercholesterolemia, systemic hypertension, cigarette smoking, diabetes mellitus, obesity, a sedentary lifestyle, and a

family history of premature development of ischemic heart disease. Psychological factors such as type A personality and stress have also been implicated. Patients with ischemic heart disease can have chronic stable angina or an acute coronary syndrome (ACS) at presentation. The latter includes ST-segment elevation myocardial infarction (STEMI) and unstable angina/non–ST-segment elevation myocardial infarction (UA/NSTEMI).

STABLE ANGINA PECTORIS

The coronary artery circulation normally supplies sufficient blood flow to meet the demands of the myocardium in

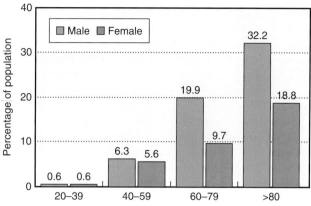

FIG. 5.1 Prevalence of coronary heart disease by age and gender in the United States (2009–2012). (Data from the National Center for Health Statistics and National Heart, Lung, and Blood Institute.)

TABLE 5.1	Risk Factors for Development of Ischemic Heart Disease

Male gender
Increasing age
Hypercholesterolemia
Hypertension
Cigarette smoking
Diabetes mellitus
Obesity
Sedentary lifestyle
Genetic factors/family history

TABLE 5.2	Common Causes of Acute Chest Pain
System	Condition
Cardiac	Angina Rest or unstable angina Acute myocardial infarction Pericarditis
Vascular	Aortic dissection Pulmonary embolism Pulmonary hypertension
Pulmonary	Pleuritis and/or pneumonia Tracheobronchitis Spontaneous pneumothorax
Gastrointestinal	Esophageal reflux Peptic ulcer Gallbladder disease Pancreatitis
Musculoskeletal	Costochondritis Cervical disk disease Trauma or strain
Infectious	Herpes zoster
Psychological	Panic disorder

response to widely varying workloads. An imbalance between coronary blood flow (supply) and myocardial oxygen consumption (demand) can precipitate ischemia, which frequently manifests as chest pain (i.e., *angina pectoris*). Stable angina typically develops in the setting of partial occlusion or significant (>70%) chronic narrowing of a segment of coronary artery. When the imbalance becomes extreme, congestive heart failure, electrical instability with cardiac dysrhythmias, and MI may result. Angina pectoris reflects intracardiac release of adenosine, bradykinin, and other substances during ischemia. These substances stimulate cardiac nociceptive and mechanosensitive receptors whose afferent neurons converge with the upper five thoracic sympathetic ganglia and somatic nerve fibers in the spinal cord and ultimately produce thalamic and cortical stimulation that results in the typical chest pain of angina pectoris. These substances also slow atrioventricular conduction and decrease cardiac contractility, which improves the balance between myocardial oxygen supply and demand. Atherosclerosis is the most common cause of impaired coronary blood flow resulting in angina pectoris, but it may also occur in the absence of coronary obstruction as a result of myocardial hypertrophy, severe aortic stenosis, or aortic regurgitation. It may also occur with paroxysmal tachydysrhythmias, marked anemia, or hyperthyroidism. Syndrome X is a rare cause of angina, and in this situation the chest pain is thought to be due to microvascular dysfunction of the coronary circulation.

Diagnosis

Angina pectoris is typically described as retrosternal chest discomfort, pain, pressure, or heaviness that may radiate to any dermatome from C8–T4. This chest discomfort often radiates to the neck, left shoulder, left arm, or jaw and occasionally to the back or down both arms. Angina may also be perceived as epigastric discomfort resembling indigestion. Some patients describe angina as shortness of breath, mistaking a sense of chest constriction as dyspnea. The need to take a deep breath rather than breathe rapidly often identifies shortness of breath as an anginal equivalent. Angina pectoris usually lasts several minutes and is crescendo-decrescendo in nature. A sharp pain that lasts only a few seconds or a dull ache that lasts for hours is rarely caused by myocardial ischemia. Physical exertion, emotional tension, and cold weather may induce angina. Rest and/or nitroglycerin relieve it. *Chronic stable angina* refers to chest pain or discomfort that does not change appreciably in frequency or severity over 2 months or longer. *Unstable angina,* by contrast, is defined as angina at rest, angina of new onset, or an increase in the severity or frequency of previously stable angina without an increase in levels of cardiac biomarkers. Sharp retrosternal pain exacerbated by deep breathing, coughing, or change in body position suggests pericarditis. There are many causes of noncardiac chest pain (Table 5.2). Noncardiac chest pain is often exacerbated by chest wall movement and is associated with tenderness over the involved area, which is often a costochondral junction. Esophageal spasm can produce severe substernal pressure that may be confused with angina pectoris and may also be relieved by administration of nitroglycerin.

Electrocardiography

The resting electrocardiogram (ECG) may be normal in patients with angina, or it may show nonspecific ST-T wave changes or abnormalities related to an old MI. During myocardial ischemia, the standard 12-lead ECG demonstrates *ST-segment depression* (characteristic of subendocardial ischemia) that coincides in time with the anginal chest pain. This may be accompanied by transient symmetric T-wave inversion. Patients with chronically inverted T waves resulting from previous MI may show a return of the T waves to the normal upright position (*pseudonormalization* of the T wave) during myocardial ischemia. These ECG changes are seen in about half of patients. Variant angina—that is, angina that results from coronary vasospasm rather than occlusive coronary artery disease—is diagnosed by *ST-segment elevation* during an episode of angina pectoris.

Exercise ECG is useful for detecting signs of myocardial ischemia and establishing their relationship to chest pain. The test also provides information about exercise capacity. Exercise testing is often combined with imaging studies (nuclear, echocardiographic, or magnetic resonance imaging [MRI]) to demonstrate areas of ischemic myocardium. Exercise testing is not always feasible, however, because of the inability of a patient to exercise owing to peripheral vascular or musculoskeletal disease, deconditioning, dyspnea on exertion, prior stroke, or the presence of chest pain at rest or with minimal activity. The presence of conditions that interfere with interpretation of the exercise ECG (e.g., paced rhythm, left ventricular hypertrophy, digitalis administration, or a preexcitation syndrome) also limit the utility of exercise stress testing. The risk of MI or death related to exercise testing is about 1/1000 tests. Contraindications to exercise stress testing include severe aortic stenosis, severe hypertension, acute myocarditis, uncontrolled heart failure, and infective endocarditis.

The exercise ECG is most likely to indicate myocardial ischemia when there is at least 1 mm of horizontal or downsloping ST-segment depression during or within 4 minutes after exercise. The greater the degree of ST-segment depression, the greater the likelihood of significant coronary artery disease. When the ST-segment abnormality is associated with angina pectoris and occurs during the early stages of exercise and persists for several minutes after exercise, significant coronary artery disease is *very likely*. Exercise ECG is less accurate but more cost-effective than imaging tests for detecting ischemic heart disease. A negative stress test result does not exclude the presence of coronary artery disease, but it makes the likelihood of three-vessel or left main coronary disease *extremely low*. Exercise ECG is less sensitive and specific in detecting ischemic heart disease than nuclear cardiology techniques.

Nuclear Cardiology Techniques

Nuclear stress imaging is useful for assessing coronary perfusion. It has greater sensitivity than exercise testing for detection of ischemic heart disease. It can define vascular regions in which stress-induced coronary blood flow is limited and can estimate left ventricular systolic size and function. Tracers such as thallium and technetium can be detected over the myocardium by single-photon emission computed tomography (SPECT) techniques. A significant coronary obstructive lesion causes a reduction in blood flow, and thus less tracer activity is present in that area. Exercise perfusion imaging with simultaneous ECG testing is superior to exercise ECG alone. Exercise increases the difference in tracer activity between normal and underperfused regions because coronary blood flow increases markedly with exercise *except* in those regions distal to a coronary artery obstruction. Imaging is carried out in two phases: the first is immediately after cessation of exercise to detect regional ischemia, and the second is hours later to detect reversible ischemia. Areas of persistently absent uptake signify an old MI. The *size* of the perfusion abnormality is the most important indicator of the significance of the coronary artery disease detected.

Alternative methods of "exercise testing" are available when exercise ECG is not possible or interpretation of ST-segment changes would be difficult. Administration of atropine, infusion of dobutamine, or institution of artificial cardiac pacing produces a rapid heart rate to create cardiac stress. Alternatively, cardiac stress can be produced by administering a coronary vasodilator such as adenosine or dipyridamole. These drugs dilate normal coronary arteries but evoke minimal or no change in the diameter of atherosclerotic coronary arteries. After cardiac stress is induced by these interventions, radionuclide tracer scanning is performed to assess myocardial perfusion.

Echocardiography

Echocardiographic *regional wall motion analysis* can be performed immediately after stressing the heart either pharmacologically or with exercise. New ventricular wall motion abnormalities induced by stress correspond to sites of myocardial ischemia, thereby localizing obstructive coronary lesions. In contrast, exercise ECG can indicate only the presence of ischemic heart disease but does not reliably predict the location of the obstructive coronary lesion. One can also visualize *global wall motion* under baseline conditions and under cardiac stress. Valvular function can be assessed as well. Limitations imposed by poor visualization have been improved by newer contrast-assisted technologies.

Stress Cardiac MRI

Pharmacologic stress imaging with cardiac MRI compares favorably with other methods and is being used clinically in some centers, especially when other modalities cannot be used effectively.

Electron Beam Computed Tomography

Calcium deposition occurs in atherosclerotic blood vessels. Coronary artery calcification can be detected by electron beam computed tomography (EBCT). Although the sensitivity of EBCT is high, it is not a very specific test and yields many false-positive results. Its routine use is not recommended.

CT Angiography

The heart and coronary arteries can be visualized with contrast medium and multislice CT scanning. This modality is most useful in ruling out coronary artery disease in patients with a low likelihood for significant coronary artery disease. The role of CT angiography in routine clinical practice has yet to be defined.

Coronary Angiography

Coronary angiography provides the best information about the condition of the coronary arteries. It is indicated in patients with known or possible angina pectoris who have survived sudden cardiac death, those who continue to have angina pectoris despite maximal medical therapy, those who are being considered for coronary revascularization, those who develop a recurrence of symptoms after coronary revascularization, those with chest pain of uncertain cause, and those with a cardiomyopathy of unknown cause. It can also be used for the definitive diagnosis of coronary disease for occupational reasons (e.g., in airline pilots). Coronary angiography is also useful for establishing the diagnosis of *nonatherosclerotic coronary artery disease,* such as coronary artery spasm, Kawasaki disease, radiation-induced vasculopathy, and primary coronary artery dissection. A narrowing of coronary luminal diameter by 50% is considered hemodynamically and clinically significant. Intravascular ultrasound is an invasive diagnostic method to determine the extent of intraluminal disease when the angiogram is equivocal. It can also help assess the results of angioplasty or stenting.

The important prognostic determinants in patients with coronary artery disease are the anatomic extent of the atherosclerotic disease, the state of left ventricular function (ejection fraction), and the stability of the coronary plaque. Left main coronary artery disease is the most dangerous anatomic lesion and is associated with an unfavorable prognosis when managed with medical therapy alone. A stenosis of greater than 50% of the left main coronary artery is associated with an annual mortality rate of 15%.

Unfortunately, coronary angiography cannot predict which plaques are most likely to rupture and initiate acute coronary syndromes. *Vulnerable plaques*—that is, those most likely to rupture and form an occlusive thrombus—have a thin fibrous cap and a large lipid core containing a large number of macrophages. The presence of vulnerable plaque predicts a greater risk of MI regardless of the degree of coronary artery stenosis. Indeed, AMI most often results from rupture of a plaque that had produced less than 50% stenosis of a coronary artery. Currently there is no satisfactory test to measure the stability of plaques.

Treatment

Comprehensive management of ischemic heart disease has five aspects: (1) identification and treatment of diseases that can precipitate or worsen myocardial ischemia, (2) reduction of risk factors for progression of coronary artery disease,

(3) lifestyle modification, (4) pharmacologic management of angina, and (5) revascularization by coronary artery bypass grafting (CABG) or percutaneous coronary intervention (PCI) with or without placement of intracoronary stents. The goal of treatment of patients with chronic stable angina is to achieve complete or almost complete elimination of anginal chest pain and a return to normal activities with minimal side effects.

Treatment of Associated Diseases

Conditions that increase oxygen demand or decrease oxygen delivery may contribute to an exacerbation of previously stable angina. These conditions include fever, infection, anemia, tachycardia, thyrotoxicosis, heart failure, and cocaine use. Treatment of these conditions is critical to the management of stable ischemic heart disease.

Reduction of Risk Factors and Lifestyle Modification

The progression of atherosclerosis may be slowed by cessation of smoking, maintenance of an ideal body weight by consumption of a low-fat, low-cholesterol diet, regular aerobic exercise, and treatment of hypertension. Hypercholesterolemia is an important modifiable risk factor and should be controlled by diet and/or drugs such as statins. Drug treatment is appropriate in patients with clinical atherosclerosis or when the low-density lipoprotein (LDL) cholesterol level exceeds 160 mg/dL. Hypertension increases the risk of coronary events as a result of direct vascular injury, left ventricular hypertrophy, and increased myocardial oxygen demand. Lowering the blood pressure from hypertensive levels to normal levels decreases the risk of MI, congestive heart failure, and stroke. In combination with lifestyle modifications, an angiotensin-converting enzyme (ACE) inhibitor or angiotensin receptor blocker (ARB), β-blockers, and calcium channel blockers are especially useful in managing hypertension in patients with angina pectoris.

Medical Treatment of Myocardial Ischemia

Antiplatelet drugs, nitrates, β-blockers, ranolazine, calcium channel blockers, and ACE inhibitors are used in the medical treatment of angina pectoris.

Antiplatelet drugs are widely used in the management of ischemic heart disease: aspirin, thienopyridines (clopidogrel and prasugrel), reversible platelet inhibitors (cangrelor and ticagrelor), and platelet glycoprotein IIb/IIIa inhibitors (eptifibatide, tirofiban, and abciximab). (See Chapter 24, "Hematologic Disorders," for a detailed discussion of platelet inhibition.)

Aspirin inhibits the enzyme cyclooxygenase (COX)-1. This results in inhibition of thromboxane A_2, which plays an important role in platelet aggregation. This inhibition is *irreversible,* lasts for the duration of platelet lifespan ($\approx$7 days), and can be produced by low dosages of aspirin. Daily aspirin therapy (75–325 mg/d) decreases the risk of cardiac events in patients with stable or unstable angina pectoris and is recommended for all patients with ischemic heart disease. Clopidogrel inhibits the adenosine diphosphate (ADP) receptor $P2Y_{12}$ and inhibits platelet aggregation in response to ADP release from activated platelets. Clopidogrel-induced inhibition of ADP receptors is *irreversible* and also lasts for the duration of the platelet's lifespan. Seven days after cessation of this drug, 80% of platelets will have recovered normal aggregation function. Clopidogrel is a prodrug that is metabolized into an active compound in the liver. Owing to genetic differences in the enzymes that metabolize clopidogrel to the active drug, significant variability in its activity has been observed. By some estimates, 10%–20% of patients taking aspirin and clopidogrel demonstrate resistance or hyperresponsiveness. Furthermore, some drugs (e.g., proton pump inhibitors) can affect the enzyme that metabolizes clopidogrel to its active compound and thereby can reduce the effectiveness of clopidogrel. Clopidogrel can be used in patients who have a contraindication to or are intolerant of aspirin. Prasugrel also inhibits the ADP $P2Y_{12}$ receptor *irreversibly*. However, the pharmacokinetics of prasugrel are more predictable. It is rapidly absorbed, has a faster onset of action, and demonstrates less individual variability in platelet responses compared with clopidogrel. It also is more potent than clopidogrel, and a higher risk of bleeding has been associated with its use. Ticagrelor and its equipotent metabolite *reversibly* interact with the platelet $P2Y_{12}$ ADP receptor, thereby preventing signal transduction and platelet activation and aggregation. Though ticagrelor and prasugrel have been shown to be more effective after ACS or stent placement, they are associated with an increased risk of bleeding. Platelet glycoprotein IIb/IIIa receptor antagonists (abciximab, eptifibatide, tirofiban) inhibit platelet activation, adhesion, and aggregation. Limited-term administration of antiplatelet drugs is particularly useful after placement of an intracoronary stent.

Organic nitrates decrease the frequency, duration, and severity of angina pectoris and increase the amount of exercise required to produce ST-segment depression. The antianginal effects of nitrates are greater when these drugs are used in combination with β-blockers or calcium channel blockers. Nitrates dilate coronary arteries and collateral blood vessels and thereby improve coronary blood flow. Nitrates also decrease peripheral vascular resistance, which reduces left ventricular afterload and myocardial oxygen consumption. The venodilating effect of nitrates decreases venous return and hence left ventricular preload and myocardial oxygen consumption. They also have potential antithrombotic effects. Nitrates are contraindicated in the presence of hypertrophic cardiomyopathy or severe aortic stenosis and *should not* be used within 24 hours of sildenafil, tadalafil, or vardenafil use because this combination may produce severe hypotension. Administration of sublingual nitroglycerin by tablet or spray produces prompt relief of angina pectoris. The most common side effect of nitrate treatment is headache. Hypotension may occur after nitrate administration in hypovolemic patients. For long-term therapy, long-acting nitrate preparations (e.g., isosorbide tablets and nitroglycerin ointment or patches) are equally effective. The therapeutic value of organic nitrates can be compromised by the development of tolerance. To avoid nitrate tolerance, *a daily 8- to 12-hour interval free of nitrate exposure* is recommended.

β-Blockers are the only drugs that have been shown to prolong life in patients with coronary artery disease. They have antiischemic, antihypertensive, and antidysrhythmic properties. Long-term administration of β-blockers decreases the risk of death and myocardial reinfarction in patients who have had an MI, presumably by decreasing myocardial oxygen demand. This benefit is present even in patients in whom β-blockers were traditionally thought to be contraindicated, such as those with congestive heart failure, pulmonary disease, or advanced age. Drug-induced *blockade of β_1-adrenergic receptors* by atenolol, metoprolol, acebutolol, or bisoprolol results in heart rate slowing and decreased myocardial contractility that are greater during activity than at rest. The result is a decrease in myocardial oxygen demand with a subsequent decrease in ischemic events during exertion. The decrease in heart rate also increases the length of diastole and thus coronary perfusion time. *β_2-Adrenergic blockers* (propranolol, nadolol) can increase the risk of bronchospasm in patients with reactive airway disease. *Despite differences between β_1 and β_2 effects, all β-blockers seem to be equally effective in the treatment of angina pectoris.* The most common side effects of β-blocker therapy are fatigue and insomnia. Heart failure may be intensified. β-Blockers are *contraindicated* in the presence of severe bradycardia, sick sinus syndrome, severe reactive airway disease, second- or third-degree atrioventricular heart block, and uncontrolled congestive heart failure. Diabetes mellitus is not a contraindication to β-blocker therapy, although these drugs may mask signs of hypoglycemia. Abrupt withdrawal of β-blockers after prolonged administration can worsen ischemia in patients with chronic stable angina.

Ranolazine is a cardioselective antiischemic agent. It interacts with sodium and potassium channels, though the exact mechanism of action for its antiischemic and antianginal effects is unclear. *It is indicated for chronic angina only and should not be used for the management of acute episodes of angina pectoris.* It is excreted by the kidney and can cause significant QTc prolongation and should be avoided in patients with kidney and/or liver disease.

Long-acting calcium channel blockers are comparable to β-blockers in relieving anginal pain. However, *short-acting calcium channel blockers* such as verapamil, diltiazem, and nifedipine are not. Calcium channel blockers are uniquely effective in decreasing the frequency and severity of angina pectoris due to coronary artery spasm (Prinzmetal or variant angina). *They are not as effective as β-blockers in decreasing the incidence of myocardial reinfarction.* The effectiveness of calcium channel blockers is due to their ability to decrease vascular smooth muscle tone, dilate coronary arteries, decrease myocardial contractility and myocardial oxygen consumption, and decrease systemic blood pressure. Many calcium channel blockers such as amlodipine, nicardipine, isradipine, felodipine, and long-acting nifedipine are potent vasodilators and are useful in treating both hypertension and angina. Common side effects of calcium channel blocker therapy include hypotension, peripheral edema, and headache. Calcium channel blockers are contraindicated in patients with severe congestive heart failure or severe aortic stenosis. They must be used cautiously if given in combination with β-blockers, because both classes of drugs have significant depressant effects on heart rate and myocardial contractility.

Excessive angiotensin II plays a significant role in the pathophysiology of cardiac disorders. It can lead to development of myocardial hypertrophy, interstitial myocardial fibrosis, increased coronary vasoconstriction, and endothelial dysfunction. Angiotensin II also promotes inflammatory responses and atheroma formation. ACE inhibitors are important not only in the treatment of heart failure but also in the treatment of hypertension and in cardiovascular protection. ACE inhibitors are recommended for patients with coronary artery disease, especially those with hypertension, left ventricular dysfunction, or diabetes mellitus. ARBs offer similar benefits. Contraindications to ACE inhibitor use include documented intolerance or allergy, hyperkalemia, bilateral renal artery stenosis, and renal failure.

Revascularization

Revascularization by CABG or PCI with or without placement of intracoronary stents is indicated when optimal medical therapy fails to control angina pectoris. Revascularization is also indicated for specific anatomic lesions, in particular, left main coronary artery stenosis of more than 50% or a 70% or greater stenosis in an epicardial coronary artery. Revascularization is also indicated in patients with significant coronary artery disease with evidence of impaired left ventricular contractility (ejection fraction of <40%). However, the presence of hypokinetic or akinetic areas in the left ventricle connotes a poor prognosis. Extensive myocardial fibrosis from a prior MI is unlikely to be improved by revascularization. However, some patients with ischemic heart disease have *chronically impaired myocardial function (hibernating myocardium)* that demonstrates improvement in contractility after surgical revascularization. In patients with stable angina pectoris and significant one- or two-vessel coronary artery disease, a PCI, with or without stent placement, or surgical CABG may be used for revascularization. CABG is preferred over PCI in patients with significant left main coronary artery disease, those with three-vessel coronary artery disease, and patients with diabetes mellitus who have two- or three-vessel coronary artery disease. Operative mortality rates for CABG surgery currently range from 1.5%–2% in younger patients but increase to 4%–8% in older individuals (>80 years) and in those who have had prior CABG.

ACUTE CORONARY SYNDROME

ACS represents an acute or worsening imbalance of myocardial oxygen supply to demand. It typically occurs as a result of focal disruption of an atheromatous plaque that triggers the coagulation cascade, with subsequent generation of thrombin and partial or complete occlusion of the coronary artery by a thrombus. Rarely it may result from prolonged

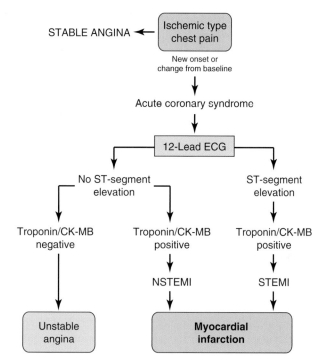

FIG. 5.2 Terminology of acute coronary syndrome. *CK-MB,* Creatine kinase, myocardial-bound isoenzyme; *ECG,* electrocardiogram; *NSTEMI,* non–ST-segment elevation myocardial infarction; *STEMI,* ST-segment elevation myocardial infarction. (Adapted from Alpert JS, Thygesen K, Antman E, et al. Myocardial infarction redefined—a consensus document of the Joint European Society of Cardiology/American College of Cardiology Committee for the redefinition of myocardial infarction. *J Am Coll Cardiol.* 2000;36:959-969.)

coronary vasospasm, embolic occlusion, vasculitis, or aortic root/coronary artery dissection. Imbalance of myocardial oxygen supply and demand leads to ischemic chest pain. ACS can be classified into three categories based on the findings of a 12-lead ECG and the levels of cardiac-specific biomarkers (troponins). Patients with ST elevation at presentation are considered to have STEMI. Patients who have ST-segment depression or nonspecific changes on the ECG are categorized based on the levels of cardiac-specific troponins or myocardial creatine kinase (CK)-MB. Elevation of cardiac-specific biomarker levels in this situation indicates NSTEMI. If levels of cardiac-specific biomarkers are normal, unstable angina (UA) is present (Fig. 5.2). STEMI and UA/NSTEMI syndromes are managed differently and have different prognoses. Many more patients have UA/NSTEMI than have STEMI at presentation.

ST-Segment Elevation Myocardial Infarction

Mortality rates from STEMI have declined steadily because of early therapeutic interventions such as angioplasty, thrombolysis and aspirin, heparin, and statin therapy. However, the mortality rate of acute STEMI remains significant. The short-term mortality rate in patients who undergo reperfusion therapy is about 6.5%. Data from the general medical community show a mortality rate of 15%–20% in patients who have not received reperfusion therapy. Advanced age consistently emerges as one of the principal determinants of early mortality in patients with STEMI. Coronary angiography has documented that nearly all STEMIs are caused by thrombotic occlusion of a coronary artery.

The long-term prognosis after an acute STEMI is determined principally by the severity of residual left ventricular dysfunction, the presence and degree of residual ischemia, and the presence of malignant ventricular dysrhythmias. Most deaths that occur during the first year after hospital discharge take place within the first 3 months. Ventricular function can be substantially improved during the first few weeks after an AMI, particularly in patients in whom early reperfusion was achieved. Therefore measurement of ventricular function 2–3 months after an MI is a more accurate predictor of long-term prognosis than measurement of ventricular function during the acute phase of the infarction.

Pathophysiology

Atherosclerosis is being increasingly recognized as an *inflammatory* disease. The presence of inflammatory cells in atherosclerotic plaques suggests that inflammation is important in the cascade of events leading to plaque rupture. Indeed, serum markers of inflammation such as C-reactive protein and fibrinogen are increased in those at greatest risk of developing coronary artery disease.

STEMI occurs when coronary blood flow decreases abruptly. This decrease in blood flow is attributable to acute thrombus formation at a site where an atherosclerotic plaque fissures, ruptures, or ulcerates. This creates a local environment that favors thrombogenesis. Typically, vulnerable plaques—that is, those with rich lipid cores and thin fibrous caps—are most prone to rupture. A platelet monolayer forms at the site of ruptured plaque, and various chemical mediators such as collagen, ADP, epinephrine, and serotonin stimulate platelet aggregation. The potent vasoconstrictor thromboxane A_2 is released, which further compromises coronary blood flow. Glycoprotein IIb/IIIa receptors on the platelets are activated, which enhances the ability of platelets to interact with adhesive proteins and other platelets and causes growth and stabilization of the thrombus. Further activation of coagulation leads to strengthening of the clot by fibrin deposition. This makes the clot more resistant to thrombolysis. It is rather paradoxical that plaques that rupture and lead to acute coronary occlusion are rarely of a size that causes significant coronary obstruction. By contrast, flow-restrictive plaques that produce chronic stable angina and stimulate development of collateral circulation are *less likely* to rupture. Rarely, STEMI develops as a result of acute coronary spasm or coronary artery embolism.

Diagnosis

The criteria for the definition of an AMI have been revised (Table 5.3). Now this diagnosis requires detection of a rise and/or fall in cardiac biomarkers (preferably troponin with at least one value above the 99th percentile of the upper reference

TABLE 5.3	Criteria for Diagnosis of Acute Myocardial Infarction

The term *myocardial infarction* should be used when there is evidence of myocardial necrosis in a clinical setting consistent with myocardial ischemia. Under these conditions any one of the following criteria meets the diagnosis for myocardial infarction:
- Detection of rise and/or fall of cardiac biomarkers, preferably troponin (with at least one value above the 99th percentile of the upper reference limit) **AND** evidence of myocardial ischemia indicated by at least one of the following:
- Symptoms of ischemia
- ECG changes indicative of new ischemia (new ST-T changes, new left bundle branch block)
- Development of pathologic Q waves on the ECG
- Imaging evidence of new loss of viable myocardium or new regional wall motion abnormality

From Thygesen K, Alpert JS, Jaffe AS, et al. Third universal definition of myocardial infarction. *Circulation*. 2012;126:2020-2035.

limit) *and* evidence of myocardial ischemia by one of the following: (1) symptoms of ischemia, (2) ECG changes indicative of new ischemia, such as new ST-T changes or new left bundle branch block (LBBB), (3) development of pathologic Q waves on the ECG, or (4) imaging evidence of a new loss of viable myocardium or a new regional wall motion abnormality.

Almost two-thirds of patients describe new-onset angina pectoris or a change in their anginal pattern during the 30 days preceding an AMI. The pain is often more severe than the previous angina pectoris and does not resolve with rest. Other potential causes of severe chest pain (pulmonary embolism, aortic dissection, spontaneous pneumothorax, pericarditis, cholecystitis) should be considered. About a quarter of patients, especially the elderly and those with diabetes, have no or only mild pain at the time of an AMI. Sometimes STEMI may masquerade as acute heart failure, syncope, stroke, or shock, with the patient's ECG showing ST-segment elevation or a new LBBB.

On physical examination, patients typically appear anxious, pale, and diaphoretic. Sinus tachycardia is usually present. Hypotension caused by left or right ventricular dysfunction or cardiac dysrhythmias may be present. Rales signal congestive heart failure due to left ventricular dysfunction. A cardiac murmur may indicate ischemic mitral regurgitation.

Laboratory Studies

Troponin is a cardiac-specific protein and biochemical marker for AMI. An increase in the circulating concentration of troponin occurs early after myocardial injury. Levels of cardiac troponins (troponin T or I) increase within 3 hours after myocardial injury and remain elevated for 7–10 days. Elevated troponins and the ECG are powerful predictors of adverse cardiac events in patients with anginal pain. Troponin is more specific than CK-MB for determining myocardial injury. The currently accepted definition of an AMI recommends assessing the magnitude of the infarction by measuring how much the cardiac biomarker level is elevated above the normal reference range (Fig. 5.3).

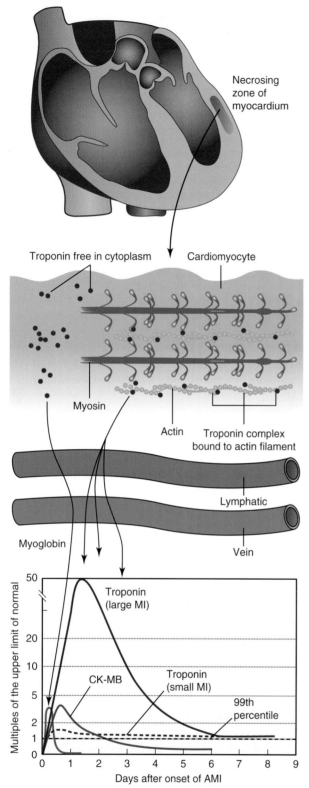

FIG. 5.3   Rate and extent of rise of cardiac troponin and myocardial creatine kinase (CK-MB) levels after a typical acute myocardial infarction (AMI). Cardiac microinfarctions can raise troponin levels without increasing CK-MB levels. (From Antman EM. ST-segment myocardial infarction: pathology, pathophysiology, and clinical features. In: Bonow RO, Mann DL, Zipes DP, et al., eds. *Braunwald's Heart Disease*. Philadelphia: Saunders; 2012: Fig. 54-14.)

Imaging Studies

Patients with typical ECG evidence of AMI do not require evaluation with echocardiography. However, echocardiography is useful in patients with LBBB or an abnormal ECG in whom the diagnosis of AMI is uncertain and in patients with suspected aortic dissection. Echocardiography will demonstrate regional wall motion abnormalities in most patients with AMI. The time required to perform myocardial perfusion imaging and the inability to differentiate between new and old MI limits the utility of radionuclide imaging in the early diagnosis of AMI.

Treatment

Early treatment of AMI reduces morbidity and mortality. Initial steps include administering oxygen to all patients. Pain relief, usually provided by intravenous (IV) morphine and/or sublingual nitroglycerin, is necessary to reduce catecholamine release and the resultant increase in myocardial oxygen requirements. All patients with suspected or definite AMI should receive aspirin. Patients with allergy to aspirin should receive a $P2Y_{12}$ inhibitor (clopidogrel, prasugrel, or ticagrelor). The combination of aspirin and $P2Y_{12}$ inhibitors improves outcomes and should be administered for at least 14 days and potentially continued for 1 year. Alternatively platelet glycoprotein IIb/IIIa inhibitors can be used even if urgent CABG is likely. Unfractionated heparin is frequently used in combination with antiplatelet drugs, especially if thrombolytic therapy or PCI is planned. β-Blockers relieve ischemic chest pain, infarct size, and life-threatening dysrhythmias. β-Blockers are administered to patients in hemodynamically stable condition who are not in heart failure, not in a low cardiac output state, and not at risk of cardiogenic shock. β-Blockers are not given to those with heart block. *The primary goal in management of STEMI is to reestablish blood flow in the obstructed coronary artery as soon as possible.* This can be achieved by thrombolytic therapy or coronary angioplasty with or without placement of an intracoronary stent. The time from the onset of symptoms to reperfusion strongly influences the outcome of an acute STEMI.

Reperfusion Therapy

Thrombolytic therapy with tissue plasminogen activator (tPA), alteplase, reteplase, or tenecteplase should be initiated within 30–60 minutes of hospital arrival and within 12 hours of symptom onset. Thrombolytic therapy restores normal antegrade blood flow in the occluded coronary artery. Dissolution of the clot by thrombolytic therapy becomes much more difficult if therapy is delayed. The most feared complication of thrombolytic therapy is intracranial hemorrhage. This is most likely in elderly patients (>75 years) and in those with uncontrolled hypertension. Patients who have gastrointestinal bleeding or have recently undergone surgery are also at increased risk of bleeding complications with thrombolysis. Contraindications to fibrinolytic therapy include hemorrhagic strokes within the previous year, known intracranial neoplasm, recent head trauma, active or recent internal bleeding (within 3 weeks), or suspected aortic dissection.

Percutaneous Coronary Intervention

PCI may be preferable to thrombolytic therapy for restoring flow to an occluded coronary artery if appropriate resources are available. Ideally, angioplasty should be performed within 90 minutes of arrival at the healthcare facility and within 12 hours of symptom onset. It is the treatment of choice in patients with a contraindication to thrombolytic therapy and those with severe heart failure and/or pulmonary edema. About 5% of patients who undergo immediate PCI require emergency cardiac surgery because of failed angioplasty or because the coronary artery anatomy precludes an intervention. The combined use of intracoronary stents and antiplatelet drugs (aspirin, clopidogrel or prasugrel, and/or a platelet glycoprotein IIb/IIIa inhibitor) during emergency PCI provides the maximum chance of achieving normal antegrade coronary blood flow and decreases the need for a subsequent revascularization procedure.

Coronary Artery Bypass Graft Surgery

CABG can restore blood flow in an occluded coronary artery, but reperfusion is achieved faster with thrombolytic therapy or coronary angioplasty. Emergency CABG is reserved for patients in whom angiography reveals coronary anatomy that precludes PCI, patients with a failed angioplasty, and those with evidence of infarction-related ventricular septal rupture or mitral regurgitation. Patients with ST-segment elevation who develop cardiogenic shock, LBBB, or a posterior wall MI within 36 hours of an acute STEMI are also candidates for early revascularization. Mortality from CABG is significant during the first 3–7 days after an AMI.

Adjunctive Medical Therapy

Intravenous heparin therapy is commonly administered for 48 hours after thrombolytic therapy to decrease the risk of thrombus regeneration. A disadvantage of unfractionated heparin is the variability in the dose response due to its binding with plasma proteins other than antithrombin. Low-molecular-weight heparin (LMWH) provides a more predictable pharmacologic effect, a long plasma half-life, and a more practical means of administration (subcutaneous), without the need to monitor the activated partial thromboplastin time. Thus LMWH is an excellent alternative to unfractionated heparin. Direct thrombin inhibitors such as bivalirudin can be used in patients with a history of heparin-induced thrombocytopenia. Administration of β-blockers is associated with a significant decrease in early (in-hospital) and long-term mortality and myocardial reinfarction. Early administration of β-blockers can decrease infarct size by decreasing heart rate, blood pressure, and myocardial contractility. In the absence of specific contraindications, it is recommended that patients receive β-blockers as early as possible after an AMI. β-Blocker therapy should be continued indefinitely.

All patients with a large anterior wall MI, clinical evidence of left ventricular failure, an ejection fraction of less than 40%, or diabetes should be treated with ACE inhibitors or angiotensin II receptor blockers.

In the absence of significant ventricular dysrhythmias, prophylactic administration of lidocaine or another antidysrhythmic drug is not recommended. Calcium channel blockers *should not be administered routinely* but should be reserved for patients with persistent myocardial ischemia despite optimal use of aspirin, β-blockers, nitrates, and heparin. Glycemic control is part of the standard care of diabetic patients with an AMI. Routine administration of magnesium is not recommended, but magnesium therapy is indicated in patients with torsade de pointes ventricular tachycardia. Statins have strong immune-modulating effects and should be started as soon as possible after MI, especially in patients on long-term statin therapy.

Unstable Angina/Non–ST-Segment Elevation Myocardial Infarction

UA/NSTEMI results from a reduction in myocardial oxygen supply. Typically, five pathophysiologic processes may contribute to the development of UA/NSTEMI: (1) rupture or erosion of a coronary plaque that leads to *nonocclusive* thrombosis, (2) dynamic obstruction due to *vasoconstriction* (Prinzmetal-variant angina, cold, cocaine use), (3) worsening coronary luminal narrowing due to progressive atherosclerosis, in-stent restenosis, or narrowing of CABGs, (4) inflammation (vasculitis), or (5) myocardial ischemia due to increased oxygen demand (sepsis, fever, tachycardia, anemia). Embolization of platelets and clot fragments into the coronary microvasculature leads to *microcirculatory* ischemia and infarction that can result in elevation of cardiac biomarker levels without elevation of the ST segments.

Diagnosis

UA/NSTEMI has three principal presentations: angina at rest (typically lasting >20 minutes unless interrupted by antianginal medication), chronic angina pectoris that becomes more frequent and more easily provoked, and new-onset angina that is severe, prolonged, or disabling. UA/NSTEMI can also present with hemodynamic instability or congestive heart failure. Signs of congestive heart failure (S_3 gallop, jugular venous distention, rales, peripheral edema) or ischemia-induced papillary muscle dysfunction causing acute mitral regurgitation may be evident. Fifty percent of patients with UA/NSTEMI have significant ECG abnormalities, including transient ST-segment elevation, ST depression, and/or T-wave inversion. Significant ST-segment depression in two or more contiguous leads and/or deep symmetric T-wave inversion, especially in the setting of chest pain, is highly consistent with a diagnosis of myocardial ischemia and UA/NSTEMI. Elevated levels of cardiac biomarkers or a new regional wall motion abnormality on echocardiogram establish the diagnosis of AMI. Approximately two-thirds of patients who would have been classified as having unstable angina have now been found to show evidence of myocardial necrosis based on sensitive cardiac enzyme assays. They should be classified as having NSTEMI.

Treatment

Management of UA/NSTEMI is directed at decreasing myocardial oxygen demand and limiting thrombus formation by inhibiting platelet activation and aggregation. Bed rest, supplemental oxygen, analgesia, and β-blocker therapy are indicated. Calcium channel blockers can also be used. Sublingual or IV nitroglycerin may improve myocardial oxygen supply. Aspirin, clopidogrel, prasugrel, or ticagrelor and heparin therapy (unfractionated heparin or LMWH) are strongly recommended to decrease further thrombus formation. Fondaparinux, a specific factor Xa inhibitor, can also be used as an anticoagulant. Glycoprotein IIb/IIIa agents may be used as an alternative or in addition to other antiplatelet drugs in certain clinical situations. *Thrombolytic therapy is not indicated in UA/NSTEMI and has been shown to increase mortality.* Older age (>65 years), positive finding for cardiac biomarkers, rales, hypotension, tachycardia, and decreased left ventricular function (ejection fraction < 40%) are associated with increased mortality. Patients at high risk include the elderly, those with ischemic symptoms in the preceding 48 hours, those with prolonged chest pain (>20 minutes), those with heart failure or hemodynamic instability, those with sustained ventricular dysrhythmias, those who had a PCI within the past 6 months or had prior CABG surgery, those with elevated troponin levels, and those with angina at low-level activity. These patients should be considered for early invasive evaluation, which includes coronary angiography and revascularization by PCI or CABG if needed. Patients with mild to moderate renal insufficiency (creatinine clearance > 30 mL/min) may also benefit from early invasive treatment. Patients at lower risk can be treated medically and undergo stress testing at a later time. Coronary angiography often follows the demonstration of significant ischemia on stress testing.

COMPLICATIONS OF ACUTE MYOCARDIAL INFARCTION

Postinfarction Ischemia

Myocardial ischemia occurs in about one-third of patients after MI. It is more common after STEMI compared to NSTEMI. It is typically managed with β-blockers, nitrovasodilators, antiplatelet agents, and anticoagulants. If medical management does not control the symptoms, patients may require early catheterization and revascularization by PCI or surgery.

Cardiac Dysrhythmias

Cardiac dysrhythmias, especially ventricular dysrhythmias, are a common cause of death during the early period following AMI.

Ventricular fibrillation occurs in 3%–5% of patients with AMI, usually during the first 4 hours after the event. Rapid defibrillation with 200–300 J of energy is necessary when ventricular fibrillation occurs. Amiodarone is regarded as one of the most effective antidysrhythmic drugs available for control of ventricular tachydysrhythmias, especially after AMI. Administration of β-blockers may decrease the early occurrence of ventricular fibrillation. Hypokalemia is a risk factor for ventricular fibrillation and should be treated. Ventricular fibrillation is often fatal when it occurs in patients with hypotension and/or congestive heart failure.

Ventricular tachycardia is common in AMI. Short periods of *nonsustained* ventricular tachycardia *do not* appear to predispose a patient to *sustained* ventricular tachycardia or ventricular fibrillation. Sustained or hemodynamically significant ventricular tachycardia must be treated promptly with electrical cardioversion. Asymptomatic ventricular tachycardia can be treated with IV amiodarone or lidocaine. Implantation of a cardioverter-defibrillator may be indicated in patients who experience recurrent ventricular tachycardia or ventricular fibrillation despite adequate revascularization.

Atrial fibrillation and atrial flutter are the most common atrial dysrhythmias seen with AMI. They occur in about 20% of patients. Precipitating factors include hypoxia, acidosis, heart failure, pericarditis, and sinus node ischemia. Atrial fibrillation may also result from atrial ischemia or from an acute increase in left atrial pressure as a result of left ventricular dysfunction. The incidence of atrial fibrillation is decreased in patients who receive thrombolytic therapy. When atrial fibrillation is hemodynamically significant, cardioversion is necessary. If atrial fibrillation is well tolerated, β-blockers or calcium channel blockers can be used to control the ventricular response.

Sinus bradycardia is common after AMI, particularly in patients with inferior wall MI. This may reflect increased parasympathetic nervous system activity or acute ischemia of the sinus node or atrioventricular node. Treatment with atropine and/or a temporary cardiac pacemaker is *needed only when* there is hemodynamic compromise from the bradycardia. First-degree block (prolonged PR interval) is common and does not require treatment. Second- or third-degree atrioventricular heart block occurs in about 20% of patients with inferior wall MI and requires treatment if accompanied by severe bradycardia. Complete heart block occurs in about 5% of patients with acute inferior infarction and often requires temporary or permanent cardiac pacing.

Pericarditis

Acute pericarditis is a common complication that occurs a few days after MI in 10%–15% of patients. It may cause chest pain that can be confused with continuing or recurrent angina. However, in contrast to the pain of myocardial ischemia, the pain of pericarditis is pleuritic, gets worse with inspiration or lying down, and may be relieved by changes in posture. It typically presents 2–7 days after an MI. A pericardial friction rub can be heard but is often transient and positional. Diffuse ST-segment and T-wave changes may be present on the ECG. In the absence of a significant pericardial effusion, treatment of pericarditis is aimed at relieving the chest pain.

Aspirin is recommended initially. Although indomethacin and corticosteroids can relieve the symptoms of pericarditis dramatically, they should be avoided because they impair infarct healing and predispose to myocardial rupture. It is recommended that steroid therapy be deferred for at least 4 weeks after an AMI. Dressler syndrome (post-MI syndrome) is a delayed form of pericarditis developing several weeks to months after an AMI. It is thought to be immune mediated and is typically managed with nonsteroidal antiinflammatory drugs or corticosteroids.

Mitral Regurgitation

Mitral regurgitation due to ischemic injury to a papillary muscle and/or the ventricular muscle to which the papillary muscles attach can occur 3–7 days after AMI. Severe mitral regurgitation is rare and usually results from rupture of a papillary muscle. Severe mitral regurgitation is 10 times more likely to occur after an inferior wall MI than after an anterior wall MI. Severe acute mitral regurgitation typically results in pulmonary edema and cardiogenic shock. Total papillary muscle rupture usually leads to death within 24 hours. Prompt surgical repair is required. Treatments that decrease left ventricular afterload and improve coronary perfusion, such as intraaortic balloon counterpulsation, can decrease the regurgitant volume and increase forward flow and cardiac output until surgery can be accomplished.

Ventricular Septal Rupture

Ventricular septal rupture is more likely after an *anterior wall MI*. The characteristic holosystolic murmur of ventricular septal rupture may be difficult to distinguish from the murmur of severe mitral regurgitation. The diagnosis is made by echocardiography. As soon as the diagnosis of ventricular septal rupture is made, intraaortic balloon counterpulsation should be initiated. Emergency surgical repair is necessary if the ventricular defect is associated with hemodynamic compromise. The mortality rate associated with surgical repair of a post-MI ventricular septal defect is about 20%. It is better to wait at least 1 week before surgical repair of the ventricular septal defect is undertaken in patients in hemodynamically stable condition. If the defect is left untreated, mortality approaches 90%.

Myocardial Dysfunction

AMI is often complicated by some degree of left ventricular dysfunction. Dyspnea, orthopnea, rales, and arterial hypoxemia indicate this left ventricular dysfunction. It is typically managed with supplemental oxygen, diuretics, morphine, and nitrovasodilators (nitroglycerin in IV, sublingual, or transdermal forms). Nitroglycerin helps reduce preload and pulmonary congestion and improves left ventricular function. If blood pressure is acceptable, inotropes are typically avoided, since they can increase myocardial oxygen demand.

Cardiogenic Shock

The term *cardiogenic shock* is restricted to an advanced form of acute heart failure in which the cardiac output is insufficient to maintain adequate perfusion of the brain, kidneys, and other vital organs. Hypotension and oliguria persist after relief of anginal pain, abatement of excess sympathetic nervous system activity, correction of hypovolemia, and treatment of dysrhythmias. Systolic blood pressure is low, and there may be associated pulmonary edema and arterial hypoxemia. Cardiogenic shock is usually a manifestation of infarction of more than 40% of the left ventricular myocardium. In the setting of an AMI, the mortality of cardiogenic shock exceeds 50%.

Important in the management of cardiogenic shock is the diagnosis and prompt treatment of potentially reversible *mechanical* complications of MI. These include (1) rupture of the left ventricular free wall, septum, or papillary muscles; (2) cardiac tamponade; and (3) acute, severe mitral regurgitation. Echocardiography is extremely helpful in diagnosing and quantifying these pathologic conditions. Treatment of cardiogenic shock depends on blood pressure and peripheral perfusion. Norepinephrine, vasopressin, dopamine, or dobutamine may be administered in an attempt to improve blood pressure and cardiac output. If the blood pressure is adequate, nitroglycerin can be used to decrease left ventricular preload and afterload. Concomitant pulmonary edema may require the use of morphine, diuretics, and mechanical ventilation. Restoration of some coronary blood flow to the zone around the infarcted area by thrombolytic therapy, PCI, or surgical revascularization may be indicated. Circulatory assist devices can help sustain viable myocardium and support cardiac output until revascularization can be performed. Left ventricular assist devices (LVADs) improve cardiac output much more than intraaortic balloon counterpulsation does. Intraaortic balloon pumps are easier to place and are more generally available than LVADs, but they have not been shown to improve mortality in cardiogenic shock. Infusion of a combination of inotropic and vasodilator drugs may serve as a pharmacologic alternative to mechanical counterpulsation. Emergent cardiac catheterization with revascularization may offer the best chance of survival.

Myocardial Rupture

Myocardial rupture occurs in fewer than 1% of patients and usually causes acute cardiac tamponade and death. This typically occurs within the first week after an MI and presents with sudden hemodynamic collapse or sudden death. In only an extremely small percentage of cases, is it possible to have time for medical stabilization and emergency surgery.

Right Ventricular Infarction

Right ventricular infarction occurs in about one-third of patients with acute inferior wall MI. Isolated right ventricular infarction is very unusual. The right ventricle has a more favorable oxygen supply/demand ratio than the left ventricle. This is because of its smaller muscle mass and low intracavitary pressures during systole, which allows coronary blood flow during both systole and diastole. *The clinical triad of hypotension, increased jugular venous pressure, and clear lung fields in a patient with an inferior wall MI is virtually pathognomonic for right ventricular infarction.* Kussmaul sign (distention of the internal jugular vein on inspiration) is often seen. Right ventricular dilation, right ventricular asynergy, and abnormal motion of the interventricular septum can be seen on echocardiography.

Recognition of right ventricular infarction is important because some pharmacologic treatments for left ventricular failure may worsen right ventricular failure. In particular, administration of vasodilators and diuretics is very dangerous. Initial therapy for right ventricular failure consists of IV fluid administration. If hypotension persists, inotropic support, with or without intraaortic balloon counterpulsation, may be necessary. Cardiogenic shock, although uncommon, is the most serious complication of right ventricular infarction. Improvement in right ventricular function generally occurs over time, which suggests reversal of "ischemic stunning" of the right ventricular myocardium. About one-third of patients with right ventricular infarction develop atrial fibrillation. Heart block may occur in as many as 50% of these patients. Both of these situations may produce severe hemodynamic compromise. Third-degree atrioventricular heart block should be treated promptly with temporary atrioventricular pacing, in recognition of the value of atrioventricular synchrony in maintaining ventricular filling in the ischemic, and therefore noncompliant, right ventricle.

Mural Thrombus and Stroke

Infarction of the anterior wall and apex of the left ventricle results in thrombus formation at the location of the infarction in as many as one-third of patients. The risk of systemic embolization and the possibility of an ischemic stroke are then very significant in these patients. Echocardiography is used to detect a left ventricular thrombus. The presence of such a thrombus is an indication for immediate anticoagulation with heparin followed by 3 months of anticoagulation with warfarin.

Thrombolytic therapy is associated with hemorrhagic stroke in 0.3%–1% of patients. The stroke is usually evident within the first 24 hours after the thrombolytic treatment and is associated with high mortality.

PERIOPERATIVE IMPLICATIONS OF PERCUTANEOUS CORONARY INTERVENTION

Percutaneous transluminal coronary angioplasty (PTCA) was introduced as an alternative to CABG to mechanically open a coronary artery stenosis. It was effective, but restenosis at the angioplasty site occurred in 15%–60% of patients within a few months. To solve the problem of abrupt coronary closure after angioplasty, bare-metal stents were introduced. However,

coronary restenosis due to neointimal hyperplasia was observed in 10%–30% of patients with bare-metal stents. Stents coated with drugs (drug-eluting stents) were then introduced to reduce neointimal hyperplasia. The drugs in these stents do this by preventing cell division. Early-generation stents released sirolimus or paclitaxel and had stainless steel platforms, whereas new-generation stents release everolimus or zotarolimus and feature cobalt-chrome or platinum-chrome platforms with thinner strut thickness and more biocompatible, durable polymer coatings. These new-generation stents have almost completely replaced the older coated stents. The two principal issues related to PCI with stent placement now are thrombosis and an increased risk of bleeding due to dual antiplatelet therapy.

Percutaneous Coronary Intervention and Thrombosis

Mechanically opening a coronary artery by angioplasty causes vessel injury, especially destruction of the endothelium. This makes the area prone to thrombosis. It takes about 2–3 weeks for the vessel to reendothelialize after balloon angioplasty. After bare-metal stent placement, reendothelialization can take up to 12 weeks, and a drug-eluting stent may not be completely endothelialized even after a full 1 year. Thus thrombosis after angioplasty and stent placement is a major concern.

Stent thrombosis is categorized by the time interval between its occurrence and the date of the PCI: *acute* (within 24 hours), *subacute* (between 2 and 30 days), *late* (between 30 days and a year), and *very late* (after a year). Early stent thrombosis is usually mechanical in origin and due to coronary artery dissection or underexpansion of the stent. In contrast, late stent thrombosis is typically related to stent malposition, abnormal reendothelialization, or hypersensitivity to the stent. Platelets play an important role in the pathophysiology of stent thrombosis, and use of antiplatelet drugs is critical until the stent becomes less prone to thrombosis. Platelets can be activated by many triggers, and there is significant redundancy and crosstalk between these pathways. Thus multiple pathways must be blocked to achieve clinically effective platelet inhibition.

Discontinuation of antiplatelet therapy increases the risk of stent thrombosis. Dual antiplatelet therapy (aspirin with a $P2Y_{12}$ inhibitor) is better in preventing stent thrombosis compared to aspirin alone. $P2Y_{12}$ inhibitor discontinuation is the most significant independent predictor of stent thrombosis. The probability of a thrombotic event is increased more than 14-fold after discontinuation of these drugs. Current recommendations for dual antiplatelet therapy are the following: it is needed *for at least 2 weeks* after balloon angioplasty without stenting, for at least 6 weeks after bare-metal stent placement, and *for at least 1 year* after drug-eluting stent placement. Some observational studies suggest that earlier discontinuation of dual antiplatelet therapy might be safe after implantation of either zotarolimus or everolimus drug-eluting stents.

Other factors can predispose to stent thrombosis, and these may be important in the perioperative period. Patients at risk for stent thrombosis include those with ACS, a low ejection fraction, diabetes, renal impairment, advanced age, prior brachytherapy, and cancer. Factors related to coronary anatomy (stent length, placement of multiple stents, bifurcated lesions) may also predispose to stent thrombosis. Both elective surgery and emergency surgery increase the risk of stent thrombosis because of the prothrombotic state present during the perioperative period.

Surgery and Risk of Stent Thrombosis

Surgery and Bare-Metal Stents

The frequency of major adverse cardiovascular events (death, MI, stent thrombosis, or the need for repeat revascularization) was about 10% when noncardiac surgery was performed within 4 weeks of PCI. This risk decreased to about 4% when surgery was performed between 31 and 90 days after PCI and to about 3% when surgery was performed more than 90 days after PCI. The risk of death, MI, stent thrombosis, and urgent revascularization is increased by 5%–30% if surgery is performed within the first 6 weeks after bare-metal stent placement.

Surgery and Drug-Eluting Stents

The absolute risk of thrombosis during noncardiac surgery 6 weeks after drug-eluting stent implantation is low but higher than in the absence of surgery. This is attributed to the delayed endothelialization seen with drug-eluting stents. The incidence of major adverse cardiac events is quite significant if dual antiplatelet therapy is discontinued and noncardiac surgery is performed within 1 year of drug-eluting stent placement. This is particularly true for the older coated stents.

The risk of adverse events is higher in patients who undergo emergency surgery. In patients with bare-metal stents, emergency surgery increases the adverse event rate threefold compared to elective surgery. For patients with drug-eluting stents, there is a 3.5-fold increase in adverse events.

Risk of Bleeding Related to Antiplatelet Drugs

It is predictable that patients who are taking antiplatelet drugs will have a higher chance of bleeding, which can be of major concern in the perioperative period. It has been shown that continuing aspirin therapy increases the risk of bleeding by a factor of 1.5, but the severity of adverse events is not increased. The addition of clopidogrel to aspirin increases the relative risk of bleeding by 50%. So far no increase in mortality has been noted except with intracranial surgery. In patients who have received coronary stents and must undergo surgical procedures that mandate discontinuation of $P2Y_{12}$ platelet receptor–inhibitor therapy, it is recommended that aspirin be continued if possible and that the $P2Y_{12}$ platelet receptor–inhibitor be discontinued preoperatively and restarted as soon as possible after surgery.

Bleeding Versus Stent Thrombosis in the Perioperative Period

Discontinuing antiplatelet therapy causes a significant increase in coronary, cerebrovascular, and peripheral vascular events. However, in the perioperative patient the risk of bleeding has to be weighed against the risk of thrombosis. In many situations the risk of coronary thrombosis is high and the consequences of coronary thrombosis could be catastrophic; on the other hand, although the risk of bleeding is increased, bleeding could be manageable and may not contribute to significant morbidity and mortality. In such cases it may be prudent to continue antiplatelet therapy. However, some individuals are more prone to bleeding or need to undergo procedures in which bleeding can have severe consequences. These include neurosurgery, spinal cord decompression, aortic aneurysm surgery, and prostatectomy, among others. In such cases the risk of bleeding may outweigh the risk of thrombosis, so antiplatelet therapy should be stopped before these operations (at least 5 days before surgery for clopidogrel or ticagrelor and 7 days for prasugrel) and resumed as soon as feasible postoperatively. Some patients come for surgery receiving antiplatelet therapy for secondary prevention of cardiovascular events. These patients have no stents, so the risk of bleeding will outweigh the risk of cardiovascular events. In this situation the antiplatelet drugs can be temporarily withheld for high-risk surgery.

Perioperative Management of Patients With Stents

Five factors should be considered when caring for a patient with a coronary stent: (1) timing of the operation after PCI, also called the *PCI-to-surgery interval,* (2) continuation of dual antiplatelet therapy, (3) perioperative monitoring strategies, (4) anesthetic technique, and (5) immediate availability of an interventional cardiologist.

PCI-to-Surgery Interval

The risk of stent thrombosis is significant in the first month after stent placement and progressively decreases as the time from PCI to surgery increases. The longer one waits after stent placement, the better it is. For patients with bare-metal stents, waiting *at least 30 days* (preferably 90 days) before elective surgery is recommended. In patients with drug-eluting stents, waiting *at least 1 year* before elective noncardiac surgery is recommended (Table 5.4).

TABLE 5.4	Recommended Time Intervals to Wait for Elective Noncardiac Surgery After Coronary Revascularization
Procedure	Time to Wait for Elective Surgery
Angioplasty without stenting	2–4 weeks
Bare-metal stent placement	At least 30 days; 12 weeks preferable
Coronary artery bypass grafting	At least 6 weeks; 12 weeks preferable
Drug-eluting stent placement	At least 12 months

Continuation of Dual Antiplatelet Therapy

Dual antiplatelet therapy should be continued for *at least 6 weeks* after bare-metal stent placement and *1 year* after drug-eluting stent placement. If dual antiplatelet therapy must be stopped, at least the aspirin portion of the therapy should be continued. Aspirin should be stopped before elective surgery only when absolutely indicated. Although less than 6 weeks after bare-metal stent placement and less than 1 year after drug-eluting stent placement is considered a highly vulnerable period for stent thrombosis, stent thrombosis can occur at any time. Intraoperative and postoperative monitoring should be based on the risk of the particular surgery, overall patient condition, and the interval between PCI and surgery. Patients who are in the vulnerable period should be monitored very closely, especially if antiplatelet therapy was discontinued for the surgery. In a bleeding patient, platelets can be administered to counteract the effects of antiplatelet drugs, but the effectiveness of the platelet infusions will depend on the timing of the last dose of antiplatelet drug. For example, platelet transfusions can be administered as soon as 4 hours after discontinuation of clopidogrel, but they will be most effective 24 hours after the last dose of clopidogrel.

Perioperative Monitoring Strategies

Practitioners should have a high index of suspicion for cardiac events and concentrate on monitoring for myocardial ischemia and infarction. Intraoperative continuous ECG monitoring with ST-segment analysis is very helpful in monitoring for myocardial ischemia. Any angina in a patient with a stent should initiate an evaluation to rule out AMI, and an urgent cardiology evaluation should be sought.

Anesthetic Technique

Use of neuraxial anesthetic techniques in patients who are receiving dual antiplatelet therapy is controversial. However, both the American Society of Regional Anesthesia (ASRA) and the European Society of Anaesthesiologists have adopted a conservative approach in this matter. Use of neuraxial blockade is not encouraged in patients who are receiving dual antiplatelet therapy. The risk of developing a spinal hematoma exists not only at the time of placement of the catheter but also at the time of its removal. The most up-to-date recommendations regarding waiting times before placement or removal of an epidural catheter and administration of antiplatelet agents are available online at www.asra.com.

Immediate Availability of an Interventional Cardiologist

Although many MIs in the perioperative period are silent, *any angina* in a patient with a stent should prompt evaluation to rule out AMI. There should be immediate access to interventional cardiology services. Once the diagnosis of AMI or acute stent thrombosis is made or considered, triage to interventional cardiology within 90 minutes is strongly recommended. Mortality increases substantially if reperfusion is delayed. Ambulatory surgical facilities, endoscopy suites, and other non–hospital-based operating locations without these resources on site must develop a relationship with interventional cardiologists that can facilitate rapid transfer if needed.

PERIOPERATIVE MYOCARDIAL INFARCTION

The incidence of perioperative cardiac injury is a cumulative result of the patient's preoperative medical condition, the specific surgical procedure, the expertise of the surgeon, the diagnostic criteria used to define MI, and the overall medical care at a particular institution. The risk of perioperative death due to cardiac causes is less than 1% in patients who do not have ischemic heart disease. The incidence of perioperative MI (PMI) in patients who undergo elective high-risk vascular surgery is 5%–15%. This risk is even higher for emergency surgery. Patients who undergo *urgent hip surgery* have an incidence of PMI of 5%–7%, whereas fewer than 3% of patients who undergo elective total hip or knee arthroplasty have a PMI. Early mortality after a PMI ranges from 3.5%–25% and is higher in patients with marked troponin elevations compared to patients with minor troponin elevation.

Pathophysiology

Myocardial ischemia occurs whenever myocardial oxygen supply does not match myocardial oxygen demand. PMI is one of the most important predictors of short- and long-term morbidity and mortality associated with noncardiac surgery. Unfortunately the exact mechanism for PMI remains uncertain and a subject of debate and controversy. The interaction between morphologic and functional factors is unpredictable. Some older pathologic and angiographic studies suggested that the etiology of PMI resembles that in the nonsurgical setting—that is, plaque rupture was the cause of PMI in 50% of the cases. Endothelial injury at the site of a plaque rupture triggers the cascade of platelet aggregation and release of mediators. Aggregation of platelets and activation of other inflammatory and noninflammatory mediators potentiates thrombus formation and leads to dynamic vasoconstriction distal to the thrombus. The combined effects of dynamic and physical blood vessel narrowing cause ischemia and/or infarction. In the postoperative period, changes in blood viscosity, catecholamine concentrations, cortisol levels, endogenous tPA concentrations, and plasminogen activator inhibitor levels create a prothrombotic state. Changes in heart rate and blood pressure as a result of the stress response can increase the propensity for a plaque to fissure and develop endothelial damage. In combination these factors can precipitate thrombus formation in an atherosclerotic coronary artery and lead to the development of STEMI. However, newer analysis suggests that myocardial oxygen supply/demand imbalance predominates as the cause of cardiac injury during the first 3–4 postoperative days. Patients suffer demand ischemia.

The high incidence of histologically confirmed perioperative transmural MIs seems to be contradictory to the ECG finding of almost exclusively *non-Q-wave MIs*. On the other hand, the presence of subendocardial myocardial injury is consistent with a myocardial oxygen supply/demand mismatch being the main trigger of myocardial injury. However, myocardial oxygen supply/demand mismatch and plaque rupture are not mutually exclusive mechanisms, and MIs may develop by different mechanisms at different locations in the same patient.

Most PMIs occur soon after surgery (1–4 days), and 90% occur within 7 days. Most are *asymptomatic,* of the non–Q–wave type (60%–100%), and are commonly preceded by ST-segment *depression* rather than ST-segment *elevation.* Long-duration ST-segment changes (a single episode lasting >20–30 minutes or a cumulative duration >1–2 hours, either intraoperatively or postoperatively) seem to be more important than just the presence of postoperative ST-segment depression in the evolution of adverse cardiac outcomes (Fig. 5.4).

Diagnosis

In the perioperative period, ischemic episodes often are not associated with chest pain. In addition, many postoperative ECGs are not diagnostic. Nonspecific ECG changes, new-onset dysrhythmias, and noncardiac hemodynamic instability can further obscure the clinical picture of ACS in the perioperative period. Therefore the diagnosis of PMI may be quite difficult.

An acute increase in troponin levels does indicate MI in the perioperative setting. The increase in cardiac troponin levels is a marker of myocardial injury, and there is a good correlation between the duration of myocardial ischemia and the increase in the level of cardiac-specific troponin. There is also a significant association between increased troponin levels and short- and long-term morbidity and mortality in surgical patients. This association exists for cardiac death, MI, myocardial ischemia, congestive heart failure, cardiac dysrhythmias, and stroke. Even relatively minor cardiovascular complications such as uncontrolled hypertension, palpitations, increased fatigue, and shortness of breath can be correlated with increased levels of cardiac-specific troponins. An increase in troponin level postoperatively, even in the absence of clear cardiovascular signs and symptoms, is an important finding that requires careful attention and management. A new wall motion abnormality on echocardiography associated with a rise in troponin confirms the diagnosis of PMI.

PREOPERATIVE ASSESSMENT OF PATIENTS WITH KNOWN OR SUSPECTED ISCHEMIC HEART DISEASE

History

Preoperative history taking is meant to elicit the severity, progression, and functional limitations imposed by ischemic heart disease. It should focus on determining the presence of clinical risk factors in a particular patient (Table 5.5). Myocardial ischemia, left ventricular dysfunction, and cardiac dysrhythmias are usually responsible for the signs and symptoms of ischemic heart disease. Symptoms such as angina and

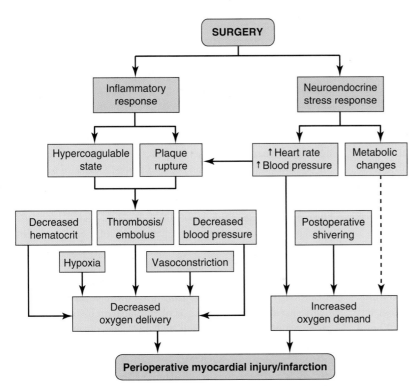

FIG. 5.4 Factors that can contribute to perioperative myocardial infarction. ↑, Increased.

TABLE 5.5	Clinical Predictors of Increased Perioperative Cardiovascular Risk

Unstable coronary syndromes
Acute or recent MI with evidence of important ischemic risk based on clinical symptoms or noninvasive study
Unstable or severe angina
Decompensated heart failure
Significant dysrhythmias
High-grade atrioventricular block
Symptomatic ventricular dysrhythmias in the presence of underlying heart disease
Supraventricular dysrhythmias with uncontrolled ventricular rate
Severe valvular heart disease
Mild angina pectoris
Previous MI based on history or Q waves on ECG
Compensated or previous heart failure
Diabetes mellitus (particularly insulin dependent)
Renal insufficiency
Age
Pulmonary hypertension

dyspnea may be absent at rest, which emphasizes the importance of evaluating the patient's response to various physical activities such as walking or climbing stairs. Limited exercise tolerance in the absence of significant lung disease is good evidence of decreased cardiac reserve. If a patient can climb two to three flights of stairs without symptoms, it is likely that cardiac reserve is adequate. Dyspnea after the onset of angina pectoris suggests the presence of acute left ventricular dysfunction caused by myocardial ischemia. In some patients, myocardial ischemia does not evoke chest pain or discomfort. *This silent myocardial ischemia usually occurs at a heart rate and blood pressure substantially lower than that present during exercise-induced ischemia.* It is estimated that nearly three-quarters of ischemic episodes in patients with symptomatic ischemic heart disease are not associated with angina pectoris, and 10%–15% of AMIs are silent. It is important to recognize the presence of incipient congestive heart failure, because the added stresses of anesthesia, surgery, fluid replacement, and pain may result in overt congestive heart failure.

A history of MI is an important piece of information. Using a discharge database of more than a half-million patients, it was shown that the postoperative MI rate in patients with a recent MI decreased substantially as the length of time from the prior MI to the time of surgery increased: less than 1 month = 32.8%, 1–2 months = 18.7%, 2–3 months = 8.4%, and 3–6 months = 5.9%. The 30-day mortality also decreased as time since the recent MI increased.

The importance of the timing of a recent MI in relation to the proposed surgery may, however, be changing in this era of thrombolytic therapy, angioplasty/stents, and risk stratification. Although many patients with a history of MI continue to have myocardium at risk, others may not. If a stress test does not indicate residual myocardium at risk, the likelihood of reinfarction is low. The current American Heart Association/American College of Cardiology (AHA/ACC) guidelines for perioperative cardiovascular evaluation suggest that more

than 60 days should elapse after an MI before noncardiac surgery is undertaken in the absence of coronary intervention.

It is important to determine whether a patient has undergone cardiac revascularization with PCI and stent placement or CABG. Stent placement (drug-eluting or bare-metal stent) is routinely followed by postprocedure dual antiplatelet therapy to prevent acute coronary thrombosis and maintain the long-term patency of the stent. It is prudent to delay elective noncardiac surgery for 4–6 weeks after PCI with bare-metal stent placement and as long as 12 months with drug-eluting stent placement. Ideally, elective noncardiac surgery should be delayed for 6 weeks after CABG surgery.

The presence of aortic stenosis is associated with a twofold to threefold increase in perioperative cardiac morbidity and mortality. Patients with *critical* aortic stenosis have the highest risk of cardiac decompensation after noncardiac surgery. Mitral valve disease is associated with a lesser risk. Regurgitant valve lesions have less risk than stenotic lesions. The presence of prosthetic heart valves should be noted, since patients with these valves will require perioperative endocarditis prophylaxis and adjustment of their anticoagulation regimens.

The history should also elicit information relevant to co-existing noncardiac disease. For example, patients with ischemic heart disease are likely to have peripheral vascular disease. A history of syncope may reflect cerebrovascular disease, a seizure disorder, or cardiac dysrhythmias. Cough is often pulmonary rather than cardiac in origin. It may be difficult to differentiate dyspnea caused by cardiac dysfunction from that caused by chronic lung disease, although patients with ischemic heart disease more often complain of orthopnea and paroxysmal nocturnal dyspnea. Chronic obstructive pulmonary disease is likely in patients with a long history of cigarette smoking. Diabetes mellitus often co-exists with ischemic heart disease. Renal insufficiency (creatinine level > 2.0 mg/dL) increases the risk of perioperative cardiac events.

A history of pulmonary hypertension should also be determined. Patients with pulmonary artery hypertension are at an increased risk of cardiopulmonary complications after noncardiac surgery. Mortality rates of 4%–26% and cardiorespiratory morbidity rates of 6%–42% have been reported.

Medical treatment of ischemic heart disease is designed to decrease myocardial oxygen requirements, improve coronary blood flow, stabilize plaque, prevent thrombosis, and remodel the injured myocardium. These goals are achieved by the use of β-blockers, nitrates, calcium entry blockers, statins, antiplatelet drugs, and ACE inhibitors. Effective β-blockade is suggested by a resting heart rate of 50–60 beats per minute. Routine physical activity is expected to increase the heart rate by 10%–20%. There is no evidence that β-blockers enhance the negative inotropic effects of volatile anesthetics. *β-Blocker therapy should be continued throughout the perioperative period.* Atropine or glycopyrrolate can be used to treat excessive bradycardia caused by β-blockers during the perioperative period. Isoproterenol is the specific pharmacologic antagonist for excessive β-blocker activity. The postoperative period is a time when inadvertent withdrawal of β-blocker therapy may occur and result in rebound hypertension and tachycardia.

Significant hypotension has been observed in patients receiving long-term treatment with ACE inhibitors who undergo general anesthesia. Many recommend withholding ACE inhibitors for 24 hours before surgery involving significant fluid shifts or blood loss. Hypotension attributable to ACE inhibitors is usually responsive to fluids or sympathomimetic drugs. If hypotension is refractory to these measures, treatment with vasopressin or one of its analogues may be required.

Antiplatelet drugs are an essential component in the pharmacotherapy of ACS and long-term management of ischemic heart disease. The use of dual antiplatelet therapy precludes neuraxial anesthesia and increases the risk of perioperative bleeding, which may then require platelet transfusion.

Physical Examination

The physical examination of patients with ischemic heart disease often yields normal findings. Nevertheless, signs of right and left ventricular dysfunction must be sought. A carotid bruit may indicate cerebrovascular disease. Orthostatic hypotension may reflect attenuated autonomic nervous system activity because of treatment with antihypertensive drugs. Jugular venous distention and peripheral edema are signs of right ventricular dysfunction. Auscultation of the chest may reveal evidence of left ventricular dysfunction such as an S_3 gallop or rales.

Specialized Preoperative Testing

Specialized preoperative testing should be limited to circumstances in which the results will affect perioperative patient management and outcomes. A conservative approach is recommended. Coronary revascularization before noncardiac surgery to enable the patient to "get through" the noncardiac procedure is inappropriate. However, in a high-risk subset of patients, such as those with left main coronary artery disease, severe multivessel coronary artery disease, severe aortic stenosis, and or ejection fraction less than 20%, coronary revascularization/valve replacement might be indicated. Currently there is overwhelming agreement that aggressive medical management to provide myocardial protection during the perioperative period is a critical element in the reduction of perioperative cardiovascular complications.

Specialized preoperative cardiac testing might include exercise ECG, stress ECG, radionuclide scintigraphy, and cardiac catheterization. Radionuclide ventriculography is rarely performed now, and high-speed CT, MRI, and positron emission tomography scanning *do not* have an established role in preoperative cardiac risk stratification algorithms.

Exercise Electrocardiography

Physiologic exercise provides an estimate of functional capacity, blood pressure, and heart rate response to stress and detection of myocardial ischemia by ST-segment changes.

A preoperative exercise stress test is appealing because perioperative increases in myocardial oxygen consumption and the development of myocardial ischemia are often accompanied by tachycardia. However, the utility of the exercise ECG can vary significantly. Preexisting ST-segment abnormalities hamper reliable ST-segment analysis, and treadmill testing has a rather low sensitivity (74%) and specificity (69%), comparable with information gleaned from daily clinical practice. Preoperative exercise stress testing is *not indicated* in patients with stable coronary artery disease and acceptable exercise tolerance.

Stress Echocardiography and Stress Nuclear Imaging

Pharmacologic stress testing with dobutamine, dipyridamole, adenosine, or regadenoson, and myocardial perfusion imaging with thallium 201 and/or technetium 99m and rubidium 82, can be used in patients undergoing noncardiac surgery who cannot perform enough exercise to detect stress-induced myocardial ischemia. *Reversible wall motion abnormalities* on echocardiography or *reversible perfusion defects* on radionuclide imaging suggest ischemia.

Myocardial perfusion imaging and dobutamine stress echocardiography before vascular surgery predict PMI or death with a positive predictive value of only 12%–14% but a negative predictive value of 88%–94%. Thus patients with a *normal scan/echo* have an excellent prognosis.

Selection of a noninvasive stress test should be based primarily on patient characteristics, local availability, and expertise in interpretation. Dobutamine stress echocardiography is the preferred test if there is an additional question regarding valvular function or LV function.

Computed Tomography and Magnetic Resonance Imaging

High-speed CT can visualize coronary artery calcification. Intravenous administration of radiographic contrast media enhances the clarity of the images. MRI provides even greater image clarity and can delineate the proximal portions of the coronary arterial circulation. However, there are currently no data regarding the place of these modalities in preoperative risk stratification. Furthermore, CT and MRI are more expensive and less mobile than other modalities of cardiac evaluation.

MANAGEMENT OF ANESTHESIA IN PATIENTS WITH KNOWN OR SUSPECTED ISCHEMIC HEART DISEASE UNDERGOING NONCARDIAC SURGERY

Preoperative management of patients with ischemic heart disease or risk factors for ischemic heart disease is geared toward the following goals: (1) determining the extent of ischemic heart disease and any previous interventions (CABG, PCI), (2) assessing the severity and stability of the disease, and (3) reviewing medical therapy and noting any drugs that can increase the risk of surgical bleeding or contraindicate use of a particular anesthetic technique. The first two goals are important in risk stratification.

TABLE 5.6	Cardiac Risk Factors in Patients Undergoing Elective Major Noncardiac Surgery

1. High-risk surgery
   Abdominal aortic aneurysm
   Peripheral vascular operation
   Thoracotomy
   Major abdominal operation
2. Ischemic heart disease
   History of myocardial infarction
   History of a positive finding on exercise testing
   Current complaints of angina pectoris
   Use of nitrate therapy
   Presence of Q waves on ECG
3. Congestive heart failure
   History of congestive heart failure
   History of pulmonary edema
   History of paroxysmal nocturnal dyspnea
   Physical examination showing rales or S_3 gallop
   Chest radiograph showing pulmonary vascular redistribution
4. Cerebrovascular disease
   History of stroke
   History of transient ischemic attack
5. Insulin-dependent diabetes mellitus
6. Preoperative serum creatinine concentration > 2 mg/dL

Adapted from Lee TH, Marcantonio ER, Mangione CM, et al. Derivation and prospective validation of a simple index for prediction of cardiac risk of major noncardiac surgery. *Circulation*. 1999;100:1043-1049.

Risk Stratification

For patients in stable condition undergoing elective major noncardiac surgery, six independent predictors of major cardiac complications have been identified and included in the Lee Revised Cardiac Risk Index (RCRI) (Table 5.6). These six predictors are (1) high-risk surgery, (2) history of ischemic heart disease, (3) history of congestive heart failure, (4) history of cerebrovascular disease, (5) preoperative insulin-dependent diabetes mellitus, and (6) preoperative serum creatinine over 2.0 mg/dL. The more risk factors present in a patient, the greater the probability of perioperative cardiac complications such as cardiac death, cardiac arrest or ventricular fibrillation, complete heart block, AMI, and pulmonary edema (Fig. 5.5). These risk factors have been incorporated into the ACC/AHA guidelines for perioperative cardiovascular evaluation for noncardiac surgery. A principal theme of these guidelines is that preoperative intervention is rarely necessary simply to lower the risk of surgery. An intervention is indicated or not indicated regardless of the need for surgery. Preoperative testing should be performed only if the result is likely to influence perioperative management. Although no prospective randomized study has been conducted to prove the efficacy of these guidelines, they offer a paradigm that has been widely adopted by clinicians. The 2014 ACC/AHA guidelines have been simplified from earlier versions. Rather than classifying patients into 9 groups based on 3 clinical risk groups and 3 surgical risk groups, the 2014 ACC/AHA guidelines categorize patients into only 2 groups—low risk and elevated risk—based on the presence of clinical risk factors and the risk of the surgery. Patients with a less than 1% chance of major adverse cardiac events are categorized as low risk, whereas patients with a cumulative risk of major adverse cardiac events greater than 1% are categorized as elevated risk. Patients who have more than 2 RCRI risk factors are considered to be elevated risk.

Two other indices for risk stratification are the American College of Surgeons' (ACS) National Surgical Quality Improvement Program (NSQIP) Myocardial Infarction and Cardiac Arrest (MICA) Risk Calculator, and the ACS NSQIP Surgical Risk Calculator (http://riskcalculator.facs.org/). Both can be used to evaluate patients preoperatively.

Though the new ACC/AHA guidelines do not categorize clinical predictors of major adverse cardiac events into major, intermediate, and minor factors, some of the following clinical factors may significantly increase the risk of perioperative adverse cardiac events:

- **Unstable coronary syndromes:** acute (MI ≤ 7 days before examination) or recent MI (>7 days but ≤ 1 month ago) with evidence of important ischemic risk by clinical symptoms or noninvasive study. It is suggested that more than 60 days should elapse after a recent MI before noncardiac surgery is undertaken (in the absence of coronary intervention).
- **Unstable or severe angina** (angina causing a marked limitation of ordinary physical activity at a normal pace or angina so severe as to prevent any physical activity without discomfort)
- **Decompensated heart failure:** patients with active heart failure have a significantly higher risk of postoperative death than do patients with coronary artery disease but no heart failure.
- **Severe valvular heart disease:** severe aortic stenosis or severe mitral stenosis. Left-sided regurgitant lesions convey an increased cardiac risk during noncardiac surgery but are better tolerated than stenotic valvular lesions.
- **Significant dysrhythmias:** High-grade atrioventricular block, Mobitz type II atrioventricular block, third-degree heart block, and symptomatic supraventricular and ventricular tachydysrhythmias may increase operative risk.
- **Age** is considered a risk factor, especially when it is associated with frailty. However, its exact role needs to be refined.

The ACC/AHA guidelines provide an algorithm for determining the need for preoperative cardiac evaluation. The first step assesses the urgency of the surgery. The need for emergency surgery takes precedence over the need for any additional workup (Fig. 5.6). Subsequent steps of the ACC/AHA guidelines integrate risk stratification according to risk classification, unstable clinical risk factors, and functional capacity. Patients who present for elective surgery and have any of the unstable clinical risk factors (unstable coronary syndrome, decompensated heart failure, significant dysrhythmias, severe valvular heart disease) may require delay of elective surgery, cardiologic evaluation, and optimization prior to elective surgery. Intensive preoperative management is necessary if surgery is urgent or emergent. For patients classified as low risk,

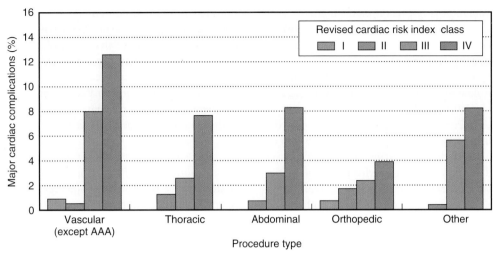

FIG. 5.5 Rates of major cardiac complications in patients in various Revised Cardiac Risk Index risk classes according to the type of surgery performed. Note that by definition, patients undergoing abdominal aortic aneurysm (AAA), thoracic, and abdominal procedures are excluded from risk class I because these operations are all considered high-risk surgery. In all subsets there was a statistically significant trend toward greater risk with higher risk class. (Adapted from Lee TH, Marcantonio ER, Mangione CM, et al. Derivation and prospective validation of a simple index for prediction of cardiac risk of major noncardiac surgery. *Circulation.* 1999;100:1043-1049.)

	Unstable clinical risk factors	Stable clinical factors	
Elevated risk (>1%)	Emergency surgery or further evaluation	<4 METs or indeterminate functional capacity + 2 or more RCRI - Further evaluation	>4 METs functional capacity - Proceed to surgery
Low risk (<1%)	Emergency surgery or further evaluation	Proceed to surgery	Proceed to surgery

FIG. 5.6 Algorithm for preoperative assessment of patients with ischemic heart disease. The need for emergency surgery takes precedence over the need for additional workup. Patients who have any of the unstable clinical risk factors (unstable coronary syndrome, decompensated heart failure, significant dysrhythmias, severe valvular heart disease) may require delay of elective surgery, cardiologic evaluation, and optimization prior to elective surgery. Subsequent steps of the ACC/ AHA guidelines integrate risk stratification according to risk classification, number of clinical risk factors, and functional capacity. For patients classified as low risk, further cardiac evaluation is not recommended, and they can proceed to surgery. For patients who are stratified into elevated-risk category and presenting for elective surgery, the next step is to determine their functional capacity. Patients stratified into elevated-risk category with good functional capacity (>4 METs) can proceed to surgery without further testing. Patients stratified into elevated-risk category with low functional capacity and/or in whom functional capacity cannot be determined can be referred for pharmacologic stress testing if the testing will impact further management. *MET,* Metabolic equivalent of the task; *RCRI,* Revised Cardiac Risk Index.

further cardiac evaluation is not recommended and patients can proceed to surgery. Patients stratified into the elevated-risk category and scheduled for elective surgery need to have their functional capacity determined.

Functional capacity or *exercise tolerance* can be expressed in metabolic equivalent of the task (MET) units. Oxygen consumption in a 70-kg, 40-year-old man in a resting state is 3.5 mL/kg/min or 1 MET. Perioperative cardiac risk is increased in patients with poor functional capacity—that is, those who are unable to meet a 4-MET demand during normal daily activities. These individuals may be able to perform some activities, such as baking, slow ballroom dancing, golfing (riding in a cart), or walking at a speed of approximately 2–3 mph, but are unable to perform more strenuous activity without developing chest pain or significant shortness of breath. The ability to participate in activities requiring more than 4 METs indicates good functional capacity.

According to the most recent ACC/AHA guidelines, patients stratified into the elevated-risk category but with a good functional capacity (>4 METs) can proceed to surgery without further testing. Patients stratified into the elevated-risk category but with a low functional capacity or in whom functional capacity cannot be determined can be referred for pharmacologic stress testing if the testing will impact further management. If such testing is negative, this elevated-risk patient can proceed to surgery. If the stress test is abnormal, coronary angiography and revascularization can be considered, depending on the degree that the test is abnormal, or the patient can proceed to surgery with *maximum medical management.* Preoperative coronary angiography is most suitable for patients with stress test results suggesting significant myocardium at risk. The aim of the angiographic study would be to identify very significant coronary artery disease (i.e., left main or severe multivessel coronary artery disease). Further management in such a patient would be dictated by the patient's clinical condition, the overall risk of an intervention, and available resources.

Management After Risk Stratification

The fundamental reason for risk stratification is to identify patients at increased risk so as to manage them with pharmacologic and other perioperative interventions that can lessen the risk and/or severity of perioperative cardiac events. Three therapeutic options are available prior to elective noncardiac surgery: (1) revascularization by cardiac surgery, (2) revascularization by PCI, and (3) optimal medical management.

In nonoperative settings, treatment strategies such as PCI (with or without stenting), CABG surgery, and medical therapy have proven efficacious in improving long-term morbidity and mortality. Patients with significant ischemic heart disease who come for noncardiac surgery are likely to be candidates for one or more of these therapies *regardless of their need for surgery.* Coronary interventions should be guided by the patient's cardiac condition and by the potential consequences of delaying surgery for recovery from the revascularization.

Coronary Artery Bypass Grafting

For CABG surgery to be beneficial before noncardiac surgery, the institutional risk of that particular noncardiac operation should be greater than the combined risk of coronary catheterization and coronary revascularization plus the generally reported risk of that noncardiac operation. The indications for preoperative surgical coronary revascularization are the same as those in the nonoperative setting.

Percutaneous Coronary Intervention

It was thought that PCI before elective noncardiac surgery could improve perioperative outcomes. However, PCI, which is now often accompanied by stenting and dual antiplatelet therapy, poses its own unique set of problems that need to be considered in patients who are scheduled to undergo elective noncardiac surgery. *There is no value in preoperative coronary intervention in a patient with stable ischemic heart disease.*

Pharmacologic Management

In view of the serious perioperative problems that PCIs pose and the lack of utility of CABG or PCI in patients with stable coronary artery disease, very few patients with stable coronary artery disease will undergo revascularization before surgery. Most patients with stable coronary artery disease and/or risk factors for coronary artery disease will be managed pharmacologically, as will patients with significant ischemic heart disease who come for emergent or urgent surgery.

Several drugs have been used to reduce perioperative myocardial injury. These are drugs that have demonstrated efficacy in the management of coronary ischemia in the nonsurgical setting. Nitroglycerin may be helpful in the management of active perioperative ischemia. However, prophylactic use of nitroglycerin has not been shown to be efficacious in reducing perioperative morbidity and mortality.

β-Blockers reduce myocardial oxygen consumption, improve coronary blood flow by prolonging diastole, improve the supply/demand ratio, stabilize cellular membranes, improve oxygen dissociation from hemoglobin, and inhibit platelet aggregation. β-Blockers suppress perioperative tachycardia and appear most efficacious in preventing perioperative myocardial ischemia. In view of all of these beneficial effects, prophylactic use of β-blockers to decrease PMI has been explored in many trials. In 2014 the ACC/AHA conducted a systematic review on this topic. The main findings were: (1) preoperative use of β-blockers was associated with a reduction in cardiac events, but there were little data to support the effectiveness of preoperative administration of β-blockers to reduce the risk of *surgical death;* and (2) a clear association exists between β-blocker administration and adverse outcomes such as bradycardia and stroke.

Currently the only class I recommendation by the ACC/AHA for perioperative β-blockers is to continue their use in the patients who are already on β-blockers. β-Blockers can be used in patients with elevated risk, especially in those with ischemia on preoperative stress testing or those with three or more RCRI risk factors. If β-blockers are to be used for pro-phylactic purposes, they should be slowly titrated (over 2–7 days prior to elective surgery), and acute administration of high-dose β-blockers in high-risk patients undergoing low-risk surgery is not recommended. Questions regarding the choice of β-blocker and the target heart rate are still unresolved. For ease of dosing and consistency of effect, longer-acting β-blockers, such as atenolol or bisoprolol, may be more efficacious in the perioperative period.

α2-Agonists such as clonidine decrease sympathetic out-flow, blood pressure, and heart rate. Older studies suggested a possible beneficial effect of clonidine perioperatively, but more recent trials failed to show any statistically significant benefits of clonidine in reducing 30-day mortality or the risk of nonfa-tal MI in patients with atherosclerosis undergoing noncardiac surgery. Based on the ACC/AHA guidelines, α2-agonists for prevention of cardiac events are not recommended in patients undergoing noncardiac surgery.

Statins are used for their *lipid-lowering effects* and are widely prescribed in patients with or at risk of ischemic heart disease. Statins also induce coronary plaque stabilization by decreas-ing lipid oxidation, inflammation, matrix metalloproteinase, and cell death. These so-called *nonlipid or pleiotropic effects* may prevent plaque rupture and subsequent MI in the peri-operative period. Trials show that statins can reduce mortality significantly in noncardiac surgery (by 44%) and in vascular surgery (by 59%). Evidence to date suggests a protective effect of perioperative statin use on cardiac complications during noncardiac surgery. The ACC/AHA guidelines recommend continuing statin therapy in patients scheduled for noncardiac surgery.

Controlling hyperglycemia in patients undergoing cardiac surgery and in patients in intensive care units has been asso-ciated with improved outcomes. Recognizing that insulin has some beneficial nonmetabolic effects and noting the harm-ful effects of hyperglycemia, it is prudent to actively manage hyperglycemia with insulin during noncardiac surgery. This is especially important in patients who are at high risk of cardiac injury. The goal in this situation is to keep the perioperative glucose below 180 mg/dL.

Because several pathophysiologic mechanisms can trigger a PMI, it seems reasonable to think that multimodal therapy with β-blockers, statins, and insulin may be more beneficial than treatment with any single drug (Fig. 5.7).

Intraoperative Management

The basic challenges during induction and maintenance of anesthesia in patients with ischemic heart disease are (1) to prevent myocardial ischemia by optimizing myocardial oxy-gen supply and reducing myocardial oxygen demand, (2) to monitor for ischemia, and (3) to treat ischemia if it develops. Intraoperative events associated with persistent tachycardia, systolic hypertension, sympathetic nervous system stimula-tion, arterial hypoxemia, or hypotension can adversely affect the patient with ischemic heart disease (Table 5.7). Periop-erative myocardial injury is closely associated with heart rate in vascular surgery patients. A rapid heart rate increases

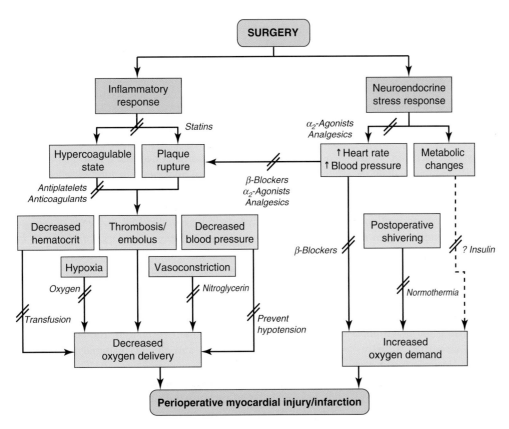

FIG. 5.7 Interventions that can modulate triggers of perioperative myocardial injury. ↑, Increased.

TABLE 5.7	Intraoperative Events That Influence the Balance Between Myocardial Oxygen Delivery and Myocardial Oxygen Requirements

DECREASED OXYGEN DELIVERY

Decreased coronary blood flow
Tachycardia
Hypotension
Hypocapnia (coronary artery vasoconstriction)
Coronary artery spasm
Decreased oxygen content
Anemia
Arterial hypoxemia
Shift of the oxyhemoglobin dissociation curve to the left

INCREASED OXYGEN REQUIREMENTS

Sympathetic nervous system stimulation
Tachycardia
Hypertension
Increased myocardial contractility
Increased afterload
Increased preload

myocardial oxygen requirements and decreases diastolic time for coronary blood flow and therefore oxygen delivery. The increased oxygen requirements produced by hypertension are offset to some degree by improved coronary perfusion. Hyperventilation must be avoided because hypocapnia may cause coronary artery vasoconstriction. Maintenance of the balance between myocardial oxygen supply and demand is more important than which specific anesthetic technique or drugs are selected to produce anesthesia and muscle relaxation.

It is important to avoid persistent and excessive changes in heart rate and blood pressure. A common recommendation is to keep the heart rate and blood pressure within 20% of the normal awake value for that patient. However, many episodes of intraoperative myocardial ischemia occur in the absence of hemodynamic changes. These episodes may be due to regional decreases in myocardial perfusion. It is unlikely that this form of ischemia can be prevented by the anesthesiologist.

Induction of anesthesia in patients with ischemic heart disease can be accomplished with an IV induction drug. A meta-analysis of more than 6000 patients undergoing noncardiac surgery failed to demonstrate a difference in PMI rates between patients who received volatile anesthesia and patients who received total IV anesthesia. Tracheal intubation can be facilitated by administration of succinylcholine or a nondepolarizing muscle relaxant.

Myocardial ischemia may accompany the sympathetic stimulation that results from direct laryngoscopy and endotracheal intubation. Keeping the duration of direct laryngoscopy short (≤15 seconds) is useful in minimizing the magnitude and duration of the circulatory changes associated with tracheal intubation. If the duration of direct laryngoscopy is not likely to be brief or if hypertension already exists, it is reasonable to consider administering drugs to minimize the sympathetic response. Laryngotracheal lidocaine, IV lidocaine,

esmolol, fentanyl, remifentanil, and dexmedetomidine have all been shown to be useful for blunting the increase in heart rate evoked by tracheal intubation.

In patients with normal left ventricular function, tachycardia and hypertension are likely to develop in response to intense stimulation, such as during direct laryngoscopy or painful surgical stimulation. Achieving controlled myocardial depression using a volatile anesthetic may be useful in such patients to minimize the increase in sympathetic nervous system activity. Overall, volatile anesthetics may be beneficial in patients with ischemic heart disease, because they decrease myocardial oxygen requirements and may precondition the myocardium to tolerate ischemic events, or they may be detrimental because they lead to a decrease in blood pressure and an associated reduction in coronary perfusion pressure. The current AHA guidelines state that "use of either a volatile anesthetic agent or total intravenous anesthesia is reasonable for patients undergoing noncardiac surgery, and the choice is determined by factors other than the prevention of myocardial ischemia and MI."

The use of nitrous oxide in patients with a history of coronary artery disease has been questioned since the early 1990s when animal and human studies showed an increase in pulmonary vascular resistance, diastolic dysfunction, and myocardial ischemia with its use. However, subsequent data showed that nitrous oxide did *not* increase the risk of death and cardiovascular complications or surgical site infection. Thus the use of nitrous oxide in patients with coronary artery disease is not contraindicated.

Patients with severely impaired left ventricular function may not tolerate anesthesia-induced myocardial depression. Opioids may then be selected as the principal anesthetic. The addition of nitrous oxide, a benzodiazepine, or a low dose of volatile anesthetic may be needed to supplement the opioid because amnesia cannot be insured with an opioid anesthetic.

Regional anesthesia is an acceptable technique in patients with ischemic heart disease. However, the decrease in blood pressure associated with epidural or spinal anesthesia must be controlled. Prompt treatment of hypotension that exceeds 20% of the preblock blood pressure is necessary. Potential benefits from the use of a regional anesthetic include excellent pain control, a decreased incidence of deep venous thrombosis in some patients, and the opportunity to continue the block into the postoperative period. However, *the incidence of perioperative cardiac morbidity and mortality does not appear to be significantly different for general and regional anesthesia.* The current guidelines recommend that the choice of anesthesia is best left to the discretion of the anesthesia care team, who will consider the need for postoperative mechanical ventilation, pulmonary/neuromuscular comorbidities, cardiovascular effects (including myocardial depression), the consequences of sympathetic blockade, and the dermatomal level of the procedure.

Muscle relaxants with minimal or no effect on heart rate and systemic blood pressure (vecuronium, rocuronium, cisatracurium) are attractive choices for patients with ischemic

TABLE 5.8	Relationship of ECG Leads to Areas of Myocardial Ischemia	
ECG Lead	Coronary Artery Responsible for Ischemia	Area of Myocardium That May Be Involved
II, III, aVF	Right coronary artery	Right atrium Right ventricle Sinoatrial node Inferior aspect of left ventricle Atrioventricular node
I, aVL	Circumflex coronary artery	Lateral aspect of left ventricle
V_3-V_5	Left anterior descending coronary artery	Anterolateral aspect of left ventricle

heart disease. The histamine release and resulting decrease in blood pressure caused by atracurium and the increase in heart rate caused by pancuronium make these drugs less desirable choices.

Reversal of neuromuscular blockade with an anticholinesterase-anticholinergic drug combination can be safely accomplished in patients with ischemic heart disease. Glycopyrrolate, which has much less chronotropic effect and central effect than atropine, is preferred in these patients.

Monitoring

The type of perioperative monitoring is influenced by the complexity of the operative procedure and the severity of the ischemic heart disease. The most important goal in selecting monitoring methods is to select those that allow *early detection of myocardial ischemia*. Since most myocardial ischemia occurs in the absence of hemodynamic alterations, one should be cautious in endorsing routine use of expensive or complex monitors to detect myocardial ischemia.

The simplest, most cost-effective method for detecting perioperative myocardial ischemia is standard ECG. The diagnosis of myocardial ischemia focuses on changes in the ST segment, characterized as elevation or depression of at least 1 mm and T-wave inversions. The degree of ST-segment depression parallels the severity of myocardial ischemia. Because visual detection of ST-segment changes can be unreliable, computerized ST-segment analysis has been incorporated into ECG monitors. Traditionally, monitoring of two leads (leads II and V_5) has been the standard, but it appears that monitoring three leads (leads II, V_4, and V_5, or else V_3, V_4, and V_5) may improve the ability to detect ischemia. There is also a correlation between the lead of the ECG that detects myocardial ischemia and the anatomic distribution of the diseased coronary artery (Table 5.8). For example, the V_5 lead (fifth intercostal space in the anterior axillary line) reflects myocardial ischemia in the portion of the left ventricle supplied by the left anterior descending coronary artery (Fig. 5.8). Lead II is more likely to detect myocardial ischemia occurring in the distribution of the right coronary artery. Lead II is also very useful for analysis of cardiac rhythm disturbances.

Events other than myocardial ischemia that can cause ST-segment abnormalities include cardiac dysrhythmias, cardiac conduction disturbances, digitalis therapy, electrolyte abnormalities, and hypothermia. However, in patients with known or suspected coronary artery disease, it is reasonable to assume that intraoperative ST-segment changes represent myocardial ischemia. The occurrence and duration of intraoperative ST-segment changes in high-risk patients are linked to an increased incidence of PMI and adverse cardiac events. Interestingly *the overall incidence of myocardial ischemia is lower in the intraoperative period than in the preoperative or postoperative period.*

If pulmonary artery catheter monitoring is being used, intraoperative myocardial ischemia can manifest as an acute increase in pulmonary artery occlusion pressure (PAOP) due to changes in left ventricular compliance and left ventricular systolic performance. If myocardial ischemia is global or involves the papillary muscle, V waves may appear in the PAOP waveform. If only small regions of left ventricular myocardium become ischemic, overall ventricular compliance and pulmonary artery occlusion pressure will remain unchanged, so the pulmonary artery catheter is a relatively *insensitive* method of monitoring for myocardial ischemia. The pulmonary artery diastolic pressure is even less sensitive than the pulmonary artery occlusion pressure in detecting a change in left ventricular compliance. Right heart catheterization is therefore not recommended as an intraoperative ischemia monitor.

The development of new regional ventricular wall motion abnormalities seen on transesophageal echocardiography (TEE) is the accepted standard for the intraoperative diagnosis of myocardial ischemia. These regional wall motion abnormalities can occur before ECG changes are seen. However, segmental wall motion abnormalities may also occur in response to events other than myocardial ischemia. The limitations of TEE include its cost, the need for extensive training in interpreting the images, and the fact that the transducer cannot be inserted until after induction of anesthesia. There is then a critical period during which myocardial ischemia may develop, but this monitor is not in place to detect it. The ACC/AHA guidelines recommend the use of TEE intraoperatively or perioperatively to determine the cause of an acute, persistent, and life-threatening hemodynamic abnormality. However, its use as an ischemia monitor in noncardiac surgery is less validated and should only be considered in patients at high risk for developing myocardial ischemia during major noncardiac surgery. Routine use of intraoperative TEE during noncardiac surgery to monitor for myocardial ischemia is not recommended.

Intraoperative Management of Myocardial Ischemia

Treatment of myocardial ischemia should be instituted when there are 1-mm ST-segment changes on ECG. Prompt drug treatment of adverse changes in heart rate and/or blood pressure is indicated. Nitroglycerin is an appropriate choice when myocardial ischemia is associated with a normal or modestly elevated blood pressure. In this situation the

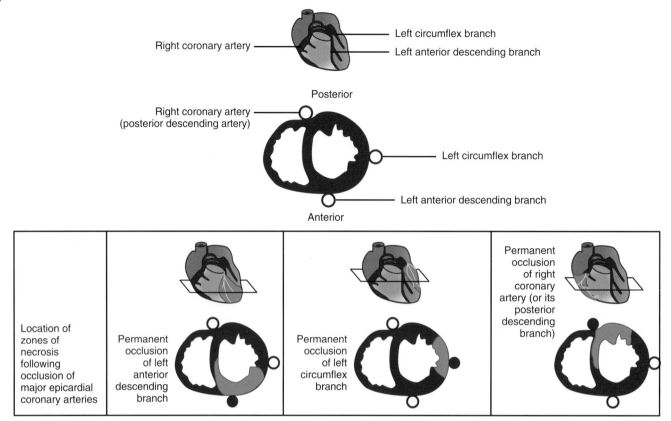

FIG. 5.8 Correlation of sites of coronary occlusion and zones of necrosis. (From Antman EM. ST-segment myocardial infarction: pathology, pathophysiology, and clinical features. In: Bonow RO, Mann DL, Zipes DP, et al., eds. *Braunwald's Heart Disease*. Philadelphia: Saunders; 2012: Fig. 54-4.)

nitroglycerin-induced coronary vasodilation and decrease in preload improve subendocardial blood flow, but the nitroglycerin-induced decrease in afterload does not decrease systemic blood pressure to the point that coronary perfusion pressure is jeopardized. A persistent increase in heart rate in the setting of normal or high blood pressure can also be treated by administration of a β-blocker such as esmolol.

Hypotension is treated with sympathomimetic drugs to restore coronary perfusion pressure. In addition to administration of vasoconstrictor drugs, fluid infusion can be useful to help restore blood pressure. Regardless of the treatment, prompt restoration of blood pressure is necessary to maintain pressure-dependent flow through narrowed coronary arteries. In an unstable hemodynamic situation, circulatory support with inotropes or an intraaortic balloon pump may be necessary. It may also be necessary to plan for early postoperative cardiac catheterization.

Postoperative Management

Although significant advances have been made in researching and refining preoperative evaluation and risk management strategies, evidence-based strategies that can be adopted in the postoperative period to improve outcome have not yet been developed.

The goals of postoperative management are the same as those for intraoperative management: prevent ischemia, monitor for myocardial injury, and treat myocardial ischemia or infarction. Any situation that leads to prolonged and significant hemodynamic perturbations can stress the heart. Intraoperative hypothermia may predispose to shivering on awakening, leading to abrupt and dramatic increases in myocardial oxygen requirements. Pain, hypoxemia, hypercarbia, sepsis, and hemorrhage also lead to increased myocardial oxygen demand. The resulting oxygen supply/demand imbalance in patients with ischemic heart disease can precipitate myocardial ischemia, infarction, or death. Although most adverse cardiac events occur within the first 48 hours postoperatively, delayed cardiac events can occur within the first 30 days and can be the result of secondary stresses. It is imperative that patients taking β-blockers and statins continue to receive these drugs throughout the perioperative period.

Prevention of hypovolemia and hypotension is necessary postoperatively, and not only an adequate intravascular volume but also an adequate hemoglobin concentration must be maintained (>7 g/dL [>8 g/dL in patients > 80 years]). Oxygen content and oxygen delivery depend significantly on the concentration of hemoglobin in blood. The degree of anemia that can be safely tolerated in patients with ischemic heart disease remains to be defined.

The timing of weaning from mechanical ventilation and tracheal extubation requires careful consideration. Early extubation is possible and desirable in many patients so long as they fulfill the criteria for extubation. However, patients with ischemic heart disease can become ischemic during emergence from anesthesia and/or weaning from mechanical ventilation. Any increase in heart rate and/or blood pressure must be managed promptly. Pharmacologic therapy with a β-blocker or a combined α- and β-blocker (e.g., labetalol) or a calcium channel blocker (e.g., nicardipine) can be very helpful.

Continuous ECG monitoring is useful for detecting postoperative myocardial ischemia, which is often silent. Postoperative myocardial ischemia predicts adverse in-hospital and long-term cardiac events. It should be identified, evaluated, and managed, preferably in consultation with a cardiologist.

CARDIAC TRANSPLANTATION

Cardiac transplantation is most often performed in patients with end-stage heart failure due to an ischemic or nonischemic cardiomyopathy, adult congenital heart disease, valvular heart disease, or a failing prior heart transplant. Preoperatively the ejection fraction is often less than 20%. *Irreversible pulmonary hypertension is a contraindication to cardiac transplantation,* and most centers do not consider candidates older than age 65 or with a life expectancy less than 2 years. Active infection, recent pulmonary thromboembolism with pulmonary infarction, irreversible renal or hepatic dysfunction, and active or recent (<5 years) solid organ or hematologic cancer are additional contraindications to heart transplantation.

Management of Anesthesia

Patients may come for cardiac transplantation with inotropic, vasodilator, or mechanical circulatory support. Additionally, they may have implanted antidysrhythmic devices (pacemaker, automatic implantable cardioverter-defibrillator [AICD]) and invasive hemodynamic monitors. Antidysrhythmic devices should be interrogated and reprogrammed to a mode that is not affected by electrical cautery. Most patients will not be in a fasting state and should be considered as having a full stomach. Patients can be anesthetized using a balanced anesthetic technique. Nitrous oxide is rarely used because significant pulmonary hypertension is often present, and there is concern about air embolism because large blood vessels are opened during the surgical procedure. Nondepolarizing neuromuscular blocking drugs that do not cause histamine release are usually selected. Many patients undergoing cardiac transplantation have coagulation disturbances due to passive congestion of the liver as a result of chronic congestive heart failure, or they may be on warfarin. Fresh frozen plasma may be required to normalize the coagulopathy and international normalized ratio (INR).

The operative technique includes cardiopulmonary bypass and anastomosis of the aorta, pulmonary artery, and left and right atria. Immunosuppressive drugs are usually begun during the preoperative period. *Intravascular catheters must be placed using strict aseptic technique.* It is necessary to withdraw the central venous or pulmonary artery catheter into the superior vena cava when the native heart is removed. The catheter can then be repositioned into the donor heart. These catheters are often inserted into the central circulation *via the left internal jugular vein* so that the right internal jugular vein is available when needed to perform endomyocardial biopsies during the postoperative period. TEE is used to monitor cardiac function intraoperatively.

After cessation of cardiopulmonary bypass, an inotropic drug may be needed briefly to maintain myocardial contractility and heart rate. Therapy to lower pulmonary vascular resistance may also be necessary and may include administration of a pulmonary vasodilator such as nitric oxide, isoproterenol, a prostaglandin, or a phosphodiesterase inhibitor. The denervated transplanted heart initially assumes an intrinsic heart rate of about 110 beats per minute, which reflects the absence of normal vagal tone. Stroke volume responds to an increase in preload by the Frank-Starling mechanism. *These patients tolerate hypovolemia poorly.* The transplanted heart does respond to direct-acting catecholamines, but drugs that act by indirect mechanisms, such as ephedrine, have a much less intense effect. Vasopressin may be needed to treat severe hypotension unresponsive to catecholamines. The heart rate does not change in response to administration of anticholinergic or anticholinesterase drugs. About 25% of patients develop bradycardia after cardiac transplantation that requires insertion of a permanent cardiac pacemaker.

Postoperative Complications

Right heart failure after cardiac transplantation occurs frequently and is responsible for approximately 20% of the early deaths after this procedure. Acute right heart failure may require urgent mechanical circulatory support and pulmonary vasodilation to prevent further hemodynamic compromise.

Cardiac transplant patients may require *β-adrenergic stimulants* for 3–4 days after transplantation. Early postoperative morbidity related to heart transplantation surgery usually involves sepsis and/or rejection. The most common early cause of death is opportunistic infection as a result of immunosuppressive therapy. Transvenous right ventricular endomyocardial biopsies are performed to provide early warning of asymptomatic allograft rejection. Congestive heart failure and development of dysrhythmias are late signs of rejection. Immunotherapy after cardiac transplantation typically involves corticosteroids and calcineurin inhibitors like cyclosporine or tacrolimus. Cyclosporine treatment can be associated with drug-induced hypertension that is often resistant to antihypertensive therapy. Nephrotoxicity is another complication of cyclosporine and tacrolimus therapy. Long-term corticosteroid use may result in skeletal demineralization and glucose intolerance.

Late complications of cardiac transplantation include development of coronary artery disease in the allograft and an increased incidence of cancer. Diffuse obliterative coronary arteriopathy affects cardiac transplant recipients over time, and the ischemic sequelae of this form of coronary artery disease are the principal limitations to long-term survival. This arterial disease is restricted to the allograft and is present in about half of cardiac transplant recipients after 5 years. The accelerated appearance of this coronary artery disease likely reflects a chronic rejection process in the vascular endothelium. This process is not unique to cardiac allografts and is thought to be analogous to the chronic immunologically mediated changes seen in other organ allografts (bronchiolitis obliterans in the lungs, vanishing bile duct syndrome in the liver). The clinical sequelae of this obliterative coronary artery disease include myocardial ischemia, left ventricular dysfunction, cardiac dysrhythmias, and sudden death. The prognosis for transplant recipients with angiographically established obliterative coronary artery disease is poor.

Any medical regimen involving long-term immunosuppression is associated with an increased incidence of cancer, especially lymphoproliferative and cutaneous cancers. Malignancy is responsible for a significant portion of the mortality of heart transplant patients. Most posttransplantation lymphoproliferative disease is related to infection with the Epstein-Barr virus.

Anesthetic Considerations in Heart Transplant Recipients

Heart transplant patients present unique anesthetic challenges because of the hemodynamic function of the transplanted denervated heart, the side effects of immunosuppressive therapy, the risk of infection, the potential for drug interactions (given the complex drug regimens), and the potential for allograft rejection.

Allograft rejection results in progressive deterioration of cardiac function. The presence and degree of rejection should be noted preoperatively. The presence of infection must also be noted because infection is a significant cause of morbidity and mortality in these patients. *Invasive monitoring requires the use of strict aseptic technique.* When hepatic and renal function are normal, there is no contraindication to the use of any anesthetic drug.

The transplanted heart has no sympathetic, parasympathetic, or sensory innervation, and the loss of vagal tone results in a higher-than-normal resting heart rate. Two P waves may be detectable on the ECG. The native sinus node remains intact if a cuff of atrium is left in place to permit surgical anastomosis to the grafted heart. Because the native P wave cannot traverse the suture line, it has no influence on the chronotropic activity of the heart. Carotid sinus massage and the Valsalva maneuver have no effect on heart rate. There is no sympathetic response to direct laryngoscopy and tracheal intubation, and the denervated heart has a blunted heart rate response to light anesthesia or intense pain. The transplanted heart is unable to increase its heart rate immediately in response to hypovolemia or hypotension but responds instead with an increase in

stroke volume via the Frank-Starling mechanism. The needed increase in cardiac output is dependent on venous return until the heart rate increases after several minutes in response to the effect of circulating catecholamines. Because α- and β-adrenergic receptors are intact on the transplanted heart, the heart will eventually respond to circulating catecholamines.

Cardiac dysrhythmias may occur in heart transplant patients, perhaps reflecting a lack of vagal innervation and/or increased levels of circulating catecholamines. At rest the heart rate reflects the intrinsic rate of depolarization of the donor sinoatrial node in the absence of any vagal tone. First-degree atrioventricular block (an increased PR interval) is common after cardiac transplantation. Some patients may require a cardiac pacemaker for treatment of bradydysrhythmias. A surgical transplantation technique that preserves the anatomic integrity of the right atrium by using anastomoses at the level of the superior and inferior vena cava rather than at the midatrial level results in better preservation of sinoatrial node and tricuspid valve function. Afferent denervation renders the cardiac transplant patient incapable of experiencing angina pectoris in response to myocardial ischemia.

Response to Drugs

Catecholamine responses are different in the transplanted heart because the intact sympathetic nerves required for normal uptake and metabolism of catecholamines are absent. The density of α and β receptors in the transplanted heart is unchanged, however, and responses to direct-acting sympathomimetic drugs are intact. Epinephrine, isoproterenol, and dobutamine have similar effects in normal and denervated hearts. Indirect-acting sympathomimetics such as ephedrine have a blunted effect in denervated hearts.

Vagolytic drugs such as atropine do not increase the heart rate. Pancuronium does not increase the heart rate, and neostigmine and other anticholinesterases do not slow the heart rate of denervated hearts.

Preoperative Evaluation

At presentation, heart transplant recipients may have ongoing rejection manifesting as myocardial dysfunction, accelerated coronary atherosclerosis, or dysrhythmias. All preoperative drug therapy must be continued, and proper functioning of a cardiac pacemaker must be confirmed. Cyclosporine-induced hypertension may require treatment with calcium channel–blocking drugs or ACE inhibitors. Cyclosporine or tacrolimus-induced nephrotoxicity may present as an increased creatinine concentration. In such cases, anesthetic drugs excreted mainly by renal clearance mechanisms should be avoided. Proper hydration is important and should be confirmed preoperatively because heart transplant patients are preload dependent.

Management of Anesthesia

Experience suggests that heart transplant recipients undergoing noncardiac surgery have monitoring and anesthetic requirements similar to those of other patients undergoing the same surgery. Intravascular volume must be maintained because these patients are *preload dependent* and the denervated heart is unable to respond to sudden shifts in blood volume with an increase in heart rate. TEE may be considered if the planned procedure is associated with large fluid shifts. General anesthesia is usually selected because there may be an impaired response to the hypotension associated with neuraxial anesthesia. Anesthetic management must include avoidance of significant vasodilation and acute reductions in preload. Although volatile anesthetics may produce myocardial depression, they are usually well tolerated in heart transplant patients who do not have significant heart failure. Despite reports of cyclosporine-induced enhanced neuromuscular blockade, it does not appear that these patients require different dosing of muscle relaxants than normal patients. Monitoring of neuromuscular blockade with a peripheral nerve stimulator will clarify any unusual dosing requirements. Careful attention must be paid to appropriate aseptic technique because of the increased susceptibility to infection.

KEY POINTS

- The exercise ECG is most likely to indicate myocardial ischemia when there is at least 1 mm of horizontal or downsloping ST-segment depression during or within 4 minutes after exercise. The greater the degree of ST-segment depression, the greater the likelihood of significant coronary disease. When the ST-segment abnormality is associated with angina pectoris and occurs during the early stages of exercise and persists for several minutes after exercise, significant coronary artery disease is very likely.

- Noninvasive imaging tests for the detection of ischemic heart disease are used when exercise ECG is not possible or interpretation of ST-segment changes would be difficult. Administration of atropine, infusion of dobutamine, institution of cardiac pacing, or administration of a coronary vasodilator such as adenosine or dipyridamole creates cardiac stress. After stress is induced, either echocardiography to assess myocardial function or radionuclide imaging to assess myocardial perfusion is performed.

- β-Blockers are the principal drug treatment for patients with angina pectoris. Long-term administration of β-blockers decreases the risk of death and myocardial reinfarction in patients who have had an MI, presumably by decreasing myocardial oxygen demand.

- Patients with acute coronary syndrome (ACS) can be categorized based on a 12-lead ECG. Patients with ST-segment elevation at presentation are considered to have STEMI. Patients who have ST-segment depression or nonspecific ECG changes can be classified based on the level of cardiac-specific troponins. Elevation of cardiac-specific biomarkers indicates NSTEMI. If levels of cardiac-specific biomarkers are normal, unstable angina (UA) is present.

- STEMI occurs when coronary blood flow decreases abruptly. This decrease in blood flow is attributable to acute thrombus formation at a site where an atherosclerotic plaque fissures, ruptures, or ulcerates, creating a local environment that favors thrombogenesis. Typically, vulnerable plaques—that is, those with rich lipid cores and thin fibrous caps—are most prone to rupture. The plaques that rupture are rarely of a size that causes significant coronary obstruction. By contrast, flow-restrictive plaques that produce stable angina pectoris and stimulate development of collateral circulation are less likely to rupture.

- The primary management goal of STEMI is reestablishment of blood flow in the obstructed coronary artery as soon as possible. This can be achieved by reperfusion therapy or coronary angioplasty with or without placement of an intracoronary stent.

- Administration of β-blockers after an AMI is associated with a significant decrease in early (in-hospital) and long-term mortality and myocardial reinfarction. Early administration of β-blockers can decrease infarct size by decreasing heart rate, blood pressure, and myocardial contractility. In the absence of specific contraindications, it is recommended that all patients receive intravenous β-blockers as soon as possible after AMI.

- NSTEMI and UA result from a reduction in myocardial oxygen supply. With an NSTEMI, rupture or erosion of an atherosclerotic coronary plaque leads to thrombosis, inflammation, and vasoconstriction. Embolization of platelets and clot fragments into the coronary microvasculature leads to microcirculatory ischemia and infarction and results in elevation of cardiac biomarker levels.

- Most postoperative MIs are NSTEMIs and can be diagnosed by ECG changes and/or release of cardiac biomarkers. Two different pathophysiologic mechanisms may be responsible for perioperative MI (PMI). One is related to acute coronary thrombosis, and the other, which is more common, is the consequence of increased myocardial oxygen demand in the setting of compromised myocardial oxygen supply.

- AMI (1–7 days previously), recent MI (8–30 days previously), and UA are associated with the highest risk of PMI, MI, and cardiac death.

- Coronary artery stent placement (drug-eluting or bare-metal stent) is routinely followed by dual antiplatelet therapy to prevent acute coronary thrombosis and maintain long-term patency of the stent. Elective noncardiac surgery should be delayed for at least 30 days after PCI with bare-metal stent placement and for at least 12 months after PCI with drug-eluting stent placement to allow endothelialization of the stent and completion of the course of dual antiplatelet therapy.

- Preoperative use of β-blockers has been associated with a reduction in cardiac events in the perioperative period, but little data support the effectiveness of administration of β-blockers to reduce the risk of surgical death. A clear association exists between β-blocker administration and adverse outcomes such as bradycardia and stroke. Currently the only class I recommendation for perioperative β-blocker use by the AHA/ACC is to continue their use in patients who are already taking them. β-Blockers can also be used in patients with elevated risk, especially those who have demonstrated ischemia on preoperative stress testing and those with three or more RCRI risk factors.

- Current AHA/ACC guidelines state that "use of either a volatile anesthetic agent or total intravenous anesthesia is reasonable for patients undergoing noncardiac surgery, and the choice is determined by factors other than the prevention of myocardial ischemia and MI."

- The transplanted heart has no sympathetic, parasympathetic, or sensory innervation, and the loss of vagal tone results in a higher-than-normal resting heart rate. Carotid sinus massage and the Valsalva maneuver have no effect on heart rate. There is no sympathetic response to direct laryngoscopy and tracheal intubation, and the denervated heart has a blunted heart rate response to light anesthesia or intense pain. The transplanted heart is unable to increase its heart rate immediately in response to hypovolemia or hypotension. It responds instead with an increase in stroke volume via the Frank-Starling mechanism. The needed increase in cardiac output is then dependent on venous return. After several minutes the heart rate increases in response to the effect of circulating catecholamines. Because α- and β-adrenergic receptors are intact on the transplanted heart, it eventually responds to circulating catecholamines.

RESOURCES

Antman EM, Loscalzo J. ST-segment elevation acute coronary syndrome. In: Braunwald E, Fauci AS, Kasper DL, et al. eds. *Harrison's Principles of Internal Medicine*. 19th ed. New York: McGraw-Hill; 2015:1599-1611.

Barash P, Akhtar S. Coronary stents: factors contributing to perioperative major adverse cardiovascular events. *Br J Anaesth*. 2010;105(suppl 1):i3-i15.

Cannon CP, Braunwald E. Non ST-segment elevation acute coronary syndrome. In: Braunwald E, Fauci AS, Kasper DL, et al. eds. *Harrison's Principles of Internal Medicine*. 19th ed. New York: McGraw-Hill; 2015:1593-1598.

Devereaux PJ, Yang H, Yusuf S, et al. Effects of extended-release metoprolol succinate in patients undergoing non-cardiac surgery (POISE trial): a randomized controlled trial. *Lancet*. 2008;371:1839-1847.

Devereaux PJ, Sessler DI, Leslie K, et al. Clonidine in patients undergoing noncardiac surgery. *N Engl J Med*. 2014;370:1504-1513.

Devereaux PJ, Mrkobrada M, Sessler DI, et al. Aspirin in patients undergoing noncardiac surgery. *N Engl J Med*. 2014;370:1494-1503.

Fischer S, Glas KE. A review of cardiac transplantation. *Anesthesiol Clin*. 2013;31:383-403.

Fleisher LA, Fleischmann KE, Auerbach AD, et al. 2014 ACC/AHA guideline on perioperative cardiovascular evaluation and management of patients undergoing noncardiac surgery: a report of the American College of Cardiology/American Heart Association Task Force on practice guidelines. *J Am Coll Cardiol*. 2014;64:e77-137.

Kristensen SD, Knuuti J, Saraste A, et al. Authors/Task Force Members: 2014 ESC/ESA Guidelines on non-cardiac surgery: cardiovascular assessment and management: the Joint Task Force on non-cardiac surgery: cardiovascular assessment and management of the European Society of Cardiology (ESC) and the European Society of Anaesthesiology (ESA). *Eur Heart J*. 2014;35:2383-2431.

Maurice-Szamburski A, Auquier P, Viarre-Oreal V, et al. Effect of sedative premedication on patient experience after general anesthesia: a randomized clinical trial. *JAMA*. 2015;313:916-925.

Myles PS, Leslie K, Chan MTV, et al. The safety of addition of nitrous oxide to general anaesthesia in at-risk patients having major non-cardiac surgery (ENIGMA-II): a randomized, single-blind trial. *Lancet*. 2014;384:1446-1454.

Opie L, Poole-Wilson P. Beta-blocking agents. In: Opie L, Gersh BJ, eds. *Drugs for the Heart*. Philadelphia: Saunders; 2009.

Ohman EM. Chronic stable angina. *N Engl J Med*. 2016;374:1167-1176.

Porter TR, Shillcutt SK, Adams MS, et al. Guidelines for the use of echocardiography as a monitor for therapeutic intervention in adults: a report from the American Society of Echocardiography. *J Am Soc Echocardiogr*. 2015;28:40-56.

Thygesen K, Alpert JS, Jaffe AS, et al. Third universal definition of myocardial infarction. *Circulation*. 2012;126:2020-2035.

Valvular Heart Disease

ADRIANA HERRERA

The prevalence of valvular heart disease in the United States is currently about 2.5% and is expected to increase significantly with the aging of the population. This will impact the healthcare system with an increasing demand for cardiac valvular surgery and percutaneous cardiac valvular interventions. Ethical issues about patient selection for these procedures may become significant matters. This form of heart disease continues to be an important cause of perioperative morbidity and mortality. In the past 30 years there have been major advances in understanding the natural history of valvular heart disease and improving cardiac function in patients with valvular disorders. Development of better noninvasive methods of monitoring ventricular function,

improved prosthetic heart valves, and better techniques for valve reconstruction, as well as the formulation of guidelines for selecting the proper timing for surgical intervention, have resulted in better outcomes.

Valvular heart disease places a hemodynamic burden on the left and/or right ventricle that is initially tolerated as a result of various compensations of the cardiovascular system. However, hemodynamic overload eventually leads to cardiac muscle dysfunction, congestive heart failure (CHF), or even sudden death. Management of patients with valvular heart disease during the perioperative period requires an understanding of the hemodynamic alterations that accompany valvular dysfunction. The most frequently encountered cardiac valve lesions produce pressure overload (mitral stenosis, aortic stenosis) or volume overload (mitral regurgitation, aortic regurgitation) on the left atrium or left ventricle. Anesthetic management during the perioperative period is based on the likely effects of drug-induced changes in cardiac rhythm and rate, preload, afterload, myocardial contractility, systemic blood pressure, systemic vascular resistance, and pulmonary vascular resistance relative to the pathophysiology of the specific valvular lesion.

PREOPERATIVE EVALUATION

Preoperative evaluation of patients with valvular heart disease includes assessment of (1) the severity of the cardiac disease, (2) the degree of impaired myocardial contractility, and (3) the presence of associated major organ system disease. Recognition of compensatory mechanisms for maintaining cardiac output, such as increased sympathetic nervous system activity and cardiac hypertrophy, as well as consideration of current drug therapy, are important. The presence of a prosthetic heart valve introduces special considerations in the preoperative evaluation, especially if noncardiac surgery is planned.

History and Physical Examination

Questions designed to define exercise tolerance are necessary to evaluate cardiac reserve in the presence of valvular heart disease and to provide a functional classification according to the criteria established by the New York Heart Association (NYHA) (Table 6.1). When myocardial contractility is impaired, patients complain of dyspnea, orthopnea, and easy fatigability. A compensatory increase in sympathetic nervous system activity may manifest as anxiety, diaphoresis, and resting tachycardia. CHF is a frequent companion of chronic valvular heart disease, and its presence is detected by noting basilar chest rales, jugular venous distention, and a third heart sound. Typically, elective surgery is deferred until CHF can be treated and myocardial contractility optimized.

Disease of a cardiac valve rarely occurs without an accompanying murmur, reflecting turbulent blood flow across the valve. The character, location, intensity, and direction of radiation of a heart murmur provide clues to the location and severity of the valvular lesion. During systole the aortic and pulmonic valves are open and the mitral and tricuspid valves are closed. Therefore a heart murmur that occurs during systole is due to stenosis of the aortic or pulmonic valves or incompetence of the mitral or tricuspid valves. During diastole

TABLE 6.1	New York Heart Association Functional Classification of Patients With Heart Disease

Class	Description
I	Asymptomatic
II	Symptoms with ordinary activity but comfortable at rest
III	Symptoms with minimal activity but comfortable at rest
IV	Symptoms at rest

the aortic and pulmonic valves are closed and the mitral and tricuspid valves are open. Therefore a diastolic heart murmur is due to stenosis of the mitral or tricuspid valves or incompetence of the aortic or pulmonic valves.

Cardiac dysrhythmias are seen with all types of valvular heart disease. Atrial fibrillation is common, especially with mitral valve disease associated with left atrial enlargement. Atrial fibrillation may be paroxysmal or chronic.

Angina pectoris may occur in patients with valvular heart disease, even in the absence of coronary artery disease. This usually reflects increased myocardial oxygen demand due to ventricular hypertrophy. The demands of this thickened muscle mass may exceed the ability of even normal coronary arteries to deliver adequate amounts of oxygen. Valvular heart disease and ischemic heart disease frequently co-exist; 50% of patients with aortic stenosis who are older than 50 years have associated ischemic heart disease. The presence of coronary artery disease in patients with mitral or aortic valve disease worsens the long-term prognosis, and mitral regurgitation due to ischemic heart disease is associated with increased mortality.

Drug Therapy

Modern drug therapy for valvular heart disease may include β-blockers, calcium channel blockers, and digitalis for heart rate control; angiotensin-converting enzyme (ACE) inhibitors, angiotensin receptor blockers (ARBs), and vasodilators to control blood pressure and afterload; and diuretics, inotropes, and vasodilators as needed to control heart failure. In addition to their immediate effects in terms of afterload reduction, it has been shown that attenuation or even reversal of hypertrophic remodeling and left ventricular dysfunction can occur in patients with aortic stenosis who are using ACE inhibitors or ARBs. Antidysrhythmic therapy may also be necessary. Certain cardiac lesions, such as aortic and mitral stenosis, require a slow heart rate to prolong the duration of diastole and improve left ventricular filling and coronary blood flow. The regurgitant valvular lesions such as aortic and mitral regurgitation require afterload reduction and a somewhat faster heart rate to shorten the time for regurgitation. Atrial fibrillation requires a controlled ventricular response so that activation of the sympathetic nervous system, as during tracheal intubation or in response to surgical stimulation, does not result in sufficient tachycardia to significantly decrease diastolic filling time and stroke volume.

Laboratory Data

The electrocardiogram (ECG) often exhibits characteristic changes due to valvular heart disease. Broad and notched P waves (P mitrale) suggest the presence of left atrial enlargement typical of mitral valve disease. Left and right ventricular hypertrophy can be diagnosed by the presence of left or right axis deviation and high voltage. Other common ECG findings include dysrhythmias, conduction abnormalities, and evidence of active ischemia or previous myocardial infarction.

The size and shape of the heart and great vessels and pulmonary vascular markings can be evaluated by chest radiography.

On a posteroanterior chest radiograph, cardiomegaly can be established if the heart size exceeds 50% of the internal width of the thoracic cage. Abnormalities of the pulmonary artery, left atrium, and left ventricle can be noted along the left heart border, and right atrial and right ventricular enlargement along the right heart border. Enlargement of the left atrium can result in elevation of the left mainstem bronchus. Valvular calcifications may be identified. Vascular markings in the peripheral lung fields are sparse in the presence of significant pulmonary hypertension.

Echocardiography with color flow Doppler imaging is essential for noninvasive evaluation of valvular heart disease (Table 6.2). It is particularly useful in evaluating the significance of cardiac murmurs such as systolic ejection murmurs when aortic stenosis is suspected and in detecting the presence of mitral stenosis. It permits determination of cardiac anatomy and function, the presence of hypertrophy, cavity dimensions, valve area, transvalvular pressure gradients, and the magnitude of valvular regurgitation.

Cardiac magnetic resonance imaging (CMRI) may be useful when echocardiographic images are suboptimal.

Computed tomography (CT) is another alternative modality useful when assessing valve area and valve calcification in aortic stenosis.

Cardiac catheterization can provide information about the presence and severity of valvular stenosis and/or regurgitation, coronary artery disease, and intracardiac shunting and can help resolve discrepancies between clinical and echocardiographic findings. Transvalvular pressure gradients determined at the time of cardiac catheterization indicate the severity of valvular heart disease. Mitral and aortic stenosis are considered to be severe when transvalvular pressure gradients are more than 10 mm Hg and 50 mm Hg, respectively. However, when CHF accompanies aortic stenosis, transvalvular pressure gradients may be smaller because of the inability of the dysfunctional left ventricular muscle to generate a large gradient. In patients with mitral stenosis or mitral regurgitation, measurement of pulmonary artery pressure and right ventricular filling pressure may provide evidence of pulmonary hypertension and right ventricular failure.

Presence of Prosthetic Heart Valves

Prosthetic heart valves may be mechanical or bioprosthetic. Mechanical valves are composed primarily of metal or carbon alloys and are classified according to their structure, such as caged-ball, single tilting-disk, or bileaflet tilting-disk valves. Bioprostheses may be heterografts composed of porcine or bovine tissues mounted on metal supports, or homografts, which are preserved human aortic valves.

Prosthetic valves differ from one another with regard to durability, thrombogenicity, and hemodynamic profile. Mechanical valves are very durable, lasting at least 20–30 years, whereas bioprosthetic valves last about 10–15 years. However, mechanical valves are highly thrombogenic and require long-term anticoagulation. Because bioprosthetic valves have a low thrombogenic potential, long-term anticoagulation often is not necessary. Mechanical valves are preferred in patients who are young, have a life expectancy of more than 10–15 years, or require long-term anticoagulation therapy for another reason, such as chronic atrial fibrillation. Bioprosthetic valves are preferred in elderly patients and in those who cannot tolerate anticoagulation.

Assessment of Prosthetic Heart Valve Function

Prosthetic heart valve dysfunction is suggested by a change in the intensity or quality of prosthetic valve clicks, the appearance of a new murmur, or a change in the characteristics of an existing murmur. *Transthoracic echocardiography* (TTE) can be used to assess sewing ring stability and leaflet motion of bioprosthetic valves, but mechanical valves may be difficult to evaluate with this method because of echo reverberations from the metal. *Transesophageal echocardiography* (TEE) may provide higher-resolution images, especially of a prosthetic valve in the mitral position. MRI can be used if prosthetic valve regurgitation or a paravalvular leak is suspected but not adequately visualized by echocardiography. Cardiac catheterization permits measurement of transvalvular pressure gradients and effective valve area of bioprosthetic valves.

Complications Associated With Prosthetic Heart Valves

Prosthetic heart valves can be associated with significant complications whose presence should be considered during the preoperative evaluation (Table 6.3). Because of the risk of thromboembolism, patients with mechanical prosthetic heart valves require long-term anticoagulant therapy. Subclinical intravascular hemolysis, evidenced by an increased serum lactate dehydrogenase concentration, decreased serum haptoglobin concentration, and reticulocytosis, is noted in many patients with normally functioning mechanical heart valves. The incidence of pigmented gallstones is increased in patients with prosthetic heart valves, presumably as a result of chronic

TABLE 6.2	Utility of Echocardiography in Evaluation of Valvular Heart Disease

Determine significance of cardiac murmurs
Identify hemodynamic abnormalities associated with physical findings
Determine transvalvular pressure gradient
Determine valve area
Determine ventricular ejection fraction
Diagnose valvular regurgitation
Evaluate prosthetic valve function

TABLE 6.3	Complications Associated With Prosthetic Heart Valves

Valve thrombosis
Systemic embolization
Structural failure
Hemolysis
Paravalvular leak
Endocarditis

low-grade intravascular hemolysis. Severe hemolytic anemia is uncommon, and its presence usually indicates valvular dysfunction or endocarditis. Antibiotic prophylaxis is necessary in patients with prosthetic heart valves to decrease the perioperative risk of infective endocarditis.

Management of Anticoagulation in Patients With Prosthetic Heart Valves

Patients may need to discontinue anticoagulation before surgery. However, this temporary discontinuation of anticoagulant therapy puts patients with mechanical heart valves or atrial fibrillation at risk of arterial or venous thromboembolism due to a rebound hypercoagulable state and to the prothrombotic effects of surgery. The risk of thromboembolism is estimated to be about 5%–8%. Anticoagulation may be continued in patients with prosthetic heart valves who are scheduled for minor surgery in which blood loss is expected to be minimal. When major surgery is planned, however, warfarin is typically discontinued 3–5 days preoperatively. Intravenous (IV) unfractionated heparin or subcutaneous low-molecular-weight heparin (LMWH) is administered after discontinuation of warfarin and continued until the day before or the day of surgery. The heparin can be restarted postoperatively when the risk of bleeding has lessened and can be continued until effective anticoagulation is again achieved with oral therapy. When possible, elective surgery should be avoided in the first month after an acute episode of arterial or venous thromboembolism.

Anticoagulant therapy is particularly important in parturients with prosthetic heart valves; the incidence of arterial embolization is greatly increased during pregnancy. However, warfarin administration during the first trimester can be associated with fetal defects and fetal death. Therefore warfarin is discontinued during pregnancy, and subcutaneous standard or LMWH is administered until delivery. Low-dose aspirin therapy is safe for the mother and fetus and can be used in conjunction with heparin therapy.

Prevention of Bacterial Endocarditis

The American Heart Association (AHA) has made recommendations for prevention of infective endocarditis for the past half-century. The most recent guidelines (2007) represent a radical departure from prior recommendations and dramatically reduce the indications for antibiotic prophylaxis. These guidelines are based on the best available evidence regarding this medical problem. Current scientific data suggest that infective endocarditis is more likely to result from frequent exposure to bacteremia associated with daily activities than from bacteremia associated with dental, gastrointestinal, or genitourinary tract procedures. For example, maintenance of good oral health and oral hygiene reduces bacteremia associated with normal daily activities (chewing, teeth brushing, flossing, use of toothpicks, etc.) and is more important than prophylactic antibiotics in reducing the risk of endocarditis. Endocarditis prophylaxis may prevent an exceedingly small number of cases of endocarditis, if any, in at-risk patients.

TABLE 6.4	Cardiac Conditions Associated With the Highest Risk of Adverse Outcomes From Endocarditis for Which Prophylaxis for Dental Procedures Is Reasonable

1. Prosthetic cardiac valve or prosthetic material used for cardiac valve repair
2. Previous infective endocarditis
3. Congenital heart disease:
   Unrepaired cyanotic congenital heart disease, including palliative shunts and conduits
   Completely repaired congenital heart defect with prosthetic material or device, whether placed by surgery or by catheter intervention, during the first 6 months after the procedure[a]
   Repaired congenital heart disease with residual defects at the site or adjacent to the site of a prosthetic patch or prosthetic device (which inhibit endothelialization)
4. Cardiac transplantation recipients who develop cardiac valvulopathy

[a]Prophylaxis is reasonable because endothelialization of prosthetic material occurs within 6 months after the procedure.
From Wilson W, Taubert KA, Gewitz M, et al. Prevention of infective endocarditis: guidelines from the American Heart Association. *Circulation*. 2007;116:1736-1754, with permission.

It also appears that the risk of antibiotic-associated adverse events exceeds the benefits of endocarditis prophylaxis overall and that the common use of antibiotic prophylaxis promotes the emergence of antibiotic-resistant organisms.

Experts feel that infective endocarditis prophylaxis should be administered *not* to individuals with a high cumulative lifetime risk of contracting endocarditis but rather to individuals *at highest risk of adverse outcomes if they develop endocarditis*. It appears that only a very small group of patients with heart disease is likely to have the most severe forms and complications of endocarditis. The conditions associated with this high risk are listed in Table 6.4. AHA guidelines target endocarditis prophylaxis *only to patients with these conditions*. The recommendations regarding which antibiotic to use for endocarditis prophylaxis are not dissimilar from previous recommendations.

In summary, the major recommendations in the AHA guidelines for infective endocarditis prophylaxis are: (1) antibiotic prophylaxis for infective endocarditis is recommended *only under a very few conditions;* (2) antibiotic prophylaxis *is* recommended for dental procedures that involve manipulation of gingival tissues or the periapical regions of the teeth or perforation of the oral mucosa; (3) antibiotic prophylaxis *is* recommended for invasive procedures (i.e., those that involve incision or biopsy of the respiratory tract or *infected* skin, skin structures, or musculoskeletal tissue); (4) antibiotic prophylaxis *is not* recommended for genitourinary or gastrointestinal tract procedures.

MITRAL STENOSIS

Mitral stenosis is quite rare in the United States, affecting only 1:100,000 people. The most common cause is rheumatic heart disease. The incidence of mitral stenosis used to be much higher when rheumatic fever was a common problem in this country. However, the incidence of rheumatic fever in developed countries is now very low, though rheumatic fever continues to be common in developing countries. Mitral stenosis primarily affects women. Diffuse thickening of the mitral leaflets and subvalvular apparatus, commissural fusion, and calcification of the annulus and leaflets are typically present. This process occurs slowly, and many patients do not become symptomatic for 20–30 years after the initial episode of rheumatic fever. Over time the mitral valve becomes stenotic and CHF, pulmonary hypertension, and right ventricular failure may develop.

Much less common causes of mitral stenosis include carcinoid syndrome, left atrial myxoma, severe mitral annular calcification, endocarditis, cor triatriatum, rheumatoid arthritis, systemic lupus erythematosus, congenital mitral stenosis, and iatrogenic mitral stenosis after mitral valve repair. Patients with mitral stenosis typically exhibit dyspnea on exertion, orthopnea, and paroxysmal nocturnal dyspnea as a result of high left atrial pressure. Left ventricular contractility is usually normal. Rheumatic heart disease presents as isolated mitral stenosis in about 40% of patients. If aortic and/or mitral regurgitation accompany mitral stenosis, there is often evidence of left ventricular dysfunction.

Pathophysiology

The normal mitral valve orifice area is 4–6 cm^2. Mitral stenosis is characterized by mechanical obstruction to left ventricular filling due to a progressive decrease in the size of the mitral valve orifice. This valvular obstruction produces an increase in left atrial volume and pressure. With mild mitral stenosis, left ventricular filling and stroke volume are maintained at rest by an increase in left atrial pressure. However, stroke volume will decrease during stress-induced tachycardia or when effective left atrial contraction is lost, as with atrial fibrillation. Symptoms usually develop when the mitral valve area is less than 1.5 cm^2. As the disease progresses the pulmonary venous pressure is increased in association with the increase in left atrial pressure. The result is transudation of fluid into the pulmonary interstitial space, decreased pulmonary compliance, and increased work of breathing, which leads to progressive dyspnea on exertion. Overt pulmonary edema is likely when the pulmonary venous pressure exceeds plasma oncotic pressure. If the increase in left atrial pressure is gradual, there is an increase in lymphatic drainage from the lungs and thickening of the capillary basement membrane that enables patients to tolerate an increased pulmonary venous pressure without development of pulmonary edema. Over time, changes in the pulmonary vasculature result in pulmonary hypertension, and eventually right-sided heart failure may occur. Left ventricular function is usually preserved. Episodes of pulmonary edema typically occur with atrial fibrillation, sepsis, pain, and pregnancy.

Diagnosis

Echocardiography is used to assess the anatomy of the mitral valve, including the degree of leaflet thickening, calcification, changes in mobility, and extent of involvement of the subvalvular apparatus. The severity of mitral stenosis is assessed by calculation of mitral valve area and measurement of the transvalvular pressure gradient. Echocardiography also allows evaluation of cardiac chamber dimensions, pulmonary hypertension, left and right ventricular function and other valvular disease, and examination of the left atrial appendage for the presence or absence of thrombus. Patients with mitral stenosis usually become symptomatic when the size of the mitral valve orifice has decreased at least 50%. When the mitral valve area is less than 1 cm^2, a mean atrial pressure of about 25 mm Hg is necessary to maintain adequate left ventricular filling and resting cardiac output. Pulmonary hypertension is likely if the left atrial pressure is above 25 mm Hg over the long term. When the mitral transvalvular pressure gradient is higher than 10 mm Hg (normal, <5 mm Hg), it is likely that mitral stenosis is severe. When mitral stenosis is severe, any additional stress such as fever or sepsis may precipitate pulmonary edema.

Stress testing is recommended when there is inconsistency between resting Doppler echocardiographic findings and clinical presentation. CMRI can also help determine the severity of the mitral stenosis.

Clinically, mitral stenosis is recognized by the characteristic opening snap that occurs early in diastole and by a rumbling diastolic heart murmur best heard at the apex or in the left axilla. Vibrations set in motion by the opening of the mobile but stenosed valve cause the opening snap. Calcification of the valve and greatly reduced leaflet mobility result in disappearance of the opening snap as the disease progresses. Left atrial enlargement is often visible on chest radiographs as straightening of the left heart border and elevation of the left mainstem bronchus. The "double density" of an enlarged left atrium, mitral calcification, and evidence of pulmonary edema or pulmonary vascular congestion may also be seen. Broad notched P waves on the ECG suggest left atrial enlargement. Atrial fibrillation is present in about one-third of patients with severe mitral stenosis.

Stasis of blood in the distended left atrium predisposes patients with mitral stenosis to a high risk of *arterial* thromboembolism. *Venous* thrombosis is also more likely because of the decreased physical activity of these patients.

Treatment

When symptoms of mild mitral stenosis develop, diuretics can decrease the left atrial pressure and relieve symptoms. If atrial fibrillation occurs, heart rate control may be achieved with β-blockers, calcium channel blockers, digoxin, or a combination of these medications. Control of the heart rate is critical because tachycardia impairs left ventricular filling and increases left atrial pressure. Anticoagulation is required in patients with mitral stenosis and atrial fibrillation, because the risk of embolic stroke in such patients is about 7%–15% per year. Warfarin is administered to a target international normalized ratio (INR) of 2.5–3.0. Surgical correction of mitral stenosis is indicated when symptoms worsen and pulmonary hypertension develops.

Mitral stenosis can sometimes be corrected by percutaneous balloon valvotomy. If heavy valvular calcification or valve deformity is present, surgical commissurotomy, valve reconstruction, or valve replacement is performed. In patients with concomitant severe tricuspid regurgitation (due to pulmonary hypertension), tricuspid valvuloplasty or ring annuloplasty can be performed at the same time as the mitral valve surgery.

Management of Anesthesia

Management of anesthesia for noncardiac surgery in patients with mitral stenosis includes prevention and treatment of events that can decrease cardiac output or produce pulmonary edema (Table 6.5). Development of atrial fibrillation with a rapid ventricular response significantly decreases cardiac output and can produce pulmonary edema. Treatment consists of cardioversion or IV administration of amiodarone, β-blockers, or calcium channel blockers. Excessive perioperative fluid administration, placement in Trendelenburg position, or autotransfusion via uterine contraction increases central blood volume and can precipitate CHF. In patients with severe mitral stenosis, a sudden decrease in systemic vascular resistance may not be tolerated, because the normal response to hypotension—that is, a reflex increase in heart rate—itself decreases cardiac output. If necessary, systemic blood pressure and systemic vascular resistance can be maintained with vasoconstrictor drugs such as phenylephrine. Use of vasopressin may also be considered, since it has minimal effect on pulmonary artery pressure. Pulmonary hypertension and right ventricular failure may be precipitated by numerous factors, including hypercarbia, hypoxemia, lung hyperinflation, and an increase in lung water. Right ventricular failure may require support with inotropic and pulmonary vasodilating drugs.

Drugs used for heart rate control should be continued until the time of surgery. Diuretic-induced hypokalemia can be detected and treated preoperatively. Orthostatic hypotension may be evidence of diuretic-induced hypovolemia. It may be acceptable to continue anticoagulant therapy for minor surgery, but major surgery associated with significant blood loss requires discontinuation of anticoagulation.

TABLE 6.5	Intraoperative Events That Have a Significant Impact on Mitral Stenosis

Sinus tachycardia or a rapid ventricular response during atrial fibrillation

Marked increase in central blood volume, as associated with overtransfusion or head-down positioning

Drug-induced decrease in systemic vascular resistance

Hypoxemia and hypercarbia that may exacerbate pulmonary hypertension and evoke right ventricular failure

Neuraxial anesthesia is an acceptable technique in the absence of anticoagulation. Other regional techniques such as peripheral nerve blocks may also be used safely. The ASRA publication *Regional Anesthesia in the Patient Receiving Antithrombotic or Thrombolytic Therapy: American Society of Regional Anesthesia and Pain Medicine Evidence-Based Guidelines* should be consulted and followed as needed. Use of neuraxial anesthesia requires measures to avoid hypotension, maintain adequate preload, and avoid tachycardia. Compared with spinal anesthesia, epidural anesthesia may allow better control of the level of sympathectomy and reduction in blood pressure.

Induction of general anesthesia can be achieved using any IV induction drug, with the exception of ketamine, which should be avoided because of its propensity to increase the heart rate. Tracheal intubation and muscle relaxation should be accomplished by administration of neuromuscular blockers that do not induce either tachycardia or hypotension from histamine release. Short-acting β-blockers may be necessary to treat episodes of tachycardia during induction. Cardioversion to treat new-onset atrial fibrillation with hemodynamic instability may be needed.

Maintenance of anesthesia is best accomplished using drugs with minimal effects on heart rate, myocardial contractility, and systemic and pulmonary vascular resistance. Often a nitrous/narcotic anesthetic or a balanced anesthetic that includes a low concentration of a volatile anesthetic can achieve this goal. Nitrous oxide can evoke pulmonary vasoconstriction and increase pulmonary vascular resistance if pulmonary hypertension is present.

Pharmacologic reversal of the effects of nondepolarizing muscle relaxants should be accomplished slowly to help ameliorate any drug-induced tachycardia caused by the anticholinergic drug in the mixture. Light anesthesia and/or surgical stimulation can result in sympathetic stimulation, producing tachycardia and systemic and pulmonary hypertension. Pulmonary vasodilator therapy may be necessary if pulmonary hypertension is severe. Intraoperative fluid replacement must be carefully titrated because these patients are very susceptible to volume overload and development of pulmonary edema.

Monitoring

Use of invasive monitoring depends on the complexity of the operative procedure and the magnitude of physiologic impairment caused by the mitral stenosis. Monitoring of asymptomatic patients without evidence of pulmonary congestion need be no different from monitoring of patients without valvular heart disease. On the other hand, TEE can be useful in patients with symptomatic mitral stenosis undergoing major surgery, especially if significant blood loss is expected. Continuous monitoring of intraarterial pressure, pulmonary artery pressure, and left atrial pressure (pulmonary artery occlusion pressure) should be considered. Such monitoring helps confirm the adequacy of cardiac function, intravascular fluid volume, ventilation, and oxygenation. Patients with significant pulmonary hypertension are at greater risk of pulmonary artery rupture from manipulation of a pulmonary artery catheter, so measurement of pulmonary artery occlusion pressure in this situation should be done infrequently and very carefully.

Postoperative Management

In patients with mitral stenosis the risk of pulmonary edema and right heart failure continues into the postoperative period, so cardiovascular monitoring should continue as well. Pain and hypoventilation with subsequent respiratory acidosis and hypoxemia may be responsible for increasing heart rate and pulmonary vascular resistance. Decreased pulmonary compliance and increased work of breathing may necessitate a period of mechanical ventilation, particularly after major thoracic or abdominal surgery. Relief of postoperative pain with neuraxial opioids can be very useful in selected patients. Anticoagulation should be restarted as soon as the risk of perioperative bleeding has diminished.

MITRAL REGURGITATION

Mitral regurgitation is much more common than mitral stenosis, affecting about 2% of the US population. It is one of the two most common forms of valvular heart disease in the elderly. Mitral regurgitation due to rheumatic fever is uncommon and is usually associated with some degree of mitral stenosis. Isolated mitral regurgitation can be associated with ischemic heart disease or result from papillary muscle dysfunction, mitral annular dilatation, or rupture of chordae tendineae. Other causes of mitral regurgitation include endocarditis, mitral valve prolapse (MVP), trauma, congenital heart disease (e.g., endocardial cushion defect), left ventricular hypertrophy, cardiomyopathy, myxomatous degeneration, systemic lupus erythematosus, rheumatoid arthritis, ankylosing spondylitis, and carcinoid syndrome.

Pathophysiology

The basic hemodynamic derangement in mitral regurgitation is a decrease in forward left ventricular stroke volume and cardiac output. A portion of every stroke volume is regurgitated through the incompetent mitral valve back into the left atrium. This results in left atrial volume overload and pulmonary congestion. Patients with a regurgitant fraction of more than 60% are considered to have severe mitral regurgitation. The fraction of left ventricular stroke volume that regurgitates into the left atrium depends on (1) the size of the mitral valve orifice, (2) the heart rate, which determines the duration of ventricular ejection, and (3) the pressure gradient across the mitral valve. Such gradients are related to left ventricle compliance and impedance to left ventricular ejection into the aorta. Pharmacologic interventions that increase or decrease systemic vascular resistance have a major impact on the regurgitant fraction in patients with mitral regurgitation.

Patients with isolated mitral regurgitation are less dependent on properly timed left atrial contraction for left ventricular filling than are patients with co-existing mitral or aortic stenosis. Patients with rheumatic fever–induced mitral regurgitation are most likely to exhibit marked left atrial enlargement and atrial fibrillation. Myocardial ischemia as a result of mitral regurgitation is uncommon because the increased left ventricular wall tension is quickly dissipated as the stroke volume is rapidly ejected into the aorta and left atrium. When mitral regurgitation develops gradually, the volume overload produced by mitral regurgitation transforms the left ventricle into a larger, more compliant chamber that is able to deliver a larger stroke volume. This occurs through a dissolution of collagen weave, remodeling of the extracellular matrix, rearrangement of myocardial fibers, and addition of new sarcomeres with the development of ventricular hypertrophy. Development of ventricular hypertrophy and increased compliance of the left atrium permit the accommodation of the regurgitant volume without a major increase in left atrial pressure. This allows patients to maintain cardiac output and remain free of pulmonary congestion and, indeed, to be asymptomatic for many years. However, because there has been no time for development of left atrial or left ventricular compensation, *acute* mitral regurgitation presents as pulmonary edema and/or cardiogenic shock.

The combination of mitral regurgitation and mitral stenosis results in volume and pressure overload of the left atrium and a markedly increased left atrial pressure. Atrial fibrillation, pulmonary edema, and pulmonary hypertension develop much earlier in these patients than in those with isolated mitral regurgitation.

Diagnosis

Mitral regurgitation is recognized clinically by the presence of a holosystolic apical murmur with radiation to the axilla. Cardiomegaly can also be detected on physical examination. Severe mitral regurgitation can produce left atrial and left ventricular hypertrophy detectable on ECG and chest radiograph. Echocardiography confirms the presence, severity, and often the cause of the mitral regurgitation. Left atrial size and pressure, left ventricular wall thickness, cavitary dimensions, ventricular function, and pulmonary artery pressure can be measured. In addition, the left atrial appendage can be evaluated for the presence of thrombus. Many methods exist to determine the severity of mitral regurgitation. These include color flow and pulsed wave Doppler examination of the mitral valve, with calculation of the regurgitant volume and the regurgitant fraction and measurement of the area of the regurgitant jet. The presence of a V wave in a pulmonary artery occlusion pressure waveform reflects regurgitant flow through the mitral valve, and the size of this V wave correlates with the magnitude of the mitral regurgitation.

There are situations where three-dimensional (3D) echocardiography is indicated because it can allow a better assessment of the mitral valve apparatus. CMRI can be used to assess left ventricular and right ventricular size and function and the severity of the mitral regurgitation when echocardiographic data is limited. CT has also been shown to be as accurate as echocardiography and CMRI when assessing mitral regurgitation, though it is not a preferred modality owing to radiation exposure and the need for contrast use.

If the severity of mitral regurgitation is in doubt, or mitral valve surgery is planned, cardiac catheterization, including coronary angiography, is necessary.

Treatment

Unlike stenotic valve lesions, regurgitant cardiac valve lesions often progress insidiously, causing left ventricular remodeling and damage before symptoms develop. Early surgery may be warranted to prevent left ventricular dysfunction from becoming severe or irreversible. Survival may be prolonged if surgery is performed before the ejection fraction is less than 60% or before the left ventricle is unable to contract to an end-systolic dimension of 45 mm (normal, <40 mm). Patients with an ejection fraction of less than 30% or a left ventricular end-systolic dimension of more than 55 mm *do not* experience improvement with mitral valve surgery. *Symptomatic* patients should undergo mitral valve surgery even if the ejection fraction is normal. Mitral valve repair, if possible, is preferred to mitral valve replacement because it restores valve competence and maintains the functional aspects of the mitral valve apparatus. The mitral valve apparatus is very important in supporting left ventricular function. The absence of the subvalvular apparatus causes distortion of left ventricular contractile geometry and impairment of left ventricular ejection. In patients in whom the valve and its apparatus cannot be preserved, valve replacement is done, but there is a postoperative decline in left ventricular ejection fraction.

Although vasodilators are useful in the medical management of acute mitral regurgitation, there is no apparent benefit to long-term use of these drugs in *asymptomatic* patients with chronic mitral regurgitation. For *symptomatic* patients, ACE inhibitors or β-blockers (particularly carvedilol) and biventricular pacing have all been shown to decrease functional mitral regurgitation and improve symptoms and exercise tolerance.

Over the past decade, percutaneous valve repair has appeared as a new treatment option for elderly high-risk patients with severe mitral regurgitation. The MitraClip device was approved for use in the United States in 2013. It is indicated for treatment of patients with degenerative mitral regurgitation of grades 3+ or 4+ who are considered to be very high risk for surgery. More clinical trials are needed to determine its efficacy in functional mitral regurgitation. Excellent cardiac imaging is essential for patient selection, anatomy evaluation, and sizing of the device. Echocardiography, especially TEE with 2D and 3D capacity, and fluoroscopy are necessary for deployment of the device, assessment of device position, seating, and stability of the device. Assessment for left ventricular outflow tract obstruction and central or paravalvular mitral regurgitation are crucial after the procedure (Fig. 6.1).

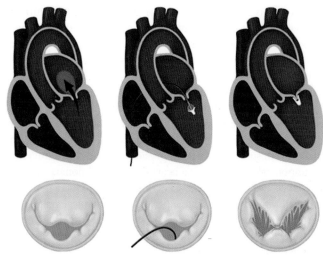

FIG. 6.1 Percutaneous MitraClip system for treatment of mitral regurgitation. The left images show that there is severe mitral regurgitation and that the mitral leaflets do not coapt. The middle images show the positioning of the MitraClip device just below the mitral valve in the area where the leak is the greatest. The right images show the MitraClip in position on the mitral valve and the two orifices (rather than the original one) that have been created by the clip for blood flow through the repaired mitral valve. (From Athappan G, Raza MQ, Kapadia SR. MitraClip therapy for mitral regurgitation. *Interv Cardiol Clin.* 2016;5:71-82. Copyright © 2016 Elsevier.)

TABLE 6.6	Anesthetic Considerations in Patients With Mitral Regurgitation

Prevent bradycardia
Prevent increases in systemic vascular resistance
Minimize drug-induced myocardial depression
Monitor the magnitude of regurgitant flow with a pulmonary artery catheter (size of the V wave) and/or echocardiography

Management of Anesthesia

Management of anesthesia for noncardiac surgery in patients with mitral regurgitation includes prevention and treatment of events that may further decrease cardiac output (Table 6.6). The goal is to improve forward left ventricular stroke volume and decrease the regurgitant fraction. Maintenance of a normal to slightly increased heart rate is recommended. Bradycardia may result in severe left ventricular volume overload. An increase in systemic vascular resistance can also cause decompensation of the left ventricle. Afterload reduction with a vasodilator drug such as nitroprusside, with or without an inotropic drug, will improve left ventricular function. In most patients, cardiac output can be maintained or improved with modest increases in heart rate and modest decreases in systemic vascular resistance. The decrease in systemic vascular resistance caused by regional anesthesia may be beneficial in some patients.

Induction of anesthesia can be achieved with an IV induction drug. Dosing should be adjusted to prevent an increase in systemic vascular resistance or a decrease in heart rate, because both of these hemodynamic changes reduce cardiac output. Selection of a muscle relaxant should follow the same principles. Pancuronium produces a modest increase in heart rate that can contribute to maintenance of forward left ventricular stroke volume.

Volatile anesthetics can be administered to attenuate the undesirable increases in systemic blood pressure and systemic vascular resistance that can accompany surgical stimulation. The increase in heart rate and decrease in systemic vascular resistance plus the minimal negative inotropic effects associated with isoflurane, desflurane, and sevoflurane make them all acceptable choices for maintenance of anesthesia. When myocardial function is severely compromised, use of an opioid-based anesthetic is another excellent option because of the minimal myocardial depression that opioids produce. However, potent narcotics can produce significant bradycardia, and this could be very deleterious in the presence of severe mitral regurgitation. Mechanical ventilation should be adjusted to maintain near-normal values on acid-base and respiratory parameters. The pattern of ventilation must provide sufficient time between breaths for adequate venous return. Maintenance of intravascular fluid volume is very important for maintaining left ventricular volume and cardiac output.

Neuraxial techniques may result in afterload reduction, decreasing the regurgitant volume. Other regional techniques can also be considered safe for these patients. ASRA guidelines for regional anesthesia in patients receiving anticoagulation therapy should be followed.

Monitoring

Anesthesia for surgery in patients with asymptomatic mitral regurgitation does not require invasive monitoring. However, in the presence of severe mitral regurgitation, the use of invasive monitoring is helpful for detecting the adequacy of cardiac output and the hemodynamic response to anesthetic and vasodilating drugs and to facilitate fluid replacement. Mitral regurgitation produces a V wave on the pulmonary artery occlusion pressure waveform. Changes in V wave amplitude can assist in estimating the magnitude and direction of changes in the degree of mitral regurgitation. However, pulmonary artery occlusion pressure may be a poor measure of left ventricular end-diastolic volume in patients with *chronic* mitral regurgitation because of the stiffer hypertrophied left ventricle. With *acute* mitral regurgitation, pulmonary artery occlusion pressure does correlate with left atrial and left ventricular end-diastolic pressure. TEE is another useful technique for monitoring mitral valve and left ventricular function during major surgery.

MITRAL VALVE PROLAPSE

MVP is defined as the prolapse of one or both mitral leaflets into the left atrium during systole, with or without mitral regurgitation. It is associated with the auscultatory findings of a midsystolic click and a late systolic murmur. MVP is the most common form of valvular heart disease, affecting about 2%–3% of the US population. It is more common in young women. MVP can be associated with Marfan syndrome, rheumatic carditis, myocarditis, thyrotoxicosis, and systemic lupus erythematosus. Although it is usually a benign condition, MVP can have devastating complications such as cerebral embolic events, infective endocarditis, severe mitral regurgitation requiring surgery, dysrhythmias, and sudden death. Patients with MVP and abnormal mitral valve morphology appear to be the subset of patients at risk for these complications.

Diagnosis

The definitive diagnosis of MVP is based on echocardiographic findings. It has been defined as valve prolapse of 2 mm or more above the mitral annulus. MVP can occur with or without leaflet thickening and with or without mitral regurgitation. Patients with redundant and thickened leaflets have a primary (anatomic) form of MVP. This form of MVP typically occurs in patients with connective tissue diseases or in elderly men. Patients with mild bowing and normal-appearing leaflets have a normal variant (functional) form of MVP, and their risk of adverse events is probably no different from that of the general population.

Patients with MVP may experience anxiety, orthostatic symptoms, palpitations, dyspnea, fatigue, and atypical chest pain. Cardiac dysrhythmias, both supraventricular and ventricular, may occur and respond well to β-blocker therapy. Cardiac conduction abnormalities are not uncommon.

Management of Anesthesia

Management of anesthesia for noncardiac surgery in patients with MVP follows the same principles as for patients with mitral regurgitation. Management is influenced primarily by the degree of mitral regurgitation. Interestingly the degree of MVP can be affected by left ventricular dimensions and is more dynamic than mitral valvular disease. A larger ventricle will often have less prolapse (and regurgitation) than a smaller ventricle. So events that affect how much the left ventricle fills or empties with each cardiac cycle will affect the amount of mitral regurgitation. Perioperative events that enhance left ventricular *emptying* (i.e., reduce left ventricular overall size) include (1) increased sympathetic activity that increases myocardial contractility, (2) decreased systemic vascular resistance, and (3) assumption of the upright posture. Hypovolemia reduces left ventricular *filling* (i.e., keeps left ventricular size small). Events that *decrease* left ventricular emptying and *increase* left ventricular volume (i.e., keep the left ventricle larger in size) may *decrease* the degree of MVP. These include hypertension or vasoconstriction, drug-induced myocardial depression, and volume resuscitation.

Preoperative Evaluation

In the absence of symptoms, the finding of a systolic click and murmur *does not* warrant a preoperative cardiologic consultation.

Preoperative evaluation of patients with a diagnosis of MVP should focus on distinguishing patients with purely functional disease from those with significant mitral regurgitation. Functional MVP is most often present in women younger than 45 years. Some patients may be taking β-blockers to control dysrhythmias, and these drugs should be continued throughout the perioperative period. Patients with a history of transient neurologic events who are in sinus rhythm with no atrial thrombi are likely to be taking daily aspirin therapy (81–325 mg/day), whereas patients with atrial fibrillation and/or left atrial thrombus and/or previous stroke are likely to be taking warfarin or another anticoagulant. Although the ECG frequently shows premature ventricular contractions, repolarization abnormalities, and QT interval prolongation, there is no evidence that these findings predict or are associated with adverse intraoperative events.

Older men with an anatomic form of MVP can have symptoms of mild to moderate CHF, including exercise intolerance, orthopnea, and dyspnea on exertion. These patients may be taking diuretics and ACE inhibitors. Physical examination often reveals a midsystolic to holosystolic murmur, an S_3 gallop, and signs of pulmonary congestion.

Most patients with MVP have normal left ventricular function and tolerate all forms of general and regional anesthesia. Volatile anesthetic–induced myocardial depression can be useful for offsetting the vasodilation that could decrease left ventricular volume and increase mitral prolapse and/or regurgitation. There is no contraindication to the use of regional anesthesia in patients with MVP. The decrease in systemic vascular resistance should be anticipated, and administration of fluids should offset any changes in left ventricular volume that could affect the degree of prolapse and regurgitation.

When an IV induction drug is selected, the need to avoid a significant or prolonged decrease in systemic vascular resistance must be considered. Etomidate causes minimal myocardial depression and minimal alterations in sympathetic nervous system activity, so it is an attractive choice for induction of anesthesia in the presence of hemodynamically significant MVP. Ketamine is generally a poor choice because of its ability to stimulate the sympathetic nervous system and enhance left ventricular emptying, causing an increase in prolapse and regurgitation.

Maintenance of anesthesia must minimize sympathetic nervous system activation resulting from painful intraoperative stimuli. Volatile anesthetics combined with nitrous oxide and/or opioids are useful for attenuating sympathetic nervous system activity, but their doses must be titrated to minimize the decrease in systemic vascular resistance.

Patients with hemodynamically significant MVP may not tolerate the dose-dependent myocardial depression of volatile anesthetics. However, low concentrations (≈0.5 minimum alveolar concentration) of isoflurane, desflurane, and sevoflurane can decrease the regurgitant fraction. In patients with severe mitral regurgitation, vasodilators such as nitroprusside or nitroglycerin may be carefully titrated to maximize forward left ventricular flow and decrease left ventricular end-diastolic volume and left atrial pressure. There are no clinical data to support the use of one muscle relaxant over another in the presence of MVP, but drug-induced hemodynamic alterations such as vagolysis or histamine release deserve consideration when selecting a specific drug.

Unexpected ventricular dysrhythmias can occur during anesthesia, especially during operations performed with the patient in the head-up or sitting position. Presumably, in these positions, there is an increase in left ventricular emptying and accentuation of MVP. Lidocaine and β-blockers can treat these dysrhythmias.

Maintenance of proper fluid balance blunts the decrease in venous return caused by positive pressure ventilation. Proper fluid balance also helps prevent an increase in the degree of prolapse. If vasopressors are needed, an α-agonist such as phenylephrine is acceptable. Use of an anesthetic technique that includes controlled hypotension would be unwise because the change in systemic vascular resistance would enhance the degree of MVP.

Monitoring

Routine monitoring is all that is necessary in the majority of patients with MVP. An intraarterial catheter and pulmonary artery catheter or TEE are needed only in patients with significant mitral regurgitation and left ventricular dysfunction.

AORTIC STENOSIS

Aortic stenosis is a common valvular lesion in the United States. Its incidence is increasing as the US population grows older. It affects about 10% of octogenarians. It is anticipated that the prevalence of aortic stenosis is likely to double in the next 20 years.

Two factors are associated with development of aortic stenosis. The *first factor* is a process of aging that results in degeneration and calcification of the aortic leaflets. The leaflets can then cause narrowing of the aortic valve orifice. This is called *calcific aortic stenosis*. It is estimated that this process affects as many as 25% of all adults older than age 65, though to varying degrees. Of this group, only about 2%–5% will develop significant aortic stenosis. Many more will develop *aortic sclerosis with mild aortic stenosis* over time. This degenerative process of the aortic valve has been compared with atherosclerosis with endothelial dysfunction, lipid deposition, and oxidative changes that stimulate inflammation and lead to fibrosis and calcification (Fig. 6.2). Not surprisingly, calcific aortic stenosis is associated with risk factors similar to those of atherosclerosis, such as systemic hypertension, hypercholesterolemia, diabetes mellitus, smoking, and male gender.

The *second factor* is the presence of a *bicuspid aortic valve* (BAV). BAV is the most common congenital valvular abnormality, and it affects 1%–2% of the population. The combination of an abnormal valve and the abnormal mechanical stresses on it promotes fibrosis and calcification, with subsequent stenosis. *Aortic stenosis often develops earlier in life (age 30–50) in individuals with BAV than in those with a tricuspid aortic valve (age 60–80).*

BAV is also associated with dilatation of the aortic root and/or ascending aorta that occurs at a younger age compared to that seen with a stenotic tricuspid aortic valve. As a result of this aortopathy, aortic aneurysms grow faster in patients with BAV, and there is a higher risk of aortic dissection and rupture. The 2014 ACC/AHA guidelines for the management of patients with valvular heart disease highly recommend surgical repair of the aortic root and/or the ascending aorta in patients with BAV and an aortic diameter greater than 55 mm. Surgery should be considered when the aortic diameter is greater than 50 mm and associated with other risk factors such as a family history of aortic dissection or rapid growth of the aorta (Fig. 6.3).

Pathophysiology

Obstruction to ejection of blood into the aorta caused by the decrease in aortic valve area necessitates an increase in left ventricular pressure to maintain stroke volume. The normal aortic valve area is $2.5–3.5$ cm^2. Transvalvular pressure gradients higher than 50 mm Hg and an aortic valve area of less than 0.8 cm^2 are characteristic of *severe aortic stenosis*. Aortic stenosis is almost always associated with some degree of aortic regurgitation.

Angina pectoris may occur in patients with aortic stenosis, despite the absence of coronary artery disease. This is due to the increase in myocardial oxygen requirements secondary to concentric left ventricular hypertrophy and the increase in

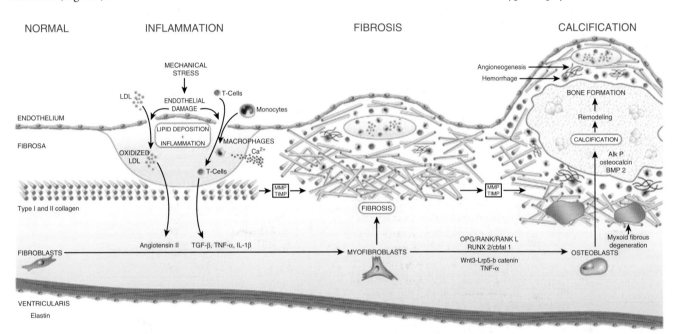

FIG. 6.2 Summary of the pathological processes occurring within the valve during aortic stenosis. Mechanical stress results in endothelial damage that allows infiltration of lipid and inflammatory cells into the valve. Lipid oxidization further increases inflammatory activity within these lesions and the secretion of proinflammatory and profibrotic cytokines. The latter drives the differentiation of fibroblasts into myofibroblasts that secrete increased collagen under the influence of angiotensin. In combination with the action of matrix metalloproteinases (MMPs) and tissue inhibitors of metalloproteinases (TIMPs), disorganized fibrous tissue accumulates within the valve. This leads to thickening and increased stiffness of the valve and in the latter stages the development of myxoid fibrous degeneration. Microcalcification begins early in the disease, driven by microvesicle secretion by macrophages. However, calcification accelerates in a proportion of patients because of the differentiation of myofibroblasts into osteoblasts. This occurs under the influence of several procalcific pathways, including osteoprotegerin (OPG)/receptor activator of nuclear factor (NF)-κB (RANK)/ RANK ligand (RANKL), Runx 2-cbfal 2, Wnt3-Lrp5-b catenin, and tumor necrosis factor (TNF)-α. Osteoblasts subsequently coordinate calcification of the valve as part of a highly regulated process akin to skeletal bone formation, with expression of many of the same mediators, such as osteocalcin, alkaline phosphatase (Alk P), and bone morphogenic protein (BMP)-2. With time, maturation of valvular calcification occurs so that by the end stages of the disease, lamellar bone, microfractures, and hemopoietic tissue can all be observed within the valve. These pathogenic processes are sustained by angioneogenesis, with new vessels localizing in particular to regions of inflammation surrounding calcific deposits. Hemorrhage in relation to these vessels has also been demonstrated in severe disease and may have a role in accelerating disease progression. *IL,* Interleukin; *LDL,* low-density lipoprotein; *TGF,* transforming growth factor. (From Dweck MR, Boon NA, Newby DE. Calcific aortic stenosis: a disease of the valve and the myocardium. *J Am Coll Cardiol.* 2012; 60:1854-1863. Copyright © 2012 American College of Cardiology Foundation, with permission.)

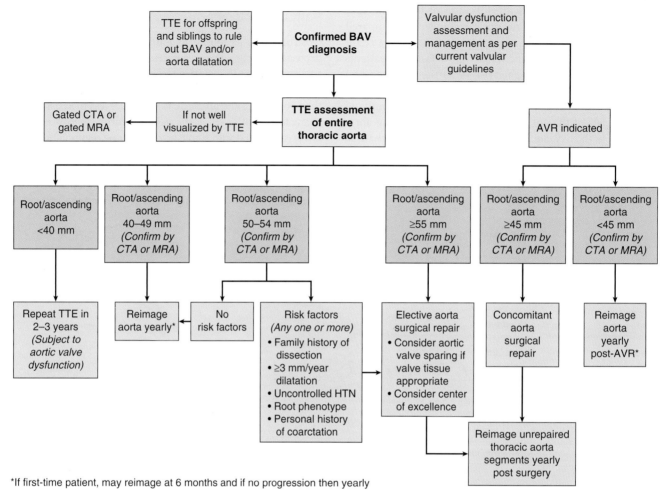

*If first-time patient, may reimage at 6 months and if no progression then yearly

FIG. 6.3 Bicuspid aortic valve (BAV) aortopathy management algorithm. An aortic root or ascending tubular aorta 55 mm or greater with no risk factors or 50 mm or greater with any one or more risk factors should prompt referral for elective surgical aorta repair regardless of aortic valve function. If the aortic valve does not have degeneration features (no calcium deposits, good mobility, no significant thickening), a valve-sparing aortic repair should be considered, and patient referral to a center of excellence may be warranted. Patients undergoing primary AVR for valvular dysfunction should have their root and/or ascending tubular aorta concomitantly repaired if these measure 45 mm or greater. Patients who undergo isolated AVR without aorta repair should continue to be followed with yearly thoracic aorta diameter assessments. (From Michelena HI, Della Corte A, Prakash SK, et al. Bicuspid aortic valve aortopathy in adults: incidence, etiology, and clinical significance. *Int J Cardiol.* 2015; 201:400-407. Copyright © 2015 Elsevier Ireland Ltd., with permission.)

myocardial work necessary to offset the afterload produced by the stenotic valve. In addition, myocardial oxygen delivery is decreased because of compression of subendocardial blood vessels by the increased left ventricular pressure.

Since the initial study by Goldman and colleagues in 1977 showing that patients with aortic stenosis had an increased risk of perioperative cardiac complications, many studies have demonstrated that patients with aortic stenosis have an increased risk of perioperative mortality and nonfatal myocardial infarction regardless of the presence or absence of risk factors for coronary artery disease. The perioperative risk attributable to aortic stenosis is independent of the risk attributable to coronary artery disease.

The origin of syncope in patients with aortic stenosis is controversial but may reflect an exercise-induced decrease in systemic vascular resistance that remains uncompensated because cardiac output is limited by the stenotic valve. CHF can be due to systolic and/or diastolic dysfunction (Fig. 6.4).

Diagnosis

The classic symptoms of *critical aortic stenosis* are angina pectoris, syncope, and dyspnea on exertion, a manifestation of CHF. The onset of these symptoms has been shown to correlate with an average time to death of 5, 3, and 2 years, respectively. *About 75% of symptomatic patients (i.e., patients with critical aortic*

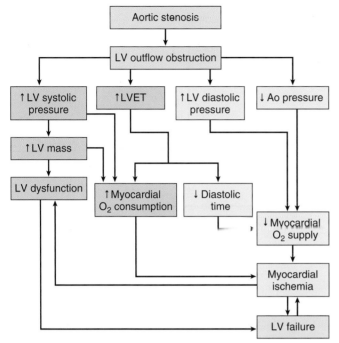

FIG. 6.4 Pathophysiology of aortic stenosis. Left ventricular (LV) outflow obstruction results in an increased LV systolic pressure, increased LV ejection time (LVET), increased LV diastolic pressure, and decreased aortic (Ao) pressure. Increased LV systolic pressure with LV volume overload increases LV mass, which may lead to LV dysfunction and failure. Increased LV systolic pressure, LV mass, and LVET increase myocardial O_2 consumption. Increased LVET results in a decrease of diastolic time (myocardial perfusion time). Increased LV diastolic pressure and decreased aortic diastolic pressure decrease coronary perfusion pressure. Decreased diastolic time and coronary perfusion pressure decrease myocardial O_2 supply. Increased myocardial O_2 consumption and decreased myocardial O_2 supply produce myocardial ischemia, which causes LV function to deteriorate further. ↑, Increased; ↓, decreased. (From Boudoulas H, Gravanis MB. Valvular heart disease. In: Gravanis MB, ed. *Cardiovascular Disorders: Pathogenesis and Pathophysiology.* St Louis, MO: Mosby; 1993:64.)

stenosis) will die within 3 years if they do not have a valve replacement. On physical examination, auscultation reveals a characteristic systolic murmur heard best in the aortic area. This murmur may radiate to the neck and mimic a carotid bruit. Confirmation by echocardiography is necessary to evaluate the presence and severity of suspected aortic valve disease. Because patients with aortic stenosis frequently have concomitant carotid artery disease, this finding deserves special attention. Because many patients with aortic stenosis are asymptomatic, it is important to listen for the systolic murmur of aortic stenosis in older patients scheduled for surgery. Chest radiography may show a prominent ascending aorta due to poststenotic aortic dilation. The ECG may demonstrate left ventricular hypertrophy.

Echocardiography with Doppler examination of the aortic valve provides a more accurate assessment of the severity of aortic stenosis than does clinical evaluation, and patients can be followed echocardiographically to assess the progression of their disease. Findings include identification of a trileaflet versus a bileaflet aortic valve, thickening and calcification of the aortic valve, decreased mobility of the aortic valve leaflets, left ventricular hypertrophy, and left ventricular systolic or diastolic dysfunction. Aortic valve area and transvalvular pressure gradients can be measured. Cardiac catheterization (and coronary angiography) may be necessary when the severity of aortic stenosis cannot be clearly determined by echocardiography.

CMRI is an option for evaluation of aortic valve disease when echocardiography is suboptimal or there is a discrepancy with clinical findings. It can be very helpful in differentiating a bicuspid from a tricuspid valve and in evaluating aortic root and ascending aortic dimensions in patients with BAV. It can also assess peak flow velocity through the valve. CT imaging allows evaluation of the valve area and the degree of calcification.

Exercise stress testing may be an additional strategy to evaluate asymptomatic patients with known moderate to severe aortic stenosis to identify those with poor exercise tolerance and/or an abnormal blood pressure response to exercise. Patients with exercise-induced symptoms may benefit from aortic valve replacement (AVR). However, exercise echocardiography is often a better option for this kind of evaluation.

B-type natriuretic peptide (BNP) levels may be helpful in deciding whether symptoms such as dyspnea on exertion are of cardiac origin. Precise parameters for elevated BNP levels are not yet defined, but an increased BNP in asymptomatic patients might help predict symptom onset, functional status, left ventricular function, and overall survival. In the asymptomatic elderly population with severe aortic stenosis, elevated levels of BNP may suggest early clinical decompensation. In symptomatic patients with a decreased ejection fraction, elevated BNP has been associated with decreased 1-year survival after AVR.

Treatment

Once patients with aortic stenosis develop symptoms, AVR is recommended unless a patient is considered inoperable due to extremes of age or other very serious comorbidities. In *asymptomatic* patients with aortic stenosis it appears to be safe to continue medical management and delay valve replacement surgery until symptoms develop. However, there is a small risk of sudden death or rapid onset and progression of symptoms and then sudden death. Risk stratification by additional testing in combination with assessment of the severity of the stenosis over time may help identify patients who might benefit from AVR *before* symptoms develop (Fig. 6.5; Tables 6.7 and 6.8). Mortality approaches 75% within 3 years after development of critical aortic stenosis unless the aortic valve is replaced. Even though many patients with aortic stenosis are quite elderly, the risks of valve replacement surgery are generally acceptable. AVR dramatically relieves the symptoms of aortic stenosis. There is regression of left ventricular hypertrophy, and the ejection fraction increases. Coronary revascularization is often done at the same time as AVR in patients with both aortic stenosis and significant coronary artery disease.

Percutaneous aortic balloon valvotomy can be beneficial in adolescents and young adults with congenital or rheumatic aortic stenosis. However, adults with acquired aortic stenosis experience only temporary relief of symptoms with this

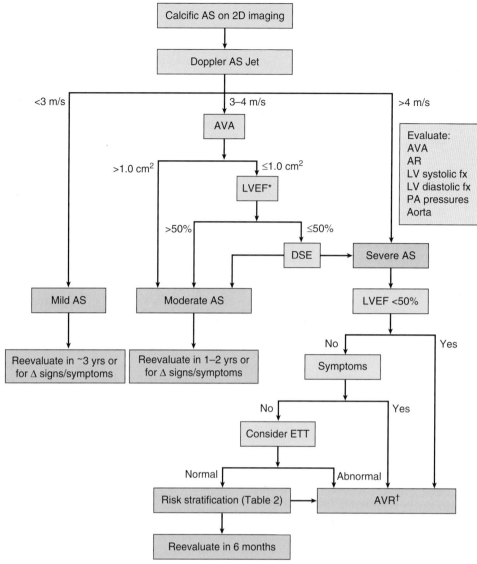

FIG. 6.5 Approach to the diagnosis of aortic stenosis (AS). *A subset of patients presents with low flow, low gradient, severe AS with preserved ejection fraction, characterized by a stroke volume index less than 35 mL/m² and usually accompanied by left ventricular hypertrophy (LVH), a very calcified valve, small LV chamber, and reduced longitudinal systolic strain. See text for details. †Surgical aortic valve replacement (SAVR) is appropriate in most patients. Transcatheter AVR (TAVR) is recommended in inoperable patients and may be reasonable in patients with high surgical risk. *2D*, Two-dimensional; *AVA*, aortic valve area; *AR*, aortic regurgitation; *DSE*, dobutamine stress echocardiography; *ETT*, exercise treadmill testing; *LV*, left ventricular; *LVEF*, left ventricular ejection fraction; *PA*, pulmonary artery. (From Lindman BR, Bonow RO, Otto CM. Current management of calcific aortic stenosis. *Circ Res.* 2013;113: 223-237, with permission.)

TABLE 6.7	Markers of Increased Rate of Disease Progression and Decreased Event-Free Interval in Asymptomatic Patients With Aortic Stenosis

Abnormal stress test
Elevated B-type natriuretic peptide
Moderate to severe valve calcification
Very high aortic velocity (5 or 5.5 m/s)
Rapid increase in aortic velocity
Increased hypertrophic left ventricular remodeling
Reduced left ventricular longitudinal systolic strain
Myocardial fibrosis
Pulmonary hypertension

Adapted from Lindman BR, Bonow RO, Otto CM. Current management of calcific aortic stenosis. *Circ Res.* 2013;113:223-237, with permission.

TABLE 6.8	Markers of Increased Risk and Potential Futility in Patients Undergoing Aortic Valve Intervention

Lack of contractile reserve in patients with low flow
Low ejection fraction
Very low mean aortic valve gradient (<20 mm Hg)
Very elevated B-type natriuretic peptide
Severe ventricular fibrosis
Oxygen-dependent lung disease
Advanced renal dysfunction
Very high Society of Thoracic Surgeons score
Frailty

Adapted from Lindman BR, Bonow RO, Otto CM. Current management of calcific aortic stenosis. *Circ Res.* 2013;113:223-237, with permission.

TABLE 6.9	Anesthetic Considerations in Patients With Aortic Stenosis

Maintain normal sinus rhythm
Avoid bradycardia or tachycardia
Avoid hypotension
Optimize intravascular fluid volume to maintain venous return and left ventricular filling

procedure. Balloon valvotomy may occasionally be useful for palliation of aortic stenosis in patients who are not candidates for AVR. It can also be used in selected patients as a bridge procedure before performing either surgical or transcatheter AVR.

Over the last decade, *transcatheter aortic valve replacement* (TAVR), also called *transcatheter aortic valve implantation* (TAVI), has become a viable treatment alternative to surgical aortic valve replacement (SAVR). It was approved by the US Food and Drug Administration (FDA) in 2011 for patients with severe symptomatic aortic stenosis who were considered inoperable. In 2012 the FDA extended its approval to use in very high-risk patients. When choosing between SAVR and TAVR in high-risk surgical patients, certain factors must be considered: (1) there is an increased risk of bleeding and atrial fibrillation with SAVR, and (2) there is an increased risk of stroke, vascular damage, complete heart block, left bundle branch block, and paravalvular regurgitation with TAVR. In the appropriately selected patient, TAVR offers a decrease in symptoms and an increase in life expectancy. Currently TAVR is contraindicated in patients with BAV, owing to concerns of malfunction and malposition because of the abnormal valve anatomy. There is a higher risk of incomplete sealing of the valve, paravalvular leak, and aortic regurgitation.

Management of Anesthesia

Patients with aortic stenosis coming for noncardiac surgery are at high risk of perioperative cardiac complications, and the risk of these complications increases with the complexity of the surgery. Hence it is important to ascertain the severity of the aortic stenosis preoperatively. Management of anesthesia in patients with aortic stenosis includes prevention of hypotension and any other hemodynamic change that will decrease cardiac output (Table 6.9).

Normal sinus rhythm should be maintained if possible because the left ventricle is dependent on a properly timed atrial contraction to produce an optimal left ventricular end-diastolic volume. Loss of atrial contraction, as with a junctional rhythm or atrial fibrillation, may produce a dramatic decrease in stroke volume and blood pressure. The overall heart rate is important because it determines the time available for ventricular filling, ejection of the stroke volume, and coronary perfusion. A sustained increase in heart rate decreases the time for left ventricular filling and ejection and reduces cardiac output. A decrease in heart rate can cause overdistention of the left ventricle. Hypotension reduces coronary blood flow and results in myocardial

ischemia and further deterioration in left ventricular function and cardiac output. Aggressive treatment of hypotension is mandatory to prevent cardiogenic shock and/or cardiac arrest. *Cardiopulmonary resuscitation is typically ineffective in patients with aortic stenosis because it is essentially impossible to create an adequate stroke volume across a stenotic aortic valve with cardiac compressions done either externally or internally.*

General anesthesia is often selected in preference to epidural or spinal anesthesia because the sympathetic blockade produced by regional anesthesia can lead to significant hypotension.

Induction of anesthesia can be accomplished with an IV induction drug that does not decrease systemic vascular resistance. An opioid induction agent may be useful if left ventricular function is compromised. Other good choices include benzodiazepines and etomidate. Ketamine may induce tachycardia and should be avoided.

Maintenance of anesthesia can be accomplished with a combination of nitrous oxide and volatile anesthetic and opioids or with opioids alone. The primary goal is to maintain systemic vascular resistance and cardiac output. Drugs that depress sinus node automaticity can produce junctional rhythm and loss of properly timed atrial contraction, which can cause a significant reduction in cardiac output. If left ventricular function is impaired, it is prudent to avoid any drugs that can cause additional depression of myocardial contractility. A decrease in systemic vascular resistance is also very undesirable. Maintenance of anesthesia with nitrous oxide plus opioids or with opioids alone in high doses is recommended for patients with marked left ventricular dysfunction. Neuromuscular blocking drugs with minimal hemodynamic effects are best. Intravascular fluid volume should be maintained at normal levels, since these patients are preload dependent.

Hypotension should be treated aggressively with α-agonists such as phenylephrine that do not cause tachycardia and therefore maintain diastolic filling time. The onset of junctional rhythm or bradycardia requires prompt treatment with ephedrine, atropine, or glycopyrrolate. Persistent tachycardia can be treated with β-blockers such as esmolol. Supraventricular tachycardia should be promptly terminated by cardioversion. Lidocaine, amiodarone, and a defibrillator should be immediately available, since these patients have a propensity to develop ventricular dysrhythmias.

Monitoring

Intraoperative monitoring of patients with aortic stenosis must include ECG leads that reliably detect cardiac rhythm and left ventricular myocardial ischemia. The complexity of the surgery and the severity of the aortic stenosis influence the decision to use an intraarterial catheter, a central venous catheter, a pulmonary artery catheter, or TEE. Such monitoring techniques help determine whether intraoperative hypotension is due to hypovolemia or heart failure. It is important to remember that pulmonary artery occlusion pressure may *overestimate* left ventricular end-diastolic volume because of the decreased compliance of the hypertrophied left ventricle.

AORTIC REGURGITATION

Aortic regurgitation results from failure of aortic leaflet coaptation caused by disease of the aortic leaflets or aortic root. Common causes of leaflet abnormalities include infective endocarditis, rheumatic fever, BAV, and the use of anorexigenic drugs. Abnormalities of the aortic root causing aortic regurgitation include idiopathic aortic root dilatation, hypertension-induced aortoannular ectasia, aortic dissection, syphilitic aortitis, Marfan syndrome, Ehlers-Danlos syndrome, rheumatoid arthritis, ankylosing spondylitis, and psoriatic arthritis. Acute aortic regurgitation is usually the result of endocarditis or aortic dissection.

Pathophysiology

The basic hemodynamic derangement in aortic regurgitation is a decrease in cardiac output due to regurgitation of a part of the ejected stroke volume from the aorta back into the left ventricle during diastole. This results in combined pressure and volume overload on the left ventricle. The magnitude of the regurgitant volume depends on (1) the time available for the regurgitant flow to occur, which is determined by the heart rate, and (2) the pressure gradient across the aortic valve, which is dependent on the systemic vascular resistance. The magnitude of aortic regurgitation is decreased by tachycardia and peripheral vasodilation. With aortic regurgitation the entire stroke volume is ejected into the aorta. Because the pulse pressure is proportional to the stroke volume and aortic elastance, the increased stroke volume increases systolic blood pressure and systolic hypertension increases afterload. The left ventricle compensates by developing hypertrophy and enlarging to accommodate volume overload. Because of the increased oxygen requirements necessitated by left ventricular hypertrophy and the decrease in aortic diastolic pressure that reduces coronary blood flow, angina pectoris may occur in the absence of coronary artery disease.

The left ventricle can usually tolerate chronic volume overload. However, if left ventricular failure occurs, left ventricular end-diastolic volume increases dramatically and pulmonary edema develops. A helpful indicator of left ventricular function in the presence of aortic regurgitation is the echocardiographically determined end-systolic volume and ejection fraction, both of which remain normal until left ventricular function becomes impaired. Indeed, surgery is recommended before the ejection fraction decreases to less than 55% and left ventricular end-systolic volume increases to more than 55 mL.

Compared to patients with chronic aortic regurgitation, patients with acute aortic regurgitation experience severe volume overload in a ventricle that has not had time to compensate. This typically results in coronary ischemia, rapid deterioration in left ventricular function, and heart failure (Fig. 6.6).

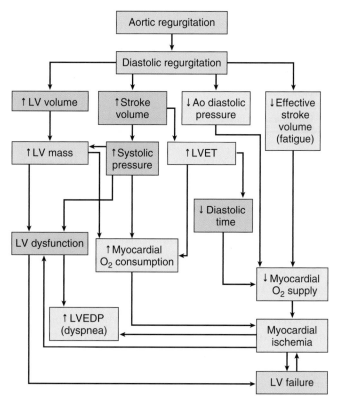

FIG. 6.6 Pathophysiology of aortic regurgitation. Aortic regurgitation results in an increased left ventricular (LV) volume, increased stroke volume, increased aortic (Ao) systolic pressure, and decreased effective stroke volume. Increased LV volume results in an increased LV mass, which may lead to LV dysfunction and failure. Increased LV stroke volume increases systolic pressure and prolongs LV ejection time (LVET). Increased LV systolic pressure results in a decrease in diastolic time. Decreased diastolic time (myocardial perfusion time), diastolic aortic pressure, and effective stroke volume reduce myocardial O_2 supply. Increased myocardial O_2 consumption and decreased myocardial O_2 supply produce myocardial ischemia, which causes further deterioration in LV function. ↑, Increased; ↓, decreased; *LVEDP*, left ventricular end-diastolic pressure. (From Boudoulas H, Gravanis MB. Valvular heart disease. In: Gravanis MB, ed. *Cardiovascular Disorders: Pathogenesis and Pathophysiology.* St Louis, MO: Mosby; 1993:64.)

Diagnosis

Aortic regurgitation is recognized clinically by its characteristic diastolic murmur, heard best along the right sternal border, and peripheral signs of a hyperdynamic circulation, including a widened pulse pressure, decreased diastolic blood pressure, and bounding pulses. In addition to the typical murmur of aortic regurgitation, there may be a low-pitched diastolic rumble (Austin-Flint murmur) that results from fluttering of the mitral valve caused by the regurgitant jet from the leaking aortic valve. As with mitral regurgitation, symptoms of aortic regurgitation may not appear until left ventricular dysfunction is present. Symptoms at this stage are manifestations of left ventricular failure (dyspnea, orthopnea, fatigue) and coronary ischemia. With chronic aortic regurgitation, evidence of left ventricular enlargement and left ventricular hypertrophy may be seen on the chest radiograph and ECG. Echocardiography will reveal any anatomic abnormalities of the aortic valve, including leaflet perforation or prolapse, and will identify any abnormalities in the aortic root and aortic annulus. Left ventricular size, volume, and ejection fraction can be measured, and Doppler examination can be used to identify the presence and severity of aortic regurgitation. Many methods exist to quantify aortic regurgitation. These include regurgitant jet width as a percentage of overall left ventricular outflow tract width, pressure half-time, and diastolic flow reversal in the descending aorta. Cardiac catheterization and CMRI may be useful for grading aortic regurgitation if echocardiography is inadequate.

Treatment

Surgical replacement of a diseased aortic valve is recommended before the onset of permanent left ventricular dysfunction, even if patients are asymptomatic. The operative mortality for isolated AVR is approximately 4%. It is higher if there is concomitant aortic root replacement or coronary artery bypass grafting or if there are substantial comorbidities. The mortality rate in *asymptomatic* patients with aortic insufficiency who have normal left ventricular size and function is less than 0.2% per year. In contrast, *symptomatic* patients have a mortality rate greater than 10% per year. In acute aortic regurgitation, immediate surgical intervention is necessary because the acute volume overload results in heart failure. Alternatives to AVR with a prosthetic valve include a pulmonic valve autograft (Ross procedure) and aortic valve reconstruction.

Medical treatment of aortic regurgitation is designed to decrease systolic hypertension and left ventricular wall stress and improve left ventricular function. Intravenous infusion of a vasodilator such as nitroprusside and an inotropic drug such as dobutamine may be useful for improving left ventricular stroke volume and reducing regurgitant volume. Long-term therapy with nifedipine or hydralazine can be beneficial and may delay the need for surgery in asymptomatic patients with good left ventricular function.

Management of Anesthesia

Management of anesthesia for noncardiac surgery in patients with aortic regurgitation is designed to maintain forward left ventricular stroke volume (Table 6.10). The heart rate must be kept above 80 beats per minute because bradycardia, by increasing the duration of diastole and thereby the time for aortic regurgitation, produces acute left ventricular volume overload. An abrupt increase in systemic vascular resistance can also precipitate left ventricular failure. The compensations for aortic regurgitation may be tenuous, and anesthetic-induced myocardial depression may upset this delicate balance. If left ventricular failure occurs, it is treated with a vasodilator to reduce afterload and an inotrope to increase contractility.

TABLE 6.10	Anesthetic Considerations in Patients With Aortic Regurgitation

Avoid bradycardia
Avoid increases in systemic vascular resistance
Minimize myocardial depression

Overall, modest increases in heart rate and modest decreases in systemic vascular resistance are reasonable hemodynamic goals during anesthesia. General anesthesia is the usual choice for patients with aortic regurgitation.

Induction of anesthesia in the presence of aortic regurgitation can be achieved with an inhaled anesthetic or an IV induction drug. Ideally the induction drug should not decrease the heart rate or increase systemic vascular resistance.

In the absence of severe left ventricular dysfunction, maintenance of anesthesia is often provided with nitrous oxide plus a volatile anesthetic and/or opioid. The increase in heart rate, decrease in systemic vascular resistance, and minimal myocardial depression associated with isoflurane, desflurane, and sevoflurane make these drugs excellent choices in patients with aortic regurgitation. In patients with severe left ventricular dysfunction, high-dose opioid anesthesia may be preferred. Bradycardia and myocardial depression from concomitant use of nitrous oxide or a benzodiazepine are risks of the high-dose narcotic technique. Neuromuscular blockers with minimal or no effect on blood pressure and heart rate are typically used, although the modest increase in heart rate associated with pancuronium administration could be helpful in patients with aortic regurgitation.

Mechanical ventilation should be adjusted to maintain normal oxygenation and carbon dioxide elimination and provide adequate time for venous return. Intravascular fluid volume should be maintained at normal levels to provide adequate preload. Bradycardia and junctional rhythm require prompt treatment with IV atropine.

Monitoring

Surgery in patients with *asymptomatic* aortic regurgitation may not require invasive monitoring. Standard monitors should be adequate to detect rhythm disturbances or myocardial ischemia. In the presence of severe aortic regurgitation, monitoring with a pulmonary artery catheter or TEE is helpful in detecting myocardial depression, facilitating intravascular volume replacement, and measuring the response to administration of a vasodilating drug.

TRICUSPID REGURGITATION

Tricuspid regurgitation is usually *functional,* caused by tricuspid annular dilatation secondary to right ventricular enlargement or pulmonary hypertension. Other causes include infective endocarditis (typically associated with IV drug abuse), carcinoid syndrome, rheumatic heart disease, tricuspid valve prolapse, and Ebstein anomaly. Tricuspid valve disease is often associated with mitral or aortic valve disease. Mild tricuspid regurgitation can be a normal finding at any age and is very commonly seen in highly trained athletes.

Pathophysiology

The basic hemodynamic consequence of tricuspid regurgitation is right atrial volume overload. The high compliance of the right atrium and vena cava result in only a minimal increase in right atrial pressure even in the presence of a large regurgitant volume. Even surgical removal of the tricuspid valve can be well tolerated. Signs of tricuspid regurgitation include jugular venous distention, hepatomegaly, ascites, and peripheral edema. Treatment of functional tricuspid regurgitation is aimed at the cause of the lesion—that is, improving lung function, relieving left-sided heart failure, or reducing pulmonary hypertension. Surgical intervention for isolated tricuspid valve disease is rarely done. However, currently it is suggested that tricuspid valve repair is indicated in any patient with severe tricuspid regurgitation with concomitant mitral valve disease for which they are to undergo mitral valve surgery. It has also been recommended in patients with significant pulmonary hypertension or tricuspid annular dilatation. Data show better outcomes and an improvement in functional class and survival. Tricuspid annuloplasty is a better and more durable procedure than tricuspid valvuloplasty. Replacement of the tricuspid valve is rarely performed. Percutaneous treatment of tricuspid valve dysfunction is still in its developmental phase.

Management of Anesthesia

Management of anesthesia in patients with tricuspid regurgitation includes maintenance of intravascular fluid volume and central venous pressure in the high-normal range to facilitate adequate right ventricular preload and left ventricular filling. Positive pressure ventilation and vasodilating drugs may be particularly deleterious if they significantly reduce venous return. Events known to increase pulmonary artery pressure (e.g., hypoxemia, hypercarbia) must also be avoided.

A specific anesthetic drug combination or technique cannot be recommended for management of patients with tricuspid regurgitation. Agents that produce some pulmonary vasodilation and those that maintain venous return are best. Nitrous oxide can be a weak pulmonary artery vasoconstrictor and could increase the degree of tricuspid regurgitation, so it is best avoided. Intraoperative monitoring should include measurement of right atrial pressure to guide IV fluid replacement and to detect changes in the amount of tricuspid regurgitation in response to administration of anesthetic drugs. With high right atrial pressures, the possibility of right-to-left intracardiac shunting through a patent foramen ovale must be considered. Meticulous care must be taken to avoid infusion of any air through the IV fluid system to reduce the potential of a systemic embolism.

TRICUSPID STENOSIS

Tricuspid stenosis is rare in the adult population. The most common cause in adults is rheumatic heart disease with co-existing tricuspid regurgitation and often mitral or aortic valve disease. Carcinoid syndrome and endomyocardial fibrosis are even rarer causes of tricuspid stenosis. Tricuspid stenosis increases right atrial pressure and increases the pressure gradient between the right atrium and right ventricle. Right atrial dimensions are increased, but the right ventricular dimensions are determined by the degree of volume overload from concomitant tricuspid regurgitation. Evaluation by echocardiography and color flow Doppler imaging helps estimate the severity of the stenosis.

PULMONIC VALVE REGURGITATION

Pulmonic valve regurgitation results from pulmonary hypertension with annular dilatation of the pulmonic valve. Other causes include connective tissue diseases, carcinoid syndrome, infective endocarditis, and rheumatic heart disease. Pulmonary regurgitation is rarely symptomatic and can be tolerated for long periods.

PULMONIC STENOSIS

Pulmonic stenosis is usually congenital (either as part of a complex congenital cardiac lesion or as an isolated congenital defect) and detected and corrected in childhood. An acquired form can be due to rheumatic fever, carcinoid syndrome, infective endocarditis, previous surgery, or other interventions. Significant obstruction can cause syncope, angina, right ventricular hypertrophy, and right ventricular failure. Surgical valvotomy can be used to relieve the obstruction. Since its introduction in 2000, percutaneous pulmonic valve implantation has evolved as an alternative to open heart surgery and as an option to delay "redo" operations for right ventricular outflow tract dysfunction in children and adults with congenital heart disease. This procedure prolongs the duration of the surgical pulmonic conduits from the prior operation. Echocardiography is essential for evaluation and management during this procedure.

PERCUTANEOUS TREATMENT OF VALVULAR HEART DISEASE

Aortic Valve Procedures

AVR in patients with critical aortic stenosis can be lifesaving. AVR has traditionally been accomplished via open heart surgery and the use of cardiopulmonary bypass. Patients who are deemed to be at very high risk or even inoperable because of age and multiple comorbid conditions have been treated medically or by balloon aortic valvotomy. Balloon valvotomy provides short-term relief of symptoms but does not alter the natural history of severe aortic stenosis. The need for alternative treatment options for this population of patients with valvular heart disease is now being addressed. During the last decade, several different procedures have been developed to treat aortic valvular heart disease without open heart surgery and cardiopulmonary bypass.

Transcatheter aortic valve replacement (TAVR or TAVI) is a procedure that can be performed percutaneously via the femoral artery (retrograde and less invasive) or via puncture of the apex of the left ventricle (antegrade and more invasive) or via a transaortic approach (less morbidity and fewer postoperative complications) (Fig. 6.7). (An article by Leon and colleagues with a link to a video animation of this procedure is listed in the Resources section at the end of the chapter.) The approach for percutaneous AVR is chosen after consideration of iliac artery size, the presence of aortic or iliac disease, pathologic changes in the left ventricular apex, pericardial disease, and any history of left thoracotomy or mediastinal or chest radiation. General anesthesia may be used for the transfemoral approach and is essential for the transapical and transaortic approaches. TEE is used initially to determine the pathologic features of the aortic valve, the annulus size, and left ventricular function, and to detect the presence of mitral regurgitation and aortic atheromas. After implantation of the valve, echocardiography is used to assess prosthesis position, determine the degree of aortic regurgitation, if any, and detect the presence of perivalvular leaks, aortic dissection, mitral regurgitation, left ventricular dysfunction, or new regional wall motion abnormalities. Further research is needed to develop less traumatic devices with features providing cerebral protection to reduce the frequency of neurologic complications, which is currently rather high, higher than with open heart surgery.

Compared with medical therapy or balloon valvotomy, transcatheter aortic valve implantation is associated with a lower 30-day and 1-year mortality from all causes, a greater improvement in cardiac symptoms, and a reduced need for repeat hospitalization for cardiac reasons. Major complications of TAVR include stroke, cognitive dysfunction, aortic dissection, bleeding, mediastinal hematoma, femoral or iliac artery injury, valve size mismatch, conduction system problems, and perivalvular leaks. Less common complications include annular rupture, coronary artery obstruction, myocardial infarction, valve malposition, esophageal perforation, and renal failure.

Mitral Valve Procedures

Percutaneous balloon valvotomy has been used for some time to correct mitral stenosis. For mitral regurgitation, however, the recommendation for symptomatic patients and those with evidence of left ventricular dysfunction is mitral valve repair (ring annuloplasty) or mitral valve replacement. This is typically performed via open heart surgery and cardiopulmonary bypass. Medical management only improves symptoms; it does not affect the progression of the disease. Percutaneous transcatheter mitral valve repair with the MitraClip is currently a viable alternative treatment for selected patients with *degenerative* severe mitral regurgitation. Additional clinical

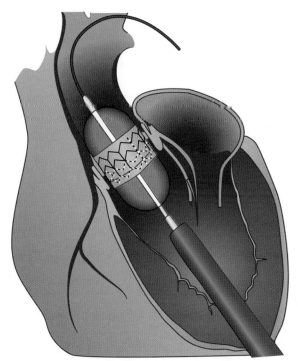

FIG. 6.7   Schematic illustration of transapical aortic valve implantation. The prosthesis is being dilated at the annular level within the native aortic valve cusps. Transapical sheath insert is secured with a purse-string suture. (From Walther T, Falk V, Borger MA, et al. Minimally invasive transapical beating heart aortic valve implantation—proof of concept. *Eur J Cardiothorac Surg*. 2007;31:9-15, with permission.)

trials are needed to determine the efficacy of this procedure in *functional* mitral regurgitation. This percutaneous procedure is associated with a low risk of stroke, myocardial infarction, and death. Bleeding and vascular problems are its most common complications. There is evidence of improvement in the degree of mitral regurgitation, NYHA functional class, quality of life, and left ventricular dimensions. (A link to an animation video of the MitraClip insertion process is noted in the Resources section of this chapter.)

Pulmonic Valve Procedures

Transcatheter pulmonic valve placement has been used in selected patients with pulmonary insufficiency and right ventricular outflow tract problems. Successful percutaneous placement of a pulmonic valve is associated with a reduction in right ventricular outflow tract obstruction, improved right ventricular pressure and/or volume unloading, and improved overall right ventricular function, biventricular function, and functional capacity. The procedure has been performed under general anesthesia with minimal hemodynamic instability. TEE is very helpful during this procedure.

Additional randomized clinical trials are needed to compare all of these new treatments for valvular heart disease with traditional methodologies and to measure the long-term outcomes in terms of both longevity and quality of life.

Left Atrial Appendage Closure

The majority of strokes that occur in patients with atrial fibrillation are a result of embolism from a thrombus in the left atrial appendage. In patients older than age 80, atrial fibrillation accounts for almost 30% of strokes. The conventional treatment of most of these patients has been oral anticoagulation with warfarin. While taking this drug, frequent monitoring and dose adjustments are necessary. In addition, drug interactions and the risk of bleeding have to be considered. When a stroke does occur in a patient taking anticoagulation therapy, mortality is substantially higher. Because of these considerations, there is a group of patients who do not take anticoagulants even though they are in atrial fibrillation.

Left atrial appendage closure (LAAC) devices, such as the Watchman LAAC device, have appeared as an alternative to oral anticoagulation for stroke prevention in selected high-risk patients with nonvalvular atrial fibrillation (Fig. 6.8). Two randomized trials (PROTECT AF and PREVAIL) have shown the LAAC has a benefit similar in efficacy to warfarin in regard to the incidence of stroke, systemic embolism, and cardiovascular death. It appears that the efficacy of percutaneous closure of the LAA is not inferior to warfarin therapy in the long term, though there are complications related to the procedure. Patient selection remains critical when deciding long-term anticoagulation versus the use of an LAAC device. (A link to an implant animation video of the Watchman device is noted in the Resources section of this chapter.)

KEY POINTS

- The most frequently encountered cardiac valve lesions produce pressure overload (mitral stenosis, aortic stenosis) or volume overload (mitral regurgitation, aortic regurgitation) on the left atrium or left ventricle.
- Angina pectoris may occur in patients with valvular heart disease even in the absence of coronary artery disease. This usually reflects increased myocardial oxygen demand due to ventricular hypertrophy. The demands of this thickened muscle mass may exceed the ability of even normal coronary arteries to deliver adequate amounts of oxygen.
- Certain cardiac lesions, such as aortic and mitral stenosis, require a slow heart rate to prolong the duration of diastole and improve left ventricular filling and coronary blood flow. The regurgitant valvular lesions such as aortic and mitral regurgitation require afterload reduction and a somewhat faster heart rate to shorten the time for regurgitation.
- Prosthetic valves differ from one another in regard to durability, thrombogenicity, and hemodynamic profile. Mechanical valves are very durable, lasting at least 20–30 years, whereas bioprosthetic valves last about 10–15 years. Mechanical valves are highly thrombogenic and require long-term anticoagulation. Because bioprosthetic valves have a low thrombogenic potential, long-term anticoagulation is often not necessary.

- In 2007, major changes were made in the AHA guidelines for prevention of infective endocarditis. Antibiotic prophylaxis is now recommended *only for those patients who are at highest risk of adverse outcomes if they were to develop infective endocarditis.*
- Management of anesthesia for noncardiac surgery in patients with mitral stenosis includes prevention and treatment of events that can decrease cardiac output or produce pulmonary edema. The development of atrial fibrillation with a rapid ventricular response significantly decreases cardiac output and can produce pulmonary edema. Excessive perioperative fluid administration, placement in Trendelenburg position, or autotransfusion via uterine contraction increases central blood volume and can precipitate congestive heart failure. A sudden decrease in systemic vascular resistance may not be tolerated, because the normal response to hypotension (i.e., a reflex increase in heart rate) decreases cardiac output in this situation.
- The basic hemodynamic derangement in mitral regurgitation is a decrease in forward left ventricular stroke volume and cardiac output. A portion of every stroke volume is regurgitated through the incompetent mitral valve back into the left atrium, which results in left atrial volume overload and pulmonary congestion. Patients with a regurgitant fraction of more than 60% have severe mitral regurgitation. Pharmacologic interventions that increase or decrease systemic vascular resistance have a major impact on the regurgitant fraction in patients with mitral regurgitation.
- *Mitral valve prolapse* (MVP) is defined as the prolapse of one or both mitral leaflets into the left atrium during systole, with or without mitral regurgitation. It is associated with the auscultatory findings of a midsystolic click and a late systolic murmur. MVP is the most common form of valvular heart disease, affecting 1%–2.5% of the US population. It is usually a benign condition.
- Calcific aortic stenosis and bicuspid aortic valve (BAV) are associated with development of aortic stenosis.
- BAV is the most common congenital valvular abnormality and is associated with aortic root dilatation and/or dilatation of the ascending aorta. Aortic stenosis in patients with BAV occurs at a younger age compared to aortic stenosis in a tricuspid aortic valve. The aortopathy associated with BAV causes aortic aneurysms to grow faster than normal, and there is a higher risk of aortic dissection and rupture than in the general population.
- Management of anesthesia in patients with aortic stenosis includes prevention of hypotension and any hemodynamic change that will decrease cardiac output. Normal sinus rhythm must be maintained because the left ventricle is dependent on a properly timed atrial contraction to produce an optimal left ventricular end-diastolic volume. Loss of atrial contraction may produce a dramatic decrease in stroke volume and blood pressure. The heart rate is important because it determines the time available for ventricular filling, ejection of the stroke volume, and coronary perfusion. A sustained increase in heart rate decreases the time

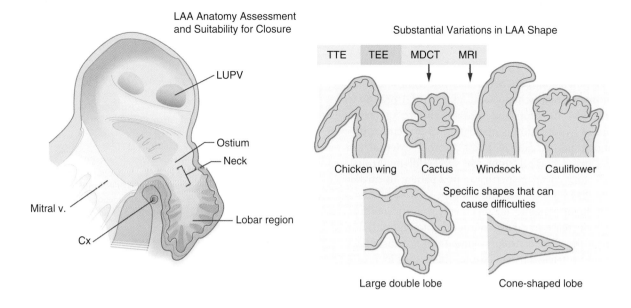

LAA Anatomy Assessment and Suitability for Closure

- LUPV
- Ostium
- Neck
- Lobar region
- Mitral v.
- Cx

Substantial Variations in LAA Shape

| TTE | TEE | MDCT | MRI |

Chicken wing Cactus Windsock Cauliflower

Specific shapes that can cause difficulties

Large double lobe Cone-shaped lobe

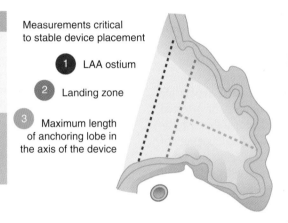

ENDOLUMINAL LAA DEVICES

LAA Occluder Device
First- and Second-Generation
LAA Plug
Flexible LAA Occlusion Device

2D TEE + 3D TEE

- Evaluation of contraindications
- LAA dimensions
- Surrounding anatomic landmarks

Measurements critical to stable device placement

1. LAA ostium
2. Landing zone
3. Maximum length of anchoring lobe in the axis of the device

EPICARDIAL LAA DEVICES

LAA Ligation Device

Spiral CT

TEE

- Evaluation of contraindications
- LAA ostium and anatomic assessments
- Magnetic wire placement within LAA during procedure

Periprocedural Echocardiographic Guidance

2D TEE + 3D TEE + Fluoroscopy

- Transseptal puncture
- Placement of delivery sheath
- Correct device positioning

Postprocedural Echocardiographic Follow-Up

2D TEE + 3D TEE

- Iatrogenic ASD
- Peridevice leakage
- Thrombi
- Device position

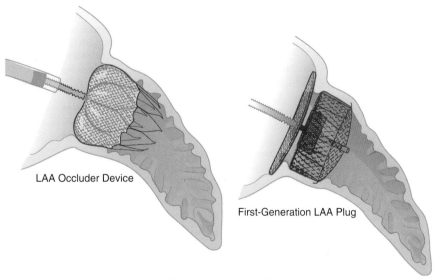

LAA Occluder Device

First-Generation LAA Plug

FIG. 6.8 Imaging approach to left atrial appendage closure: an overview. Top left panel shows a cross section of the left atrium and the orientation of the LAA, left circumflex coronary artery, mitral valve, as well as the left upper pulmonary vein. Top right panel depicts the various LAA morphologies and shapes. Middle panel demonstrates the critical locations where measurements need to be made for optimal sizing of the LAA occlusion device. Bottom left panel illustrates the optimal placement of LAA occluder device and first-generation LAA plug for LAA occlusion. *ASD,* Atrial septal defect; *CT,* computed tomography; *Cx,* circumflex coronary artery; *LAA,* left atrial appendage; *LUPV,* left upper pulmonary vein; *MDCT,* multidetector computed tomography; *MRI,* magnetic resonance imaging; *TEE,* transesophageal echocardiography; *TTE,* transthoracic echocardiography. (From Wunderlich NC, Beigel R, Swaans MJ, et al. Percutaneous interventions for left atrial occlusion. *JACC Cardiovasc Imaging.* 2015;8:472-478. Copyright © 2015 American College of Cardiology, with permission.)

for left ventricular filling and ejection and reduces cardiac output. Hypotension reduces coronary blood flow and can result in myocardial ischemia and further deterioration in left ventricular function and cardiac output. Aggressive treatment of hypotension is mandatory to prevent cardiogenic shock and/or cardiac arrest. Neither external nor internal cardiac compressions are successful in producing satisfactory coronary perfusion in a patient in cardiac arrest who has significant aortic stenosis.

- The basic hemodynamic derangement in aortic regurgitation is a decrease in cardiac output due to regurgitation of a part of the ejected stroke volume from the aorta back into the left ventricle during diastole. This results in a combined pressure and volume overload on the left ventricle. The magnitude of the regurgitant volume depends on (1) the time available for the regurgitant flow to occur, which is determined by the heart rate, and (2) the pressure gradient across the aortic valve, which is dependent on systemic vascular resistance. The magnitude of aortic regurgitation is decreased by tachycardia and peripheral vasodilation.

- Percutaneous valve replacement for severe aortic stenosis or pulmonic stenosis, and percutaneous valve repair for severe mitral regurgitation are now options in selected high-risk patients or those considered inoperable. Multimodal imaging is necessary for preprocedural assessment of the valvular lesions and proper patient selection, postprocedure evaluation of the newly inserted device, and long-term follow up.

- The majority of strokes that occur in patients with atrial fibrillation are a result of embolism from a thrombus in the left atrial appendage. The conventional treatment for most of these patients has been oral anticoagulation with warfarin. For patients who cannot tolerate anticoagulation, left atrial appendage closure (LAAC) devices have been developed as an alternative to chronic oral anticoagulation for stroke prevention in selected high-risk patients with *non-valvular* atrial fibrillation.

RESOURCES

Badheka Ao, Singh V, Patel NJ, et al. Trends of hospitalizations in the United States from 2000 to 2012 of patients older than 60 years with aortic valve disease. *Am J Cardiol.* 2015;116:132-141.

Billings FT, Kodali SK, Shanewise JS. Transcatheter aortic valve implantation: anesthetic considerations. *Anesth Analg.* 2009;108:1453-1462.

Cullen MW, Cabalka AK, Alli OO, et al. Transvenous, antegrade Melody® valve-in-valve implantation for bioprosthetic mitral and tricuspid valve dysfunction: a case series in children and adults. *JACC Cardiovasc Interv.* 2013;6:598-605.

Downs EA, Lim DS, Saji M, et al. Current state of transcatheter mitral valve repair with the MitraClip®. *Ann Cardiothorac Surg.* 2015;4:335-340.

Feldman T, Foster E, Glower DG, et al. Percutaneous repair or surgery for mitral regurgitation. *N Engl J Med.* 2011;364:1395-1406.

Holmes DR, Doshi SK, Kar S, et al. Left atrial appendage closure as an alternative to warfarin for stroke prevention in atrial fibrillation. *J Am Coll Cardiol.* 2015;65:2614-2623.

Kertai MD, Bountioukos M, Boersma E, et al. Aortic stenosis: an underestimated risk factor for peri-operative complications in patients undergoing noncardiac surgery. *Am J Med.* 2004;116:8-13.

Leon MB, Smith CR, Mack M, et al. Transcatheter aortic-valve implantation for aortic stenosis in patients who cannot undergo surgery. *N Engl J Med.* 2010;363:1597-1607. Associated link to an animation of the transcatheter aortic valve implantation (TAVI) procedure. http://www.nejm.org/doi/full/10.1056/NEJMoa1008232.

Lindman BR, Bonow RO, Otto CM. Current management of calcific aortic stenosis. *Circ Res.* 2013;113:223-237.

McElhinney DB, Hellenbrand WE, Zahn EM, et al. Short- and medium-term outcomes after transcatheter pulmonary valve placement in the expanded multicenter US Melody® valve trial. *Circulation.* 2010;122:507-516.

MitraClip® Procedural Animation Video. www.mitraclip.com.

Nishimura RA, Otto CM, Bonow RO, et al. 2014 AHA/ACC guidelines for the management of patients with valvular heart disease: executive summary: a report of the American College of Cardiology/American Heart Association Task Force on Practice Guidelines. *J Am Coll Cardiol.* 2014;63:2438-2488.

Nkomo VT, Gardin JM, Skelton TN, et al. Burden of valvular heart diseases: a population-based study. *Lancet.* 2006;368:1005-1011.

Perrino AC, Reeves ST. *A Practical Approach to Transesophageal Echocardiography.* Philadelphia, PA: Lippincott Williams & Wilkins; 2014.

Rogers JH, Bolling SF. Surgical approach to functional tricuspid regurgitation: should we be more aggressive? *Curr Opin Cardiol.* 2014;29:133-139.

Ruiz CE, Kliger C, Perk G, et al. Transcatheter therapies for the treatment of valvular and paravalvular regurgitation in acquired and congenital valvular heart disease. *J Am Coll Cardiol.* 2015;66:169-183.

Singh SP, Alli O, Melby S, et al. TAVR: imaging spectrum of complications. *J Thorac Imaging.* 2015;30:359-377.

Walther T, Volkman F, Borger MA, et al. Minimally invasive transapical heart aortic valve implantation—proof of concept. *Eur J Cardiothorac Surg.* 2007;31:9-15.

Watchman® Procedural Animation Video. www.watchmandevice.com.

Wilson W, Taubert KA, Gewitz M, et al. Prevention of infective endocarditis: guidelines from the American Heart Association. *Circulation.* 2007;116:1736-1754.

Wong MCG, Clark DJ, Horrigan HE, et al. Advances in percutaneous treatment of adult valvular heart disease. *Intern Med J.* 2009;39:465-474.

Congenital Heart Disease

JOCHEN STEPPAN, BRYAN G. MAXWELL

Congenital heart disease is the most common congenital abnormality, accounting for 4–10 cases per 1000 live births (clustering around 8). These numbers do not include bicuspid aortic valves, which would double or triple the incidence. Overall, congenital heart disease accounts for approximately a third of all congenital defects. Moreover, in developed countries, congenital heart disease has become the principal cause of heart disease in children, with 10%–15% having associated congenital anomalies of the skeletal, genitourinary, or gastrointestinal system. The incidence of congenital heart disease in children has remained constant over the last few decades. However, because therapeutic options have improved, the number of adults with congenital heart disease has steadily increased. It is estimated that in the United States, more adults than children are currently living with congenital heart disease. This trend is reflected in an ever-rising number of patients presenting for cardiac surgery, including primary repair, revision of a prior operation, conversion to a more modern operation, treatment of long-term sequelae of congenital heart disease,

or for noncardiac surgery that is unrelated to their congenital cardiac defect; it can be quite daunting to familiarize oneself with them all. However, fewer than a dozen lesions, most of them acyanotic, comprise almost 90% of congenital heart diseases encountered (Table 7.1).

Over the last few decades, physicians have become more and more facile at diagnosing congenital heart disease earlier in life. It is not uncommon now for physicians to diagnose even subtle congenital cardiovascular lesions in utero using ultrasonography.

Diagnosing congenital heart disease post utero has also evolved from fairly crude methods (auscultation, chest x-rays, and phenotypic appearance) to highly sophisticated imaging modalities such as ultrasonography, cardiac catheterization, and magnetic resonance imaging (MRI). These techniques have made it possible to go beyond simply diagnosing a lesion to (1) accurately visualizing minute details of cardiac function, blood flow, and driving pressures and (2) predicting (to a certain extent) the perioperative course and long-term prognosis. It is therefore not surprising that these techniques allow almost half of patients with congenital heart disease to

TABLE 7.1	Classification and Incidence of Congenital Heart Disease	
Disease		Incidence (%)
ACYANOTIC DEFECTS		
Shunting lesions		
Ventricular septal defect		37
Atrial septal defect		9
Patent ductus arteriosus		8
Atrioventricular septal defect		4
Stenotic lesions		
Pulmonary stenosis		8
Aortic stenosis		4
Coarctation of the aorta		4
CYANOTIC DEFECTS		
Tetralogy of Fallot		4
Transposition of the great vessels		3
Hypoplastic left heart		3
Hypoplastic right heart		2

be diagnosed within the first week of life. Most of the remaining patients are diagnosed before their fifth birthday, often by the accidental finding of a heart murmur or when the child presents with signs and symptoms of congenital heart disease like feeding problems, failure to thrive, growth retardation, dyspnea, or even cyanosis. In addition to these presenting symptoms the anesthesiologist faces a long list of cardiac and noncardiac sequelae that occur with higher frequency in patients with congenital heart disease (Table 7.2). Therefore

TABLE 7.2	Common Problems Associated With Congenital Heart Disease

CARDIAC
Dysrhythmias
Conduction defects
Pulmonary hypertension (Eisenmenger syndrome)
Endocarditis
Heart failure

PULMONARY
Cyanosis
Altered response to hypoxia or hypercarbia
Decreased lung compliance
Chronic lung disease
Hemoptysis
Airway compression

VASCULAR
Prior cannulation sites complicating the ability to gain vascular access

RENAL
Chronic renal insufficiency
Renal failure

HEPATOBILIARY
Cholelithiasis
Hepatic congestion
Protein-losing enteropathy

CENTRAL NERVOUS SYSTEM
Brain abscesses
Seizures
Strokes
Paradoxical emboli
Developmental status

PERIPHERAL NERVOUS SYSTEM
Phrenic nerve paralysis
Recurrent nerve paralysis

HEMATOLOGIC
Erythrocytosis (hyperviscosity syndrome)
Abnormal coagulation studies
Thromboembolism
Coagulopathy

MUSCULOSKELETAL
Higher incidence of scoliosis

MISCELLANEOUS
Decreased exercise tolerance
Failure to thrive and feeding difficulties in children

the selection of induction drugs and monitoring methods should take into account not only the patient's overall health status, cardiac defect, and planned intervention but also changes in major organ systems (heart, vasculature, lungs, kidneys, etc.).

CONGENITAL HEART LESIONS

Acyanotic Congenital Heart Disease

Shunting Lesions

Acyanotic shunting lesions are principally characterized by blood flow that shunts from left to right inside the heart or proximal great vessels (Table 7.3). This shunting leads to increased pulmonary blood flow that increases pulmonary vascular resistance, leading to intimal hyperplasia and vascular remodeling. All these effects culminate in pulmonary hypertension, right ventricular hypertrophy, and eventually congestive heart failure (CHF). In general the younger the patient at the time of surgical repair, the greater the likelihood that pulmonary vascular resistance will normalize. Survival in such patients is usually excellent, especially if shunting is minor. However, if the defect is not repaired and shunting involves more than one-third of cardiac output, long-term sequelae are highly likely, including the development of pulmonary hypertension, ventricular remodeling, and CHF.

Atrial Septal Defect

Atrial septal defects (ASDs), although less prevalent in children than other acyanotic shunt lesions, account for the majority of congenital heart lesions detected in adults. Ventricular septal defects (VSDs) occur more commonly than ASDs, but they have a high spontaneous closure rate (almost 70%). Moreover, small ASDs can remain asymptomatic for decades. Consequently they are more commonly diagnosed in adults.

Depending on the embryologic origin and location of the defect in the interatrial septum and the specific point of shunting, one can differentiate four different types of ASDs (Fig. 7.1). An *ostium primum defect* occurs when the ostium primum fails to fuse with the endocardial cushions. The result

TABLE 7.3	Congenital Heart Defects Resulting in Left-to-Right Shunting

Atrial septal defect
    Ostium primum defect
    Ostium secundum defect
    Sinus venosus defect
    Unroofed coronary sinus
Ventricular septal defect (VSD)
    Subarterial VSD
    Perimembranous VSD
    Inlet VSD
    Muscular VSD
Patent ductus arteriosus
Aortopulmonary fenestration

is a defect in the interatrial septum that is located caudally just above the atrioventricular valves. The most common type of ASD, the *ostium secundum defect* (75% of all ASDs) is located in the middle of the interatrial septum in the same location as the foramen ovale and can vary from a single opening to a fenestrated septum. The two remaining ASDs, the *sinus venosus defect* (located at either the superior vena cava or the inferior vena cava junction) and the *unroofed coronary sinus* (opening of the coronary sinus into the left atrium via its crossing behind the heart), occur with the least frequency. These defects do not always present in isolation but can be part of more complex syndromes, each of which is associated with other specific lesions. Specifically, ostium primum defects are associated with a cleft mitral valve and/or mitral regurgitation, the ostium secundum defect is associated with mitral valve prolapse and/or regurgitation, sinus venous defects are associated with anomalous right pulmonary venous return, and an unroofed coronary sinus is associated with a persistent left superior vena cava.

Regardless of the type of ASD, the resulting physiologic changes depend on the degree of net blood shunting from the left to the right atrium. The degree of shunting in turn depends not simply on the pressure difference between the two chambers but also on the size of the lesion and the relative compliance of the ventricles. The resulting mostly left-to-right shunt increases pulmonary blood flow and causes volume overloading of the right ventricle and right atrium. Smaller defects

result in minor or negligible shunts that are mostly without hemodynamic consequences. Larger ASDs that allow more than a 50% increase in pulmonary blood flow can have severe hemodynamic consequences that produce pulmonary hypertension, ventricular remodeling, and supraventricular tachydysrhythmias such as atrial fibrillation.

Similar to many other congenital heart lesions, diagnosis in asymptomatic patients is often initiated after auscultation of a heart murmur. In patients with an ASD it is usually a systolic murmur with a split second heart sound due to delayed pulmonary valve closure secondary to increased flow across the pulmonary valve. This finding can then be followed up by an electrocardiogram (ECG), which might reveal signs of right axis deviation and an incomplete right bundle branch block from right ventricular strain. A chest x-ray may show enlarged pulmonary arteries, prominent lung vasculature, and cardiomegaly. Ultimately the diagnosis is confirmed by using echocardiography with color Doppler to determine the location of the ASD, the degree of shunting, the direction of blood flow, and associated cardiac anomalies.

Signs and Symptoms. Patients can present with increasing dyspnea on exertion, decreased exercise tolerance, fatigue, heart failure, palpitations, or embolic stroke. However, many patients with ASDs will remain asymptomatic for years and the diagnosis made only accidentally after evaluation of a heart murmur. Smaller defects with a ratio of pulmonary to systemic blood flow (Qp:Qs ratio) of less than 1.5:1 usually

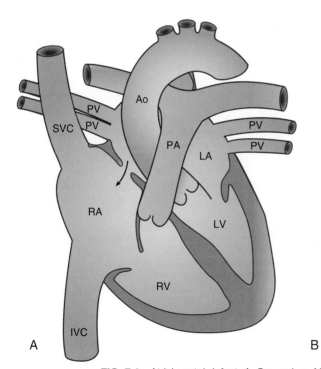

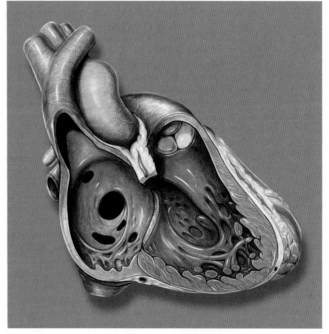

FIG. 7.1   Atrial septal defect. A, Secundum ASD, in which blood flows left to right across the atria along a pressure gradient. B, Schematic drawing of the locations of ASDs. *1*, Septum primum defect; *2*, septum secundum defect; *3*, sinus venosus defects; *4*, unroofed coronary sinus. *Ao*, Aorta; *IVC*, inferior vena cava; *LA*, left atrium; *LV*, left ventricle; *PA*, pulmonary artery; *PV*, pulmonary vein; *RA*, right atrium; *RV*, right ventricle; *SVC*, superior vena cava. (http://radiopaedia.org/images/25224 by Patrick Lynch).

remain asymptomatic and do not require further intervention. Shunt lesions with a Qp:Qs ratio greater than 1.5:1 should be considered for closure to prevent long-term sequelae. Depending on the location and size of the ASD, it can be closed percutaneously using a septal occlusion device or surgically with either a full sternotomy or a minimally invasive approach via thoracotomy.

Management of Anesthesia. For general management strategies and anesthetic management, please see "Balancing Pulmonary and Vascular Resistance (Qp:Qs)" later in the chapter. For patients undergoing ASD closure, management depends on the chosen approach. A percutaneous ASD closure can be conducted with minimal or noninvasive monitoring under general anesthesia or deep sedation, whereas a surgical ASD repair requires all of the monitors and access needed for cardiopulmonary bypass and the capacity to treat/manage potential postoperative heart block.

Ventricular Septal Defect

With an incidence of more than 30%, excluding bicuspid aortic valves, VSDs are the most prevalent form of congenital heart disease in children. However, because of the high spontaneous closure rate, especially for muscular septal defects, they are more rare in adults. The classification of VSDs can be confusing because there are multiple names for each of the four different lesions, which are classified according to their location in the interventricular septum (Fig. 7.2). According to the Congenital Heart Surgery Nomenclature and Database project, a *VSD type I*, also called *subarterial, supracristal, outlet, subpulmonic,* or *infundibular VSD,* is located high in the interventricular septum just below the pulmonic valve above the crista terminalis. The most common VSD (more than two-thirds of all VSDs) is the *type II VSD,* also called the *perimembranous* or *infracristal VSD,* which is located lower in the septum just below the crista terminalis. A *type III VSD,* also called *inlet of canal–type VSD,* is located just below the mitral and tricuspid valve. The last type of VSD, *type IV* or *muscular VSDs,* are located deep in the muscular portion of the ventricular septum and can range from a single perforation to a multitude of holes with different sizes. Similar to ASDs, certain types of VSDs are associated with different lesions. Type I VSDs are associated with aortic insufficiency caused by prolapse of the aortic valve cusp, and type II VSDs are associated with tricuspid valve aneurysms or insufficiency caused by entrapment of the valve leaflets. Type III VSDs are associated with a cleft mitral valve or tricuspid valve and are part of the complete atrioventricular canal defect. Lastly, type IV VSDs can be associated with a multitude of different lesions but do have the highest probability of closing spontaneously during aging.

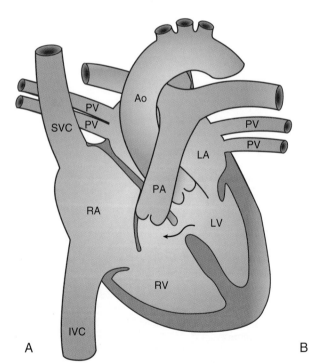
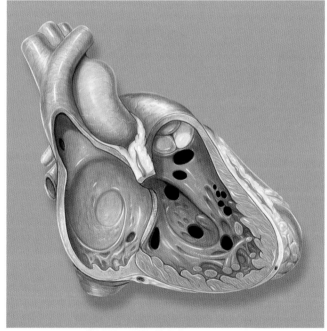

FIG. 7.2 Ventricular septal defect. A, Schematic depiction of a VSD resulting in a left-to-right shunting lesion. B, Locations of the different types of VSDs. *1,* Subarterial; *2,* perimembranous; *3,* inlet; *4,* muscular. *Ao,* Aorta; *IVC,* inferior vena cava; *LA,* left atrium; *LV,* left ventricle; *PA,* pulmonary artery; *PV,* pulmonary vein; *RA,* right atrium; *RV,* right ventricle; *SVC,* superior vena cava. (Patrick J. Lynch; illustrator; C. Carl Jaffe; MD; cardiologist Yale University Center for Advanced Instructional Media Medical Illustrations by Patrick Lynch, generated for multimedia teaching projects by the Yale University School of Medicine, Center for Advanced Instructional Media, 1987-2000. Patrick J. Lynch, http://patricklynch.net. http://commons.wikimedia.org/wiki/File:Heart_right_vsd.jpg.)

Signs and Symptoms. The severity of signs and symptoms depends on the size of the defect, the pressure difference between the ventricles, and the ratio of pulmonary to systemic vascular resistance. Small defects with a resulting Qp:Qs ratio of 1.4:1 or less usually remain asymptomatic and do not result in major hemodynamic compromise (e.g., pulmonary hypertension or heart failure). These defects are usually referred to as *restrictive VSDs* because the amount of shunting is restricted by the size of the defect. Moderately restrictive VSDs with a Qp:Qs ratio of 1.4–2.2:1 or nonrestrictive VSDs with a Qp:Qs ratio greater than 2.2:1 can result in an equalization of left and right ventricular systolic pressure that causes both volume and pressure overload of the pulmonary circulation. This overload can in turn lead to pulmonary hypertension. Over time the pulmonary vasculature starts to remodel, resulting in increased pulmonary vascular resistance and a decrease in the Qp:Qs ratio that ultimately can lead to shunt reversal (see "Eisenmenger Syndrome"). Patients become progressively hypoxic as more blood bypasses the lungs. Such patients are no longer candidates for a VSD closure because this would inevitably lead to right heart failure. Over time, even in the absence of advanced disease and Eisenmenger syndrome, patients with moderately restrictive or unrestrictive VSDs develop left ventricular failure and pulmonary hypertension, putting them at increased perioperative risk. Therefore it is important to diagnose patients early and perform a VSD closure before pulmonary vascular resistance increases to such high levels that closure is no longer possible.

Clinically, patients with a VSD have a holosystolic murmur that is loudest at the left sternal border. With increasing size of the defect the ECG can demonstrate signs of left atrial and left ventricular hypertrophy as well as right ventricular strain. Similarly, chest x-rays will show an enlarged cardiac silhouette in advanced disease. Echocardiography (two-dimensional [2D] and color Doppler) is the imaging modality most commonly used to evaluate the presence, directionality, and severity of a VSD. Other more invasive techniques include cardiac catheterization and angiography to measure the amount of intracardiac shunting, intravascular and intracavitary pressures, and pulmonary and systemic vascular resistance.

Management of Anesthesia. The most conservative summary would probably be to treat a patient with a VSD of unknown severity like a patient with CHF and pulmonary hypertension. For general management strategies and anesthetic management, please see "Balancing Pulmonary and Vascular Resistance (Qp:Qs)."

A VSD can be closed percutaneously in older children and adults, especially if it is small. Alternatively, surgical VSD closure is now performed in children of all ages. Thus it is rare for a provider to encounter a newborn undergoing pulmonary artery banding to reduce left-to-right shunting–induced pulmonary overcirculation in anticipation of a VSD closure later in life. However, in the uncommon situation of band placement, tight placement of the pulmonary band can lead to bradycardia and systemic hypotension and should be corrected by prompt removal of the band. Furthermore, positive end-expiratory pressure is often discontinued after placement of the pulmonary artery band to facilitate optimal tightness. Most children will undergo surgical VSD closure, which is generally very well tolerated. Common postsurgical complications include atrioventricular block, ventricular tachycardia, and CHF (especially with the development of pulmonary hypertension).

Patent Ductus Arteriosus (PDA)
During fetal development the ductus arteriosus connects the left pulmonary artery and descending aorta just below the left subclavian artery. It allows shunting of blood from right (pulmonary artery) to left (descending aorta), bypassing the nonventilated lungs. Within the first 24 hours after delivery the ductus begins to close and is completely sealed off within the first month of life. However, in some patients (especially preterm babies) the ductus remains open beyond that time frame (Fig. 7.3). This connection causes left-to-right blood flow from the high-pressure aorta to the low-pressure pulmonary artery. The amount of blood shunting left to right depends on the size of the ductus (diameter and length), the pressure difference between the aorta and the pulmonary artery, and the ratio between pulmonary and systemic vascular resistance.

Signs and Symptoms. Most patients with a PDA have only mild to moderate shunting and remain asymptomatic. It is

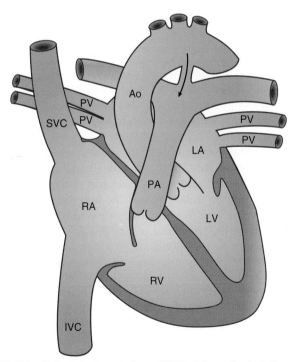

FIG. 7.3 Patent ductus arteriosus (PDA). Schematic depiction of a PDA connecting the distal aortic arch to the pulmonary artery (PA). This connection results in a left-to-right shunt, with blood flowing from the aorta (Ao) to the pulmonary artery. *IVC,* Inferior vena cava; *LA,* left atrium; *LV,* left ventricle; *PV,* pulmonary vein; *RA,* right atrium; *RV,* right ventricle; *SVC,* superior vena cava.

not uncommon for those patients to be diagnosed incidentally during a routine physical in which auscultation of a heart murmur triggers further workup. In the rare incidences that the shunt is large and left-to-right shunting is substantial, the patient can show signs of ventricular hypertrophy and pulmonary hypertension that lead to heart failure, failure to thrive, aneurysmal dilatation of the ductus, and in long-standing disease, Eisenmenger syndrome. The classic auscultatory finding is a continuous systolic and diastolic murmur that is best heard at the left infraclavicular area or the left upper sternal border. Definite diagnosis and quantification can then be established with 2D and Doppler echocardiography or cardiac catheterization and angiography.

Management of Anesthesia. Most patients in whom the ductus fails to close spontaneously will be operated on during the neonatal period. Minimally invasive duct closure by interventional cardiology is not yet widely practiced and is usually performed in older children and young adults. This age range represents a second period for surgery, given that most patients who have not been diagnosed in the perinatal period remain asymptomatic until adolescence, at which point they may present with heart failure or pulmonary hypertension. This condition should prompt immediate action because development of severe pulmonary hypertension can be a contraindication for duct closure.

Most infants born before 28 weeks' gestation will require treatment to facilitate duct closure. Of those, the vast majority can be treated medically with a continuous infusion of the cyclooxygenase inhibitor indomethacin, which decreases the production of prostaglandins that are required to keep the ductus open. Indomethacin is considered the first-line treatment for a PDA.

If medical treatment fails or is contraindicated, the duct is generally closed surgically during the neonatal period. The procedure can be performed off bypass via left thoracotomy either in the operating room or at the bedside in the neonatal intensive care unit, with low morbidity (<1%).

For general management strategies and anesthetic management, please see "Balancing Pulmonary and Vascular Resistance (Qp:Qs)." During the dissection phase of the operation, the surgeon usually pushes the lung out of his field. This action can lead to a temporary drop in oxygen saturation, given the high incidence of lung disease with poor lung compliance in premature infants, and may require multiple adjustments of the ventilator settings to optimize oxygenation. Additionally, the patient may require lung recruitment at the conclusion of the surgery. Ligation of the ductus can result in significant hypertension. Other adverse events include hoarseness (due to recurrent laryngeal nerve injury), hemidiaphragm paralysis (due to phrenic nerve paralysis), chylothorax (due to injury of the thoracic duct), and reopening of the ductus over time.

Obstructive Lesions

Obstructive lesions are characterized by increased resistance to blood flow around the level of the cardiac valves or outflow tracts. Importantly there is no shunting in purely obstructive lesions. In this section we will discuss aortic stenosis, the major left-sided obstructive lesion of the heart; its counterpart pulmonic stenosis on the right side of the heart; and coarctation of the aorta (preductal and postductal). As a result of obstruction, increased pressure is required to overcome the stenosis, which leads to either left- or right-sided concentric hypertrophy and ultimately heart failure.

Aortic Stenosis

Stenosis of the left ventricular outflow tract (LVOT) can be due to subvalvular, valvular, or supravalvular aortic stenosis. Valvular aortic stenosis is frequently the result of a bicuspid aortic valve, which is present in approximately 2% of all newborns in the United States. Because of that extreme high frequency, almost 10 times more frequent than VSDs and at least twice as frequent as all congenital heart lesions combined, and because it very rarely becomes symptomatic until patients reach adulthood, it is usually not counted in the statistics on congenital heart disease. However, it is frequently associated with other vascular abnormalities, such as a PDA or coarctation of the aorta.

Patients with bicuspid aortic valves are not born with a stenosed valve. Rather, because the aortic valve has two instead of the normal three cusps, blood flow is more turbulent, resulting in endothelial disruption and local inflammation, a predisposition for calcification. These factors all culminate in premature aortic stenosis. Severity is commonly determined by the pressure gradient across the aortic valve. A mean gradient of 20 mm Hg is considered mild, but more than 40 mm Hg is considered severe.

Signs and Symptoms. Most patients with bicuspid aortic valves remain asymptomatic until adulthood. Infants with severe (more likely subvalvular) aortic stenosis suffer from feeding difficulties, poor growth, and heart failure. Supravalvular aortic stenosis is much less common and can be associated with a typical phenotype (round forehead, prominent facial bones, pursed upper lip). During anesthesia, patients with supravalvular aortic stenosis are at high risk of sudden death, likely caused by myocardial ischemia. The same is true for patients with subvalvular aortic stenosis, which can be due to either a fixed stenosis (membrane, fibromuscular ridge, etc.) or a dynamic component of left ventricular outflow obstruction.

The classic symptoms of patients with aortic stenosis are syncope, angina, and dyspnea. In such patients the left ventricle must generate higher-than-normal pressures to overcome the stenotic lesion, which is not reflected by a normal systemic blood pressure measured poststenosis. The logical consequence is concentric hypertrophy of the left ventricle, which over time increases oxygen requirements, decreases myocardial compliance and thereby left ventricular filling, and reduces the gradient required for the coronary arteries to perfuse the left ventricular myocardium, leading to angina in the absence of coronary artery disease. Because of the high blood flow velocity and turbulent flow poststenosis, the aortic root and ascending aorta can respond with poststenotic dilation, necessitating the repair of not only the valve but also the root and maybe even the ascending aorta.

Patients with aortic stenosis have a characteristic and fairly easy-to-identify systolic murmur. It is loudest at the second intercostal space and radiates to the neck. The ECG can demonstrate left ventricular hypertrophy with strain—especially during exercise. Chest x-rays show an enlarged left ventricular silhouette ("boot-shaped heart") and potentially a prominent ascending aorta. Ultimately the diagnosis will be confirmed with echocardiography using 2D imaging, continuous wave Doppler, and color Doppler to evaluate the exact location of the stenosis, its severity, associated lesions or changes, and ventricular function. Similarly, cardiac catheterization and angiography can be used to assess severity and associated lesions not easily detectable with echocardiography (e.g., concomitant coronary artery disease). Recently, cardiac MRI has become more and more frequent to combine all evaluation options into one comprehensive study.

Management of Anesthesia. See Chapter 6, "Valvular Heart Disease," and the section about aortic stenosis for details on anesthetic management.

Pulmonic Stenosis

Many of the concepts for aortic stenosis can be extrapolated to pulmonary stenosis, with the main difference being that the right ventricle is much more sensitive to increases in afterload. Similar to aortic stenosis, pulmonary stenosis is mainly valvular in origin rather than supravalvular or subvalvular. Associated lesions, especially of supravalvular pulmonic stenosis, include ASDs, VSDs, a PDA, and tetralogy of Fallot. Subvalvular pulmonic stenosis is typically associated with a VSD, whereas valvular pulmonic stenosis tends to occur in isolation or sometimes in combination with a VSD. Interestingly, peak pressure gradients are frequently used for the classification of pulmonic stenosis (as opposed to mean gradients), with less than 36 mm Hg being mild and more than 64 mm Hg being considered severe.

Signs and Symptoms. Symptoms depend on the severity and associated defects (e.g., cyanosis in severe cases with an associated VSD). In general, patients will present with signs of right heart failure, including dyspnea, jugular venous distension, peripheral edema, and ascites. On auscultation a systolic ejection murmur, best heard at the second left intercostal space, might be found. The ECG may reveal signs of right ventricular hypertrophy and strain. Echocardiography or MRI can be used to confirm and classify the type and severity of the lesion.

Management of Anesthesia. Pulmonary stenosis can be treated with open surgery that requires cardiopulmonary bypass or percutaneously via balloon valvuloplasty. For any patient with pulmonary stenosis undergoing cardiac or noncardiac surgery, the anesthetic goals are to avoid increases in right ventricular oxygen requirements. See Chapter 6, "Valvular Heart Disease," and the section about pulmonic stenosis for details on anesthetic management.

Coarctation of the Aorta

Coarctation of the aorta is more common in male than in female patients. It consists of a narrowing of the aorta in close proximity to the ductus arteriosus and can be preductal, juxtaductal, or postductal. Depending on its location, symptoms and age at diagnosis tend to vary. The most common form, postductal coarctation, lies beyond the ductus arteriosus and is more commonly diagnosed in older children. A preductal coarctation is located proximal to the ductus and is most likely to manifest in infants.

Signs and Symptoms. All forms of aortic coarctation share the common adverse outcomes of systolic hypertension, CHF, aortic dissection, premature coronary artery disease, and intracerebral hemorrhage caused by aneurysm rupture.

Signs and symptoms depend not only on the severity of the coarctation but also on its location (preductal vs. postductal). In general, presenting symptoms include headache, dizziness, palpitations, and epistaxis. Children or adults with postductal aortic coarctation usually remain asymptomatic and come to medical attention for the workup of headaches or for an incidental finding on a routine physical exam, namely a blood pressure difference between the upper (hypertensive) and lower (normotensive or hypotensive) extremities or weak and delayed femoral pulses. In severe cases of diminished lower extremity blood flow, the initial presenting symptom can be lower extremity claudication. Patients tend to have isolated systolic hypertension with normal diastolic blood pressure and consequently widened pulse pressure. Infants with preductal aortic coarctation, on the other hand, tend to become symptomatic earlier in life. Newborns whose ductus is still open have selective cyanosis of the lower extremity, with a pink face and upper extremities. If this coarctation is not diagnosed at that time, the difference in blood pressure between the upper and lower extremities tends to disappear later in life as those children develop extensive collateral blood flow involving the internal thoracic, intercostal, and subclavian arteries.

On physical exam a systolic ejection murmur can be auscultated along the left sternal boarder. It can also be auscultated in the back and over the area of the coarctation, especially if sufficient collateral blood flow is present. The ECG shows the classic signs of left ventricular hypertrophy. Chest x-ray can also reveal notching in the posterior parts of the ribs as a sign of increased collateral blood flow in the intercostal arteries. This notching is visible only posteriorly because the anterior intercostal arteries lie in the costal grooves. Sometimes the actual coarctation and its poststenotic dilatation can also be visualized ("reversed E sign"). The definitive diagnosis can be made with ultrasonography, computed tomography (CT), or MRI, which can classify the location and severity of the stenosis. The latter two techniques can be used to quantify the degree of collateral flow.

Management of Anesthesia. Coarctation ideally should be repaired in infancy or early childhood before patients develop systemic hypertension. Once hypertension develops, the risk is high that it will persist despite an adequate repair. Although coarctation can be repaired percutaneously by a balloon dilation and stent placement, surgical resection of the coarctation and open repair with either a patch or an end-to-end anastomosis remains a popular treatment option. Both approaches are successful in most patients and pose little risk of subsequent aortic aneurysms or recurrent coarctation.

Surgical repair generally does not involve cardiopulmonary bypass, but it does require a high (proximal) aortic cross-clamp. Placement of the cross-clamp necessitates the management of two circulations (proximal and distal to the clamp) with very different pressures. Importantly the tighter the aortic stenosis, the fewer hemodynamic perturbations arise during placement of the cross-clamp. The proximal circulation (especially the heart, head, and upper extremity) are exposed to a relatively high pressure that has the potential to cause heart failure and cerebral hemorrhage. The distal circulation (especially the gut, kidneys, spinal cord, and lower extremities) are faced with the opposite problem, profound hypotension and hypoperfusion (depending on the amount of collateral blood flow), potentially leading to gut ischemia, renal failure, or in rare cases paraplegia. Blood pressure should be monitored continuously above the cross-clamp, which leaves only the right arm as a reliable source of measurement (blood supply to the left arm can be compromised during the repair). Blood pressure should also be monitored below the level of the cross-clamp to ensure adequate perfusion via the collaterals during cross-clamping and to verify the absence of a pressure gradient after the repair. Alternatively, partial circulatory bypass might be needed. Blood pressure proximal to the aortic cross-clamp is usually easier to control. Nevertheless, increases in systemic pressure should be avoided.

Besides the complications mentioned, patients have a postoperative risk of paradoxical hypertension, which might be triggered by a baroreceptor reflex, activation of the renin-angiotensin-aldosterone system, or excessive release of catecholamines. Initial treatment includes infusion of vasoactive medications. The most common nerve injury is damage to the left laryngeal nerve, leading to stridor or hoarseness. Phrenic nerve damage is less common but could result in the need for prolonged respiratory support.

Ebstein Anomaly

Ebstein anomaly is rare (<1%) and produces an acyanotic lesion if it occurs as an isolated entity. However, it can be associated with other shunting lesions that in combination with right ventricular outflow tract (RVOT) obstruction render those patients cyanotic. Patients with Ebstein anomaly have an atrialized ventricle with a malformed and caudally displaced tricuspid valve. Frequently the anterior cusp is sail-like in structure with multiple fenestrations, resulting in tricuspid insufficiency and rarely stenosis. With the tricuspid valve displaced downward the effective right ventricle is relatively small and inefficient.

Signs and Symptoms. Severity of symptoms is proportional to the degree of tricuspid valve displacement and function. Symptoms can range from CHF, syncope, and dysrhythmias to an incidental finding without any symptoms at all. If patients do have an associated shunting lesion, they are at risk for paradoxical emboli and hypoxia, depending on the extent of the right-to-left shunt.

The ECG can show right ventricular hypertrophy and conduction abnormalities, such as a right bundle branch block or first-degree atrioventricular block. Some may also have signs of paroxysmal supraventricular or ventricular tachydysrhythmias, or preexcitation syndromes. Chest x-rays can show right ventricular and atrial enlargement, which might compress lung tissue. The actual right ventricular cavity, however, remains small and inefficient. In severe disease the shape of the heart approximates a sphere filling a significant portion of the chest cavity ("wall-to-wall heart"). More information can be obtained by using echocardiography to visualize the extent of atrial dilatation, tricuspid valve anatomy, and tricuspid regurgitation, as well as associated shunting lesions and their severity.

Management of Anesthesia. Symptomatic treatment includes pharmacologic therapy for heart failure and dysrhythmias, as well as catheter-based ablation of accessory pathways to treat excitation syndromes. Surgical repair can be quite complex. If primary repair of the valve (plus shunt closure if applicable) is not feasible, a staged procedure and ultimately a Fontan palliation might be required.

Management of anesthesia depends on the severity of right ventricular dysfunction, functional status of the tricuspid valve, presence of dysrhythmias, and presence or absence of associated shunting lesions. General management strategies and anesthetic management are discussed later under "Important Management Strategies for Adults With Congenital Heart Disease."

Cyanotic Congenital Heart Disease

The major characteristic finding in patients with cyanotic heart disease is a predominantly right-to-left shunt that results in decreased pulmonary blood flow and hypoxemia. Children with cyanotic heart disease have a low likelihood of surviving into adulthood unless they receive surgical correction of the defect. Severity of hypoxemia is mainly determined by the ratio of blood flowing through the lungs to that flowing through the systemic circulation (Qp:Qs < 1). Chronic hypoxemia also results in many secondary changes, such as erythrocytosis and associated hyperviscosity syndrome (headaches, lightheadedness, thromboembolism). Often patients with extremely high hematocrits are found to have abnormal coagulation studies. The condition is not a true coagulopathy but rather the result of measuring technique. Other common problems in cyanotic heart disease include heart failure, pulmonary hypertension, dysrhythmias, decreased lung compliance, altered response to hypoxia and hypercarbia, and renal insufficiency.

Tetralogy of Fallot

Among cyanotic congenital lesions, tetralogy of Fallot is the most common, accounting for 7%–10% of all congenital heart lesions. The four components of this lesion are (1) a perimembranous VSD, (2) an aorta that overrides the VSD, (3) RVOT obstruction, and (4) right ventricular hypertrophy (Fig. 7.4). Almost a quarter of patients will also have an ASD, sometimes

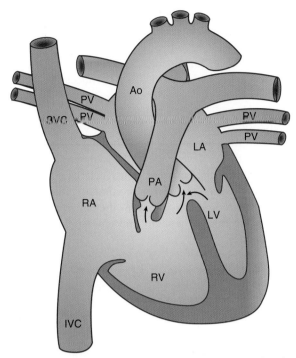

FIG. 7.4 Tetralogy of Fallot. The components associated with tetralogy of Fallot are (1) VSD, (2) aorta (Ao) overriding the VSD, (3) right ventricular outflow tract obstruction, and (4) right ventricular hypertrophy. *IVC,* Inferior vena cava; *LA,* left atrium; *PV,* pulmonary vein; *RA,* right atrium; *SVC,* superior vena cava.

referred to as *pentalogy of Fallot.* The key lesions of tetralogy of Fallot that determine its severity are the size of the VSD and the magnitude of the RVOT obstruction (subvalvular, valvular, supravalvular, or involving the main pulmonary arteries). The resultant pressure and volume overload lead to right ventricular hypertrophy, and the right-to-left shunt leads to hypoxia of varying degrees. Increases in systemic vascular resistance or pressure (either pharmacologically or physically [squatting]) can decrease the amount of right-to-left shunt, forcing more blood through the pulmonary circulation and improving oxygen saturation. The opposite is also true; systemic hypotension (e.g., with induction of anesthesia) facilitates right-to-left blood flow and therefore hypoxia.

Signs and Symptoms

Newborns with mild to moderate disease tend to become cyanotic during the first few months of life, but severe forms can cause profound cyanosis in the newborn period. Patients with mild disease might remain acyanotic and can present with heart failure later in life.

The classic presentation is a hypercyanotic spell ("tet spell") during which profound cyanosis develops rapidly, accompanied by hyperpnea, possible loss of consciousness, stroke, seizures, or even death. Generally, those attacks occur during periods of stress (exercise, feeding) or agitation (crying), but they can also occur without obvious provocation. The proposed mechanisms include spasms of the infundibular portion of the RVOT, peripheral vasodilation, and hyperventilation. The most susceptible period

appears to be 2–3 months of age, but hypercyanotic spells can occur anytime during the first year of life, after which they strike with less frequency. Children often squat down during hypercyanotic spells, thereby increasing peripheral vascular resistance, presumably by kinking the large vessels in the groin, ameliorating the right-to-left shunt and cyanosis. Treatment focuses on relieving the RVOT obstruction and reversing (or ameliorating) the right-to-left shunt. Preventive treatment includes administration of a long-acting β-blocker. Acute or emergent treatment entails (in escalating order) administration of 100% oxygen, fluid administration, and positioning (bending at the hip or gentle pressure on the abdomen). A systemic vasoconstrictor should be administered because it will minimize right-to-left shunting by reversing systemic vasodilatation. The next steps would be to administer a short-acting β-blocker followed by deepening of sedation to relieve the potential for spastic RVOT obstruction. Should these attacks recur frequently, a surgical intervention to repair the lesion is likely indicated sooner rather than later.

Other associated symptoms could include cyanosis, hyperviscosity syndrome, and paradoxical emboli (including cerebral abscesses, seizures, and strokes); infectious agents can more readily reach the brain via the bloodstream. The underlying reason for these abscesses is that lung vasculature of all children with a right-to-left shunt loses the ability to filter out small clots and infectious agents. Paradoxical emboli are therefore common, and cerebrovascular accidents occur more frequently. These events cannot be explained only by the propensity for paradoxical emboli. They also occur secondary to local thrombosis, especially in children with very high hematocrits (60% and beyond).

On auscultation, one appreciates a systolic ejection murmur at the left sternal border as a result of the RVOT obstruction. This murmur becomes shorter and less intense with worsening RVOT obstruction and can disappear during hypercyanotic spells. The VSD can further lead to a holosystolic murmur at the left sternal border. The ECG shows mainly right axis deviation and hypertrophy. Chest x-rays show decreased pulmonary vascularity, a boot-shaped heart, an elevated right ventricular apex, and a concave pulmonary artery. The final diagnosis is made by using echocardiography. Additional hemodynamic data can be obtained invasively with cardiac catheterization, which can provide information on the severity of the shunt and RVOT obstruction, anatomy of the pulmonary circulation, and origin of the coronary arteries.

Management of Anesthesia

Without surgical repair, only 25% of children survive to adolescence and only 3% will survive to age 40. Surgical repair at an early age has a great survival benefit, with almost 90% of patients still alive in their 30s. Repair entails VSD closure and widening of the RVOT to relieve the obstruction of blood flow into the lungs. Occasionally, repair of the pulmonary valve is required during the same operation.

One of the most frequent adverse outcomes after surgery is pulmonic regurgitation. It is not uncommon for those patients to return to the operating room or the cardiac catheterization lab to have surgical repair/replacement of the valve or to have a valve placed percutaneously. Another potential adverse event after the operation is right-to-left shunting via the foramen ovale, which is often left open to serve as a "pop-up valve" that will relieve high right ventricular pressures in case of right ventricular failure. A right bundle branch block caused by injury to the cardiac conduction system is common immediately after surgery, but it usually remains asymptomatic.

Historically, patients with tetralogy of Fallot were palliated with a systemic arterial-to-pulmonary artery shunt like the Waterson shunt (ascending aorta to right pulmonary artery), the Potts shunt (descending aorta to left pulmonary artery), or the Blalock-Taussig shunt (subclavian artery to pulmonary artery). Although these operations relieve the cyanosis, they do not address the fundamental problems (VSD and RVOT obstruction) and result in multiple long-term complications such as pulmonary hypertension, CHF, or pulmonary artery distortion. Today a primary repair is the accepted first-line management. If the child's size precludes a primary repair, a balloon pulmonary valvuloplasty can be used to temporarily relieve the RVOT obstruction. This procedure allows further development and growth of the pulmonary vasculature and possibly the left ventricle in anticipation of a subsequent primary repair.

Preoperative preparation: The major preoperative considerations focus on measures that are known to decrease the incidence of hypercyanotic spells. Perioperative fasting should be kept to a minimum because patients need to be well hydrated to avoid hypotension, which favors a right-to-left shunt. Also, stressful situations and crying should be avoided, with premedications if necessary; catecholamine release can trigger infundibular spasms. Patients on β-blockers should take them the morning of surgery.

Induction and maintenance of anesthesia: There is no single best induction agent for children with tetralogy of Fallot, nor is there a single best method to maintain anesthesia that will guarantee stable hemodynamic conditions. Intravenous (IV) or inhalational techniques are acceptable, but care should be taken to choose drugs that favor pulmonary blood flow and manage the Qp:Qs ratio. For management strategies and anesthetic management, please see "Balancing Pulmonary and Vascular Resistance (Qp:Qs)" later in the chapter.

Eisenmenger Syndrome

Eisenmenger syndrome is basically the development of severe pulmonary hypertension (leading to shunt reversal) as a result of a left-to-right intracardiac shunt. Theoretically it can affect all patients with a significant left-to-right shunt, regardless of the underlying cause. Prolonged exposure of the pulmonary vascular bed to volume and pressure overload leads to remodeling of both the muscle layer and the extracellular matrix of the pulmonary arteries and veins. The result is a slow but steady increase in pulmonary vascular resistance that ultimately leads to a flow reversal of the left-to-right shunt, which now becomes predominantly right to left. A common cause of Eisenmenger syndrome is an unrestricted and unrepaired VSD, half of which will ultimately result in Eisenmenger syndrome.

Signs and Symptoms

With progressive development of a right-to-left shunt, patients become more and more hypoxic and experience decreased exercise tolerance. Enlargement of the right ventricle and atrium lead to dysrhythmias such as atrial fibrillation or flutter, which the patient may experience in the form of palpitations. Progressive hypoxia also stimulates erythrocytosis, leading to hyperviscosity syndrome.

It is interesting to note that the associated cardiac murmurs disappear with the development of Eisenmenger syndrome. The ECG shows signs of right ventricular hypertrophy and strain. Chest x-rays can reveal prominent pulmonary vessels, and echocardiography can show the underlying shunting lesion, the direction of the shunt, and a measure of pulmonary artery pressures.

Management of Anesthesia

Treatments that are widely used for patients with pulmonary arterial hypertension seem to be less effective in patients with Eisenmenger syndrome. Adjunct treatment focuses on amelioration of associated symptoms. Phlebotomy can be used to treat hyperviscosity syndrome, and oxygen administration can counteract hypoxia. The only definite treatment in selected patients is combined heart and lung transplant or a lung transplant with a surgical repair of the underlying shunting lesion. Surgical repair of the underlying defect without lung transplant is contraindicated because this would result in right heart failure and death.

Management of anesthesia in patients with Eisenmenger syndrome who are undergoing noncardiac surgery closely reflects the management of anesthesia in patients with other forms of severe pulmonary hypertension. The general wisdom that every procedure is better done with minimally invasive laparoscopy does not necessarily apply to patients with Eisenmenger syndrome. This approach necessitates insufflation of the abdominal cavity with carbon dioxide, which increases intraabdominal pressures and raises the $Paco_2$. As a result the patient experiences hypotension (due to lower right ventricular preload), acidosis and hypercarbia (due to increased $Paco_2$ levels), higher intrathoracic pressures (to counteract the increased abdominal pressure, which gets exaggerated by the Trendelenburg position), and the propensity for dysrhythmias (high $Paco_2$ and atrial distension). All of these effects worsen right-to-left shunting, hypoxia, and effective cardiac output. Therefore, doing the procedure open instead of laparoscopically, while still striving for early extubation and pain control, might be preferred in these patients.

The anesthesiologist might consider using a neuraxial technique for either the primary anesthetic or intraoperative and postoperative analgesia. The major concern is the sudden drop in blood pressure, especially with a spinal. An epidural, however, is not necessarily contraindicated in patients with Eisenmenger syndrome; they are actually used frequently for the reasons stated earlier. However, one needs to be cognizant about the potential for systemic hypotension and worsening right-to-left shunting.

By definition, pulmonary vascular resistance is fixed and cannot decrease in response to changes in systemic vascular resistance. To minimize the gradient driving the right-to-left shunt, practitioners should maintain systemic vascular levels at preoperative levels or slightly above. A sudden drop in oxygen saturation without changes in ventilation can be a first sign that systemic vascular resistance has decreased. For general management strategies and anesthetic management, please see "Management of Pulmonary Hypertension" and "Balancing Pulmonary and Vascular Resistance (Qp:Qs)" later in the chapter.

Tricuspid Atresia

As the name suggests, the key feature of tricuspid atresia is the absence or permanent closure of the tricuspid valve. This closure blocks blood flow into the right ventricle, necessitating additional lesions for at least temporary survival. For example, blood flows from the right atrium to the left atrium either via a patent foramen ovale or an ASD, where it mixes with oxygenated blood. It then flows across the mitral valve into the left ventricle, where a variable portion crosses a VSD into the right ventricle and the pulmonary circulation; the rest is ejected into the systemic circulation across the aortic valve. Alternatively, if no VSD is present, pulmonary blood flow can be established across a PDA or bronchial vessels. Patients with tricuspid atresia are cyanotic and have a small right ventricle, a normal or enlarged left ventricle, and decreased pulmonary blood flow. Additionally, tricuspid atresia can be subclassified according to the position of the great vessels: type I, normal relationship; type II, dextrotransposition; type III, nondextrotransposition (levotransposition or double outlet); type IV, truncus arteriosus. Patients with normally related great arteries tend to have the obstruction at the level of the VSD, whereas patients with transposition tend to have either subvalvular or valvular stenosis.

Signs and Symptoms

Severity and timing of symptoms depends on the complexity of the cumulative lesions as well as the severity of obstruction to pulmonary blood flow.

Approximately 50% of patients develop symptoms by 24 hours of life, and 80% by the end of the first month. Decreased levels of pulmonary blood flow with a right-to-left shunt lead to cyanosis (clubbing in older children), tachypnea, prominent a waves (due to interatrial obstruction), and failure to thrive, all in the absence of abnormal pulses, hepatic enlargement, or overt heart failure. The subset of patients with increased pulmonary blood flow will present with minimal cyanosis, tachypnea, tachycardia, hepatomegaly, prominent a waves, feeding difficulties, and signs of heart failure.

Auscultation can reveal the holosystolic murmur of a VSD or the continuous murmur of a PDA over the left lower sternal border—if either one is present. The ECG reveals signs of left axis deviation (especially in patients with type I tricuspid atresia), left ventricular hypertrophy, and right atrial enlargement. The final diagnosis can be made by echocardiography, which will demonstrate the absent or closed tricuspid valve,

the enlarged chambers (with the exception of the right ventricle), the flow characteristics across the VSD, the magnitude of RVOT obstruction, and the magnitude of pulmonary artery pressures. Similar results can also be obtained by cardiac catheterization and angiography.

Management of Anesthesia

Management of anesthesia varies slightly depending on the stage of palliation the child is undergoing. For general management strategies and anesthetic management, please see "The Univentricular Heart During Different Stages of Repair" later in this chapter. Long-term survival is very good and depends in part on the anatomic origin of the systemic ventricle, with the left ventricle having a better long-term prognosis.

Transposition of the Great Arteries

Transposition of the great arteries can be divided into two separate forms: D-transposition and L-transposition, also referred to as *congenitally corrected transposition of the great arteries (a misnomer)*.

D-transposition (dextrotransposition) is the more common form and is generally implied if someone refers to transposition of the great arteries without a qualifier. D-transposition results when the truncus arteriosus (the common origin of the aorta and pulmonary artery) fails to divide properly (Fig. 7.5).

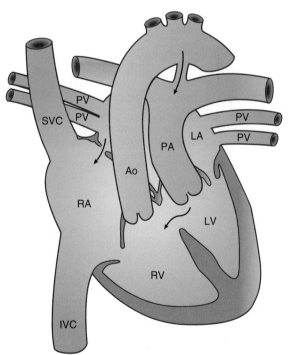

FIG. 7.5 Transposition of the great arteries. Schematic depiction of transposition of the great arteries. The right ventricle (RV) and left ventricle (LV) are connected in parallel to each other, creating independent circulations, with the aorta (Ao) arising from the RV and the pulmonary artery (PA) arising from the LV. Survival depends on mixing of blood between the two circulations through an ASD, VSD, or PDA. *IVC,* Inferior vena cava; *LA,* left atrium; *PV,* pulmonary vein; *RA,* right atrium; *SVC,* superior vena cava.

This arrangement results in two parallel circulations, and unless there is an additional communication between the pulmonary circulation and systemic circulation (e.g., ASD, VSD, PDA), it is incompatible with life.

L-transposition (levotransposition) results from a misdirected folding of the embryonic heart tube. Instead of folding toward the right side, the embryonic heart tube folds toward the left side, thereby switching the position of the genetically right and left ventricle without affecting the connection to the great vessels. Blood then flows from the right atrium across the mitral valve into the left ventricle, out of the pulmonic valve into the pulmonary circulation, then into the left atrium across the tricuspid valve into the right ventricle, from which it is ejected across the aortic valve into the systemic circulation. Because the two circulations are in series, patients remain acyanotic and generally asymptomatic until later in life when the genetically right ventricle (now the systemic ventricle) starts to fail prematurely.

Signs and Symptoms

Symptoms depend on the type of transposition; children diagnosed with L-transposition are generally asymptomatic at birth. Neonates who have D-transposition of the great arteries and no associated shunting lesions become profoundly cyanotic within the first week of life and worsen as the ductus arteriosus closes. Neonates with large associated shunting lesions may be asymptomatic initially but then start to develop signs and symptoms of heart failure, tachypnea, tachycardia, feeding intolerance, and respiratory distress without overt cyanosis. These symptoms result from left ventricular volume overload and failure caused by the left-to-right shunting.

Auscultatory findings are determined by the associated shunting lesions and can range from no murmur at all to a loud systolic ejection murmur. The ECG shows right axis deviation and right ventricular hypertrophy. Chest x-rays demonstrate an "egg-shaped heart with a narrow stalk."

Management of Anesthesia

Neonates with D-transposition of the great arteries and insufficient associated shunting lesions require some variety of intracardiac shunt. Initially a prostaglandin infusion can be used to maintain patency of the ductus arteriosus, as can stent placement. Alternatively, a balloon septostomy can be used to either create or increase the size of an ASD, thereby creating an atrial-level shunt. Symptomatic treatment includes administration of oxygen, medical management of heart failure, and lowering of pulmonary artery pressures.

Definitive surgical correction has been achieved historically with either the Mustard or Senning procedure, or more recently with the arterial switch operation. Both the Mustard and Senning procedures involve the creation of an interatrial baffle to redirect blood from the vena cava to the left ventricle. In the Mustard procedure the baffle is created with synthetic material, whereas the Senning procedure creates the baffle with the patient's own tissue. Blood then flows through the pulmonary circulation back into the left atrium via a newly created septectomy into the right atrium and then into the right ventricle,

from which it is ejected into the aorta. One of the major downsides of these operations is that the genetically right ventricle becomes the systemic ventricle, making it prone to heart failure later in life. In addition, there is a significant dysrhythmia burden, given the long suture lines in the atria. Today most children undergo the arterial switch operation, which involves transecting the pulmonary artery and aorta and reanastomosing them with the right and left ventricle, respectively. This procedure is followed by reimplantation of the coronary arteries into the aortic root using coronary buttons so as not to directly suture the tiny coronary ostia. Outcomes are generally excellent, with good long-term survival. Patients experience less dysrhythmia burden and a lower rate of right ventricular failure than they do with the Mustard or Senning procedure.

Anesthetic management for patients with transposition of the great arteries will depend on the degree of separation of the circulations and the amount of shunting. For general management strategies and anesthetic management, please see "Balancing Pulmonary and Vascular Resistance (Qp:Qs)" later in the chapter. Postoperatively, patients are at increased risk of atrial dysrhythmias and conduction defects.

Truncus Arteriosus

Patients with truncus arteriosus have a single vessel originating from the heart that gives rise to both the aorta and pulmonary artery (Fig. 7.6). This vessel overrides a large VSD and

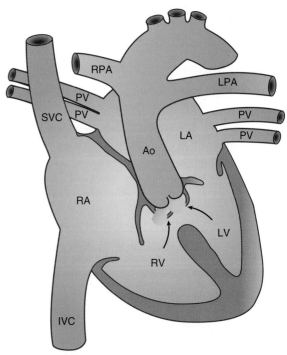

FIG. 7.6 Truncus arteriosus. In patients with truncus arteriosus, a single vessel arises from the heart, overrides the left ventricle (LV) and right ventricle (RV), and gives rise to the aorta and pulmonary arteries. *IVC,* Inferior vena cava; *LA,* left atrium; *LPA,* left pulmonary artery; *PV,* pulmonary vein; *RA,* right atrium; *RPA,* right pulmonary artery; *SVC,* superior vena cava.

thereby both ventricles. Unoperated, prognosis is poor, with a median survival of only about 6 weeks.

Signs and Symptoms

Depending on the location of the pulmonary artery origins from the truncus, truncus arteriosus can be divided into different types using either the Van Praagh or Collett and Edwards classification. According to Collett and Edwards, *type I truncus arteriosus* is defined by a main pulmonary artery arising from the base of the truncus. *Type II truncus arteriosus* is defined by the branch pulmonary arteries arising separately from the truncus in close proximity to each other (likely posterior). *Type III truncus arteriosus* is defined by the pulmonary arteries rising on opposite sides of the truncus, and *type IV* is defined by the pulmonary arteries arising from the descending aorta. All forms result in mixing of the oxygenated and deoxygenated blood, left-to-right shunting, and consequently pulmonary overcirculation. Infants can present with cyanosis, failure to thrive, and CHF. During diastole, blood escapes into the pulmonary circulation, resulting in low diastolic pressures and a high pulse pressure, which can be felt as accentuated peripheral pulses.

There are no characteristic auscultatory or ECG findings in patients with truncus arteriosus. Chest x-rays can show an enlarged cardiac silhouette and a plumb pulmonary vasculature. Diagnosis can be made angiographically by catheterization or with CT.

Management of Anesthesia

Definitive surgical correction involves patch closure of the VSD, disconnecting the pulmonary arteries from the truncus, and placing a graft between the right ventricle and pulmonary artery to provide pulmonary blood flow. The magnitude of pulmonary blood flow is the main determinant of anesthetic management. For general management strategies and anesthetic management, please see "Balancing Pulmonary and Vascular Resistance (Qp:Qs)" later in the chapter.

Partial Anomalous Pulmonary Venous Return

Partial anomalous pulmonary venous return, a milder form of total anomalous pulmonary venous return (see later), occurs when one (most likely) or more pulmonary veins drain into either the venous or right side of the heart instead of the left atrium. In the most common form of partial anomalous pulmonary venous return, the drainage is into the superior vena cava, resulting in a left-to-right shunt at the atrial level and consequent right heart dilatation.

Only a few patients with large increases in pulmonary blood flow present with symptoms (e.g., dyspnea on exertion, fatigue). Severe symptoms like cyanosis and CHF are relatively rare. In addition to right ventricular failure, patients also present with right atrial dilatation and a high dysrhythmia burden. Definite treatment is by open surgical repair to redirect pulmonary venous blood flow back to the left atrium.

Visualization of the pulmonary veins and their drainage can be challenging with transesophageal echocardiography (TEE), but angiography and transthoracic echocardiography (TTE) or CT are often used to establish the diagnosis. Cardiac catheterization can demonstrate elevated filling pressures as well as oxygen saturations of the cardiac chambers and large vessels.

Total Anomalous Pulmonary Venous Return

In patients with total anomalous pulmonary venous return, all four pulmonary veins drain either separately or via a common confluence into the right atrium or the systemic venous tributaries proximal to the lungs. Most frequently (50% of cases) this connection occurs above the level of the heart (supracardiac) into the left innominate vein, which is associated with a left-sided superior vena cava. Cardiac connections occur in approximately 25% of cases and are characterized by either direct connections of the pulmonary veins to the right atrium or a connection of the confluence of all four pulmonary veins to the coronary sinus. Infracardiac total pulmonary venous return results from a connection of the pulmonary vein confluence directly to either the inferior vena cava or the portal venous system. In either case, for blood to reach the systemic circulation an additional shunt in the form of an ASD, VSD, or PDA must be present. Any of these shunts will cause mixing of oxygenated and deoxygenated blood and systemic hypoxia of varying degrees.

Signs and Symptoms

Patients tend to present early in life—half within the first month and almost 90% by age 1 year. The most frequent presentations are CHF, cyanosis, respiratory distress, and tachypnea. Mortality is high if the condition is left untreated. Approximately 80% of patients die before the age of 1.

Auscultation reveals the typical findings of the associated shunting lesion, which in most cases is an ASD. The ECG shows signs of right atrial and ventricular enlargement. Chest x-rays also demonstrate cardiomegaly and possibly pulmonary edema. Echocardiography can be helpful in detecting the origin and magnitude of the shunting lesion, as well as cardiac enlargement and ventricular function.

Management of Anesthesia

Definitive treatment is by surgical correction. The common pulmonary venous confluence or the individual pulmonary veins are mobilized and reconnected to the back of the left atrium. All associated shunting lesions (mostly ASD) are closed with a patch closure. This approach restores normal blood flow and eliminates volume overload and hypoxia.

Anesthesia can be induced with a wide variety and combination of IV or inhaled medications. Intraoperative management focuses on managing pulmonary blood flow and balancing the Qp:Qs ratio (see later). Practitioners should follow a restrictive strategy for fluid administration, because fluid overload could result in elevated right atrial pressure and pulmonary edema as the pressure is transmitted directly to the pulmonary veins.

Hypoplastic Left Heart Syndrome

Hypoplastic left heart syndrome (HLHS) is the most common cyanotic heart lesion destined for Fontan palliation and single ventricle physiology. The key pathology includes left ventricular and mitral valve hypoplasia and hypoplasia of the aortic valve (Fig. 7.7). HLHS is not associated with any extracardiac syndromes. Blood mixes inside the remaining chambers of the heart and then gets ejected mainly into the pulmonary artery and via an open ductus into the systemic circulation. A lesser portion of blood is ejected directly into the aorta. The ratio of blood supplied to the pulmonary versus systemic circulation depends on the resistance between those two vascular beds and on the patency of the ductus arteriosus.

Signs and Symptoms

Newborns with HLHS show signs and symptoms of heart failure, shock, and cardiovascular collapse in the immediate perinatal period. The degree of cyanosis tends to be mild but varies with changes in pulmonary vascular resistance. Pulses are weak according to the degree of ductal resistance, without any difference between extremities.

Auscultation reveals a normal first heart sound, a prominent second heart sound, and in a minority of children a gallop. Some patients do have an apical diastolic rumble, but this is not specific. The ECG demonstrates right axis deviation, signs of right ventricular hypertrophy, and low voltages. Chest x-ray reveals signs of cardiomegaly and prominent pulmonary vascular markings. An echocardiogram will identify the exact pathology, intracardiac pressures, shunts, and function.

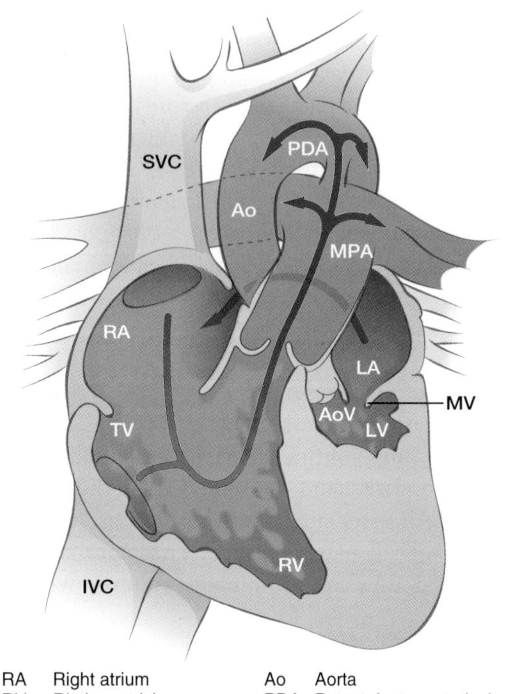

Management of Anesthesia

Newborns with suspected HLHS will require IV prostaglandins to maintain duct patency. This treatment will ensure systemic and coronary artery perfusion and thereby prevent progressive acidosis, cardiovascular collapse, and imminent death. Definitive therapy requires a multistage operation over the next few years, ultimately culminating in a Fontan palliation and single ventricle physiology. Consequently, management of anesthesia for patients with HLHS varies depending on which stage of palliation patients are currently experiencing.

Mechanical Obstruction of the Trachea

Children with mechanical obstruction of the trachea present with stridor and upper airway obstruction. Mechanical obstruction of the trachea is frequently the result of an enlarged vessel that is compromising tracheal patency. This can be due to circular anomalies that result in a ring around the trachea (double aortic arch, aberrant left pulmonary artery) or to an enlarged, dilated pulmonary artery (e.g., from pulmonary valve atresia). Children can present with symptoms of stridor and signs of mechanical obstructions after nasogastric tube placement, even without any apparent airway compromise at baseline.

Double Aortic Arch

A persistent right aortic arch or double aortic arch is rare, but it leads to a complete vascular ring (Fig. 7.8). Pressure exerted

RA	Right atrium	Ao	Aorta
RV	Rigth ventricle	PDA	Patent ductus arteriosis
LA	Left atrium	TV	Tricuspid valve
LV	Left ventrticle	MV	Mitral valve
SVC	Superior vena cava	PV	Pulmonary valve
IVC	Inferior vena cava	AoV	Aortic valve
MPA	Main pulmomary artery		

FIG. 7.7 Hypoplastic left heart. (https://www.cdc.gov/ncbddd/heartdefects/hlhs.html)

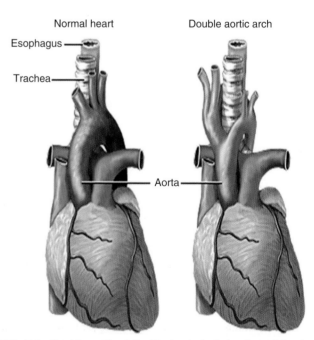

FIG. 7.8 Double aortic arch. Mechanical obstruction of the trachea secondary to a double aortic arch. (http://www.nlm.nih.gov/medlineplus/ency/article/007316.htm)

by these vessels compresses the trachea and esophagus, and children present with inspiratory stridor, dysphagia, and difficulty mobilizing secretions.

Treatment of choice is surgical resection of the smaller part of the arch. It is important to place the endotracheal tube distal to the tracheal compression to ensure adequate ventilation while avoiding a mainstem intubation. Nasogastric tubes and even temperature probes should not be advanced beyond the obstruction before intubation; they can worsen tracheal compression. Prolonged tracheal compression places patients at risk for postoperative tracheomalacia, which could endanger tracheal patency even after successful surgery.

NONCARDIAC SURGERY IN THE ADULT PATIENT WITH CONGENITAL HEART DISEASE

Our understanding of congenital heart disease and care for affected patients have improved dramatically over the last 30 years. Major strides have been made in long-term medical treatment, surgical techniques and skills, percutaneous interventions, intraoperative and perioperative care, and critical care management. These improvements have led to an increased likelihood of survival for children born with congenital heart disease. Based on data from Canada, 85% survive to adulthood, and it is now estimated that at least as many adults as children are living with congenital heart disease. For the United States that would mean that more than 1 million adults with congenital heart disease may present not only for cardiac surgery (primary repair, revision, or conversion to a more modern operation) but also for surgery that is completely unrelated to their cardiac disease. Indeed, admissions of adults with congenital heart disease for noncardiac surgery have been increasing steadily and more than doubled over the last decade. Moreover, though the age distribution of all patients with congenital heart disease was heavily skewed toward children only 30 years ago, new data show that it now almost perfectly resembles the age distribution of the general population.

Although many patients who survive into adulthood are considered cured or palliated, they do experience a high morbidity burden. The list of cardiovascular complications of long-standing congenital heart disease includes pulmonary hypertension, systemic hypertension, heart failure (especially right heart failure), cyanosis, residual shunts, dysrhythmias, conduction defects, and valvular lesions (see Table 7.2). The probability of developing heart failure increases in almost all patients with congenital heart disease over their lifetime, but the magnitude depends on the type of lesion. Similarly the cumulative incidence of any type of dysrhythmia increases steadily over time. The majority of patients with congenital heart disease who are over age 65 experience some kind of dysrhythmia. Moreover, cardiac lesions such as valvular stenosis or regurgitation, residual shunts, outflow tract obstructions, and dysrhythmias will cause these patients to return to the cardiac operating room or electrophysiology suite for treatment of these long-term sequelae.

Noncardiac long-term complications can occur in multiple organ systems (see Table 7.2). It is helpful to categorize the possible symptoms according to organ system and think about how the specific form of congenital heart disease can influence that particular system. Congenital heart disease–specific comorbidities occur in addition to changes of aging not related to congenital heart disease. The adult with congenital heart disease therefore combines two phenotypes into one: an anatomic phenotype that is similar to that of a pediatric patient and a physiologic phenotype that is similar to that of a geriatric patient. This analogy has been very nicely demonstrated previously in a study showing that adult patients with congenital heart disease (mean age, 33) had the exact same exercise tolerance as a group of heart failure patients (mean age, 59) stratified by New York Heart Association class.

Preoperative Evaluation

Evaluation of adult patients with congenital heart disease can be very complex. These patients represent a wide variety of congenital lesions at different stages of repair and with different comorbidities. Patients can present with an uncorrected lesion, a partially corrected lesion, a lesion that is between repair stages, or a failed lesion repair attempt. Moreover, adult congenital heart disease is not an isolated well-described entity but rather a multisystem disease with a broad range of severity. Consequently, no single best risk index delineates perioperative risk and stratifies the contributions of comorbidities in these patients. The American College of Cardiology and the American Heart Association (ACC/AHA) made a cautious attempt to categorize severity and perioperative risk according to the type of lesion. They considered low-risk patients to be those with a small ASD or PDA, an isolated VSD, or those who were status post complete ASD, VSD, or PDA repair. Moderate-risk lesions are aortic coarctation, complete atrioventricular canal, Ebstein anomaly, and tetralogy of Fallot, among others. Lastly, high-risk patients are those with any form of cyanotic heart disease (with the exception of tetralogy of Fallot), conduits, Eisenmenger syndrome, single ventricle physiology, and transposition of the great arteries, among others. In addition to this general assessment, perioperative risk increases with the patient's comorbidities and symptoms (e.g., heart failure, pulmonary hypertension, poor exercise tolerance, renal insufficiency, cyanosis, etc.). Patients usually undergo an extensive workup, and multiple functional and imaging modalities are available. Besides the standard workup for all patients, preoperative evaluation should include detailed knowledge of the patient's current anatomy, physiology at rest, and—importantly—a thorough understanding of any changes in pulmonary and vascular resistance. Particular focus is placed on preoperative exercise tolerance as an indicator of cardiovascular reserve.

Premedication: The use of preoperative anxiolytics is beneficial in many adults with congenital heart disease insofar as they often have had multiple prior operations and hospitalizations. Furthermore a subset of patients will present with developmental delay (e.g., trisomy 21) or cognitive impairment from prior strokes or cerebral abscesses. Administration of any preoperative sedation must take into account the potential consequence that hypercapnia- or hypoxia-induced increases in pulmonary pressure can pose—especially in patients with pulmonary hypertension or shunting lesions.

Endocarditis prophylaxis: The AHA/ACC have updated their guidelines to recommend endocarditis prophylaxis only in the highest-risk patients undergoing a high-risk procedure (see later). Therefore not every patient with congenital heart disease will qualify for routine endocarditis prophylaxis.

Vascular access: It can be very challenging to obtain vascular access in adults with congenital heart disease, given multiple prior cannulations of vessels. Alternatively, patients might exhibit a blood pressure difference between extremities. The femoral vessels or internal jugular veins can also be thrombosed or scarred after prior cannulation attempts. Also, in patients with a Glenn shunt or Fontan circulation, a central venous catheter might inadvertently be placed in the right main pulmonary artery, and a thrombosed catheter tip might block the only route for blood flow to the lungs.

Dysrhythmias: Although most adult patients with congenital heart disease experience at least one form of dysrhythmia during their lifetime, atrial reentry tachycardia is especially prevalent. Many patients present after multiple electrophysiologic studies to ablate those dysrhythmias, and a substantial number have a pacemaker or defibrillator that might require interrogation.

Pulmonary hypertension: Development of pulmonary hypertension secondary to volume or pressure overload can substantially increase perioperative risk. Patients with left-to-right shunting lesions can also develop Eisenmenger syndrome. It is of particular importance to avoid medications and maneuvers that increase pulmonary artery pressures (Table 7.4). Low exercise tolerance, syncope, atrial dysrhythmias, high atrial pressures, cyanosis, right ventricular dysfunction, and renal insufficiency are all predictors of worse outcomes in patients with severe pulmonary hypertension.

Heart failure: The prevalence of heart failure, especially right-sided heart failure caused by volume or pressure overload, increases with age and is highest in patients with single ventricle physiology. Patients with heart failure should be medically optimized and might require preoperative diuresis to optimize volume status.

Bleeding diathesis: Patients with hyperviscosity syndrome from elevated hemoglobin levels often present with abnormal coagulation studies. Also, although a subset of patients will have low levels of von Willebrand factor and vitamin K–dependent clotting factors, bleeding time in the remaining patients will be normal despite an abnormal prothrombin time or partial thromboplastin time. Nevertheless, patients with hyperviscosity are at increased risk for thrombosis, and adequate preoperative hydration is necessary (avoid long preoperative fasting).

Intraoperative Management

No one management strategy is applicable to all adults with congenital heart disease, and no one anesthetic technique has proven to be superior in those patients. As discussed previously, this is a multisystem disease with varying anatomy; management will depend on the patient's functional status, comorbidities, and specific anatomy and on the type and urgency of the procedure. Many patients with noncomplex congenital heart disease who are undergoing low- to moderate-risk surgery will do fine with standard monitoring and care. However, patients with moderate to severe forms of congenital heart disease will require special attention even for seemingly minor surgery. Many physicians will have a low threshold to place invasive monitoring, especially an arterial catheter in patients presenting with severe pulmonary hypertension (or Eisenmenger syndrome), unrestricted or long-standing shunting lesions, heart failure, or severely depressed exercise tolerance. Central venous access is less often used, especially in patients with Fontan palliation in whom the central access catheter will measure pulmonary artery pressures, or in patients with shunting lesions in whom the catheter might end up in the systemic circulation. Interpretation of the central venous pressure can also be misleading in patients with altered right heart compliance or shunting lesions. Practitioners are increasingly using TEE to monitor those patients intraoperatively and to help guide fluid therapy and administration of inotropic or vasoactive medications.

Intraoperative management focuses on optimization of oxygen delivery to all organs. Maintaining cardiac contractility (especially of the right ventricle), balancing the Qp:Qs ratio, treating dysrhythmias, and maintaining systemic blood pressure and oxygen saturation remain key components in anesthetic management (see later).

Postoperative Management

Similar to preoperative and intraoperative management, decisions regarding postoperative management depend on multiple factors, including the type of procedure performed,

TABLE 7.4	Patient Groups at Highest Risk for Developing Endocarditis

History of endocarditis
Prosthetic heart valve (prosthetic material used for valve repair)
Status post heart transplant with valvulopathy
Congenital heart disease–associated conditions:
    Unrepaired cyanotic congenital heart lesion (including palliative shunts and conduits)
    Completely repaired congenital heart lesion, during the first 6 months after the procedure (if prosthetic materials or device were used)
    Repaired congenital heart lesion with a residual defect (at or adjacent to the site of a prosthetic patch or prosthetic device)

the patient's comorbidities, and the intraoperative course. In general, many providers have a low threshold for utilizing an intensive care bed, at least for the first day, to monitor for and treat common complications such as bleeding, changes in volume status, hypotension, increasing pulmonary artery pressures, dysrhythmias, and thrombosis.

IMPORTANT MANAGEMENT STRATEGIES FOR ADULTS WITH CONGENITAL HEART DISEASE

Infective Endocarditis Prophylaxis

The ACC/AHA jointly updated their recommendation on endocarditis prophylaxis for patients with congenital heart disease in 2007. After reviewing the literature they restricted their recommendations of antibiotic use for endocarditis prevention to only patients at highest risk undergoing a high-risk procedure. Patients at high risk for endocarditis include those with a previous history of endocarditis, those with a prosthetic cardiac valve or in whom prosthetic material was used for cardiac valve repair, and those who received a heart transplant and developed cardiac valvulopathy. In addition to those patients, the recommendations contain a separate section that focuses on congenital heart disease. It states that only the following patients with congenital heart disease are at highest risk: patients with unrepaired cyanotic congenital heart disease (including palliative shunts and conduits), patients during the first 6 months after complete repair of a congenital heart lesion who have prosthetic material or a prosthetic device, and patients with a repaired lesion who have a residual defect at or adjacent to a prosthetic patch or device that inhibits endothelialization (see Table 7.4).

Endocarditis prophylaxis for these patients is reasonable if they undergo dental procedures involving gingival tissue manipulation, manipulation of the periapical region of the teeth, or perforation of the oral mucosa. The guidelines specifically *do not* recommend using endocarditis prophylaxis for nondental procedures, such as colonoscopy or esophagogastroduodenoscopy, if the patient is not actively infected. However, they state that it is reasonable to consider endocarditis prophylaxis in selected patients for vaginal delivery at the time of membrane rupture if the patient has a prosthetic cardiac valve or if prosthetic material was used to repair a cardiac valve, and in patients with unrepaired or palliated cyanotic congenital heart disease (including surgical palliative shunts and conduits).

Management of Pulmonary Hypertension

The key element to managing patients with pulmonary hypertension is lowering pulmonary resistance (Table 7.5) while supporting right ventricular function. For a more in-depth description of the options for managing pulmonary hypertension, please refer to Chapter 9, "Systemic and Pulmonary Arterial Hypertension," of this text.

Balancing Pulmonary and Vascular Resistance (Qp:Qs)

The anesthetic management of patients with shunting lesions who are undergoing noncardiac surgery varies with the severity of the lesion. Usually there is a component of bidirectional blood flow; however, the net amount of shunting in patients without Eisenmenger syndrome is left to right. Patients with minor shunting (e.g., a small ASD and a Qp:Qs ratio < 1.5:1) will likely require only minor anesthetic adjustments. However, for all patients with a shunting lesion, care should be taken to meticulously avoid air bubbles in all IV lines, because they can result in paradoxical emboli that can lead to heart attacks and strokes. With increasing degrees of left-to-right shunting and a Qp:Qs ratio greater than 1.5:1, it is increasingly important to manage and limit pulmonary blood flow to prevent right ventricular failure secondary to volume overload.

Modifying pulmonary and systemic vascular resistance: Some congenital heart lesions (e.g., unrestricted VSDs) are very responsive to changes in the ratio of pulmonary to systemic vascular resistance. In general, drugs and maneuvers that increase systemic vascular resistance (hypothermia, sympathetic stimulation, vasoconstrictive drugs) and lower pulmonary vascular resistance will promote left-to-right shunting. The same is true for drugs (e.g., nitric oxide, milrinone) and nonpharmacologic measures that decrease pulmonary vascular resistance. Examples of such measures include hyperventilation with a high inspired oxygen concentration, alkalosis, minimizing positive pressure ventilation or positive end-expiratory pressure (opening the chest decreases

TABLE 7.5	Factors That Change Pulmonary and Systemic Vascular Resistance	
Decrease Pulmonary Vascular Resistance	**Increase Pulmonary Vascular Resistance**
100% inspired oxygen concentration	Hypoxia
Hypocarbia	Hypercarbia (e.g., hypoventilation due to premedication or sedation)
Alkalosis	Acidosis
Normothermia	Hypothermia
Low mean airway pressures or spontaneous ventilation	High mean airway pressures (positive pressure ventilation, positive end-expiratory pressure)
Avoidance of catecholamine release (avoid pain, anxiety, light anesthesia)	Catecholamine release (due to pain, anxiety, light anesthesia)
Medications (inhaled nitric oxide, prostaglandins, milrinone, others)	Medications (phenylephrine, all α_1-agonists, nitrous oxide, ketamine, others)
Increase systemic vascular resistance	Decrease systemic vascular resistance
Sympathetic stimulation	β_2-Agonists
α_1-Agonists	Neuraxial anesthesia
Hypothermia	Deep general anesthesia

intrapulmonary pressures intraoperatively), maintaining normothermia, and lowering catecholamine levels (deep anesthesia, avoiding pain and anxiety). These measures produce higher pulmonary blood flow (improved oxygen saturation) but also have the potential to cause CHF. In contrast, measures that increase pulmonary vascular resistance (positive pressure ventilation with room air, drugs [nitrous oxide], volatile anesthetics) or that decrease systemic vascular resistance (anesthetics agents, histamine [drugs, anaphylaxis], α-blockers, ganglionic blockers) will promote a decrease in left-to-right shunting (see Table 7.5).

Onset of IV and inhaled agents: There is ongoing but mostly academic concern that the induction of anesthesia is altered by left-to-right shunt lesions, given the brief transit time in the pulmonary circulation. However, even in patients with highly elevated pulmonary blood flow, which could theoretically dilute IV anesthetic agents and cause slow transit to the brain because of recirculation, there is usually little or no effect on induction speed. Similarly the induction speed with volatile agents is unaffected as long as cardiac output is maintained. In contrast, patients with a right-to-left shunting lesion tend to have a more rapid onset of action after IV drug administration. Because the drug bypasses the lungs, it gets relatively less diluted and reaches its targets (e.g., brain) faster and at a higher concentration than it does in patients without a shunting lesion. The reverse is true for inhaled anesthetics, which exhibit a slower induction speed as blood concentrations rise more slowly.

Left-to-right shunts: Patients with elevated pulmonary blood flow benefit from medications and maneuvers that maintain or slightly increase pulmonary artery pressure, which can lessen the symptoms of CHF. Patients with a mainly left-to-right shunting lesion (high oxygen saturations at baseline) usually tolerate a balanced anesthetic with positive pressure ventilation, a low inspired concentration of oxygen, and use of vapor anesthetics to decrease systemic vascular resistance, which will facilitate right-to-left shunting or at least decrease the amount of left-to-right shunting. Practitioners should minimize the use of drugs or interventions that increase systemic vascular resistance or decrease pulmonary vascular resistance (see Table 7.5).

Right-to-left shunts: In patients with a significant component of right-to-left shunting, (low oxygen saturations at baseline), scenarios that favor right-to-left shunting include (1) increased pulmonary vascular resistance, (2) increased RVOT obstruction (infundibula spasm), and (3) decreased systemic vascular resistance. In patients with a fixed RVOT obstruction, changes in pulmonary vascular resistance are not able to modify the Qp:Qs ratio, and changes in systemic vascular resistance become much more important. In general, practitioners can use ketamine for IV induction in patients with right-to-left shunts. Although it probably increases pulmonary vascular resistance, ketamine still leads to an improvement of oxygenation. The improvement is most likely due to the increased inotropy and contractile force of the right ventricle helping to push blood across the obstruction and the similarly increased systemic vascular resistance that offsets pulmonary vascular increases.

THE UNIVENTRICULAR HEART DURING DIFFERENT STAGES OF REPAIR

Surgical Management

Surgical repair of infants with single-ventricle physiology is completed in stages to accomplish the following goals: (1) maintain duct patency as needed, (2) balance pulmonary-to-systemic blood flow, (3) unload the systemic ventricle, and (4) fully separate the circulations, culminating in single-ventricle palliation with Fontan completion.

The initial concern in the neonate is to determine what the ratio of pulmonary to systemic blood flow is and how much of it depends on a PDA. If pulmonary blood flow is diminished (e.g., tricuspid atresia with intact ventricular septum or severe RVOT obstruction), a significant contribution of pulmonary blood flow stems from the ductus arteriosus. It is therefore imperative to maintain duct patency with a prostaglandin infusion to ensure peripartum survival.

The goal of the first operation is to eliminate the need for a PDA and to provide adequate pulmonary and systemic blood flow. If both the aorta and pulmonary artery are of sufficient size, the first surgical intervention is usually a modified Blalock-Taussig shunt (subclavian artery to main branch pulmonary artery), which provides adequate pulmonary circulation at an age when pulmonary pressures are still elevated, necessitating a high (arterial) driving pressure. The Blalock-Taussig shunt allows the child to grow and the pulmonary vascular resistance to fall until venous pressure suffices to move blood across the vascular bed of the lungs. The other scenario is the neonate with single-ventricle physiology and no obstruction in pulmonary blood flow. These neonates can suffer from too much pulmonary blood flow and overcirculation of the lungs. They present not with cyanosis but with signs and symptoms of heart failure. Therefore they require medical management of heart failure first. The first surgical intervention in this cohort is often a pulmonary artery band to limit pulmonary blood flow and prevent pulmonary vascular remodeling and volume overload of the heart. Alternatively, if the pulmonary artery or aorta is of insufficient size or patency, a Norwood procedure might be required at this stage (Fig. 7.9A). The Norwood procedure consists of an atrial septectomy to achieve maximal mixing of blood inside the heart; transection and ligation of the main pulmonary artery to direct all blood from the heart into the aorta; reconstruction of the aorta, the hypoplastic arch, and possibly a coarctation to ensure unimpeded systemic blood flow; and lastly, placement of either a systemic-to-pulmonary shunt (e.g., modified Blalock-Taussig shunt) or a conduit from the right ventricle to the pulmonary artery (Sano modification) to provide pulmonary blood flow (see Fig. 7.9). This extensive operation is performed with the

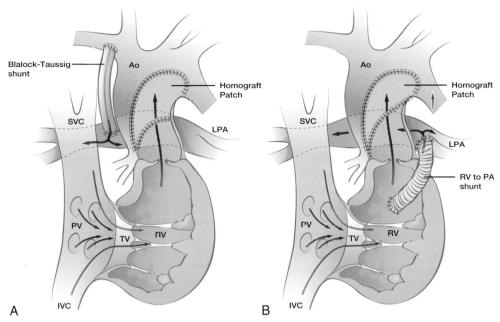

FIG. 7.9 The Norwood procedure for hypoplastic left heart syndrome. The figure shows the two variants in surgical technique according to the way in which pulmonary blood flow is established. A, The classical procedure with a systemic pulmonary artery shunt (Blalock-Taussig). B, Modification with a right ventricle–pulmonary artery conduit. *Ao,* Aorta; *IVC,* inferior vena cava; *LPA,* left pulmonary artery; *PA,* pulmonary artery; *PV,* pulmonary valve; *RPA,* right pulmonary artery; *RV,* right ventricle; *SVC,* superior vena cava; *TV,* tricuspid valve. (From Barron DJ, Kilby MD, Davies B, Wright JGC, Jones TJ, Brawn WJ. *The Lancet,* August 15, 2009. Volume 374, Issue 9689, Pages 551-564.)

patient on cardiopulmonary bypass and in deep hypothermia and circulatory arrest during reconstruction of the aorta. At the conclusion of the Norwood procedure with Sano modification, a single right ventricle ejects blood into both the systemic and pulmonary circulation in parallel. If the Norwood operation is done without a Sano modification and uses a Blalock-Taussig shunt instead, the right ventricle ejects blood only into the aorta, and pulmonary blood flow occurs via the subclavian-to-pulmonary artery shunt downstream of the aorta.

Regardless of the type of initial operation (or no intervention in the case of balanced blood flow), the child is allowed to grow until he or she is large enough for the next step of the palliation. Over the next few months the Sano or modified Blalock-Taussig shunt becomes relatively too small for adequate pulmonary blood flow because the shunts do not grow with the child, and cyanosis begins to worsen slowly. However, pulmonary vascular resistance continues to decline, making venous pressure sufficient to drive blood across the lungs. Therefore the next step of the palliation, at the age of 4–6 months, aims to improve pulmonary blood flow and begin to unload the right ventricle, which would not be able to supply both the pulmonary and systemic circulation over decades to come. These goals can be accomplished with a bidirectional cavopulmonary anastomosis (Glenn shunt) and takedown of the modified Blalock-Taussig shunt or Sano modification (see Fig. 7.9B).

The superior vena cava is anastomosed with the right pulmonary artery, which allows for venous blood from the upper part of the body to passively flow into the lungs. This anastomosis can grow with the child, directs more than 30% of the cardiac output away from the ventricle, and reduces the risk of heart failure. It also allows the ventricle to remodel over time from a volume-overloaded state in which it has to provide both the full systemic and full pulmonary blood flow, to a state in which it has to provide the full systemic and half of the pulmonary blood flow. However, given that the venous blood flowing through the inferior vena cava from the lower part of the body now bypasses the lungs completely, arterial oxygen saturation in children after a Glenn shunt is low (75%–85%) but generally well tolerated. The child is discharged to home. After a few years with the Glenn shunt, during which the child can grow and the heart remodel, he or she is brought back for the final stage of the palliation, the completion of the Fontan.

Timing of the last step of the operation varies from institution to institution but is generally between 2 and 6 years of age, with a trend toward performing the operation on the earlier side in recent years. Furthermore, if the child starts to become symptomatic and shows signs of heart failure, such as increased shortness of breath or fatigue, the operation might need to proceed sooner. Before going to the operating room, children will require cardiac catheterization to ensure that the pulmonary pressures have decreased sufficiently and the systemic venous-to-atrial pressure gradient (transpulmonary pressure) is high enough to allow for passive blood flow through the lungs. After that has been verified, the child can undergo the final stage, the Fontan completion, in which the pulmonary and systemic circulations are completely separated. This last stage of the Fontan palliation has evolved significantly over the years and now has two main surgical approaches: (1) the lateral tunnel and (2) the extracardiac conduit. The lateral tunnel approach has been performed for a little longer and entails placement of an intraatrial baffle that shunts blood through the right atrium and via an anastomosis to the right pulmonary artery directly into the pulmonary circulation. In the newer lateral tunnel procedure, a conduit is placed from the inferior vena cava below the right atrium to the right pulmonary artery, and both superior and inferior vena cava connections of the right atrium are severed. In either case, the Glenn shunt remains in place, draining the upper body via the superior vena cava directly into the right pulmonary artery. Blood flows across a pressure gradient between the venous circulation and the left atrium passively to the lungs, into the left atrium, and then into the systemic ventricle, where it gets ejected into the aorta. This flow restores normal arterial oxygenation and unloads the heart, which now only needs to provide a single cardiac output to the systemic circulation while the pulmonary circulation is fed passively. Of note, in patients with a marginal transpulmonary pressure gradient, the surgeon might elect to create a fenestration between the inferior vena cava conduit and the right atrium. This fenestration serves as a small left-to-right shunt that is inconsequential for the child under normal circumstances. However, during times of increased pulmonary vascular resistance (exercise, straining), pulmonary pressure might be too high to allow passive pulmonary blood flow, in which case blood can flow across the fenestration (right-to-left shunt). This shunting results in a small drop in oxygen saturation (well tolerated) but ensures adequate ventricular preload and prevents dangerous levels of hypotension.

KEY POINTS

- Congenital heart disease is the most common congenital abnormality, accounting for 5–10 cases per 1000 live births, not including bicuspid aortic valves, which would double or even triple the incidence.
- The most prevalent congenital heart defect in children and infants is a ventricular septal defect (VSD).
- Noninvasive imaging, especially echocardiography, is the cornerstone of diagnosis and classification of congenital heart lesions.
- Congenital heart disease is not an isolated entity but affects many other organs, making it a multiorgan disease.
- Balancing pulmonary and systemic blood flow and supporting the right ventricle are key management features.
- Selectively modifying systemic and pulmonary vascular resistance can be accomplished by changing the Po_2, the Pco_2, the pH, the patient's temperature, intrathoracic

pressures, controlling catecholamine release, and by administering certain medications.
- Adults with congenital heart disease outnumber children with congenital heart disease in developed countries. They can present not only for cardiac surgery but increasingly for noncardiac surgery that is completely unrelated to their congenital heart lesion. Furthermore, they present at different stages of repair or palliation and with a broad set of comorbidities (congestive heart failure, pulmonary hypertension, dysrhythmias, thrombosis, bleeding diathesis, etc.) that pose a unique challenge to the anesthesiologist.
- The ACC/AHA have jointly published guidelines that limit antibiotic endocarditis prophylaxis to only patients at highest risk undergoing high-risk procedures.

RESOURCES

Andropoulos DB, Stayer SA, Skjonsby BS, et al. Anesthetic and perioperative outcome of teenagers and adults with congenital heart disease. *J Cardiothorac Vasc Anesth.* 2002;16:731-736.

Baum VC, Perloff JK. Anesthetic implications of adults with congenital heart disease. *Anesth Analg.* 1993;76:1342-1358.

Bouchardy J, Therrien J, Pilote L, et al. Atrial arrhythmias in adults with congenital heart disease. *Circulation.* 2009;1201679–1686.

Burch TM, McGowan FX, Kussman BD, et al. Congenital supravalvular aortic stenosis and sudden death associated with anesthesia: what's the mystery? *Anesth Analg.* 2008;107:1848-1854.

Cannesson M, Earing MG, Collange V, et al. Anesthesia for noncardiac surgery in adults with congenital heart disease. *Anesthesiology.* 2009;111:432-440.

Diller GP, Dimopoulos K, Okonko D, et al. Exercise intolerance in adult congenital heart disease: comparative severity, correlates, and prognostic implication. *Circulation.* 2005;112:828-835.

Dimopoulos K, Diller GP, Koltsida E, et al. Prevalence, predictors, and prognostic value of renal dysfunction in adults with congenital heart disease. *Circulation.* 2008;117:2320-2328.

Eagle SS, Daves SM. The adult with Fontan physiology: systematic approach to perioperative management for noncardiac surgery. *J Cardiothorac Vasc Anesth.* 2011;25:320-334.

Gratz A, Hess J, Hager A. Self-estimated physical functioning poorly predicts actual exercise capacity in adolescents and adults with congenital heart disease. *Eur Heart J.* 2009;30:497-504.

Hoffman JI, Kaplan S. The incidence of congenital heart disease. *J Am Coll Cardiol.* 2002;39:1890-1900.

Hoffman JI, Kaplan S, Liberthson RR. Prevalence of congenital heart disease. *Am Heart J.* 2004;147:425-439.

Jacobs ML. Congenital Heart Surgery Nomenclature and Database Project: truncus arteriosus. *Ann Thorac Surg.* 2000;69(4 Suppl):S50-S55.

Khairy P, Poirier N, Mercier LA. Univentricular heart. *Circulation.* 2007; 115:800-812.

Khairy P, Ionescu-Ittu R, Mackie AS, et al. Changing mortality in congenital heart disease. *J Am Coll Cardiol.* 2010;56:1149-1157.

Khairy P, Aboulhosn J, Gurvitz MZ, et al. Arrhythmia burden in adults with surgically repaired tetralogy of Fallot: a multi-institutional study. *Circulation.* 2010;122:868-875.

Maxwell BG, Steppan J, Cheng A. Complications of catheter-based electrophysiology procedures in adults with congenital heart disease: a national analysis. *J Cardiothorac Vasc Anesth.* 2015;29:258-264.

Maxwell BG, Wong JK, Kin C, Lobato RL. Perioperative outcomes of major noncardiac surgery in adults with congenital heart disease. *Anesthesiology.* 2013;119:762-769.

Maxwell BG, Wong JK, Lobato RL. Perioperative morbidity and mortality after noncardiac surgery in young adults with congenital or early acquired heart disease: a retrospective cohort analysis of the National Surgical Quality Improvement Program database. *Am Surg.* 2014;80:321-326.

Minette MS, Sahn DJ. Ventricular septal defects. *Circulation*. 2006;114:2190-2197.

Mullen MP. Adult congenital heart disease. *Sci Am Med*. 2000:1-10.

Mylotte D, Pilote L, Ionescu-Ittu R, et al. Specialized adult congenital heart disease care: the impact of policy on mortality. *Circulation*. 2014;129:1804-1812.

Perloff JK, Warnes CA. Challenges posed by adults with repaired congenital heart disease. *Circulation*. 2001;103:2637-2643.

Sommer RJ, Hijazi ZM, Rhodes Jr JF. Pathophysiology of congenital heart disease in the adult: part I: shunt lesions. *Circulation*. 2008;117:1090-1099.

Sommer RJ, Hijazi ZM, Rhodes JF. Pathophysiology of congenital heart disease in the adult: part III: complex congenital heart disease. *Circulation*. 2008;117:1340-1350.

Stumper O. Hypoplastic left heart syndrome. *Heart*. 2010;96:231-236.

Triedman JK. Arrhythmias in adults with congenital heart disease. *Heart*. 2002;87:383-389.

Twite MD, Ing RJ. Tetralogy of Fallot: perioperative anesthetic management of children and adults. *Semin Cardiothorac Vasc Anesth*. 2012;16:97-105.

Van Overmeire B, Smets K, Lecoutere D, et al. A comparison of ibuprofen and indomethacin for closure of patent ductus arteriosus. *N Engl J Med*. 2000;343:674-681.

Warnes CA, Liberthson R, Danielson GK, et al. Task force 1: the changing profile of congenital heart disease in adult life. *J Am Coll Cardiol*. 2001;37:1170-1175.

Warnes CA, Williams RG, Bashore TM, et al. ACC/AHA 2008 guidelines for the management of adults with congenital heart disease: a report of the American College of Cardiology/American Heart Association Task Force on Practice Guidelines (Writing Committee to Develop Guidelines on the Management of Adults with Congenital Heart Disease). *Circulation*. 2008;118:e714-e833.

Wilson W, Taubert KA, Gewitz M, et al. Prevention of infective endocarditis: guidelines from the American Heart Association: a guideline from the American Heart Association Rheumatic Fever, Endocarditis, and Kawasaki Disease Committee, Council on Cardiovascular Disease in the Young, and the Council on Clinical Cardiology, Council on Cardiovascular Surgery and Anesthesia, and the Quality of Care and Outcomes Research Interdisciplinary Working Group. *Circulation*. 2007;116:1736-1754.

Abnormalities of Cardiac Conduction and Cardiac Rhythm

KELLEY TEED WATSON

HISTORICAL ROOTS OF DYSRHYTHMIA DETECTION

Around 466 BC, Hippocrates wrote, "Those who are subject to frequent and severe fainting attacks without obvious cause die suddenly." His writings describe recurrent syncope in otherwise normal individuals. His notations may be the first documentation of fatal dysrhythmogenic cardiac disease. His observations could be attributed to electrophysiologic diseases such as long-QT syndrome, Wolff-Parkinson-White syndrome, or dilated cardiomyopathy.

Practitioners in Hippocrates' era lacked the tools we have today, like the simple electrocardiogram (ECG), to evaluate cardiac rhythm disturbances. Instead, they relied upon information obtained from manual palpation of the pulse to make cardiac diagnoses. They believed that the qualities of the pulse, such as strength, rate, and regularity, were indicative of the health of the heart. Hippocrates' observations inspired many scientists to investigate the mechanisms, treatment, and prevention of sudden death. Centuries later we are as captivated by the heart and its mysteries as our scientific forerunners, and we must agree with their basic idea that the rate and quality of the pulse are an indication of the health and strength of the heart.

THE ECG AS A MONITOR

The pulse, as manually palpated or electronically sensed, is detected owing to the pressure wave transmission of the forward flow of blood ejected from the heart during systole and the force it exerts on the compliant arteries of the body. These properties create a palpable pressure wave. In the absence of routine monitors, palpation of a pulse can give us an idea of the regularity of the heart rhythm and the overall heart rate. However, the essential monitor for diagnosis of cardiac conduction abnormalities and rhythm disturbances is the ECG.

The ECG machine uses electrodes placed on the skin to amplify the movement of electrical potentials through the heart and record the electrical signal deflections (waves). The direction of the electrical signal relative to a ground electrode determines the direction of the deflection seen on the ECG. Positive signals are represented by deflections above an isoelectric line, and negative signals are represented as deflections below an isoelectric line. The type and configuration of the deflections determine the type of rhythm.

As perioperative clinicians, anesthesiologists must be proficient in recognizing normal and abnormal ECG findings. The ECG is considered the single most important clinical test to diagnose dysrhythmias and to diagnose myocardial ischemia and infarction. However, it is seldom feasible to monitor all 12 leads simultaneously and continuously in the operating room or other acute monitoring situation. As clinicians caring for patients in the operating room, we are often faced with treating dysrhythmias and ST-segment changes without being able to obtain a full confirmatory 12-lead ECG.

In the acute setting a 5-lead continuous ECG is most often available to monitor heart rate, rhythm, and ST-segment trends. The two most common leads monitored are leads II and V$_5$. Lead II represents the inferior wall of the left ventricle and the right ventricle. This distribution is perfused by the right coronary artery. Lead II is superior to other lead choices for the detection of atrial dysrhythmias. Lead V$_5$ represents the lateral wall of the left ventricle, perfused by the left circumflex coronary artery. For monitoring of ST-segment trends, studies have shown that V$_5$ detects 90% of ischemic changes.

At a minimum, it is helpful to have a baseline ECG prior to moderate- or high-risk surgery in all patients with evidence-based indicators of perioperative cardiovascular risk such as age older than 65 years, known coronary artery disease, hyperlipidemia, history of significant dysrhythmia, peripheral arterial disease, cerebrovascular disease, or significant structural heart disease. The utility and cost-effectiveness of preoperative ECGs in patients undergoing surgeries classified as "low risk" has been questioned because there is a lack of evidence that the test improves intraoperative safety or clinical outcome. There are some variations in what is considered low-, moderate- and high-risk surgery, but for the most part, cataract, breast, endoscopic, and superficial plastic

surgery are considered low (<1%) risk of myocardial infarction (MI) or death. Procedures considered intermediate risk (1%–5%) for MI or death include intraperitoneal, intrathoracic, head and neck, orthopedic, and prostate surgery, and carotid endarterectomy. Noncardiac procedures considered high risk (>5%) for MI and death are aortic, major vascular, and peripheral vascular surgery.

CONDUCTION SYSTEM OF THE HEART

The cardiac conduction system is a complex group of specialized cells within the heart that initiate and conduct electrical signals with great precision and speed. The myocardial cells in the heart are arranged in a functional syncytium. The cells are interconnected by a specialized membrane with gap junctions that are synchronized electrically during an action potential. As an electrical impulse moves along the conduction system, a coordinated wave of depolarization is propagated through the heart, causing progressive contraction of the myocardium (Fig. 8.1).

In the resting (polarized) state the inside of a myocardial cell is negative relative to the outside. Cardiac muscle cells have a resting membrane potential of −80 to −90 mV. The resting gradient is maintained by membrane-bound sodium-potassium adenosinetriphosphatase (Na$^+$,K$^+$-ATPase) that concentrates potassium intracellularly and extrudes sodium extracellularly. The membrane potential increases when the sodium and calcium channels open in response to shifts in the charge on neighboring cell membranes. At the point at which the membrane potential reaches +20 mV, an action potential (or depolarization) occurs. After depolarization, cells are refractory to subsequent action potentials for a period of time corresponding to phase 4 of the depolarization potential (Fig. 8.2).

The sinoatrial (SA) node is the primary site for impulse initiation and is considered the major intrinsic pacemaker of the heart. The SA node is located at the junction of the superior vena cava and the right atrium and is richly innervated by sympathetic and parasympathetic nerve endings. It is perfused by the right coronary artery in 60% of individuals. Most of the remaining 40% of people receive their blood supply to the SA node from the left circumflex coronary artery. An impulse generated by the SA

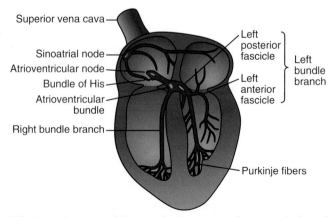

FIG. 8.1 Anatomy of the conduction system for transmission of cardiac electrical impulses.

node spreads rapidly across the right and left atria, causing them to contract. This portion of the electrical signal coincides with the P wave on an ECG. After passing through the atria, the electrical impulse travels between the fibrous atrioventricular (AV) rings of the tricuspid and mitral valves to the AV node.

The AV node is a secondary pacemaker for the heart, located in the septal wall of the right atrium anterior to the coronary sinus and above the insertion of the septal leaflet of the tricuspid valve. The blood supply to the AV node comes from the right coronary artery in 85%–90% of the population and from the left circumflex coronary artery in the remaining 10%–15%. Like the SA node, it is innervated by both parasympathetic and sympathetic nerves.

Normally when the electrical impulse reaches the AV node, it slows down. This is due to a long refractory period characteristic of the AV node commonly called the "AV delay." The AV delay prevents overstimulation of the ventricles in the event of abnormally rapid atrial impulses. Hemodynamically significant dysrhythmias with rapid ventricular

responses can occur when the AV node is bypassed through an accessory pathway.

After exiting the AV node, the impulse continues down the proximal ventricular conduction system within the interventricular septum. This part of the conduction system, the *bundle of His,* splits into right and left portions called *bundle branches.* Movement through the bundle branches coincides with the isoelectric PR interval on the ECG tracing. The normal reference range for the PR interval is 120–200 ms.

The left bundle branch (LBB) divides into two fascicles: the left anterior superior fascicle and the left posterior inferior fascicle. The right bundle branch (RBB) is a relatively thin bundle of fibers that courses down the right ventricle and then branches late in its course near the right ventricular apex. The right and left bundle branches terminate in an interlacing network of small fibers called the *His-Purkinje system.*

After the electrical impulse exits the AV node and travels through the bundle branches, the first portion of the ventricles to depolarize is the septum. This causes a minor ECG deflection called the *Q wave.* It is followed by depolarization of the apex and the bulk of the ventricular free walls, as reflected in the R wave of the ECG. The last area to be depolarized is the superior portion of the left ventricular free wall and the right ventricular outflow tract. Depending on the bulk of the left ventricular free wall, this vector may show up as a negative deflection, the S wave.

The interval from the Q wave through the R wave to the end of the S wave is called the *QRS complex.* Normal QRS duration varies depending on age and gender. However, as a general guideline, abnormal intraventricular conduction is suggested by a QRS complex that exceeds 110 ms in adults.

The portion of the ECG between the S and T waves (ST segment) is normally isoelectric and represents the time between ventricular *depolarization* and the start of ventricular *repolarization.* Ventricular repolarization is represented by the T wave. After the T wave, there is another isoelectric period until the depolarization process begins again. The T-wave deflection should be in the same direction as the QRS complex and should not exceed 5 mm in amplitude in standard limb leads or 15 mm in precordial leads. T waves should be upright in all leads except aVR and V_1.

Changes in ST segments trending down (depression) or up (elevation) can be due to many factors. The differential diagnosis for elevation or depression of the ST segment includes myocardial ischemia/infarction, but there are many other causes of ST-segment changes besides ischemia. ECG changes that occur with acute ischemia and infarction include peaked T waves (hyperacute T wave changes), ST-segment elevation and/or depression, changes in the QRS complex, and inverted T waves. Ischemic ST-segment changes are produced by injury currents as depolarization spreads across areas in the myocardium where injury has occurred.

ST-segment elevation is commonly seen with pericarditis, hyperkalemia, acute myocarditis, cardiac tumors, Osborne waves, and a normal variant called *early repolarization.* An Osborne wave, also called a *J wave,* is a positive deflection at the J point where the QRS complex meets the ST segment and is most prominent in the precordial leads. Osborne waves are

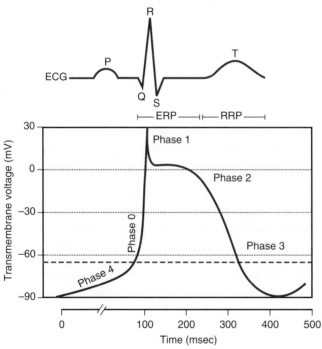

FIG. 8.2 Transmembrane action potential occurring in an automatic cardiac cell and the relationship of this action potential to events depicted on the electrocardiogram (ECG). Phase 4 is characterized by spontaneous depolarization from the resting membrane potential (–90 mV) until the threshold potential *(broken line)* is reached. Depolarization (phase 0) occurs when the threshold potential is reached and corresponds to the QRS complex on the ECG. Phases 1 through 3 represent repolarization, with phase 3 corresponding to the T wave on the ECG. The effective refractory period (ERP) is the time during which cardiac impulses cannot be conducted, regardless of the intensity of the stimulus. During the relative refractory period (RRP), a strong stimulus can initiate an action potential. The action potential developed in a contractile cardiac cell differs from that occurring in an automatic cardiac cell in that phase 4 is not characterized by spontaneous depolarization.

characteristically seen in hypothermia (typically, body temperature < 30°C). ST-segment depression is often seen in left ventricular hypertrophy ("LV strain"), with certain cardioactive drugs (digoxin), and hypokalemia.

The QT interval is the time from the start of the Q wave to the end of the T wave. It represents the time taken for full ventricular depolarization and repolarization. The QT shortens at faster heart rates and lengthens at slower heart rates. An abnormally prolonged QT is associated with an increased risk of ventricular dysrhythmias, especially torsades de pointes (TdP). Normal values for the QT interval should be corrected for the heart rate (QTc) because the QT interval varies inversely with heart rate. QTc is prolonged if it exceeds 440 ms in men or 460 ms in women. QTc over 500 ms is associated with an increased risk of TdP. As a general rule the QT interval is less than half of the preceding R-R interval. Causes of a prolonged QTc (>440 ms) include hypokalemia, hypomagnesemia, hypocalcemia, hypothermia, myocardial ischemia, raised intracranial pressure, congenital long QT syndrome, and certain drugs. A QTc below 350 ms is abnormally short. *Short QT syndrome* has been discovered within the past 20 years. It is an inherited primary electrical disease of the heart associated with paroxysmal atrial fibrillation, ventricular tachycardia, ventricular fibrillation, syncope, and sudden cardiac death.

CARDIAC CONDUCTION DISTURBANCES

An intact cardiac conduction system normally ensures conduction of each sinus node impulse from the atria to the ventricles. Abnormalities of the conduction system can disrupt this process and lead to heart block. The classification of conduction block is by the site and degree of blockade. Knowing the type of heart block from the ECG gives the clinician an idea of the risk of worsening heart block and what treatment strategies and equipment need to be available.

A variety of acute and chronic conditions can cause or contribute to heart block. Disease processes such as acute MI (especially in the distribution of the right coronary artery), myocarditis, rheumatic fever, mononucleosis, Lyme disease, and infiltrative diseases such as sarcoidosis and amyloidosis can contribute to heart block. Iatrogenic causes for heart block include traumatic injury from monitoring or ablation catheters or cardiac surgery, and drug effects such as digitalis toxicity or excessive β-blockade or calcium channel blockade.

First-Degree Atrioventricular Heart Block

A delay in passage of the cardiac impulse through the AV node resulting in a PR interval of longer than 200 ms is called *first-degree AV block.* Although the PR interval is extended, each P wave has a corresponding QRS complex of normal duration. First-degree AV block can be found in patients with and without structural heart disease. Patients are usually asymptomatic.

Commonly, this is a result of minor degenerative changes in the cardiac conduction system that accompany normal aging.

Other causes of first-degree heart block include myocardial ischemia (involving blood supply to the AV node), inferior wall MI, drugs affecting AV node conduction (digitalis and amiodarone), and processes that enhance parasympathetic nervous system activity and increase vagal tone.

Anesthetic management of the patient with first-degree heart block should be aimed at avoiding any clinical situation or drug that increases vagal tone or further slows AV conduction. Atropine administration can speed conduction of cardiac impulses through the AV node. However, in patients with significant coronary heart disease the increase in heart rate produced by atropine may contribute to myocardial ischemia. In patients with risk factors for first-degree heart block (e.g., coronary ischemia, systemic infection) these clinical conditions should be treated and medically optimized prior to surgery. Digoxin levels should be checked before surgery, and serum potassium should be maintained at normal levels.

Second-Degree Atrioventricular Heart Block

Second-degree AV block can be suspected when a P wave is present without a corresponding QRS complex. Second-degree AV heart block can be categorized as Mobitz type I (Wenckebach) block or Mobitz type II block. Mobitz type I block shows progressive prolongation of the PR interval until a beat is entirely blocked (dropped beat), followed by a repeat of this sequence. In contrast, Mobitz type II block is characterized by sudden and complete interruption of conduction (dropped QRS) without PR prolongation. Mobitz type II block is considered more serious and is much more likely to be associated with permanent damage to the conduction system. Mobitz Type II block is more likely to progress to third-degree block, especially in the setting of acute MI.

Mobitz type I (Wenckebach) block demonstrates progressive prolongation of the PR interval until a beat is dropped. It is thought to occur because each successive depolarization produces a prolongation of the refractory period of the AV node. This process continues until an atrial impulse reaches the AV node during its absolute refractory period and conduction of that impulse is blocked completely. A pause allows the AV node to recover, and then the process resumes.

This type of block is often transient, *asymptomatic,* and rarely progresses to third-degree heart block. Since secondary pacemakers in the AV node usually take over pacing duties and maintain adequate cardiac output, Mobitz type I block does not usually require treatment unless the decreased ventricular rate results in signs of hemodynamic compromise. Symptomatic patients may be treated with atropine as needed. If atropine is unsuccessful, pacing may be indicated. Mobitz type I block can be the result of myocardial ischemia or infarction, myocardial fibrosis or calcification, or infiltrative or inflammatory diseases of the myocardium, or it can occur after cardiothoracic surgery. It can also be associated with the use of certain drugs such as calcium channel blockers, β-blockers, digoxin, and sympatholytic drugs.

Mobitz type II block is a complete interruption in the conduction of a cardiac impulse, usually at a point below the AV node in the bundle of His or in a bundle branch. Mobitz type II block is usually *symptomatic,* with palpitations and near-syncope being common complaints. Mobitz type II block has a less favorable prognosis because there is a substantial risk of progression to third-degree AV block. Reliable secondary pacemakers are not present in Mobitz type II block or in third-degree heart block, because these disorders are associated with serious disease involving the infranodal conduction system.

Therapeutic decisions for patients with second-degree heart block depend on the ventricular response and the patient's symptoms. In the presence of an acceptable ventricular rate and an adequate cardiac output, no treatment is needed. Mobitz type II block has a high rate of progression to third-degree heart block and can manifest as a slow escape rhythm insufficient to sustain an acceptable cardiac output. Placement of a cardiac pacemaker is necessary under these circumstances. Temporizing treatment for Mobitz type II block includes transcutaneous or transvenous cardiac pacing until a permanent pacemaker is in place. Atropine is unlikely to improve bradycardia in this situation, but an isoproterenol infusion acting as a "chemical pacemaker" may be helpful as a temporizing measure prior to pacemaker placement.

Bundle Branch Blocks

Conduction disturbances at various levels of the His-Purkinje system are called *bundle branch blocks.* The left and right bundles both receive blood supply from branches of the left anterior descending coronary artery. Infarction in the territory of the left anterior descending coronary artery can often affect the left anterior superior fascicle and the RBB. The left posterior inferior fascicle is usually spared because it receives additional blood supply from the posterior descending coronary artery, a branch of the right coronary artery. This redundant blood supply to the LBB explains why complete disruption of the LBB, as indicated by a left bundle branch block (LBBB) on ECG, usually indicates more extensive cardiac disease or damage than a right bundle branch block (RBBB). Bundle branch blocks can be chronic or intermittent.

Right Bundle Branch Block

RBBB is present in approximately 1% of hospitalized adult patients. The conduction delay resulting from RBBB is seldom symptomatic and rarely progresses to advanced AV block. It does not always imply cardiac disease and is often of no clinical significance in patients without structural heart disease. RBBB is more common than LBBB.

RBBB is due to a disruption of the cardiac impulse as it travels over the RBB. It is recognized by a widened QRS complex (≥120 ms in adults) and an rSR′ configuration in leads V_1 and V_2. There is also a deep S wave (>40 ms) in leads I and V_6. If the QRS is between 110 and 120 ms, with the other criteria for RBBB fulfilled, it is considered an *incomplete RBBB.*

Bifascicular heart block is present when RBBB exists in combination with block of either the left anterior or left posterior fascicle of the LBB. RBBB in association with left anterior hemiblock is more common than RBBB with left posterior hemiblock. Indications of RBBB with left anterior hemiblock are present on approximately 1% of all adult ECGs. The combination of RBBB and left posterior hemiblock is much less frequent, and each year approximately 1%–2% of patients with this form of block progress to third-degree heart block.

Acute treatment of RBBB or RBBB with left anterior hemiblock consists of observation and elimination of drugs or clinical factors known to contribute to conduction disturbances. Pacing capability should be available in the event of progression to complete heart block. A theoretical concern in patients with bifascicular heart block is that perioperative events (changes in blood pressure, arterial oxygenation, serum electrolyte concentrations) might compromise impulse conduction in the remaining fascicle and lead to third-degree heart block. There is, however, no evidence that surgery performed with general or regional anesthesia predisposes patients with preexisting bifascicular heart block to the development of third-degree heart block. Prophylactic placement of a cardiac pacemaker is *not* necessary.

Left Bundle Branch Block

The LBB of the bundle of His is composed of two components, the left anterior fascicle and the left posterior fascicle. A complete LBBB is recognized as a QRS complex of longer than 120 ms in duration in the absence of Q waves in leads I and V_5 and V_6, a broad notched or slurred R wave in leads I, aVL, V_5, and V_6. The S and T waves are usually opposite in direction to the QRS.

If one of the two fascicles of the LBB fails to conduct for whatever reason, this is called a *hemiblock* (HB). Block of the left anterior fascicle (LAHB) is the most common hemiblock. Left posterior hemiblock (LPHB) is uncommon because the posterior fascicle of the LBB is larger and better perfused than the anterior fascicle. Although hemiblock is a form of *intraventricular heart block,* the duration of the QRS complex is normal or only minimally prolonged. The direction of deviation of the QRS axis is the main criterion for determining which fascicle is involved. Left axis deviation is associated with LAHB, and right axis deviation is associated with LPHB.

The LBB is more richly perfused than the RBB. This is due to the redundant blood supply to the LBB and the fact that it branches early and widely into anterior and posterior fascicles during its course down the left ventricular septum. The appearance of LBBB on ECG is often an indication of serious heart disease (e.g., hypertension, coronary artery disease, aortic valve disease, cardiomyopathy). Isolated LBBB is often asymptomatic, and some patients have LBBB only after a critical heart rate is reached.

The appearance of LBBB has been observed during anesthesia, particularly during hypertensive or tachycardic episodes, and may be a sign of myocardial ischemia. It is very difficult to diagnose MI in the presence of a LBBB, because ST-segment and T-wave changes (repolarization abnormalities) are already present as part of the bundle branch block pattern. A supraventricular tachycardia in a patient with LBBB can be mistaken for ventricular tachycardia, because the QRS complex is already widened from the LBBB. The presence of LBBB has special implications if insertion of a pulmonary artery catheter is planned. Third-degree heart block can occur if the catheter induces RBBB in a patient with preexisting LBBB. RBBB (usually transient) occurs during insertion of a pulmonary artery catheter in approximately 2%–5% of patients.

Third-Degree Atrioventricular Heart Block

Third-degree AV heart block, also known as *complete heart block,* is complete interruption of AV conduction. There is no conduction of cardiac impulses from the atria to the ventricles. Continued activity of the ventricles is due to impulses from an ectopic pacemaker distal to the site of the conduction block. If the conduction block is near the AV node, the heart rate is usually 45–55 beats per minute (bpm) and the QRS complex is narrow. When the conduction block is below the AV node (infranodal), the heart rate is usually 30–40 bpm and the QRS complex is wide.

Onset of third-degree AV block in an awake patient may be signaled by vertigo or syncope. Syncope attributed to third-degree heart block is called a *Stokes-Adams attack.* Congestive heart failure (CHF) with symptoms such as weakness and dyspnea can also occur from the bradycardia-induced reduction in cardiac output that can accompany third-degree AV block. In patients with isolated chronic RBBB, the progression to complete AV block is rare. Patients with bifascicular block (RBBB and left anterior or posterior fascicular block) or complete LBBB have a 6% incidence of progression to complete heart block. Approximately 8% of patients with acute inferior wall MI develop complete heart block. It is usually transient, although it may last for several days. Development of new bifascicular block plus first-degree AV block is associated with a very high risk (40%) of progression to complete heart block. ECG evidence of alternating bundle branch blocks, even if asymptomatic, is a sign of advanced conduction system disease and is an indication for permanent pacing.

The most common cause of third-degree AV block in adults is fibrotic degeneration of the distal conduction system associated with aging (Lenègre disease). Degenerative and calcific changes in more proximal conduction tissue adjacent to the mitral valve annulus can also interrupt cardiac conduction (Lev disease).

In anesthetized patients, third-degree heart block can be due to cardiac ischemia, metabolic or electrolyte abnormalities, infection or inflammation near the conduction system, reperfusion injury, or stunned myocardium after cardiac surgery. Treatment of third-degree AV block occurring during anesthesia consists of transcutaneous or transvenous cardiac pacing. An intravenous (IV) isoproterenol infusion may also be helpful in maintaining an acceptable heart rate by acting as a "chemical pacemaker."

Caution must be exercised when administering antidysrhythmic drugs to patients with third-degree AV block before permanent pacemaker placement. Such drugs may suppress the only remaining functioning ectopic pacemaker responsible for maintaining the heart rate.

Preoperative placement of a transvenous pacemaker or the availability of transcutaneous cardiac pacing is necessary before an anesthetic is administered for insertion of a permanent cardiac pacemaker.

CARDIAC DYSRHYTHMIA OVERVIEW

Cardiac rhythms that have abnormalities in rate, interval length, or conduction path are referred to as *dysrhythmias.* The significance of these abnormalities for the anesthesiologist depends on the clinical effect the dysrhythmias have on vital signs and on the potential to deteriorate into a life-threatening dysrhythmia. However, even the occurrence of an occasional benign ectopic beat deserves notice and a consideration of possible causes. In healthy adults a wide variation in heart rate can be tolerated because normal compensatory mechanisms serve to maintain cardiac output and blood pressure. In patients with cardiac disease, dysrhythmias and conduction abnormalities that might be benign in one patient may be catastrophic in another. Each disturbance has the potential to lead to hemodynamic instability, cardiac ischemia, CHF, and end-organ dysfunction or even death.

Sinus dysrhythmia is a normal variant encountered in patients who exhibit normal sinus rhythm with a normal sinus rate (>60 bpm and <100 bpm), normal PR interval, normal QRS length and normal ST intervals, but an *irregular R-R interval length.* Variation in the R-R is usually due to a physiologic phenomenon known as the *Bainbridge reflex,* which accelerates the heart rate when intrathoracic pressure is increased during inspiration and slows the heart rate when the intrathoracic pressure decreases during expiration. The occurrence of sinus dysrhythmia carries no increased risk of deterioration into a dangerous rhythm. It is most commonly seen in children and young people and tends to decrease with age.

MECHANISMS OF TACHYDYSRHYTHMIAS

A cardiac rhythm greater than 100 bpm is considered a tachydysrhythmia. Tachydysrhythmias can be generated from sources above or below the bundle of His. Those whose mechanism involves tissue above the bundle of His are called *supraventricular tachycardias* (SVTs). Tachydysrhythmias originating at or above the AV node usually have a narrow QRS complex. The differential for a *narrow complex tachycardia* includes sinus tachycardia, atrial flutter, atrial fibrillation (AF), junctional tachycardia, paroxysmal atrial tachycardia, and accessory pathway–mediated reentrant tachycardias.

Tachydysrhythmias generated from below the AV node have a wide QRS complex. The differential diagnosis for a *wide QRS complex tachycardia* includes ventricular tachycardia, SVT with an intraventricular conduction defect or bundle branch block, SVT with aberrant conduction, SVT with wide

QRS due to a metabolic or electrolyte disorder, and SVT with conduction over a preexcitation (accessory) pathway.

Tachydysrhythmias can result from three mechanisms: (1) increased automaticity in normal conduction tissue or in an ectopic focus, (2) reentry of electrical potentials through abnormal pathways, and (3) triggering of abnormal cardiac potentials due to afterdepolarizations.

Increased Automaticity

The fastest pacemaker in the heart is normally the SA node. The SA node spontaneously discharges at a rate of 60–100 bpm. Other pacemakers can be accelerated and overdrive the SA node as a result of disease states or iatrogenic influences such as drug toxicity. Cardiac dysrhythmias caused by enhanced automaticity result from repetitive firing of a focus other than the sinus node. Dysrhythmias resulting from an ectopic focus often have a gradual onset and termination.

A sustained rhythm resulting from accelerated firing of a pacemaker other than the SA node is called an *ectopic rhythm.* Automaticity is not confined to secondary pacemakers within the conduction system; virtually any myocardial cell can exhibit automaticity under certain circumstances and is therefore capable of initiating cardiac depolarization.

The automaticity of cardiac tissue changes when the slope of phase 4 depolarization shifts or the resting membrane potential changes. Sympathetic stimulation causes an increase in heart rate by increasing the slope of phase 4 of the action potential and by decreasing the resting membrane potential. Conversely, parasympathetic stimulation results in a decrease in the slope of phase 4 depolarization and an increase in resting membrane potential to slow the heart rate.

Reentry Pathways

Reentry pathways account for most premature beats and tachydysrhythmias. Reentry or triggered dysrhythmias require two pathways over which cardiac impulses can be conducted at different velocities (Fig. 8.3). Extra pathways called *accessory tracts* can exist around the AV node and can conduct impulses to the ventricles bypassing the AV node and normal infranodal conduction tract.

The AV node is normally the slowest portion of the conduction system. In a reentry circuit there is anterograde (forward) conduction over the slower normal conduction pathway and retrograde (backward) conduction over a faster accessory pathway. Pharmacologic or physiologic events may alter the balance between conduction velocities and refractory periods of the dual pathways, resulting in the initiation or termination of reentrant dysrhythmias. Reentrant dysrhythmias tend to be paroxysmal with abrupt onset and termination.

Triggering by Afterdepolarizations

Afterdepolarizations are oscillations in membrane potential that occur during or after repolarization. Normally these

membrane oscillations dissipate. However, under certain circumstances they can trigger a complete depolarization. Once triggered, the process may continue and result in a self-sustaining dysrhythmia.

Triggered dysrhythmias associated with *early* afterdepolarizations are enhanced by a slow heart rate and are treated by accelerating the heart rate with positive chronotropic drugs or pacing. Conversely, triggered dysrhythmias associated with *delayed* afterdepolarizations are enhanced by fast heart rates and can be suppressed with drugs that lower the heart rate.

SUPRAVENTRICULAR DYSRHYTHMIAS

Sinus Tachycardia

Normal sinus rhythm in a patient at rest is under the control of the sinus node, which fires at a rate of 60–100 bpm. When sinus rhythm exceeds 100 bpm, it is considered *sinus tachycardia.* The ECG shows a normal P wave before every QRS complex. The PR interval is normal unless a co-existing conduction block exists. Sinus tachycardia is caused by acceleration of SA node discharge due to either sympathetic stimulation or parasympathetic suppression. Typically it is a nonparoxysmal increase in heart rate that speeds up and slows down gradually. It is the most common supraventricular dysrhythmia in the operating room.

Sinus tachycardia without hemodynamic instability is not life-threatening. It can occur in an awake patient as part of the normal physiologic response to stimuli (e.g., fear, pain, anxiety) or as a pharmacologic response to medications such as atropine, ephedrine, or other vasopressors. Intake of

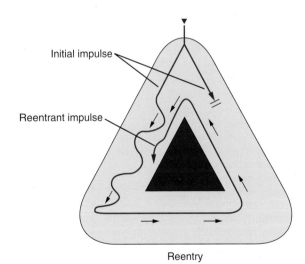

FIG. 8.3 The essential requirement for initiation of reentry excitation is a unilateral block that prevents uniform anterograde propagation of the initial cardiac impulse. Under appropriate conditions, this same cardiac impulse can traverse the area of blockade in a retrograde direction and become a reentrant cardiac impulse. (Adapted from Akhtar M. Management of ventricular tachyarrhythmias. *JAMA.* 1982;247:671-674.)

substances such as caffeine and cocaine may also cause sinus tachycardia.

Sinus tachycardia is usually well tolerated in young healthy patients. Treatment of sinus tachycardia is directed toward correcting the underlying cause. If a specific cause of sinus tachycardia can be determined, it should be treated. Reasons for sinus tachycardia range from simple to complex. Potential intraoperative causes include sympathetic stimulation, vagolytic drug administration, hypovolemia, "light" anesthesia, hypoxia, hypercarbia, heart failure, cardiac ischemia, fever, and infection. In patients with ischemic heart disease, diastolic dysfunction, or CHF, the heart rate increase above normal sinus rhythm can lead to significant clinical deterioration because of increased oxygen demand, increased wall stress, and a decrease in coronary perfusion. During tachycardia the length of diastole is shortened more than the length of systole, so the time for coronary artery blood flow is decreased at the same time as cardiac work is increased by the tachycardia.

Strategies to decrease the likelihood of sinus tachycardia include avoidance of vagolytic drugs such as pancuronium, ensuring adequate anesthetic depth, maintenance of euvolemia, correction of hypercarbia, avoidance of hypoxemia, antibiotic treatment of suspected infection, use of the lowest effective dose of inotropic support for heart failure (many inotropes increase heart rate), and prompt treatment of myocardial ischemia (Table 8.1).

Treatment may include IV administration of a β-blocker to lower the heart rate and decrease myocardial oxygen demand. However, β-blockers must be used with caution in patients

TABLE 8.1 | Perioperative Causes of Sinus Tachycardia

PHYSIOLOGIC INCREASE IN SYMPATHETIC TONE
Pain
Anxiety or fear
Light anesthesia
Hypovolemia or anemia
Arterial hypoxemia
Hypotension
Hypoglycemia
Fever or infection

PATHOLOGIC INCREASE IN SYMPATHETIC TONE
Myocardial ischemia or infarction
Congestive heart failure
Pulmonary embolus
Hyperthyroidism
Pericarditis
Pericardial tamponade
Malignant hyperthermia
Ethanol withdrawal

DRUG-INDUCED INCREASE IN HEART RATE
Atropine or glycopyrrolate
Sympathomimetic drugs
Caffeine
Nicotine
Cocaine or amphetamines

susceptible to bronchospasm and in patients with impaired cardiac function. Patients with a low ejection fraction may be unable to increase their stroke volume to compensate for the reduction in heart rate, and as a result the β-blocker–mediated decrease in heart rate can cause an abrupt and dangerous decrease in blood pressure.

Premature Atrial Beats

Premature atrial contractions (PACs) are early (premature) ectopic beats. The P wave of the PAC originates from an ectopic focus in the atria. The PR interval is variable. Most often the corresponding QRS complex is narrow because activation of the ventricles following the ectopic P wave occurs through the normal conduction pathway. However, aberrant conduction of atrial impulses can occur, resulting in a widened QRS complex that may resemble a premature ventricular contraction (PVC). There is typically a slight pause after the PAC before the next sinus beat.

Symptoms of PACs in an awake patient include an awareness of a "fluttering" in the chest or a "heavy" heart beat. PACs are common in patients of all ages, with or without heart disease. They often occur at rest and become less frequent with exercise. Precipitating factors include sympathetic stimulation from excessive caffeine, emotional stress, alcohol, nicotine, recreational drugs, and hyperthyroidism. They are more common in patients with chronic lung disease, ischemic heart disease, and digitalis toxicity. PACs are usually hemodynamically insignificant and do not require therapy unless they are associated with initiation of a tachydysrhythmia. In this situation, treatment is directed at controlling or converting the tachydysrhythmia. Underlying predisposing conditions should also be treated if possible.

Strategies for the management of patients with PACs include avoidance of excessive sympathetic stimulation and drugs that might induce PACs, suppression of PACs with calcium channel blockers or β-blockers, treatment of secondary dysrhythmias with drugs, or maneuvers that improve heart rate control and/or convert the dysrhythmia to sinus rhythm.

Paroxysmal Supraventricular Tachycardia

Paroxysmal supraventricular tachycardia (PSVT) is a tachydysrhythmia (average heart rate, 160–220 bpm) initiated and sustained by tissue at or above the AV node. Unlike sinus tachycardia, PSVT usually begins and ends abruptly. The incidence of PSVT in the US population is 2.25 per 1000 persons. It is estimated there will be approximately 89,000 new cases of PSVT per year. Women are more likely than men to have PSVT, and the most common type of PSVT is AV nodal reentry tachycardia (AVNRT). Individuals older than 65 years have a 5 times greater risk of developing PSVT than younger patients.

AVNRT is most commonly due to a reentry circuit in which there is anterograde conduction over the slower AV nodal pathway and retrograde conduction over a faster accessory pathway. Other mechanisms for PSVT include enhanced automaticity of secondary pacemaker cells and triggered impulse initiation by afterdepolarizations.

Common symptoms in an awake patient experiencing PSVT include light-headedness, dizziness, fatigue, chest discomfort, and dyspnea. Up to 15% of patients with PSVT may experience syncope. PSVT often occurs in individuals without structural heart disease.

Strategies for clinical care of a patient with a history of PSVT should include avoiding factors known to increase ectopy, such as increased sympathetic tone, electrolyte imbalances, and acid-base disturbances. Because PSVT is paroxysmal, monitoring of vital signs to detect any progression to hemodynamic instability and verbal reassurance (if the patient is awake) is usually all that is needed until an episode of PSVT terminates. One should evaluate and treat any potential aggravating factors and anticipate the potential need for antidysrhythmics and/or cardioversion. If the patient is in hemodynamically stable

condition, the initial treatment of PSVT can consist of vagal maneuvers such as carotid sinus massage or a Valsalva maneuver. Termination by a vagal maneuver suggests reentry as the causative mechanism. If conservative treatment is not effective, pharmacologic treatment directed at blocking AV nodal conduction is indicated. Clinical factors guide the choice of drug treatment, but adenosine, calcium channel blockers, and β-blockers are commonly used to terminate PSVT (Fig. 8.4).

Adenosine has an advantage over other IV drugs used to treat PSVT; it has a very rapid onset (15–30 seconds) and very brief duration of action (10 seconds). Most AVNRT episodes can be terminated by a single dose of adenosine. Multifocal atrial tachycardia, atrial flutter, and AF *do not* respond to adenosine. Heart transplant recipients require a reduction in adenosine dosage because of denervation hypersensitivity. Conversely, methylxanthines such as theophylline act as adenosine receptor antagonists, so a higher dose of adenosine will likely be needed to produce a therapeutic effect.

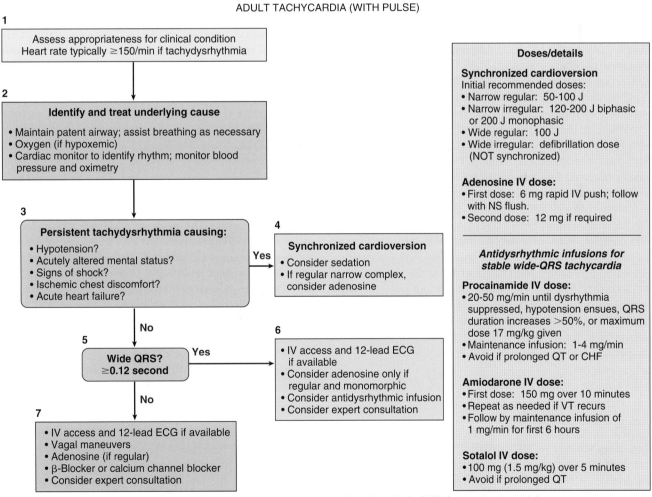

FIG. 8.4   Algorithm for treatment of adult tachycardia (with pulse). *CHF,* Congestive heart failure; *ECG,* electrocardiogram; *IV,* intravenous; *NS,* normal saline; *VT,* ventricular tachycardia. (American Heart Association. Web-based Integrated Guidelines for Cardiopulmonary Resuscitation and Emergency Cardiovascular Care—Part 7: Adult Advanced Cardiovascular Life Support. ECCguidelines. heart.org [Copyright 2015 American Heart Association, Inc.].)

Intravenous administration of calcium channel blocking drugs such as verapamil and diltiazem can also be useful for terminating PSVT. These drugs have a longer duration of action than adenosine. However, side effects, including peripheral vasodilation and negative inotropy, can contribute to an undesirable degree of hypotension. Intravenous β-blockers can be used to control or convert PSVT. Digoxin is not clinically useful in acute control of PSVT because IV digoxin has a delayed peak effect and a narrow therapeutic window. Electrical cardioversion is indicated for PSVT unresponsive to drug therapy or PSVT associated with hemodynamic instability. Long-term medical treatment of patients with repeated episodes of PSVT includes calcium channel blockers, digoxin, and/or β-blockers. Radiofrequency catheter ablation may be used in patients with recurrent or recalcitrant AVNRT.

Wolff-Parkinson-White Syndrome

Wolff-Parkinson-White (WPW) syndrome is an inherited disorder characterized by reentrant tachycardias. The diagnosis of WPW syndrome is reserved for conditions characterized by both preexcitation and tachydysrhythmia. Ventricular preexcitation causes an earlier-than-normal deflection of the QRS complex called a *delta wave*. These preexcitation ECG changes are a form of conduction block. The ECG criteria in adults are PR interval less than 120 ms, slurring of the initial portion of the QRS (delta wave), QRS longer than 120 ms in adults, and secondary ST-segment and T-wave changes.

AVNRT is the most common tachydysrhythmia seen in patients with WPW syndrome. It accounts for 95% of the dysrhythmias seen with this syndrome. This tachydysrhythmia is usually triggered by a premature atrial contraction. AVNRT is classified as either orthodromic (narrow QRS complex) or antidromic (wide QRS complex). *Orthodromic* AVNRT is much more common (90%–95% of cases) and has a narrow QRS complex because the cardiac impulse is conducted from the atrium through the normal AV node–His-Purkinje system. These impulses return from the ventricle to the atrium using the accessory pathway. Treatment of orthodromic AVNRT in conscious patients in stable condition should begin with vagal maneuvers such as carotid sinus massage or a Valsalva maneuver. If vagal maneuvers are unsuccessful, adenosine, verapamil, β-blockers, or amiodarone may be used as clinically appropriate.

In the less common *antidromic* form of AVNRT the cardiac impulse is conducted from the atrium to the ventricle through the accessory pathway and returns from the ventricles to the atria via the normal AV node. The wide QRS complex seen in antidromic AVNRT makes it difficult to distinguish this dysrhythmia from ventricular tachycardia. Treatment of antidromic AVNRT is intended to block conduction of the cardiac impulse along the accessory pathway. Drugs that slow AV nodal conduction (e.g., adenosine, calcium channel blockers, β-blockers, lidocaine, digoxin) may *increase* conduction along the accessory pathway and are *contraindicated*. Facilitation of conduction over the accessory pathway may produce a marked increase in ventricular rate.

Treatment of antidromic AVNRT in patients with stable vital signs includes IV administration of procainamide 10 mg/kg IV infused at a rate not to exceed 50 mg/min. Procainamide slows conduction of cardiac impulses along the accessory pathway and may slow the ventricular response and terminate the wide-complex tachydysrhythmia. Electrical cardioversion is indicated if the ventricular response cannot be controlled by drug therapy.

Atrial fibrillation and atrial flutter are uncommon in WPW syndrome but are potentially lethal because they can result in very rapid heart rates and deteriorate into ventricular fibrillation. The mechanism responsible is anterograde conduction from the atria to the ventricles *through the accessory pathway*. There is no mechanism along an accessory pathway to slow the conduction speed. The result is extremely rapid ventricular rates that often degenerate into ventricular fibrillation and death. Atrial fibrillation in the setting of WPW syndrome can be treated with IV procainamide. Verapamil and digoxin are *contraindicated* in this situation because they accelerate conduction through the accessory pathway. Electrical cardioversion is preferred in the presence of hemodynamic instability. Long-term management of tachydysrhythmias in patients with WPW syndrome usually involves radiofrequency catheter ablation of the accessory pathway. The procedure is curative in 95% of patients and has a low complication rate. Antidysrhythmic drugs may be used as adjuvant therapy.

The preexcitation changes of WPW on ECG occur in 0.1%–0.3% of the general population. However, not all these individuals develop PSVT. The presence of ECG changes does not mean that the patient will ever develop a dysrhythmia, but it suggests the risk of this. There is a bimodal age distribution in initial symptoms, with the first peak in early childhood, then a second in young adulthood. Some women experience their initial manifestation of WPW syndrome during pregnancy. Other patients may have the first manifestation of WPW syndrome during the perioperative period. The incidence of sudden cardiac death in patients with WPW syndrome is 0.15%–0.39% per patient-year, but it is very unusual for sudden death to be the initial manifestation of WPW syndrome. WPW is more common in patients with Ebstein malformation of the tricuspid valve, hypertrophic cardiomyopathy, and transposition of the great vessels. Paroxysmal palpitations with or without dizziness, syncope, dyspnea, or angina pectoris are common during the tachydysrhythmias associated with this syndrome.

Patients with known WPW syndrome coming for surgery should continue to receive their antidysrhythmic medications. The goal during management of anesthesia is to avoid any event (e.g., increased sympathetic nervous system activity due to pain, anxiety, or hypovolemia) or drug (digoxin, verapamil) that could enhance anterograde conduction of cardiac impulses through an accessory pathway. Appropriate antidysrhythmic drugs and equipment for electrical cardioversion-defibrillation must be immediately available.

Multifocal Atrial Tachycardia

Multifocal atrial tachycardia (MAT) is a form of SVT that demonstrates the presence of multiple ectopic atrial pacemakers.

The ECG shows P waves with three or more different morphologies, and the PR intervals vary. This rhythm is frequently confused with atrial fibrillation, but unlike AF, the rate is not excessively rapid, and each QRS is associated with a P wave. (Fig. 8.5). The atrial rhythm is usually between 100 and 180 bpm.

MAT is most commonly seen in patients experiencing an acute exacerbation of chronic lung disease. It can also be associated with methylxanthine (theophylline and caffeine) toxicity, CHF, sepsis, metabolic derangements, and electrolyte abnormalities. It usually responds to treatment of the underlying pulmonary decompensation with supplemental oxygen and bronchodilators. An improvement in arterial oxygenation decreases the activity of the ectopic foci that cause MAT.

Patients with MAT who must undergo urgent surgery benefit from optimization of their pulmonary function and arterial oxygenation prior to surgery. Intraoperative avoidance of medications or procedures that could worsen the pulmonary status and avoidance of hypoxemia are the main strategies to avoid worsening of MAT in susceptible patients. Pharmacologic treatment of MAT has limited success and is considered secondary to improvement in oxygenation.

Magnesium sulfate 2 g IV over 1 hour followed by 1–2 g IV per hour by infusion has shown some success in decreasing atrial ectopy and converting MAT to sinus rhythm. Verapamil 5–10 mg IV over 5–10 minutes slows the ventricular rate and will convert to sinus rhythm in some patients. Likewise, β-blockers such as esmolol or metoprolol can decrease the ventricular rate but at the risk of provoking bronchospasm in susceptible patients. Theophylline use can exacerbate this condition. Cardioversion has *no effect* on the multiple sites of ectopy that produce this dysrhythmia.

Atrial Fibrillation

AF is the most common sustained cardiac dysrhythmia in the general population. In 2005 there were about 3 million Americans with AF. This number is expected to nearly triple by 2050. The incidence of AF increases with age: it is present in 1% of individuals younger than 60 years and increases to 12% of patients aged 70–84 years. One-third of patients with AF are older than 80 years. For individuals of Northern European descent the lifetime risk for developing AF after age 40 is 26% for men and 23 % for women. African Americans tend to have more risk factors for developing AF but a lower incidence of occurrence. AF is the most common postoperative tachydysrhythmia and often occurs early in the postoperative period (first 2–4 days), especially in elderly patients following cardiothoracic surgery.

AF is a type of supraventricular dysrhythmia characterized on ECG by chaotic atrial activity with no discernible P waves and irregular R-R intervals (see Fig. 8.5). The resulting heart rate can be normal or rapid depending on the status of the conduction system and the use of drugs that affect AV conduction. AF may be identified on physical examination or ECG in a patient with no associated symptoms. However,

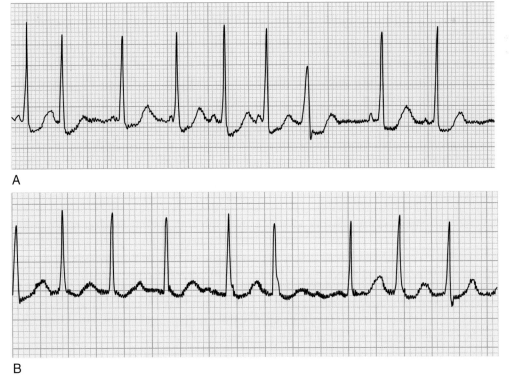

FIG. 8.5 Comparison of the ECG appearance of multifocal atrial tachycardia (A) and atrial fibrillation (B). Both rhythms are irregular. However, note several distinct P-wave morphologies and varying PR intervals with multifocal atrial tachycardia. There are no distinct P waves with atrial fibrillation.

most patients are symptomatic. The most common complaint is fatigue. Other common signs and symptoms are generalized weakness, palpitations, hypotension, syncope, angina pectoris, shortness of breath, orthopnea, and hypotension.

The most common underlying comorbid disease conditions associated with AF are systemic hypertension, ischemic heart disease, hyperlipidemia, heart failure, diabetes, anemia, arthritis, chronic kidney disease, and chronic obstructive lung disease. AF occurs with structural and/or electrophysiologic abnormalities that promote abnormal impulse generation or propagation. The causes of these abnormalities are diverse but include medical issues commonly encountered in the anesthetic patient, such as obesity, sleep apnea, hypertension, recreational drug use, hyperthyroidism, rheumatic heart disease (especially mitral valve disease), ischemic heart disease, chronic obstructive pulmonary disease, alcohol intake (holiday heart syndrome), pericarditis, pulmonary embolus, and atrial septal defect. In some instances, treating the underlying disorder eliminates the AF permanently.

Although AF is a common chronic medical problem, a large proportion of patients with new-onset AF experience spontaneous conversion to sinus rhythm within 24–48 hours. After conversion to sinus rhythm, β-blockers are often useful in preventing recurrent AF episodes and reduce symptoms should subsequent episodes occur.

If new-onset AF occurs before induction of anesthesia, surgery should be postponed if possible until the ventricular rate is controlled or conversion to sinus rhythm has been achieved. Intraoperative management of AF depends on the hemodynamic stability of the patient. If the AF is hemodynamically significant, the treatment is synchronized cardioversion at 100–200 J (biphasic).

Electrical cardioversion is the most effective method for converting AF to normal sinus rhythm and is indicated in patients with co-existing symptoms of heart failure, angina pectoris, or hemodynamic instability. If vital signs are stable, the primary goal should be rate control with a β-blocker or calcium channel blocker if there are no clinical contraindications. Digoxin can be useful to control ventricular rate but is not effective for conversion of AF to sinus rhythm. In the acute setting the usefulness of digoxin is limited because its peak therapeutic effects are delayed by several hours. Side effects associated with digitalis therapy are dose related and most commonly include AV block and ventricular ectopy.

The drugs of choice for rate control in patients with AF and a known or suspected accessory pathway and preexcitation are procainamide or amiodarone.

In the operating room or other acute settings, amiodarone is a good choice for chemical cardioversion and rate control. The efficacy of IV amiodarone in producing chemical cardioversion ranges from 34%–69% for a bolus dose of the drug and 55%–95% when the bolus is followed by a continuous drug infusion. Amiodarone also suppresses atrial ectopy and thus recurrent AF and improves the success rate of electrical cardioversion. It is the preferred drug for patients with significant heart disease, including ischemic heart disease, left ventricular hypertrophy, left ventricular dysfunction, and heart failure. Adverse effects of short-term amiodarone administration include bradycardia, hypotension, and phlebitis at the site of administration. Potential long-term side effects include visual disturbances, thyroid dysfunction, pulmonary toxicity, and skin discoloration.

Patients with chronic AF are usually treated with anticoagulants. The loss of coordinated atrial contraction promotes stasis of blood within the left atrium and can lead to formation of atrial thrombi. As a result, AF is associated with a fivefold increase in the risk of embolic stroke. AF is also associated with a threefold increase in the risk of heart failure and a twofold increase in the risk of dementia and death.

Long-term anticoagulation for AF is most often accomplished with warfarin, a vitamin K antagonist with a narrow therapeutic window that necessitates frequent monitoring and measurement of its clinical effect. Warfarin drug levels can be affected by numerous foods and medications. Newer drugs for long-term anticoagulation include dabigatran (Pradaxa), rivaroxaban (Xarelto), apixaban (Eliquis), and clopidogrel (Plavix). They inhibit other portions of the coagulation cascade. Their principal benefit is that they do not require monitoring of drug effect.

Patients coming for elective surgery who are taking anticoagulants typically have their anticoagulant stopped for 3–7 days before surgery, depending on the pharmacokinetics of the particular drug. The goal is normal coagulation on the day of surgery. Patients having urgent or emergent surgery present a dilemma. Warfarin's effects can be "reversed" by administration of vitamin K, fresh frozen plasma, and/or 4-factor prothrombin complex concentrates to facilitate production and replacement of the clotting factors suppressed by warfarin. Until recently there were no antidotes for reversal of the anticoagulation effects of the other anticoagulants such as dabigatran, rivaroxaban, apixaban, and clopidogrel. In 2015 the US Food and Drug Administration (FDA) approved a reversal agent for dabigatran called *Praxbind* (idarucizumab). Idarucizumab is a monoclonal antibody fragment that binds to dabigatran and reverses its clinical effects within minutes to a few hours. As such, it is very useful for emergency surgery or urgent procedures and in life-threatening bleeding due to dabigatran. Its effects appear to last for 12–24 hours. More studies and clinical experience will be needed to clarify its safety profile, with both one-time and repeat administration.

Regimens for prophylaxis against perioperative stroke are determined by risk stratification for stroke based on one of two major stratification systems that have weighted scores for patient comorbidities such as CHF, hypertension, age older than 75 years, diabetes mellitus, previous embolic event (stroke or transient ischemic attack), sex, and evidence of vascular disease.

Intravenous standard heparin or low-molecular-weight heparin are used most often for this perioperative prophylaxis. They can be administered as needed and then as a bridge until long-term anticoagulation can be safely reestablished.

Catheter ablation can be used in patients who cannot tolerate drug therapy for maintenance of sinus rhythm. If the patient is undergoing cardiac surgery for other indications, a surgical Maze procedure and left atrial appendage exclusion may be done to convert AF and eliminate a site of blood stasis site in the heart.

Atrial Flutter

Atrial flutter is characterized by an organized atrial rhythm with an atrial rate of 250–350 bpm with varying degrees of AV block. The rapid P waves create a sawtooth appearance on ECG and are called *flutter waves.* Flutter waves are particularly noticeable in leads II, III, aVF, and V_1. The flutter waves are not separated by an isoelectric baseline. The ventricular rate may be regular or irregular depending on the rate of conduction. Most commonly, patients have 2:1 AV conduction; an atrial rate of 300 bpm with 2:1 conduction, for example, results in a ventricular rate of 150 bpm. Characteristically the ventricular rate is about 150 bpm. Atrial flutter frequently occurs in association with other dysrhythmias such as AF. It occurs in approximately 30% of patients with AF and may be associated with more intense symptoms than AF because of the more rapid ventricular response. About 60% of patients experience atrial flutter in association with an acute exacerbation of a chronic condition such as pulmonary disease, acute MI, ethanol intoxication, thyrotoxicosis, or after cardiothoracic surgery. In many instances, treatment of the underlying disease process restores sinus rhythm.

Ventricular response rates as high as 180 bpm can occur in patients with normal AV node function. Extremely rapid ventricular responses in excess of 180 bpm can be seen in patients with accessory AV nodal bypass tracts. In this situation the QRS complex is often wide, and the ECG can resemble ventricular tachycardia or ventricular fibrillation.

If atrial flutter is hemodynamically significant, the treatment is cardioversion. Often less than 50 J (monophasic) is adequate to convert the rhythm to sinus. If the patient is hemodynamically stable, overdrive pacing using transesophageal or atrial electrodes may be helpful to convert atrial flutter to sinus rhythm. Patients with atrial flutter lasting longer than 48 hours should receive anticoagulant therapy.

Pharmacologic control of the ventricular response and conversion to sinus rhythm can be challenging in patients with atrial flutter. Ventricular rate control should be the initial goal of therapy. This is done to prevent deterioration in AV conduction from 2:1 to 1:1, which would represent a doubling of the heart rate. Such an increase in heart rate can cause severe hemodynamic instability. If there is 1:1 conduction with a ventricular rate of 300 bpm or faster, reentry is the most likely mechanism and procainamide administration should be considered. Drug therapy for ventricular rate control includes amiodarone, diltiazem, and verapamil. All these drugs are helpful in controlling the ventricular rate, but none of them is likely to convert atrial flutter to sinus rhythm.

If atrial flutter occurs before induction of anesthesia, surgery should be postponed if possible until control of the dysrhythmia has been achieved. Management of atrial flutter occurring during anesthesia or surgery depends on the hemodynamic stability of the patient. If the atrial flutter is hemodynamically significant, treatment requires cardioversion. Synchronized cardioversion starting at 50 J (monophasic) is indicated. Pharmacologic control of the ventricular response with IV amiodarone, diltiazem, or verapamil may be attempted if vital signs are stable. The choice of drug depends on the co-existing medical conditions of the patient.

VENTRICULAR DYSRHYTHMIAS

Ventricular Ectopy (Premature Ventricular Beats)

Premature ventricular beats (PVCs) can arise from single (unifocal) or multiple (multifocal) foci located below the AV node. Characteristic ECG findings include a premature and wide QRS complex, no preceding P wave, ST-segment and T-wave deflections opposite the QRS deflection, and a *compensatory pause* before the next sinus beat. PVCs can be benign and self-limiting or progressive and detrimental.

Ventricular ectopy can occur as short episodes with spontaneous termination or as a sustained pattern. Two or three PVCs—called a *couplet* or *triplet,* respectively—separated by one or more regular sinus beats is called *bigeminy* or *trigeminy.* The occurrence of more than three consecutive PVCs is considered ventricular tachycardia.

PVCs can be dangerous when they occur during the vulnerable period in the cardiac cycle during the middle third of the T wave. This clinical situation is known as the *R-on-T phenomenon.* This point in the T wave represents a relative refractory period during the cardiac action potential. Initiation of PVCs during this time may initiate repetitive beats that can deteriorate into sustained ventricular tachycardia or ventricular fibrillation.

The most common symptoms in patients experiencing ventricular ectopy are palpitations, near-syncope, and syncope. The volume of blood ejected during a PVC is smaller than that ejected during a sinus beat because of the lack of the atrial contribution to ventricular filling during the PVC. This can account for the presyncope and syncope that can occur with frequent PVCs. After a PVC there is a compensatory pause before the P wave of the next sinus beat. The stroke volume of the sinus beat following the compensatory pause is usually larger than normal. Ejection of that extra volume can cause the feeling of a prominent heart beat or palpitation in some patients.

The prognostic significance of ventricular ectopy depends on the presence and severity of co-existing structural heart disease. The incidence of PVCs in a healthy population ranges from 0.5% in those younger than 20 years to 2.2% in those older than 50. In the absence of structural heart disease, asymptomatic ventricular ectopy is benign with no demonstrable risk of sudden death. Benign ventricular premature beats occur at rest and disappear with exercise; however, an increased frequency of PVCs with exercise may be an indication of underlying heart disease.

The differential diagnosis of causes of PVCs includes acidosis, electrolyte imbalances (e.g., hypokalemia, hypomagnesemia), use of prodysrhythmic drugs, arterial hypoxemia, myocardial ischemia or infarction, valvular heart disease, cardiomyopathy, direct mechanical irritation from thoracic and/or cardiac surgery, intracardiac or intrathoracic catheters, drugs prolonging the QT interval, and digitalis toxicity. Excessive caffeine, alcohol, and cocaine use can also cause PVCs (Table 8.2).

During administration of an anesthetic, if a patient exhibits six or more PVCs per minute or repetitive or multifocal forms of ventricular ectopy, there is an increased risk of development of a life-threatening dysrhythmia. Immediate availability of a

defibrillator is a priority should the rhythm deteriorate. Other treatment includes elimination of as many causative factors as possible. Amiodarone, lidocaine, and other antidysrhythmics are indicated only if the PVCs progress to ventricular tachycardia or are frequent enough to cause hemodynamic instability. Many antidysrhythmic drugs have prodysrhythmic effects and/or prolong the QT interval and can increase the propensity for dysrhythmias. β-Blockers are the most successful drugs in suppressing ventricular ectopy and other ventricular dysrhythmias and reducing the risk of sudden cardiac death in patients with heart diseases, including heart failure.

Ventricular Tachycardia

Ventricular dysrhythmias occur in 70%–80% of persons older than age 60 and are often asymptomatic. Ventricular tachycardia (VT; also called *monomorphic ventricular tachycardia*) is present when 3 or more consecutive ventricular premature beats occur at a heart rate of more than 120 bpm (usually 150–200 bpm). VT can occur as a nonsustained paroxysmal rhythm or as a sustained rhythm. The rhythm is regular with wide QRS complexes and no discernible P waves (Fig. 8.6). A wide-complex SVT can be difficult to distinguish from VT, especially if there is aberrant conduction or if the patient has an RBBB or LBBB causing a widened QRS. A wide QRS tachycardia should be presumed to be VT if the diagnosis is unclear. DC cardioversion is recommended if at any point a patient with sustained monomorphic VT develops hemodynamic compromise.

In the perioperative environment, mechanical ventilation, drug therapy, insertion of central catheters, and other interventions can be iatrogenic causes of ventricular dysrhythmias.

TABLE 8.2	Conditions and Factors Associated With Development of Ventricular Premature Beats

Normal heart
Arterial hypoxemia
Myocardial ischemia
Myocardial infarction
Myocarditis
Sympathetic nervous system activation
Hypokalemia
Hypomagnesemia
Digitalis toxicity
Caffeine
Cocaine
Alcohol
Mechanical irritation (central venous or pulmonary artery catheter)

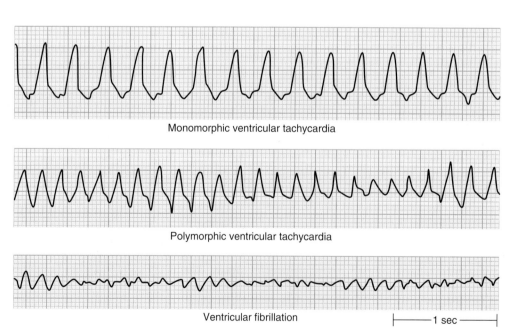

Monomorphic ventricular tachycardia

Polymorphic ventricular tachycardia

Ventricular fibrillation |————— 1 sec —————|

FIG. 8.6   Comparison of the ECG appearance of monomorphic ventricular tachycardia, polymorphic ventricular tachycardia (torsades de pointes), and ventricular fibrillation.

VT is common after an acute MI and in the presence of inflammatory or infectious diseases of the heart. It is also associated with digitalis toxicity. The occurrence of paroxysmal nonsustained VT during anesthesia should prompt an investigation into potential causes and correction of any reversible factors. Timely termination of VT is desirable even if it is well tolerated. IV procainamide is a first-line drug for patients with stable VT. Close monitoring of the blood pressure and cardiovascular status is necessary because this drug can cause hypotension.

Amiodarone may be used in patients refractory to procainamide or having recurrence after cardioversion, but it is not the first choice for chemical conversion of VT. Lidocaine is effective if the VT is related to myocardial ischemia. Transvenous catheter pacing termination of VT can be useful in patients with sustained VT refractory to cardioversion or recurrent on antidysrhythmic therapy. Calcium channel blockers should *never* be used to terminate a wide QRS complex tachycardia of unknown origin, especially in patients with a history of myocardial dysfunction.

At any point, episodic VT can progress to stable VT or deteriorate into unstable VT, pulseless VT, or ventricular fibrillation (VF). The occurrence of sustained VT with or without a pulse demands immediate action. Pulseless VT requires initiation of cardiopulmonary resuscitation (CPR) and immediate defibrillation using 360 J (monophasic).

Patients with symptomatic or unstable monomorphic or polymorphic VT should undergo cardioversion immediately. Pulseless VT of any kind requires defibrillation. Cardioversion can begin at an output of 100 J (monophasic) and increase in increments of 50–100 J as necessary. In addition to electrical therapy and drug treatment, endotracheal intubation and evaluation and correction of acid-base and electrolyte disturbances should be undertaken as clinically appropriate. If vital signs are stable but the VT is persistent or recurrent after cardioversion, administration of amiodarone 150 mg over 10 minutes is necessary. Dosing of amiodarone may be repeated as needed to a maximum total dose of 2.2 g in 24 hours. Alternative drugs include procainamide, sotalol, and lidocaine. Sotalol is effective in suppressing ventricular dysrhythmias but has significant prodysrhythmic effects and has not been shown to improve long-term survival.

Reversible factors contributing to cardiac arrest should be managed by advanced cardiac life support (ACLS), including treatment of hypoxia, electrolyte disturbances, mechanical factors, and volume depletion. Long-term treatment with a β-blocker or calcium channel blocker can suppress VT and prevent recurrence.

The prognosis for patients with VT depends on the presence or absence of structural heart disease. The risk of sudden death in patients with structurally normal hearts experiencing ventricular dysrhythmias is low. Catheter ablation of the causative ectopic pathway or implantation of a pacemaker/defibrillator are options for long-term treatment of drug-refractory VT. Implantable cardioverter-defibrillator therapy, compared with conventional antidysrhythmic therapy, has been associated with reductions in mortality ranging from 23%–55% depending on the study, and this is attributed to a reduction in sudden cardiac death from ventricular dysrhythmias. In certain circumstances, coronary revascularization may improve survival from malignant ventricular dysrhythmias, especially in patients with left main and proximal left anterior descending coronary artery disease.

Ventricular Fibrillation

VF is a rapid, grossly irregular ventricular rhythm with marked variability in QRS cycle length, morphology, and amplitude (see Fig. 8.6). It is incompatible with life because no stroke volume is generated by this rhythm.

A pulse or blood pressure *never* accompanies VF. VT often precedes the onset of VF. *Ventricular fibrillation is the most common cause of sudden cardiac death.* Most victims have underlying ischemic heart disease. Patients with acute coronary ischemia receiving β-blockers, angiotensin-converting enzyme inhibitors, or statins have VT and VF less often than those not receiving these drugs. Also, the incidence of VF occurring with acute MI has decreased due to increased β-blocker use and early revascularization. The gold standard for long-term treatment of recurrent episodic VT or VF is implantation of a permanent automatic cardioverter-defibrillator, with adjuvant drug therapy if needed as a second-line treatment.

VF during anesthesia is a critical event. CPR must be initiated immediately. Without defibrillation, cardiac output, coronary blood flow, and cerebral blood flow are extremely low even with ideally performed external cardiac compressions. Electrical defibrillation is the only effective method to convert VF to a viable rhythm. Defibrillation involves delivery of a high-energy electric current throughout the heart to depolarize all myocardial cells at once. Ideally a single intrinsic pacemaker focus will then restore myocardial synchrony. The single most important factor affecting survival in patients experiencing VF is time to defibrillation. Survival is best if defibrillation occurs within 3–5 minutes of cardiac arrest.

In any pulseless arrest, contributing factors must be sought and treated. The differential diagnosis includes hypoxia, hypovolemia, acidosis, hypokalemia, hyperkalemia, hypomagnesemia, hypoglycemia, hypothermia, drug or environmental toxins, cardiac tamponade, tension pneumothorax, coronary ischemia, pulmonary embolism, and hemorrhage.

When VF is refractory to electrical treatment, IV administration of epinephrine 1 mg or amiodarone 150–300 mg may improve the response to electrical defibrillation. Adjunctive therapy with amiodarone, lidocaine, or magnesium may be indicated. Standardized ACLS algorithms (Fig. 8.7) should be followed for electrical, pharmacologic, and adjunctive therapy.

Prolonged QT Syndromes

By definition a patient with long QT syndrome (LQTS) has a prolongation of the QTc exceeding 460 ms. There are two

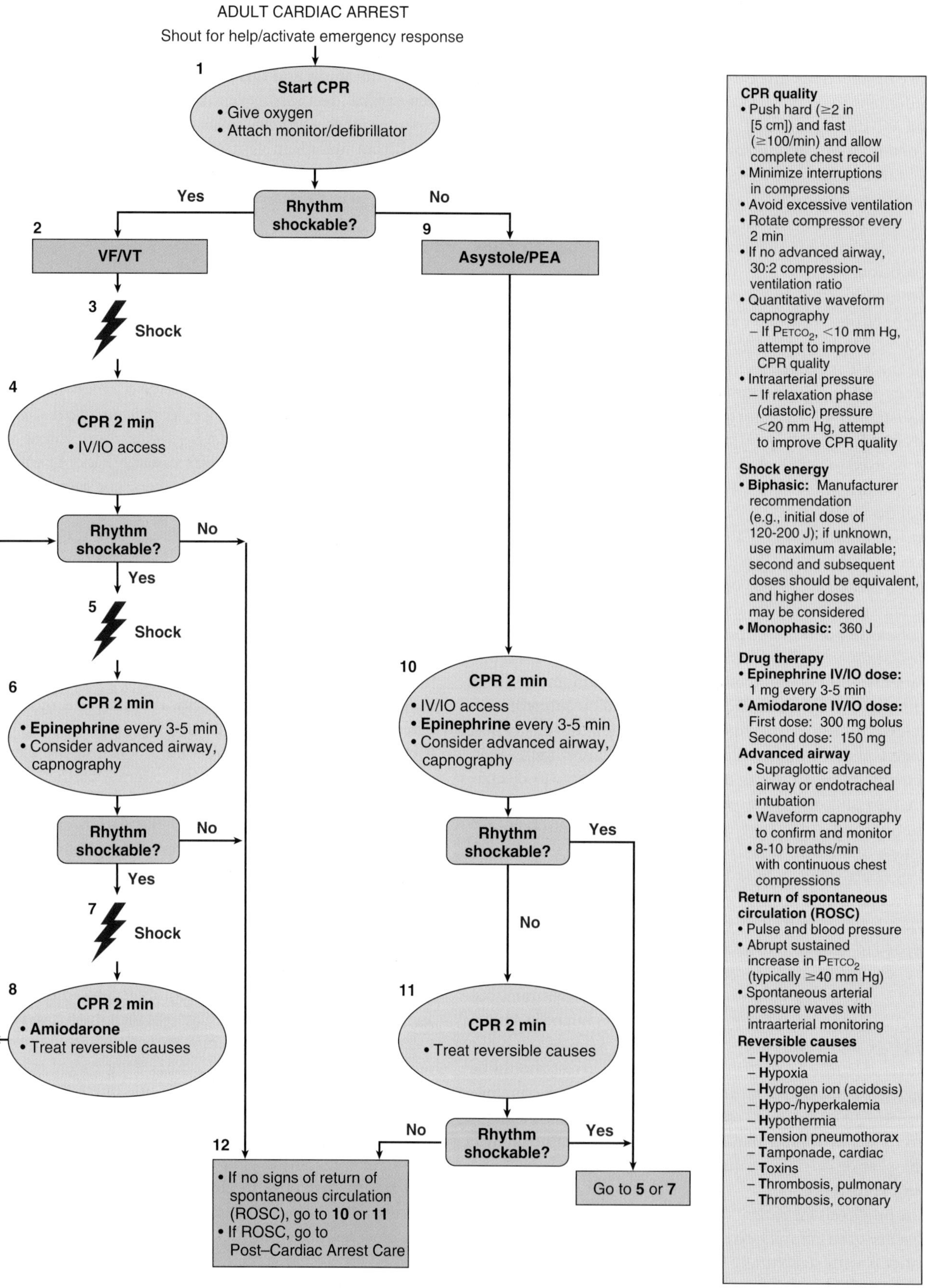

ADULT CARDIAC ARREST

Shout for help/activate emergency response

1
Start CPR
- Give oxygen
- Attach monitor/defibrillator

Rhythm shockable?

Yes → **2 VF/VT**

No → **9 Asystole/PEA**

3 ⚡ Shock

4
CPR 2 min
- IV/IO access

Rhythm shockable? — No →

Yes

5 ⚡ Shock

6
CPR 2 min
- **Epinephrine** every 3-5 min
- Consider advanced airway, capnography

Rhythm shockable? — No →

Yes

7 ⚡ Shock

8
CPR 2 min
- **Amiodarone**
- Treat reversible causes

10
CPR 2 min
- IV/IO access
- **Epinephrine** every 3-5 min
- Consider advanced airway, capnography

Rhythm shockable? — Yes →

No

11
CPR 2 min
- Treat reversible causes

Rhythm shockable? — No → / Yes →

12
- If no signs of return of spontaneous circulation (ROSC), go to **10** or **11**
- If ROSC, go to Post–Cardiac Arrest Care

Go to **5** or **7**

CPR quality
- Push hard (≥2 in [5 cm]) and fast (≥100/min) and allow complete chest recoil
- Minimize interruptions in compressions
- Avoid excessive ventilation
- Rotate compressor every 2 min
- If no advanced airway, 30:2 compression-ventilation ratio
- Quantitative waveform capnography
  – If P_{ETCO_2}, <10 mm Hg, attempt to improve CPR quality
- Intraarterial pressure
  – If relaxation phase (diastolic) pressure <20 mm Hg, attempt to improve CPR quality

Shock energy
- **Biphasic:** Manufacturer recommendation (e.g., initial dose of 120-200 J); if unknown, use maximum available; second and subsequent doses should be equivalent, and higher doses may be considered
- **Monophasic:** 360 J

Drug therapy
- **Epinephrine IV/IO dose:** 1 mg every 3-5 min
- **Amiodarone IV/IO dose:** First dose: 300 mg bolus Second dose: 150 mg

Advanced airway
- Supraglottic advanced airway or endotracheal intubation
- Waveform capnography to confirm and monitor
- 8-10 breaths/min with continuous chest compressions

Return of spontaneous circulation (ROSC)
- Pulse and blood pressure
- Abrupt sustained increase in P_{ETCO_2} (typically ≥40 mm Hg)
- Spontaneous arterial pressure waves with intraarterial monitoring

Reversible causes
- **H**ypovolemia
- **H**ypoxia
- **H**ydrogen ion (acidosis)
- **H**ypo-/hyperkalemia
- **H**ypothermia
- **T**ension pneumothorax
- **T**amponade, cardiac
- **T**oxins
- **T**hrombosis, pulmonary
- **T**hrombosis, coronary

FIG. 8.7 Algorithm for treatment of adult cardiac arrest. *CPR,* Cardiopulmonary resuscitation; *ET,* endotracheal; *IV/IO,* intravenous/intraosseous; *PEA,* pulseless electrical activity; PETCO₂, extrapolated end-tidal carbon dioxide pressure; *VF,* ventricular fibrillation; *VT,* ventricular tachycardia. (American Heart Association. Web-based Integrated Guidelines for Cardiopulmonary Resuscitation and Emergency Cardiovascular Care—Part 7: Adult Advanced Cardiovascular Life Support. ECCguidelines.heart.org [Copyright 2015 American Heart Association, Inc.].)

types of LQTS: congenital and acquired. Iatrogenic acquired LQTS is far more common than the inherited forms of LQTS. Acquired LQTS may be caused by many prescription medications such as antibiotics, antidysrhythmics, antidepressants, antiemetics, and many anesthetic drugs. LQTS can be associated with hypokalemia, hypomagnesemia, severe malnutrition, hypertrophic cardiomyopathy, and intracranial catastrophes such as subarachnoid hemorrhage.

A preoperative ECG to rule out LQTS is useful in a patient with a history of unexplained syncope or a family history of sudden death. The choice of anesthetic drugs deserves special attention in the case of LQTS, since many common anesthetic drugs cause some degree of QTc prolongation. Isoflurane and sevoflurane have both been shown to prolong the QTc in otherwise healthy children and adults. However, there is insufficient information to favor one volatile anesthetic over another at this time. Ondansetron and other antiemetic drugs also increase the QT interval. Events known to prolong the QT interval should be avoided, such as abrupt increases in sympathetic stimulation associated with preoperative anxiety and noxious stimulation intraoperatively, acute hypokalemia due to iatrogenic hyperventilation, and administration of drugs known to prolong the QTc.

Preoperative treatment of LQTS includes correction of electrolyte abnormalities, particularly those of magnesium or potassium. Any drugs associated with QT prolongation should be discontinued. Cardiac pacing is a treatment option in LQTS, because TdP is often preceded by bradycardia. Programming a pacemaker to pace at a higher backup rate than usual can prevent the bradycardia that precedes TdP and abort the dysrhythmia. Pacing is usually employed in combination with β-blocker therapy. Cardiac events and mortality in congenital LQTS patients have been reduced from 50% to less than 5% over 10 years with β-blocker therapy. Consideration should be given to establishing β-blockade before induction in patients believed to be at particular risk. A defibrillator should be available because the likelihood of perioperative VF is increased.

Typically, women have longer QT intervals than men. This difference is more pronounced at slower heart rates. The incidence of congenital and acquired prolonged QT syndromes is higher in women. The strongest predictor of the risk of syncope or sudden death in patients with congenital prolonged QT syndrome is a QTc exceeding 500 ms. The prolongation of repolarization in LQTS results in a dispersion of refractory periods throughout the myocardium. This abnormality in repolarization allows afterdepolarizations to trigger PVCs.

TdP, also called *polymorphic ventricular tachycardia,* is a distinct form of reentrant VT initiated by a PVC in the setting of abnormal ventricular repolarization (prolongation of the QT interval). TdP is characterized by a "twisting of the peaks" or rotation around the ECG baseline. In other words, there is a constantly changing cycle length, axis, and morphology of the QRS complexes around the isoelectric baseline during TdP (see Fig. 8.6). This dysrhythmia may be repetitive, episodic, or sustained and may degenerate into VF. The incidence of TdP is higher in women.

Implantable cardioverter-defibrillators (ICDs) with pacing capability have emerged as lifesaving therapy for patients with recurrent symptoms and recalcitrant TdP despite ventricular suppression therapy with β-blockers. Pacing these patients is helpful because an episode of bradycardia often precedes TdP. In addition, left cervicothoracic sympathetic ganglionectomy may assist in reducing dysrhythmogenic syncope in patients with congenital LQTS who cannot take β-blockers or have recurrent syncope despite ICD and β-blocker therapy.

There are several genetic syndromes that manifest a long QT interval. The two most common are the Romano-Ward and Timothy syndromes. These are inherited in an autosomal dominant fashion and usually present as syncope in late childhood. Manifestations can occur as early as the first year of life or as late as the sixth decade. A rarer autosomal recessive form of prolonged QT syndrome called *Jervell and Lange-Nielsen syndrome* is associated with congenital deafness. Syncope is the hallmark symptom of the inherited forms of prolonged QT syndrome. These syncopal events are commonly associated with stress, emotion, exercise, or other situations that lead to increased sympathetic stimulation.

In pregnancy, women with unstable VT or VF should be cardioverted or defibrillated. β_1-Selective blockers, amiodarone, or both in combination with an ICD may be considered. Pregnant women with LQTS with symptoms should be on β-blockers unless contraindicated. VT in the absence of structural heart disease may be due to elevated catecholamine levels. β-Blockers are particularly effective in this circumstance. If VT presents in the last 6 weeks of pregnancy or in the postpartum period, the possibility of postpartum cardiomyopathy should be considered.

MECHANISMS OF BRADYDYSRHYTHMIAS

Bradycardia is defined as a heart rate less than 60 bpm (Table 8.3). The SA node normally fires between 60 and 100 times per minute and therefore overdrives other potential

TABLE 8.3	Perioperative Causes of Sinus Bradycardia

Vagal stimulation
    Oculocardiac reflex: traction on eye muscles
    Celiac plexus stimulation: traction on the mesentery
    Laryngoscopy
    Abdominal insufflation
    Nausea
    Pain
    Electroconvulsive therapy
Drugs
    β-Blockers
    Calcium channel blockers
    Opioids (fentanyl, sufentanil)
    Succinylcholine
Hypothermia
Hypothyroidism
Athletic heart syndrome
Sinoatrial nodal disease or ischemia

pacemakers in the heart. However, if the SA node does not fire, other slower pacemaker cells may take over primary intrinsic pacemaker function. There is normally a pause in electrical activity before a secondary slower pacemaker begins to fire. Each group of potential pacemaker cells has an intrinsic rate. Cells near the AV node, so-called junctional pacemakers, fire at 40–60 bpm. Ventricular cells below the AV node can act as ectopic pacemakers but fire at a very slow rate in the range of 30–45 bpm.

Sinus Bradycardia

The ECG during sinus bradycardia demonstrates a regular rhythm with a normal-appearing P wave before each QRS complex and a heart rate less than 60 bpm. Trained athletes often exhibit resting sinus bradycardia, as do many normal individuals during sleep. Sinus bradycardia is due to decreased sympathetic stimulation or increased parasympathetic stimulation, as in deep relaxation, sleep, the Valsalva maneuver, carotid sinus massage, gut traction, and vomiting. Noncardiac causes of sinus bradycardia include hyperkalemia, increased intracranial pressure, hypothyroidism, and hypothermia.

Sinus bradycardia may be asymptomatic or symptomatic. In asymptomatic patients, no treatment is required. However, these patients should be monitored for worsening bradycardia or hemodynamic deterioration. In mildly symptomatic patients, any potential contributing factors such as excess vagal tone or drugs should be eliminated. In severely symptomatic patients (i.e., those with chest pain or syncope), immediate transcutaneous or transvenous pacing is indicated. Atropine 0.5 mg IV every 3–5 minutes (to a maximum of 3 mg) may be given to increase heart rate but should not delay initiation of pacing. It should be noted that small doses of atropine (<0.5 mg IV) can cause a further *slowing* of the heart rate. In the event that cardiac pacing is delayed or pacing capabilities are limited, an epinephrine or dopamine infusion may be titrated to response while cardiac pacing is awaited. If atropine is ineffective, glucagon may be useful if the bradycardia is due to β-blocker or calcium channel blocker overdose. Glucagon stimulates glucagon-specific receptors on the myocardium that increase cyclic adenosine monophosphate (cAMP) levels and increase myocardial contractility, heart rate, and AV conduction. Suggested dosing of glucagon is 50–70 μg/kg (3–5 mg in a 70-kg patient) every 3–5 minutes until clinical response is achieved or a total dose of 10 mg is reached. To maintain clinical effect a continuous infusion at 2–10 mg/h should be maintained.

Bradycardia during neuraxial blockade can occur in patients of any age and any American Society of Anesthesiologists (ASA) physical status class, whether or not they are sedated. The incidence of profound bradycardia and cardiac arrest during neuraxial anesthesia is approximately 1.5 per 10,000 cases. By contrast, cardiac arrest during general anesthesia occurs at a rate of 5.5 per 10,000 cases.

Bradycardia or asystole may develop suddenly (within seconds or minutes) in a patient with a previously normal or even increased heart rate, or the heart rate slowing may be progressive. Bradycardia can occur at any time during neuraxial blockade but most often occurs approximately an hour after anesthetic administration. The risk of bradycardia and asystole may persist into the postoperative period even after the sensory and motor blockade has diminished. Oxygen saturation is usually normal before the onset of bradycardia. Approximately half of patients who experience cardiac arrest during neuraxial anesthesia complain of shortness of breath, nausea, restlessness, light-headedness, or tingling of the fingers and manifest deterioration in mental status before the arrest.

The exact mechanism responsible for bradycardia and asystole during spinal and epidural anesthesia is not known. One proposed mechanism is termed the *Bezold-Jarisch response*. This is a paradoxical reflex-induced bradycardia resulting from decreased venous return and activation of vagal reflex arcs mediated by baroreceptors and stretch receptors. Another possible mechanism is the unopposed parasympathetic nervous system activity that results from the anesthetic-induced sympathectomy. Blockade of cardiac accelerator fibers originating from thoracic sympathetic ganglia (T1–T4) may alter the balance of autonomic nervous system input to the heart and lead to relatively unopposed parasympathetic influences on the SA node and AV node.

Bradydysrhythmias associated with spinal or epidural anesthesia should be treated aggressively. Bradycardia can occur despite prophylactic therapy with atropine and/or IV fluids. Recalcitrant bradycardia necessitates transcutaneous or transvenous pacing. Secondary factors such as hypovolemia, opioid administration, sedation, hypercarbia, concurrent medical illnesses, and long-term use of medications that slow the heart rate can contribute to the development of bradycardia. In the clinical setting of severe bradycardia, preparation should be made for management of asystole, which is treated with CPR. Pharmacologic management should follow ACLS protocols and include treatment with atropine, epinephrine, and/or dopamine as appropriate (Fig. 8.8).

Junctional Rhythm

Junctional or nodal rhythm is due to the activity of a cardiac pacemaker in the tissues surrounding the AV node. Junctional pacemakers usually have an intrinsic rate of 40–60 bpm. The impulse initiated by a junctional pacemaker travels to the ventricles along the normal conduction pathway but can also be conducted retrograde into the atria. The site of the junctional pacemaker determines whether the P wave precedes the QRS complex (with a shortened PR interval), follows the QRS complex, or is buried within the QRS complex and is not visible. The diagnosis of junctional rhythm may be an incidental finding on ECG. Junctional rhythm can be suspected if on physical examination the jugular venous pulsation shows *cannon "a" waves*.

If the junctional rhythm has an accelerated rate, it is called a *junctional tachycardia* or *accelerated nodal (junctional) rhythm*. Junctional tachycardia is a narrow-complex tachycardia at a

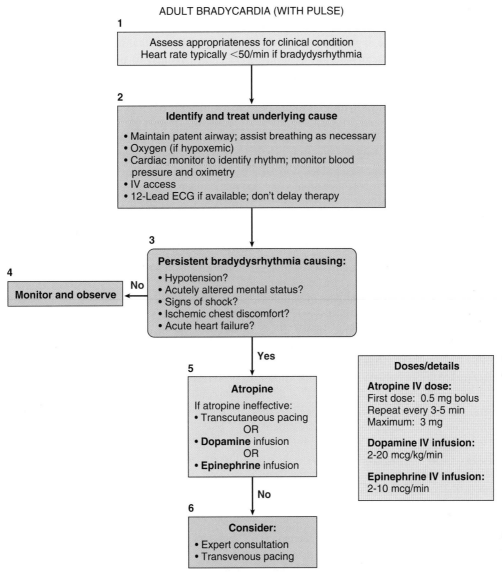

FIG. 8.8 Algorithm for treatment of adult bradycardia (with pulse). *ECG,* Electrocardiogram; *IV,* intravenous. (American Heart Association. Web-based Integrated Guidelines for Cardiopulmonary Resuscitation and Emergency Cardiovascular Care—Part 7: Adult Advanced Cardiovascular Life Support. ECCguidelines.heart.org [Copyright 2015 American Heart Association, Inc.].)

rate usually less than 120 bpm. Junctional rhythms can cause AV dyssynchrony, loss of atrial kick, and in some circumstances rapid ventricular rates. This can result in symptoms such as fatigue, generalized weakness, angina pectoris, impaired cardiac output, CHF, pulmonary edema, and hypotension.

Junctional rhythm can occur in association with many different disorders. It is often an escape rhythm because of depressed sinus node function, SA node block, or delayed conduction in the AV node. Junctional tachycardia can result from increased automaticity of junctional tissue in the setting of digitalis toxicity or cardiac ischemia. Junctional rhythm that occurs in association with myocarditis, myocardial ischemia, or digitalis toxicity should be managed by treating the underlying disorder. Junctional rhythms are not uncommon during general anesthesia using halogenated vapor anesthetics and in

this setting require no treatment. Even in the setting of acute MI, junctional rhythms are usually considered benign and require no treatment. However, in certain patients the loss of AV synchrony during a junctional rhythm will result in myocardial ischemia, heart failure, or hypotension. Atropine at a dose of 0.5 mg IV (repeatable every 3-5 minutes up to a total dose of 3.0 mg) can be used to accelerate the heart rate if a slow junctional rhythm becomes hemodynamically significant.

TREATMENT OF CARDIAC DYSRHYTHMIAS

Antidysrhythmic Drugs

Antidysrhythmic drugs are administered when correction of identifiable precipitating events is insufficient to suppress dysrhythmias. The majority of antidysrhythmic drugs work by one of three mechanisms: (1) suppressing automaticity in pacemaker cells by decreasing the slope of phase 4 depolarization, (2) prolonging the effective refractory period to eliminate reentry circuits, or (3) facilitating impulse conduction along normal conduction pathways to prevent conduction over a reentrant pathway. These antidysrhythmic modes of action can be seen on ECG as an increased PR interval or a prolonged QRS duration.

Prior to initiating antidysrhythmic drug therapy or inserting a cardiac pacemaker, physiologic acid-base values, normal serum electrolyte concentrations, and stable autonomic nervous system activity should be established to maximize the likelihood of reestablishing normal sinus rhythm.

Adenosine

Adenosine is a nucleoside and the drug of choice for pharmacologic termination of AVNRT. Sixty percent of patients respond at a dose of 6 mg, and an additional 32% of patients respond at a dose of 12 mg. Adenosine has an extremely short half-life (≈10 seconds) owing to rapid active transport of the drug into red blood cells and endothelial cells, where it is metabolized. To be effective, adenosine should be injected rapidly and flushed quickly through the IV tubing with saline.

Several drugs influence the clinical effectiveness of adenosine. Caffeine and theophylline antagonize the actions of adenosine. On the other hand, dipyridamole pretreatment increases the potency of adenosine. Carbamazepine also potentiates the action of adenosine. Patients with a heart transplant require only one-third to one-fifth the usual dose of adenosine because the transplanted heart is denervated. Administration of adenosine is contraindicated in patients with sick sinus syndrome and second- or third-degree heart block unless the patient has a functioning cardiac pacemaker. Common side effects of adenosine in the awake patient include facial flushing, dyspnea, and chest pressure. Generally these effects are transient, lasting less than 60 seconds. Less common side effects include nausea, light-headedness, headache, sweating, palpitations, hypotension, and blurred vision.

Atropine

Atropine sulfate is a vagolytic drug that is a competitive antagonist at muscarinic cholinergic receptor sites. It is used to increase heart rate and blood pressure. Potential adverse side effects of atropine administration include tachycardia, sedation (especially in the elderly), urinary retention, and increased intraocular pressure in patients with closed-angle glaucoma.

Atropine is recommended in the treatment of symptomatic bradycardia as a temporizing measure while awaiting initiation of transcutaneous or transvenous pacing. The recommended dose is 0.5 mg IV every 3–5 minutes as needed to a maximum total dose of 3 mg. Doses of less than 0.5 mg in adults can worsen bradycardia. Heart rate effects appear within seconds of administration and last 15–30 minutes. Atropine is not effective in patients who have undergone cardiac transplantation.

Amiodarone

Amiodarone is an antidysrhythmic structurally similar to thyroxine and procainamide. It acts on sodium, potassium, and calcium channels to produce α- and β-blocking effects that result in prolongation of the refractory period in myocardial cells. Amiodarone is useful in controlling ventricular rate in patients with AF. It is also indicated for treatment of VF and pulseless VT unresponsive to defibrillation, CPR, and vasopressors. In this situation, amiodarone improves the likelihood of successful defibrillation.

Amiodarone is metabolized in the liver and slows the metabolism and increases the blood levels of other drugs metabolized by the liver, such as warfarin, digoxin, diltiazem, quinidine, procainamide, disopyramide, and propafenone. The dose recommended for cardiac arrest unresponsive to CPR, defibrillation, and vasopressor therapy is an initial dose of 300 mg IV. It can be followed by a second dose of 150 mg IV.

β-Adrenergic Blockers

β-Blockers counteract the effects of circulating catecholamines and decrease heart rate and blood pressure. These cardioprotective effects are particularly important in patients with acute coronary syndromes. β-Blockers are indicated in patients with preserved left ventricular function who require ventricular rate control in AF, atrial flutter, and narrow-complex tachycardias originating at or above the AV node.

Side effects of β-blockade include bradycardia, AV conduction delays, and hypotension. Contraindications to β-blocker therapy include second- or third-degree heart block, hypotension, severe CHF, and reactive airway disease. β-Blockers should not be used in the treatment of AF or atrial flutter associated with WPW syndrome, since they may decrease conduction through the AV node and speed conduction through the accessory bypass tract, resulting in an increased ventricular response.

Calcium Channel Blockers

Calcium channel blockers (e.g., verapamil, diltiazem) inhibit the influx of extracellular calcium across myocardial and vascular smooth muscle cell membranes. They inhibit vascular smooth muscle contraction and cause vasodilation in coronary and other peripheral vascular beds. Calcium channel blockers are contraindicated in patients with an accessory bypass tract, such as those with WPW syndrome, since they can accelerate conduction through the accessory tract and thereby increase the ventricular rate to dangerously high levels. Calcium channel blockers have negative inotropic properties and should be avoided in patients with left ventricular dysfunction. If they are administered to patients already receiving β-blockers, additive effects can result in iatrogenic second- or third-degree heart block.

Verapamil is indicated for the treatment of narrow-complex tachycardia (SVT) in patients in whom vagal maneuvers and adenosine therapy have failed. It is also indicated for ventricular rate control with atrial flutter or fibrillation. Verapamil slows conduction and increases the refractoriness of the AV node and is useful in controlling ventricular rate in patients with atrial tachydysrhythmias and in terminating reentrant dysrhythmias. Diltiazem has a similar mechanism of action and similar clinical indications as verapamil. However, diltiazem has less negative inotropic effect and causes less peripheral vasodilation than verapamil. The degree of AV node inhibition is similar for both drugs.

Verapamil can prolong the PR interval and is *not* effective in treating tachycardias originating below the AV node. The initial dose of verapamil is typically 2.5–5 mg IV over 2 minutes. This can be repeated if needed to a maximum total dose of 0.15 mg/kg. Hemodynamic effects peak in 5 minutes and persist for 20–30 minutes. The recommended dose for diltiazem is 0.25 mg/kg IV over 2 minutes. This can be repeated if needed. Successful dysrhythmia treatment can be followed by a maintenance infusion at 5–15 mg/h.

Digoxin

Digoxin is a cardiac glycoside used for the treatment of CHF and AF. Digoxin inhibits the myocardial cell membrane Na^+,K^+-ATPase pump. Useful pharmacologic effects include positive inotropy, slowing of conduction through the AV node, and lengthening of the refractory period of the AV node.

The inotropic effects of digoxin are due to an increase in intracellular calcium that allows for greater activation of contractile proteins. In addition to having positive inotropic effects, digoxin also increases phase 4 depolarization and shortens the action potential. This decreases conduction velocity through the AV node and prolongs the AV nodal refractory period.

Digoxin is effective in controlling the ventricular rate in AF, although it does not convert AF to sinus rhythm. Onset of therapeutic effect after IV administration of digoxin occurs in 5–30 minutes, with the peak effect at 2–6 hours after injection. Digoxin has a narrow therapeutic index, especially in the presence of hypokalemia.

High serum digoxin levels can cause a variety of symptoms and signs, including life-threatening dysrhythmias. Coexisting disease states that can contribute to digitalis toxicity include hypothyroidism, hypokalemia, and renal dysfunction. A digoxin-specific antibody is available for treatment of significant digitalis toxicity.

Dopamine

Dopamine is a precursor to the catecholamines norepinephrine and epinephrine and is present in nerve terminals and the adrenal medulla. It has direct dose-related effects on α, β, and dopaminergic receptors. At low doses (3–5 μg/kg/min), dopamine increases renal, mesenteric, coronary, and cerebral blood flow through the activation of dopaminergic receptors. At moderate doses (5–7 μg/kg/min), β-effects predominate, producing an increase in heart rate, contractility, and cardiac output with a decrease in systemic vascular resistance. At high doses (>10 μg/kg/min), α-receptor stimulation causes peripheral vasoconstriction and a reduction in renal blood flow.

Dopamine is a second-line drug for the treatment of symptomatic bradycardia unresponsive to atropine. In this clinical scenario it should be considered a temporizing measure while awaiting initiation of transcutaneous or transvenous pacing. The dose is 2–20 μg/kg/min titrated to the heart rate response. Caution must be exercised if infusion is through a peripheral IV line, because skin necrosis can result from extravasation at the injection site.

Epinephrine

Epinephrine is a catecholamine produced by the adrenal medulla. Epinephrine is a potent mast cell stabilizer and bronchodilator and is useful in the treatment of severe bronchospasm and anaphylactic reactions. It is also a potent inotrope, chronotrope, and vasopressor. Increased contractility and heart rate occur at all dosages, but the effect on systemic vascular resistance is dose-dependent. At low dosages (10–100 μg/min) the systemic vascular resistance may decrease or stay the same, but at high dosages (>100 μg/min) the systemic vascular resistance increases.

Epinephrine is indicated in the treatment of cardiac arrest because of its α-adrenergic vasoconstrictor properties. The α effects of epinephrine can be beneficial during CPR by increasing coronary and cerebral perfusion. There is a higher likelihood of return to spontaneous circulation in patients treated with epinephrine during cardiac arrest from VF, pulseless electrical activity, or asystole. The suggested dose is 1 mg IV every 3–5 minutes during adult cardiac arrest. Occasionally, larger doses may be needed to treat cardiac arrest resulting from β-blocker or calcium channel blocker overdose. Epinephrine is a second-line drug in the treatment of symptomatic bradycardia unresponsive to atropine. The recommended dosage is an infusion of 2–10 μg/min titrated to heart rate response. Like atropine, it should be considered a temporizing measure while awaiting initiation of transcutaneous or transvenous pacing.

Epinephrine should be given through central venous catheters if at all possible, because extravasation from a peripheral IV line can cause tissue necrosis. Epinephrine can also be administered by the intratracheal route. The dose for intratracheal use is 2–2.5 mg diluted in 5 to 10 mL of sterile water (which provides better drug absorption than saline). Other drugs that may be given intratracheally include lidocaine, atropine, naloxone, and vasopressin.

Isoproterenol

Isoproterenol is a potent bronchodilator and sympathomimetic structurally similar to epinephrine. Functionally it has potent $β_1$- and $β_2$-agonist actions but lacks any α-adrenergic properties. The actions of isoproterenol are mediated intracellularly by cAMP. Stimulation of $β_1$ receptors produces positive inotropic and chronotropic effects. Isoproterenol increases myocardial excitability and automaticity, which potentially favors dysrhythmias.

Isoproterenol administration causes the systolic blood pressure to increase and the diastolic blood pressure to decrease. This is attributed to drug-induced peripheral vasodilation. This vasodilatory effect does increase coronary blood flow, but the increased oxygen demand resulting from a higher heart rate outweighs the potential benefit of any increase in myocardial blood flow. Isoproterenol is a second-line drug in the treatment of symptomatic bradycardia unresponsive to atropine. The recommended dosage is 2–10 μg/min by continuous infusion titrated to heart rate effect. Because of its direct action on β receptors, isoproterenol is useful to treat symptomatic bradycardia in heart transplant recipients. An initial IV dosage of 1 μg/min is titrated slowly upward until the desired effect is achieved.

Lidocaine

Lidocaine is an amide local anesthetic commonly employed in regional anesthetic nerve blockade. However, the same sodium channel blocking effects that make it a good local anesthetic also make it a useful antidysrhythmic drug when administered intravenously. Lidocaine may be used in the treatment of cardiac arrest associated with VF or pulseless VT *if amiodarone is not available*. The recommended dose is 1–1.5 mg/kg IV. If VF or pulseless VT persists, half this dose can be repeated at 5- to 10-minute intervals to a maximum total dose of 3 mg/kg. Therapeutic doses of lidocaine have minimal negative inotropic effects. When administered in combination with other antidysrhythmic drugs, lidocaine can cause some myocardial depression or sinus node dysfunction.

During lidocaine therapy, monitoring of mental status is desirable because the first signs of lidocaine toxicity are usually central nervous system symptoms such as tinnitus, drowsiness, dysarthria, or confusion. At higher blood levels, signs of central nervous system depression such as sedation and respiratory depression predominate and may be accompanied by seizures. Lidocaine undergoes extensive first-pass hepatic metabolism, so clinical conditions that result in decreased hepatic blood flow (e.g., general anesthesia, CHF, liver disease, advanced age) can result in higher-than-normal blood levels. Certain drugs such as cimetidine can also cause an increase in the plasma concentration of lidocaine.

Lidocaine is rapidly redistributed out of the plasma and myocardium, so multiple loading doses may be needed to achieve therapeutic blood levels. Clinical duration of action is 15–30 minutes after a loading dose. To sustain therapeutic effect, lidocaine must be administered by continuous infusion. The recommended infusion dose is 1–4 mg/min.

Magnesium

Magnesium functions in the body as a cofactor in the control of sodium and potassium transport. With regard to its antidysrhythmic properties, there are a few observational studies supporting the use of magnesium in the termination of TdP ventricular tachycardia associated with QT prolongation. However, there is *no evidence* that magnesium is effective in treating VT associated with a normal QT interval. In VF or pulseless VT associated with TdP, magnesium can be given in a dose of 1–2 g over 5 minutes. If a pulse is present, the same dose can be administered but more slowly.

Procainamide

Procainamide is an antidysrhythmic drug that slows conduction, decreases automaticity, and increases the refractoriness of myocardial cells. It can be used in patients with preserved ventricular function to treat the following conditions: VT with a pulse, atrial flutter or fibrillation, AF in WPW syndrome, and SVT resistant to adenosine and vagal maneuvers.

Procainamide can be administered at a rate of 50 mg/min IV until the dysrhythmia is suppressed, significant hypotension occurs, or the duration of the QRS complex is prolonged by 50%. The duration of action after a bolus dose is 2–4 hours. Procainamide must be used with caution in patients with QT prolongation and in combination with other drugs that prolong the QT interval. To maintain therapeutic effect, procainamide can be given as a maintenance infusion at a rate of 1–4 mg/min. Dosage should be reduced in renal failure.

Sotalol

Sotalol is a nonselective β-blocker. It prolongs the duration of the action potential and increases the refractoriness of cardiac cells. Sotalol can be used in the treatment of VT and AF or atrial flutter in patients with WPW syndrome. The dose is 1.5 mg/kg IV over 5 minutes. Potential side effects include bradycardia, hypotension, and QT prolongation.

Vasopressin

Vasopressin is a potent peripheral vasoconstrictor that works independently of α- or β-adrenergic mechanisms. It is an endogenous antidiuretic hormone that in high concentrations produces direct peripheral vasoconstriction by activating smooth muscle vasopressin (V_1) receptors. Prior ACLS guidelines listed epinephrine and vasopressin as recommended interchangeably to treat cardiac arrest. However, the most recent ACLS guidelines no longer support the use of vasopressin in cardiac arrest. However, vasopressin therapy may be useful in maintaining systemic vascular resistance in patients who have severe sepsis or acidosis or have undergone cardiopulmonary bypass when other drug treatments have failed.

Twenty-Percent Lipid Emulsion

Infusion of 20% lipid emulsion is used in the clinical scenario of bupivacaine or other local anesthetic overdose. The first reported case of its use in an adult human to successfully treat a bupivacaine-related cardiac arrest was in 2006. Since then, with accumulation of more data and experience, "lipid rescue" had become a widely accepted treatment. The suggested initial dose is 1 mL/kg over 1 minute while chest compressions and related ACLS maneuvers are continued. The dose can be repeated every 3–5 minutes to a maximum of 3 mL/kg. After conversion to sinus rhythm, a maintenance infusion of 0.25 mL/kg/min is suggested until hemodynamic recovery occurs.

Transcutaneous Pacing

Transcutaneous pacing is an effective temporizing measure to treat bradydysrhythmias until a transvenous pacemaker can be placed or a more permanent mode of cardiac pacing can be implemented. If transcutaneous pacing is needed, pacer/defibrillator electrodes are placed on the chest and back, and electrical impulses are delivered through the chest wall to pace the heart. The device is impractical for long-term use because of the high current required, the skin irritation caused by the delivery pads, and significant patient discomfort during pacing.

Electrical Cardioversion

Electrical cardioversion is the delivery of an electrical discharge synchronized to the R wave of the ECG. The purpose of cardioversion is to recoordinate the electrical pathways of the heart by delivering a single dominant burst of electricity on the R wave of the ECG. The electrical discharge or "shock" is transmitted through two chest electrodes configured as hand-held paddles or adhesive pads on the chest in the anterior and apical positions or in the anterior and posterior positions. The shock is coordinated with the R wave on the ECG so that the stimulus is not delivered during the relative refractory period during the T wave. This is to avoid the R-on-T phenomenon, which could produce VT or VF.

Synchronized cardioversion is used to treat acute unstable SVTs such as PSVT, atrial flutter, and AF and to convert chronic stable rate-controlled atrial flutter or fibrillation to sinus rhythm. Cardioversion can also be used to treat monomorphic VT *with a pulse.* Cardioversion is only useful if there is an R wave on ECG to synchronize the shock. Without an organized rhythm and therefore no R wave, defibrillation (unsynchronized shock) is necessary to depolarize the entire myocardium at once in the hope that a normal pacemaker will take over and restore a functional rhythm.

Digitalis-induced dysrhythmias are refractory to cardioversion, and attempts at cardioversion in this situation could trigger more serious ventricular dysrhythmias. Digitalis-induced dysrhythmias should be treated by correction of acid-base status and electrolyte abnormalities, and administration of digitalis-binding antibody if needed.

Defibrillation

In contrast to cardioversion, *electrical defibrillation* is used to correct dysrhythmias when it is not possible to synchronize the electric current to the ECG because there is no R wave (no defined QRS complex). The position of the paddles or pads is the same as for cardioversion. Defibrillation-cardioversion electrodes *should not* be placed directly over pacemakers or ICD pulse generators. Delivery of a high current near a pacemaker or ICD can cause the device to malfunction and can block and/or divert the current path and result in suboptimal current delivery to the myocardium. All permanently implanted cardiac devices should be evaluated after defibrillation or cardioversion to ensure proper function.

Modern defibrillators are classified according to the type of waveform delivered and may be monophasic or biphasic. The first-generation defibrillators were monophasic. Most modern defibrillators are biphasic devices. Neither type of defibrillator has been shown to be more successful in terminating pulseless rhythms or improving survival. A current dose of 360 J is indicated for transthoracic defibrillation using a monophasic defibrillator.

Biphasic defibrillators deliver lower currents (120–200 J) than monophasic devices. The optimal energy dose delivered by a biphasic defibrillator is not standardized; the manufacturer of each device has suggestions specific to its equipment. In the absence of a generally recommended dose, 200 J should be used. The electric current delivered encounters some increase in impedance from air spaces within the lung tissue in the current path. Therefore the defibrillator current is ideally delivered when the lungs are deflated (i.e., during exhalation). The single most important factor determining survival after cardiac arrest due to VF is the time between arrest and the first defibrillation attempt. In witnessed cardiac arrest due to VF, patients who undergo defibrillation within the first 3 minutes have a survival rate of 74%.

Radiofrequency Catheter Ablation

Radiofrequency catheter ablation refers to a procedure in which an intracardiac electrode catheter is inserted percutaneously under local anesthesia through a large vein (femoral, subclavian, internal jugular, or cephalic). This electrode is then used to produce small, well-demarcated areas of thermal injury that destroy the myocardial tissue responsible for initiation or maintenance of dysrhythmias. Cardiac dysrhythmias amenable to radiofrequency catheter ablation include reentrant supraventricular dysrhythmias and some ventricular dysrhythmias. Radiofrequency catheter ablation is usually considered after pharmacologic therapy has failed or has not been well tolerated. The procedure is typically performed under conscious sedation with routine monitoring.

CARDIAC IMPLANTED ELECTRONIC DEVICES

Cardiac implanted electronic devices (CIEDs) are implanted cardiac rhythm management devices. CIEDs include permanent pacemakers, implantable cardioverter-defibrillators (ICDs), and cardiac resynchronization devices. Although not specified in the name, all ICDs include pacing and shock therapies for the management of bradydysrhythmias and tachydysrhythmias.

All implanted cardiac devices are designed to detect and respond to low-amplitude electrical signals. Extraneous signals produced by external electric or magnetic fields can influence the function of CIEDs. These signals are known as *electromagnetic interference* (EMI). There are no known CIED concerns involving exposure to plain x-rays, ultrasonography, fluoroscopy, mammography, or electroconvulsive therapy (ECT). However, there are reports of EMI associated with electrocautery, radiofrequency ablation, magnetic resonance imaging (MRI), radiation therapy, and lithotripsy.

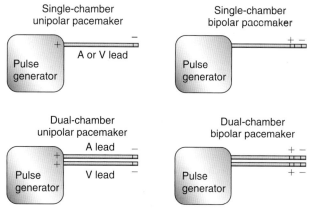

FIG. 8.9   Unipolar and bipolar lead systems. *A,* Atrial; *V,* ventricular. (From Stone ME, Apinis A. Current perioperative management of the patient with a cardiac rhythm management device. *Semin Cardiothorac Vasc Anesth.* 2009;13:32.)

EMI can be any strong external electrical or magnetic force in close proximity to a CIED. EMI signals enter device circuits primarily through the leads. Unipolar systems are more prone to EMI because there is a larger separation between the positive and negative poles. In a bipolar lead system there are two separate electrodes (positive and negative) in the same chamber in very close proximity to each other, so the distance the current travels to complete the circuit is very small, and hence there is very little chance that extraneous signals will intrude into or affect the lead circuit (Fig. 8.9).

Other factors influencing the susceptibility of a device to EMI include field strength, patient body mass, and the proximity and orientation of the implanted electronic device to the EMI field. Potential effects of EMI depend on the pacing mode and the lead(s) involved but range from cessation of pacing to inappropriate triggering of pacemaker activity. Improved shielding of pacemakers and use of mostly bipolar lead systems has eliminated many problems related to EMI.

Permanently Implanted Cardiac Pacemakers

Bradycardia associated with symptoms such as syncope, dizziness, and chest pain; inability to increase the heart rate adequately during exercise; or a heart rate of less than 40 bpm in the absence of physical conditioning or sleep is considered abnormal. The prevalence of sinus node dysfunction may be as high as 1 in 600 patients older than 65 years. Many patients with sick sinus syndrome are asymptomatic; others experience syncope or palpitations. Episodes of SVT may be interspersed with periods of bradycardia. This accounts for another common name for sinus node dysfunction, *tachycardia-bradycardia (tachy-brady) syndrome.* In patients with ischemic heart disease, periods of bradycardia may contribute to the development of CHF, whereas periods of tachycardia can contribute to the development of hypertension and angina pectoris. The rate of progression to second- or third-degree AV block in patients with sick sinus syndrome is approximately 1%–5% per year. Sick sinus syndrome with *symptomatic bradycardia* is the most common reason for insertion of a permanent cardiac pacemaker.

Permanently implanted cardiac pacemakers are CIEDs composed of a pulse generator, one or more sensing and pacing electrodes (usually located in the right atrium and right ventricle), and a battery power source. Electrical impulses originating in the pulse generator are transmitted through specialized leads to excite endocardial cells and produce a propagating wave of depolarization in the myocardium. The pulse generator is powered by a small lithium-iodide battery. The lithium-iodide batteries used in pulse generators can last up to 10 years, but battery depletion requires surgical replacement of the entire pulse generator. The pulse generator for endocardial leads is usually implanted in a subcutaneous pocket below the clavicle.

Endocardial leads can be unipolar or bipolar. In a unipolar pacing system there is one electrode that is an active lead. Current flows from the negative pole (active lead) to stimulate the heart and then returns to the positive pole (the casing of the pulse generator). The current returns to the positive pole by traveling through myocardium to complete the circuit.

Pacing Modes

A five-letter generic code is used to describe the various characteristics of cardiac pacemakers. The first letter denotes the cardiac chamber(s) being paced (A, atrium; V, ventricle; D, dual-chamber). The second letter denotes the cardiac chamber(s) in which electrical activity is being sensed or detected (O, none; A, atrium; V, ventricle; D, dual). The third letter indicates the response to sensed signals (O, none; I, inhibition; T, triggering; D, dual—inhibition and triggering). The fourth letter, R, denotes activation of rate response features, and the fifth position denotes the chamber(s) in which multisite pacing is delivered. The most common pacing modes are AAI, VVI, and DDD.

Asynchronous Pacing

Asynchronous pacing is the simplest form of pacing. It can be AOO, VOO, or DOO. In this mode, the lead(s) fire at a fixed rate regardless of the patient's underlying rhythm. This pacing mode can be used safely in patients with no intrinsic ventricular activity, because there is no risk of the R-on-T phenomenon. Asynchronous pacing could compete with a patient's intrinsic rhythm, and the continuous pacing activity decreases battery life and necessitates more frequent battery/pulse generator replacement.

Single-Chamber Pacing

The choice of pacing mode depends on the primary indication for the artificial pacemaker. Single-chamber pacemakers can be atrial or ventricular. If the patient has SA node disease and no evidence of disease in the AV node or bundle of His, an atrial pacemaker (AAI) can be placed. Use of atrial pacing modes requires a functioning AV node, and then AAI pacing can maintain AV synchrony. However, it has been estimated that approximately 8% of patients with SA node dysfunction will progress to AV node dysfunction within 3 years.

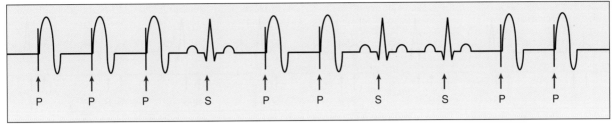

FIG. 8.10 ECG evidence of pacemaker function with a VVI (ventricular pacing, ventricular sensing, inhibition) pacemaker. *P,* Paced beat; *S,* sensed beat. (From Allen M. Pacemakers and implantable cardioverter defibrillators. *Anaesthesia.* 2006;61:885.)

Individuals experiencing episodes of symptomatic bradycardia caused by SA node or AV node disease may benefit from placement of a single-chamber ventricular (VVI) pacemaker. This mode of pacing senses the native R wave, and if it is present, pacemaker discharge is inhibited (Fig. 8.10). It is often used in patients with complete heart block with chronic atrial flutter or fibrillation and in patients with long ventricular pauses. A factor to consider in the patient with a single-chamber ventricular pacemaker is the potential for pacemaker syndrome.

Pacemaker syndrome is a constellation of symptoms caused by the loss of AV synchrony. Symptoms include syncope, weakness, lethargy, cough, orthopnea, paroxysmal nocturnal dyspnea, hypotension, and pulmonary edema. DDD pacing can be used to alleviate symptoms of pacemaker syndrome by restoring AV synchrony.

Dual-Chamber Pacing

Cardiac pacing is the only long-term treatment for symptomatic bradycardia, regardless of cause. Disease of the AV node or His bundle, or ongoing drug treatment to slow AV nodal conduction, requires a dual-chamber (DDD or DDI) system. Disorders such as neurogenic syncope (resulting from carotid sinus hypersensitivity), vasovagal syncope, and hypertrophic cardiomyopathy can also be successfully treated with a dual-chamber pacemaker.

Dual-chamber pacing is also known as *physiologic pacing* because it maintains AV synchrony. This improves cardiac output by maintaining the contribution of atrial systole to ventricular filling. AV synchrony also maintains appropriate valve closure timing, which reduces the risk of significant mitral and/or tricuspid insufficiency. Several studies suggest that patients receiving dual-chamber pacing have a decreased risk of AF and heart failure.

DDD Pacing. Dual-chamber pacemakers have two leads, one placed in the right atrium and one located in the right ventricle. DDD pacing is based on electrical feedback from the leads in the atrium and ventricle. If a native atrial signal is sensed, the atrial pacemaker output is inhibited, and if no intrinsic atrial signal is sensed, the pacemaker output is triggered. Likewise, if intrinsic ventricular activity is sensed at the end of a programmable AV interval, the intrinsic ventricular activity inhibits pacemaker output. If intrinsic ventricular activity is not sensed, the pacemaker triggers a spike (Fig. 8.11).

The DDD pacing mode permits the pacemaker to respond to increases in sinus node discharge rate, such as occurs during exercise.

Programming the dual-chamber leads to have an adjustable AV interval provides an important benefit in maintaining AV synchrony over a wide range of heart rates. Loss of AV synchrony has many deleterious effects, including reducing cardiac output by 20%–30% or more, increasing atrial pressure resulting from contraction of the atria against closed mitral and tricuspid valves, and activation of baroreceptors that may induce reflex peripheral vasodilation.

DDI Pacing. In the DDI pacing mode, there is sensing in both the atrium and ventricle, but the only response to a sensed event is inhibition (inhibited pacing of the atrium and ventricle). DDI pacing is useful when there are frequent atrial tachydysrhythmias that might be inappropriately tracked by a DDD pacemaker and result in rapid ventricular rates.

Rate-Adaptive Pacemakers

Rate-adaptive pacing is considered for patients who do not have an appropriate heart rate response to exercise (*chronotropic incompetence*). This syndrome can be caused by drug treatment with negative chronotropic drugs such as β-blockers or calcium channel blockers or by pathologic processes such as sick sinus syndrome.

Normally, AV synchrony contributes more to cardiac output at rest and at low levels of exercise, whereas rate adaptation (i.e., a higher heart rate) is more important at higher levels of exercise. Sensors within rate-adaptive pacemakers detect changes in movement (using a piezoelectric crystal) or minute ventilation (by transthoracic impedance) as physical or physiologic signs of exercise. In response the device makes rate adjustments to mimic the response of a normal sinus node.

Anesthesia for Cardiac Pacemaker Insertion

Most pacemakers are inserted under conscious sedation in the cardiac catheterization laboratory or under monitored anesthesia care in the operating room. Routine anesthetic monitoring is employed. A functioning cardiac pacemaker should be in place or transcutaneous cardiac pacing available before administration of anesthetic drugs. Drugs such as atropine and isoproterenol should be available should a decrease in heart rate compromise hemodynamics before the new pacemaker is functional.

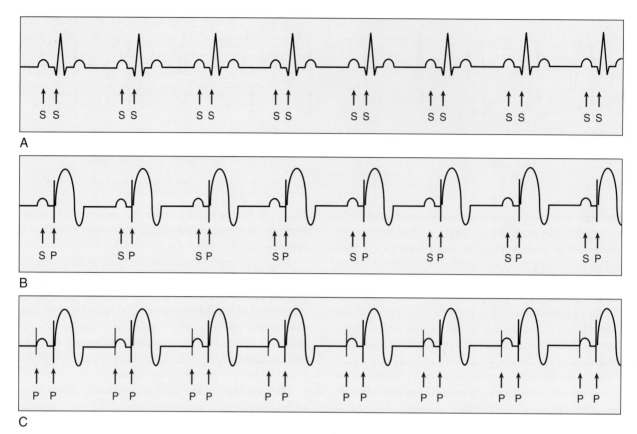

FIG. 8.11 ECG evidence of pacemaker function with a DDD (dual pacing, dual sensing, inhibition and triggering) pacemaker. A, Patient has intrinsic atrial and ventricular activity that is sensed by the pacemaker. B, Patient has intrinsic activity that is not conducted to the ventricle, so the pacemaker senses the atrial activity and paces the ventricle. C, Patient has no atrial or ventricular activity sensed by the pacemaker, so the pacemaker paces both the atrium and the ventricle. *P,* Paced beat; *S,* sensed beat. (From Allen M. Pacemakers and implantable cardioverter defibrillators. *Anaesthesia.* 2006;61:886.)

The incidence of complications related to pacemaker insertion is approximately 5%. An artificial cardiac pacemaker can be inserted intravenously using endocardial leads or via a subcostal incision or median sternotomy (after cardiac surgery) using epicardial or myocardial leads. Early complications are often associated with the venous access and/or surgical access necessary to place the leads. Perioperative complications include pneumothorax, hemothorax, and air embolism. Pneumothoraces are often small and asymptomatic. However, tension pneumothorax should always be considered if hypotension or pulseless electrical activity develops during or immediately after pacemaker placement. Hemothorax can result from trauma to the great vessels or other vascular structures. Arterial cannulation must be immediately recognized and treated with manual compression or arterial repair. Arterial damage can be minimized by placing a small guidewire under fluoroscopic guidance before placing the much larger introducer sheath. Variable amounts of air can be introduced into the low-pressure venous system during the procedure. Small amounts of air are generally well tolerated, but larger amounts can result in oxygen desaturation, hypotension, and cardiac arrest.

Permanently Implanted Cardioverter-Defibrillators

The ICD system consists of a pulse generator and leads for dysrhythmia detection and current delivery. In addition to internal defibrillation, an ICD can deliver antitachycardia or antibradycardia pacing and synchronized cardioversion. Detailed diagnostic data concerning intracardiac electrograms and event markers are stored in the memory of the device and can be retrieved for analysis. The pulse generator is a small computer powered by a lithium battery that is sealed within a titanium case. The transvenous leads consist of pacing and sensing electrodes and one or two defibrillation coils. The defibrillation circuit is completed by the titanium case of the pulse generator, which acts as a defibrillation electrode. The pulse generator is usually implanted into a subcutaneous pocket. The position of the pulse generator is important because the position affects the defibrillation wave front. The left pectoral region is the ideal location for the pulse generator. Right-sided implantation can result in a significantly higher defibrillation threshold. ICDs employ electrical defibrillation as the sole method for treatment of VF.

The ICD uses a specialized lead in the right ventricle that senses ventricular depolarization. It amplifies, filters, and rectifies the signal and then compares it with the programmed sensing thresholds and the R-R interval algorithms. If the device detects VF, the capacitor charges, a secondary algorithm is fulfilled by signal analysis to confirm the rhythm, and then the shock is delivered. This secondary confirmatory process prevents inappropriate shocks in response to self-terminating events or spurious signals. The process takes approximately 10 to 15 seconds from dysrhythmia detection to shock delivery. During this time the patient may experience presyncope or syncope.

A defibrillator coding system exists similar to the one used for pacemakers. The first letter is the chamber shocked (O, none; A, atrium; V, ventricle; D, dual). The second letter indicates the antitachycardia pacing chamber (O, none; A, atrium; V, ventricle; D, dual). The third position indicates the tachycardia detection mechanism (E, electrogram; H, hemodynamic). The fourth position denotes the antibradycardia pacing chamber (O, none; A, atrium; V, ventricle; D, dual).

Implantable ICDs were approved by the FDA in 1985. Currently, there are over 1.5 million Americans living with a pacemaker and over 500,000 living with an ICD. The indications for implantation of an ICD have changed dramatically over the past few years. An increase in ICD implantation occurred after clinical trials showed a survival benefit with ICD placement compared to antidysrhythmic drug therapy in survivors of cardiac arrest *not* caused by transient or reversible factors such as acute MI, use of prodysrhythmic drugs, or electrolyte disturbances.

Anesthesia for Insertion of Implantable Cardioverter-Defibrillators

Preparation of a patient for ICD placement is the same as that for pacemaker insertion. Some of these procedures are done under general anesthesia because of the increased risks associated with repeated defibrillation during threshold testing. The nature and severity of the patient's co-existing medical conditions dictate the extent of monitoring and the necessary clinical preparations.

Cardiac Resynchronization Devices

Cardiac resynchronization therapy (CRT) using biatrial or biventricular pacing is being employed in heart failure patients with electromechanical asynchrony and intraventricular conduction block. As CHF progresses, ventricular electrical dyssynchrony can result in mechanical dyssynchrony. As a result, left ventricular contraction becomes increasingly inefficient and cardiac output decreases. This can be further worsened by a prolongation of AV conduction, which leads to AV dyssynchrony and a decrease in the atrial contribution to left ventricular filling.

Cardiac resynchronization therapy uses three pacing leads: right atrial, right ventricular, and a coronary sinus lead (or an additional atrial or ventricular lead depending on the sites of

dysfunction). By adjusting the timing of each lead, AV synchrony is optimized. Cardiac resynchronization therapy is now a mainstay of treatment in patients who have left ventricular dysfunction (ejection fraction ≤ 35%), QRS prolongation (≥120 ms), and moderate to severe heart failure symptoms (New York Heart Association [NYHA] functional class III or IV) while receiving optimal medical therapy. Cardiac resynchronization therapy with or without a defibrillator component has been shown to reduce hospitalizations and all-cause mortality in these patients.

SURGERY IN PATIENTS WITH CARDIAC IMPLANTABLE ELECTRONIC DEVICES

The presence of any type of CIED—whether an artificial cardiac pacemaker or ICD for any indication; whether pacing, cardioversion, defibrillation, or resynchronization—in a patient scheduled for surgery unrelated to the device introduces special considerations for preoperative evaluation and subsequent management of anesthesia to ensure patient safety and preservation of proper device function. These CIED recommendations apply to all forms of anesthetic care, from conscious sedation and monitored anesthesia care to regional and general anesthesia; there are no clear data regarding the effect of anesthetic technique on CIED function.

Potential adverse patient outcomes associated with perioperative CIED-related issues include hypotension, tachydysrhythmias or bradydysrhythmias, myocardial damage, and myocardial ischemia or infarction. In addition, adverse outcomes related to the functionality of the device are also important. The CIED device may be affected by perioperative EMI, resulting in damage to the pulse generator or leads (circuitry), damage to the tissue around the device (burns, thermal changes affecting impedance), failure of the device to pace or defibrillate, inappropriate pacing or defibrillation, and inadvertent electrical reset to backup pacing modes. Other undesirable outcomes from the interaction of CIEDs and EMI during medical procedures include delay or cancellation of surgery, readmission to a healthcare facility for management of device malfunction, extended hospital stay, and increased patient and hospital costs.

Preoperative Evaluation

A patient with a preexisting CIED coming for surgery has at least one of three underlying cardiac problems: sustained or intermittent bradydysrhythmia, tachydysrhythmia, and/or heart failure. Regardless of the indication for the device, any patient with a CIED requiring anesthetic care must undergo a detailed systematic preoperative evaluation. This preoperative evaluation should include determination of the type of device present, identification of the clinical indication for the device, appraisal of the patient's degree of dependence on the device, and assessment of device function.

Strong evidence indicating that a patient is CIED dependent includes a history of bradycardia symptoms, a history of

AV node ablation, and an ECG showing a majority of paced beats. Also, pacemaker dependence is indicated by a lack of ventricular activity during CIED interrogation when the pacemaker function is programmed to VVI at the lowest programmable rate. A preoperative history of presyncope or syncope in a patient with a pacemaker could reflect pacemaker dysfunction.

The best way to determine CIED function preoperatively is CIED interrogation by a qualified consultant. However, in the event this is not possible, clinical evidence such as pacing spikes present on the ECG that successfully create paced beats may suffice. The ECG is not a diagnostic aid if the intrinsic heart rate is greater than the preset pacemaker rate. In such cases, proper function of a ventricular synchronous or sequential cardiac pacemaker is best confirmed by electronic evaluation. Beyond the routine indications for antibradycardia pacing or antitachycardia defibrillation, many pacemaker-defibrillators are implanted for resynchronization therapy to treat heart failure. This has made management decisions increasingly complex, so early involvement of a qualified consultant is desirable. Ideally, perioperative assessment and planning for the patient with a CIED should be coordinated with a cardiologist and the pacemaker representative for that specific device. All major CIED manufacturers have developed proprietary systems to allow patients to have their devices interrogated remotely, and many use wireless cellular technology to extend the bidirectional telemetry links to the patient's location.

There are several major areas of concern that must be addressed regarding the CIED to ensure safety during the administration of anesthesia. Is EMI likely to occur during the surgery? Does the CIED need to be reprogrammed to asynchronous mode? Is there a need to disable any special algorithms such as rate adaptive functions or to suspend antitachycardia functions? Are temporary pacing equipment and a defibrillator immediately available? Can bipolar cautery or a Harmonic scalpel be used in place of monopolar cautery?

The most common CIED-related problem encountered in the perioperative period is interference with device function resulting from EMI. Improved shielding of cardiac pacemakers has reduced the problems associated with EMI from electrocautery, but the use of monopolar electrocautery remains the principal intraoperative concern in patients with CIEDs. The care team involved in the procedure needs to be aware of these issues and plan accordingly.

Use of "coagulation" settings in monopolar electrocautery causes more EMI problems than use of "cutting" settings. The cautery tool and return pad should be positioned so the current pathway does not pass near the CIED pulse generator or leads. It is beneficial to keep the electrocautery current as low as possible and to apply electrocautery in short bursts, especially if current is being applied in close proximity to the pulse generator. It is recommended to avoid using cautery in the area of the pulse generator and leads if at all possible. The cautery device generating the EMI field need not actually touch the patient to adversely affect the CIED. Use of bipolar electrocautery or the ultrasonic Harmonic scalpel is associated with lower rates of EMI interference on the pulse generator and leads. Even with the utmost caution, problems can arise. There is at least one case report of pacemaker failure in a procedure using bipolar cautery.

The current return pad (grounding pad) of the electrocautery system should be placed so that the current path does not cross the chest or CIED system. The grounding electrode should be as far as possible from the pulse generator to minimize detection of the cautery current by the pulse generator.

Recommendations for patients with ICDs who undergo a procedure with a high risk of EMI include suspending the antitachycardia function—that is, turning off the defibrillator—and electronically adjusting the pacing modes as appropriate in pacemaker-dependent individuals. This can be accomplished by applying a magnet over certain devices. In others it may require reprogramming. The routine application of a magnet over a CIED is discouraged. Application of a magnet to a cardioverter-defibrillator often results in asynchronous pacing at a predetermined rate without rate responsiveness. The magnet-adjusted rate varies by manufacturer and can be affected by remaining battery life. The default magnet rate may be excessive for some patients. Some ICDs have no magnet response; others can be permanently disabled by magnet exposure. By whatever means necessary, the antitachycardia function of the CIED should be suspended and the bradycardia functions adjusted by programming.

Management of Anesthesia

The choice of drugs for anesthesia is not altered by the presence of a properly functioning CIED, nor is there any evidence that anesthetic drugs alter the stimulation threshold of CIEDs (Table 8.4). However, sequelae of anesthetic management such as hyperventilation, acid-base disturbances, electrolyte abnormalities, significant volume loads, blood transfusion, myocardial ischemia, and a high blood

TABLE 8.4	Factors That Can Alter the Depolarization Threshold of Cardiac Pacemakers
Factors Increasing the Threshold	**Factors Decreasing the Threshold**
Hyperkalemia	Hypokalemia
Acidosis or alkalosis	Increased catecholamine levels
Antidysrhythmic medication (e.g., quinidine, procainamide, lidocaine, propafenone)	Sympathomimetic drugs
Hypoxia	Anticholinergics
Hypoglycemia	Glucocorticoids
Local anesthetics (lidocaine)	Stress or anxiety
Myocardial ischemia	Hyperthyroidism
Myocardial infarction (scar tissue)	Hypermetabolic states
Acute inflammation around lead tip during first month after implantation	
Hypothermia	

concentration of local anesthetic can alter capture thresholds and lead impedance. Conceivably, succinylcholine could increase the stimulation threshold because of the associated acute increase in serum potassium concentration. In addition, succinylcholine could inhibit a normally functioning cardiac pacemaker by causing contraction of skeletal muscle groups (myopotentials) that the pulse generator could interpret as intrinsic R waves. Clinical experience suggests that succinylcholine is usually a safe drug for use in patients with cardiac pacemakers and that if myopotential inhibition does occur, it is generally transient.

Monitoring of the patient with a CIED should always follow the ASA standards and should include continuous ECG monitoring and continuous monitoring of a peripheral pulse. This can be done with a pulse oximeter, manual palpation of a pulse, auscultation of heart sounds, or intraarterial catheterization. *Verification of the presence of a pulse* is necessary to confirm continued cardiac activity in the event of disruption of the ECG signal by EMI. Temporary pacing and defibrillation equipment should be immediately available before during and after procedures in CIED patients.

No special laboratory testing or radiographs are needed for CIED patients undergoing surgery unless otherwise clinically indicated. At times a chest radiograph can be useful to evaluate the location and external condition of pacemaker electrodes. Most current CIEDs have an x-ray code that can be used to identify the manufacturer of the device. If the patient is known to have a biventricular pacemaker, a chest radiograph to confirm the position of the coronary sinus lead is helpful when insertion of a central line or pulmonary artery catheter is planned. There have been reports of coronary sinus and endocardial lead dislodgement in association with central venous catheterization. The danger of lead dislodgment is minimal a month or more after lead implantation.

MRI scanning of patients with CIEDs is controversial and is generally regarded as contraindicated. However, 50%–75% of patients with cardiac devices will likely need to undergo MRI at some point in their lifetimes, so this is becoming an important concern. There is insufficient evidence at present to standardize management of the patient with a CIED needing MRI scanning. If MRI must be performed, care should be coordinated among the ordering physician, radiologist, and pacemaker specialist or cardiologist.

Management of EMI associated with radiofrequency ablation includes keeping the radiofrequency current path, which runs from the electrode tip to the current return pad, as far away from the pulse generator as possible. Some suggest keeping the ablation electrode at least 5 cm away from the pacer leads.

Recommendations for patients undergoing lithotripsy include keeping the focus of the lithotripsy beam away from the pulse generator. If the lithotripsy triggers on the R wave, it may be necessary to disable atrial pacing before the procedure.

There is insufficient evidence to standardize care for CIED patients needing radiation therapy. It is preferable to keep the device out of the radiation field. Most manufacturers recommend verification of appropriate pulse generator function at the completion of radiation therapy.

No clinical studies have reported EMI or permanent CIED malfunction in association with electroconvulsive therapy, but care should be coordinated with a cardiologist. The device should be interrogated and the antitachycardia functions suspended. Because electroconvulsive therapy can be associated with considerable swings in blood pressure and heart rate, a backup external defibrillator and temporary pacing capability should be immediately available. In pacemaker-dependent patients, programming to asynchronous mode is recommended, since the myopotentials produced by the seizure may inhibit pacemaker activity.

If emergency defibrillation is necessary in a patient with a CIED (permanent cardiac pacemaker or ICD that is turned off), an effort should be made to keep the defibrillation current away from the pulse generator and lead system. The recommended position of the electrode pads is the anterior-posterior position. An acute increase in pacing threshold and loss of capture by the CIED may follow external defibrillation. If this occurs, transcutaneous cardiac pacing or temporary transvenous pacing may be required.

It has been suggested that before performing defibrillation or cardioversion in a patient with an ICD in a magnet-disabled treatment mode, all sources of EMI be eliminated and the magnet be removed to reactivate the antitachycardia capabilities of the device. The patient can then be observed for appropriate CIED function. The primary goal is care of the patient, with care of the CIED being secondary, but in most circumstances these two goals are not mutually exclusive.

Postoperative management of the patient with a CIED consists of interrogating the device and restoring appropriate baseline settings, including antitachycardia therapy in patients with ICDs. This should be done as soon as possible after the procedure, either in the postanesthesia care unit or the intensive care unit. All major CIED manufacturers have developed proprietary systems to allow remote interrogation of devices. The information from the device is accessible to clinicians via the internet. Information available to them includes battery voltage, charge time, pacing and sensing thresholds, percent pacing, pacing and shock impedance, and stored dysrhythmia events with electrograms. These developments greatly facilitate the possibilities for preprocedure and postprocedure interrogation of CIEDs, particularly in clinical situations where there is no immediate availability of an electrophysiologist or other qualified device interrogator. Nevertheless, cardiac rate and rhythm should be monitored throughout the immediate postoperative period, including during transport from the anesthetizing location to the recovery area. Backup cardioversion-defibrillation and pacing equipment should be immediately available. Postoperative CIED checks may not be needed if surgery did not include use of EMI-generating devices, no electronic preoperative device reprogramming was done, no blood transfusions were administered, and no intraoperative problems were identified that related to CIED function.

KEY POINTS

- The cardiac conduction system is a complex group of specialized cells within the heart that initiate and conduct electrical signals with great precision and speed. The myocardial cells in the heart are arranged in a functional syncytium. The cells are interconnected by a specialized membrane with gap junctions that are synchronized electrically during an action potential.

- A variety of acute and chronic conditions can cause or contribute to heart block. Disease processes such as acute myocardial infarction (especially in the distribution of the right coronary artery), myocarditis, rheumatic fever, mononucleosis, Lyme disease, and infiltrative diseases such as sarcoidosis and amyloidosis can contribute to heart block. Iatrogenic causes of heart block include traumatic injury from monitoring or ablation catheters or cardiac surgery, and drug effects such as digitalis toxicity and excessive β-blockade or calcium channel blockade.

- Cardiac rhythms that have abnormalities in rate, interval length, or conduction path are referred to as *dysrhythmias*. The significance of these abnormalities for the anesthesiologist depends on the clinical effect the dysrhythmias have on vital signs and on their potential to deteriorate into life-threatening dysrhythmias.

- A cardiac rhythm greater than 100 beats per minute is considered a tachycardia. Tachydysrhythmias can be generated from sources above or below the bundle of His. Those whose mechanism involves tissue above the bundle of His are called *supraventricular tachycardias* (SVTs). Tachydysrhythmias originating at or above the AV node tend to have a narrow QRS complex. Tachydysrhythmias generated from below the AV node have a wide QRS complex.

- Cardiac dysrhythmias caused by enhanced automaticity result from repetitive firing of a focus other than the sinus node. Reentry pathways account for most premature beats and tachydysrhythmias. Reentry or triggered dysrhythmias require two pathways over which cardiac impulses can be conducted at different velocities. Afterdepolarizations are oscillations in membrane potential that occur during or after repolarization. Normally these membrane oscillations dissipate. However, under special circumstances they can trigger a complete depolarization. Once triggered, the process may continue and result in a self-sustaining dysrhythmia.

- Atrial fibrillation (AF) is the most common sustained cardiac dysrhythmia in the general population. In 2005 it affected about 3 million adults in the United States. That number is expected to nearly triple by 2050. The incidence of AF increases with age: it is present in 1% of individuals younger than 60 years and increases to 12% in patients aged 70–84 years. One-third of patients with AF are older than age 80.

- Ventricular fibrillation (VF) is a rapid, grossly irregular ventricular rhythm with marked variability in QRS cycle length, morphology, and amplitude. It is incompatible with life because no stroke volume is generated by this rhythm. A pulse or blood pressure *never* accompanies VF. Ventricular tachycardia (VT) often precedes the onset of ventricular fibrillation. VF is the most common cause of sudden cardiac death.

- Bradycardia during neuraxial blockade can occur in patients of any age and any American Society of Anesthesiologists (ASA) physical status class, whether or not they are sedated. The incidence of profound bradycardia and cardiac arrest during neuraxial anesthesia is approximately 1.5 per 10,000 cases. By contrast, cardiac arrest during general anesthesia occurs at a rate of 5.5 per 10,000 cases.

- A patient with a preexisting CIED coming for surgery has at least one of three underlying cardiac problems: sustained or intermittent bradydysrhythmia, tachydysrhythmia, and/or heart failure. Regardless of the indication for the device, any patient with a CIED requiring anesthetic care must undergo a detailed systematic preoperative evaluation. This should include determination of the type of device present, identification of the clinical indication for the device, appraisal of the patient's degree of dependence on the device, and assessment of device function.

RESOURCES

American Heart Association. Web-based Integrated Guidelines for Cardiopulmonary Resuscitation and Emergency Cardiovascular Care—Part 7: Adult Advanced Cardiovascular Life Support. ECCguidelines.heart.org (Copyright 2015 American Heart Association, Inc.).

Apfelbaum JL, Belott P, Connis RT, et al. Practice advisory for the perioperative management of patients with cardiac implantable electronic devices: pacemakers and implantable cardioverter-defibrillators: an updated report by the American Society of Anesthesiologists Task Force on Perioperative Management of Patients with Cardiac Implantable Electronic Devices. *Anesthesiology*. 2011;114:247-261.

Correll DJ, Hepner DL, Chang C, et al. Preoperative electrocardiograms: patient factors predictive of abnormalities. *Anesthesiology*. 2009;110:1217-1222.

Crossley GH, Poole JE, Rozner MA, et al. The Heart Rhythm Society (HRS)/American Society of Anesthesiologists (ASA) expert consensus statement on the perioperative management of patients with implantable defibrillators, pacemakers and arrhythmia monitors: facilities and patient management. *Heart Rhythm*. 2011;8(7):1114-1154.

Drew BJ, Ackerman MJ, Funk M, et al. On behalf of the American Heart Association Acute Cardiac Care Committee of the Council on Clinical Cardiology, the Council on Cardiovascular Nursing, and the American College of Cardiology Foundation. Prevention of torsade de pointes in hospital settings: a scientific statement from the American Heart Association and the American College of Cardiology Foundation. *Circulation*. 2010;121:1047-1060.

Fleisher LA, Fleischmann KE, Auerbach AD, et al. ACC/AHA guideline on perioperative cardiovascular evaluation and management of patients undergoing noncardiac surgery: a report of the American College of Cardiology/American Heart Association Task Force on Practice Guidelines. *Circulation*. 2014;130:e278-e333.

Hancock EW, Deal BJ, Mirvis DM, et al. AHA/ACCF/HRS recommendations for the standardization and interpretation of the electrocardiogram, part V: electrocardiogram changes associated with cardiac chamber hypertrophy: a scientific statement from the American Heart Association Electrocardiography and Arrhythmias Committee, Council on Clinical Cardiology; the American College of Cardiology Foundation; and the Heart Rhythm Society. *Circulation*. 2009;119:e251-e261.

January CT, Wann LS, Alpert JS, et al. AHA/ACC/HRS guideline for the management of patients with atrial fibrillation: a report of the American College of Cardiology/American Heart Association Task Force on Practice Guidelines and the Heart Rhythm Society. *Circulation.* 2014;130:e199-e267.

Lüderitz B. Historical perspectives of cardiac electrophysiology. *Hellenic J Cardiol.* 2009;50:3-16.

Page RL, Joglar JA, Al-Khatib SM, et al. ACC/AHA/HRS guideline for the management of adult patients with supraventricular tachycardia: a report of the American College of Cardiology/American Heart Association Task Force on Clinical Practice Guidelines and the Heart Rhythm Society. *Circulation.* 2015;132:e000-e000.

Pollack Jr CV, Reilly PA, Eikelboom J, et al. Idarucizumab for dabigatran reversal. *N Engl J Med.* 2015;373:511-520.

Rautaharju PM, Surawicz B, Gettes LS. AHA/ACCF/HRS recommendations for the standardization and interpretation of the electrocardiogram, part IV: the ST segment, T and U waves, and the QT interval: a scientific statement from the American Heart Association Electrocardiography and Arrhythmias Committee, Council on Clinical Cardiology; the American College of Cardiology Foundation; and the Heart Rhythm Society. *Circulation.* 2009;119:e241-e250.

Stone ME, Salter B, Fischer A. Perioperative management of patients with cardiac implantable electronic devices. *Br J Anaesth.* 2011;107(S1):i16-i26.

Surawicz B, Childers R, Deal BJ, Gettes LS. AHA/ACCF/HRS recommendations for the standardization and interpretation of the electrocardiogram, part III: intraventricular conduction disturbances: a scientific statement from the American Heart Association Electrocardiography and Arrhythmias Committee, Council on Clinical Cardiology; the American College of Cardiology Foundation; and the Heart Rhythm Society. *Circulation.* 2009;119:e235-e240.

Wagner GS, Macfarlane P, Wellens H, et al. AHA/ACCF/HRS recommendations for the standardization and interpretation of the electrocardiogram: part VI: acute ischemia/infarction: a scientific statement from the American Heart Association Electrocardiography and Arrhythmias Committee, Council on Clinical Cardiology; the American College of Cardiology Foundation; and the Heart Rhythm Society. *Circulation.* 2009;119:e262-e270.

Zipes DP, Camm AJ, Borggrefe M, et al. CC/AHA/ESC 2006 guidelines for management of patients with ventricular arrhythmias and the prevention of sudden cardiac death—executive summary: a report of the American College of Cardiology/American Heart Association Task Force and the European Society of Cardiology Committee for Practice Guidelines (Writing Committee to Develop Guidelines for Management of Patients With Ventricular Arrhythmias and the Prevention of Sudden Cardiac Death). *Circulation.* 2006;114:1088-1132.

Systemic and Pulmonary Arterial Hypertension

MANUEL FONTES, PAUL M. HEERDT

SYSTEMIC HYPERTENSION

Defined as a sustained systolic blood pressure above 140 mm Hg or a diastolic pressure above 90 mm Hg, *hypertension* affects about one-quarter of the global population. In the United States alone this includes approximately 75 million people, most of whom are older than 50 years. In adult surgical patients, nearly one-third presenting for noncardiac surgery and two-thirds presenting for coronary bypass have a preexisting history of hypertension. Occurring more frequently in African Americans than non-Hispanic whites, the incidence of hypertension increases with age. More prevalent in men until age 45, the gender disparity dissipates at age 64, after which elevated blood pressure is present in a much higher percentage of women than men.

Public Health Implications

Worldwide, hypertension is the leading risk factor for morbidity and mortality, accounting for 7% of disability-adjusted life-years and 9.4 million deaths in 2010. It has been estimated that in the United States the lifetime risk of developing hypertension is close to 90%. The clinical consequences of chronically elevated blood pressure have been well characterized and underscore a high age-related association with ischemic heart disease and stroke (Fig. 9.1), as well as renal failure, retinopathy, peripheral vascular disease, and overall mortality. In the surgical population, multiple studies have found hypertension to be a common risk factor for perioperative morbidity and mortality, particularly in untreated or poorly treated patients. It is not clear, however, that increased blood pressure alone increases surgical risk or that normalization of blood pressure preoperatively significantly reduces these risks. Furthermore, chronic hypertension represents a dynamic spectrum spanning so-called prehypertension to severe disease (Table 9.1), with risk assessment often not clearly differentiating subtypes: isolated systolic hypertension (systolic > 140 mm Hg and diastolic < 90 mm Hg), *isolated diastolic* hypertension (systolic < 140 mm Hg with diastolic > 90 mm Hg), and *combined systolic and diastolic* hypertension (systolic > 140 mm Hg and diastolic > 90 mm Hg). As noted in the Eighth Joint National Committee Report on the Treatment of Hypertension (JNC 8), age dependence, risk association, pharmacologic therapy, and treatment goals can vary among subtypes. In addition to systolic and diastolic pressure abnormalities, an increase in their difference—*pulse pressure*—has been shown to be a risk factor for cardiovascular morbidity. Considered to be an index of vascular remodeling and "stiffness," some studies have linked increased pulse pressure with intraoperative hemodynamic instability and adverse postoperative outcomes.

Pathophysiology

Given the physiologic importance and complexity of blood pressure regulation, hypertension can result from a wide range of primary and secondary processes that increase cardiac output, peripheral vascular resistance, or both. For primary hypertension (often referred to as *essential hypertension*) a specific etiology is unclear, but contributing factors include sympathetic nervous system activity, dysregulation of the renin-angiotensin-aldosterone system, and deficient production of endogenous vasodilators (Table 9.2). Importantly, blood pressure elevation is often coincident with other morbidities and may occur in a constellation of symptoms

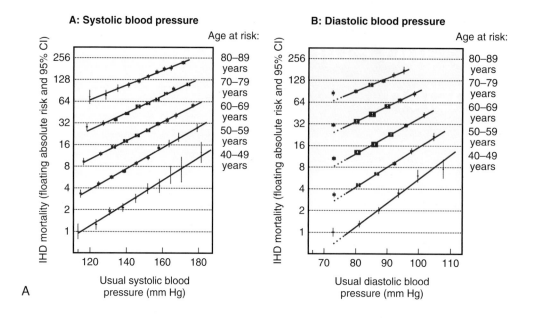

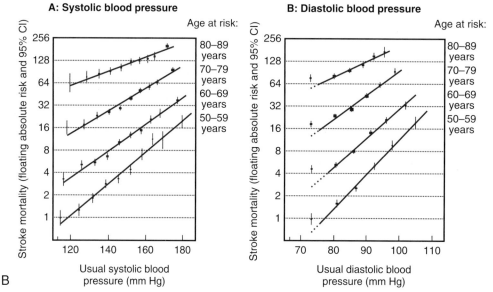

FIG. 9.1   Ischemic heart disease mortality (A) and stroke mortality (B) rates in each decade of age versus usual blood pressure at the start of that decade. Mortality rates are termed *floating* because multiplication by a constant appropriate for a particular population would allow prediction of the absolute rate in that population. *CI,* Confidence interval; *IHD,* ischemic heart disease. (Data from Lewington S, Clarke R, Qizilbash N, et al. Age-specific relevance of usual BP to vascular mortality: a meta-analysis of individual data for one million adults in 61 prospective studies. *Lancet.* 2002;360:1903-1913.)

TABLE 9.1	Classification of Systemic Blood Pressure in Adults	
Category	Systolic BP (mm Hg)	Diastolic BP (mm Hg)
Normal	<120	<80
Prehypertension	120–139	80–89
Stage 1 hypertension	140–159	90–99
Stage 2 hypertension	≥160	≥100

Data from Chobanian AV, Bakris GL, Black HR, et al; Joint National Committee on Prevention, Detection, Evaluation, and Treatment of High BP; National Heart, Lung, and Blood Institute; National High BP Education Program Coordinating Committee. Seventh report of the Joint National Committee on Prevention, Detection, Evaluation and Treatment of High BP. *Hypertension.* 2003;42:1206-1252.

TABLE 9.2	Pathophysiology of Primary Hypertension

AUTONOMIC NERVOUS SYSTEM

Normal: Integration of input from cardiac stretch receptors, vascular baroreceptors, and peripheral chemoreceptors with central regulatory processes and emotional stress. Provides acute control of cardiac output, vascular resistance, and blood volume.

Abnormal: Hypertension associated with dysregulation of baroreflex and chemoreflex pathways both peripherally and centrally

New concepts:
- Evidence for a novel renin-angiotensin system within the brain
- Activation of this pathway in response to oxidative stress and inflammation increases sympathetic nervous system output and arginine vasopressin release and inhibits baroreflex regulation.

CLASSICAL RENIN-ANGIOTENSIN-ALDOSTERONE SYSTEM

Normal: Provides acute and sustained control of extracellular fluid volume, peripheral resistance, and blood pressure based largely on peripheral sensors and effectors. Renin released from the kidney in response to decreased blood pressure hydrolyzes angiotensinogen → angiotensin I that is then cleaved to angiotensin II by angiotensin-converting enzyme (ACE) located on vascular endothelium in the lung. Angiotensin II → vasoconstriction, adrenal release of aldosterone → kidney reabsorption of salt and water.

Abnormal: Dysregulated renin release leads to elevated renin levels, angiotensin II overproduction, increased aldosterone, and hypertension.

New concepts:
- Local production of angiotensin II occurs in various tissues including fat, blood vessels, heart, adrenals, and brain.
- AI to AII cleavage by non-ACE enzymes including the serine protease chymase
- A recently described counterregulatory renin-angiotensin pathway that decreases blood pressure and target organ damage

ENDOGENOUS VASODILATOR/VASOCONSTRICTOR BALANCE

Normal: The vascular endothelium produces a range of vasoactive substances in response to pressure and the shear force imparted by pulsatile blood flow. Nitric oxide (dilation) and endothelin (constriction/dilation) in particular are major regulators of vascular tone. Other vasoactive substances include the peptides atrial natriuretic peptide (ANP), brain natriuretic peptide (BNP), and urodilatin. ANP and BNP are released from myocardium, and urodilatin is renal in origin. These peptides exert vasodilation along with natriuresis and blunting of renin-angiotensin-aldosterone responsiveness by activation of the NP receptors.

Abnormal: With hypertension, oxidative stress in particular has been linked to impaired endothelial function, leading to "feedforward" changes in vascular tone, vascular reactivity, and coagulation and fibrinolytic pathways. Disruption of NP release or receptor response may be present.

New concepts:
- The NPs are degraded by the enzyme neprilysin, and endothelin-1 formation requires endothelin-converting enzyme.
- Therapy directed toward neprilysin inhibition in combination with an endothelin-converting enzyme inhibitor or angiotensin receptor blocker may promote vasodilator/natriuretic effects of the natriuretic peptides while reducing the deleterious vasoconstrictor/proinflammatory effects of endothelin 1 and angiotensin II.

TABLE 9.3	Causes of Secondary Hypertension

DRUG-INDUCED SECONDARY HYPERTENSION

Class	Example
Estrogen	Oral contraceptives
Herbal	Ephedra, ginseng, ma huang
Illicit	Amphetamines, cocaine
Nonsteroidal antiinflammatory	Cyclooxygenase-2 inhibitors, ibuprofen, naproxen (Naprosyn)
Steroid	Methylprednisolone (Depo-Medrol), prednisone
Psychiatric	Buspirone (Buspar), carbamazepine (Tegretol), clozapine (Clozaril), fluoxetine (Prozac), lithium, tricyclic antidepressants

AGE DEPENDENCE OF NONDRUG-INDUCED SECONDARY HYPERTENSION

Age Group	% Secondary Hypertension	Most Common Etiologies
Children (birth to 12 years)	70–85	Renal parenchymal disease Coarctation of the aorta
Adolescents (12–18 years)	10–15	Coarctation of the aorta
Young adults (19–39 years)	5	Thyroid dysfunction Fibromuscular dysplasia Renal parenchymal disease
Middle-aged adults (40–64 years)	8–12	Aldosteronism Thyroid dysfunction Obstructive sleep apnea Cushing syndrome Pheochromocytoma
Older adults (65 years and older)	17	Atherosclerotic renal artery stenosis Renal failure Hypothyroidism

Adapted from Viera AJ, Neutze DM. Diagnosis of secondary hypertension: an age-based approach. *Am Fam Physician.* 2010;82:1471-1478.

associated with oxidative stress and systemic inflammation. There are now defined genetic risk factors and lifestyle choices such as obesity, alcohol consumption, and tobacco use that are associated with an increased incidence of hypertension.

Only about 5% of patients with elevated blood pressure have *secondary hypertension* resulting from a demonstrable potentially correctable cause that may be physiologic or pharmacologic (Table 9.3). Both the common etiologies and prevalence of secondary hypertension are age dependent. For example, in children younger than age 12 years, 70%–85% of hypertension is secondary to renal parenchymal disease. In contrast, for middle-aged adults, only about 10% of hypertension is deemed secondary, most often as a consequence of hyperaldosteronism, thyroid dysfunction, obstructive sleep apnea, Cushing syndrome, or pheochromocytoma.

TABLE 9.4	End-Organ Damage in Hypertension

VASCULOPATHY
Endothelial dysfunction
Remodeling
Generalized atherosclerosis
Arteriosclerotic stenosis
Aortic aneurysm

CEREBROVASCULAR DAMAGE
Acute hypertensive encephalopathy
Stroke
Intracerebral hemorrhage
Lacunar infarction
Vascular dementia
Retinopathy

HEART DISEASE
Left ventricular hypertrophy
Atrial fibrillation
Coronary microangiopathy
Coronary heart disease, myocardial infarction
Heart failure

NEPHROPATHY
Albuminuria
Proteinuria
Chronic renal insufficiency
Renal failure

Data from Schmieder RE. End organ damage in hypertension. *Dtsch Arztebl Int.* 2010;107:866-873.

Regardless of the underlying cause, chronic hypertension leads to remodeling of small and large arteries, endothelial dysfunction, and potentially irreversible end-organ damage (Table 9.4). Overall, disseminated vasculopathy plays a major role in ischemic heart disease, left ventricular hypertrophy, congestive heart failure, cerebrovascular disease and stroke, peripheral vascular disease and aortic aneurysm, and nephropathy. The degree to which some abnormalities are reversible is controversial, but early and effective intervention is essential. Improved diagnostic techniques may help provide a more detailed assessment than just blood pressure alone. Ultrasonic measurement of common carotid artery intimal-medial thickness and arterial pulse-wave velocity can provide early diagnosis of vasculopathy, and echocardiographic and electrocardiographic indices may track progression of left ventricular hypertrophy. Early signs of hypertensive nephropathy have become easier to detect, and magnetic resonance imaging (MRI) can be used to follow microangiopathic changes indicative of cerebrovascular damage.

Current Treatment of Hypertension

The general therapeutic goal for hypertension treatment is a blood pressure less than 140/90 mm Hg, although some experts believe this is still too high. However, a substantial number of people with hypertension are not attaining this goal due to nondiagnosis or misdiagnosis, minimal or adverse responses to medications, or noncompliance with prescribed treatment. In fact, approximately 35 million people in the United States alone have poorly controlled blood pressure, with an estimated 13 million people unaware of their hypertension. *Resistant hypertension,* defined as uncontrolled blood pressure despite three or more antihypertensive drugs of different classes, including a nonpotassium-sparing diuretic, or the need for four or more drugs to achieve control is present in 10%–15% of the hypertensive population. *Refractory hypertension,* defined as uncontrolled blood pressure on five or more drugs, is present in 0.5%. Even more common is intolerance to antihypertensive drugs or simple noncompliance. A study of patients with apparent treatment-resistant hypertension who had been prescribed three to five antihypertensive medications revealed that nearly a quarter of the study subjects had no detectable drug in blood or urine samples.

Lifestyle Modification

Lifestyle modifications of proven value in lowering blood pressure include weight reduction, moderation of alcohol intake, increased aerobic exercise, and smoking cessation. Weight loss may be the most effective nonpharmacologic intervention, with a 10-kg reduction decreasing systolic and diastolic blood pressures by an average of 6.0 and 4.6 mm Hg, respectively. Weight loss also enhances the efficacy of antihypertensive drug therapy. Excessive alcohol consumption can be associated with increased hypertension and may cause resistance to antihypertensive drugs.

There is an inverse relationship between dietary potassium and calcium intake and blood pressure in the general population. Salt restriction (e.g., Dietary Approaches to Stop Hypertension [DASH] eating plan) is associated with small but consistent decreases in systemic blood pressure. Sodium restriction appears to be most beneficial in lowering blood pressure in the elderly and African Americans, patient populations with low renin activity.

Pharmacologic Therapy

With continual research regarding the physiology and public health implications of hypertension, as well as identification of new cellular and molecular targets for pharmacologic intervention, treatment guidelines remain fluid. It is clear, however, that optimal drug therapy needs to consider ethnicity, advanced age, comorbidities, and end-organ function. The most recent evidence-based guidelines for the management of high blood pressure in adults (the JNC 8 in 2014) outlined several broad conclusions:

1. There is strong evidence to support treating hypertensive persons aged 60 years or older to a blood pressure goal of less than 150/90 mm Hg, and hypertensive persons 30 through 59 years of age to a diastolic goal of less than 90 mm Hg.

2. There is insufficient evidence in hypertensive persons younger than 60 years for a systolic goal, or in those younger than 30 years for a diastolic goal; a blood pressure of less than 140/90 mm Hg for those groups was recommended.

3. The same thresholds and goals are recommended for hypertensive adults with diabetes or nondiabetic chronic kidney disease as for the general hypertensive population younger than 60 years.
4. There is moderate evidence to support initiating drug treatment with angiotensin-converting enzyme (ACE) inhibitors, angiotensin receptor blockers (ARBs), calcium channel blockers, or thiazide-type diuretics in the nonblack hypertensive population, including those with diabetes.
5. In the black hypertensive population, including those with diabetes, a calcium channel blocker or thiazide-type diuretic is recommended as initial therapy.
6. There is moderate evidence to support initial or add-on antihypertensive therapy with an ACE inhibitor or ARB in persons with chronic kidney disease to improve kidney outcomes.

As noted in the guidelines, first-line antihypertensive therapy consists of diuretics, calcium channel blockers, ACE inhibitors, and ARBs. Notably absent from first-line therapy are β-blockers, which tend to be reserved for patients with coronary artery disease or tachydysrhythmia, or as a component of multidrug therapy in resistant hypertension. A wide range of antihypertensive drugs are in common use (Table 9.5). A recent review noted that drugs in 15 different classes have been approved for the treatment of hypertension in the United States, many of which are also available in single-pill combinations with other compounds. Importantly, although all the available drugs can reduce blood pressure, their disparate pharmacology is evident in the reported relative risk reduction of hypertension-related events. For example, calcium channel blockers may lower the risk of stroke but not heart failure or mortality, whereas a Cochrane review found that in patients with uncomplicated hypertension, low-dose thiazides reduce mortality and cardiovascular morbidity. Nonetheless, across the range of hypertension etiology and severity, the varying pharmacology of available medications allows for combining drugs with different and potentially beneficial properties in terms of optimizing end-organ function (Table 9.6). Despite the plethora of treatment options already available, the public health burden of hypertension continues to drive research into new pharmacologic targets and therapies including vaccines and surgical interventions (Table 9.7).

Treatment of Secondary Hypertension

Treatment of secondary hypertension is often interventional, including correction of renal artery stenosis via angioplasty or direct arterial repair, and adrenalectomy for adrenal adenoma or pheochromocytoma. For patients in whom renal artery repair is not possible, blood pressure control may be accomplished with ACE inhibitors alone or in combination with diuretics. Primary hyperaldosteronism in women can be treated with an aldosterone antagonist such as spironolactone, whereas amiloride is often used in men owing to the potential for spironolactone-induced gynecomastia. Certain disease entities, such as pheochromocytoma, may require a combined pharmacologic and surgical approach for optimal outcome.

TABLE 9.5 Commonly Used Antihypertensive Drugs

Class	Subclass	Generic Name	Trade Name
Diuretics	Thiazides	Chlorothiazide	Diuril
		Hydrochlorothiazide	HydroDiuril, Microzide
		Indapamide	Lozol
		Metolazone	Zaroxolyn, Mykrox
	Loop	Bumetanide	Bumex
		Furosemide	Lasix
		Torsemide	Demadex
	Potassium sparing	Amiloride	Midamor
		Spironolactone	Aldactone
		Triamterene	Dyrenium
Adrenergic antagonists	β-Blockers	Atenolol	Tenormin
		Bisoprolol	Zebeta
		Metoprolol	Lopressor
		Nadolol	Corgard
		Propranolol	Inderal
		Timolol	Blocadren
	α₁-Blockers	Doxazosin	Cardura
		Prazosin	Minipress
		Terazosin	Hytrin
	Combined α- and β-blockers	Carvedilol	Coreg
		Labetalol	Normodyne, Trandate
	Centrally acting	Clonidine	Catapres
		Methyldopa	Aldomet
Vasodilators		Hydralazine	Apresoline
Angiotensin-converting enzyme inhibitors		Benazepril	Lotensin
		Captopril	Capoten
		Enalapril	Vasotec
		Fosinopril	Monopril
		Lisinopril	Prinivil, Zestril
		Moexipril	Univasc
		Quinapril	Accupril
		Ramipril	Altace
		Trandolapril	Mavik
Angiotensin receptor blockers		Candesartan	Atacand
		Eprosartan	Teveten
		Irbesartan	Avapro
		Losartan	Cozaar
		Olmesartan	Benicar
		Telmisartan	Micardis
		Valsartan	Diovan
Calcium channel blockers	Dihydropyridine	Amlodipine	Norvasc
		Felodipine	Plendil
		Isradipine	DynaCirc
		Nicardipine	Cardene
		Nifedipine	Adalat, Procardia
		Nisoldipine	Sular
		Clevidipine	Cleviprex
	Nondihydropyridine	Diltiazem	Cardizem, Dilacor, Tiazac
		Verapamil	Calan, Isoptin SR, Covera

TABLE 9.6	Drug Combinations With End-Organ Damage
SUBCLINICAL END-ORGAN DAMAGE	
Left ventricular hypertrophy	ACEIs, ARBs, CAs
Elevated albuminuria	ACEIs, ARBs
Renal dysfunction	ACEIs, ARBs
IRREVERSIBLE HYPERTENSIVE END-ORGAN DAMAGE	
Prior stroke	Any antihypertensive
Prior MI	BBs, ACEIs, ARBs
Angina pectoris, CHD	BBs, CAs
Heart failure	Diuretics, BBs, ACEIs, ARBs, MR antagonists
Left ventricular dysfunction	ACEIs, ARB
Atrial fibrillation	
• Prevention, recurrence	ARBs, ACEIs
• Permanent	BBs, nondihydropyridine calcium antagonists
Tachydysrhythmia	BBs
Chronic renal insufficiency, proteinuria	ACEIs, ARBs, loop diuretics
Peripheral arterial occlusive disease	CA

ACEIs, Angiotensin-converting enzyme inhibitors; *ARBs,* angiotensin receptor blockers; *BBs,* β-blockers; *CAs,* calcium antagonists; *CHD,* coronary heart disease; *MI,* myocardial infarction; *MR,* mineralocorticoid.
Adapted from Schmieder RE. End organ damage in hypertension. *Dtsch Arztebl Int.* 2010;107:866-873.

TABLE 9.7	New Treatment Approaches for Hypertension

NEW DRUGS
Mineralocorticoid receptor antagonists
Aldosterone synthase inhibitors
Activators of the ACE2/angiotensin-(1–7)/Mas receptor axis
Centrally acting aminopeptidase inhibitors
Vasopeptidase inhibitors
Dual-acting angiotensin receptor–neprilysin inhibitors
Dual-acting endothelin-converting enzyme–neprilysin inhibitors
Natriuretic peptide receptor agonists
Vasoactive intestinal peptide receptor agonist
Soluble epoxide hydrolase inhibitors
Intestinal Na^+/H^+ exchanger 3 inhibitor
Dopamine β-hydroxylase (DβH) inhibitor

VACCINES
Vaccine against angiotensin II
Vaccine against angiotensin II type 1 receptor

NOVEL APPROACHES TO PREECLAMPSIA TREATMENT
Antidigoxin antibody fragment
Recombinant antithrombin

INTERVENTIONAL PROCEDURES
Renal denervation
Baroreflex activation therapy
Carotid body ablation
Arteriovenous fistula creation
Neurovascular decompression
Renal artery stenting (revascularization)

ACE, Angiotensin-converting enzyme.
Adapted from Oparil S, Schmeider RE. New approaches in the treatment of hypertension. *Circ Res.* 2015;116:1074-1095.

Perioperative Implications of Hypertension

Preoperative Evaluation

Both the adequacy of blood pressure control in known hypertensives and the potential for previously undiagnosed hypertension need to be considered with the caveat of a "white coat" effect (anxiety-related hypertensive response). Current guidelines indicate that a definitive diagnosis of hypertension requires multiple elevated blood pressure readings over time, so making a new diagnosis based upon a single measurement in a preoperative clinic is problematic. Nonetheless, when considered along a spectrum from normal to prehypertension to stage 2 disease, there may be incremental risk. For patients with long-standing and/or poorly controlled hypertension, additional consideration of vasculopathy and end-organ function is important. In general, elevated blood pressure per se is not a direct prompt to delay surgery for cardiac evaluation in asymptomatic patients without other risk factors. In fact, unless there is marked hypertension (systolic > 180 mm Hg and/or diastolic > 110 mm Hg) or end-organ dysfunction that can be ameliorated by aggressive blood pressure control, delaying surgery is not generally recommended.

A possible exception to the "no delay" concept is suspicion that previously undiagnosed or untreated hypertension observed during a preoperative evaluation is secondary in nature; there have been multiple reports of a pheochromocytoma being "diagnosed" by induction of general anesthesia for an incidental procedure. A secondary etiology may be indicated by symptoms (e.g., flushing, sweating suggestive of pheochromocytoma), physical examination (e.g., a renal bruit suggestive of renal artery stenosis), laboratory abnormalities (e.g., hypokalemia suggestive of hyperaldosteronism), or age (most hypertension in children <12 years of age is secondary).

Once the decision is made to proceed with surgery, it is now common practice to continue antihypertensive medications, with the possible exception of high-dose angiotensin II receptor antagonists and ACE inhibitors. Some authors advocate discontinuing these drugs at least 10 hours prior to surgery owing to concerns about refractory hypotension. In contrast, others believe there is little direct association between chronic use of angiotensin II receptor antagonists and ACE inhibitors and sustained hypotension and therefore support continuing these drugs up to the time of surgery, especially in ambulatory patients. In addition, cessation of β-adrenergic antagonists or clonidine can be associated with rebound effects.

Intraoperative Considerations

Although guidelines do not support delaying surgery for poorly controlled blood pressure, perioperative hypertension increases blood loss as well as the incidence of myocardial ischemia and cerebrovascular events. Furthermore, owing to a combination of physiologic factors (volume depletion, loss of vascular elasticity, baroreceptor desensitization) in combination with antihypertensive treatment, hypertensive patients are prone to intraoperative hemodynamic volatility. When superimposed on organ damage

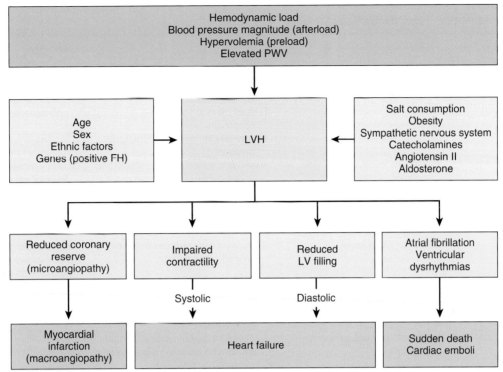

FIG. 9.2 Pathogenetic factors and clinical presentation of hypertensive heart disease. *FH,* Family history; *LV,* left ventricle; *LVH,* LV hypertrophy; *PWV,* pulse wave velocity. (From Schmieder RE. End organ damage in hypertension. *Dtsch Arztebl Int.* 2010;107:866-873.)

from chronic hypertensive disease, even transient hypotension can impart renal and myocardial injury. Ultimately, regardless of treatment efficacy at the time of surgery, hypertension as a disease entity has long been known to be an independent predictor for adverse perioperative cardiovascular events, especially when combined with other risk factors. Accordingly, clinicians need to consider acute intraoperative changes in blood pressure in the context of alterations in end-organ functional reserve brought about by chronic disease. Particular emphasis has been placed upon ischemic heart disease, and more recently the implications of left ventricular hypertrophy on cardiac relaxation and filling during diastole (Fig. 9.2).

Induction of Anesthesia and Monitoring

As already noted, hypertensive patients can be hemodynamically volatile, with induction of anesthesia producing hypotension and subsequent laryngoscopy and tracheal intubation eliciting hypertension and tachycardia. To lessen this risk it has been suggested that placement of an intraarterial catheter followed by a multimodal induction that includes transient β-blockade with esmolol may be beneficial. Poorly controlled hypertension is often accompanied by relative volume depletion, especially if a diuretic is part of chronic therapy. In some patients, modest volume loading prior to induction of anesthesia may provide hemodynamic stability. Although recommended for situations such as pheochromocytoma, this approach may be counterproductive in patients with marked left ventricular hypertrophy and significant diastolic dysfunction.

As with any procedure, a management plan for hemodynamic monitoring and vasoactive drug therapy for hypertensive patients should consider age, functional reserve, preoperative pharmacotherapy, and the planned operation. For example, intention-to-treat thresholds for patients undergoing repair of aortic dissection or women with peripartum hypertension will be lower than for the general surgical population. Arterial catheterization provides useful continuous information, but clinicians should keep in mind the potential for differences between peripheral (radial) and more central (femoral) blood pressures. Assessment of fluid status can be challenging in patients with long-standing hypertension, especially those with a history of heart failure with preserved ejection fraction (HFpEF). Left ventricular hypertrophy reduces chamber compliance such that with volume infusion, right heart pressures rise despite the fact that the left ventricle is relatively underfilled. Ultimately, intraoperative use of a pulmonary artery catheter is controversial, and pressure measurements from a central venous catheter may not provide a clear representation of volume status. Overall, for the patient with HFpEF, echocardiographic evaluation of cardiac volumes may be the most useful.

Maintenance of Anesthesia

Achieving hemodynamic stability may be more important than targeting an arbitrary intraoperative blood pressure, especially given the influence of other comorbidities, surgical procedure and position, volume status, mechanical ventilation, and depth of anesthesia. The management of intraoperative blood pressure over the wide range of potential clinical

TABLE 9.8	Treatment for Hypertensive Emergencies		
Cause/Manifestation	Primary Agents	Cautions	Comments
Encephalopathy and intracranial hypertension	Clevidipine, nitroprusside, labetalol, nicardipine	Cerebral ischemia may result from lower BP due to altered autoregulation. Risk of cyanide toxicity with nitroprusside Nitroprusside increases intracranial pressure.	Lower BP may lessen bleeding in intracerebral hemorrhage. Elevated BP often resolves spontaneously.
Aortic dissection	Clevidipine, nicardipine, esmolol, labetalol	Vasodilators may cause marked drop in blood pressure that can result in end-organ ischemia.	Goal is lessening of pulsatile force of left ventricular contraction
Acute kidney injury	Clevidipine, nicardipine, labetalol	Same as above	May require emergent hemodialysis if it progresses to renal failure
Preeclampsia and eclampsia	Labetalol, nicardipine	β-Blockers may reduce uterine blood flow and inhibit labor.	Definitive therapy is delivery. ACE inhibitors and ARBs are teratogenic and contraindicated during pregnancy.
Pheochromocytoma	Phentolamine, phenoxybenzamine, propranolol, labetalol	Unopposed α-adrenergic stimulation following β-blockade worsens hypertension.	
Cocaine intoxication	Labetalol, dexmedetomidine, clevidipine	Unopposed α-adrenergic stimulation following β-blockade worsens hypertension.	

scenarios is beyond the scope of this review. However, it is important to consider that although high-dose anesthetics can acutely control blood pressure in many patients, this approach can have side effects, slows emergence, and cannot be continued into the postoperative phase. Accordingly, addition of sympathomodulators (esmolol, metoprolol, labetalol) or titrated calcium channel blocker therapy can facilitate the transition from the operating room to postanesthesia care unit (PACU) or intensive care unit (ICU).

Hypertensive Crises

Hypertensive crises are categorized as either urgent or emergent, based on the presence or absence of progressive organ damage. Patients with chronic hypertension tend to tolerate a higher systemic blood pressure than previously normotensive individuals and are more likely to require urgent (as opposed to emergent) intervention. Emergencies that may present in the perioperative setting include manifestations of *central nervous system injury* (hypertensive encephalopathy, intracerebral hemorrhage, subarachnoid hemorrhage, acute stroke); *kidney injury* (hypertension-induced acute renal dysfunction); and *cardiovascular insult* (hypertension associated with unstable angina, acute myocardial infarction, acute heart failure, and acute aortic dissection). In addition, women with *pregnancy-induced hypertension* may show evidence of end-organ dysfunction, in particular encephalopathy, with a diastolic blood pressure of less than 100 mm Hg. Current guidelines for peripartum hypertension recommend immediate intervention for a systolic pressure above 160 mm Hg and/or diastolic pressure above 110 mm Hg.

Given the familiarity of perioperative physicians with vasoactive drug infusions and invasive monitoring, intervention for severe hypertension can generally be accomplished quickly, but care must be taken to titrate blood pressure down slowly to avoid overshoot hypotension. Placement of an intra-arterial catheter to continuously monitor blood pressure can facilitate this process. Multiple vasodilator drugs are available, with different pharmacologic properties preferable under certain circumstances (Table 9.8). Labetalol has been described as the first-line drug for peripartum hypertension, whereas the addition of a β-blocker (esmolol, labetalol) to an arteriolar dilator is especially desirable in aortic dissection. For rapid arterial dilation and blood pressure reduction, sodium nitroprusside infusion has long been the standard, since it offers fast onset and dose titration, but cost constraints have lessened drug availability. More recently, clevidipine, a third-generation dihydropyridine calcium channel blocker with an ultra-short duration of action (≈1 minute half-life) and selective arteriolar vasodilating properties has become available. Nicardipine, a second-generation dihydropyridine calcium channel blocker, can also be used but has a longer half-life (≈30 minutes), making it less titratable than clevidipine.

Acute Postoperative Hypertension

Acute postoperative hypertension (APH) has been described as a significant elevation in blood pressure during the immediate postoperative period that may lead to serious neurologic, cardiovascular, or surgical site complications requiring urgent management. Although APH is widely recognized, there is no standardized definition for this disorder. Some authors suggest APH can be characterized by a progressive rise in systolic pressure to a level more than 20% above that measured upon admission to the PACU or ICU, or an increase in diastolic blood pressure to above 110 mm/Hg. Others have defined APH as a systolic pressure above 190 mm Hg and/or a diastolic pressure above 100 mm Hg on two consecutive postoperative measurements. APH usually develops shortly after surgery (1–2 hours) and subsequently resolves over several hours. Complications associated with APH can be both technical (surgical site bleeding, disruption of vascular anastomoses) and physiologic (myocardial ischemia, dysrhythmia, congestive heart failure with pulmonary edema, intracranial hemorrhage, cerebral ischemia, stroke, and encephalopathy).

Given the interplay of preexisting pathophysiology and withdrawal of chronic antihypertensive therapy, surgical stress, and pain, the cause of APH is undoubtedly multifactorial: autonomic nervous system activation at multiple levels, stress-induced disruption/activation of the renin-angiotensin-aldosterone system, emergence delirium and anxiety, and shivering. A study of nearly 20,000 general surgical patients found that about 2% developed APH and were at increased risk for hospital mortality. Other studies have reported the overall incidence of PACU hypertension in general surgical patients to be 0.6%–1.1%. The highest incidence (20%–60%) is following carotid endarterectomy, abdominal aortic surgery, radical neck dissection, and intracranial surgery, suggesting that disruption of normal homeostatic mechanisms regulated by perivascular structures (baroreceptors, chemoreceptors) may play a role.

Treatment of APH is generally a clinical decision based on the surgery (noncardiac vs. cardiac, presence of vascular anastomoses, intracranial), underlying comorbidities, and risks of treatment. For cardiac surgical patients in closely monitored postoperative settings, relatively tight limits for blood pressure have been incorporated into care plan protocols. For general surgical patients, the risk/benefit of aggressive postoperative blood pressure control in a PACU environment remains unclear. Common factors (pain, anxiety, hypoxemia, hypercarbia, shivering, bladder distension) should be addressed before administration of specific antihypertensive therapy. When no identifiable treatable cause is apparent, titration of a short-acting intravenous drug is recommended because of the risk of hypotension as the hypertensive stimulus abates. Sympatholysis with esmolol or labetalol is often the first-line choice, with clevidipine or nicardipine as alternatives or adjuncts. Escalating doses of ACE inhibitor or ARB can also be used, as can hydralazine, but the longer half-life of these drugs may complicate management should secondary hypotension occur.

Although rare, withdrawal from clonidine (a centrally acting α_2-agonist) can present as marked postoperative hypertension and often tachycardia. Occurring 18–24 hours after clonidine cessation, the greatest risk of rebound hypertension is in patients taking more than 1 mg/d. Prevention is accomplished by switching to a clonidine patch preoperatively.

Although predominantly the result of excessive sympathetic nervous activity, hypertension may be aggravated by simultaneous use of a nonselective β-blocker (e.g., propranolol) that blocks vasodilatory β_2 receptors without affecting vasoconstrictive α receptors. There is no parenteral replacement for clonidine, but dexmedetomidine, a rapid-acting intravenous α_2-adrenergic agonist, may have utility in patients with clonidine withdrawal syndrome.

PULMONARY ARTERIAL HYPERTENSION

Unlike systemic hypertension that can be diagnosed with a noninvasive blood pressure cuff, and efficacy of treatment monitored on a daily basis, the diagnosis and treatment of chronic pulmonary hypertension (PH) is more complex. Defined as a mean pulmonary artery pressure (mPAP) over 25 mm Hg, right heart catheterization is generally required for a definitive PH diagnosis and formulation of an optimal therapeutic plan. Importantly, whereas systemic hypertension tends to reflect arterial pathology, PH can result from abnormalities in either arterial or venous components of the lung circulation, sometimes including contributions from both. Improved understanding of the pathogenesis and pathophysiology of PH in combination with new drug therapies for PH of arterial origin has led to improved survival. At the same time, a clear association between the increasing obesity rate and the potential for more widespread PH has emerged. Ultimately the likelihood of patients with PH—treated or untreated—presenting for anesthesia and surgery is increasing.

The impact of PH on cardiac surgical outcome has been relatively well described in large measure because PH is often identified with routine preoperative testing. Furthermore, cardiac surgical patients are more prone to be managed in a perioperative setting where insertion of a pulmonary artery catheter is commonplace and ICU admission routine. In contrast, specific risk factors for PH patients undergoing noncardiac surgery are less well defined, possibly reflecting the fact that across the etiologic spectrum and need for invasive diagnosis, PH may be occult or undertreated preoperatively. This section will first review the diagnosis and classification of PH in general and then focus upon perioperative implications of precapillary pulmonary arterial hypertension (PAH) in noncardiac surgery.

Definitions and Classification

Definition

As noted earlier, *pulmonary hypertension* as a broad entity is defined as mPAP over 25 mm Hg measured by right heart catheterization. It is important to understand, however, that mPAP can be increased by a variety of mechanisms: (1) elevated resistance to blood flow within the arterial circulation, (2) increased pulmonary venous pressure from left heart disease, (3) chronically increased pulmonary blood flow, or (4) a combination of these processes. Importantly, PH is not always associated with increased pulmonary vascular resistance

(PVR). Calculated from right heart catheterization data as (mPAP-pulmonary capillary wedge pressure)/cardiac output, PVR is commonly expressed either as Wood units (mm Hg/L/min) or in dyne/s/cm^5 (Wood units × 80) and may be normal despite increased mPAP.

Hemodynamic Classification

Owing to the ease and noninvasive nature of echocardiography, it is commonly used to estimate pulmonary arterial systolic pressure (PASP) as a screening tool for PH. However, although echocardiographic PASP above 45 mm Hg is quite specific for PH, it is relatively insensitive and cannot provide the accurate mPAP measurement needed for definitive diagnosis. Once right heart catheterization is performed, severity of PH based upon measurements obtained at rest is characterized as mild (mPAP = 25–40 mm Hg), moderate (mPAP = 41–55 mm Hg), or severe (mPAP > 55 mm Hg). It is important to note that the normal pulmonary circulation can accommodate approximately a fourfold increase in cardiac output without a marked change in mPAP. Studies conducted under high altitude conditions have shown that when the pulmonary circulation is constricted by hypoxia, there is a much greater rise in mPAP with increased flow, but that the normal right ventricle can acutely adapt to the added load.

It is useful to consider the physiologic mechanisms responsible for the hemodynamic response. *Precapillary PH* is defined as PVR of 3.0 or more Wood units without significant elevation of the left atrial pressure or more commonly its surrogate, pulmonary capillary wedge pressure (PCWP). In general a PCWP below 15 mm Hg is considered normal. *Postcapillary PH* results from increased pulmonary venous pressure, most commonly the result of elevated left atrial pressure secondary to valve disease or inotropic/lusitropic dysfunction of the left ventricle. Pure postcapillary PH is characterized by a PCWP above 15 mm Hg, with normal values for PVR and the transpulmonary gradient (mPAP – PCWP, the numerator in the PVR calculation). *Mixed PH* reflects chronic pulmonary venous hypertension with secondary pulmonary arterial vasoconstriction and remodeling. This is also known as *reactive PH* and most commonly related to left heart failure. The mixed variety is characterized by a PCWP above 15 mm Hg in combination with a transpulmonary pressure gradient above 12–15 mm Hg and ultimately a PVR more than 2.5–3.0 Wood units. Mixed PH can be subcategorized as fixed or vasoreactive depending on the response to vasodilators, diuretics, or mechanical assistance. *High-flow PH* occurs without an elevation in PCWP or PVR and results from increased pulmonary blood flow secondary to systemic-to-pulmonary shunt or high cardiac output states.

WHO Clinical Classification

The World Health Organization (WHO) clinical classification of PH was updated in 2008 and refined in 2013 (Table 9.9). *PAH (WHO group 1)* is a relatively rare disease with a prevalence of approximately 15 cases per million people per year. *Idiopathic PAH* (IPAH)—cases with no familial context

TABLE 9.9	Updated Classification of Pulmonary Hypertension

1. **Pulmonary arterial hypertension (PAH)**
   1.1 Idiopathic PAH
   1.2 Heritable PAH
      1.2.1 BMPR2
      1.2.2 ALK-1, ENG, SMAD9, CAV1, KCNK3
      1.2.3 Unknown
   1.3 Drug and toxin induced
   1.4 Associated with:
      1.4.1 Connective tissue disease
      1.4.2 HIV infection
      1.4.3 Portal hypertension
      1.4.4 Congenital heart diseases
      1.4.5 Schistosomiasis
   1′ Pulmonary venoocclusive disease and/or pulmonary capillary hemangiomatosis
   1″ Persistent pulmonary hypertension of the newborn (PPHN)
2. **Pulmonary hypertension due to left heart disease**
   2.1 Left ventricular systolic dysfunction
   2.2 Left ventricular diastolic dysfunction
   2.3 Valvular disease
   2.4 Congenital/acquired left heart inflow/outflow tract obstruction and congenital cardiomyopathies
3. **Pulmonary hypertension due to lung diseases and/or hypoxia**
   3.1 Chronic obstructive pulmonary disease
   3.2 Interstitial lung disease
   3.3 Other pulmonary diseases with mixed restrictive and obstructive pattern
   3.4 Sleep-disordered breathing
   3.5 Alveolar hypoventilation disorders
   3.6 Chronic exposure to high altitude
   3.7 Developmental lung diseases
4. **Chronic thromboembolic pulmonary hypertension (CTEPH)**
5. **Pulmonary hypertension with unclear multifactorial mechanisms**
   5.1 Hematologic disorders: chronic hemolytic anemia, myeloproliferative disorders, splenectomy
   5.2 Systemic disorders: sarcoidosis, pulmonary histiocytosis, lymphangioleiomyomatosis
   5.3 Metabolic disorders: glycogen storage disease, Gaucher disease, thyroid disorders
   5.4 Others: tumoral obstruction, fibrosing mediastinitis, chronic renal failure, segmental PH

From Simonneau G, Gatzoulis MA, Adatia I, et al. Updated clinical classification of pulmonary hypertension. *J Am Coll Cardiol.* 2013;62:D34-41.

and no identifiable risk factor—accounts for nearly half of all PAH diagnoses. Roughly 3% of PAH diagnoses are deemed *heritable PAH,* with mutations in bone morphogenetic protein receptor type 2 *(BMPR2)* most prominent. The majority of remaining cases are designated as "associated PAH," since they can be ascribed to manifestations of drugs, toxins, or other diseases. Etiology remains unclear for less than 1% of diagnoses. Traditionally characterized primarily as a disease of young women, with median survival from time of PAH diagnosis of about 3 years, current data indicate a demographic shift, with older patients and more men being diagnosed. Overall, despite improved diagnosis and therapy, 1-year mortality is estimated to be 15%. The poorest prognosis is in patients with PAH associated with scleroderma, and/or a reduced distance on a 6-minute walk test (<300 meters), right ventricular (RV) enlargement/dysfunction, central venous pressure above 20 mm Hg, cardiac index below 2 L/min/m², and elevated brain natriuretic peptide. The impact of *pulmonary venous hypertension (WHO group 2 PH)* on morbidity and mortality in cardiac surgical patients is well described. *Pulmonary hypertension secondary to lung disease and/or hypoxia (WHO group 3)* may represent an emerging focus for perioperative physicians, since it includes obesity-related PH. Recent data indicate that about 60% of the US population is overweight or frankly obese. The associated rise in obesity-related obstructive sleep apnea (OSA) and obesity hypoventilation syndrome (OHS) may impact PH-related perioperative morbidity; it is estimated that PH is present in 20% of OSA patients and 50% of those with OHS. *Patients with chronic thromboembolic PH (WHO group 4)* are generally refractory to medical management and require high-risk surgery, and those in *WHO group 5 (multifactorial)* may present with occult disease.

When all PH etiologies are considered, prevalence in the surgical population is probably substantial. Using echocardiographic estimates of PASP as a screening tool, investigators found that 25% of the residents in a Minnesota county had a PASP above 30 mm Hg, and that the magnitude of rise was age dependent. Using an estimated PASP threshold of 40 mm Hg, 9.1% of over 10,000 residents in western Australia were found to have PH. Overall, elevated PASP was more prominent in women and primarily related to left heart disease.

Pathophysiology and Pharmacologic Treatment

The development of PAH seems to involve multiple events accumulating on top of a genetic predisposition to generate complex changes in the expression of genes that promote cell proliferation and altered metabolism. Ultimately, sustained vasoconstriction and proremodeling processes lead to pathologic distortion of small pulmonary arteries (intimal hyperplasia, medial hypertrophy, adventitial thickening, and in situ thrombosis). Current theories indicate that PAH may be associated with a proapoptotic insult to the vascular endothelium, resulting in endothelial dysfunction and selection of apoptosis-resistant cell populations that go on to form the *plexiform lesions* characteristic of the disease. It has been suggested that PAH exhibits a neoplastic-like pathobiology.

Pharmacologic targets for PAH treatment continue to emerge, with a range of new therapeutic options under investigation. In addition to adjuncts such as diuretics and anticoagulants, and nonspecific calcium channel blockers in a relatively small subset, there are currently three main classes of pulmonary vasodilator drugs used for the treatment of PAH: prostanoids, endothelin receptor antagonists (ERAs), and those working through nitric oxide/guanylate cyclase pathways. Given the different mechanisms of action, it is not uncommon for patients to receive combination therapy.

Prostanoids

Prostanoids mimic the effect of prostacyclin to produce vasodilation while inhibiting platelet aggregation. They also have antiinflammatory effects and may reduce proliferation of vascular smooth muscle cells. Currently available drugs include epoprostenol (intravenous), iloprost (inhaled), treprostinil (subcutaneous, intravenous, inhaled, oral), and most recently the oral drug beraprost. All have been shown to provide symptomatic improvement, but only epoprostenol has been proven to reduce mortality.

Endothelin Receptor Antagonists

The vascular endothelial dysfunction associated with PAH involves an imbalance between vasodilating (nitric oxide) and vasoconstricting (endothelin) substances. Currently available ERAs are all oral drugs and include bosentan, ambrisentan, and most recently macitentan. As a class, ERAs have been shown to improve hemodynamics and exercise capacity.

Nitric Oxide/Guanylate Cyclase

When endogenously released by endothelial cells or exogenously inhaled, nitric oxide produces pulmonary vasodilation by stimulating guanylate cyclase activity and subsequent cyclic guanosine monophosphate (cGMP) formation in smooth muscle cells. This effect is transient because nitric oxide is quickly bound by hemoglobin and other molecules, and cGMP is rapidly degraded by phosphodiesterase type 5 (PDE5). Continuously inhaled nitric oxide has been widely used in both perioperative and critical care settings, and preparations for home use have become available. More commonly, chronic therapy has been directed toward PDE5 inhibition with the oral drugs sildenafil and tadalafil. Multiple randomized controlled trials have confirmed efficacy of these drugs. Recently the oral guanylate cyclase stimulant riociguat was introduced. This drug both augments nitric oxide activation of soluble guanylate cyclase and stimulates the enzyme directly.

Perioperative Considerations

Preoperative Evaluation

It is important to consider that the specifics of many surgical procedures may not be known to some physicians asked to provide preoperative clearance. While all should be familiar with the ACC/AHA guidelines defining high-risk procedures (emergent major operations, aortic and major vascular surgery, peripheral vascular surgery, and prolonged procedures associated with the potential for large blood loss or fluid shifts), "high-risk" takes on a somewhat different connotation for patients with PAH. Particular consideration needs to be given to procedures with the potential for venous embolism (air, fat, cement), elevations in venous and/or airway pressure (laparoscopy, Trendelenburg positioning), hypoxic pulmonary vasoconstriction (HPV) or reduction in pulmonary vascular volume (single-lung ventilation, lung compression, or resection), a profound perioperative systemic inflammatory response, and emergency procedures.

Identifying patients at risk for PH of any etiology that has gone underappreciated or undiagnosed is especially important. Patients suffering from PAH often present with nonspecific symptoms of fatigue and dyspnea. With more advanced disease, angina pectoris, presyncope, and syncope can occur with exercise because coronary blood flow cannot meet supply/demand needs of a markedly hypertrophied right ventricle, and cardiac output cannot increase to meet metabolic demands. The New York Heart Association (NYHA) functional heart failure classification has been adapted for PH, with *class 1* representing no symptoms with physical activity, and at the other end of the spectrum, *class 4* exhibiting symptoms with minimal or no exertion. On physical examination, patients—especially those with uncompensated PAH and RV dysfunction—may exhibit a parasternal lift, an S_3 gallop, jugular venous distention, peripheral edema, hepatomegaly, and ascites. Rarely, hoarseness due to left recurrent laryngeal nerve paralysis secondary to compression by a dilated pulmonary artery (Ortner syndrome) may be present.

Assessing Risk Factors

A known or suspected history of PH should prompt further evaluation of functional status (exercise capacity, often a 6-minute walk), cardiac performance (especially RV function), and pulmonary function tests. For patients with moderate or severe PH by history or transthoracic echocardiography, or for those with related comorbidities, a right heart catheterization prior to high- or moderate-risk surgery is recommended. Owing to the potential for discrepancies between PCWP and actual left ventricular end-diastolic pressure, left heart catheterization should also be performed in patients with co-existing left heart disease, because inaccurate estimation of left ventricular end-diastolic pressure may lead to misclassification of PH and inappropriate application of treatment paradigms. Vasoreactivity testing, often with inhaled nitric oxide, is performed during right heart catheterization in PAH patients to determine responsiveness to vasodilator therapy. A substantial number of patients with PAH show little response (85%–90% are deemed nonresponders), but those found responsive to inhaled nitric oxide (defined as a >10 mm Hg decline in mPAP to <40 mm Hg, along with no change or increase in cardiac output) tend to also respond to calcium channel blockers and/or may benefit from advancing other targeted therapy (inhaled, parenteral, or oral) preoperatively (Fig. 9.3).

Outcome Studies

Interpretation of studies analyzing outcomes for PAH patients undergoing noncardiac surgery is complicated by inconsistency in how the disease was diagnosed and categorized (echo vs. right heart catheterization), how severity of disease was defined, and use of modern vasodilator therapy. Nonetheless, it is clear that PAH is associated with a high rate (up to 42% in one study) of perioperative morbidity (respiratory failure, dysrhythmia, heart failure, hemodynamic instability, prolonged intubation) and mortality (3.5%–18%). In a recent prospective survey of 114 well-characterized PAH patients undergoing surgery in the era of current vasodilator therapy, there was a 6.1% major complication rate and perioperative mortality of 3.5%. Importantly, mortality was higher for emergency procedures (15%) than nonemergent (2%), and risk was not different between general or spinal anesthesia. Recognized risk factors are summarized in Table 9.10.

Perioperative Physiology

Appreciation of the risk associated with PAH and the specific challenges presented to anesthetic management has prompted publication of reviews in the anesthesiology, cardiology, critical care, and surgical literature. Ultimately all emphasize the primary goal of maintaining optimal "mechanical coupling" between the right ventricle and pulmonary circulation to promote adequate left-sided filling and systemic perfusion. Any intervention that may affect RV preload, inotropy, afterload (including contributions from both small and large vessels), and oxygen supply/demand relationships needs to be considered. This takes on added complexity in the perioperative environment, where relatively common and generally benign events (transient hypotension, mechanical ventilation, modest hypercarbia, small bubbles in an intravenous line, Trendelenburg position, pneumoperitoneum, single-lung ventilation) can have potentially serious consequences.

Right Ventricular Afterload

A hallmark of PAH is increased RV afterload, leading to RV dilation, increased wall stress, and in the more chronic state, RV hypertrophy. Although often described simply as PVR (the *steady-state* mean pressure/mean flow relationship largely dictated by small vessels), the true interaction between the right ventricle and the pulmonary circulation is pulsatile and *dynamic* and involves the compliance and "stiffness" of large vessels as well as the resistance of small ones. This is particularly relevant to acute insults that may occur during surgery and affect RV pulsatile load. For example, large vessel compliance may be altered by events such as a change to prone or Trendelenburg positions, pneumoperitoneum during a laparoscopic procedure, or direct compression or displacement of the large pulmonary artery branches. In addition, ventilator management can have distinct effects on RV afterload via addition of positive end-expiratory pressure (PEEP), hypoventilation with hypercarbia and acidosis, and promotion of atelectasis.

Right Ventricular Inotropy

Some authors have advocated that for patients with PAH, attempts should be made to maintain the heart in a hypercontractile state. However, aspects of anesthetic care and intraoperative course can affect myocardial contractile performance via both direct and indirect mechanisms. Many of the drugs used for induction and maintenance of anesthesia have dose-related negative inotropic effects and also tend to depress the autonomic nervous system. Alternatively, high neuraxial anesthesia can produce an acute cardiac sympathectomy.

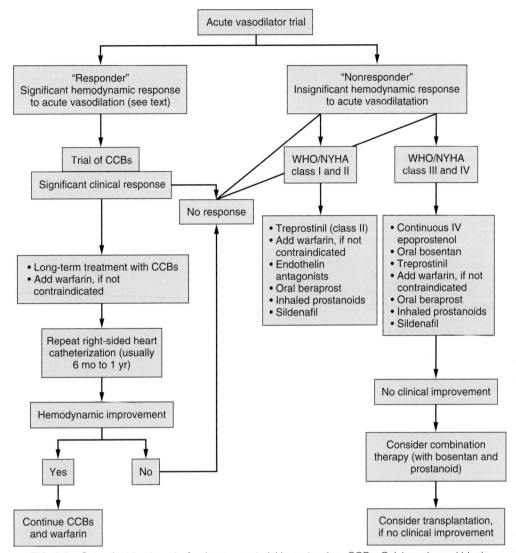

FIG. 9.3 Outpatient treatment of pulmonary arterial hypertension. *CCBs,* Calcium channel blockers; *IV,* intravenous; *NYHA,* New York Heart Association; *WHO,* World Health Organization. (Data from Dincer HE, Presberg KW. Current management of pulmonary hypertension. *Clin Pulm Med.* 2004;11:40-53.)

Nonetheless, acute RV decompensation from direct myocardial depression and/or sympatholysis has not been featured in outcome studies. Clinical and basic science investigations have suggested that the impact of negative inotropy on pump function of the left ventricle is offset to some degree by a simultaneous decline in afterload. Intriguingly, studies of the inhaled anesthetics isoflurane and desflurane have indicated a different effect on the RV. For example, data show that when the pulmonary circulation is normal, isoflurane increases total RV afterload. Whether the same response occurs in the setting of PAH is unclear, but clinical experience has not suggested that isoflurane or other volatile anesthetics are contraindicated. In contrast, acidosis is clearly detrimental both for effects on afterload and contractility. Even modest reductions in extracellular pH can negatively affect inotropy, and this effect becomes hemodynamically more pronounced when cardiac performance is tenuous to begin with.

Myocardial Supply and Demand

In contrast to the left ventricle, the thinner-walled right ventricle is subjected to greater wall tension for the same degree of increase in end-diastolic volume, leading to increased RV myocardial oxygen demand. Under normal circumstances the RV intramyocardial pressure is lower than the aortic root pressure, and the RV coronary perfusion occurs throughout the cardiac cycle. However, owing to the elevated RV intramyocardial pressure present in PAH, more coronary flow occurs during diastole, making the RV vulnerable to systemic hypotension, which worsens the mismatch between oxygen demand and supply and can precipitate ischemia even in the absence of coronary occlusive disease.

Interventricular Dependence

Systemic hypotension in combination with RV ischemia and high afterload may result in the "lethal combination" of RV

TABLE 9.10	Risk Factors for Morbidity and Mortality in Noncardiac Surgery in Patients With Pulmonary Arterial Hypertension

PATIENT FACTORS

History of PE, CAD, chronic renal disease
NYHA/WHO FC ≥ II
Higher ASA class
RAD on ECG
Echo parameters: RVH, RVMPI ≥ 0.75
Hemodynamics: higher PAP, RVSP/SBP ratio > 0.66

OPERATIVE FACTORS

Emergency surgery
Intermediate- or high-risk operations
   High risk for venous embolism (air, fat, cement)
   Elevation in venous pressure (Trendelenburg positioning, insufflation)
   Reduction in lung vascular volume (lung compression or resection)
   Induction of severe systemic inflammatory response
Longer duration of anesthesia
Intraoperative vasopressor use

ASA, American Society of Anesthesiologists; *CAD*, coronary artery disease; *ECG*, electrocardiogram; *FC*, functional class; *NYHA*, New York Heart Association; *PAP*, pulmonary artery pressure; *PE*, pulmonary embolism; *RAD*, right axis deviation; *RVH*, right ventricular hypertrophy; *RVMPI*, right ventricular myocardial performance index; *RVSP*, right ventricular systolic pressure; *SBP*, systolic blood pressure; *WHO*, World Health Organization.
Adapted from Goldsmith YB, Ivascu N, McGlothlin D, Heerdt PM, Horn EM. Perioperative management of pulmonary hypertension. In Klinger JR, Frantz RP, eds: *Diagnosis and Management of Pulmonary Hypertension.* New York: Springer; 2015:437-464.

dilatation, interventricular septal bulging, insufficient left ventricular filling, reduced stroke volume, and further systemic hypotension.

Procedural Considerations

Although the added risk of PAH in labor and delivery is understood by all clinicians involved with the parturient's care, the potential interaction of PH in general with aspects of other procedures may be underappreciated. This takes on added importance given recent data showing a shift in PH demographics toward an older population with more comorbidities.

Orthopedics

Although many procedures are amenable to regional or neuraxial anesthesia, concomitant intraoperative sedation can promote hypoventilation and hypercarbia. Superimposed on this is the added potential for embolic sequelae during major joint repair or replacement. Echocardiography studies have indicated embolic "showers" produced by different stages of joint replacement procedures that can acutely increase RV afterload. Consistent with these observations, database analysis has demonstrated a substantial increase in risk of perioperative morbidity and mortality in patients with PH undergoing hip and knee replacement.

Laparoscopy

Although laparoscopy has clear benefits in terms of postoperative pain and recovery time, the required carbon dioxide pneumoperitoneum has an acute impact on biventricular load and pump function. For the right ventricle in particular the combination of pneumoperitoneum, head-down position, and the increased inspiratory pressure required for mechanical ventilation and prevention of atelectasis affects filling pressures and both the magnitude and character of afterload. Even in otherwise healthy individuals, pneumoperitoneum can reduce cardiac output and produce an increase in pulmonary arterial pressure that may not immediately decline when the pneumoperitoneum is relieved. This has been linked to retained carbon dioxide and hypercarbia. Overall, although laparoscopy is generally well tolerated in normal individuals, it may not be in patients with PH and poorly compensated RV function.

Thoracic Surgery

The postoperative benefits of minimally invasive thoracoscopy are becoming increasingly clear, but the short-term stresses on the RV can be profound. Although thoracoscopy does not universally entail sustained pressurization of the chest similar to that produced in the abdomen during laparoscopy, it does involve nonventilation and atelectasis of the operative lung. Three features of this intentional lung collapse are particularly relevant to the PH patient: (1) some centers *transiently* pressurize the chest to facilitate onset of atelectasis; (2) there is a potential for systemic hypoxia; and (3) HPV will further increase RV afterload. To facilitate perioperative care, patients with PAH are often converted from oral to inhaled or parenteral pulmonary vasodilator therapy. Although the specific effect of parenteral pulmonary vasodilators on HPV during single-lung ventilation is not well described, to lessen the potential for HPV inhibition and systemic hypoxia, it has been recommended that inhaled pulmonary vasodilators be administered during single-lung ventilation to allow for limiting or even discontinuing intravenous therapy for a period of time. Finally, removal of lung tissue will decrease pulmonary vascular surface area, raising the probability that mPAP and PVR will remain increased from preoperative levels even when the operative lung is reexpanded.

KEY POINTS

- Hypertension is a significant risk factor for cardiovascular disease, stroke, and renal disease. The goal of antihypertensive therapy is to decrease the systemic blood pressure to less than 140/90 mm Hg, but a high percentage of patients remain poorly controlled.
- Hypertensive patients coming for surgery can pose management dilemmas for the anesthesiologist. However, the relationship between blood pressure control and perioperative complications is unclear, and clinical practices vary widely.

- Preoperative evaluation of a patient with hypertension should focus on the adequacy of blood pressure control, the antihypertensive drug regimen, and most importantly the presence of end-organ damage.
- There is no clear evidence that the incidence of postoperative complications is increased when patients with uncomplicated hypertension undergo elective surgery. However, hypertension associated with end-organ damage does increase surgical risk.
- Hemodynamic instability is common during anesthesia and surgery in hypertensive patient, even those patients effectively treated with antihypertensive drugs.
- Defined as a mean pulmonary artery pressure (mPAP) above 25 mm Hg, *pulmonary hypertension* (PH) can result from a range of processes that directly constrict and remodel arteries, elevate pulmonary venous pressure, or chronically increase blood flow to initiate vascular remodeling.
- Pulmonary arterial hypertension (PAH) represents one of five PH groups defined by the World Health Organization. Patients with PAH exhibit endothelial dysfunction, maladaptive arterial remodeling and cell proliferation, and in situ thrombosis.
- Right heart catheterization is required to provide a definitive PAH diagnosis and guide treatment. Only a small percentage respond to calcium channel blockade. Most current pulmonary vasodilator therapy consists of prostacyclin analogues, endothelin receptor antagonists, and drugs activating the guanylate cyclase pathway. PAH is the only class of PH found to exhibit therapeutic benefit in response to pulmonary vasodilator treatment. Although quality of life and survival have improved with increased vasodilator options, the prognosis for PAH patients remains poor.
- PH in general and PAH in particular increase the risk of perioperative morbidity and mortality. PAH patients receiving vasodilator therapy should have it continued intraoperatively and postoperatively, with plans made to convert from oral to parenteral or inhaled drugs when necessary.

RESOURCES

American College of Obstetrics and Gynecology. Committee on Obstetric Practice. *Emergent Therapy for Acute-Onset, Severe Hypertension During Pregnancy and the Postpartum Period*. Number. 623, February 2015.

Archer SL, Weir EK, Wilkins MR. Basic science of pulmonary arterial hypertension for clinicians: new concepts and experimental therapies. *Circulation*. 2010;121:2045-2066.

Aronson S, Fontes ML, Miao Y, Mangano DT. Investigators of the Multicenter Study of Perioperative Ischemia Research Group; Ischemia Research and Education Foundation. Risk index for perioperative renal dysfunction/failure: critical dependence on pulse pressure hypertension. *Circulation*. 2007;115:733-742.

Aronson S, Fontes ML. Hypertension: a new look at an old problem. *Curr Opin Anaesthesiol*. 2006;19:59-64.

Dodson GM, Bentley WE 4th, Awad A, Muntazar M, Goldberg ME. Isolated perioperative hypertension: clinical implications & contemporary treatment strategies. *Curr Hypertens Rev*. 2014;10:31-36.

Fleisher LA, Beckman JA, Brown KA, et al. American College of Cardiology/American Heart Association Task Force on Practice Guidelines (Writing Committee to Revise the 2002 Guidelines on Perioperative Cardiovascular Evaluation for Noncardiac Surgery); American Society of Echocardiography; American Society of Nuclear Cardiology; Heart Rhythm Society; Society of Cardiovascular Anesthesiologists; Society for Cardiovascular Angiography and Interventions; Society for Vascular Medicine and Biology; Society for Vascular Surgery. ACC/AHA 2007 guidelines on perioperative cardiovascular evaluation and care for noncardiac surgery: executive summary: a report of the American College of Cardiology/American Heart Association Task Force on Practice Guidelines. *Anesth Analg*. 2008;106:685-712.

Friedman SE, Andrus BW. Obesity and pulmonary hypertension: a review of pathophysiologic mechanisms. *J Obes*. 2012;2012:505274.

Gei A, Montúfar-Rueda C. Pulmonary hypertension and pregnancy: an overview. *Clin Obstet Gynecol*. 2014;57:806-826.

Goldman L, Caldera DL. Risks of general anesthesia and elective operation in the hypertensive patient. *Anesthesiology*. 1979;50:285-292.

Goldsmith YB, Ivascu N, McGlothlin D, Heerdt PM, Horn EM. Perioperative management of pulmonary hypertension. In: Klinger JR, Frantz RP, eds. *Diagnosis and Management of Pulmonary Hypertension*. New York: Springer; 2015:437-464.

Grassi G, Ram VS. Evidence for a critical role of the sympathetic nervous system in hypertension. *J Am Soc Hypertens*. 2016;10:457-466.

Harris SN, Ballantyne GH, Luther MA, et al. Alterations of cardiovascular performance during laparoscopic colectomy: a combined hemodynamic and echocardiographic analysis. *Anesth Analg*. 1996;83:482-487.

Friedman SE, Andrus BW. Obesity and pulmonary hypertension: a review of pathophysiologic mechanisms. *J Obes*. 2012;2012:505274.

James PA, Oparil S, Carter BL, et al. 2014 evidence-based guideline for the management of high blood pressure in adults. Report from the panel members appointed to the Eighth Joint National Committee (JNC 8). *JAMA*. 2014;311:507-520.

Laurent S, Boutouyrie P. The structural factor of hypertension: large and small artery alterations. *Circ Res*. 2015;116:1007-1021.

Lonjaret L, Lairez O, Minville V, Geeraerts T. Optimal perioperative management of arterial blood pressure. *Integr Blood Press Control*. 2014;7:49-59.

McGlothlin D, Ivascu N, Heerdt PM. Anesthesia and pulmonary hypertension. *Prog Cardiovasc Dis*. 2012;55:199-217.

McLaughlin VV, Archer SL, Badesch DB, Barst RJ, Farber HW, Lindner JR, et al. for the American College of Cardiology Foundation Task Force on Expert Consensus Documents and the American Heart Association. ACCF/AHA 2009 expert consensus document on pulmonary hypertension developed in collaboration with the American College of Chest Physicians, American Thoracic Society, and the Pulmonary Hypertension Association. *Circulation*. 2009;119:2250-2294.

Memtsoudis SG, Ma Y, Chiu YL, Walz JM, Voswinckel R, Mazumdar M. Perioperative mortality in patients with pulmonary hypertension undergoing major joint replacement. *Anesth Analg*. 2010;111:1110-1116.

Meyer S, McLaughlin VV, Seyfarth HJ, et al. Outcomes of noncardiac, nonobstetric surgery in patients with PAH: an international prospective survey. *Eur Respir J*. 2013;41:1302-1307.

Minai OA, Yared JP, Kaw R, Subramaniam K, Hill NS. Perioperative risk and management in patients with pulmonary hypertension. *Chest*. 2013;144:329-340.

Oparil S, Schmieder RE. New approaches in the treatment of hypertension. *Circ Res*. 2015;116:1074-1095.

Osseyran Samper F, Vicente Guillen R. Severe pulmonary hypertension: implications for anesthesia in laparoscopic surgery. *Rev Esp Anestesiol Reanim*. 2008;55:438-441.

Pilkington SA, Taboada D, Martinez G. Pulmonary hypertension and its management in patients undergoing non-cardiac surgery. *Anaesthesia*. 2015;70:56-70.

Rahimi K, Emdin CA, MacMahon S. The epidemiology of blood pressure and its worldwide management. *Circ Res*. 2015;116(6):925-936.

Schmieder RE. End organ damage in hypertension. *Dtsch Arztebl Int*. 2010;107:866-873.

Sear JW. Perioperative control of hypertension: when will it adversely affect perioperative outcome? *Curr Hypertens Rep.* 2008;10:480-487.

Sharma M, Pinnamaneni S, Aronow WS, Jozwik B, Frishman WH. Existing drugs and agents under investigation for pulmonary arterial hypertension. *Cardiol Rev.* 2014;22:297-305.

Simonneau G, Gatzoulis MA, Adatia I, et al. Updated clinical classification of pulmonary hypertension. *J Am Coll Cardiol.* 2013;62:D34-D41.

Solak Y, Afsar B, Vaziri ND, Aslan G, Yalcin CE, Covic A, Kanbay M. Hypertension as an autoimmune and inflammatory disease. *Hypertens Res.* 2016 Apr 7. http://dx.doi.org/10.1038/hr.2016.35. [Epub ahead of print].

Szelkowski LA, Puri NK, Singh R, Massimiano PS. Current trends in preoperative, intraoperative, and postoperative care of the adult cardiac surgery patient. *Curr Probl Surg.* 2015;52:531-569.

Heart Failure and Cardiomyopathies

WANDA M. POPESCU, ADNAN MALIK

HEART FAILURE

Definition

Heart failure is a complex pathophysiologic state characterized by the inability of the heart to fill with or eject blood at a rate appropriate to meet tissue requirements. Symptoms of dyspnea and fatigue and signs of circulatory congestion and/or hypoperfusion are the clinical features of the heart failure syndrome. This clinical syndrome of heart failure may result from *structural* or *functional* impairment of the pericardium, myocardium, endocardium, heart valves, great vessels, or certain metabolic abnormalities. However, the majority of heart failure cases are caused by impaired left ventricular (LV) myocardial function.

Epidemiology and Costs

Heart failure is a major health problem in the United States, affecting about 5 million adults; each year an additional 550,000 patients are diagnosed. Heart failure is responsible for about 287,000 deaths per year. This is mainly a disease of the elderly, so aging of the population is contributing to its increased incidence. In the population of patients 65–69 years, its incidence is approximately 20 per 1000 individuals, and in the population older than 85 years, it is over 80 per

1000 individuals. About 23 million people worldwide carry a diagnosis of heart failure, and the prevalence is expected to increase over the coming years. The epidemiology of heart failure varies based on race and gender, with black males having the highest risk of developing heart failure. *Systolic heart failure* is more common among *middle-aged men* because of its association with coronary artery disease. *Diastolic heart failure* is usually seen in *elderly women* because of its association with hypertension, obesity, and diabetes mellitus after menopause.

In the United States, more than 1 million hospitalizations per year list heart failure as the primary diagnosis. The 30-day readmission rate for patients with heart failure is the highest of all diagnoses and approaches 25%. Heart failure is the most common Medicare hospital discharge diagnosis. More Medicare dollars are spent on the diagnosis and treatment of heart failure than on any other disease. It is estimated that the annual total direct and indirect cost of heart failure in the United States is $32 billion and is expected to increase to roughly $70 billion by 2030.

Etiology

Heart failure is a clinical syndrome arising from diverse heart failure causes that may co-exist and interact with each other. The principal pathophysiologic feature of heart failure is the inability of the heart to fill or empty the ventricles. Heart failure is most often a result of (1) impaired myocardial contractility caused by ischemic heart disease or cardiomyopathy, (2) cardiac valve abnormalities, (3) systemic hypertension, (4) diseases of the pericardium, or (5) pulmonary hypertension (cor pulmonale). The most common cause of right ventricular failure is left ventricular failure.

FORMS OF VENTRICULAR DYSFUNCTION

Heart failure may be described in various ways: systolic or diastolic, acute or chronic, left sided or right sided, high output or low output. Early in the course of heart failure, the various categories may have different clinical and therapeutic implications. Ultimately, however, *all forms* of heart failure are characterized by a high ventricular end-diastolic pressure due to altered ventricular function and neurohormonal regulation.

Systolic and Diastolic Heart Failure

Decreased ventricular systolic wall motion reflects systolic dysfunction, whereas diastolic dysfunction is characterized by abnormal ventricular relaxation and reduced compliance. There are differences in both myocardial architecture and function in systolic and diastolic heart failure, but clinical signs and symptoms cannot reliably differentiate between these two entities.

Systolic Heart Failure
Causes of systolic heart failure include coronary artery disease, dilated cardiomyopathy, chronic pressure overload from aortic stenosis or chronic hypertension, and chronic volume overload from regurgitant valvular lesions or high-output cardiac failure. Coronary disease typically results in *regional defects* in ventricular contraction that may become global over time, whereas all other causes of systolic heart failure produce *global* ventricular dysfunction. Ventricular dysrhythmias are common in patients with LV dysfunction. Patients with left bundle branch block and systolic heart failure are at high risk of sudden death.

A decreased ejection fraction (EF), the hallmark of chronic LV systolic dysfunction, is closely related to the increase in the diastolic volume of the LV (Fig. 10.1). Measuring the LVEF via echocardiography, magnetic resonance imaging (MRI), radionuclide imaging, or ventriculography provides the data necessary to document the severity of ventricular systolic dysfunction.

Diastolic Heart Failure
Symptomatic heart failure in patients with normal or near-normal LV systolic function is most likely due to diastolic dysfunction. However, diastolic heart failure may co-exist with systolic heart failure. The prevalence of diastolic heart failure is age dependent, increasing from less than 15% in patients younger than 45 years to 35% in those between the ages of 50 and 70 to more than 50% in patients older than 70 years. Diastolic heart failure can be classified into four stages. Class I is characterized by an abnormal LV relaxation pattern with normal left atrial pressure. Classes II, III, and IV are characterized by abnormal relaxation and reduced LV compliance resulting in an increase in LV end-diastolic pressure (LVEDP). As a compensatory mechanism the pressure in the left atrium increases so that LV filling can occur despite the increase in LVEDP. Factors that predispose to decreased ventricular distensibility include myocardial edema, fibrosis, hypertrophy, aging, and pressure overload. Ischemic heart disease, long-standing systemic hypertension, and progressive aortic stenosis are the most common causes of diastolic heart failure. In contrast to systolic heart failure, diastolic heart failure affects women more than men. Hospitalization and mortality rates are similar in patients with systolic and diastolic heart failure. The major differences between systolic and diastolic heart failure are presented in Table 10.1.

Acute and Chronic Heart Failure

Acute heart failure is defined as a change in the signs and symptoms of heart failure requiring *emergency* therapy. Chronic heart failure is present in patients with *long-standing* cardiac disease. Typically, chronic heart failure is accompanied by venous congestion, but blood pressure is maintained. In acute heart failure due to a sudden decrease in cardiac output, systemic hypotension is often present without signs of peripheral edema. Acute heart failure encompasses three entities: (1) worsening chronic heart failure, (2) new-onset heart failure (such as that caused by cardiac valve rupture, large myocardial infarction [MI], or severe hypertensive crisis), and (3) terminal heart failure that is refractory to therapy.

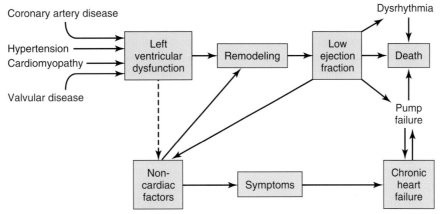

FIG. 10.1 Left ventricular dysfunction, regardless of cause, results in progressive remodeling of the ventricular chamber leading to dilation and a low ejection fraction. Cardiac dysrhythmias, progressive cardiac failure, and premature death are likely. Noncardiac factors such as neurohormonal stimulation, vasoconstriction, and renal sodium retention may be stimulated by left ventricular dysfunction and ultimately contribute to remodeling of the left ventricle and to the symptoms (dyspnea, fatigue, edema) considered characteristic of the clinical syndrome of congestive heart failure. (Adapted from Cohn JN. The management of chronic heart failure. *N Engl J Med.* 1996;335: 490-498. Copyright 1996 Massachusetts Medical Society. All rights reserved.)

TABLE 10.1	Characteristics of Patients With Diastolic Heart Failure and Patients With Systolic Heart Failure	
Characteristic	Diastolic Heart Failure	Systolic Heart Failure
Age	Frequently elderly	Typically 50–70 yr
Sex	Frequently female	More often male
Left ventricular ejection fraction	Preserved, ≥40%	Depressed, ≤40%
Left ventricular cavity size	Usually normal, often with concentric left ventricular hypertrophy	Usually dilated
Chest radiograph	Congestion ± cardiomegaly	Congestion and cardiomegaly
Gallop rhythm present	Fourth heart sound	Third heart sound
Hypertension	+++	++
Diabetes mellitus	+++	++
Previous myocardial infarction	+	+++
Obesity	+++	+
Chronic lung disease	++	0
Sleep apnea	++	++
Dialysis	++	0
Atrial fibrillation	+ Usually paroxysmal	+ Usually persistent

Left-Sided and Right-Sided Heart Failure

Increased ventricular pressures and subsequent fluid accumulation upstream from the affected ventricle produce the clinical signs and symptoms of heart failure. In left-sided heart failure, high LVEDP promotes pulmonary venous congestion. The patient complains of dyspnea, orthopnea, and paroxysmal nocturnal dyspnea, which can evolve into pulmonary edema. Right-sided heart failure causes systemic venous congestion. Peripheral edema and congestive hepatomegaly are the most prominent clinical manifestations. Right-sided heart failure may be caused by pulmonary hypertension or right ventricular (RV) myocardial infarction, but the most common cause is left-sided heart failure.

Low-Output and High-Output Heart Failure

The *normal cardiac index* varies between 2.2 and 3.5 L/min/m². It may be difficult to diagnose low-output heart failure, because a patient may have a cardiac index that is nearly normal in the resting state but shows an inadequate response to stress or exercise. The most common causes of low-output heart failure are coronary artery disease, cardiomyopathy, hypertension, valvular disease, and pericardial disease.

Causes of high cardiac output include anemia, pregnancy, arteriovenous fistulas, severe hyperthyroidism, beriberi, and Paget's disease. The ventricles fail not only because of increased hemodynamic burden but also because of direct myocardial toxicity (thyrotoxicosis and beriberi) or myocardial hypoxia caused by severe and prolonged anemia.

PATHOPHYSIOLOGY OF HEART FAILURE

Heart failure is a complex phenomenon at both the clinical and cellular levels. Our understanding of the pathophysiology of heart failure is evolving. The initiating mechanisms are pressure overload (aortic stenosis, systemic hypertension), volume overload (mitral or aortic regurgitation), myocardial ischemia or infarction, myocarditis, and restricted diastolic filling (constrictive pericarditis, restrictive cardiomyopathy). In the failing ventricle, various adaptive mechanisms are initiated to help maintain a normal cardiac output. These include (1) increases in stroke volume according to the Frank-Starling relationship, (2) activation of the sympathetic nervous system, (3) alterations in the inotropic state, heart rate, and afterload, and (4) humorally mediated responses. In more advanced stages of heart failure, these mechanisms become maladaptive and ultimately lead to *myocardial remodeling,* which is the key pathophysiologic change responsible for the development and progression of heart failure.

Frank-Starling Relationship

The Frank-Starling relationship describes the increase in stroke volume that accompanies an increase in LV end-diastolic volume and pressure (Fig. 10.2). Stroke volume increases because the tension developed by contracting muscle is greater when the resting length of that muscle is increased. Constriction of venous capacitance vessels shifts blood centrally, increases preload, and helps maintain cardiac output by the Frank-Starling relationship. The magnitude of the increase in stroke volume produced by changing the tension of ventricular muscle fibers depends on myocardial contractility. When myocardial contractility is decreased, as in the presence of heart failure, a lesser increase in stroke volume is achieved relative to any given increase in LVEDP.

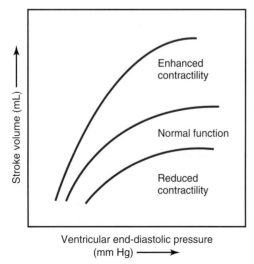

FIG. 10.2 The Frank-Starling relationship states that stroke volume is directly related to ventricular end-diastolic pressure.

Activation of the Sympathetic Nervous System

Activation of the sympathetic nervous system promotes arteriolar and venous constriction. Arteriolar constriction serves to maintain systemic blood pressure despite a decrease in cardiac output. Increased venous tone shifts blood from peripheral sites to the central circulation, thereby enhancing venous return and maintaining cardiac output by the Frank-Starling relationship. Furthermore, arteriolar constriction causes redistribution of blood from the kidneys, splanchnic circulation, skeletal muscles, and skin to maintain coronary and cerebral blood flow despite an overall decrease in cardiac output. The decrease in renal blood flow activates the renin-angiotensin-aldosterone system (RAAS), which increases renal tubular reabsorption of sodium and water and thus results in an increase in blood volume and ultimately cardiac output by the Frank-Starling relationship. These compensatory responses may be effective in the short term, but they contribute to the deterioration of heart failure in the long term. For example, fluid retention, increased venous return, and increased afterload impose more work on the failing myocardium, increase myocardial energy expenditure, and further reduce cardiac output and tissue perfusion. Interruption of this vicious circle is the purpose of the current therapeutic strategies for heart failure.

Although heart failure is associated with sympathetic activation, a downregulation of β-adrenergic receptors is observed. Plasma and urinary concentrations of catecholamines are increased, and these elevated levels correlate with worse clinical outcomes. High plasma levels of norepinephrine are directly cardiotoxic and promote myocyte necrosis, which leads to ventricular remodeling. Therapy with β-blockers is aimed at decreasing the deleterious effects of catecholamines on the heart.

Alterations in Inotropy, Heart Rate, and Afterload

The *inotropic state* describes myocardial contractility as reflected by the velocity of contraction developed by cardiac muscle. The maximum velocity of contraction is referred to as V_{max}. When the inotropic state of the heart is increased, as in the presence of catecholamines, V_{max} is increased. Conversely, V_{max} is decreased when myocardial contractility is impaired, as in heart failure.

Afterload is the tension the ventricular muscle must develop to open the aortic or pulmonic valve. The afterload presented to the left ventricle is increased in the presence of systemic arteriolar constriction and hypertension. Administration of vasodilating drugs can increase LV stroke volume in patients with heart failure.

In the presence of systolic heart failure and low cardiac output, stroke volume is relatively fixed, and any increase in cardiac output depends on an increase in heart rate. Tachycardia is an expected finding in the presence of systolic heart failure with a low EF and reflects activation of the sympathetic nervous system. In the presence of diastolic heart failure, however, tachycardia can produce a decrease in cardiac output resulting from inadequate ventricular relaxation and filling time. Therefore heart rate control is an important goal in the treatment of diastolic heart failure.

Humorally Mediated Responses and Biochemical Pathways

As heart failure progresses, various neurohumoral pathways are activated to maintain adequate cardiac output during exercise and ultimately even at rest. Generalized vasoconstriction is initiated via several mechanisms, including increased activity of the sympathetic nervous system and the RAAS, parasympathetic withdrawal, high levels of circulating vasopressin, endothelial dysfunction, and release of inflammatory mediators.

In an attempt to counterbalance these mechanisms, the heart evolves into an "endocrine" organ. This concept emerged more than 20 years ago when the presence of a potent diuretic and vasodilator was found in the atria of rats. Atrial natriuretic peptide (ANP) is stored in atrial muscle and released in response to increases in atrial pressure, such as are produced by tachycardia or hypervolemia. B-type natriuretic peptide (BNP) is secreted by both the atrial and ventricular myocardium. In the failing heart the ventricle becomes the principal site of BNP production. The natriuretic peptides promote blood pressure control and protect the cardiovascular system from the effects of volume and pressure overload. Physiologic effects of the natriuretic peptides include diuresis, natriuresis, vasodilation, antiinflammatory effect, and inhibition of the RAAS and the sympathetic nervous system. Both ANP and BNP inhibit cardiac hypertrophy and fibrosis and therefore limit remodeling. The response to elevated levels of *endogenous* natriuretic peptides is blunted over time in heart failure. However, *exogenous* administration of BNP can be useful in the treatment of acute heart failure. More recently, other protective neurohumoral pathways have been described. *Chromogranin A* and its derived peptides *catestatin* and *vasostatin* appear to counteract the negative effects of excessive sympathetic stimulation on the myocardium.

Myocardial Remodeling

Myocardial remodeling is the result of the various *endogenous* mechanisms the body uses to maintain cardiac output. *It is the process by which mechanical, neurohormonal, and genetic factors change LV size, shape, and function.* The process includes myocardial hypertrophy, myocardial dilatation and wall thinning, increased interstitial collagen deposition, myocardial fibrosis, and scar formation resulting from myocyte death. Myocardial hypertrophy represents the compensatory mechanism for chronic pressure overload. The effects of this mechanism are limited, however, because hypertrophied cardiac muscle functions at a lower inotropic state than normal cardiac muscle. Cardiac dilatation occurs in

response to volume overload and increases cardiac output by the Frank-Starling relationship. However, the increased cardiac wall tension produced by an enlarged ventricular radius is associated with increased myocardial oxygen requirements and decreased pumping efficiency. Ischemic injury is the most common cause of myocardial remodeling and encompasses both hypertrophy and dilatation of the left ventricle. Angiotensin-converting enzyme (ACE) inhibitors and aldosterone inhibitors (spironolactone and eplerenone) have been proven to promote a *"reverse remodeling"* process. Therefore they are indicated as first-line therapy for heart failure. Several studies have also documented that cardiac resynchronization therapy has beneficial reverse remodeling effects, not only in patients with advanced heart failure but also in patients with milder forms of heart failure who exhibit wide QRS complexes.

SYMPTOMS AND SIGNS OF HEART FAILURE

The hemodynamic consequences of heart failure include decreased cardiac output, increased LVEDP, peripheral vasoconstriction, retention of sodium and water, and decreased oxygen delivery to the tissues with a widened arterial-venous oxygen difference. LV failure results in signs and symptoms of pulmonary edema, whereas RV failure results in systemic venous hypertension and peripheral edema. Fatigue and organ system dysfunction are related to inadequate cardiac output.

Symptoms

Dyspnea reflects the increased work of breathing caused by stiffness of the lungs produced by interstitial pulmonary edema. It is one of the earliest subjective findings of LV failure and initially occurs only with exertion. Dyspnea can be quantified by asking the patient how many flights of stairs can be climbed or the distance that can be walked at a normal pace before symptoms begin. Some patients experiencing angina pectoris may interpret substernal discomfort as breathlessness. Dyspnea can be caused by many other diseases, including asthma, chronic obstructive pulmonary disease (COPD), airway obstruction, anxiety, and neuromuscular weakness. Dyspnea related to heart failure will be linked to other supporting evidence such as a history of orthopnea, paroxysmal nocturnal dyspnea, a third heart sound, rales on physical examination, and elevated BNP levels.

Orthopnea reflects the inability of the failing LV to handle the increase in venous return associated with the recumbent position. Clinically, orthopnea is manifested as a dry nonproductive cough that develops in the supine position and is relieved by sitting up. The orthopneic cough differs from the productive morning cough characteristic of chronic bronchitis and must be differentiated from the cough produced by ACE inhibitors. Paroxysmal nocturnal dyspnea is shortness of breath that awakens a patient from sleep. This symptom must be differentiated from anxiety-provoked hyperventilation or wheezing resulting from accumulation of secretions in patients with chronic bronchitis. Paroxysmal nocturnal dyspnea and wheezing caused by pulmonary congestion *(cardiac asthma)* are accompanied by radiographic evidence of pulmonary congestion.

Hallmarks of decreased cardiac reserve and low cardiac output include fatigue and weakness at rest or with minimal exertion. During exercise the failing ventricle is unable to increase its output to deliver adequate amounts of oxygen to muscles. These symptoms of fatigue and weakness, although nonspecific, are very common in patients with heart failure.

Heart failure patients may complain of anorexia, nausea, or abdominal pain related to liver congestion or prerenal azotemia. Decreases in cerebral blood flow may produce confusion, difficulty concentrating, insomnia, anxiety, or memory deficits. Anemia is frequently encountered in patients with advanced stages of heart failure. The cause of this anemia appears to be related to the decrease in cardiac output and therefore a decrease in renal blood flow. The subsequent RAAS activation leads to increased erythropoietin production. However, in these patients the bone marrow is less sensitive to this hormone and does not respond with increased production of red blood cells.

Signs

The classic physical findings in patients with LV failure are tachypnea and moist rales. These rales may be confined to the lung bases with mild heart failure, or they may be diffuse in those with pulmonary edema. Other findings of heart failure include a resting tachycardia and a third heart sound (S_3

gallop). This heart sound is produced by blood entering and distending a relatively noncompliant left ventricle. Despite peripheral vasoconstriction, severe heart failure may manifest as *systemic hypotension* with cool and pale extremities. Lip and nail bed cyanosis may be present. A narrow pulse pressure with a high diastolic pressure reflects a decreased stroke volume. Marked weight loss, also known as *cardiac cachexia,* is a sign of severe chronic heart failure. This weight loss is caused by a combination of factors, including an increase in the metabolic rate, anorexia, nausea, decreased intestinal absorption of food due to splanchnic venous congestion, and the presence of high levels of circulating cytokines.

With right-sided heart failure or biventricular failure, jugular venous distention may be present or may be inducible by pressing on the liver *(hepatojugular reflux).* The liver is typically the first organ to become engorged with blood in the presence of right-sided or biventricular failure. The hepatic engorgement may be associated with right upper quadrant pain and tenderness or even jaundice in severe cases. Pleural effusions (usually right sided) may be present. Bilateral pitting pretibial edema is typically present and reflects both venous congestion and sodium and water retention.

DIAGNOSIS OF HEART FAILURE

The diagnosis of heart failure is based on the history, physical examination findings, and results of laboratory and diagnostic tests. Various criteria for the diagnosis of heart failure have been developed; the most commonly used are presented in Table 10.2.

TABLE 10.2	Diagnostic Criteria for Heart Failure		
Framingham Criteria	**Boston Criteria**	**ESC Criteria**	
Major criteria	*History*	1. Symptoms of heart failure	
PND or orthopnea	Rest dyspnea, 4p		
Neck vein distension	Orthopnea, 4p	*and*	
Rales	PND, 3p		
Cardiomegaly	Dyspnea while walking on level area, 2p	2. Signs of cardiac dysfunction	
Acute pulmonary edema	Dyspnea while climbing, 1p		
Third heart sound	*Physical examination*	*and*	
Increased central venous pressure	Heart rate abnormality, 1–2p		
Circulation time > 25 s	Jugular venous distension, 1–2p	3. Demonstration of an underlying cardiac cause	
Hepatojugular reflux	Lung crackles, 1–2p		
Weight loss > 4.5 kg in 5 days with treatment			
Minor criteria	Wheezing, 3p		
Bilateral ankle edema	Third heart sound, 3p		
Nocturnal cough	*Chest radiography*		
DOE	Alveolar pulmonary edema, 4p		
Hepatomegaly	Interstitial pulmonary edema, 3p		
Pleural effusion	Bilateral pleural effusion, 3p		
	Cardiothoracic ratio > 0.5, 3p		
Reduction in vital capacity by 1/3	Upper zone flow redistribution, 2p		
Tachycardia > 120 bpm			
Heart failure present if:	Definite heart failure: 8–12p	Criteria 1 and 2 should always be fulfilled	
2 major criteria or	Possible heart failure: 5–7p		
1 major + 2 minor criteria	Unlikely heart failure: <4p		

bpm, Beats per minute; *DOE,* dyspnea on exertion; *ESC,* European Society of Cardiology; *p,* points; *PND,* paroxysmal nocturnal dyspnea.

Laboratory Tests

The differential diagnosis of dyspnea continues to be challenging both in the urgent/emergent setting and in the primary care setting. The use of serum levels of BNP and its associated N-terminal fragment NT-proBNP as biomarkers for heart failure can help establish the cause of dyspnea. Plasma BNP levels below 100 pg/mL indicate that heart failure is unlikely (90% negative predictive value). BNP levels in the range of 100–500 pg/mL suggest an intermediate probability of heart failure. Levels above 500 pg/mL are consistent with the diagnosis of heart failure (90% positive predictive value). An NT-proBNP level of 300 pg/mL appears to be a sensitive cutoff point for detecting dyspnea of cardiac origin. Plasma levels of BNP and NT-proBNP may be affected by other factors such as gender, advanced age, renal function, obesity, pulmonary embolism, atrial fibrillation, and other tachydysrhythmias. Therefore the interpretation of BNP levels requires a clinical context. Both the 2013 American College of Cardiology/American Heart Association (ACC/AHA) guidelines for the management of heart failure and the 2014 Canadian Cardiovascular Society heart failure management guidelines recommend use of these biomarkers for the purpose of confirming the diagnosis of heart failure, risk stratification, and to guide therapeutic management.

Recently, additional biomarkers have evolved into useful adjuncts in the diagnosis and risk stratification of patients with heart failure. With systolic heart failure, increased circulating levels of high-sensitivity cardiac troponins correlate with more severe disease. These biomarkers represent a powerful predictor of mortality and cardiovascular events in both ambulatory and acutely decompensating patients. Soluble toll-like receptor 2 (ST2) is a transmembrane receptor that regulates inflammation and immunity. In the heart it promotes cardiac hypertrophy, fibrosis, and ventricular dysfunction. Its release into the circulation is stimulated by myocyte stress and an increased diastolic workload. Increased circulating levels of soluble ST2 are independently associated with higher mortality and disease progression and offer additive information to NT-proBNP measurement. Neutrophil gelatinase-associated lipocalin (NGAL) and cystatin C are renal function biomarkers. The use of such biomarkers in clinical practice may allow for earlier and more sensitive detection of a deterioration in renal function and improve risk stratification. However, there is no evidence that the use of renal biomarkers improves clinical outcomes in heart failure patients.

A complete metabolic profile should be obtained. Decreases in renal blood flow may lead to prerenal azotemia, characterized by a disproportionate increase in blood urea nitrogen concentration relative to serum creatinine concentration. When moderate liver congestion is present, liver enzyme levels may be mildly elevated, and when liver engorgement is severe, the prothrombin time may be prolonged. Hyponatremia, hypomagnesemia, and hypokalemia may also be present.

Electrocardiography

Patients with heart failure usually have abnormalities on the 12-lead electrocardiogram (ECG). Therefore the *ECG has a low predictive value for the diagnosis of heart failure.* The ECG may show evidence of previous MI, LV hypertrophy, conduction abnormalities (left bundle branch block, widened QRS complex), or various dysrhythmias, especially atrial fibrillation and ventricular dysrhythmias.

Chest Radiography

Chest radiography (posteroanterior and lateral views) may detect the presence of pulmonary disease, cardiomegaly, pulmonary venous congestion, and interstitial or alveolar pulmonary edema. An early radiographic sign of LV failure and associated pulmonary venous hypertension is distention of the pulmonary veins in the upper lobes of the lungs. Perivascular edema appears as hilar or perihilar haze. The hilum appears large with ill-defined margins. Kerley's lines, which reflect edematous interlobular septae in the upper lung fields (Kerley's A lines), lower lung fields (Kerley's B lines), or basilar regions of the lungs (Kerley's C lines) and produce a honeycomb pattern, may also be present. Alveolar edema produces homogeneous densities in the lung fields, typically in a butterfly pattern. Pleural effusion and pericardial effusion may be observed. Radiographic evidence of pulmonary edema may lag behind the clinical evidence of pulmonary edema by up to 12 hours. Likewise, radiographic patterns of pulmonary congestion may persist for several days after normalization of cardiac filling pressures and resolution of symptoms.

Echocardiography

Echocardiography is the most useful test in the diagnosis of heart failure. Comprehensive two-dimensional echocardiography coupled with Doppler flow examination can assess whether any abnormalities of the myocardium, cardiac valves, or pericardium are present. This examination can evaluate left and right ventricular structure and function in both systole and diastole, as well as valvular function, and can detect the presence of pericardial disease. This information is presented as numerical estimates of EF, LV size and wall thickness, left atrial size, and pulmonary artery pressure, as well as a description of anatomic structures and wall motion. Assessment of diastolic function provides information regarding LV filling and left atrial pressure. A preoperative echocardiographic evaluation provides information useful in guiding perioperative management and serves as a baseline for comparison if the patient's condition changes.

CLASSIFICATION OF HEART FAILURE

Heart failure has been classified in various ways. The most commonly used classification is that of the New York Heart Association (NYHA) and is based on the functional status of the patient at a particular time. Functional status may worsen or improve. The classification is intended for patients who have structural heart disease and symptoms of heart failure. There are four functional classes:

Class I: Ordinary physical activity does not cause symptoms.
Class II: Symptoms occur with ordinary exertion.
Class III: Symptoms occur with less-than-ordinary exertion.
Class IV: Symptoms occur at rest.

This classification is useful because the severity of the symptoms has an excellent correlation with quality of life and survival.

The 2005 ACC/AHA guideline update for the diagnosis and management of chronic heart failure introduced a new classification based on progression of the disease. This classification is meant to be complementary to the NYHA classification and to be used in guiding therapy. The ACC/AHA classification of heart failure stratifies patients into four disease stages:

Stage A: Patients at high risk of heart failure but without structural heart disease or symptoms of heart failure

Stage B: Patients with structural heart disease but without symptoms of heart failure

Stage C: Patients with structural heart disease with previous or current symptoms of heart failure

Stage D: Patients with refractory heart failure requiring specialized interventions

MANAGEMENT OF HEART FAILURE

Current therapeutic strategies are aimed at reversing the pathophysiologic alterations present in heart failure and interrupting the vicious circle of maladaptive mechanisms (Fig. 10.3). Short-term therapeutic goals include relieving symptoms of circulatory congestion, increasing tissue perfusion, and improving quality of life. However, management of heart failure involves more than symptomatic treatment. The processes that contributed to the LV dysfunction may progress independently of the development of symptoms. *Therefore the long-term therapeutic goal is to prolong life by slowing or reversing the progression of ventricular remodeling.*

Management of Chronic Heart Failure

Current therapeutic protocols are based on the results of large, adequately powered randomized trials and on the ACC/AHA and European Society of Cardiology (ESC) guidelines for the diagnosis and treatment of chronic heart failure. According to these guidelines, treatment options include lifestyle modification, patient and family education, medical therapy, corrective surgery, implantation of cardiac devices, and cardiac transplantation (Fig. 10.4).

Lifestyle modifications are aimed at decreasing the risk of heart disease and include smoking cessation, adherence to a healthy diet with moderate sodium restriction, weight control, exercise, moderation of alcohol consumption, and adequate glycemic control. It is estimated that a decrease of 30% in the incidence of obesity would reduce the incidence of heart

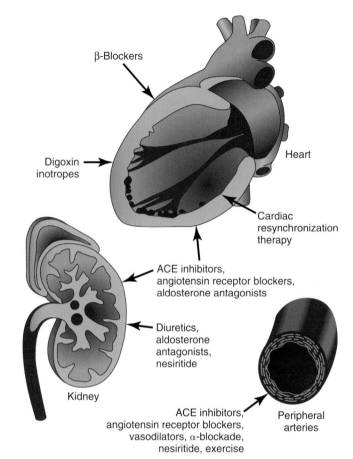

FIG. 10.3 Primary targets of treatment in heart failure. Treatment options for patients with heart failure affect the pathophysiologic mechanisms that are stimulated in heart failure. Angiotensin-converting enzyme (ACE) inhibitors and angiotensin II receptor blockers decrease afterload by interfering with the renin-angiotensin-aldosterone system, which results in peripheral vasodilation. They also affect left ventricular hypertrophy, remodeling, and renal blood flow. Aldosterone production by the adrenal glands is increased in heart failure. It stimulates renal sodium retention and potassium excretion and promotes ventricular and vascular hypertrophy. Aldosterone antagonists counteract the many effects of aldosterone. Diuretics decrease preload by stimulating natriuresis in the kidneys. Digoxin affects the sodium-potassium adenosinetriphosphatase (Na^+,K^+-ATPase) pump in the myocardial cell, increasing contractility. Inotropes such as dobutamine and milrinone increase myocardial contractility. β-blockers inhibit the sympathetic nervous system and adrenergic receptors. They slow the heart rate, decrease blood pressure, and have a direct beneficial effect on the myocardium by enhancing reverse remodeling. Selected agents that also block α-adrenergic receptors can cause vasodilation. Vasodilator therapy such as combination therapy with hydralazine and isosorbide dinitrate decreases afterload by counteracting peripheral vasoconstriction. Cardiac resynchronization therapy with biventricular pacing improves left ventricular function and favors reverse remodeling. Nesiritide (B-type natriuretic peptide) decreases preload by stimulating diuresis and decreases afterload by vasodilation. Exercise improves peripheral blood flow by eventually counteracting peripheral vasoconstriction. It also improves skeletal muscle physiology. (Reproduced with permission from Jessup M, Brozena S. Heart failure. *N Engl J Med.* 2003;348:2007-2018. Copyright © 2003 Massachusetts Medical Society. All rights reserved.)

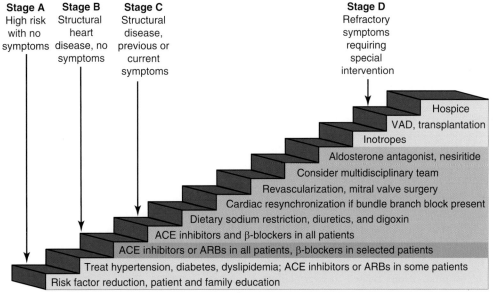

FIG. 10.4 Stages of heart failure and treatment options for systolic heart failure. Patients with stage A heart failure are at high risk of heart failure but do not yet have structural heart disease or symptoms of heart failure. This group includes patients with hypertension, diabetes, coronary artery disease, previous exposure to cardiotoxic drugs, or a family history of cardiomyopathy. Patients with stage B heart failure have structural heart disease but no symptoms of heart failure. This group includes patients with left ventricular hypertrophy, previous myocardial infarction, left ventricular systolic dysfunction, or valvular heart disease, all of whom would be considered to have New York Heart Association (NYHA) class I symptoms. Patients with stage C heart failure have known structural heart disease and current or previous symptoms of heart failure. Their current symptoms may be classified as NYHA class I, II, III, or IV. Patients with stage D heart failure have refractory symptoms of heart failure at rest despite maximal medical therapy, are hospitalized, and require specialized interventions or hospice care. All such patients would be considered to have NYHA class IV symptoms. *ACE,* Angiotensin-converting enzyme; *ARB,* angiotensin receptor blocker; *VAD,* ventricular assist device. (Reproduced with permission from Jessup M, Brozena S. Heart failure. *N Engl J Med.* 2003;348:2007-2018. Copyright © 2003 Massachusetts Medical Society. All rights reserved.)

failure by 8.5%. An even more impressive result can be seen with reductions in the incidence of diabetes mellitus.

Management of Systolic Heart Failure

The major classes of drugs used for medical management of systolic heart failure include inhibitors of the RAAS, β-blockers, diuretics, digoxin, vasodilators, and statins. Most heart failure patients are treated with a combination of drugs. *Therapy with ACE inhibitors and β-blockers favorably influences long-term outcome.*

Inhibitors of the Renin-Angiotensin-Aldosterone System
Inhibition of the RAAS can be performed at several levels: by inhibiting the enzyme that converts angiotensin I to angiotensin II, by blocking the angiotensin II receptor, or by blocking the aldosterone receptor.

Angiotensin-Converting Enzyme Inhibitors
ACE inhibitors block the conversion of angiotensin I to angiotensin II. This decreases the activation of the RAAS and decreases the degradation of bradykinin. Beneficial effects

include promoting vasodilation, reducing sodium and water reabsorption, and supporting potassium conservation. *This class of drugs has been proven to decrease ventricular remodeling and even to potentiate the reverse remodeling phenomenon.* ACE inhibitors have consistently been shown to reduce morbidity and mortality in patients *at any stage of heart failure.* Therefore they are considered first-line treatment in all heart failure patients. It appears, however, that the African American population does not derive as much clinical benefit from ACE inhibitor therapy as does the white population. Side effects of ACE inhibitors include hypotension, syncope, renal dysfunction, hyperkalemia, and development of a nonproductive cough and/or angioedema. Treatment with ACE inhibitors should be started at a low dosage to avoid significant hypotension. Then the dosage can be gradually increased until the target dosage is reached.

Angiotensin II Receptor Blockers
Angiotensin receptor blockers (ARB) block angiotensin II receptors. The efficacy of these drugs is similar but not superior to that of ACE inhibitors. Currently, ARBs are recommended only for patients who cannot tolerate ACE inhibitors. In some

patients treated with ACE inhibitors, angiotensin levels may gradually return to normal because of alternative pathways of angiotensin production. Such patients may benefit from the addition of an angiotensin receptor blocker to their medical therapy.

Aldosterone Antagonists

In advanced stages of heart failure there are high circulating levels of aldosterone. Aldosterone stimulates sodium and water retention, hypokalemia, and ventricular remodeling. Aldosterone antagonists reverse all these effects and therefore improve the cardiovascular milieu in patients with heart failure. There is strong clinical evidence showing reduced mortality and hospitalization rates with use of a low dosage of an aldosterone antagonist in patients with NYHA class III or IV heart failure. More recently, eplerenone has been demonstrated to reduce the rate of death from cardiovascular events and the number of hospitalizations related to heart failure, even in patients with NYHA class II heart failure. In patients being treated with aldosterone antagonists, renal function and potassium levels should be monitored and the medication dosage adjusted accordingly. *Currently it is recommended that aldosterone antagonists be incorporated as first-line therapy in all patients with heart failure.*

β-Blockers

β-Blockers are used to reverse the harmful effects of sympathetic nervous system activation in heart failure. Clinical trials have consistently shown that use of β-blockers reduces morbidity and the number of hospitalizations and improves both quality of life and length of survival. β-Blockers increase the EF and decrease ventricular remodeling. The 2013 ACC/AHA guidelines for management of heart failure recommend the use of β-blockers as an integral part of therapy. However, caution must be used when administering β-blockers to patients with reactive airway disease, diabetic patients with frequent hypoglycemic episodes, and patients with bradydysrhythmias or heart block.

Statins

Because of their antiinflammatory and lipid-lowering effects, statins have been proven to decrease morbidity and mortality in patients with systolic and diastolic heart failure. Therefore the most recent guidelines recommend the use of statins in *all* patients with heart failure.

Diuretics

Diuretics can relieve circulatory congestion and its accompanying pulmonary and peripheral edema and do so more rapidly than any other drugs. Symptomatic improvement can be noted within hours. Diuretic-induced decreases in ventricular diastolic pressure will decrease diastolic ventricular wall stress and prevent the persistent cardiac distention that interferes with subendocardial perfusion and negatively affects myocardial metabolism and function. Thiazide and/or loop diuretics are recommended as an essential part of the therapy for heart failure. Potassium and magnesium supplementation may be needed in patients on long-term treatment with diuretics to prevent cardiac dysrhythmias. Excessive dosages of diuretics may cause hypovolemia, prerenal azotemia, or an undesirably low cardiac output and are associated with worse clinical outcomes.

Vasodilators

Vasodilator therapy relaxes vascular smooth muscle, decreases resistance to LV ejection, and increases venous capacitance. In patients with a dilated left ventricle, administration of vasodilators results in increased stroke volume and decreased ventricular filling pressures. African Americans seem to respond very well to vasodilator therapy and show improved clinical outcomes when treated with a combination of hydralazine and nitrates.

Novel Therapies

Impaired nitric oxide–mediated pulmonary vascular tone is frequently encountered in patients with heart failure. This is associated with impaired LV function and decreased exercise tolerance. Udenafil, a new long-acting phosphodiesterase type 5 inhibitor, when used in combination with optimal medical therapy, improves both systolic and diastolic function as measured by improvements in EF and decreases in left atrial volume and BNP levels. Exercise tolerance is improved. However, this drug is not yet available in the United States.

Cardiopoietic stem cell therapy is gaining popularity in patients with end-stage heart failure. A recent small multicenter trial evaluated the feasibility and effects of infusing autologous bone marrow–derived "cardiogenically oriented" mesenchymal stem cells into patients with ischemic or nonischemic heart failure. It was concluded that this therapy is safe. All patients who received these stem cell infusions had a significantly improved EF as compared to baseline. This treatment modality is still in its infancy and requires definitive clinical evaluation.

Management of Diastolic Heart Failure

Management of systolic heart failure is based on the results of large-scale randomized trials, but treatment of diastolic heart failure remains mostly empirical. It is generally accepted that the best treatment strategy for diastolic heart failure is prevention. ACC/AHA guidelines recommend that patients at risk of developing diastolic heart failure be treated preemptively. Unfortunately there are no drugs that selectively improve diastolic distensibility. Current treatment options include consumption of a low-sodium diet, cautious use of diuretics to relieve pulmonary congestion without an excessive decrease in preload, maintenance of normal sinus rhythm at a heart rate that optimizes ventricular filling, and correction of precipitating factors such as acute myocardial ischemia and systemic hypertension. Long-acting nitrates and diuretics may alleviate the symptoms of diastolic heart failure but do not alter the natural history of the disease.

Early statin therapy may play an important role in decreasing ventricular remodeling and reducing disease progression. The general concepts of managing patients with diastolic heart failure are outlined in Table 10.3.

Surgical Management of Heart Failure

Cardiac resynchronization therapy (CRT) is aimed at patients with heart failure who have a ventricular conduction delay (QRS prolongation on ECG). Such a conduction delay creates a mechanical dyssynchrony that impairs ventricular function and worsens prognosis. CRT, also known as *biventricular pacing*, consists of placement of a dual-chamber cardiac pacemaker (right atrial and right ventricular leads), with an additional lead introduced via the coronary sinus into an epicardial coronary vein and advanced until it reaches the lateral wall of the left ventricle. With this lead in place and the timing adjusted, the heart can contract more efficiently and eject a larger cardiac output. Classically, CRT has been recommended for patients with NYHA class III or IV disease with an LVEF less than 35% and a QRS duration of 120–150 milliseconds. Recent trials suggest a benefit of CRT in heart failure patients with an EF above 30% and even mild symptoms. Patients who undergo CRT have fewer symptoms of heart failure, better exercise tolerance, improved ventricular function, fewer hospitalizations, and decreased mortality compared with similar patients receiving drug therapy alone. The reverse remodeling process induced by CRT appears to be the main reason for the improved survival seen in some patients. However, this form of therapy fails to produce an improvement in about one-third of patients.

Implantable hemodynamic monitoring has emerged as a novel approach to ambulatory monitoring of intracardiac pressures. A device for pulmonary artery pressure monitoring, the CardioMEMS Heart Failure System has received regulatory approval in the United States. This system allows for management of LV filling pressures with proactive titration of medications based on daily measurement of pulmonary artery pressure (PAP) obtained noninvasively at home by the patient and then uploaded to the physician managing the heart failure. The sensor unit contains a wireless system to measure PAP that does not require battery power for operation, nor does it have any replaceable parts. It is implanted via right heart catheterization into the pulmonary artery, and an external antenna allows for determination of the resonant frequency of the device, which is converted to a pressure waveform. Data indicate that use of this device may result in fewer hospitalizations for heart failure.

Implantable cardioverter-defibrillators (ICDs) are used for prevention of sudden death in patients with advanced heart failure. Approximately one-half of deaths in heart failure patients are sudden and due to cardiac dysrhythmias. Current recommendations for the use of ICDs in patients at risk of sudden death are listed in Table 10.4. Recent studies have demonstrated that patients treated with a combination of CRT and ICD placement have fewer hospitalizations and better survival rates at 2 years than patients who receive only ICD therapy. However, this advantage comes at the cost of higher device-related complication rates in the first 30 days after implantation.

Part of the overall management of heart failure includes strategies aimed at eliminating the cause of the disease responsible for the heart failure. Ischemic heart disease may be treated with percutaneous coronary intervention or coronary artery bypass surgery. Severe heart failure in the presence of correctable cardiac valve lesions may be alleviated by surgical correction of the valve pathology. *Ventricular aneurysmectomy* may be useful in patients with large ventricular scars. The definitive treatment for heart failure is *cardiac transplantation*. Currently, worldwide there are over 50,000 patients listed as

TABLE 10.3	Management Strategies for Diastolic Heart Failure
Goals	Management Strategies
Prevent development of diastolic heart failure by decreasing risk factors.	Treatment of coronary artery disease Treatment of hypertension Control of weight gain Treatment of diabetes mellitus
Allow adequate filling time for left ventricle by decreasing heart rate.	β-Blockers, calcium channel blockers
Control volume overload.	Diuretics, long-acting nitrates, consumption of low-sodium diet
Restore and maintain sinus rhythm.	Cardioversion, amiodarone
Decrease ventricular remodeling.	Angiotensin-converting enzyme inhibitors, statins
Correct precipitating factors.	Aortic valve replacement Coronary revascularization

TABLE 10.4	Indications for Implantation of a Cardioverter-Defibrillator for Prevention of Sudden Death
Cause of Heart Failure	Condition
Coronary artery disease	Structural heart disease with sustained VT Syncope of undetermined origin, inducible VT or VF at EPS LVEF < 35%, NYHA class II or III LVEF < 30% due to prior MI, at least 40 days post MI EF < 40% due to prior MI *and* inducible VT or VF at EPS
All other causes	After first episode of syncope or aborted ventricular tachycardia/ventricular fibrillation

EF, Ejection fraction; *EPS,* electrophysiologic study; *LV,* left ventricular; *MI,* myocardial infarction; *NYHA,* New York Heart Association classification of the functional status of heart failure patients; *VF,* ventricular fibrillation; *VT,* ventricular tachycardia.

candidates for cardiac transplantation, but only about 5000 hearts are available per year. About 2000 heart transplants are being performed annually in the United States. From 2006-2013, approximately 3% of patients with a transplanted heart underwent retransplantation. The limited supply of donors renders cardiac transplantation unattainable for most patients.

Patients in the terminal stages of heart failure may benefit from *mechanical support of the circulation* by a device such as a ventricular assist device (VAD) or a total artificial heart. Studies have demonstrated not only increased survival but also improved quality of life in heart failure patients treated with VADs compared to those treated with medical therapy alone. These mechanical pumps can take over partial or total function of the damaged ventricle and facilitate restoration of normal hemodynamics and tissue blood flow. A VAD drains blood returning to the failed side of the heart and pumps it downstream of the failed ventricle. These devices are useful in patients who require temporary ventricular assistance to allow the heart to recover its function *(bridge to recovery)*, in patients who are awaiting cardiac transplantation *(bridge to therapy)*, in patients who are on inotropic drugs or intraaortic balloon pump counterpulsation with potentially reversible medical conditions *(bridge to decision)*, and in patients with advanced heart failure who are not transplant candidates *(destination therapy)*. First-generation left ventricular assist devices (LVADs) captured the entire cardiac output and ejected it in a pulsatile fashion into the ascending aorta to simulate the work of the native left ventricle. This pulsatile flow required a complicated mechanism that included valves preventing systolic retrograde blood flow. As a result, first-generation LVADs were noisy, fairly large, and prone to significant complications due to mechanical pump failure and thromboembolic events. With the advent of modern miniaturization technology and a general acceptance by the medical community that nonpulsatile flow can be well tolerated, second and third generations of LVADs have been developed.

Second-generation LVADs are axial flow pumps. Third-generation LVADs are centrifugal electromagnetically powered pumps. These devices generate nonpulsatile flow, are smaller and quieter, and have a lower incidence of thromboembolic events. Therefore they have become an attractive therapeutic option for an increasing number of patients with heart failure.

Patients with *fixed pulmonary hypertension requiring biventricular support* for extended periods of time may benefit from implantation of a *total artificial heart*. A total artificial heart can be implanted in the chest in lieu of the native heart. Such a device generates pulsatile flow and consists of two mechanical pumps, each operating as a "ventricle," with each pump having two valves. Currently the SynCardia Total Artificial Heart is approved as a bridge to cardiac transplantation and has received designation as a humanitarian use device (HUD), so it can also be used as destination therapy. The maximum dynamic stroke volume of each "ventricle" in this system is 70 mL, allowing generation of flow rates (cardiac output) of up to 9.5 L/min. It also comes in a 50-mL size intended for most women, small adults, and adolescents.

Anesthetic Considerations for Patients With Implantable Nonpulsatile Ventricular Assist Devices

As more and more VADs are being inserted, a growing number of patients with VADs will likely be undergoing noncardiac surgery. The anesthesiologist needs to understand the features of nonpulsatile devices and the potential mishaps that can occur during anesthesia and surgery. The most commonly used VAD in the United States is the HeartMate II, a second-generation continuous-flow device. The pump is implanted extraperitoneally in the left upper abdomen, draining blood from the LV apex via the inflow cannula and ejecting it into the ascending aorta via the outflow cannula (Fig. 10.5). A drive line connects the pump to electrical power as well as to an external console that displays pump flows and other system information. The drive line crosses the abdomen and exits the skin in the right upper

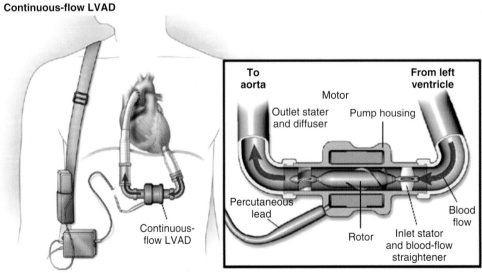

FIG. 10.5   HeartMate II left ventricular assist device (LVAD). Blood is drawn through the inflow cannula attached to the ventricular apex into the pump and is ejected into the ascending aorta through the outflow cannula. The percutaneous lead is the drive line, which exits the right side of the abdomen and connects the pump to the external console and power source.

quadrant, and this is the site most likely to become infected. However, the drive line cannot be prepped with povidone-iodine solutions because this leads to breakdown of its plastics. If possible, the drive line can be draped out of the surgical field.

Anesthetic considerations for patients with VADs include perioperative management of anticoagulation therapy (patients with HeartMate devices are on antiplatelet drugs), management of cardiac rhythm devices, provision of suitable antibiotic prophylaxis, confirmation that the device is plugged into an electrical outlet, and avoidance of chest compression to prevent dislodgement of the VAD cannulae. Use of surgical electrocautery can cause electromagnetic interference that can affect pump flow and induce device reprogramming. Therefore bipolar cautery should be used when feasible, or the grounding electrode of monopolar cautery should be placed to direct the current *away from* the VAD generator.

Hemodynamic monitoring of a patient with an implantable nonpulsatile device represents a particular challenge. Neither a noninvasive blood pressure monitor nor a pulse oximeter can be used reliably, since the majority of these patients have nonpulsatile flow. A small number of patients will intermittently eject some blood from their ventricle, and this can allow for measurement of oxygen saturation via pulse oximetry. As a substitute for pulse oximetry a cerebral oximeter that does not rely on pulsatile flow can be used. Intermittent monitoring of oxygen saturation can also be accomplished by arterial blood gas analysis. An intraarterial catheter is *required* for measurement of *mean arterial pressure*. However, placement of an arterial catheter into a nonpulsatile artery can be very difficult and is usually facilitated by ultrasonographic guidance. Transesophageal echocardiography (TEE) represents one of the most useful monitoring techniques for patients with VADs, since it provides real-time information regarding volume status, RV function, and inflow-outflow cannulae function.

The three main causes of hypotension occurring in patients with continuous-flow LVADs are decreased preload, RV failure, and increased afterload. Intravascular volume optimization is a major concern in patients with all types of VADs, but this is particularly important with nonpulsatile devices because continuous drainage of an underfilled left side of the heart will eventually lead to *LV suck-down*. Leftward shift of the interventricular septum due to suck-down alters RV geometry and thereby increases RV compliance and decreases RV contractility. This results in a dramatic decrease in cardiac output. Fortunately this situation can be rapidly diagnosed by TEE. It is treated by temporarily decreasing the VAD pump speed and then by volume expansion. *Good RV function is critical for optimal LVAD flow.* Factors that increase pulmonary vascular resistance, such as hypercarbia or vasoconstrictor drugs, will impair RV function and impede blood flow to the left side of the heart. Spontaneous ventilation can result in hypercarbia, which can increase pulmonary artery pressure and worsen RV strain. Therefore some advocate for controlled ventilation for any general anesthetic. Both decreases and increases in afterload can significantly impact LVAD flow. Small doses of vasopressor medications that have less impact on pulmonary vascular resistance (e.g., vasopressin) may be used to counteract the decrease

in afterload seen with general anesthesia. However, high doses of vasopressors, especially in the presence of hypovolemia, will invariably lead to a decrease in LVAD flow. High output from an LVAD can paradoxically increase RV preload and worsen RV failure in susceptible patients. Excellent communication among the entire perioperative team (anesthesiologist, surgeon, cardiologist, nurses, VAD personnel) is essential for good outcomes.

Management of Acute Heart Failure

Patients may experience new acute heart failure or decompensated chronic heart failure. Anesthesiologists often deal with acute heart failure in patients who undergo emergency surgery or in patients who experience cardiac decompensation during elective surgery. Acute heart failure therapy has three phases: the emergency phase, the in-hospital management phase, and the predischarge phase. For the anesthesiologist, the emergency phase is of most interest. High ventricular filling pressures, low cardiac output, and hypertension or hypotension characterize the hemodynamic profile of acute heart failure. Traditional therapies include diuretics, vasodilators, inotropic drugs, mechanical assist devices (intraaortic balloon counterpulsation, VADs) and emergency cardiac surgery. Newer therapies include calcium sensitizers, exogenous BNP, and nitric oxide synthase inhibitors.

Diuretics and Vasodilators
Loop diuretics can improve symptoms rapidly. A poor diuretic response is associated with hypotension, renal impairment, low urine output, and an increased risk of death or rehospitalization early after discharge. Another therapeutic alternative is a combination of a low dose of loop diuretic and an intravenous vasodilator. Nitroglycerin and nitroprusside reduce LV filling pressure and systemic vascular resistance and increase stroke volume. However, nitroprusside may have a negative impact on clinical outcome in patients with acute MI.

Inotropic Support
Inotropic drugs have been the mainstay of treatment for patients in cardiogenic shock. The positive inotropic effect is produced via an increase in cyclic adenosine monophosphate (cAMP), which promotes an increase in intracellular calcium and an improvement in excitation-contraction coupling. Catecholamines (epinephrine, norepinephrine, dopamine, dobutamine) do this by direct β-receptor stimulation, whereas phosphodiesterase inhibitors (e.g., milrinone) block the degradation of cAMP. Side effects of inotropic drugs include tachycardia, increased myocardial oxygen consumption, dysrhythmias, worsening of diastolic heart failure, and downregulation of β-receptors. Long-term use of these drugs may result in cardiotoxicity and accelerate myocardial cell death.

Calcium Sensitizers
Myofilament calcium sensitizers are a new class of positive inotropic drugs that increase contractility *without* increasing intracellular levels of calcium. As a result there is no significant increase in myocardial oxygen consumption or heart rate and no propensity for dysrhythmias. The most widely used

medication in this class is *levosimendan*. It is an *inodilator*—that is, it increases myocardial contractile strength and promotes dilation of systemic, pulmonary, and coronary arteries. It does not worsen diastolic function. Studies have shown that levosimendan may be particularly useful in the setting of myocardial ischemia. Use of levosimendan is included in the European guidelines for treatment of acute heart failure, but the drug is not yet approved for use in the United States.

Exogenous B-Type Natriuretic Peptide

Nesiritide is recombinant BNP that binds to both the A- and B-type natriuretic receptors. By inhibiting the RAAS and sympathetic tone, this natriuretic peptide promotes arterial, venous, and coronary vasodilation, thereby decreasing LVEDP and improving dyspnea. It also induces diuresis and natriuresis, can relax cardiac muscle, and lacks any prodysrhythmic effects. Its effects are quite similar to those of nitroglycerin, but nesiritide generally produces less hypotension and more diuresis than nitroglycerin. Intravenous nesiritide has been studied extensively in large clinical trials but may not offer advantages over traditional treatments for acute heart failure and may be associated with worsening renal function. Current research is evaluating the use of *subcutaneous* BNP in patients with acute heart failure and an EF below 35%. Preliminary results indicate an increase in cardiac output, a decrease in mean arterial pressure, no change in heart rate, a decrease in RAAS activity, and increased diuresis and natriuresis. Its place in clinical practice remains to be defined.

Nitric Oxide Synthase Inhibitors

The inflammatory cascade stimulated by heart failure results in production of a large amount of nitric oxide in the heart and vascular endothelium. These high levels of nitric oxide have a negative inotropic effect and a *profound* vasodilatory effect that can lead to cardiogenic shock and vascular collapse. Inhibition of nitric oxide synthase should decrease these harmful effects. *L-NAME* (N^G-nitro-L-arginine methyl ester) is the principal drug in this class currently under investigation for treatment of cardiogenic shock. It seems to cause a rapid, progressive, and durable increase in mean arterial pressure and urine output. It is not approved for clinical use at this time.

Mechanical Devices

If the cause of acute heart failure is an extensive MI, insertion of an intraaortic balloon pump should be considered. This pump is a mechanical device inserted via the femoral artery and positioned just below the left subclavian artery. Its balloon inflates in diastole, increasing aortic diastolic blood pressure and coronary perfusion pressure. The balloon deflates in systole, creating a suction effect that enhances LV ejection. Complications of intraaortic balloon counterpulsation include femoral artery or aortic dissection, bleeding, thrombosis, and infection.

In cases of severe cardiogenic shock, emergency insertion of a left and/or right VAD may be necessary for survival. Percutaneously inserted ventricular assist devices (pVADs) have been developed and successfully inserted into patients with acute heart failure. These devices can restore normal hemodynamics and maintain vital organ perfusion. More importantly these devices "unload" the left ventricle, thereby reducing LV strain and myocardial work and improving the remodeling process seen in acute heart failure. The pVADs offer *temporary* circulatory support in cardiogenic shock and can be used for up to 14 days as a transition to recovery or as a bridge to a definitive cardiac procedure (coronary artery stenting, coronary artery bypass grafting, VAD insertion, or heart transplantation). Trials comparing the efficacy of a pVAD to intraaortic balloon counterpulsation in patients with severe acute heart failure have demonstrated a better metabolic profile and superior hemodynamic support in patients with pVAD therapy but have failed to show a decrease in 30-day mortality with the use of a pVAD. Two percutaneous VAD devices designed for short-term circulatory support are available: the Impella system and the TandemHeart.

The Impella system consists of a miniaturized axial-flow rotary blood pump that is inserted via the femoral artery and advanced under fluoroscopic or TEE guidance until it passes through the aortic valve and is situated in the LV cavity (Fig. 10.6). The pump draws blood continuously from the LV through the distal port and ejects it into the ascending aorta through the proximal port of the device. A device for use in right heart failure would be inserted via a central vein into the RV, and ejection of blood from the distal port would go

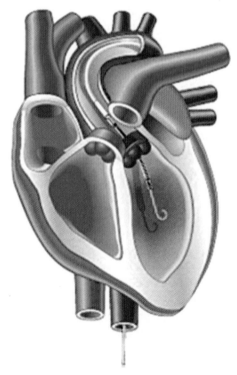

FIG. 10.6 Impella Recover 2.5 percutaneous ventricular assist device. The pump is percutaneously placed in the femoral artery, advanced through the aortic valve, and situated in the left ventricular cavity. The Impella 5.0 has a similar design.

into the pulmonary arteries. These pumps can generate cardiac outputs of up to 5 L/min. Placement of an Impella device is contraindicated in the presence of a prosthetic aortic valve, severe aortic stenosis or aortic regurgitation, or peripheral vascular disease. Relative contraindications to insertion of the Impella system include thoracoabdominal or abdominal aortic aneurysms or an aortic dissection. However, in such cases the axillary artery could serve as the insertion site of the pump. Complications of this device include stroke, aortic insufficiency, aortic valve injury, dysrhythmias, atrial fibrillation, cardiac tamponade, vascular injury with limb ischemia, thrombocytopenia, and infection. Because of the centrifugal nature of the pump, hemolysis and thrombocytopenia typically develop.

The TandemHeart is a system consisting of an extracorporeal centrifugal continuous-flow pump and inflow and outflow cannulae. The inflow cannula is placed percutaneously in the femoral vein, advanced to the right atrium, and then positioned transseptally into the left atrium. The outflow cannula is placed in the femoral artery (Fig. 10.7). Oxygenated blood is drained from the left atrium via the inflow cannula and ejected retrograde into the abdominal aorta via the outflow cannula. This system generates cardiac outputs similar to those of the Impella system. However, optimal functioning of the TandemHeart *depends on good RV function.* In

situations of acute right-sided heart failure, the system can be configured as a right-sided VAD, pumping blood from the right atrium into the pulmonary artery. Unique complications of use of this device include paradoxical embolism, a right-to-left intracardiac shunt manifested as hypoxemia, and coronary sinus or right atrial injury with subsequent cardiac tamponade. The most devastating complication is inflow cannula dislodgement with mitral valve entrapment. This situation leads to a sudden decrease in cardiac output and requires immediate diagnosis and repositioning of the cannula.

Prognosis

Despite advances in therapy, the number of heart failure deaths continues to increase steadily in the United States. Mortality during the first 5 years after the diagnosis of heart failure approaches 50%. Factors associated with a poor prognosis include increased blood urea nitrogen and creatinine levels, hyponatremia, hypokalemia, severely depressed EF, high levels of endogenous BNP, very limited exercise tolerance, and the presence of multifocal premature ventricular contractions. In heart failure patients the prognosis depends on the underlying heart disease and the presence or absence of a specific precipitating factor. If a correctable cause of heart failure can be effectively eliminated, prognosis improves.

MANAGEMENT OF ANESTHESIA

Preoperative Evaluation and Management

The presence of heart failure has been described as the single most important risk factor for predicting perioperative cardiac morbidity and mortality. Data showed that heart failure patients had an increased risk of developing renal failure, sepsis, pneumonia, and cardiac arrest; required longer periods of mechanical ventilation; and had an increased 30-day mortality. Interestingly the risk of perioperative MI was similar in the two groups. Thus all precipitating factors for heart failure should be sought and aggressively treated *before proceeding with elective surgery.*

Patients treated for heart failure usually take several medications that may affect anesthetic management. It is generally accepted that diuretics may be discontinued on the day of surgery. Maintaining β-blocker therapy is *essential,* since many studies have shown that β-blockers reduce perioperative morbidity and mortality. Owing to inhibition of the RAAS, ACE inhibitors may put patients at increased risk of intraoperative hypotension. This hypotension can be treated with a sympathomimetic drug such as ephedrine, an α-agonist such as phenylephrine, or vasopressin. Despite the known hypotensive effect of both ACE inhibitors and ARBs, the 2014 ACC/AHA guidelines on perioperative cardiovascular evaluation and management of patients undergoing noncardiac surgery recommend maintaining this therapy in the perioperative period.

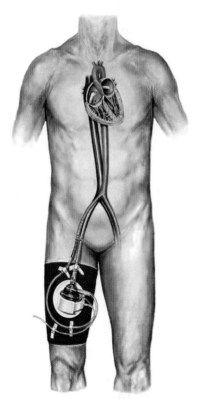

FIG. 10.7 TandemHeart percutaneous ventricular assist device. The inflow cannula is placed in the femoral vein and advanced into the right atrium. It then pierces the interatrial septum to draw oxygenated blood from the left atrium. The outflow cannula pumps blood retrograde into the aorta via the femoral artery.

Results of recent electrolyte, renal function, and liver function tests and the most recent ECG and echocardiogram should be reviewed.

Intraoperative Management

All types of general anesthetics have been successfully used in patients with heart failure. However, drug dosages often need to be adjusted. Opioids seem to have a particularly beneficial effect in heart failure patients because of their effect on the δ receptor, which inhibits adrenergic activation. Positive pressure ventilation and positive end-expiratory pressure may be beneficial in decreasing pulmonary congestion and improving arterial oxygenation.

Monitoring is based on the complexity of the surgery. Intra-arterial pressure monitoring is justified when major surgery is required. Monitoring of ventricular filling and fluid status is a more challenging task. Fluid overload during the perioperative period may contribute to the development or worsening of heart failure. Intraoperative use of a pulmonary artery catheter may help in evaluation of optimal fluid loading, but in patients with diastolic heart failure and poor ventricular compliance, accurate assessment of LV end-diastolic volume may be quite difficult. TEE may be a better alternative, and this monitor can evaluate not only ventricular filling but also ventricular wall motion and valvular function. However, TEE requires trained personnel to perform the study and interpret the results and may not be readily available in all circumstances. More recently, multiple noninvasive and minimally invasive devices for continuous monitoring of cardiac output have become available in clinical practice. The esophageal Doppler monitor is a noninvasive device composed of a small probe placed in the esophagus parallel to the blood flow in the descending aorta; it is connected to a monitor that shows *continuous data* on stroke volume and cardiac output and offers an estimation of systemic vascular resistance. Use of this device requires minimal training and expertise. It has been validated for fluid optimization in multiple clinical situations.

Other minimally invasive devices include the FloTrac, the LiDCO, the PiCCO and others. The FloTrac provides flow-based hemodynamic parameters measured through an existing arterial line. The LiDCO system measures cardiac output by the dye dilution method, using lithium solution as the "dye." This measurement can be made through *peripheral* venous catheters. The PiCCO (pulse index continuous cardiac output) device requires both an arterial catheter and a central venous catheter. It combines pulse contour analysis and trans-cardiopulmonary thermodilution techniques and can measure cardiac output, preload, afterload, contractility, volume responsiveness, and bedside assessment of lung water.

Regional anesthesia is acceptable in heart failure patients. Indeed the modest decrease in systemic vascular resistance due to sympathetic blockade may increase cardiac output. However, this decrease in systemic vascular resistance is not always predictable or easy to control. The pros and cons of regional anesthesia must be carefully weighed in each heart failure patient.

Special consideration must be given to patients who have undergone cardiac transplantation and now require other surgery. These patients are receiving long-term immunosuppressive therapy and are at very high risk of infection. *Strict aseptic technique* is necessary when performing any invasive procedure such as central line placement or neuraxial blockade. The transplanted heart is denervated. Therefore an increase in heart rate can best be achieved by administering direct-acting β-adrenergic agonists such as isoproterenol and epinephrine. A blunted response to indirect-acting α-adrenergic agonists is observed. A change in heart rate will *not* occur with administration of atropine or pancuronium. The transplanted heart increases cardiac output by increasing stroke volume. Therefore these patients are *preload dependent* and require adequate intravascular volume. However, diastolic dysfunction can be a result of chronic graft rejection. Therefore intraoperative fluid administration decisions must be made knowing that adequate preload is a requirement for optimal function of the transplanted heart, but excessive fluid administration incurs the risk of pulmonary edema.

Postoperative Management

Patients who have evidence of acute heart failure during surgery should be transferred to an intensive care unit postoperatively so that invasive monitoring and intensive treatment can be continued as long as needed. Pain should be adequately treated, since its presence and hemodynamic consequences may worsen heart failure. Home medications should be restarted as soon as possible.

CARDIOMYOPATHIES

The definition of *cardiomyopathies* used by the AHA expert consensus panel in its 2006 document entitled "Contemporary Definition and Classification of the Cardiomyopathies" reads as follows:

> *Cardiomyopathies are a heterogeneous group of diseases of the myocardium associated with mechanical and/or electrical dysfunction that usually (but not invariably) exhibit inappropriate ventricular hypertrophy or dilation and are due to a variety of causes that frequently are genetic. Cardiomyopathies either are confined to the heart or are part of generalized systemic disorders, often leading to cardiovascular death or progressive heart failure-related disability.*

Cardiomyopathies can be divided into two groups: primary cardiomyopathies and secondary cardiomyopathies. *Primary cardiomyopathies* are those exclusively (or predominantly) confined to heart muscle; they can be genetic, acquired, or of mixed origin. *Secondary cardiomyopathies* demonstrate pathophysiologic involvement of the heart in the context of a multiorgan disorder. Tables 10.5 and 10.6 list the most common cardiomyopathies. It is important to emphasize that the previously used terms *ischemic cardiomyopathy, restrictive cardiomyopathy,* and *obliterative cardiomyopathy* do not appear

TABLE 10.5	Classification of Primary Cardiomyopathies
Genetic	Hypertrophic cardiomyopathy
	Dysrhythmogenic right ventricular cardiomyopathy
	Left ventricular noncompaction
	Glycogen storage disease
	Conduction system disease (Lenègre disease)
	Ion channelopathies: long QT syndrome, Brugada syndrome, short QT syndrome
Mixed	Dilated cardiomyopathy
	Primary restrictive nonhypertrophic cardiomyopathy
Acquired	Myocarditis (inflammatory cardiomyopathy): viral, bacterial, rickettsial, fungal, parasitic (Chagas disease)
	Stress cardiomyopathy
	Peripartum cardiomyopathy

TABLE 10.6	Classification of Secondary Cardiomyopathies
Infiltrative	Amyloidosis
	Gaucher disease
	Hunter syndrome
Storage	Hemochromatosis
	Glycogen storage disease
	Niemann-Pick disease
Toxic	Drugs: cocaine, alcohol
	Chemotherapy drugs: doxorubicin, daunorubicin, cyclophosphamide
	Heavy metals: lead, mercury
	Radiation therapy
Inflammatory	Sarcoidosis
Endomyocardial	Hypereosinophilic (Löffler) syndrome
	Endomyocardial fibrosis
Endocrine	Diabetes mellitus
	Hyperthyroidism or hypothyroidism
	Pheochromocytoma
	Acromegaly
Neuromuscular	Duchenne-Becker dystrophy
	Neurofibromatosis
	Tuberous sclerosis
Autoimmune	Lupus erythematosus
	Rheumatoid arthritis
	Scleroderma
	Dermatomyositis
	Polyarteritis nodosa

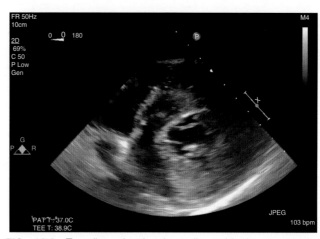

FIG. 10.8 Two-dimensional echocardiographic image showing a transgastric short-axis view of the left ventricle in a patient with hypertrophic cardiomyopathy. Note the concentric thickness of the left ventricular walls.

in this new classification. The following sections address the cardiomyopathies most often seen by an anesthesiologist: hypertrophic cardiomyopathy (HCM), dilated cardiomyopathy, peripartum cardiomyopathy, and secondary cardiomyopathies with restrictive physiology.

Hypertrophic Cardiomyopathy

HCM is a complex cardiac disease with unique pathophysiologic characteristics and a great diversity of morphologic, functional, and clinical features. The disease can affect patients of all ages and has a prevalence in the general population of about 1 in 500 persons. *It is the most common genetic cardiovascular disease* and is transmitted as an autosomal dominant trait with variable penetrance. This cardiomyopathy is characterized by LV hypertrophy in the absence of any other cardiac disease capable of inducing ventricular hypertrophy (e.g., hypertension, aortic stenosis). The most common form of HCM presents as hypertrophy of the interventricular septum and anterolateral free wall. However, in other types of HCM the hypertrophy can be concentric (Fig. 10.8) or may involve both ventricles, only the LV free wall, or only the apex of the heart. Histologic features include hypertrophied myocardial cells and areas of patchy myocardial scarring.

The pathophysiology of HCM is related to the following features: myocardial hypertrophy, dynamic left ventricular outflow tract (LVOT) obstruction, systolic anterior movement of the mitral valve causing mitral regurgitation, diastolic dysfunction, myocardial ischemia, and dysrhythmias. During systole, contraction of the hypertrophied septum accelerates blood flow through the narrowed LVOT, which creates a Venturi effect on the anterior leaflet of the mitral valve and induces anterior movement of the anterior mitral valve leaflet during systole. The presence of this systolic anterior movement accentuates the dynamic LVOT obstruction and causes significant mitral regurgitation. LVOT obstruction can be present at rest or can be induced by the Valsalva maneuver. Situations that worsen LVOT obstruction are listed in Table 10.7. However, it must be noted that *not all* patients with HCM have LVOT obstruction. Based on the obstruction pattern, the HCM can be classified as *nonobstructive* (with peak pressure gradients across the LVOT < 30 mm Hg), *obstructive* (peak pressure gradients > 30 mm Hg), and *latent* (exercise-induced pressure gradients > 30 mm Hg). Diastolic dysfunction is seen more often than LVOT obstruction. The hypertrophied myocardium has a prolonged relaxation time and decreased compliance. *Myocardial ischemia is present in patients with HCM whether or not they have coronary artery disease.* Myocardial ischemia is caused by several factors, including abnormal coronary arteries, a mismatch between ventricular mass and coronary artery size, increased

TABLE 10.7	Factors Influencing Left Ventricular Outflow Tract Obstruction in Patients With Hypertrophic Cardiomyopathy

EVENTS THAT INCREASE OUTFLOW OBSTRUCTION
Increased myocardial contractility
  β-Adrenergic stimulation (catecholamines)
  Digitalis
Decreased preload
  Hypovolemia
  Vasodilators
  Tachycardia
  Positive pressure ventilation
Decreased afterload
  Hypotension
  Vasodilators

EVENTS THAT DECREASE OUTFLOW OBSTRUCTION
Decreased myocardial contractility
  β-Adrenergic blockade
  Volatile anesthetics
  Calcium entry blockers
Increased preload
  Hypervolemia
  Bradycardia
Increased afterload
  Hypertension
  α-Adrenergic stimulation

LVEDP that compromises subendocardial coronary perfusion, decreased diastolic filling time, increased oxygen consumption caused by the hypertrophy, and the presence of a metabolic derangement in the use of oxygen at the cellular level. Dysrhythmias in patients with HCM result from the disorganized cellular architecture, myocardial scarring, and expanded interstitial matrix. Dysrhythmias are the cause of sudden death in young adults with this cardiomyopathy.

Signs and Symptoms
The clinical course of HCM varies widely. Most patients remain asymptomatic throughout their lives. Some, however, have symptoms of severe heart failure and others experience sudden death. The principal symptoms of HCM include angina pectoris, fatigue, syncope (which may represent aborted sudden death), tachydysrhythmias, and heart failure. Interestingly, lying down often relieves the angina pectoris of HCM. Presumably the change in LV size that accompanies this positional change decreases LV outflow obstruction.

Physical examination may reveal a double apical impulse, gallop rhythm, and cardiac murmurs and thrills. The murmurs can result from LV outflow obstruction or mitral regurgitation and can be confused with aortic or intrinsic mitral valve disease. The intensity of these murmurs can change markedly with certain maneuvers. For example, the Valsalva maneuver, which increases LV outflow obstruction, will enhance the systolic murmur, heard best along the left sternal border. The murmur of mitral regurgitation also intensifies with the Valsalva maneuver. Nitroglycerin and standing (vs. lying down) also increase the intensity of these murmurs.

Sudden death is a recognized complication of HCM. The severity of the ventricular hypertrophy is directly related to the risk of sudden death. *Young individuals with massive hypertrophy,* even if they have few or no symptoms, should be considered for an intervention to prevent sudden death. Sudden death is especially likely to occur in patients between the ages of 10 and 30 years. For this reason there is general agreement that young patients with HCM should not participate in competitive sports. Patients with mild hypertrophy are at low risk of sudden death.

Diagnosis
The ECG typically shows signs of LV hypertrophy. In asymptomatic patients, unexplained LV hypertrophy may be the only sign of the disease. The 12-lead ECG shows abnormalities in 75%–90% of patients. These abnormalities include high QRS voltage, ST-segment and T-wave alterations, abnormal Q waves resembling those seen with MI, and left atrial enlargement. The diagnosis of HCM should also be considered in any young patient whose ECG findings are consistent with previous MI, because not all patients have evidence of LV hypertrophy on ECG.

Echocardiography can demonstrate the presence of myocardial hypertrophy. Ejection fraction is usually higher than 80%, which reflects the hypercontractile state of the heart. Echocardiography can also assess the mitral valve apparatus and detect the presence of systolic anterior movement. Color flow Doppler imaging can reveal the presence of LVOT obstruction by demonstrating turbulent outflow as well as mitral regurgitation. Pressure gradients across the LVOT can be measured. Echocardiography is also useful in evaluating diastolic function.

Cardiac catheterization allows direct measurement of the increased LVEDP and the pressure gradient between the left ventricle and the aorta. Provocative maneuvers may be required to evoke evidence of LVOT obstruction. Ventriculography characteristically shows near–cavity obliteration of the left ventricle.

Definitive diagnosis of HCM is made by endomyocardial biopsy and DNA analysis, but these diagnostic modalities are usually reserved for patients in whom the diagnosis cannot be otherwise established.

Treatment
The diverse clinical and genetic features of HCM make it impossible to define precise guidelines for management of this disorder (Fig. 10.9). Some patients are at high risk of sudden death and must be treated aggressively in this regard. Pharmacologic therapy to improve diastolic filling, reduce LV outflow obstruction, and possibly decrease myocardial ischemia is the primary means of relieving the signs and symptoms of HCM. Surgery to remove the area of hypertrophy causing outflow tract obstruction is considered in the 5% of patients who have both marked outflow tract obstruction and severe symptoms unresponsive to medical therapy.

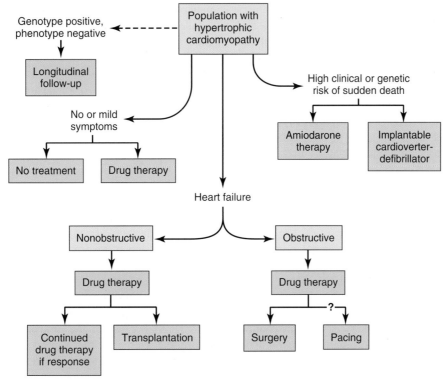

FIG. 10.9   Clinical presentations of hypertrophic cardiomyopathy and corresponding treatment strategies. (Adapted from Spirito P, Seidman CE, McKenna WJ, et al. The management of hypertrophic cardiomyopathy. *N Engl J Med.* 1997;336:775-785. Copyright 1997 Massachusetts Medical Society.)

Medical Therapy

β-Blockers and calcium channel blockers are used to treat HCM. The beneficial effects of β-blockers on dyspnea, angina pectoris, and exercise tolerance are likely due to the resulting decrease in heart rate, with consequent prolongation of diastole and lengthening of the time for passive ventricular filling. β-Blockers lessen myocardial oxygen requirements and decrease dynamic outflow tract obstruction during exercise by blunting sympathetic nervous system activity. Similarly, calcium channel blockers (e.g., verapamil, diltiazem) have beneficial effects on the symptoms of HCM because they improve ventricular filling and decrease myocardial ischemia. Patients who develop congestive heart failure despite treatment with β-blockers or calcium channel blockers may show improvement with the addition of a diuretic. Diuretic administration must be done very cautiously because of the presence of diastolic dysfunction and the requirement for relatively high ventricular filling pressures to achieve adequate cardiac output. Patients at high risk of sudden death may require amiodarone therapy or placement of an ICD.

Atrial fibrillation often develops in patients with HCM and is associated with an increased risk of arterial thromboembolism, congestive heart failure, and sudden death. Amiodarone is the most effective antidysrhythmic drug for prevention of paroxysms of atrial fibrillation in these patients. β-Blockers and calcium channel blockers can control the heart rate. Long-term anticoagulation is indicated in those with recurrent or chronic atrial fibrillation.

Surgical Therapy

The small subgroup of patients with HCM who have both large outflow tract gradients (≥50 mm Hg) and severe symptoms of congestive heart failure despite medical therapy are candidates for surgery. There are several surgical strategies. A pacemaker can be placed in an attempt to *desynchronize* the LV during contraction and thereby decrease outflow obstruction. Surgical reduction of the outflow gradient is usually achieved by removing a small amount of cardiac muscle from the ventricular septum (septal myomectomy). Surgery abolishes or greatly reduces the LVOT gradient in most patients. Intraventricular systolic and end-diastolic pressures are markedly reduced, and these changes favorably influence LV filling and myocardial oxygen requirements. Similar results can be obtained by cardiac catheterization and selective alcohol injection into the septal perforator arteries. This maneuver causes ischemic injury followed by necrosis of the interventricular septum, which results in relief of the LVOT obstruction. If patients remain symptomatic despite these therapies, a prosthetic mitral valve can be inserted in an attempt to counteract the systolic anterior motion of the mitral leaflet.

Prognosis

The overall annual mortality of patients with HCM is approximately 1%. However, the subset of patients at high risk of sudden death (family history of sudden death or history of malignant ventricular dysrhythmias) has a mortality rate of 5% per year.

Management of Anesthesia

Management of anesthesia in patients with HCM is directed toward minimizing LVOT obstruction. *Any drug or event that decreases myocardial contractility or increases preload or afterload will improve LVOT obstruction. Conversely, sympathetic stimulation, hypovolemia, and vasodilation worsen LVOT obstruction* (see Table 10.7). Intraoperatively, patients with HCM may develop severe hypotension, myocardial ischemia, acute heart failure, and supraventricular or ventricular tachy-dysrhythmias. Previously unrecognized HCM may become manifest intraoperatively as unexplained hypotension or development of a systolic murmur in association with acute hemorrhage or drug-induced vasodilation.

Preoperative Evaluation and Management

Given the prevalence of HCM in the general population, patients with this disorder will be seen regularly in the operating room. Patients already diagnosed with this disease should undergo an updated cardiac evaluation before elective surgery. Such evaluation should include a 12-lead ECG and an echocardiogram. Patients taking β-blockers or calcium channel blockers should continue these medications throughout the perioperative period. For patients with an ICD the unit should be turned off immediately before surgery, an external defibrillator should be readily available in the operating room, and the device should be reactivated in the recovery room.

A more challenging task is detecting patients with HCM in whom the diagnosis has not yet been made. These patients are often young and appear healthy. Every patient should be asked preoperatively about any possible cardiac symptoms or a family history of cardiac disease or sudden death. The presence of a systolic murmur should raise suspicion of a possible diagnosis of HCM. If the ECG shows abnormalities, cardiologic evaluation is prudent.

In patients with HCM, preoperative administration of medication to allay anxiety and its associated activation of the sympathetic nervous system may be advisable. Expansion of intravascular volume during the preoperative period may also be useful in minimizing LVOT obstruction and the adverse hemodynamic effects of positive pressure ventilation.

Intraoperative Management

Regional or general anesthesia can be selected for patients with HCM so long as the anesthesiologist is aware of the main pathophysiologic mechanisms that trigger LVOT obstruction and has developed an anesthetic plan tailored to meet these specific needs.

Induction of anesthesia with an intravenous drug is acceptable, but the importance of avoiding sudden decreases in systemic vascular resistance and increases in heart rate and contractility must be kept in mind. A modest degree of direct myocardial depression is acceptable. Administration of a volatile anesthetic or β-adrenergic antagonist before direct laryngoscopy can blunt the sympathetic response typically evoked by tracheal intubation. Positive pressure ventilation can significantly decrease preload and predispose a hypovolemic patient to dynamic LVOT obstruction. To help avoid this, smaller tidal volumes and higher respiratory rates should be used, and positive end-expiratory pressure should be avoided if possible. Preload reduction and severe hypotension due to LVOT obstruction can also be encountered when abdominal insufflation is performed for laparoscopic surgery. The surgeon should be advised about this possibility, and the abdomen should be insufflated slowly.

Nondepolarizing muscle relaxants that have only minimal effects on the systemic circulation should be used for skeletal muscle relaxation. The increased heart rate that may accompany administration of pancuronium and the histamine release associated with other neuromuscular blockers should be avoided.

Anesthesia should be maintained with drugs that produce mild depression of myocardial contractility and have minimal effects on preload and afterload. A volatile anesthetic in a moderate dose is often used for this purpose.

Invasive monitoring of blood pressure may be helpful. TEE during surgery and anesthesia is particularly useful in patients with HCM because of the unique pathophysiology of this disorder. Note that neither central venous pressure monitoring nor pulmonary artery pressure monitoring can diagnose LVOT obstruction or systolic anterior motion of the mitral valve leaflet, nor do these monitoring techniques give an accurate assessment of LV filling in patients with HCM.

Hypotension that occurs in response to a decrease in preload or afterload should be treated with an α-adrenergic agonist such as phenylephrine. Drugs with β-adrenergic agonist activity, such as ephedrine, dopamine, and dobutamine, are *contraindicated* because the drug-induced increase in myocardial contractility and heart rate *increases* LVOT obstruction. Prompt replacement of blood loss and careful titration of intravenous fluids is important for maintaining preload and blood pressure. However, because of diastolic dysfunction, aggressive fluid replacement may result in pulmonary edema. Vasodilators should *not* be used to lower blood pressure; the decrease in systemic vascular resistance will accentuate LVOT obstruction.

Maintenance of normal sinus rhythm is very important because adequate LV filling is dependent on left atrial contraction. Patients who develop intraoperative supraventricular tachydysrhythmias should undergo immediate pharmacologic or electrical cardioversion. A cardioverter-defibrillator must be readily available in the operating room. β-Blockers such as metoprolol and esmolol are indicated to slow persistently elevated heart rates.

Parturient Patients. Pregnancy is usually well tolerated in patients with HCM despite the pregnancy-induced decrease in systemic vascular resistance and the risk of impaired venous return due to aortocaval compression. Parturient women with HCM may present major anesthetic challenges because events such as labor pain, which produces catecholamine release, and bearing down (Valsalva maneuver) may increase LVOT obstruction. There is no evidence that regional anesthesia increases complication rates in parturient patients with HCM undergoing vaginal delivery. Epidural anesthesia has been successfully administered to these patients. Maintenance of euvolemia or slight hypervolemia is helpful. Should hypotension unresponsive to fluid administration occur as a result of regional anesthesia, phenylephrine should be used to increase afterload. Oxytocin must be administered carefully because of its vasodilating properties and the compensatory tachycardia it causes and because of the abrupt inflow of large amounts of blood into the central circulation as a consequence of uterine contraction.

Pulmonary edema has been observed in parturient women with HCM after delivery, a finding that emphasizes the delicate balance in fluid requirements of these patients. Treatment of pulmonary edema may include phenylephrine if hypotension is present and esmolol to slow the heart rate, prolong diastolic filling time, and decrease myocardial contractility, all of which will decrease LVOT obstruction. Diuretics and nitrates *cannot* be used to treat pulmonary edema in this setting. They worsen the situation by provoking further LVOT obstruction.

Postoperative Management

Patients with HCM must be vigilantly monitored in the recovery room or intensive care unit in the immediate postoperative period. All factors that stimulate sympathetic activity (e.g., pain, shivering, anxiety, hypoxia, hypercarbia) must be eliminated. Maintenance of euvolemia and prompt treatment of hypotension are crucial.

Dilated Cardiomyopathy

Dilated cardiomyopathy is a primary myocardial disease characterized by LV or biventricular dilatation, systolic dysfunction, and normal ventricular wall thickness. The etiology of dilated cardiomyopathy is unknown, but it may be genetic or associated with infection such as coxsackievirus B infection. There is a familial transmission pattern in some 30% of cases, usually of an autosomal dominant form. Many types of secondary cardiomyopathies have features of dilated cardiomyopathy. These include the cardiomyopathies associated with alcohol abuse, cocaine abuse, the peripartum state, pheochromocytoma, infectious diseases (human immunodeficiency virus infection), uncontrolled tachycardia, Duchenne muscular dystrophy, thyroid disease, chemotherapeutic drugs, radiation therapy, hypertension, coronary artery disease, and valvular heart disease. African American men have an increased risk of developing dilated cardiomyopathy. Dilated cardiomyopathy is the most common type of cardiomyopathy, the third most common cause of heart failure, and the most common indication for cardiac transplantation.

Signs and Symptoms

The initial manifestation of dilated cardiomyopathy is usually heart failure. Chest pain on exertion that mimics angina pectoris occurs in some patients. Ventricular dilatation may be so marked that *functional* mitral and/or tricuspid regurgitation occurs. Supraventricular and ventricular dysrhythmias, conduction abnormalities, and sudden death are common. Systemic embolization due to formation of mural thrombi in dilated and hypokinetic cardiac chambers is also common.

Diagnosis

The ECG often shows ST-segment and T-wave abnormalities and left bundle branch block. Dysrhythmias are common and include ventricular premature beats and atrial fibrillation. Chest radiography may show enlargement of all four cardiac chambers, but LV dilatation is the principal morphologic feature.

Echocardiography typically reveals dilatation of all four cardiac chambers, most especially of the left ventricle, as well as global hypokinesis. Regional wall motion abnormalities may be seen in dilated cardiomyopathy and do not necessarily imply the presence of coronary disease. Mural thrombi can be detected, and valvular regurgitation due to annular dilatation is a common finding.

Laboratory testing should be performed to eliminate other causes of cardiac dilation such as hyperthyroidism. Coronary angiography is usually normal in patients with dilated cardiomyopathy. Right-sided heart catheterization reveals high pulmonary capillary wedge pressure, high systemic vascular resistance, and low cardiac output. Endomyocardial biopsy is *not* recommended.

Treatment

Treatment of dilated cardiomyopathy includes general supportive measures such as adequate rest, weight control, a low-sodium diet, fluid restriction, abstinence from tobacco and alcohol, and decreased physical activity during periods of cardiac decompensation. Cardiac rehabilitation, if possible, will improve general conditioning.

The medical management of dilated cardiomyopathy is similar to that of chronic heart failure. Patients with dilated cardiomyopathy are at risk of systemic and pulmonary embolization because blood stasis in the hypocontractile cardiac chambers leads to activation of the coagulation cascade. The risk of cardiac embolization is greatest in patients with severe LV dysfunction, atrial fibrillation, a history of thromboembolism, or echocardiographic evidence of intracardiac thrombus. Anticoagulation with warfarin, dabigatran (direct thrombin inhibitor), rivaroxaban, or apixaban (factor Xa inhibitors) is often instituted in patients with dilated cardiomyopathy and symptomatic heart failure.

Asymptomatic nonsustained ventricular tachycardia is common. However, suppression of this dysrhythmia with drug therapy does not improve survival. Placement of an ICD can decrease the risk of sudden death in patients who have survived a previous cardiac arrest (see Table 10.4).

Dilated cardiomyopathy remains the principal indication for cardiac transplantation in adults and children. Patients most likely to benefit from a heart transplant are those formerly very active persons younger than 60 years who have intractable symptoms of heart failure despite optimal medical therapy.

Prognosis

Symptomatic patients with dilated cardiomyopathy referred to tertiary care medical centers have a 5-year mortality rate of 50%. If the cardiomyopathy involves both the left and right ventricles, the prognosis is even worse. Hemodynamic abnormalities that predict a poor prognosis include an EF lower than 25%, a pulmonary capillary wedge pressure above 20 mm Hg, a cardiac index of less than 2.5 L/min/m², *systemic hypotension, pulmonary hypertension,* and increased central venous pressure. Alcoholic cardiomyopathy is largely reversible if complete abstinence from alcohol is maintained.

Management of Anesthesia

Since dilated cardiomyopathy is a cause of heart failure, the anesthetic management of these patients is the same as that described for other patients with heart failure.

Regional anesthesia may be an alternative to general anesthesia in selected patients with dilated cardiomyopathy. However, anticoagulant therapy may limit this option.

Apical Ballooning Syndrome

Apical ballooning syndrome, also known as *takotsubo cardiomyopathy, stress-induced cardiomyopathy,* and *broken heart syndrome,* is a *temporary* cardiac condition characterized by LV apical hypokinesis with ischemic ECG changes but unobstructed coronary arteries at cardiac catheterization. There is a temporary disruption of cardiac contractility in the LV apex while the rest of the heart has normal or even enhanced contractility. The apical ballooning seen on echocardiography resembles a Japanese octopus trap, thus the name "takotsubo." The most common symptoms according to the International Takotsubo Registry study include chest pain and dyspnea. Indeed, most patients think they are having a heart attack. Stress is determined to be the main factor in the development of this cardiomyopathy. The stressor can be either a physical event (e.g., acute asthma, surgery, chemotherapy, stroke), or it can be an emotional event. Women are affected much more often than men.

Diagnosis, Treatment, and Prognosis

Mayo Clinic diagnostic criteria for confirming apical ballooning syndrome include transient LV systolic dysfunction, absence of obstructive coronary disease, new ECG abnormalities, and the absence of pheochromocytoma or myocarditis. Treatment is supportive. However, since the disease process involves a high catecholamine state, inotropes should be avoided, and instead *negative inotropes* such as β-blockers or calcium channel blockers should be used. Intraaortic balloon counterpulsation has also been demonstrated to be a successful treatment option. Prognosis is generally favorable, and most patients have complete recovery within 2 months. There is a 10% chance of recurrence.

Peripartum Cardiomyopathy

Peripartum cardiomyopathy is a rare form of dilated cardiomyopathy of unknown cause that arises during the peripartum period (i.e., third trimester of pregnancy until 5 months after delivery). It occurs in women with no history of heart disease. The estimated incidence of peripartum cardiomyopathy is 1 in 3000 to 1 in 4000 parturients. The incidence is noted to be higher in South Africa, at 1:1000, and as high as 1:300 in Haiti. Postpartum cardiomyopathy may be related to diet and lifestyle. Risk factors include hypertension, obesity, prior toxin exposure (e.g., cocaine), multiparity, age older than 30 years, multifetal pregnancy, preeclampsia, long-term oral tocolytic therapy, and African American ethnicity. Other causes may include viral myocarditis, an abnormal immune response to pregnancy, and maladaptive responses to the hemodynamic stresses of pregnancy.

Signs and Symptoms

The signs and symptoms of peripartum cardiomyopathy are those of heart failure: dyspnea, fatigue, and peripheral edema. However, these signs and symptoms are common in the final trimester of many pregnant women, and there are no specific criteria for differentiating subtle symptoms of heart failure from normal late pregnancy. Clinical conditions that may mimic heart failure, such as amniotic fluid or pulmonary embolism, should be excluded when considering the diagnosis of peripartum cardiomyopathy.

Diagnosis

The diagnosis of peripartum cardiomyopathy is based upon three clinical criteria: development of heart failure in the period surrounding delivery, absence of another explainable cause of heart failure, and LV systolic dysfunction with an LVEF generally lower than 45%. Studies that can assist in this diagnosis include ECG, BNP levels, chest radiography, echocardiography, cardiac MRI, cardiac catheterization, and endomyocardial biopsy.

Treatment

The goal of treatment is to alleviate the symptoms of heart failure. Diuretics and vasodilators can be used. ACE inhibitors are teratogenic but can be useful following delivery. During pregnancy, vasodilation is accomplished with hydralazine and nitrates. Intravenous immunoglobulin may also have a beneficial effect. Thromboembolic complications are not uncommon, and anticoagulation is often recommended. Patients in whom conservative therapy fails may be treated with mechanical circulatory support or even heart transplantation.

Prognosis

The mortality rate of peripartum cardiomyopathy ranges from 25%–50%. Higher mortality rates have been noted in African American patients. Most deaths occur within 3 months of delivery. Death is usually a result of progression of heart failure or sudden death related to cardiac dysrhythmias or thromboembolic events. The prognosis appears to depend on the degree of normalization of LV size and function within 6 months of delivery.

Management of Anesthesia

Anesthesia management in women with peripartum cardiomyopathy requires assessment of cardiac status and careful planning of the analgesia and/or anesthesia required for delivery. Regional anesthesia may provide a desirable decrease in afterload.

Secondary Cardiomyopathies With Restrictive Physiology

Secondary cardiomyopathies with restrictive physiology are due to systemic diseases that produce myocardial infiltration and severe diastolic dysfunction. The most common of these is caused by amyloidosis. Other systemic diseases such as hemochromatosis, sarcoidosis, and carcinoid may produce a similar type of cardiomyopathy. *The diagnosis should be considered in patients who have heart failure but no evidence of cardiomegaly or systolic dysfunction.* The condition results from increased stiffness of the myocardium caused by the deposition of abnormal substances. Although there is impaired diastolic function and reduced ventricular compliance, systolic function is usually normal. Cardiomyopathies with restrictive physiology must be differentiated from constrictive pericarditis, which has a similar physiology. A clinical history of pericarditis makes the diagnosis of constrictive pericarditis more likely.

Signs and Symptoms

Because cardiomyopathies with restrictive physiology can affect both ventricles, symptoms and signs of both LV and RV failure may be present. In advanced stages of this disease, *all the signs and symptoms of heart failure are present, but there is no cardiomegaly.* Amyloid cardiomyopathy often presents with thromboembolic complications. Atrial fibrillation is common. Cardiac conduction disturbances are particularly common in amyloidosis and sarcoidosis. Over time, this involvement of the conduction system can lead to heart block or ventricular dysrhythmias, resulting in sudden death.

Diagnosis

The ECG may demonstrate conduction abnormalities. The chest radiograph may show signs of pulmonary congestion and/or pleural effusion, *but cardiomegaly is absent.* Laboratory tests should be used as needed to diagnose the systemic disease responsible for the cardiac infiltration.

Echocardiography will demonstrate significant diastolic dysfunction and normal systolic function. The atria are enlarged because of the high atrial pressures, but the ventricles are normal in size. In cardiac amyloidosis, the ventricular mass appears speckled, a characteristic sign of amyloid deposition. Various echocardiographic criteria can differentiate secondary cardiomyopathy with restrictive physiology from constrictive pericarditis. Endomyocardial biopsy can help elucidate the cause of an infiltrative cardiomyopathy.

Treatment

Symptomatic treatment is similar to that for diastolic heart failure. It includes administration of diuretics to treat pulmonary and systemic venous congestion. Excessive diuresis may decrease ventricular filling pressures and cardiac output and result in hypotension and hypoperfusion. The development of atrial fibrillation with loss of the "atrial kick" may substantially worsen diastolic dysfunction, and a rapid ventricular response may further compromise cardiac output. *Maintenance of normal sinus rhythm is extremely important.* Because stroke volume tends to be fixed in the presence of cardiomyopathy with restrictive physiology, bradycardia may precipitate acute heart failure. Significant bradycardia or severe conduction system disease may require implantation of a cardiac pacemaker. With cardiac sarcoidosis, malignant ventricular dysrhythmias are common and may necessitate insertion of an ICD. Anticoagulation may be needed in patients with atrial fibrillation and/or low cardiac output. Cardiac transplantation is not a treatment option because myocardial infiltration will recur in the transplanted heart.

Prognosis

The prognosis of secondary cardiomyopathy with restrictive physiology is very poor.

Management of Anesthesia

Management of anesthesia for patients with restrictive cardiomyopathy follows the same principles as that for patients with cardiac tamponade (see Chapter 11, "Pericardial Disease and Cardiac Trauma"). Because stroke volume is relatively fixed, it is important to maintain sinus rhythm and to avoid any significant decrease in the heart rate. Maintenance of venous return and intravascular fluid volume is also necessary to maintain an acceptable cardiac output.

Cor Pulmonale

Cor pulmonale is RV enlargement (hypertrophy and/or dilatation) that may progress to right-sided heart failure. Diseases that induce *pulmonary hypertension,* such as COPD, restrictive lung disease, and respiratory insufficiency of central origin (obesity-hypoventilation syndrome), cause cor pulmonale. It can also result from idiopathic pulmonary artery hypertension—that is, pulmonary hypertension that occurs in the absence of left-sided heart disease, myocardial disease, congenital heart disease, or any other clinically significant respiratory, connective tissue, or chronic thromboembolic disease. The most common cause of cor pulmonale is COPD.

Cor pulmonale usually occurs in persons older than age 50 because of its association with COPD. Men are affected five times more often than women.

Pathophysiology

The main pathophysiologic determinant of cor pulmonale is pulmonary hypertension. By various mechanisms, chronic lung disease induces an increase in pulmonary vascular resistance.

Chronic alveolar hypoxia is the most important factor in this process. Acute hypoxia, such as seen in exacerbations of COPD or during sleep in patients with obesity-hypoventilation syndrome, causes pulmonary vasoconstriction. Chronic alveolar hypoxia promotes pulmonary vasculature remodeling and an increase in pulmonary vascular resistance. Even mild hypoxemia may result in vascular remodeling, so it appears that other factors are also involved in the development of cor pulmonale.

Pulmonary hypertension causes an increased workload for the right ventricle, and RV hypertrophy develops. Over time, RV dysfunction occurs, and eventually RV failure is present.

Signs and Symptoms

Symptoms of cor pulmonale may be obscured by the co-existing lung disease. Clinical signs occur late in the course of the disease, and the most prominent is peripheral edema. As RV function deteriorates, dyspnea increases and effort-related syncope can occur. Accentuation of the pulmonic component of the second heart sound, a diastolic murmur due to incompetence of the pulmonic valve, and a systolic murmur due to tricuspid regurgitation connote severe pulmonary hypertension. Evidence of overt RV failure consists of increased jugular venous pressure and hepatosplenomegaly.

Diagnosis

The ECG may show signs of right atrial and RV hypertrophy. Right atrial hypertrophy is suggested by peaked P waves in leads II, III, and aVF ("P pulmonale"). Right axis deviation and a partial or complete right bundle branch block are also often seen. A normal-appearing ECG, however, does not exclude the presence of pulmonary hypertension.

Radiographic signs of cor pulmonale include an increase in the width of the right pulmonary artery and a decrease in pulmonary vascular markings in the lung periphery. On a lateral chest radiograph, RV enlargement is indicated by a decrease in the retrosternal space.

Transesophageal echocardiography can provide quantitative estimates of pulmonary artery pressure, assessment of the size and function of the right atrium and ventricle, and evaluation of the presence and severity of tricuspid or pulmonic regurgitation. *Transthoracic echocardiography* (TTE) is often difficult to perform in patients with COPD, because the hyperinflated lungs impair transmission of the ultrasound waves.

Treatment

Treatment of cor pulmonale is aimed at reducing the workload of the right ventricle by decreasing pulmonary artery pressure and pulmonary vascular resistance. If the pulmonary artery vasoconstriction has a reversible component, as may occur during an acute exacerbation of COPD, this goal can be achieved by returning the PaO_2, $PaCO_2$, and arterial pH to normal.

Oxygen supplementation to maintain the PaO_2 above 60 mm Hg (oxygen saturation > 90% by pulse oximetry) is useful in both the acute and long-term treatment of right-sided heart failure. *Long-term oxygen therapy decreases the mortality of cor pulmonale and improves cognitive function and quality of life.*

Diuretics may be used to treat right-sided heart failure that does not respond to correction of hypoxia or hypercarbia. Diuretics must be administered very carefully because diuretic-induced metabolic alkalosis, which encourages CO_2 retention, may aggravate ventilatory insufficiency by depressing the effectiveness of CO_2 as a stimulus to breathing. Diuresis can also increase blood viscosity and myocardial work. Pulmonary vasodilators such as sildenafil and bosentan have been shown to improve the symptoms of cor pulmonale and reduce RV mass as well as RV remodeling.

When cor pulmonale is progressive despite maximum medical therapy, transplantation of one or two lungs or a heart-lung transplantation will provide dramatic relief of cardiorespiratory failure.

Prognosis

The prognosis of patients with cor pulmonale is dependent on the disease responsible for initiating the pulmonary hypertension. Patients with COPD in whom arterial oxygenation can be maintained at near-normal levels and whose pulmonary hypertension is relatively mild have a favorable prognosis. Prognosis is poor in patients with severe irreversible pulmonary hypertension.

Management of Anesthesia

Preoperative preparation of patients with cor pulmonale is directed toward (1) eliminating and controlling acute and chronic pulmonary infection, (2) reversing bronchospasm, (3) improving clearance of airway secretions, (4) expanding collapsed or poorly ventilated alveoli, (5) maintaining hydration, and (6) correcting any electrolyte imbalances. Preoperative measurement of arterial blood gases will provide guidelines for perioperative management.

Induction of general anesthesia can be accomplished using any available method or drug. Adequate depth of anesthesia should be present before endotracheal intubation, because this stimulus can elicit reflex bronchospasm in lightly anesthetized patients.

Anesthesia is typically maintained with a balanced anesthetic. Volatile anesthetics are effective bronchodilators. Large doses of opioids should be avoided because they can contribute to prolonged postoperative ventilatory depression. Muscle relaxants associated with histamine release should also be avoided because of the adverse effect of histamine on airway resistance and pulmonary vascular resistance.

Positive pressure ventilation improves oxygenation, presumably because of better ventilation/perfusion matching. Humidification of inhaled gases helps maintain hydration, liquefaction of secretions, and mucociliary function.

Intraoperative monitoring of patients with cor pulmonale is influenced by the complexity of the surgery. An intraarterial catheter permits frequent determination of arterial blood gases. A central venous catheter or pulmonary artery catheter may be useful depending on the surgery. Trend values of right atrial pressure can provide some information about RV function. Direct measurement of pulmonary artery pressure helps determine the time to treat pulmonary hypertension and the response to treatment. TEE is an alternative method for monitoring RV function and fluid status. An implantable pulmonary artery pressure measurement system was recently approved for the management of NYHA class III patients with heart failure.

Regional anesthesia can be used in appropriate situations in patients with cor pulmonale, but regional anesthesia is best avoided for operations that require a high level of sensory and motor block, because loss of function of the accessory muscles of respiration may be very deleterious in patients with pulmonary disease. In addition, any decrease in systemic vascular resistance in the presence of fixed pulmonary hypertension can produce very significant systemic hypotension.

The respiratory and cardiovascular status of a patient with cor pulmonale must be carefully monitored in the postoperative period, and any factors that exacerbate pulmonary hypertension (e.g., hypoxia, hypercarbia) must be avoided/treated. Oxygen therapy should be maintained as long as needed.

KEY POINTS

- Heart failure is a complex pathophysiologic state in which the heart is unable to fill with or eject blood at a rate appropriate to meet tissue requirements. Heart failure is characterized by specific symptoms (dyspnea and fatigue) and signs (circulatory congestion or hypoperfusion).
- Heart failure is associated with significant morbidity and mortality, which imposes a great financial burden on the healthcare system.
- The principal pathophysiologic derangement in the development and progression of heart failure is ventricular remodeling. The principal treatment goals in heart failure patients are avoiding or decreasing the degree of ventricular remodeling and promoting reverse remodeling. Therapies proven to be of value in this regard include ACE inhibitors, β-blockers, statins, aldosterone inhibitors, and cardiac resynchronization therapy.
- Management of acute heart failure includes the use of loop diuretics in combination with vasodilators, positive inotropic drugs, exogenous B-type natriuretic peptide (BNP), and/or insertion of mechanical devices.
- Hypertrophic cardiomyopathy (HCM) is the most common genetic cardiac disorder. Its pathophysiology is related to the development of left ventricular outflow tract (LVOT) obstruction and ventricular dysrhythmias that can cause sudden death.
- Factors that induce LVOT obstruction in HCM include hypovolemia, tachycardia, an increase in myocardial

contractility, and a decrease in afterload. Outflow tract obstruction can be managed by maintaining hydration, increasing afterload (phenylephrine), and decreasing heart rate and myocardial contractility (β-blockers or calcium channel blockers).
- Dilated cardiomyopathy is the most common form of cardiomyopathy and the second most common cause of heart failure.
- Cor pulmonale is RV enlargement (hypertrophy and/or dilatation) that may progress to right-sided heart failure. It is caused by diseases that promote development of pulmonary hypertension.
- The most important pathophysiologic determinant of the development of pulmonary hypertension and cor pulmonale in patients with chronic lung disease is alveolar hypoxia. The best available treatment to improve the prognosis in these patients is long-term oxygen therapy.

RESOURCES

Abraham WT. The role of implantable hemodynamic monitors to manage heart failure. *Heart Fail Clin.* 2015;11:183-189.

Armstrong PW. Aldosterone antagonists—last man standing? *N Engl J Med.* 2011;364:79-80.

Elliott PM, Anastasakis A, Borger MA, et al. 2014 ESC Guidelines on diagnosis and management of hypertrophic cardiomyopathy: the Task Force for the Diagnosis and Management of Hypertrophic Cardiomyopathy of the European Society of Cardiology (ESC). *Eur Heart J.* 2014;35:2733-2779.

Givertz MM. Peripartum cardiomyopathy. *Circulation.* 2013;127:e622-e626.

Japanese Circulation Society Joint Working Group. Guidelines for treatment of acute heart failure. *Circ J.* 2013;77:2157-2201.

Kutyifa V, Voors AA, Zareba W, et al. The influence of left ventricular ejection fraction on the effectiveness of cardiac resynchronization therapy. *J Am Coll Cardiol.* 2013;61:936-944.

Maile MD, Engoren MC, Tremper KK, et al. Worsening preoperative heart failure is associated with mortality and noncardiac complications, but not myocardial infarction after noncardiac surgery: a retrospective cohort study. *Anesth Analg.* 2014;119:522-532.

Moe GW, Ezekowitz JA, O'Meara E, et al. The 2014 Canadian Cardiovascular Society heart failure management guideline focus update: anemia, biomarkers, and recent therapeutic trial implications. *Can J Cardiol.* 2015;31:3-16.

Ponikowski P, Voors AA, Anker SD, et al. 2016 ESC Guidelines for the diagnosis and treatment of acute and chronic heart failure. The Task Force for the diagnosis and treatment of acute and chronic heart failure of the European Society of Cardiology (ESC). Developed with the special contribution of the Heart Failure Association of the ESC. *Eur Heart J.* 2016;37:2129-2200.

Pulido JN, Park SJ, Rihal CS. Percutaneous left ventricular assist devices: clinical uses, future applications, and anesthetic considerations. *J Cardiothorac Vasc Anesth.* 2010;24:478-486.

Roger VL. Epidemiology of heart failure. *Circ Res.* 2013;113:646-659.

Templin C, Ghadri JR, Diekmann LC, et al. Clinical features and outcomes of takotsubo (stress) cardiomyopathy. *N Engl J Med.* 2015;373:929-938.

Thunberg CA, Gaitan BD, Arabia FA, et al. Ventricular assist devices today and tomorrow. *J Cardiothorac Vasc Anesth.* 2010;24:656-680.

Yancy CW, Jessup M, Bozkurt B, et al. 2013 ACCF/AHA Guideline for the management of heart failure. A report of the American College of Cardiology Foundation/American Heart Association Task Force on Practice Guidelines. Developed in collaboration with the American College of Chest Physicians, Heart Rhythm Society and International Society for Heart and Lung Transplantation. *J Am Coll Cardiol.* 2013;62:e147-e239.

Pericardial Disease and Cardiac Trauma

RAJ K. MODAK, LUIZ MARACAJA

Although the causes of pericardial disease are diverse, the resulting clinical and pathologic manifestations are similar. The three most frequent responses to pericardial injury are acute pericarditis, pericardial effusion, and constrictive pericarditis. Cardiac tamponade may present whenever pericardial fluid accumulates under pressure. Management of anesthesia in patients with pericardial disease is facilitated by an understanding of the alterations in cardiovascular function produced by pericardial disease.

PERICARDIAL ANATOMY AND FUNCTION

The visceral pericardium is a thin layer of mesothelial cells that adheres to the epicardial surface of the heart. The parietal pericardium has a layer of serous pericardium and an outer portion composed largely of collagen that is mostly acellular. The parietal pericardium has ligamentous attachments to the mediastinum, sternum, and diaphragm to help maintain the heart's position in the thoracic cavity. The pericardial sac is the space between these two layers and contains serous fluid, which is an ultrafiltrate of plasma that comes from the visceral pericardium. Native pericardial fluid lubricates the heart and facilitates normal cardiac motion within the pericardial sac. The pericardium covers the entire heart and also extends for a distance along the proximal aorta, the proximal pulmonary artery, and the vena cava just outside the right atrium.

ACUTE PERICARDITIS

Viral infection is often presumed to be the cause of acute pericarditis when it occurs as a primary illness (Table 11.1). Most cases of acute pericarditis follow a transient and uncomplicated clinical course, and thus this entity is often termed *acute benign pericarditis*. Acute benign pericarditis is unaccompanied by either a substantial pericardial effusion or cardiac tamponade and rarely progresses to constrictive pericarditis.

Pericarditis can also occur after myocardial infarction (MI). It most commonly appears 1–3 days following a transmural MI as a result of the interaction between the healing necrotic myocardium and the pericardium. Dressler syndrome is a delayed form of acute pericarditis that may follow acute MI. It can occur weeks to months after the initial myocardial event. It is thought that Dressler syndrome is the result of an autoimmune process initiated by the entry of bits of necrotic myocardium into the circulation, where they act as antigens. Acute pericarditis occurs more commonly in adult men 20–50 years of age.

Diagnosis

The clinical diagnosis of acute pericarditis is based on the presence of chest pain, a pericardial friction rub, and changes on the electrocardiogram (ECG). The chest pain is typically acute in onset and is described as a severe pain localized over the anterior chest. This pain typically worsens with inspiration, which helps distinguish it from pain caused by myocardial ischemia. Patients often report relief when changing position from being supine to sitting forward. Low-grade fever and sinus tachycardia are also common. Auscultation of the chest often reveals a friction rub, especially when the symptoms are acute. These high-pitched scratchy sounds occur when volumes in the heart undergo the most dramatic changes, such as during early ventricular filling and ventricular ejection. Pericardial friction rubs are related to the cardiac cycle; this makes it possible to differentiate these sounds from pleural rubs, which are related to inspiration.

Inflammation of the superficial myocardium is the most likely explanation for the diffuse changes seen on ECG. Classically the ECG changes associated with acute pericarditis evolve through four stages. Stage I is characterized by diffuse ST-segment elevation and PR-segment depression. In stage II, the ST and PR segments normalize. Stage III shows widespread T-wave inversions. And stage IV is characterized by normalization of the T waves. The early ST-segment elevations are usually present in all leads, but in post-MI pericarditis the changes may be more localized. The diffuse distribution and the absence of reciprocal ST-segment depressions helps distinguish these changes from the ECG changes of MI. Depression of the PR segment reflects superficial injury of the atrial myocardium and may be the earliest sign of acute pericarditis. ECG changes are seen in 90% of patients with acute pericarditis. However, a clear evolution of ECG changes through all four stages just described is noted in somewhat more than half of all patients with acute pericarditis. Patients with uremic pericarditis frequently do not have these typical ECG abnormalities of pericarditis. Acute pericarditis in the absence of an associated pericardial effusion does not alter cardiac function.

Treatment

Salicylates or other nonsteroidal antiinflammatory drugs may be useful for decreasing pericardial inflammation. Aspirin is most commonly prescribed, although ketorolac has also been used successfully. Symptomatic relief of the pain of acute pericarditis can also be provided by oral analgesics such as codeine. In some settings, relief may be achieved with the use of colchicine. Corticosteroids such as prednisone can also relieve the symptoms of acute pericarditis. However, their use early in the course of acute pericarditis is associated with an increased incidence of relapse after discontinuation of the drug. Therefore steroid therapy is usually reserved for cases that do not respond to conventional therapy.

Relapsing Pericarditis

Acute pericarditis resulting from any cause may follow a recurrent or chronic relapsing course. Relapsing pericarditis has two clinical presentations: incessant and intermittent. *Incessant pericarditis* is diagnosed in patients in whom discontinuation of or attempts to wean from antiinflammatory drugs nearly always result in a relapse within a period of 6 weeks or less. *Intermittent pericarditis* occurs in patients who have symptom-free intervals of longer than 6 weeks without drug treatment. In many patients the symptoms of relapsing pericarditis include weakness, fatigue, and headache and are associated with chest discomfort. Although relapsing pericarditis is uncomfortable, it is rarely life threatening. Treatment may include the standard therapies for acute pericarditis and/or corticosteroids (prednisone) or immunosuppressive drugs such as azathioprine.

Pericarditis After Cardiac Surgery

Postcardiotomy syndrome presents primarily as acute pericarditis. The cause of this syndrome may be infective or autoimmune, and it may follow blunt or penetrating cardiac trauma, hemopericardium, or epicardial pacemaker implantation. Most commonly it is seen in patients undergoing cardiac surgery in which pericardiotomy is performed. The incidence of postcardiotomy syndrome associated with cardiac surgery is between 10% and 40%. It is more common in pediatric patients. The risk is lower after cardiac transplantation, presumably because of the immunosuppressed state. Cardiac tamponade is a rare complication of postcardiotomy syndrome, with an incidence ranging from 0.1%–6%. The treatment of postcardiotomy syndrome is similar to that of other forms of acute pericarditis.

PERICARDIAL EFFUSION AND CARDIAC TAMPONADE

Pericardial fluid may accumulate in the pericardial sac with virtually any form of pericardial disease. The pathophysiologic effects of a pericardial effusion reflect whether or not the fluid is under pressure. *Cardiac tamponade* occurs when the pressure of the fluid in the pericardial space impairs cardiac filling. Common causes of pericardial effusion are listed in Table 11.1. In up to 20% of cases the cause of the pericardial effusion is unknown. Neoplastic pericardial effusion is a common cause of cardiac tamponade in nonsurgical patients.

Pericardial fluid may be classified as transudative or exudative. Serosanguineous (exudative) fluid is typically seen when the pericardial disease is due to cancer, tuberculosis, or radiation exposure. Serosanguineous pericardial effusion

TABLE 11.1	Causes of Acute Pericarditis and Pericardial Effusion

Infection
  Viral
  Bacterial
  Fungal
  Tuberculous
Myocardial infarction (Dressler syndrome)
Trauma or cardiotomy
Metastatic disease
Drugs
Mediastinal radiation
Systemic disease
  Rheumatoid arthritis
  Systemic lupus erythematosus
  Scleroderma

also occurs in patients with end-stage renal disease. Traumatic injury usually presents as hemopericardium. Perforation of the heart and subsequent cardiac tamponade may also result from insertion of central venous catheters or pacemaker wires.

Signs and Symptoms

The signs and symptoms of a pericardial effusion depend on its size and duration (acute vs. chronic). The pericardial space normally holds 15–50 mL of pericardial fluid. Acute changes in

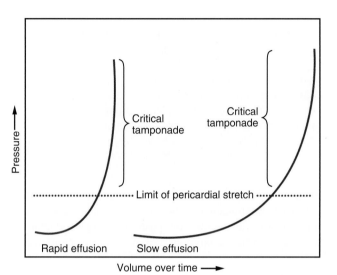

FIG. 11.1 Pericardial pressure-volume curves are shown in which the intrapericardial volume increases slowly or rapidly over time. On the left, rapidly increasing pericardial fluid quickly exceeds the limit of pericardial stretch, which causes a steep increase in pericardial pressure. On the right a slower rate of pericardial filling takes longer to exceed the limit of pericardial stretch because there is more time for the pericardium to stretch and compensatory mechanisms to become activated. (From Spodick DH. Acute cardiac tamponade. *N Engl J Med.* 2003;349:684-690. Copyright 2003 Massachusetts Medical Society, with permission.)

pericardial volume as small as 100 mL may result in increased intrapericardial pressure and development of cardiac tamponade. Conversely, large volumes can be accommodated if the pericardial effusion develops gradually. In this context the pressure-volume relationship is altered, and cardiac tamponade may not develop because the pericardium stretches to accommodate the volume of the effusion (Fig. 11.1). The development of a chronic pericardial effusion can result in effusion volumes in excess of 2 L. If the pressure in the pericardium remains low, large effusions can be tolerated without significant signs and symptoms. However, when the pericardial pressure increases, the right atrial pressure increases in parallel, so right atrial pressure becomes an accurate reflection of the intrapericardial pressure. At this point, signs and symptoms of cardiac tamponade may develop.

Cardiac Tamponade

Cardiac tamponade presents as a spectrum of hemodynamic abnormalities of varying severity rather than as an all-or-none phenomenon (Fig. 11.2). Symptoms of large pericardial effusions reflect compression of adjacent anatomic structures, specifically the esophagus, trachea, and lung. In this situation, common symptoms include anorexia, dyspnea, cough, and chest pain. Symptoms such as dysphagia, hiccups, and hoarseness may indicate higher pressure on the adjacent tissues.

Two important physical signs of cardiac tamponade and constrictive pericarditis were described by Dr. Adolf Kussmaul in 1873. *Kussmaul sign* is distention of the jugular veins during inspiration. *Pulsus paradoxus* was described by Kussmaul as "a pulse simultaneously slight and irregular, disappearing during inspiration and returning on expiration." The modern definition of pulsus paradoxus is a decrease in systolic blood pressure of more than 10 mm Hg during inspiration (Fig. 11.3). This hemodynamic change reflects selective impairment of diastolic filling of the left ventricle. Pulsus paradoxus is observed in approximately 75% of patients with acute cardiac tamponade but in only about 30% of patients with chronic pericardial

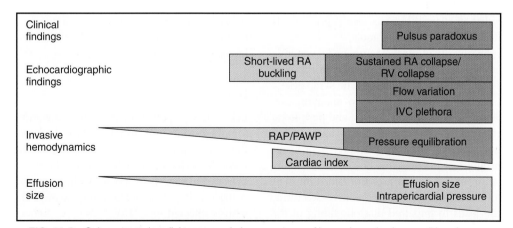

FIG. 11.2 Subacute pericardial tamponade is a spectrum of hemodynamic abnormalities. A common timeline for different findings is shown although a wide variation is possible. *IVC,* Inferior vena cava; *PAWP,* pulmonary arterial wedge pressure; *RA,* right atrium; *RAP,* right atrial pressure; *RV,* right ventricle. (From Argulian E, Messerli F. Misconceptions and facts about pericardial effusion and tamponade. *Am J Med.* 2013;126:858-861.)

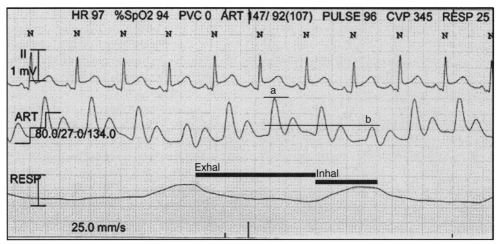

FIG. 11.3 Cyclical systolic pressure variation during tidal breathing is normal. In the presence of cardiac tamponade the arterial blood pressure decreases more than 10 mm Hg (a→b) from exhalation (Exhal) to inhalation (Inhal) as a reflection of a concomitant decrease in left ventricular stroke volume. This contrasts with the opposite response observed during inspiration in the absence of cardiac tamponade, which accounts for its designation as a paradoxical pulse (pulsus paradoxus). (From Binks A, Soar J, Cranshaw J. Pulsus paradoxus and pericardial effusion. *Resuscitation.* 2006;68:177-178.)

effusion. Kussmaul sign and pulsus paradoxus both reflect the dyssynchrony or opposing responses of the right and left ventricles to filling during the respiratory cycle. Another term for this is *ventricular discordance.*

Beck's triad consists of distant heart sounds, increased jugular venous pressure, and hypotension. Beck's triad is observed in one-third of patients with acute cardiac tamponade. Another triad consisting of quiet heart sounds, increased central venous pressure (CVP), and ascites has been described in patients with chronic pericardial effusion. More commonly, symptomatic patients with chronic pericardial effusion exhibit sinus tachycardia, jugular venous distention, hepatomegaly, and peripheral edema. *Ewart sign,* in which there is an area of bronchial breath sounds and dullness to percussion, is an uncommon sign of pericardial effusion. It is caused by compression of the left lower lobe by the pericardial effusion. When this sign is present it is observed at the inferior angle of the left scapula.

Depending on the severity of cardiac tamponade, systemic blood pressure may be decreased or maintained in the normal range. CVP is almost always increased. The sympathetic nervous system is activated in an attempt to maintain cardiac output and blood pressure by tachycardia and peripheral vasoconstriction. Cardiac output is maintained as long as CVP exceeds right ventricular end-diastolic pressure. A progressive increase in intrapericardial pressure, however, eventually results in equalization of right atrial pressure and right ventricular end-diastolic pressure. Ultimately the increased intrapericardial pressure leads to impaired diastolic filling of the heart, decreased stroke volume, and hypotension (Table 11.2). Fig. 11.4 demonstrates the effects of mechanical ventilation on hemodynamics in patients with cardiac tamponade. Changes in right and left ventricular preload/volume are reversed compared to spontaneous ventilation (Fig. 11.3).

Cardiac tamponade may be the cause of a low cardiac output syndrome during the early postoperative period after cardiac surgery. Cardiac tamponade may occur as a complication of various invasive procedures in the cardiac catheterization laboratory and intensive care unit. Acute cardiac tamponade may also be due to hemopericardium caused by aortic dissection, penetrating cardiac trauma, or acute MI.

Loculated Pericardial Effusions

Loculated pericardial effusion may selectively compress one or more cardiac chambers, producing a *localized* cardiac tamponade. This localization is most frequently observed after cardiac surgery when blood accumulates behind the sternum and selectively compresses the right ventricle and right atrium. A similar response may be seen following anterior chest wall trauma. Transesophageal echocardiography (TEE) is superior to transthoracic echocardiography (TTE) for demonstrating a localized pericardial effusion.

Diagnosis

Echocardiography is the most accurate and practical method for diagnosing pericardial effusion and cardiac tamponade. Because of this, echocardiography fulfills the class I recommendations by the 2013 Task Force of the American Society of Echocardiography, American College of Cardiology, and the American Heart Association for the evaluation of all patients with suspected pericardial disease. Echocardiography can detect pericardial effusions of as little as 20 mL. The measurement of the echo-free space between the heart and pericardium allows easy assessment of effusion size and may also provide information about the cause of the effusion. Computed tomography (CT) and magnetic resonance imaging (MRI) are

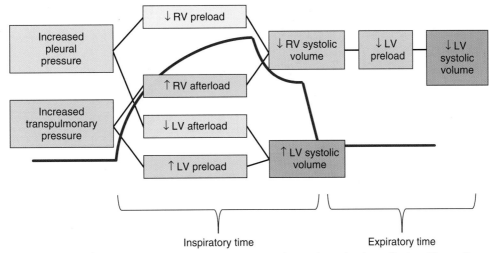

FIG. 11.4 The effects of mechanical ventilation on hemodynamics in patients with cardiac tamponade. Mechanical ventilation increases pleural pressure and transpulmonary pressure. During inspiration, left ventricular (LV) stroke volume increases because of the increase in LV preload, whereas LV afterload decreases. This leads to an increase in arterial blood pressure at the end of inspiration. In contrast, right ventricular (RV) stroke volume decreases during inspiration because of the decrease in RV preload, but RV afterload increases. Because of the pulmonary transit time of blood, the inspiratory decrease in RV output causes a decrease in LV filling and output a few heart beats later, usually during expiration. This in turn leads to a decrease in systemic blood pressure at the end of expiration. (Adapted from Carmona P, Mateo E, Casanovas I, et al. Management of cardiac tamponade after cardiac surgery. *J Cardiothorac Vasc Anesth.* 2012;26:302-311, Fig. 2; and from Michard F, Teboul JL. Using heart-lung interactions to assess fluid responsiveness during mechanical ventilation. *Crit Care.* 2000;4:282-289.)

TABLE 11.2	Signs and Symptoms of Cardiac Tamponade

Increased central venous pressure
Pulsus paradoxus
Equalization of cardiac filling pressures
Hypotension
Decreased voltage on ECG
Activation of sympathetic nervous system

also useful in detecting both pericardial effusion and pericardial thickening. The ECG may demonstrate low voltage in the presence of a large effusion. Chest radiography often shows a characteristic "water bottle heart" (Fig. 11.5). However, this is a nonspecific sign of pericardial effusion. Pericardiocentesis may be useful for diagnosing metastatic disease or infection in the pericardium.

Echocardiography, although definitive for diagnosing pericardial effusion, cannot always confirm the presence of cardiac tamponade. However, the finding of early diastolic inward wall motion of the right atrium or right ventricle ("collapse"), reflecting similar intracavitary and intrapericardial pressure, is highly suggestive of the presence of cardiac tamponade. Echocardiography can also demonstrate ventricular discordance. Pulsed wave Doppler examination

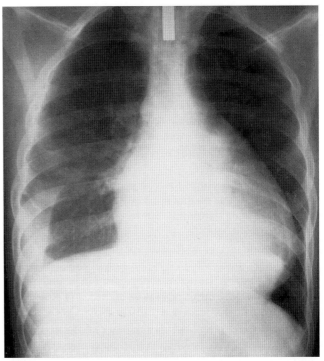

FIG. 11.5 Chest radiograph demonstrating a "water bottle" heart.

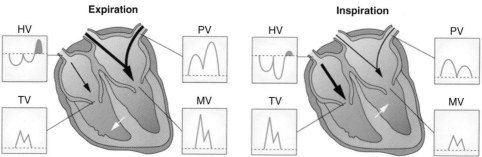

FIG. 11.6 Ventricular interdependence and dissociation of intrathoracic and intracardiac pressures in patients with constrictive pericarditis. This figure shows the typical changes during respiration in interventricular septum movement *(white arrows)* and blood flow velocity *(black arrows)*. Insets depict typical Doppler velocity (*y*-axis) versus time (*x*-axis) across the hepatic vein (HV), tricuspid valve (TV), pulmonary vein (PV), and mitral valve (MV). (From Syed FF, Schaff HV, Oh JK. Constrictive pericarditis—a curable diastolic heart failure. *Nat Rev Cardiol.* 2014;11:530-544.)

of peak mitral and tricuspid inflow velocities will show a decrease in mitral flow and an increase in tricuspid flow during inspiration if tamponade is present. Ventricular septal deviation toward the left can also be seen during inspiration (Fig. 11.6). With cardiac tamponade, the pressures within the cardiac chambers eventually equilibrate. Clinically this can be confirmed by right-sided heart catheterization. Pulmonary artery occlusion pressure and pulmonary artery diastolic pressure (both estimates of left atrial pressure and left ventricular end-diastolic pressure), right atrial pressure, and right ventricular end-diastolic pressure will be nearly equal.

Treatment

Mild cardiac tamponade can be managed conservatively in some patients. However, removal of fluid is required for definitive treatment and should be performed when CVP is increased. Pericardial fluid may be removed by pericardiocentesis or by surgical techniques, which include subxiphoid pericardiostomy, thoracoscopic pericardiostomy, and thoracotomy with pericardiostomy. Removal of even a small amount of pericardial fluid can result in a dramatic *decrease* in intrapericardial pressure.

Temporizing measures likely to help maintain stroke volume until definitive treatment of cardiac tamponade can be instituted include expanding intravascular volume, administering catecholamines to increase myocardial contractility, and correcting metabolic acidosis. Expansion of intravascular fluid volume can be achieved by infusion of either colloid or crystalloid solution. However, improvement in hemodynamic function from these measures may be limited, and pericardiocentesis must not be delayed.

Continuous intravenous infusion of a catecholamine such as isoproterenol may be effective for increasing myocardial contractility and heart rate. Atropine may be necessary to treat the bradycardia that results from vagal reflexes evoked by the increased intrapericardial pressure. Dopamine infusion, which increases systemic vascular resistance, can also be

employed to treat cardiac tamponade. As with intravascular fluid replacement, pericardiocentesis should never be delayed in deference to vasoactive drug therapy.

Correction of metabolic acidosis is essential when considering the management of cardiac tamponade. Metabolic acidosis resulting from low cardiac output must be treated to correct the myocardial depression seen with severe acidosis and to improve the inotropic effects of catecholamines.

Management of Anesthesia

General anesthesia and positive pressure ventilation in the presence of a hemodynamically significant cardiac tamponade can result in life-threatening hypotension. This hypotension may be due to anesthesia-induced peripheral vasodilation, direct myocardial depression, or decreased venous return caused by the increased intrathoracic pressure associated with positive pressure ventilation. *Pericardiocentesis performed under local anesthesia* is preferred for the initial management of hypotensive patients with cardiac tamponade (Fig. 11.7). After the hemodynamic status is improved by the percutaneous pericardiocentesis, general anesthesia and positive pressure ventilation can be instituted to permit surgical exploration and more definitive treatment of the cardiac tamponade. Induction and maintenance of anesthesia is often accomplished with ketamine. Intraoperative monitoring typically includes intraarterial and CVP monitoring.

In the unusual circumstance in which it is not possible to relieve a significant part of the cardiac tamponade before induction of anesthesia, the principal goals of the anesthesiologist must be maintenance of adequate cardiac output and blood pressure. Anesthesia-induced decreases in myocardial contractility, systemic vascular resistance, and heart rate *must* be avoided. Increased intrathoracic pressure caused by straining or coughing during induction or by mechanical ventilation may further decrease venous return and further lower the blood pressure. Some advocate preparing and draping for incision before induction of anesthesia and endotracheal intubation. This would allow for the shortest possible time from the

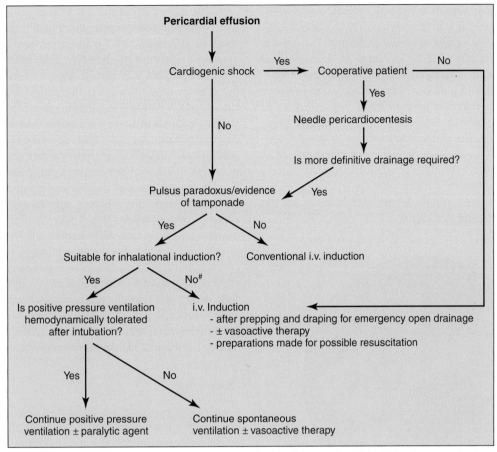

FIG. 11.7 Management strategies for patients with significant pericardial effusion/tamponade. In the absence of overt cardiogenic shock, anesthetic management of patients for pericardial effusion drainage relies on the determination of the hemodynamic significance of the effusion. When tamponade is not present, a conventional intravenous (i.v.) induction can proceed. If there is significant tamponade, consideration can be given to an inhalational induction unless specific contraindications exist. Use of positive pressure ventilation versus spontaneous ventilation will be based on the hemodynamic tolerance to either mode of ventilation. The need for vasoactive therapy should be anticipated regardless of the anesthetic technique chosen. #, Conditions that might preclude inhalational induction include significant aspiration risk, significant obesity, severe orthopnea, or an uncooperative patient. (From Grocott HP, Gulati H, Srinathan S, Mackensen GB. Anesthesia and the patient with pericardial disease. *Can J Anaesth.* 2011;58:952-966.)

adverse hemodynamic consequences of anesthetic induction and institution of mechanical ventilation to surgical relief of the tamponade. Ketamine is useful for induction and maintenance of anesthesia because it increases myocardial contractility, systemic vascular resistance, and heart rate. Preinduction arterial line placement is recommended, since significant hemodynamic instability is very likely during induction of anesthesia. Central line placement is not mandatory, but it is strong recommended. After release of a severe tamponade there is often a significant swing in blood pressure from hypotension to *marked hypertension.* This change should be anticipated, and appropriate treatment must be prompt, especially in cases of tamponade due to an aortic dissection or aneurysm. These entities could be severely or even fatally compromised by a bout of hypertension. TEE is recommended to confirm that the effusion was completely drained.

CONSTRICTIVE PERICARDITIS

Constrictive pericarditis is most often idiopathic or the result of previous cardiac surgery or exposure to radiotherapy (Fig. 11.8). Tuberculosis may also cause constrictive pericarditis. *Chronic constrictive pericarditis* is characterized by fibrous scarring and adhesions that obliterate the pericardial space, creating a rigid shell around the heart. Calcification may develop in long-standing cases. *Subacute constrictive pericarditis* is more common than chronic calcific pericarditis, and the resulting constriction in this situation is fibroelastic.

Signs and Symptoms

Pericardial constriction typically presents with symptoms and signs of a combination of increased CVP and low cardiac output. Symptoms include decreased exercise tolerance and fatigue. Jugular venous distention, hepatic congestion, ascites, and peripheral edema are signs of pericardial constriction that mimic right ventricular failure. Pulmonary congestion is typically absent. Increases in and eventual equalization of right atrial pressure, right ventricular end-diastolic pressure, and pulmonary artery occlusion pressure are features that occur in the presence of *both* constrictive pericarditis and cardiac tamponade. As pericardial pressure increases, right atrial pressure increases in parallel, and therefore CVP is an accurate reflection of intrapericardial pressure. Atrial dysrhythmias (atrial fibrillation or flutter) are often seen in patients with chronic constrictive pericarditis and are associated with the length of the disease and the amount of pericardial calcification.

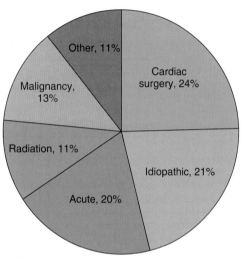

FIG. 11.8 Etiology of constrictive pericarditis among 506 patients undergoing pericardiectomy at the Mayo Clinic. Note that the two most common causes were cardiac surgery (24%) and idiopathic (21%). (From Cho YH, Schaff HV. Surgery for pericardial disease. *Heart Fail Rev.* 2013;18:375-387, Figure 3.)

Constrictive pericarditis is similar to cardiac tamponade in that both conditions impede diastolic filling of the heart and result in an increased CVP and ultimately decreased cardiac output. Diagnostic signs, however, differ in the two conditions. Pulsus paradoxus is a regular feature of cardiac tamponade but is often absent in constrictive pericarditis. Kussmaul sign (increased CVP during inspiration) occurs more frequently in patients with constrictive pericarditis than in those with cardiac tamponade. An early diastolic sound (pericardial knock) is often heard in patients with constrictive pericarditis but does not occur in cardiac tamponade. A prominent *y* descent of the jugular venous pressure waveform (Friedreich sign) reflects rapid right ventricular filling in early diastole that is seen with constrictive pericarditis. This rapid early diastolic filling is also detected by a dip in early diastolic pressure. The ventricle is completely filled by the end of the rapid filling phase, and a period of constant ventricular volume known as *diastasis* persists for the remainder of diastole. Corresponding to this prolonged diastasis, ventricular diastolic pressure remains unchanged for the latter two-thirds of diastole. This pattern of ventricular diastolic pressure in constrictive pericarditis is referred to as the *square root sign* or *dip-and-plateau morphology* (Fig. 11.9).

Diagnosis

Constrictive pericarditis is difficult to diagnose, and its signs and symptoms are often erroneously attributed to liver disease or idiopathic pericardial effusion. The clinical diagnosis of constrictive pericarditis depends on confirmation of an increased CVP without other signs or symptoms of heart disease. Heart size and lung fields appear normal on chest radiographs. However, pericardial calcification can be seen in 30%–50% of cases. The ECG may display only minor nonspecific abnormalities. Echocardiography can be quite helpful in many instances by demonstrating abnormal septal motion and pericardial thickening that suggests the presence of constrictive pericarditis.

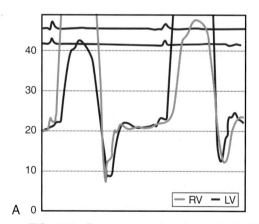
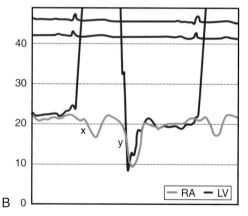

FIG. 11.9 Pressure recordings in a patient with constrictive pericarditis. A, Simultaneous right ventricular (RV) and left ventricular (LV) pressure tracings with equalization of diastolic pressure as well as dip-and-plateau morphology. B, Simultaneous right atrial (RA) and LV pressure with equalization of RA and LV diastolic pressure. Note the prominent *y* descent. (From Vaitkus PT, Cooper KA, Shuman WP, et al. Images in cardiovascular medicine: constrictive pericarditis. *Circulation.* 1996;93:834-835, with permission.)

TEE, CT of the chest, and MRI are superior to TTE for demonstrating pericardial thickening. As with cardiac tamponade, ventricular discordance is a feature of constrictive pericarditis. Pulsed wave Doppler studies often demonstrate an exaggerated respiratory variation in mitral and tricuspid diastolic flow velocities. Cardiac catheterization reveals characteristic abnormalities including increased CVP, nondilated and normally contracting right and left ventricles, near equilibration of right- and left-sided cardiac filling pressures, and a dip-and-plateau waveform in the right ventricle (see Fig. 11.9). Many features considered characteristic of constrictive pericarditis may also be present with restrictive cardiomyopathy, but several features help distinguish these two entities (Table 11.3). Pericardial calcifications, normal pulmonary artery pressures, and ventricular discordance are features of constrictive pericarditis but *not* of restrictive cardiomyopathy. Kussmaul sign and pulsus paradoxus are *present* in constrictive pericarditis but *absent* in restrictive cardiomyopathy. Two echocardiographic techniques can also help in evaluation. Pulsed wave Doppler ultrasonography demonstrates ventricular discordance in constrictive pericarditis. Tissue Doppler ultrasonography can be used to interrogate the motion of the mitral valve annulus. In restrictive cardiomyopathy the motion of the mitral annulus is *restricted*. In constrictive pericarditis the motion of the mitral annulus is *normal*. Cardiac catheterization can demonstrate ventricular discordance by looking at simultaneous recording of right and left ventricular systolic pressures. If discordance is present, right ventricular peak systolic pressure increases on inspiration, whereas left ventricular peak pressure decreases. This observation of ventricular discordance indicates the presence of constrictive pericarditis rather than restrictive cardiomyopathy. TEE is superior to TTE in measuring pericardial thickness and correlates well with CT measurements of pericardial thickness.

Treatment

Constrictive pericarditis that develops as a complication of acute pericarditis will occasionally resolve spontaneously. In most patients, however, the definitive treatment of constrictive pericarditis consists of surgical removal of the adherent constricting pericardium. This procedure may result in considerable bleeding from the epicardial surface of the heart. Cardiopulmonary bypass may occasionally be needed to facilitate pericardial stripping, especially if hemorrhage is difficult to control. Unlike the treatment of cardiac tamponade, in which hemodynamic improvement occurs immediately, surgical removal of constricting pericardium is not followed by an immediate improvement in cardiac output or a reduction in right atrial pressure. Typically, right atrial pressure returns to normal within 3 months of surgery. The absence of immediate hemodynamic improvement may be due to disuse atrophy of myocardial muscle fibers or persistent constrictive effects from sclerotic *epicardium* that is not removed with the pericardium. Inadequate long-term relief after surgical removal of constricting pericardium may reflect associated myocardial disease, especially in patients with radiation-induced pericardial disease.

Management of Anesthesia

Anesthetic drugs and techniques that minimize changes in heart rate, systemic vascular resistance, venous return, and myocardial contractility should be selected. Combinations of opioids and benzodiazepines with or without low doses of volatile anesthetics are appropriate for maintenance of anesthesia. Muscle relaxants with minimal circulatory effects are the best choices, although the modest increase in heart rate observed with administration of pancuronium is also acceptable. Preoperative optimization of intravascular volume is essential. If hemodynamic compromise (hypotension) resulting from increased intrapericardial pressure is present before surgery, management of anesthesia will be similar to that for cardiac tamponade.

Invasive monitoring of arterial pressure and CVP is helpful because removal of adherent pericardium may be a tedious and long operation and is often associated with significant fluid and blood losses. Cardiac dysrhythmias are common and

TABLE 11.3	Differentiating Constrictive Pericarditis From Restrictive Cardiomyopathy	
Feature	Constrictive Pericarditis	Restrictive Cardiomyopathy
Medical history	Previous pericarditis, cardiac surgery, trauma, radiotherapy, connective tissue disease	No such history
Mitral or tricuspid regurgitation	Usually absent	Often present
Ventricular septal movement with respiration	Movement toward left ventricle on inspiration	Little movement toward left ventricle
Respiratory variation in mitral and tricuspid flow velocity	>25% in most cases	<15% in most cases
Equilibration of diastolic pressures in all cardiac chambers	Within 5 mm Hg in nearly all cases	Present in only a small proportion of cases
Respiratory variation of ventricular peak systolic pressures	Right and left ventricular peak systolic pressures are out of phase (discordant)	Right and left ventricular peak systolic pressures are in phase
MRI/CT	Show pericardial thickening in most cases	Rarely show pericardial thickening
Endomyocardial biopsy	Normal or nonspecific findings	Amyloid present in some cases

Adapted from Hancock EW. Differential diagnosis of restrictive cardiomyopathy and constrictive pericarditis. *Heart*. 2001;86:343-349.

presumably reflect direct mechanical irritation of the heart. Intravenous administration of fluids and blood products will be necessary to treat the significant fluid and blood losses associated with pericardiectomy.

Postoperative ventilatory insufficiency may necessitate continued mechanical ventilation. Cardiac dysrhythmias and low cardiac output may require treatment during the postoperative period.

PERICARDIAL AND CARDIAC TRAUMA

Blunt injuries to the chest can result in cardiovascular injury. The severity of this injury may be as mild as bruising or as severe as death within minutes. Motor vehicle accidents are the primary cause of blunt chest trauma. The main mechanisms of injury are the rapid deceleration of the chest as it impacts the steering wheel and shear forces on internal thoracic structures. Fragile tissues can be crushed by their impact on the sternum and ribs; soft mobile tissues may tear. There may be serious cardiovascular injury despite the lack of obvious external signs of trauma. Sudden deceleration from speeds as low as 20 mph can result in serious injury. Because of its location immediately behind the sternum, the right ventricle is more likely than the left ventricle to be injured. Traumatic cardiac injury can result in a wide range of problems, including myocardial contusion or rupture and damage to internal cardiac structures (valves and conduction system) or the coronary arteries. Dysrhythmias are a frequent problem. Injuries to the aorta include aortic hematoma, dissection, and rupture. The pericardium can be lacerated or ruptured, and the heart can herniate through the pericardial defect. Blood from aortic or cardiac injury can fill the pericardial space, causing cardiac tamponade. Lacerations can be limited to the pericardium or can involve adjacent structures such as the pleura and/or diaphragm. Pulmonary contusion may also result from blunt chest trauma and can present as hypoxemia, lung consolidation, or pleural effusion. Hemorrhage into the tracheobronchial tree may accompany pulmonary contusion.

Traumatic herniation of the diaphragm can result in movement of abdominal contents into the pleural or pericardial space, or the heart can herniate into the abdomen. Small partial herniations of the heart may manifest as impaired cardiac filling or ischemia if coronary blood flow becomes impaired. Larger herniations can result in impaired ventricular filling and ejection.

Diagnosis

The nonspecific signs and symptoms of pericardial rupture and cardiac herniation make the diagnosis difficult. Suspicion of pericardial trauma or pericardial rupture should be raised when unexplained alterations in heart rate and blood pressure occur after initial trauma resuscitation, especially if a sternal fracture and/or multiple rib fractures are present. Palpation and auscultation can reveal an abnormal location of the heart. Mediastinal air on a chest radiograph must be investigated to

rule out pneumopericardium, which could indicate the presence of a pericardial laceration. Rarely, chest radiography or CT shows evidence of cardiac herniation. Two characteristic CT findings include the *collar sign* and *empty pericardial sac sign*. The collar sign is a tomographically observable "waist" around the strangled part of the heart that herniates through the pericardial defect. The empty pericardial sac sign appears as air outlining the empty pericardium as a result of displacement of the heart into the hemithorax.

Treatment

Minor injury or a small pericardial laceration can often go unnoticed. Some patients may develop an "idiopathic" pericarditis with or without pericardial effusion. Severe lacerations associated with hemodynamic instability and cardiac herniation require emergency thoracotomy. It is important to note that initiation of mechanical ventilation may precipitate hemodynamic collapse. Cardiac output should be maintained with fluids and/or inotropic drugs as needed until the herniation is released.

Myocardial Contusion

Signs and Symptoms

The symptoms of myocardial contusion include chest pain and palpitations. The chest pain can resemble angina pectoris but it is not relieved by nitroglycerin. Dysrhythmias frequently complicate myocardial contusion, but cardiac failure is uncommon.

Diagnosis

The presence of chest pain and ECG changes, especially in young patients, should prompt questions regarding recent chest trauma that might have seemed trivial at the time of its occurrence. ECG changes include ST-T wave abnormalities, supraventricular and ventricular dysrhythmias, and AV nodal dysfunction. However, diffuse nonspecific ST-T wave abnormalities are commonly noted in trauma patients, even in the absence of myocardial contusion.

Cardiac contusion can be recognized by TTE or TEE, which can demonstrate impaired ventricular wall motion, valvular regurgitation, or pericardial effusion. These wall motion abnormalities usually resolve within a few days.

Serum concentrations of creatine kinase and its MB fraction increase but are often difficult to interpret because of the release of creatine kinase from injured skeletal muscles. However, the cardiac biomarkers troponin I and T can provide specific information about myocardial injury.

Treatment

Treatment of a myocardial contusion is directed toward improving the symptoms and anticipating possible complications. Life-threatening dysrhythmias can occur within the first 24–48 hours after injury. Severely contused hearts may also require hemodynamic support. Patients with a severe myocardial contusion may have other injuries that require emergent surgical intervention. Invasive hemodynamic monitoring is prudent in this situation. Anesthetic drugs that depress myocardial function should be avoided. A cardioverter-defibrillator and medications for dysrhythmia management should be immediately available.

Commotio Cordis

Commotio cordis (from Latin "agitation of the heart") is a disturbance of cardiac rhythm resulting from precordial trauma. The mechanism of this injury is not well understood, but it is known that the myocardium is sensitive to ventricular dysrhythmias within a 10- to 20-millisecond window during ventricular repolarization, the so-called vulnerable period. A focused mechanical injury during this small window of time could stretch cardiac fibers and cause an unsynchronized impulse, a *mechanical R-on-T phenomenon* that could cause ventricular fibrillation and require defibrillation. The essential treatment for commotio cordis is defibrillation. Because of this, the syndrome must be recognized and rapid defibrillation must be available. Public awareness programs and the availability of automatic external defibrillators and rapid-response teams at sporting events are already making an impact on the survival of individuals sustaining this injury.

KEY POINTS

- Most cases of acute pericarditis are due to viral infection and follow a transient and uncomplicated clinical course. Therefore this disease process is often termed *acute benign pericarditis.*
- Postcardiotomy syndrome presents primarily as acute pericarditis. It may follow blunt or penetrating trauma, hemopericardium, or epicardial pacemaker implantation. However, it is most commonly seen after cardiac surgery in which pericardiotomy is performed.
- The pathophysiologic effects of a pericardial effusion depend on whether or not the fluid is under increased pressure. Cardiac tamponade occurs when the pressure of the fluid in the pericardial space impairs cardiac filling.
- *Pulsus paradoxus* is defined as a decrease in systolic blood pressure of more than 10 mm Hg during inspiration. This hemodynamic change reflects impairment of diastolic filling of the left ventricle. Pulsus paradoxus represents dyssynchrony or opposing responses of the right and left ventricles to filling during the respiratory cycle. Another term for this is *ventricular discordance.*
- Cardiac output is maintained during cardiac tamponade as long as central venous pressure (CVP) exceeds right ventricular end-diastolic pressure. However, a progressive increase in intrapericardial pressure will eventually result in equalization of right atrial pressure and right ventricular end-diastolic pressure. The increased intrapericardial pressure then leads to impaired diastolic filling, decreased stroke volume, and hypotension.

- Temporizing measures likely to help maintain stroke volume until definitive treatment of cardiac tamponade is undertaken include expanding intravascular volume, administering catecholamines to increase myocardial contractility, and correcting any metabolic acidosis.
- Removal of pericardial fluid is the definitive treatment of cardiac tamponade and should be performed when CVP is increased. Pericardial fluid may be removed by percutaneous pericardiocentesis or by surgical techniques. Removal of even a small amount of pericardial fluid can result in a dramatic decrease in intrapericardial pressure.
- Pericardiocentesis under local anesthesia is often preferred for initial management of hypotensive patients with cardiac tamponade. After the hemodynamic status has been improved by this percutaneous pericardiocentesis, general anesthesia and positive pressure ventilation can be instituted to permit surgical exploration and more definitive treatment of the tamponade.
- Many features considered characteristic of constrictive pericarditis may also be present in patients with restrictive cardiomyopathy, but several characteristics help distinguish between these two entities. Kussmaul sign and pulsus paradoxus are present with constrictive pericarditis but are not associated with restrictive cardiomyopathy. Ventricular discordance is a feature of constrictive pericarditis but not of restrictive cardiomyopathy.
- Trauma, especially motor vehicle trauma, is the primary cause of blunt chest injury. Rapid deceleration of the chest as it impacts the steering wheel serves as the main mechanism of cardiovascular injury. Injuries to the aorta include aortic hematoma, dissection, and rupture. The pericardium can be lacerated or ruptured, and the heart can herniate through the pericardial defect. The heart itself can be contused, ruptured, or suffer damage to its internal structures (valves) or blood supply. Because it is immediately behind the sternum, the right ventricle is more likely than the left ventricle to be seriously injured.
- *Commotio cordis* is a syndrome in which a focused high-impact injury to the chest results in a malignant ventricular dysrhythmia and sudden death.

RESOURCES

Acute pericarditis

Ariyarajah V, Spodick DH. Acute pericarditis: diagnostic clues and common electrocardiographic manifestations. *Cardiol Rev.* 2007;15:24-30.

Cosyns B, Plein S, Nihoyanopoulos P, et al. European Association of Cardiovascular Imaging (EACVI) position paper: multimodality imaging in pericardial disease. *Eur Heart J Cardiovasc Imaging.* 2015;16:12-31.

Imazio M, Brucato A, Derosa FG, et al. Etiological diagnosis in acute and recurrent pericarditis: when and how. *J Cardiovasc Med.* 2009;10:217-230.

Imazio M, Gaita F, LeWinter M. Evaluation and treatment of pericarditis: a systematic review. *JAMA.* 2015;314:1498-1506.

Peebles CR, Shambrook JS, Harden SP. Pericardial disease—anatomy and function. *Br J Radiol.* 2011;84(Spec No 3):S324-S337.

Pericardial effusion and cardiac tamponade

Carmona P, Mateo E, Casanovas I, et al. Management of cardiac tamponade after cardiac surgery. *J Cardiothorac Vasc Anesth.* 2012;26:302-311.

Cho YH, Schaff HV. Surgery for pericardial disease. *Heart Fail Rev.* 2013;18:375-387.

Cruite I, McNeely MF, Moshiri M, et al. Correlation of transesophageal ultrasound of the pericardium with computed tomography. *Ultrasound Q.* 2014;30:179-183.

Hoit BD. Pericardial disease and pericardial tamponade. *Crit Care Med.* 2007;35(8 Suppl):S355-S364.

Imazio M, Adler Y. Management of pericardial effusion. *Eur Heart J.* 2013;34:1186-1197.

Klein AL, Abbara S, Agler DA, et al. American Society of Echocardiography clinical recommendations for multimodality cardiovascular imaging of patients with pericardial disease: endorsed by the Society for Cardiovascular Magnetic Resonance and Society of Cardiovascular Computed Tomography. *J Am Soc Echocardiogr.* 2013;26:965-1012. e15.

Little WC, Freeman GL. Pericardial disease. *Circulation.* 2006;113:1622-1632.

Constrictive pericarditis

Asher CR, Klein AL. Diastolic heart failure: restrictive cardiomyopathy, constrictive pericarditis, and cardiac tamponade: clinical and echocardiographic evaluation. *Cardiol Rev.* 2002;10:218-229.

Hancock EW. Differential diagnosis of restrictive cardiomyopathy and constrictive pericarditis. *Heart.* 2001;86:343-349.

Verhaert D, Gabriel RS, Johnston D, et al. The role of multimodality imaging in the management of pericardial disease. *Circ Cardiovasc Imaging.* 2010;3:333-343.

Pericardial and cardiac trauma

Embrey R. Cardiac trauma. *Thorac Surg Clin.* 2007;17:87-93.

Gerlach R, Mark D, Poologaindran A, et al. Cardiac rupture from blunt chest trauma diagnosed on transesophageal echocardiography. *Anesth Analg.* 2015;120:293-295.

Marcolini EG, Keegan J. Blunt cardiac injury. *Emerg Med Clin North Am.* 2015;33:519-527.

Mitchell MM. Detection of occult hemopericardium using intraoperative transesophageal echocardiography. *Anesthesiology.* 1992;76:145-147.

Singh KE, Baum VC. The anesthetic management of cardiovascular trauma. *Curr Opin Anaesthesiol.* 2011;24:98-103.

Myocardial contusion

Sybrandy KC, Cramer MJ, Burgersdijk C. Diagnosing cardiac contusion: old wisdom and new insights. *Heart.* 2003;89:485-489.

Commotio cordis

Link MS. Pathophysiology, prevention, and treatment of commotio cordis. *Curr Cardiol Rep.* 2014;16:495.

Maron BJ, Estes NAM. Commotio cordis. *N Engl J Med.* 2010;362:917-927.

Vascular Disease

LORETA GRECU, NIKHIL CHAWLA

DISEASES OF THE THORACIC AND ABDOMINAL AORTA

Aneurysms, dissections, or occlusive diseases are the main pathologies that can affect arterial vessels. Whereas occlusive disease is more likely to occur in peripheral arteries, the aorta and its major branches are affected by two abnormalities that may be present simultaneously or occur at different stages of the same disease process—namely, aneurysms (more common) and dissections (Fig. 12.1 and Table 12.1). Although there can be some overlap, a clear distinction between these entities can be critical, since approach and treatment may be very different. Upon presentation, this differentiation is essential because, for example, an ascending aortic dissection is a catastrophic event that requires immediate surgical intervention and carries a mortality of 1%–2% per hour for the first 48 hours, with overall mortality between 27% and 58%. That is a very different clinical situation from aortic aneurysms that are primarily treated medically, with surgical intervention needed only when they reach a certain threshold diameter.

An *aneurysm* is a dilatation of all three layers of an artery, which appears ballooned in a certain region, such as the ascending or descending portions of the thoracic aorta or the abdominal aorta. The most common definition is a 50% increase in diameter compared with normal, or greater than 3 cm in diameter. Arterial diameter depends on age, gender, and body habitus. Aneurysms may occasionally produce symptoms because of compression of surrounding structures, but rupture with exsanguination is the most dreaded complication, since only about 25% of patients who experience rupture of an abdominal aortic aneurysm survive (Fig. 12.2).

Dissection of an artery occurs when blood enters the medial layer. The media of large arteries is made up of organized lamellar units that decrease in number with distance from the heart. The initiating event of an aortic dissection is a tear in the intima. Blood surges through the intimal tear into an extraluminal channel called the *false lumen*. Blood in the false lumen can reenter the true lumen anywhere along the course of the dissection. The origins of aortic branch arteries arising from the area involved in the dissection may be compromised and the aortic valve rendered incompetent. This sequence of events occurs over minutes to hours. A delay in diagnosis or treatment can be fatal (Fig. 12.3).

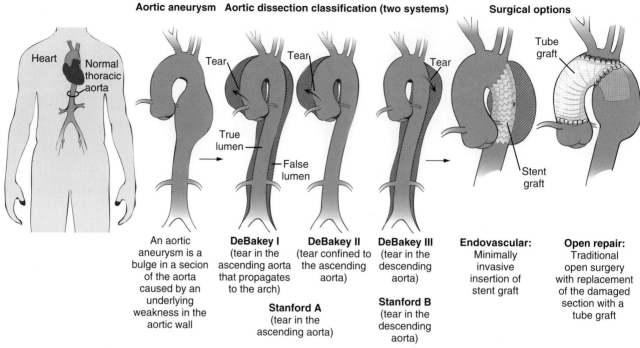

FIG. 12.1 Overview of thoracic aneurysms and dissections. (Adapted from Goldfinger JZ, Halperin JL, Marin ML, et al. Thoracic aortic aneurysms and dissection. *J Am Coll Cardiol.* 2014:64;1725-1739.)

TABLE 12.1	Comparison Between Aortic Aneurysms and Dissections	
	Aortic Aneurysm	Aortic Dissection
Definition	Dilatation of all three aortic layers	Blood entry into the media
False lumen	No	Yes
Predisposing factors	HTN, atherosclerosis, age, male, smoking, family history of aneurysm	HTN, atherosclerosis, preexisting aneurysm, inflammatory diseases, collagen diseases, family history of aortic dissection, aortic coarctation, bicuspid aortic valve, Turner syndrome, CABG, previous aortic valve replacement, cardiac catheterization, crack cocaine use, trauma
Symptoms	May be asymptomatic or present with pain mostly due to compression of adjacent structures or vessels	Severe sharp pain in the posterior chest or back pain
Diagnosis	CXR, echocardiography, CT, MRI, angiography	For patients in unstable condition, echocardiography; after patient's condition is medically stabilized, imaging can include CT, CXR, aortography, MRI, echocardiography.
Management	Elective surgical repair, whether thoracic or abdominal, for diameter > 6 cm or rapidly enlarging aneurysms with >10-mm growth over 6 mo for thoracic and diameter of >5.5 cm or >5-mm increase for abdominal; endovascular repair recommended owing to better patient outcomes, especially in patients at high risk, although no randomized trial data exist.	*Type A dissection:* Acute surgical emergency; as accurate diagnosis is made, patient will require acute medical management to decrease blood pressure and aortic wall stress. *Type B dissection:* If uncomplicated, medical management can be pursued.

CABG, Coronary artery bypass grafting; *CT,* computed tomography, *CXR,* chest x-ray; *HTN,* hypertension; *MRI,* magnetic resonance imaging.

ANEURYSMS AND DISSECTIONS OF THE THORACIC AND ABDOMINAL AORTA

Incidence

The incidence of descending thoracic aneurysms is 5.9–10.4 per 100,000 person-years, and rupture occurs at a rate of 3.5 per 100,000 person-years. Although it is commonly accepted that the threshold for repair is a diameter of 6 cm or larger,

one must be aware of the possibility of synchronous aneurysms involving the ascending aorta or arch, which occur in approximately 10% of patients. Dissection of the aorta can originate anywhere along the length of the aorta, but the most common points of origin are in the thorax, in the ascending aorta just above the aortic valve, and just distal to the origin of the left subclavian artery near the insertion of the ligamentum arteriosum.

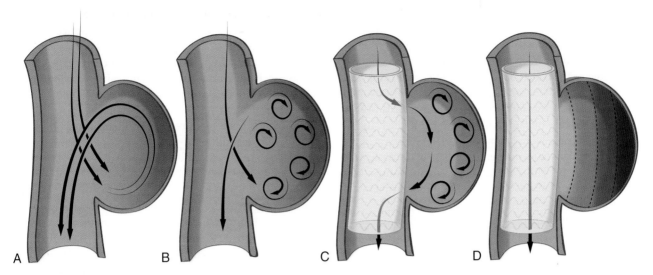

FIG. 12.2 A, Blood flow through a saccular aneurysm. B, Saccular aortic aneurysm with increased flow velocity. C, Saccular aortic aneurysm treated with a multilayer stent that decreases the flow velocity into the aneurysm. D. Saccular aneurysm that is now excluded from blood flow circulation. (Adapted from Buck DB, van Herwaarden JA, Schermerhorn ML, Moll FL. Endovascular treatment of abdominal aortic aneurysms. *Nat Rev Cardiol.* 2014;11:112-123.)

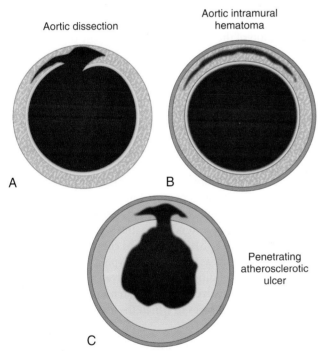

FIG. 12.3 Acute aortic syndromes. A, Classic aortic dissection. B, Aortic intramural hematoma. C, Penetrating atherosclerotic ulcer. (Adapted from Braverman AC. Diseases of the aorta. In: Mann DL, Zipes DP, Libby P, Bonow RO, eds. *Braunwald's Heart Disease: A Textbook of Cardiovascular Medicine.* 10th ed. Philadelphia: Elsevier; 2015:1277.)

Etiology

The most frequently implicated factors in the development of aortic aneurysmal disease are hypertension, atherosclerosis, older age, male sex, family history of aneurysmal disease, and smoking. Causes of aortic dissection are deceleration injuries resulting from blunt trauma and use of crack cocaine, and iatrogenic dissection may occur secondary to aortic cannulation including cardiac catheterization, cross-clamping, aortic manipulation, or arterial incision for surgical procedures such as aortic valve replacement, bypass grafting, or aneurysm operations. Systemic hypertension is a factor that can be implicated in both genetic and nongenetic causes. Aortic dissection is more common in men, but there is also an association with pregnancy. Approximately half of all aortic dissections in women younger than age 40 occur during pregnancy, usually in the third trimester.

Thoracic aortic aneurysms and dissections associated with known genetic syndromes are well described. These inherited diseases of blood vessels include both conditions affecting large arteries, such as the aorta, and those involving the microvasculature. Four major inherited disorders are known to affect major arteries: Marfan syndrome, Ehlers-Danlos syndrome, bicuspid aortic valve, and nonsyndromic familial aortic dissection. Although it was once believed that mutant connective tissue proteins corrupted proteins from the normal allele (dominant negative effect) in combination with normal wear and tear, it is now known that matrix proteins, in addition to showing specific mechanical properties, have important roles in the homeostasis of the smooth muscle cells that produce them. Matrix proteins play a key metabolic function because of their ability to sequester and store bioactive molecules and participate in their precisely controlled activation and release. In the inherited disorders associated with aortic dissection, loss of this function (biochemical rather than mechanical) is thought to alter smooth muscle cell homeostasis. The end result is a change in matrix metabolism that causes structural weakness in the aorta.

Marfan syndrome is one of the most prevalent hereditary connective tissue disorders. Its inheritance pattern is autosomal dominant. Marfan syndrome is caused by mutations in the fibrillin-1 gene. Fibrillin is an important connective tissue protein in the capsule of the ocular lens, arteries, lung, skin, and dura mater. Fibrillin mutations can result in disease manifestations in each of these tissues. Because fibrillin is an integral part of elastin, recognition of the mutations in fibrillin led to the assumption that the clinical manifestations of Marfan syndrome in the aorta were secondary to an inherent weakness of the aortic wall exacerbated by aging. However, histologic studies of the aortas of Marfan syndrome patients also demonstrate abnormalities in matrix metabolism that can result in matrix destruction.

Although the genetics of thoracic aortic aneurysm disease in patients with Marfan syndrome are well documented, less is known about familial patterns of aneurysm occurrence not associated with any particular collagen or vascular disease. Up to 19% of people with thoracic aortic aneurysm and dissection do not have syndromes traditionally considered to predispose them to aortic disease. However, these individuals often have several relatives with thoracic aortic aneurysm disease, which suggests a strong genetic predisposition.

Bicuspid aortic valve is the most common congenital anomaly resulting in aortic dilation/dissection. It occurs in 1% of the general population. Histologic studies show elastin degradation in the aorta just above the aortic valve. Echocardiography shows that aortic root dilatation is common even in younger patients with bicuspid aortic valve. Bicuspid aortic valve clusters in families and is found in approximately 9% of first-degree relatives of affected individuals.

Nonsyndromic familial aortic dissection and aneurysm is found in approximately 20% of patients referred for repair of thoracic aneurysm or dissection. Affected families do not meet the clinical criteria for Marfan syndrome and do not have biochemical abnormalities in type III collagen, as in Ehlers-Danlos syndrome. In most of these families the inheritance pattern appears to be dominant with variable penetrance. At least three chromosomal regions have so far been mapped in families with nonsyndromic thoracic aortic aneurysm disease. The specific biochemical abnormalities predisposing to thoracic aortic aneurysm disease remain to be identified.

Abdominal aortic aneurysms have traditionally been viewed as resulting from atherosclerosis. This atherosclerosis involves several highly interrelated processes, including lipid disturbances, platelet activation, thrombosis, endothelial dysfunction, inflammation, oxidative stress, vascular smooth muscle cell activation, altered matrix metabolism, remodeling, and genetic factors. Atherosclerosis represents a response to vessel wall injury caused by processes such as infection, inflammation, increased protease activity within the arterial wall, genetically regulated defects in collagen and fibrillin, and mechanical factors. A familial component has also been identified, because 12%–19% of first-degree relatives (usually men) of a patient with an abdominal aortic aneurysm will develop an aneurysm. Specific genetic markers and biochemical changes that produce this pathologic condition remain to be elucidated.

Factors that disrupt the normal integrity of the aortic wall or significant increases in shear tension may induce the occurrence of dissections. Examples of conditions associated with aortic dissection are hypertension, genetically triggered aortic disease (see earlier), bicuspid aortic valve, tetralogy of Fallot, atherosclerosis, penetrating atherosclerotic ulcer, trauma, intraaortic balloon pump, aortic/vascular surgery, coronary artery bypass graft, giant cell arteritis, aortitis, syphilis, pregnancy, and weightlifting.

Classification

Aortic aneurysms can be classified morphologically as either fusiform or saccular. In fusiform aneurysm there is a uniform dilatation involving the entire circumference of the aortic wall, whereas a saccular aneurysm is an eccentric dilatation of the aorta that communicates with the main lumen by a variably sized neck. Aneurysms can also be classified based on the pathologic features of the aortic wall (e.g., atherosclerosis or cystic medial necrosis).

Arteriosclerosis is the primary lesion associated with aneurysms in the infrarenal abdominal aorta, thoracoabdominal aorta, and descending thoracic aorta. Aneurysms affecting the ascending aorta are primarily the result of lesions that cause degeneration of the aortic media, a pathologic process termed *cystic medial necrosis.*

Aneurysms of the thoracoabdominal aorta may also be classified according to their anatomic location. Two classifications widely used for aortic dissection are the *DeBakey* and *Stanford classifications* (Fig. 12.4; also see Fig. 12.1). The DeBakey classification includes types I to III. In type I, the intimal tear originates in the ascending aorta and the dissection involves the ascending aorta, arch, and variable lengths of the descending thoracic and abdominal aorta. In DeBakey type II, the dissection is confined to the ascending aorta. In type III, the dissection is confined to the descending thoracic aorta (type IIIa) or extends into the abdominal aorta and iliac arteries (type IIIb). The Stanford classification describes thoracic aneurysms as type A or B. Type A includes all cases in which the ascending aorta is involved by the dissection, with or without involvement of the arch or descending aorta. Type B includes all cases in which the ascending aorta is not involved.

Signs and Symptoms

Many patients with thoracic aortic aneurysms are asymptomatic at the time of presentation, and the aneurysm is detected during testing for other disorders. Symptoms resulting from thoracic aneurysm typically reflect impingement of the aneurysm on adjacent structures. Hoarseness results from stretching of the left recurrent laryngeal nerve. Stridor is due to compression of the trachea. Dysphagia is due to compression of the esophagus. Dyspnea results from compression of the lungs. Plethora and edema result from compression of the superior vena cava. Patients with ascending aortic aneurysms

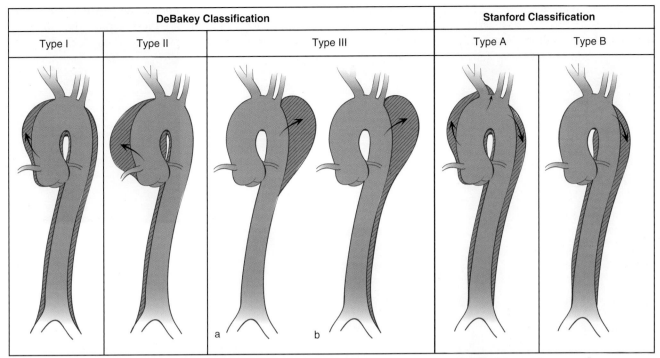

DeBakey Classification			Stanford Classification	
Type I	Type II	Type III	Type A	Type B

FIG. 12.4   The two most widely used classifications of aortic dissection: DeBakey and Stanford classifications. In DeBakey type I dissection the intimal tear usually originates in the proximal ascending aorta, and the dissection involves the ascending aorta and variable lengths of the aortic arch and descending thoracic and abdominal aorta. In DeBakey type II the dissection is confined to the ascending aorta. In DeBakey type III the dissection is confined to the descending thoracic aorta (type IIIa) or extends into the abdominal aorta and iliac arteries (type IIIb). Stanford type A dissection includes all cases in which the ascending aorta is involved by the dissection, with or without involvement of the arch or the descending aorta. Stanford type B includes cases in which the ascending aorta is not involved. (Data from Kouchoukos NT, Dougenis D. Surgery of the thoracic aorta. *N Engl J Med.* 1997;336:1876-1888. Copyright 1997 Massachusetts Medical Society.)

associated with dilatation of the aortic valve annulus may have signs of aortic regurgitation and congestive heart failure.

Acute, severe, sharp pain in the anterior chest, the neck, or between the shoulder blades is the typical presenting symptom of thoracic aortic dissection. The pain may migrate as the dissection advances along the aorta. Patients with aortic dissection often appear as if they are in shock (vasoconstricted), yet the systemic blood pressure may be quite elevated. Patients who have severe hypotension or even shock at presentation have a worse prognosis. Hypotension at presentation is more common with proximal dissections. Other symptoms and signs of acute aortic dissection, such as diminution or absence of peripheral pulses, reflect occlusion of branches of the aorta and may be followed by inadequate treatment because of falsely low blood pressure measurements. Neurologic complications of aortic dissection may include stroke caused by occlusion of a carotid artery, ischemic peripheral neuropathy associated with ischemia of an arm or a leg, and paraparesis or paraplegia caused by impairment of the blood supply to the spinal cord. Myocardial infarction (MI) may reflect occlusion of a coronary artery. Gastrointestinal ischemia may occur. Renal artery obstruction is manifested by an increase in serum creatinine concentration. Retrograde dissection into the sinus

of Valsalva with rupture into the pericardial space leading to cardiac tamponade is a major cause of death. Approximately 90% of patients with acute dissection of the ascending aorta who are not treated surgically die within 3 months.

Abdominal aortic aneurysms are usually detected as asymptomatic pulsatile abdominal masses.

Diagnosis

Widening of the mediastinum on chest radiograph may be diagnostic of a thoracic aortic aneurysm. However, enlargement of the ascending aorta may be confined to the retrosternal area, so the aortic silhouette can appear normal. Computed tomography (CT) and magnetic resonance imaging (MRI) can be used to diagnose thoracic aortic disease, but in acute aortic dissection the diagnosis is most rapidly and safely made using echocardiography with color Doppler imaging (Fig. 12.5). Although transthoracic echocardiography (TTE) is the mainstay in evaluation of the heart, including evaluation for complications of dissection like aortic insufficiency, pericardial effusions, and impaired regional left ventricular function, it is of somewhat limited value in assessment of the distal ascending, transverse, and

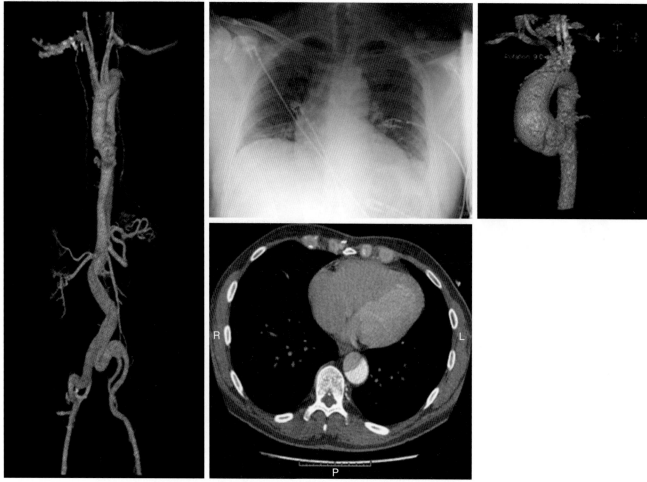

FIG. 12.5 Tomographic reconstruction of a type B aortic dissection, chest radiography showing enlarged mediastinum, and type A aortic dissections seen on image reconstruction as well as with contrast CT scanning.

descending aorta. Transesophageal echocardiography (TEE), on the other hand, plays an essential role in diagnosing aortic dissection because it is both highly sensitive and specific (98% and 95%, respectively), has the advantage of using portable equipment, and can be performed as a single study, especially in patients in unstable condition. Angiography of the aorta may be required for patients undergoing elective surgery on the thoracic aorta so that the complete extent of the dissection and the location of all compromised aortic branches can be defined.

Abdominal ultrasonography is a very sensitive test for the detection of abdominal aortic aneurysms. CT is also very sensitive and is more accurate than ultrasonography in estimating aneurysm size.

Improvements in CT technology, such as the advent of helical CT and CT angiography, have increased the role of CT imaging in the evaluation and treatment of abdominal aortic aneurysms. Helical CT provides excellent three-dimensional anatomic detail and is particularly useful for evaluating the feasibility of endovascular stent graft repair of the aneurysm.

MRI is useful for accurate measurement of aneurysm size and evaluation of relevant vascular anatomy without the need for the use of ionizing radiation or contrast medium.

Medical Management of Aortic Aneurysms

Medical management of an aortic aneurysm focuses on decreasing its expansion rate and thus potentially avoiding its evolution toward dissection and/or rupture. Careful management of blood pressure, hyperlipidemia, and smoking cessation are essential. Avoidance of strenuous exercise, stimulants such as cocaine, and overall stress are important aspects of long-term care of these patients. The most commonly used agents are β-blockers, angiotensin-converting enzyme (ACE) inhibitors, and angiotensin-II receptor blockers, as well as statins for lipid control. In addition, patients with known aneurysms should be followed at regular intervals to evaluate for possible continued expansion of their aneurysm and subsequent need for surgical intervention.

Preoperative Evaluation

Because myocardial ischemia or infarction, respiratory failure, renal failure, and stroke are the principal causes of morbidity and mortality associated with surgery of the thoracic aorta, preoperative assessment of the function of the corresponding organ systems is needed. Assessment for the presence of myocardial ischemia, previous MI, valvular dysfunction, and heart failure is important in performing risk stratification and planning maneuvers for risk reduction. A preoperative percutaneous coronary intervention or coronary artery bypass grafting may be indicated in some patients with ischemic heart disease.

Preoperative evaluation of cardiac function might include exercise or pharmacologic stress testing with or without echocardiography or radionuclide imaging. Severe reductions in vital capacity and FEV_1 (forced expiratory volume in the first second of expiration), as well as abnormal renal function, may mitigate against abdominal aortic aneurysm resection or significantly increase the risk of elective aneurysm repair.

Cigarette smoking and the presence of chronic obstructive pulmonary disease (COPD) are important predictors of respiratory failure after thoracic aorta surgery. Spirometric tests of lung function and arterial blood gas analysis may better define this risk. Reversible airway obstruction and pulmonary infection should be treated with bronchodilators, antibiotics, and chest physiotherapy. Smoking cessation is very desirable.

The presence of preoperative renal dysfunction is the single most important predictor of the development of acute renal failure after surgery on the thoracic aorta. Preoperative hydration and avoidance of hypovolemia, hypotension, low cardiac output, and nephrotoxic drugs during the perioperative period are important to decrease the likelihood of postoperative renal failure.

Duplex imaging of the carotid arteries or angiography of the brachiocephalic and intracranial arteries may be performed preoperatively in patients with a history of stroke or transient ischemic attacks (TIAs). Patients with severe stenosis of one or both common or internal carotid arteries could be considered for carotid endarterectomy before elective surgery on the thoracic aorta.

Indications for Surgery

As noted earlier, the mainstay of treatment for aortic aneurysm is medical management, so thoracic aortic aneurysm repair is an elective procedure, and surgery is contemplated only when aneurysm size exceeds a diameter of 5.5 cm. This size limit may be raised somewhat for patients with a significant family history, a previous diagnosis of any of the hereditable diseases that affect blood vessels, or an aneurysm growth rate of 10 mm or more per year. A number of important technical advances have decreased the risk of surgery on the thoracic aorta, including the use of adjuncts such as distal aortic perfusion, profound hypothermia with circulatory arrest, monitoring of evoked potentials in the brain and spinal cord, and cerebrospinal fluid (CSF) drainage, as well as the rapid increase in endovascular procedures for aortic repairs.

The recommendation for surgery for abdominal aortic aneurysms larger than 5.5 cm in diameter is based on clinical studies indicating that the risk of rupture within a 5-year period is 25%–41% for aneurysms larger than 5 cm. Smaller aneurysms are less likely to rupture, but patients with aneurysms less than 5 cm in diameter should be followed with serial ultrasonography. However, these recommendations are only guidelines. Each patient must be evaluated for the presence of risk factors for accelerated aneurysm growth and rupture, such as tobacco use and family history. If the abdominal aortic aneurysm expands by more than 0.6–0.8 cm per year, repair is usually recommended. Surgical risk and overall health are also part of the evaluation to determine the timing of aneurysm repair. Endovascular aneurysm repair is a valid alternative to surgical repair.

Rupture of Abdominal Aortic Aneurysm

The classic triad of hypotension, back pain, and a pulsatile abdominal mass is present in only about half of patients who have a ruptured abdominal aortic aneurysm. Renal colic, diverticulitis, and gastrointestinal hemorrhage may be confused with a ruptured abdominal aortic aneurysm.

Most abdominal aortic aneurysms rupture into the left retroperitoneum. Although hypovolemic shock may be present, exsanguination may be prevented by clotting and the tamponade effect of the retroperitoneum. Euvolemic resuscitation may be deferred until the aortic rupture is surgically controlled in the operating room, because euvolemic resuscitation and the resultant increase in blood pressure without surgical control of bleeding may lead to loss of retroperitoneal tamponade, further bleeding, hypotension, and death.

Patients in unstable condition who have a suspected ruptured abdominal aortic aneurysm require immediate operation and control of the proximal aorta without preoperative confirmatory testing or optimal volume resuscitation.

Aortic Dissections

Ascending and aortic arch dissection *requires* emergent or urgent surgery; however, descending thoracic aortic dissection is *rarely* treated with urgent surgery.

Type A Dissection

The International Registry of Acute Aortic Dissection is a consortium of 21 large referral centers around the world. This registry's data have shown that the in-hospital mortality rate of patients with ascending aortic dissection is approximately 27% in those who undergo timely and successful surgery. This is in contrast to an in-hospital mortality rate of 56% in those treated medically. Other independent predictors of in-hospital death include older age, visceral ischemia, hypotension, renal failure, cardiac tamponade, coma, and pulse deficits.

Long-term survival rates (i.e., survival at 1–3 years after hospital discharge) are 90%–96% in the surgically treated group and 69%–89% in those treated medically who survive initial hospitalization. Thus aggressive medical treatment and imaging surveillance of patients who for various reasons are unable to undergo surgery appears prudent.

Ascending Aorta. All patients with acute dissection involving the ascending aorta should be considered candidates for surgery. The most commonly performed procedures are replacement of the ascending aorta and aortic valve with a composite graft (Dacron graft containing a prosthetic valve) or replacement of the ascending aorta and resuspension of the aortic valve. In the last decade it appears that more centers perform valve-sparing surgical procedures that allows for re-implantation of the aortic valve.

Aortic Arch. In patients with acute aortic arch dissection, resection of the aortic arch (i.e., the segment of aorta that extends from the origin of the innominate artery to the origin of the left subclavian artery) is indicated. Surgery on the aortic arch requires cardiopulmonary bypass, profound hypothermia, and a period of circulatory arrest. With current techniques, a period of circulatory arrest of 30–40 minutes at a body temperature of 15°–18°C can be tolerated by most patients. Focal and diffuse neurologic deficits are the major complications associated with replacement of the aortic arch. These occur in 3%–18% of patients, and it appears that selective antegrade cerebral perfusion decreases but does not completely eliminate the morbidity and mortality associated with this procedure.

Type B Dissection

Descending Thoracic Aorta. Patients with an acute but uncomplicated type B aortic dissection who have normal hemodynamics, no periaortic hematoma, and no branch vessel involvement at presentation can be treated with medical therapy. Such therapy consists of (1) intraarterial monitoring of systemic blood pressure and urinary output and (2) administration of drugs to control blood pressure and the force of left ventricular contraction. Short-acting β-blockers like esmolol and nitroprusside or nicardipine, and more recently clevidipine, are commonly used for this purpose. This patient population has an in-hospital mortality rate of 10%. Long-term survival rate with medical therapy only is approximately 60%–80% at 4–5 years and 40%–50% at 10 years.

Surgery is indicated for patients with type B aortic dissection who have signs of impending rupture (persistent pain, hypotension, left-sided hemothorax); ischemia of the legs, abdominal viscera, or spinal cord; and/or renal failure. Surgical treatment of distal aortic dissection is associated with a 29% in-hospital mortality rate.

Unique Risks of Surgery
Surgical Approach

Classically the ascending aorta and aortic arch are approached via median sternotomy and require cardiopulmonary bypass. The descending thoracic aorta is repaired through a thoracotomy incision, and abdominal aneurysms are repaired via laparotomy. Endovascular repairs require groin incisions and have only minimal scars.

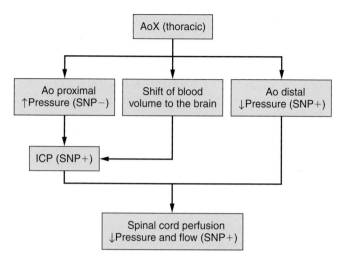

FIG. 12.6 Spinal cord blood flow and perfusion pressure during thoracic aortic occlusion, with or without sodium nitroprusside (SNP) infusion. The arrows represent the response to aortic cross-clamping (AoX) per se. ↑, Increased; ↓, decreased; *Ao*, aorta; *ICP*, intracranial pressure; *SNP+*, the effects enhanced by SNP infusion; *SNP–*, the effects counteracted by SNP infusion. (Adapted from Gelman S. The pathophysiology of aortic cross-clamping and unclamping. *Anesthesiology.* 1995;82:1026-1060. © 1995, Lippincott Williams & Wilkins.)

Surgical resection of thoracic aortic aneurysms can be associated with a number of serious, even life-threatening, complications. There is the risk of spinal cord ischemia (anterior spinal artery syndrome) with resulting paraparesis or paraplegia. Cross-clamping and unclamping the aorta introduces the potential for adverse hemodynamic responses such as myocardial ischemia and heart failure. Hypothermia, an important neuroprotective maneuver, can be responsible for the development of coagulopathy. Renal insufficiency or renal failure occurs in up to 30% of patients. Approximately 6% of patients will require hemodialysis. Pulmonary complications are common; the incidence of respiratory failure approaches 50%. Cardiac complications are the leading cause of mortality.

Anterior Spinal Artery Syndrome. Cross-clamping the thoracic aorta can result in ischemic damage to the spinal cord (see Fig. 12.2). The frequency of spinal cord injury ranges from 0.2% after elective infrarenal abdominal aortic aneurysm repair to 8% in elective thoracic aortic aneurysm repair to 40% in the setting of acute aortic dissection or rupture involving the descending thoracic aorta. Manifestations of anterior spinal artery syndrome include flaccid paralysis of the lower extremities and bowel and bladder dysfunction. Sensation and proprioception are spared.

Spinal Cord Blood Supply. The spinal cord is supplied by one anterior spinal artery and two posterior spinal arteries (Fig. 12.6). The anterior spinal artery begins at the fusion of branches of both vertebral arteries and relies on reinforcement of its blood supply by six to eight radicular arteries, the largest and most important of which is the great radicular artery of Adamkiewicz. Multiple levels of the spinal cord do not receive feeding radicular branches, which leaves watershed areas that are particularly susceptible to ischemic injury. These areas are in jeopardy during aortic occlusion or hypotension. Damage can also result from surgical resection of the artery of Adamkiewicz (because the origin is unknown) or exclusion of the origin of the artery by the cross-clamp. In this situation, not only is the anterior spinal artery blood flow reduced directly, but the potential for collateral blood flow to the spinal cord is also reduced because aortic pressure distal to the cross-clamp is very low.

Risk Factors. The risk of paraplegia during thoracic aortic surgery is determined by the interaction of four factors: (1) the decrease in spinal cord blood flow, (2) the rate of neuronal metabolism, (3) postischemia reperfusion injury, and (4) blood flow after reperfusion. The duration of aortic cross-clamping is critical in determining the risk of paraplegia. A brief period of thoracic aortic cross-clamping (<30 minutes) is usually tolerated. If cross-clamp time is more than 30 minutes, the risk of spinal cord ischemia is significant and use of techniques for spinal cord protection is indicated. These include partial circulatory assistance (left atrium–to–femoral artery bypass), reimplantation of critical intercostal arteries when possible, CSF drainage, maintenance of proximal hypertension during cross-clamping, reduction of spinal cord metabolism by moderate hypothermia (30°–32°C) including spinal cooling, avoidance of hyperglycemia, and the use of mannitol, corticosteroids, and/or calcium channel blockers.

There is debate regarding the incidence of spinal cord ischemia after endovascular repair. Although some studies report an incidence similar to that with open aortic surgery, others showed a lower rate with endovascular repair. Nevertheless, the incidence seems to be directly correlated with the severity of aortic disease. The theoretical reason is that although the respective vessel may be taken out of circulation, with endovascular repair (as opposed to open repair), there is no dissection of other vessels that may represent important collateral flow, which ensures secularization of the spinal cord.

Hemodynamic Responses to Aortic Cross-Clamping. Thoracic aortic cross-clamping and unclamping are associated with severe hemodynamic and homeostatic disturbances in virtually all organ systems because of the decrease in blood flow distal to the aortic clamp and the substantial increase in blood flow above the level of aortic occlusion. There is a substantial increase in systemic blood pressure and systemic vascular resistance, with no significant change in heart rate. A reduction in cardiac output usually accompanies these changes. Systemic hypertension is attributed to increased impedance to aortic outflow (increased afterload). In addition, there is blood volume redistribution caused by collapse and constriction of the venous vasculature distal to the aortic cross-clamp. An increase in preload results. Evidence of this blood volume redistribution can be seen as an increase in filling pressures (central venous pressure, pulmonary capillary occlusion pressure, left ventricular end-diastolic pressure). Substantial differences in the hemodynamic response to aortic cross-clamping can be seen at different levels of clamping: thoracic, supraceliac, and infrarenal. Changes in mean arterial

pressure, end-diastolic and end-systolic left ventricular area and ejection fraction, and wall motion abnormalities may be assessed by TEE or pulmonary artery catheterization and are minimal during infrarenal aortic cross-clamping but dramatic during intrathoracic aortic cross-clamping. Some of these differences result in part from different patterns of blood volume redistribution. Preload may not increase if the aorta is clamped distal to the celiac artery, because the blood volume from the distal venous vasculature may be redistributed into the splanchnic circulation. For the increase in afterload and preload to be tolerated, an increase in myocardial contractility and an autoregulatory increase in coronary blood flow are required. If coronary blood flow and myocardial contractility cannot increase, left ventricular dysfunction is likely. Indeed, echocardiography often indicates abnormal wall motion of the left ventricle during aortic cross-clamping, which suggests the presence of myocardial ischemia. Hemodynamic responses to aortic cross-clamping are blunted in patients with aortoiliac occlusive disease.

Pharmacologic interventions intended to offset the hemodynamic effects of aortic cross-clamping, especially clamping of the thoracic aorta, are related to the effects of the administered drug on arterial and/or venous capacitance. For example, vasodilators such as nicardipine, nitroprusside, and nitroglycerin often reduce the clamp-induced decrease in cardiac output and ejection fraction. The most plausible explanation for this effect is a drug-induced decrease in systemic vascular resistance and afterload, and increased venous capacitance.

It is important, however, to recognize that perfusion pressures distal to the aortic cross-clamp are decreased and are directly dependent on proximal aortic pressure—that is, the pressure above the level of aortic clamping. Blood flow to tissues distal to aortic occlusion (kidneys, liver, spinal cord) occurs through collateral vessels or through a shunt. It decreases dramatically during aortic clamping. Blood flow to vital organs distal to the aortic clamp depends on perfusion pressure, not on cardiac output or intravascular volume.

Clinically, drugs and volume replacement must be adjusted to maintain distal aortic perfusion pressure even if that results in an increase in blood pressure proximal to the clamp. Strategies for myocardial preservation during and after aortic cross-clamping include decreasing afterload and normalizing preload, coronary blood flow, and contractility. Modalities such as placement of temporary shunts, reimplantation of arteries supplying distal tissues (spinal cord), and hypothermia may influence the choice of drugs and end points of treatment.

Cross-clamping of the thoracic aorta just distal to the left subclavian artery is associated with severe decreases (≈90%) in spinal cord and renal blood flow, glomerular filtration rate, and urinary output. Infrarenal aortic cross-clamping is associated with a large increase in renal vascular resistance and a decrease (≈30%) in renal blood flow. Renal failure following aortic surgery is almost always due to acute tubular necrosis. Ischemia-reperfusion insults to the kidneys play a central role in the pathogenesis of this renal failure.

Cross-clamping of the thoracic aorta is associated not only with a decrease in distal aortic–anterior spinal artery pressure but also with an increase in CSF pressure. Presumably, intracranial hypertension resulting from systemic hypertension above the clamp produces redistribution of blood volume and engorgement of the intracranial compartment (intracranial hypervolemia). This results in redistribution of CSF into the spinal fluid space and a decrease in the compliance of the spinal fluid space. CSF drainage may increase spinal cord blood flow and decrease the incidence of neurologic complications.

Pulmonary damage associated with aortic cross-clamping and unclamping is reflected by an increase in pulmonary vascular resistance (particularly with unclamping of the aorta), an increase in pulmonary capillary membrane permeability, and development of pulmonary edema. The mechanisms involved may include pulmonary hypervolemia and the effects of various vasoactive mediators.

Aortic cross-clamping is associated with formation and release of hormonal factors (caused by activation of the sympathetic nervous system and the renin-angiotensin-aldosterone system) and other mediators (prostaglandins, oxygen free radicals, complement cascade). These mediators may aggravate or blunt the harmful effects of aortic cross-clamping and unclamping. Overall, injury to the spinal cord, lungs, kidneys, and abdominal viscera is principally due to ischemia and subsequent reperfusion injury caused by the aortic cross-clamp (local effects) and/or the release of mediators from ischemic and reperfused tissues (distant effects).

Hemodynamic Responses to Aortic Unclamping. Unclamping of the thoracic aorta is associated with substantial decreases in systemic vascular resistance and systemic blood pressure. Cardiac output may increase, decrease, or remain unchanged. Left ventricular end-diastolic pressure decreases, and myocardial blood flow increases. Gradual release of the aortic clamp is recommended to allow time for volume replacement and to slow the washout of vasoactive and cardiodepressant mediators from ischemic tissues.

The principal causes of unclamping hypotension include (1) central hypovolemia caused by pooling of blood in reperfused tissues, (2) hypoxia-mediated vasodilation, which causes an increase in vascular capacitance in the tissues below the level of aortic clamping, and (3) accumulation of vasoactive and myocardial-depressant metabolites in these tissues. Vasodilation and hypotension may be further aggravated by the transient increase in carbon dioxide release and oxygen consumption in these tissues following unclamping. Correction of metabolic acidosis does not significantly influence the degree of hypotension following aortic unclamping.

Management of Anesthesia

Management of anesthesia in patients undergoing thoracic aortic aneurysm resection requires consideration of monitoring systemic blood pressure, neurologic function, and intravascular volume and planning the pharmacologic interventions and hemodynamic management that will be needed to control hypertension during the period of aortic cross-clamping. Proper monitoring is more important than selection of anesthetic drugs in these patients.

Monitoring Blood Pressure

Surgical repair of a thoracic aortic aneurysm requires aortic cross-clamping just distal to the left subclavian artery or between the left subclavian artery and the left common carotid artery. Therefore blood pressure monitoring must be via an artery in the right arm, since occlusion of the aorta can prevent measurement of blood pressure in the left arm. Monitoring blood pressure both above (right radial artery) and below (femoral artery) the aneurysm is less commonly done but may be useful. This approach permits assessment of cerebral, renal, and spinal cord perfusion pressure during cross-clamping.

Blood flow to tissues below the aortic cross-clamp is dependent on perfusion pressure rather than on preload and cardiac output. Therefore during cross-clamping of the thoracic aorta, proximal aortic pressures should be maintained as high as the heart can safely withstand unless other modalities (e.g., temporary shunts, hypothermia) are implemented. A common recommendation is to maintain mean arterial pressure near 100 mm Hg above the cross-clamp and above 50 mm Hg in the areas distal to the cross-clamp.

Use of vasodilators to treat hypertension above the level of the aortic cross-clamp must be balanced against the likelihood of a decrease in perfusion pressure in the tissues below the clamp. Indeed, nitroprusside may decrease spinal cord perfusion pressure both by decreasing distal aortic pressure and by increasing CSF pressure as a result of cerebral vasodilation (see Fig. 12.6). It is prudent to limit the use of drugs that decrease proximal aortic pressure and cause cerebral vasodilation. Use of temporary shunts to bypass the occluded thoracic aorta (proximal aorta–to–femoral artery or left atrium–to–femoral artery shunts) may be considered when attempting to maintain renal and spinal cord perfusion. Partial cardiopulmonary bypass is another option to maintain distal aortic perfusion.

Monitoring Neurologic Function

Somatosensory evoked potentials (SEPs) and electroencephalography (EEG) are monitoring methods for evaluating central nervous system viability during the period of aortic cross-clamping. Unfortunately, intraoperative monitoring of SEPs is not completely reliable for detecting spinal cord ischemia during aortic surgery, because SEP monitoring reflects dorsal column (sensory tract) function. Ischemic changes in anterior spinal cord function (motor tracts) are not detected. Monitoring of motor evoked potentials would indicate anterior spinal cord function but is impractical, since it prohibits use of neuromuscular blocking drugs. Spinal cooling with epidural instillation of iced saline during cross-clamping in thoracic aneurysm surgery has been employed successfully for many years in some institutions across the United States on the basis that lowering the spinal cord temperature directly will improve recovery of potentially poorly perfused tissues after reimplantation of patent critical intercostal vessels by the surgeon. Nevertheless, spinal drainage has been used to decrease pressure around the spinal cord and avoid ischemia in a confined space if the spinal cord dilates after adequate perfusion is reestablished. CSF pressure is also maintained at a value of less than 10 cm H_2O in the days immediately after surgery for the same reason—namely, that an increase in pressure in the spinal canal may decrease perfusion to the spinal cord and impair motor function. This method is used successfully in both open surgical procedures and endovascular repairs of the aorta (see later). Another method that can be useful is atriofemoral bypass to maintain distal aortic perfusion.

Monitoring Cardiac Function

During operations on the thoracic aorta, TEE can provide valuable information about the presence of atherosclerosis in the thoracic aorta, the competence of cardiac valves, ventricular function, adequacy of myocardial perfusion, and intravascular volume status. A pulmonary artery catheter provides data that may complement information obtained from TEE.

Monitoring Intravascular Volume and Renal Function

Optimization of systemic hemodynamics, including circulating blood volume, represents the most effective measure for protecting the kidneys from the ischemic effects produced by aortic cross-clamping. Use of diuretics such as mannitol before aortic clamping may also be useful. Mannitol improves renal cortical blood flow and glomerular filtration rate.

Renal protection is achieved by direct instillation of renal preservation fluid (4°C lactated Ringer solution with 25 g of mannitol per liter and 1 g methylprednisolone per liter) and can be administered directly by the surgeon into the renal artery.

Induction and Maintenance of Anesthesia

Induction of anesthesia and tracheal intubation must minimize undesirable increases in systemic blood pressure that could exacerbate an aortic dissection or rupture an aneurysm. Use of a double-lumen endobronchial tube permits collapse of the left lung and facilitates surgical exposure during resection of a thoracic aneurysm.

General anesthesia can be maintained with volatile anesthetics and/or opioids. General anesthesia may cause some reduction in cerebral metabolic rate, which may be particularly desirable during this surgery. The choice of neuromuscular blocking drug may be influenced by the dependence of a particular drug on renal clearance.

Management of anesthesia for resection of an abdominal aortic aneurysm requires consideration of commonly associated medical conditions in this patient group: ischemic heart disease, hypertension, COPD, diabetes mellitus, and renal dysfunction. Monitoring intravascular volume and cardiac, pulmonary, and renal function is essential during the perioperative period. An intraarterial catheter monitors systemic blood pressure continuously. If appropriate personnel and equipment are available, echocardiography can be very useful for evaluating the cardiac response to aortic cross-clamping

and unclamping and assessing left ventricular filling volume and regional and global myocardial function. Urine output is monitored continuously.

No single anesthetic drug or technique is ideal for all patients undergoing elective abdominal aortic aneurysm repair. Combinations of volatile anesthetics and/or opioids are commonly used, with or without nitrous oxide. Continuous epidural anesthesia combined with general anesthesia may offer advantages by decreasing overall anesthetic drug requirements, attenuating the increased systemic vascular resistance associated with aortic cross-clamping, and facilitating postoperative pain management. Nevertheless, there is no evidence that the combination of epidural anesthesia and general anesthesia decreases postoperative cardiac or pulmonary morbidity compared with general anesthesia alone in high-risk patients who undergo aortic surgery. Postoperative epidural analgesia may favorably influence the postoperative course, however. Administration of anticoagulants during abdominal aortic surgery raises the controversial issue of placement of an epidural catheter and the remote risk of epidural hematoma formation.

Patients undergoing thoracoabdominal aortic aneurysm repair usually experience significant fluid and blood losses. Administration of a combination of balanced salt and colloid solutions (and blood if needed) guided by appropriate monitoring of cardiac and renal function facilitates maintenance of adequate intravascular volume, cardiac output, and urine formation. Balanced salt and/or colloid solutions should be infused during aortic cross-clamping to build up an intravascular volume reserve and thereby minimize unclamping hypotension. If urinary output is decreased despite adequate fluid and blood replacement, diuretic therapy with mannitol or furosemide might be considered. The efficacy of low-dose dopamine in preserving renal function during abdominal aortic aneurysm surgery is unproven.

Infrarenal aortic cross-clamping and unclamping are significant events during abdominal aortic surgery. The anticipated consequences of abdominal aortic cross-clamping include increased systemic vascular resistance (afterload) and decreased venous return (see earlier discussion). Often, myocardial performance and circulatory parameters remain acceptable after the aorta is clamped at an infrarenal level. An alteration in anesthetic depth or infusion of vasodilators may be necessary in some patients to maintain myocardial performance at acceptable levels.

Hypotension may occur when the aortic cross-clamp is removed (see earlier discussion). Prevention of unclamping hypotension and maintenance of a stable cardiac output can often be achieved by volume loading to pulmonary capillary occlusion pressures higher than normal before the cross-clamp is removed. Likewise, gradual opening of the aortic cross-clamp may minimize the decrease in systemic blood pressure by allowing some pooled venous blood to return to the central circulation. The washout of acid metabolites from ischemic areas below the cross-clamp when the clamp is released plays a much less important role than central hypovolemia in producing unclamping hypotension, and sodium bicarbonate pretreatment does *not* reliably blunt unclamping hypotension. If hypotension persists for more than a few minutes after removal of the cross-clamp, the presence of unrecognized bleeding or inadequate volume replacement must be considered. Echocardiography at this time may be particularly helpful in determining the adequacy of volume replacement and cardiac function.

Postoperative Management

Posterolateral thoracotomy is among the most painful of surgical incisions; major muscles are transected and ribs are removed. In addition, chest tube insertion sites can be very painful. Amelioration of pain is essential to ensure patient comfort and facilitate coughing and maneuvers designed to prevent atelectasis. Pain relief is commonly provided by neuraxial opioids and/or local anesthetics. Intrathecal or epidural catheters providing intermittent or continuous infusion of analgesic medications can be adapted to provide an element of patient-controlled analgesia as well. Inclusion of local anesthetic drugs in these solutions may produce sensory and motor anesthesia and delay recognition of anterior spinal artery syndrome. Moreover, when a neurologic deficit is recognized, the epidural drug may be implicated as the cause of the paraplegia. If neuraxial analgesia is used in the period immediately after surgery, opioids are preferred over local anesthetics to prevent masking of anterior spinal artery syndrome.

Patients recovering from thoracic aortic aneurysm resection are at risk of developing cardiac, pulmonary, and renal failure during the immediate postoperative period. In the majority of clinical series, postoperative pulmonary complications are the most common, representing 25%–45% of cases. Cerebrovascular accidents may result from air or thrombotic emboli that occur during surgical resection of the diseased aorta. Patients with co-existing cerebrovascular disease may be more vulnerable to development of new central nervous system complications. Spinal cord injury may manifest during the period immediately after surgery as paraparesis or flaccid paralysis. Delayed appearance of paraplegia (12 hours to 21 days postoperatively) has been associated with postoperative hypotension in patients with severe atherosclerotic disease in whom marginally adequate collateral circulation to the spinal cord is present.

Systemic hypertension is not uncommon and may jeopardize the integrity of the surgical repair and/or predispose to myocardial ischemia. The role of pain in the development of hypertension must be considered.

Patients recovering from abdominal aortic aneurysm repair are also at risk of developing cardiac, pulmonary, and renal dysfunction during the postoperative period. Assessment of graft patency and lower extremity blood flow is primordial. Adequate pain control accomplished with either neuraxial opioids or patient-controlled analgesia is very important in facilitating early tracheal extubation.

ENDOVASCULAR AORTIC ANEURYSM REPAIR

Endovascular placement of intraluminal stent grafts to treat patients with aneurysms of the descending thoracic and abdominal aorta may be particularly useful in the elderly and in those with co-existing medical conditions such as hypertension, COPD, and renal insufficiency that would significantly increase the risks associated with conventional operative treatment. These devices have been approved for aneurysms above 5.5 cm as well as complicated type B dissections. Endovascular devices appear to improve initial hospital morbidity and mortality, but there is a higher risk for later complications and need for reinterventions. At 5-year follow-up the mortality advantage is less evident. Endovascular treatment of aortic aneurysms is achieved by transluminal placement of one or more stent graft devices across the longitudinal extent of the lesion. The prosthesis bridges the aneurysmal sac to exclude it from high-pressure aortic blood flow, thereby allowing for sac thrombosis around the stent and possible remodeling of the aortic wall. Endovascular repair offers the benefit of aneurysm exclusion without causing the significant physiologic changes that occur during cross-clamping (see earlier discussion).

Currently, endovascular aneurysm repair of the intrathoracic aorta has been focused on the descending thoracic aorta (i.e., the portion distal to the left subclavian artery). Endovascular repair of the thoracic aorta poses several unique challenges compared with endovascular repair of the abdominal aorta. First, the hemodynamic forces are significantly more severe and place greater mechanical demands on thoracic endografts. The potential for device migration, kinking, and late structural failure are important concerns. Second, greater flexibility is required of thoracic devices to conform to the natural curvature of the proximal descending aorta and to lesions with tortuous morphology. Third, because larger devices are necessary to accommodate the diameter of the thoracic aorta, arterial access is more problematic. Fourth, as with conventional open thoracic aneurysm repair, paraplegia remains a potential complication of the endovascular approach, despite the absence of aortic cross-clamping. Fifth, visceral and renal ischemia still can occur if the graft occludes the celiac axis.

Over the past decade, many endovascular devices to repair abdominal aortic aneurysms have been developed (Fig. 12.7; also see Fig. 12.2). Endovascular repair involves gaining access to the lumen of the abdominal aorta, usually via small incisions over the femoral vessels. Although each device has unique features, all employ the same basic structural design and are composed of a metal stent covered with fabric. There are two types of devices: unibody and modular. The *unibody type* comes in one piece and is easier to deploy but requires contralateral occlusion and bypass grafting. *Modular* devices are composed of more than one piece, and the components are deployed through both groin areas. The great variability in patient anatomy makes it difficult to find a single graft that will be adequate to cover an aneurysm; thus most surgeons use multipart grafts that interlock and provide a better fit.

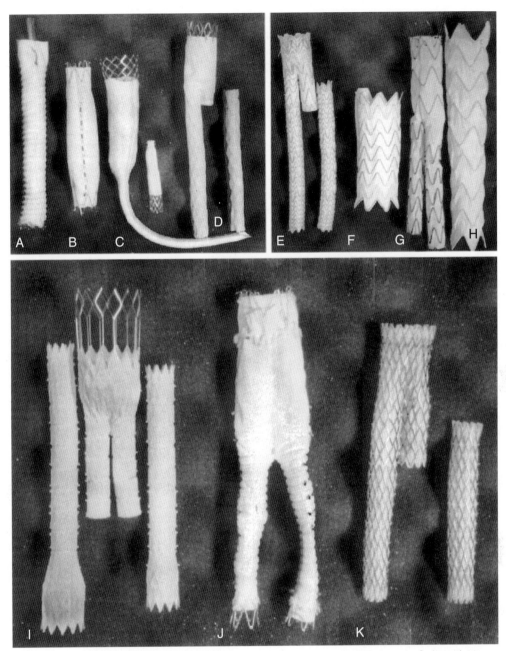

FIG. 12.7 Endovascular stent graft devices. A, Parodi graft. B, EVT Endograft. C, Investigator ESG. D, Boston Scientific Vanguard stent graft. E, W.L. Gore Excluder stent graft. F, W.L. Gore thoracic stent graft. G, Medtronic/World Medical Talent abdominal aortic stent graft. H, Medtronic/World Medical Talent thoracic aortic stent graft. I, Teramed/Cordis abdominal aortic stent graft. J, Guidant Ancure stent graft. K, Medtronic AneuRx stent graft. (From Marin ML, Hollier LH, Ellozy SH, et al. Endovascular stent graft repair of abdominal and thoracic aortic aneurysms: a ten-year experience with 817 patients. *Ann Surg.* 2003;238:586-595.)

The literature on thoracic stent grafting consists mostly of reports of small- to medium-sized case series with short- to medium-term follow-up. All these studies show a common pattern of outcomes. Overall, successful device deployment is achieved in 85%–100% of cases, and perioperative mortality ranges from 0%–14%, falling within or below elective surgery mortality rates of 5%–20%. Outcomes have improved over time with accumulated technical expertise, technologic advances in the devices, and improved patient selection criteria. Current reported experience with thoracic stent grafting demonstrates successful deployment in 87% of cases, 30-day mortality of 1.9%–2.1% in elective cases, and paraplegia and endoleak rates of 4%–9%. Survival at 1, 5, and 8 years is 82%, 49%, and 27%, respectively. Therefore mortality at 3 or 4 years is nearly identical in patients receiving stent grafts and in those undergoing open aneurysm repair. Other authors describe an approximately 98% rate of freedom from aneurysm rupture at 9 years in a cohort of 817 patients undergoing stenting, but a high rate of death (47% survival at 8 years) from comorbid medical diseases, especially cardiovascular events, even though patients were evaluated preoperatively with stress testing, and revascularization was performed if needed. There are no randomized studies comparing endovascular repair with the open procedure. Nevertheless, the overall trend is that endovascular procedures are associated with lower perioperative mortality, and the endovascular approach offers patients shorter hospital stay, quicker rehabilitation, and longer average number of months lived resulting from the decrease in preoperative mortality. Even if the results of the open procedure are more durable, it is associated with major postoperative complications. Therefore with the development of new types of grafts the endovascular approach will most probably become the primary method of aortic aneurysmal repair when anatomic conditions are optimal.

Complications

Complications associated with endografts include endoleaks, vascular injury during graft deployment, inadequate fixation and sealing of the graft to the wall (i.e., risk of graft migration), stent frame fractures, and breakdown of graft material. After the graft has been deployed, the aneurysm eventually will thrombose and decrease in diameter.

Device migration is one of the most common causes of a need for secondary intervention, because if such migration is left unmanaged, it may lead to endoleaks, aneurysm expansion, and rupture.

Reinterventions are part of late complications and although minor are more common after endovascular repair (9% of cases) than after open repair (1.7%); however, repeat laparotomy and hospitalizations are more common after open surgical repair (9.7% vs. 4.1%). Most practitioners do not consider the requirement for a secondary intervention to represent a failure. Nevertheless, patients must be aware that they will require lifelong surveillance.

Although endovascular repair does not require a period of aortic clamping, the possibility of spinal cord ischemia still exists because of exclusion of important intercostal arteries. There is no role for epidural cooling, but spinal drainage may offer some benefits in individuals at high risk. These may include patients with prior aortic repair (usually infrarenal), those with aortic dissections, and those with stable aortic ruptures. In patients in unstable condition the drain may be placed postoperatively.

Consideration of the risk of intraabdominal ischemia is an important aspect, especially when the celiac artery is occluded by the graft. Under development are bifurcated grafts that will be used in the near future to achieve aneurysm exclusion with preservation of flow to important vessels (e.g., celiac and renal arteries) when aneurysms involve their origins.

Anesthetic Management

General or regional anesthesia is acceptable for endovascular aneurysm repair. Monitoring consists of, at a minimum, intravascular blood pressure and urine output monitoring. The potential need for conversion to an open aneurysm repair must always be kept in mind. Large-bore intravenous access and availability of blood are still important concerns. Spinal drain placement is a consideration for thoracic aneurysm repair after discussion with the surgeon (see earlier discussion). Maintenance of euvolemia and normotension are important.

Administration of heparin and verification of activated clotting time are still mainstays, as in any other vascular procedure.

Postoperative Management

Postoperative management depends on numerous physiologic and procedural variables. Commonly, patients undergoing higher thoracic aortic repair will be cared for in an intensive care unit until all perioperative concerns have been resolved, including the possibility of ischemia, acidosis, ongoing respiratory failure, and cardiac problems. Patients undergoing lower abdominal aortic repair still must be followed closely, with particular attention to the development or worsening of renal dysfunction, even if it is transitory because of intravenous dye administration.

CAROTID ARTERY DISEASE AND STROKE

Cerebrovascular accidents (strokes) are characterized by sudden neurologic deficits resulting from ischemic or hemorrhagic events. Carotid artery disease is an important contributor to stroke risk. Anesthesiologists frequently manage anesthesia in patients with carotid diseases, both for carotid surgery and for other surgical procedures.

Epidemiology and Risk Factors

Approximately 3% of US adults have experienced a stroke. It is the leading cause of disability and the third leading cause of death in this country. Strokes are classified as either ischemic (most commonly thrombotic or embolic in origin) or hemorrhagic (secondary to vascular malformation, trauma, or coagulopathy). Approximately 87% of all strokes are ischemic. TIAs are a subset of self-limited ischemic strokes and present as a sudden focal neurologic deficit that resolves within 24 hours. TIAs often herald an impending ischemic stroke, and individuals experiencing TIAs have a 10-times greater risk of subsequent stroke than age- and sex-matched populations.

Neurologic deficits following intracranial arterial occlusion are often extensive, reflecting the large areas of brain supplied by the major arteries and their branches. Six months after an ischemic stroke, fully one-quarter of survivors older than age 65 will be institutionalized.

TABLE 12.2	Factors Predisposing to Stroke

INHERITED RISK FACTORS
Age
Prior history of stroke
Family history of stroke
Black race
Male gender
Sickle cell disease

MODIFIABLE RISK FACTORS
Elevated blood pressure
Smoking
Diabetes
Carotid artery disease
Atrial fibrillation
Heart failure
Hypercholesterolemia
Obesity or physical inactivity

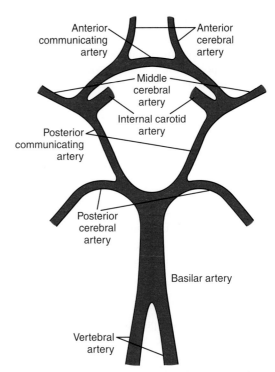

FIG. 12.8 Cerebral circulation and the circle of Willis. Cerebral blood supply comes from the vertebral arteries (arising from the subclavian arteries) and the internal carotid arteries (arising from the common carotid arteries).

Major risk factors for stroke are listed in Table 12.2. Although anesthesiologists may play a role in educating patients with modifiable health risk factors such as smoking or hypertension, the anesthetic management of patients who have already developed cerebrovascular disorders, including advanced carotid disease, is a common challenge for the specialty.

Cerebrovascular Anatomy

Blood supply to the brain (20% of cardiac output) is brought through the neck via two pairs of blood vessels: the internal carotid arteries and the vertebral arteries, which join into the basilar artery (Fig. 12.8). These vessels join in the circle of Willis to form major intracranial blood vessels (anterior cerebral arteries, middle cerebral arteries, posterior cerebral arteries). Occlusion of a specific major intracranial artery results in a constellation of predictable clinical neurologic deficits.

The major branches of the vertebral arteries are the arteries to the spinal cord and the posteroinferior cerebellar arteries that supply the inferior cerebellum and lateral medulla. The two vertebral arteries then unite to form the basilar artery. Occlusion of the vertebral arteries or basilar artery results in signs and symptoms that depend on the level of the infarction. The basilar artery terminates by dividing into two posterior cerebral arteries that supply the medial temporal lobe, occipital lobe, and parts of the thalamus.

Diagnostic Tests

Conventional angiography can demonstrate acute vascular occlusion from a thrombus or embolus lodged in the vascular tree. The vasculature can also be visualized noninvasively by CT angiography and magnetic resonance angiography. In addition to identifying ischemic stroke, these modalities can also identify aneurysms or arteriovenous malformations that may be precipitants for hemorrhagic stroke. Transcranial Doppler ultrasonography can provide indirect evidence of major vascular occlusion and offers the advantage of real-time bedside monitoring in patients undergoing thrombolytic therapy.

In the evaluation of ischemic stroke or TIA, auscultation of the carotid arteries may identify a bruit. Carotid ultrasonography can quantify carotid stenosis and may rarely identify a dissection. Carotid stenosis most commonly occurs at the bifurcation of the internal and external carotid arteries because of the tendency for turbulent flow at this branch point. Even in the presence of known carotid stenosis, workup of an intracranial embolic event includes evaluation for cardiac sources of emboli such as intraluminal thrombi (secondary to heart failure or atrial fibrillation), valvular vegetations, or paradoxical emboli in the setting of a patent foramen ovale.

Treatment of Stroke

The US Food and Drug Administration (FDA) has approved intravenous administration of recombinant *tissue plasminogen activator* (tPA) within 3 hours of stroke onset, once the diagnosis of ischemic stroke is established and in the absence of contraindications. The American Heart Association has subsequently expanded that recommended window to 4.5 hours. In qualifying patients the number needed to treat with recombinant tPA for one additional favorable outcome is approximately 10. Some stroke centers with access to interventional neuroradiology may offer intraarterial thrombolysis or endovascular clot removal, particularly in cases of persistent thrombus. Recent clinical trials have brought about a paradigm shift in managing strokes secondary to large vessel occlusion with *endovascular evacuation* of clot, showing benefit up to 8.5 hours after the initial event. Advances made with these suction systems have improved recanalization with acceptable rates of symptomatic intracerebral hemorrhage.

Regardless of thrombolytic efforts, the importance of evaluating for and avoiding hypoxia is paramount, as are the control of glycemic derangements, hyperthermia, hypotension, severe hypertension, and unstable dysrhythmias. Specific hemodynamic goals for patients with acute stroke undergoing thrombolysis or neuroradiologic procedures depend on a variety of patient-specific factors, but the overarching need to preserve or restore perfusion of at-risk brain tissue is universal. Outside the acute setting, medical management of strokes in general overlaps with the medical management of carotid stenosis discussed in the next section.

Carotid Endarterectomy

Surgical treatment of symptomatic carotid artery stenosis greatly decreases the risk of stroke compared with medical management in men with severe carotid stenosis (70%–99% luminal stenosis) and modestly reduces stroke risk in those with 50%–69% luminal narrowing. Strokes and TIAs caused by carotid stenosis occur as a result of atheroembolic phenomena or hemodynamically significant pressure drops across the stenosis in the absence of sufficient collateral cerebral blood flow.

The advisability of surgical treatment for asymptomatic carotid disease varies based on the expected periprocedural risk and associated patient comorbid conditions. The absolute risk reduction in stroke is small (≈1% per year for the first few years) but is higher with longer-term follow-up. A suggested guideline has been to recommend surgery for asymptomatic carotid disease only for patients and at centers for which the expected periprocedural complication rates are 3% or less. In patients foregoing surgical treatment, optimal medical therapy includes smoking cessation, antiplatelet therapy, aggressive blood pressure control, physical activity, and both dietary and pharmacologic lipid-lowering strategies. Hypoglycemic medications for diabetic patients, as well as ACE inhibitors, are beneficial.

Preoperative Evaluation

In addition to undergoing a neurologic evaluation, patients scheduled for carotid endarterectomy should be examined for significant comorbid conditions, particularly cardiovascular disease. Perioperative MI is a major cause of morbidity and mortality following carotid endarterectomy, and predisposing coronary artery disease is highly prevalent among patients with cerebrovascular occlusive disease. The reported incidence of perioperative MI in this population depends on the threshold and method of surveillance but was 2.3% among symptomatic patients who underwent endarterectomy in the Carotid Revascularization Endarterectomy versus Stenting Trial (CREST). Currently a follow-up trial, CREST-2, is underway to compare the outcomes in patients with asymptomatic carotid stenosis.

Chronic essential hypertension is a common finding in patients with cerebrovascular disease. It is useful to establish the usual range of blood pressure for each patient preoperatively to provide a guide for acceptable perfusion pressures during anesthesia and surgery. Intraoperative stability of chronically elevated blood pressure may be critical for maintenance of collateral blood flow through the stenotic cranial vasculature, especially during cross-clamping of the carotid artery. The effect of a change in head position on cerebral function should also be ascertained. Extreme head rotation, flexion, or extension in patients with co-existing vertebral or carotid artery disease could lead to angulation or compression of the artery. Recognition of this response preoperatively allows hazardous head positions to be avoided while patients are anesthetized.

Patients with known severe coronary artery disease and severe carotid occlusive disease present a clinical dilemma. A staged surgical approach in which carotid endarterectomy is performed first could result in significant morbidity or mortality from cardiac causes. On the other hand, performing coronary revascularization first is associated with a high incidence of stroke. Insufficient evidence exists to make general guidelines, and the timing of surgical procedures should instead be individualized based on the severity and symptomatic profile of each patient.

Management of Anesthesia

Anesthetic management for carotid endarterectomy mandates careful control of heart rate, blood pressure, pain, and stress responses so organ perfusion is maintained in patients with a high preoperative risk of cardiac and cerebral ischemic events. At the conclusion of surgery, the goal should be to awaken the patient sufficiently for a neurologic examination.

Carotid endarterectomy can be performed under regional or general anesthesia. Regional anesthesia via cervical plexus blockade allows a patient to remain awake to facilitate neurologic assessment during carotid artery cross-clamping. During establishment of the block, care should be taken to avoid vascular puncture that would obscure the surgical field or could dislodge microemboli.

Appropriate sedation during surgical preparation and draping allows many otherwise anxious patients to tolerate the procedure quite well when a regional anesthetic technique under regional blockade is used. If general anesthesia is selected, the focus should be on maintenance of hemodynamic stability and prompt emergence to allow immediate assessment of neurologic status in the operating room.

Appropriate blood pressure management is important during carotid endarterectomy and is made more crucial because of the abnormal cerebral autoregulation present in many of these patients. Elevated blood pressure during cross-clamping may facilitate collateral blood flow but after surgery may predispose to hematoma formation. Vasopressors or vasodilators are often needed to maintain an appropriate perfusion pressure during the various stages of the procedure. Surgical manipulation of the carotid sinus may cause marked alterations in heart rate and blood pressure. Carotid sinus infiltration with local anesthetic for controlling blood pressure lability has been anecdotal and yet to be proven effective.

It is generally accepted that changes in regional cerebral blood flow associated with changes in $Paco_2$ are unpredictable in these patients. Therefore maintenance of normocarbia is generally recommended.

Monitoring usually includes placement of an intraarterial catheter. As with any major vascular surgery, patients with poor left ventricular function and/or severe coronary artery disease might require a central venous or pulmonary artery catheter or TEE, but this is rarely necessary. The hemodynamic goals for cerebral and coronary perfusion are similar, and achievement of these goals will benefit both organ systems. If central venous cannulation is pursued, particular care must be taken during contralateral jugular venous access attempts to prevent inadvertent arterial or venous puncture, which could cause a hematoma that compromises collateral blood flow during carotid cross-clamping.

When carotid endarterectomy is performed under general anesthesia, monitoring for cerebral ischemia, hypoperfusion, and cerebral emboli should be strongly considered. The principal reason to monitor cerebral function in these patients is to identify patients who would benefit from use of a carotid artery shunt during carotid cross-clamping; another is to guide hemodynamic management in patients who require increased cerebral perfusion pressure. The standard EEG is a sensitive indicator of inadequate cerebral perfusion during carotid cross-clamping. Perioperative neurologic complications correlate with intraoperative EEG changes indicating cerebral ischemia. However, the utility of EEG monitoring during carotid endarterectomy is limited by several factors: (1) EEG may not detect subcortical or small cortical infarcts, (2) false-negative results are not uncommon (patients with previous strokes or TIAs have a high incidence of false-negative test results), and (3) the EEG can be affected not only by cerebral ischemia but also by changes in temperature, blood pressure, and depth of anesthesia. SEP monitoring can detect specific changes produced by decreased regional cerebral blood flow, but it can be difficult to determine whether these changes are due to anesthesia, hypothermia, changes in blood pressure, or cerebral ischemia. Stump pressure (internal carotid artery back pressure) is a poor indicator of the adequacy of cerebral perfusion. Transcranial Doppler ultrasonography allows continuous monitoring of blood flow velocity and the occurrence of microembolic events. It can be used to determine the need for shunt placement, to recognize shunt malfunction, and to manage postoperative hyperperfusion.

In situations in which general anesthesia is chosen and cerebral perfusion monitoring is unavailable, an alternative approach is to insert shunts in all patients, but placement of the shunt can itself predispose to an increased embolic load. Overall, awake neurologic assessment is the simplest, most cost-effective, and most reliable method of cerebral function monitoring during carotid endarterectomy.

Postoperative Management and Complications

In the period immediately after carotid endarterectomy, patients must be observed for cardiac, airway, and neurologic complications. These include hypertension or hypotension, myocardial ischemia or infarction, development of significant soft tissue edema or a hematoma in the neck, and the onset of neurologic signs and symptoms that signal a new stroke or acute thrombosis at the endarterectomy site.

Hypertension is frequently observed during the immediate postoperative period, often in patients with co-existing essential hypertension. The increase in blood pressure often peaks at 2–3 hours after surgery and may persist for 24 hours. Hypertension should be treated to avoid the hazards of cerebral edema, myocardial ischemia, and hematoma formation. The incidence of new neurologic deficits is increased threefold in patients who are hypertensive postoperatively. Continuous infusion of short-acting drugs such as nitroprusside, nitroglycerin, or clevidipine and the use of longer-acting drugs such as hydralazine or labetalol are options for blood pressure control. The mechanism of this postoperative hypertension may be related to altered activity of the carotid sinus or loss of carotid sinus function resulting from denervation during surgery.

Hypotension is also commonly observed during the period immediately after surgery. This hypotension can be explained based on carotid sinus hypersensitivity. The carotid sinus, previously shielded by atheromatous plaque, is now able to perceive blood pressure oscillations more clearly and goes through a period of hyperresponsiveness to these stimuli. Hypotension resulting from carotid sinus hypersensitivity is usually treated with vasopressors such as phenylephrine. It typically resolves within 12–24 hours.

Nerve dysfunction is possible after carotid endarterectomy, but most injuries are transient. Patients should be examined for evidence of hypoglossal, recurrent laryngeal, or superior laryngeal nerve injury. Such injury may produce difficulty swallowing or protecting the airway and could result in aspiration.

Carotid body denervation can also occur after carotid artery surgery and impair cardiac and ventilatory responses to hypoxemia. This can be clinically significant after bilateral carotid endarterectomy or with administration of narcotics.

Endovascular Treatment of Carotid Disease

The technique of carotid artery stenting continues to evolve as an alternative to carotid endarterectomy. The major complication of carotid stenting is stroke as a result of microembolization of atherosclerotic material into the cerebral circulation during the procedure. Embolic protection devices for use during carotid stenting have been developed, but the technology has so far failed to reduce endovascular stroke risk to that seen with the surgical approach. Nevertheless, endovascular approaches carry a lower risk of MI, and if embolic protection devices are improved, stenting may one day reemerge as a more widespread alternative to surgery.

TABLE 12.3	Peripheral Vascular Diseases

Chronic peripheral arterial occlusive disease (atherosclerosis)
    Distal abdominal aorta or iliac arteries
    Femoral arteries
    Subclavian steal syndrome
    Coronary-subclavian steal syndrome
Acute peripheral arterial occlusive disease (embolism)
Systemic vasculitis
    Takayasu arteritis
    Thromboangiitis obliterans
    Wegener granulomatosis
    Temporal arteritis
    Polyarteritis nodosa
Other vascular syndromes
    Raynaud phenomenon
    Kawasaki disease

Data comparing surgical and endovascular approaches comes from several studies. The CREST results demonstrated an increased risk of stroke and decreased risk of MI in endovascular treatment compared with endarterectomy, but the investigators also found that periprocedural stroke was more devastating to quality of life than MI. The Stent-Supported Percutaneous Angioplasty of the Carotid Artery Versus Endarterectomy (SPACE) trial also showed increased rates of ischemic stroke or death within 30 days after an endovascular repair compared with a surgical procedure. As a result of this evidence, surgical endarterectomy for symptomatic carotid stenosis remains the recommended treatment for most patients.

PERIPHERAL ARTERIAL DISEASE

Peripheral arterial disease results in compromised blood flow to the extremities. Chronic impairment of blood flow to the extremities is most often due to atherosclerosis, whereas arterial embolism is most likely to be responsible for acute arterial occlusion (Table 12.3). Vasculitis may also be responsible for compromised peripheral blood flow.

Chronic Arterial Insufficiency

The most widely accepted definition of *peripheral arterial insufficiency* is an ankle-brachial index (ABI) less than 0.9. The ABI is calculated as the ratio of the systolic blood pressure at the ankle to the systolic blood pressure in the brachial artery. An ABI below 0.9 correlates extremely well with angiogram-positive disease.

The characteristics of peripheral atherosclerosis resemble those of atherosclerosis seen in the aorta, coronary arteries, and extracranial cerebral arteries. The prevalence of peripheral atherosclerosis increases with age, exceeding 70% in individuals older than age 75. Peripheral arterial disease has been estimated to reduce quality of life in approximately 2 million symptomatic Americans, and millions more without claudication are likely to experience peripheral arterial

disease–associated impairment. Among patients who have claudication, 80% have femoropopliteal stenosis, 40% have tibioperoneal stenosis, and 30% have lesions in the aorta or iliac arteries.

Atherosclerosis is a systemic disease. Consequently, patients with peripheral arterial disease have a three to five times overall greater risk of cardiovascular ischemic events such as MI, ischemic stroke, and death than do those without this disease. Critical limb ischemia is associated with very high intermediate-term morbidity and mortality, due mostly to a high incidence of cardiovascular events in these patients. Associated cardiovascular ischemic events are much more frequent than actual ischemic limb events.

Risk Factors

Risk factors associated with development of peripheral atherosclerosis are similar to those related to ischemic heart disease: older age, family history, smoking, diabetes mellitus, hypertension, obesity, and dyslipidemia. The risk of significant peripheral arterial disease and claudication is doubled in smokers compared with nonsmokers, and continued cigarette smoking increases the risk of progression from stable claudication to severe limb ischemia and amputation.

Signs and Symptoms

Intermittent claudication and rest pain are the principal symptoms of peripheral arterial disease. Intermittent claudication occurs when the metabolic requirements of exercising skeletal muscles exceed oxygen delivery. Rest pain occurs when the arterial blood supply does not meet even the minimal nutritional requirements of the affected extremity. Even minor trauma to an ischemic foot may produce a nonhealing skin lesion.

Decreased or absent arterial pulses are the most reliable physical findings associated with peripheral arterial disease. Bruits auscultated in the abdomen, pelvis, or inguinal area and decreased femoral, popliteal, posterior tibial, or dorsalis pedis pulses may indicate the anatomic site of arterial stenosis. Less commonly, reduced lower extremity pulses may be the presenting sign of undiagnosed aortic coarctation. Signs of chronic leg ischemia include subcutaneous atrophy, hair loss, coolness, pallor, cyanosis, and dependent redness. Patients may report relief with hanging the affected extremity over the edge of the bed, a move that increases hydrostatic pressure in the arterioles of the affected limb.

Diagnosis

Doppler ultrasonography and the resulting pulse volume waveform are used to identify arterial vessels with stenotic lesions. In the presence of severe ischemia, the arterial waveform may be entirely absent. The ABI is a quantitative means of assessing the presence and severity of peripheral arterial stenosis. Duplex ultrasonography can identify areas of plaque formation and calcification as well as blood flow abnormalities caused by arterial stenoses. Transcutaneous oximetry can be used to assess the severity of skin ischemia in patients with peripheral arterial disease. Results of noninvasive tests and clinical evaluation are usually sufficient for the diagnosis of peripheral arterial disease. MRI and contrast angiography are used to guide endovascular intervention or surgical bypass.

Treatment

Medical therapy for peripheral arterial disease includes exercise programs and treatment or modification of risk factors for atherosclerosis. Supervised exercise training programs can improve the walking capacity of patients with peripheral arterial disease even though no change in ABI can be demonstrated. Patients who stop smoking have a more favorable prognosis than those who continue to smoke. Aggressive lipid-lowering therapy slows the progression of peripheral atherosclerosis, and treatment of diabetes mellitus can slow microvascular disease progression.

Treatment of hypertension results in a reduction in stroke and cardiovascular morbidity. Although β-adrenergic antagonists are a mainstay for patients who have experienced MI, their use solely as an antihypertensive agent has fallen out of favor. In sum, patients with severe arterial insufficiency benefit from effective blood pressure control because cardiovascular and stroke risk are reduced, but the presence of peripheral arterial insufficiency does not in itself govern the choice of an antihypertensive agent.

Revascularization procedures are indicated in patients with disabling claudication, ischemic rest pain, or impending limb loss. The prognosis of the limb is determined by the extent of arterial disease, the severity of limb ischemia, and the feasibility and rapidity of restoring arterial circulation. In patients with chronic arterial occlusive disease and continuous progression of symptoms (i.e., development of new wounds, rest pain, or gangrene) the prognosis is very poor unless revascularization can be accomplished. In patients who experience acute occlusive events resulting from arterial embolism in an extremity with little underlying arterial disease, the long-term prognosis of the limb is related to the rapidity and completeness of revascularization before the onset of irreversible ischemic tissue or nerve damage.

Revascularization can be achieved by endovascular interventions or surgical reconstruction. Percutaneous transluminal angioplasty of iliac arteries has a high initial success rate that is further improved by selective stent placement. Femoral and popliteal artery percutaneous transluminal angioplasty has lower success rates than iliac artery percutaneous transluminal angioplasty; however, stent placement has improved superficial femoral artery patency substantially.

Despite improvement in long-term outcome after percutaneous transluminal angioplasty and stenting of peripheral vessels, restenosis remains a significant problem, particularly in long lesions, small-diameter vessels, and recurrently stenotic lesions. Current therapies focus on the use of mechanical devices, stents, stent grafts, vascular irradiation, and drugs, although none of these approaches has yet become a definitive treatment.

The operative procedures used for vascular reconstruction depend on the location and severity of the peripheral arterial stenosis. Aortobifemoral bypass is a surgical procedure used to treat aortoiliac disease. Intraabdominal aortoiliac reconstructive surgery may not be feasible in patients with severe comorbid conditions. However, in these patients, axillobifemoral bypass can circumvent the abdominal aorta and achieve revascularization of both legs. Femorofemoral bypass can be performed in patients with unilateral iliac artery obstruction. Infrainguinal bypass procedures using saphenous vein grafts or synthetic grafts include femoropopliteal and tibioperoneal reconstruction. Amputation is frequently necessary for patients with advanced limb ischemia in whom revascularization is not possible or has failed. Lumbar sympathectomy is occasionally used to treat critical limb ischemia in cases of persistent vasospasm.

Management of Anesthesia

Management of anesthesia for surgical revascularization of the lower extremities incorporates principles similar to those described earlier for management of patients undergoing abdominal aortic aneurysm repair. For example, the principal risk during reconstructive peripheral vascular surgery is myocardial ischemia. The increased incidence of perioperative MI and cardiac death in patients with peripheral arterial disease is due to the high prevalence of coronary artery disease in this patient population. Mortality following revascularization surgery is usually a result of MI in patients with preoperative evidence of ischemic heart disease.

Because patients with claudication are usually unable to perform an exercise stress test, pharmacologic stress testing with or without echocardiography or nuclear imaging is helpful to determine the presence and severity of ischemic heart disease preoperatively in patients with multiple cardiac risk factors. Depending on the severity of coronary artery disease and claudication, treatment of the ischemic heart disease by percutaneous coronary intervention or coronary artery bypass grafting may be considered before revascularization surgery is performed. In American College of Cardiology/American Heart Association (ACC/AHA) guidelines, unstable angina is considered an active cardiac condition requiring treatment or optimization before nonemergent surgery. However, in patients with anatomically significant but stable coronary artery disease, vascular surgery can proceed, and mortality and morbidity outcomes are similar to those in patients who undergo coronary artery revascularization before elective vascular surgery.

Perioperative heart rate control (usually with carefully titrated β-blockers) in vascular surgery patients at high risk reduces the incidence of myocardial ischemia. The ACC/AHA guidelines on perioperative β-blocker therapy recommend β-blockade for patients at intermediate and high risk who are undergoing vascular surgery. For patients with low cardiac risk who are undergoing vascular surgery, β-blockers may still be considered. Both acute withdrawal of β-blockers and initiation of high-dose β-blocker therapy on the day of surgery are associated with increased mortality. Perioperative initiation of statins is also reasonable in patients undergoing vascular surgery.

The choice of anesthetic technique must be individualized for each patient. Regional anesthesia and general anesthesia each offer specific advantages and disadvantages. Patient preference for general anesthesia, patient factors such as obesity or previous spine surgery, and use of antiplatelet or anticoagulant drugs may increase the risks associated with use of a regional technique. Regional anesthesia may also be poorly tolerated in patients with severe dementia but may reduce the risk of postoperative delirium compared with general anesthesia. Epidural or spinal anesthesia offers the advantages of increased graft blood flow, postoperative analgesia, less activation of the coagulation system, and fewer postoperative respiratory complications. Intraoperative heparinization is not in itself a contraindication to epidural anesthesia, but risk of bleeding may increase when the patient is also taking other anticoagulants or antiplatelet agents. If epidural catheter placement is attempted, it should occur at least 1 hour before intraoperative heparinization. In addition, before placement of the catheter is attempted, the surgical team should be consulted regarding the possible need to delay the procedure in the event of a bloody tap.

General anesthesia may be necessary when procedures are expected to require long operative hours or when vein harvesting from the upper extremities is needed. There is no strong evidence to suggest an advantage of one particular type of general anesthetic agent over another. The possible benefits of using inhalation anesthetics in patients with high cardiac risk resulting from the cardiac preconditioning effects of these agents are the subject of ongoing investigations.

During aortoiliac or aortofemoral surgery, infrarenal aortic cross-clamping is associated with fewer hemodynamic derangements than higher aortic cross-clamping. Likewise the hemodynamic changes associated with unclamping the abdominal aorta are less with infrarenal aortic cross-clamping. Because of the comparatively benign effects of infrarenal

clamping, many practitioners place a central venous pressure catheter in lieu of a pulmonary artery catheter in these patients, especially in the absence of symptomatic left ventricular dysfunction. Monitoring of left ventricular function and intravascular volume may also be facilitated by the use of TEE.

Heparin is commonly administered before application of a vascular cross-clamp to decrease the risk of thromboembolic complications. However, distal embolization may still occur to any downstream vascular bed, including to the bowel or kidneys. Administration of heparin does not obviate the importance of surgical care when manipulating and clamping an atherosclerotic artery to minimize the likelihood of distal embolization. Spinal cord damage associated with surgical revascularization of the legs is extremely unlikely, and special monitoring for this complication is not generally pursued.

Postoperative Management
Postoperative management includes provision of analgesia, treatment of fluid and electrolyte derangements, and maintenance of oxygenation, ventilation, heart rate, and blood pressure to reduce the incidence of myocardial ischemia or infarction. As with the choice of intraoperative anesthetics, there is no strong evidence to recommend a particular postoperative medication regimen so long as the goal of patient stability and comfort is achieved.

Subclavian Steal Syndrome

Occlusion of the subclavian or innominate artery proximal to the origin of the vertebral artery may result in reversal of flow through the ipsilateral vertebral artery into the distal subclavian artery (Fig. 12.9). This reversal of flow diverts blood from the brain to supply the arm (subclavian steal syndrome). Symptoms of central nervous system ischemia (syncope, vertigo, ataxia, hemiplegia) and/or arm ischemia are usually present. Extreme neck movements or exercise of the ipsilateral arm may accentuate these hemodynamic changes and cause neurologic symptoms. There is often an absent or diminished

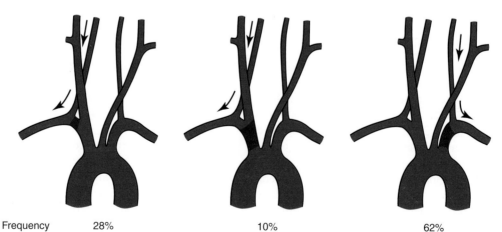

| Frequency | 28% | 10% | 62% |

FIG. 12.9   Comparison of the frequency of occurrence of left, right, and bilateral subclavian steal syndrome. (Adapted from Heidrich H, Bayer O. Symptomatology of the subclavian steal syndrome. *Angiology.* 1969;20:406-413.)

pulse in the ipsilateral arm, and systolic blood pressure is often found to be 20 mm Hg lower in that arm. A bruit may be heard over the subclavian artery. Stenosis of the left subclavian artery is responsible for this syndrome in most patients. Subclavian endarterectomy may be curative.

Coronary-Subclavian Steal Syndrome

A rare complication of using the left internal mammary artery for coronary revascularization is coronary-subclavian steal syndrome. This syndrome occurs when proximal stenosis in the left subclavian artery produces reversal of blood flow through the patent internal mammary artery graft (Fig. 12.10). This steal syndrome is characterized by angina pectoris and a 20-mm Hg or more decrease in systolic blood pressure in the ipsilateral arm. Angina pectoris associated with coronary-subclavian steal syndrome requires surgical bypass grafting.

Acute Arterial Occlusion

Acute arterial occlusion differs from the gradual development of arterial occlusion caused by atherosclerosis and is frequently the result of cardiogenic embolism. Systemic emboli may arise from a left atrial thrombus in the setting of atrial fibrillation or less commonly from an atrial myxoma. Left ventricular thrombi may develop after MI or in the setting of dilated cardiomyopathy. Other cardiac causes of systemic

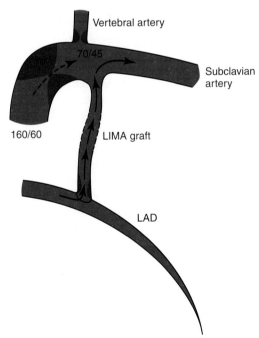

FIG. 12.10 Coronary-subclavian steal syndrome. Development of subtotal stenosis of the left subclavian artery may produce reversal of flow through a patent internal mammary graft (LIMA), which thereby diverts flow destined for the left anterior descending (LAD) coronary artery. (Adapted from Martin JL, Rock P. Coronary-subclavian steal syndrome: anesthetic implications and management in the perioperative period. *Anesthesiology.* 1988;68:933-936.)

emboli are valvular heart disease, prosthetic heart valves, infective endocarditis, and paradoxical emboli from a patent foramen ovale. Noncardiac causes of acute arterial occlusion include atheroemboli from an upstream artery, plaque rupture, and hypercoagulability derangements. Aortic dissection and trauma can acutely occlude an artery by disrupting the integrity of the vessel lumen.

Signs and Symptoms
Acute arterial occlusion in an extremity presents with signs of limb ischemia: intense pain, paresthesias, and motor weakness distal to the site of arterial occlusion. Loss of a palpable peripheral pulse, cool skin, and sharply demarcated skin color changes (pallor or cyanosis) occur distal to the arterial occlusion. Large embolic fragments often lodge at an arterial bifurcation (e.g., aortic or femoral artery bifurcations).

Diagnosis
Noninvasive tests can provide additional evidence of peripheral arterial occlusion and reveal the severity of the ischemia, but such testing should not delay definitive treatment. Arteriography may be used to define the site of acute arterial occlusion and the appropriateness of revascularization surgery.

Treatment
Surgical embolectomy is used to treat acute systemic embolism, typically thromboembolism, to a large peripheral artery. Embolectomy is rarely feasible for atheromatous embolism, because the atheromatous material usually fragments into very small pieces. However, if the primary source of atheroembolism is identified and amenable to surgical exposure, it may be resectable. Once the diagnosis of acute arterial embolism is confirmed, anticoagulation with heparin is initiated to prevent propagation of the thrombus. Intraarterial thrombolysis with urokinase or recombinant tPA may restore vascular patency in acutely occluded arteries and synthetic bypass grafts. The clinical outcome is highly dependent on the rapidity of revascularization. Amputation may be necessary in some patients.

Management of Anesthesia
Management of anesthesia in patients undergoing surgical treatment of acute arterial occlusion resulting from a systemic embolism is similar to that in patients with chronic peripheral arterial disease.

Raynaud Phenomenon

Raynaud phenomenon is episodic vasospastic ischemia of the digits. It affects women more often than men and is characterized by digital blanching or cyanosis in association with cold exposure or sympathetic activation. Vasodilation with hyperemia is often seen after rewarming and reestablishment of blood flow. The disorder is categorized as either primary (also called *Raynaud disease*) (Table 12.4) or secondary when it is associated with other diseases.

TABLE 12.4	Secondary Causes of Raynaud Phenomenon

CONNECTIVE TISSUE DISEASES
Scleroderma
Systemic lupus erythematosus
Rheumatoid arthritis
Dermatomyositis

PERIPHERAL ARTERIAL OCCLUSIVE DISEASE
Atherosclerosis
Thromboangiitis obliterans
Thromboembolism
Thoracic outlet syndrome

NEUROLOGIC SYNDROMES
Carpal tunnel syndrome
Reflex sympathetic dystrophy
Cerebrovascular accident
Intervertebral disk herniation

TRAUMA
Cold thermal injury (frostbite)
Percussive injury (vibrating tools)

DRUGS
β-Adrenergic antagonists
Tricyclic antidepressants
Antimetabolites
Ergot alkaloids
Amphetamines

TABLE 12.5	Factors Predisposing to Thromboembolism

Venous stasis
  Recent surgery
  Trauma
  Lack of ambulation
  Pregnancy
  Low cardiac output (congestive heart failure, myocardial infarction)
  Stroke
Abnormality of venous wall
  Varicose veins
  Drug-induced irritation
Hypercoagulable state
  Surgery
  Estrogen therapy (oral contraceptives)
  Cancer
  Deficiencies of endogenous anticoagulants (antithrombin III, protein C, protein S)
  Stress response associated with surgery
  Inflammatory bowel disease
History of previous thromboembolism
Morbid obesity
Advanced age

Diagnosis

The primary diagnosis of Raynaud phenomenon is based on history and physical examination findings. When the clinical diagnosis is made, it may lead to workup for associated inflammatory diseases.

Raynaud phenomenon sometimes appears as part of the constellation of symptoms seen with the scleroderma subtype known as *CREST syndrome. CREST* is an acronym for subcutaneous *c*alcinosis, *R*aynaud phenomenon, *e*sophageal dysmotility, *s*clerodactyly (scleroderma limited to the fingers), and *t*elangiectasia.

Treatment

Primary and secondary Raynaud phenomena are usually managed conservatively by protecting the hands and feet from exposure to cold. Pharmacologic intervention including calcium channel blockade or α-blockade may be helpful in some patients. In rare instances, surgical sympathectomy is considered for treatment of persistent severe digital ischemia.

Management of Anesthesia

There are no specific recommendations as to the choice of drugs to produce general anesthesia in patients with Raynaud phenomenon. Increasing the ambient temperature of the operating room and maintaining normothermia are basic considerations. Noninvasive blood pressure measurement

techniques may be strongly considered to avoid any arterial compromise of potentially affected extremities.

Regional anesthesia is acceptable for peripheral operations in patients with Raynaud phenomenon, but to avoid undesirable vasoconstriction, it may be prudent not to include epinephrine in the local anesthetic solution.

PERIPHERAL VENOUS DISEASE

Common peripheral venous diseases encountered in patients undergoing surgery include superficial thrombophlebitis, deep vein thrombosis (DVT), and chronic venous insufficiency. The most important associated complication of DVT is pulmonary embolism, a leading cause of perioperative morbidity and mortality.

The major factors predisposing to venous thrombosis, classically referred to as *Virchow's triad,* are routinely encountered in the perioperative period: (1) venous stasis (due to immobility), (2) hypercoagulability (due to inflammation and acute surgical stress), and (3) disruption of vascular endothelium (due to perioperative trauma). Table 12.5 expands on Virchow's triad to include more recently appreciated risk factors such as the use of oral contraceptives.

Superficial Thrombophlebitis and Deep Vein Thrombosis

Thrombosis of deep or superficial peripheral veins is particularly common among surgical patients, occurring in approximately 50% of patients undergoing total hip replacement. Most of these thromboses are subclinical and resolve completely when mobility is restored. Although deep and superficial venous thromboses may co-exist, isolated deep thrombosis

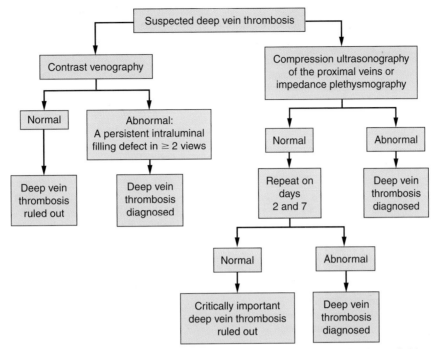

FIG. 12.11 Steps in the diagnosis of deep vein thrombosis. (Adapted from Ginsberg JS. Management of venous thromboembolism. *N Engl J Med.* 1996;335:1816-1828. Copyright 1996 Massachusetts Medical Society.)

may be distinguished from superficial venous thrombosis based on history, physical examination findings, and results of confirmatory ultrasonography.

Superficial venous thrombosis of a saphenous vein or its tributary often occurs in association with intravenous therapy, varicose veins, or systemic vasculitis and causes localized pain and superficial inflammation along the path of the involved vein. Superficial thrombophlebitis is rarely associated with pulmonary embolism. The intense inflammation that accompanies superficial thrombophlebitis rapidly leads to total venous occlusion. Typically the vein can be palpated as a cordlike structure surrounded by an area of erythema, warmth, and edema.

DVT is more often associated with generalized pain of the affected extremity, tenderness, and unilateral limb swelling, but diagnosis based on clinical signs alone is unreliable. Doppler ultrasonography with vein compression is highly sensitive for detecting proximal vein thrombosis (popliteal or femoral vein) but less sensitive for detecting calf vein thrombosis (Fig. 12.11). Venography and impedance plethysmography are also potential diagnostic modalities.

Most postoperative venous thrombi arise in the lower legs, often in the low-flow soleal sinuses and in large veins draining the gastrocnemius muscle. However, in approximately 20% of patients, thrombi originate in more proximal veins.

Prevention of Venous Thromboembolism
Clinical Risk Factors
Assessment of clinical risk factors identifies patients who can benefit from prophylactic measures aimed at reducing the risk of DVT development (Table 12.6). Patients at low risk require only minimal prophylactic measures such as early postoperative ambulation and the use of compression stockings, which augment propulsion of blood from the ankles to the knees. The risk of DVT may be much higher in patients older than age 40 who are undergoing operations lasting longer than 1 hour, especially orthopedic surgery on the lower extremities, pelvic or abdominal surgery, and surgery that requires a prolonged convalescence period with bed rest or limited mobility. The presence of cancer also increases the risk of thrombotic complications.

Subcutaneous heparin in doses of 5000 units administered twice or three times daily reduces DVT risk, as does the use of intermittent external pneumatic compression devices (see Table 12.6).

Regional Anesthesia
The incidence of postoperative DVT and pulmonary embolism in patients undergoing total knee or total hip replacement can be substantially decreased (20%–40%) by using epidural or spinal anesthesia techniques instead of general anesthesia. Postoperative epidural analgesia does not augment this benefit but may allow earlier ambulation, which can reduce the risk of DVT.

Presumably the beneficial effects of regional anesthesia compared with general anesthesia are due to (1) vasodilation, which maximizes venous blood flow, and (2) the ability to provide excellent postoperative analgesia and early ambulation.

Treatment of Deep Vein Thrombosis
Anticoagulation is the first-line treatment for all patients with a diagnosis of DVT. Therapy is initiated with heparin

TABLE 12.6   Risk and Predisposing Factors for Development of Deep Vein Thrombosis After Surgery or Trauma

Associated Conditions	Low Risk	Moderate Risk	High Risk
General surgery	Younger than age 40 Operation < 60 min	Older than age 40 Operation > 60 min	Older than age 40 Operation > 60 min Previous deep vein thrombosis Previous pulmonary embolism Extensive trauma Major fractures
Orthopedic surgery Trauma			Knee or hip replacement Extensive soft tissue injury Major fractures Multiple trauma sites
Medical conditions	Pregnancy	Postpartum period Myocardial infarction Congestive heart failure	Stroke
Incidence of deep vein thrombosis without prophylaxis	2%	10%–40%	40%–80%
Incidence of symptomatic pulmonary embolism	0.2%	1%–8%	5%–10%
Incidence of fatal pulmonary embolism	0.002%	0.1%–0.4%	1%–5%
Recommended steps to minimize deep vein thrombosis	Graduated compression stockings Early ambulation	External pneumatic compression Subcutaneous heparin Intravenous dextran	External pneumatic compression Subcutaneous heparin Intravenous dextran or vena cava filter Warfarin

Adapted from Weinmann EE, Salzman EW. Deep-vein thrombosis. *N Engl J Med*. 1994;331:1630-1642.

(unfractionated or low-molecular-weight heparin [LMWH]) because this drug produces an immediate anticoagulant effect. Heparin has a narrow therapeutic window, and the response of individual patients can vary considerably. Advantages of LMWH over unfractionated heparin include a longer half-life, a more predictable dose response without the need for serial assessment of activated partial thromboplastin time, and a lower risk of bleeding complications. Disadvantages include increased cost and lack of availability of a rapid reversal agent.

Therapy with warfarin, an oral vitamin K antagonist, is initiated during heparin treatment and adjusted to achieve a prothrombin time yielding an international normalized ratio (INR) between 2 and 3. Heparin is discontinued when warfarin has achieved its therapeutic effect. Oral anticoagulants may be continued for 3–6 months or longer. Inferior vena cava filters may be inserted into patients who experience recurrent pulmonary embolism despite adequate anticoagulant therapy or in whom anticoagulation is contraindicated.

Thrombophilia workup should be considered for patients with DVT. Laboratory abnormalities associated with initial and recurrent venous thrombosis or embolism include the presence of factor V Leiden and congenital deficiencies of antithrombin III, protein C, protein S, or plasminogen. Congenital resistance to activated protein C and increased levels of antiphospholipid antibodies are also associated with venous thromboembolism. A family history of unexplained venous thrombosis is often present.

Complications of Anticoagulation

The most obvious complication of anticoagulant therapy is bleeding. Frequent monitoring of activated partial thromboplastin time in patients receiving intravenous heparin is necessary owing to the variability in dose response. Similarly, patients receiving warfarin must be monitored closely with frequent prothrombin times and INR. Life-threatening bleeding in patients receiving warfarin might require rapid correction with vitamin K, fresh frozen plasma infusions, and factor concentrates.

A frequently encountered complication of unfractionated heparin administration is heparin-induced thrombocytopenia (HIT). HIT is classically divided into two types. HIT type 1 is a benign thrombocytopenia seen soon after initiation of heparin therapy (within the first few days) that resolves spontaneously and does not preclude continued treatment with heparin. In HIT type 1, thrombocytopenia is mild, generally staying above 100,000 platelets/mm^3. In contrast, HIT type 2 is an immune-mediated phenomenon occurring in 1%–3% of patients receiving unfractionated heparin. HIT type 2 is caused by antibodies to the heparin–platelet factor 4 complex and leads to severe thrombocytopenia and platelet activation that causes microvascular thrombosis. Identification of thrombosis in the setting of HIT type 2 necessitates treatment with a direct thrombin inhibitor such as argatroban or lepirudin to prevent further thrombosis. The diagnosis of HIT type 2 is based on the presence of heparin antibodies along with a positive result on a platelet serotonin-release assay. *Such a diagnosis mandates avoidance of all future heparin exposure* (Fig. 12.12).

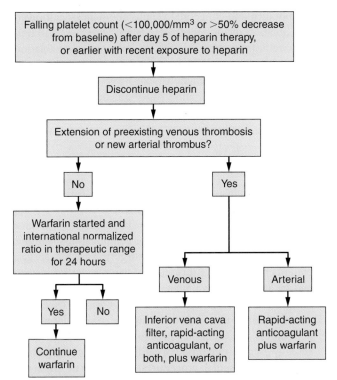

FIG. 12.12 Steps in the management of patients with venous thromboembolism and heparin-induced thrombocytopenia. (Adapted from Ginsberg JS. Management of venous thromboembolism. *N Engl J Med.* 1996;335:1816-1828. Copyright 1996 Massachusetts Medical Society.)

Text boxes in figure:
Falling platelet count (<100,000/mm³ or >50% decrease from baseline) after day 5 of heparin therapy, or earlier with recent exposure to heparin

Discontinue heparin

Extension of preexisting venous thrombosis or new arterial thrombus?

No — Yes

Warfarin started and international normalized ratio in therapeutic range for 24 hours

Yes — No

Continue warfarin

Venous — Arterial

Inferior vena cava filter, rapid-acting anticoagulant, or both, plus warfarin

Rapid-acting anticoagulant plus warfarin

SYSTEMIC VASCULITIS

Inflammatory diseases of the vasculature form a diverse and numerous group of ailments with characteristic presentations that are often grouped by the size of the vessels at the primary site of clinically apparent abnormalities. Large-artery vasculitides include Takayasu arteritis and temporal (or giant cell) arteritis. In contrast, Kawasaki disease is a vasculitis affecting medium-sized arteries, most prominently the coronary arteries. Medium- and small-artery vasculitides include thromboangiitis obliterans, Wegener granulomatosis, and polyarteritis nodosa. In addition, vasculitis can be a feature of connective tissue diseases such as systemic lupus erythematosus and rheumatoid arthritis, which are discussed in other chapters.

Temporal (Giant Cell) Arteritis

Temporal arteritis is inflammation of the arteries of the head and neck, manifesting most often as headache, scalp tenderness, or jaw claudication. This diagnosis is suspected in any patient older than age 50 complaining of a unilateral headache. Superficial branches of the temporal arteries are often tender and enlarged. Arteritis of branches of the ophthalmic artery may lead to ischemic optic neuritis and unilateral blindness. Indeed, prompt initiation of treatment with corticosteroids is indicated in patients with visual symptoms

to prevent blindness. Evidence of arteritis on a biopsy specimen of the temporal artery is present in approximately 90% of patients.

Thromboangiitis Obliterans (Buerger Disease)

Thromboangiitis obliterans is an inflammatory vasculitis leading to occlusion of small and medium-sized arteries and veins in the extremities. The disease is most prevalent in men, and the onset is typically before age 45. The most important predisposing factor is tobacco use. The disorder has been identified as an autoimmune response triggered when nicotine is present. The traditional diagnosis of Buerger disease is based on five criteria: smoking history, onset before age 50, infrapopliteal arterial occlusive disease, upper limb involvement or phlebitis migrans, and the absence of risk factors for atherosclerosis other than smoking. The diagnosis of thromboangiitis obliterans is confirmed by biopsy of active vascular lesions.

Signs and Symptoms

Involvement of extremity arteries causes forearm, calf, or foot claudication. Severe ischemia of the hands and feet can cause rest pain, ulcerations, and skin necrosis. Raynaud phenomenon is commonly associated with thromboangiitis obliterans, and cold exacerbates the symptoms. Periods of vasospasm may alternate with periods of quiescence. Migratory superficial vein thrombosis develops in approximately 40% of patients.

Treatment

The most effective treatment for patients with thromboangiitis obliterans is smoking cessation. Surgical revascularization is not usually feasible because of the involvement of small distal blood vessels. There is no proven effective drug therapy, and the efficacy of platelet inhibitors, anticoagulants, and thrombolytic therapy is not established. Recently, gene therapy with vascular endothelial growth factor was found to be helpful in healing ischemic ulcerations and relieving rest pain. Cyclophosphamide therapy has been tried because of the autoimmune nature of the disease.

Management of Anesthesia

Management of anesthesia in the presence of thromboangiitis obliterans requires avoidance of events that might damage already ischemic extremities. Positioning and padding of pressure points must be meticulous. The operating room ambient temperature should be warm, and inspired gases should be warmed and humidified to maintain normal body temperature. When feasible, systemic blood pressure should be measured noninvasively rather than by intraarterial means. Co-existing pulmonary and cardiac disease are considerations in these cigarette smokers.

Regional or general anesthetic techniques can be used in these patients. If regional anesthesia is selected, it may be prudent to omit epinephrine from the local anesthetic solution to avoid any possibility of accentuating vasospasm.

Polyarteritis Nodosa

Polyarteritis nodosa is an ANCA-negative vasculitis that sometimes occurs in association with hepatitis B, hepatitis C, or hairy cell leukemia. Males more frequently contract this disease than females. Small and medium-sized arteries are involved, with inflammatory changes resulting in glomerulonephritis, myocardial ischemia, peripheral neuropathy, and seizures. The lung vasculature is generally not affected. Hypertension is common and presumably reflects renal disease. Renal failure is the most common cause of death. Human immunodeficiency virus–associated vasculitis may present in a similar fashion.

The diagnosis of polyarteritis nodosa depends on histologic evidence of vasculitis on biopsy specimens and demonstration of characteristic aneurysms on arteriography. Treatment is empirical and usually includes corticosteroids and cyclophosphamide, removal of offending drugs, and treatment of underlying diseases such as cancer.

Management of anesthesia in patients with polyarteritis nodosa should take into consideration the likelihood of co-existing renal disease, cardiac disease, and systemic hypertension. Supplemental corticosteroids may be appropriate in patients who have been receiving these drugs as treatment for this disease.

Lower Extremity Chronic Venous Disease

Chronic venous disease includes symptoms associated with long-standing venous reflux and vein dilatation and affects approximately 50% of the population. Presentation varies from mild to severe, beginning with telangiectasias and varicose veins, to the more severe group of chronic venous insufficiency that includes clinical signs of edema, skin changes, and ultimately ulcerations.

Risk factors include advanced age, family history, pregnancy, ligamentous laxity, previous venous thrombosis as well as lower extremity injuries, prolonged standing, obesity, smoking, sedentary lifestyle, and high estrogen states.

Diagnosis includes symptoms of leg pain, fatigue, and heaviness and is confirmed by ultrasound studies that point toward *venous reflux,* which is defined by retrograde blood flow of greater than 0.5 seconds duration.

Treatment is conservative initially and includes leg elevation, exercise, weight reduction, compression therapy, skin barrier therapy, emollients, steroids in certain cases, and wound management for ulcerations. Conservative medical management may include diuretics, aspirin, systemic antibiotics, micronized purified flavonoid fraction, pentoxifylline, stanazol, escin (horse chestnut seed extract), hydroxyethylrutoside, sulodexide, prostacyclin analogues, and zinc sulfate.

If medical management fails and/or symptoms progress, ablation therapies can be performed. Indications include vein hemorrhage, superficial thrombophlebitis, and venous reflux associated with symptoms. Contraindications include pregnancy, vein thrombosis (superficial or deep), moderate to severe peripheral artery disease, joint disease that limits mobility, and congenital venous anomalies. Methods of venous ablation include thermal ablation with laser and light therapy, radiofrequency ablation, endovenous laser ablation, and sclerotherapy with chemical sclerosing agents. Surgical methods include saphenous vein inversion and removal, high saphenous ligation, ambulatory phlebectomy, transilluminated powered phlebectomy, conservative venous ligation, and perforator ligation.

KEY POINTS

- Cardiac complications are the leading cause of perioperative morbidity and mortality in patients undergoing noncardiac surgery. Compared with the general surgical population, the incidence of these complications is higher in patients undergoing vascular surgery. Vascular surgery patients have a higher incidence of coronary artery disease and are at particularly high risk of perioperative myocardial infarction (MI). However, the risk of perioperative cardiac complications differs based on the type of vascular surgery performed. For example, peripheral vascular procedures actually carry a higher rate of cardiovascular complications than central vascular procedures such as aortic aneurysm repair. The trend toward endovascular management of aortic and peripheral vascular disease may change cardiovascular risk substantially.

- Atherosclerosis is a systemic disease. Patients with peripheral arterial disease have a three to five times greater risk of cardiovascular ischemic events such as MI, ischemic stroke, and death than those without this disease. Critical limb ischemia is associated with very high intermediate-term morbidity and mortality resulting from cardiovascular events.

- Aortic cross-clamping and unclamping are associated with significant hemodynamic disturbances because of the decrease in blood flow distal to the aortic clamp and the increase in blood flow proximal to the level of aortic occlusion. There is also a substantial increase in systemic blood pressure. The hemodynamic response to aortic cross-clamping differs depending on the level of clamping: thoracic, supraceliac, or infrarenal.

- Perfusion pressures distal to the aortic cross-clamp are decreased and directly dependent on the pressure above the level of aortic clamping to aid in blood flow through collateral vessels or a shunt. Blood flow to vital organs distal to the aortic clamp depends on perfusion pressure, not on cardiac output or intravascular volume.

- Aortic cross-clamping is associated with formation and release of hormonal factors (activation of the sympathetic nervous system and the renin-angiotensin-aldosterone system) and other mediators (prostaglandins, oxygen free radicals, complement cascade). Overall, injury to the spinal cord, lungs, kidneys, and abdominal viscera is principally due to ischemia and subsequent reperfusion injury caused by the aortic cross-clamp (local effects) and/or release of mediators from ischemic and reperfused tissues (distant effects).

- The principal causes of unclamping hypotension are (1) central hypovolemia caused by pooling of blood in reperfused tissues, (2) hypoxia-mediated vasodilation causing an increase in vascular capacitance in the tissues below the level of aortic clamping, and (3) accumulation of vasoactive and myocardial-depressant metabolites in these tissues.

- Data from transcranial Doppler and carotid duplex ultrasonography studies suggest that carotid artery stenosis with a residual luminal diameter of 1.5 mm (70%–75% stenosis) represents the point at which a pressure drop occurs across the stenosis—that is, the point at which the stenosis becomes hemodynamically significant. Therefore if collateral cerebral blood flow is not adequate, transient ischemic attacks and ischemic infarction can occur.

- Both hypertension and hypotension may be observed frequently during the period immediately after carotid endarterectomy.

- Acute arterial occlusion is typically caused by cardiogenic embolism. Systemic emboli may arise from a mural thrombus in the left ventricle that develops because of MI or dilated cardiomyopathy. Other cardiac causes of systemic emboli are valvular heart disease, prosthetic heart valves, infective endocarditis, left atrial myxoma, atrial fibrillation, and atheroemboli from the aorta and iliac or femoral arteries.

- Thromboangiitis obliterans is an inflammatory vasculitis leading to occlusion of small and medium-sized arteries and veins in the extremities.

- Patients at low risk for deep vein thrombosis (DVT) require only minimal prophylactic measures such as early postoperative ambulation and use of compression stockings. The risk of DVT may be much higher in patients older than age 40 who are undergoing operations lasting longer than 1 hour, especially orthopedic surgery on the lower extremities, pelvic or abdominal surgery, and surgery that requires a prolonged convalescence with bed rest or limited mobility. The presence of cancer also increases the risk of thrombotic complications. Subcutaneous heparin (minidose heparin) and intermittent external pneumatic compression of the legs help prevent DVT in patients at moderate risk following abdominal and orthopedic surgery.

- Endovascular repair of aortic lesions is a relatively new technique for which data on long-term outcomes and randomized trials are lacking, but the significant improvement in perioperative mortality together with development of new grafts and devices has started a new era in vascular surgery. Carotid and peripheral arterial endovascular procedures have emerged as alternative, less invasive methods of arterial repair.

RESOURCES

Asymptomatic Carotid Surgery Trial (ACST) Collaborative Group. Prevention of disabling and fatal strokes by successful carotid endarterectomy in patients without recent neurological symptoms: randomized controlled trial. *Lancet.* 2004;363:1491-1502.

Brott TG, Hobson II RW, Howard G, et al. Stenting versus endarterectomy for treatment of carotid-artery stenosis. *N Engl J Med.* 2010;363:11-23. Erratum in *N Engl J Med.* 2010;363:198.

Buck DB, van Herwaarden JA, Schermerhorn ML, Moll FL, et al. Endovascular treatment of abdominal aortic aneurysms. *Nat Rev Cardiol.* 2014;11:112-123.

Chaturvedi S, Bruno A, Feasby T, et al. Carotid endarterectomy—an evidence-based review: report of the Therapeutics and Technology Assessment Subcommittee of the American Academy of Neurology. *Neurology.* 2005;65:794-801.

Conrad MF, Cambria RP. Contemporary management of descending thoracic and thoracoabdominal aortic aneurysms: endovascular versus open. *Circulation.* 2008;117:841-852.

Cremonesi A, Setacci C, Angelo Bignamini A, et al. Carotid artery stenting: first consensus document of the ICCS-SPREAD Joint Committee. *Stroke.* 2006;37:2400-2409.

EVAR trial participants. Endovascular aneurysm repair versus open repair in patients with abdominal aortic aneurysm (EVAR trial 1): randomised controlled trial. *Lancet.* 2005;365:2179-2186.

EVAR trial participants. Endovascular aneurysm repair and outcome in patients unfit for open repair of abdominal aortic aneurysm (EVAR trial 2): randomised controlled trial. *Lancet.* 2005;365:2187-2192.

Goldfinger JZ, Halperin JL, Marin ML, et al. Thoracic aortic aneurysms and dissection. *J Am Coll Cardiol.* 2014;64:1725-1739.

Grotta JC, Hacke W. Stroke Neurologist's Perspective on the New Endovascular Trials. *Stroke.* 2015 Jun;46:1447-1452.

Hirsch AT, Haskal ZJ, Hertzer NR, et al. ACC/AHA 2005 practice guidelines for the management of patients with peripheral arterial disease (lower extremity, renal, mesenteric, and abdominal aortic): a collaborative report from the American Association for Vascular Surgery/Society for Vascular Surgery, Society for Cardiovascular Angiography and Interventions, Society for Vascular Medicine and Biology, Society of Interventional Radiology, and the ACC/AHA Task Force on Practice Guidelines (Writing Committee to Develop Guidelines for the Management of Patients with Peripheral Arterial Disease): endorsed by the American Association of Cardiovascular and Pulmonary Rehabilitation; National Heart, Lung, and Blood Institute; Society for Vascular Nursing; TransAtlantic Inter-Society Consensus; and Vascular Disease Foundation. *Circulation.* 2006;113:e463-e654.

Katzen BT, Dake MD, MacLean AA, et al. Endovascular repair of abdominal and thoracic aortic aneurysms. *Circulation.* 2005;112:1663-1675.

Marin ML, Hollier LH, Ellozy SH, et al. Endovascular stent graft repair of abdominal and thoracic aortic aneurysms. A ten-year experience with 817 patients. *Ann Surg.* 2003;238:586-595.

McFalls EO, Ward HB, Moritz TE, et al. Coronary artery revascularization before elective major vascular surgery. *N Engl J Med.* 2004;351:2795-2804.

Pleis JR, Ward BW, Lucas JW. Summary health statistics for U. S. adults: National Health Interview Survey, 2009 *Vital Health Stat 10.* 2010;1-207.

Sarode R, Milling Jr TJ, Refaai MA, et al. Efficacy and safety of a 4-factor prothrombin complex concentrate in patients on vitamin K antagonists presenting with major bleeding: a randomized, plasma-controlled, phase IIIb study. *Circulation.* 2013;128:1234-1243.

Stone NJ, Robinson JG, Lichtenstein AH, et al. 2013 ACC/AHA Guideline on the treatment of blood cholesterol to reduce atherosclerotic cardiovascular risk in adults. A report of the American College of Cardiology/American Heart Association Task Force on Practice Guidelines. *J Am Coll Cardiol.* 2014;63:2889-2934.

Tang TY, Walsh SR, Gillard JH, et al. Carotid sinus nerve blockade to reduce blood pressure instability following carotid endarterectomy: a systematic review and meta-analysis. *Eur J Vasc Endovasc Surg.* 2007 Sep;34:304-311.

Trimarchi S, Nienaber CA, Rampoldi V, et al. Role and results of surgery in acute type B aortic dissection: insights from the International Registry of Acute Aortic Dissection (IRAD). *Circulation.* 2006;114:357-364.

Tsai TT, Evangelista A, Nienaber CA, et al. Long-term survival in patients presenting with type A acute aortic dissection. Insights from the International Registry of Acute Aortic Dissection (IRAD). *Circulation.* 2006;114(Suppl I):I-350-I-356.

Veith FJ, Lachat M, Mayer D, et al. Collected world and single center experience with endovascular treatment of ruptured abdominal aortic aneurysms. *Ann Surg.* 2009;250:818-824.

Yadav JS, Wholey MH, Kuntz RE, et al. Protected carotid-artery stenting versus endarterectomy in high-risk patients. *N Engl J Med.* 2004;351:1493-1501.

Diseases Affecting the Brain

JEFFREY J. PASTERNAK, WILLIAM L. LANIER, JR.

Patients with diseases affecting the brain and central nervous system (CNS) may undergo surgery to treat the neurologic condition or surgery unrelated to the nervous system disease. Regardless of the reason for surgery, co-existing nervous system diseases often have important implications for the selection of anesthetic drugs, techniques, and monitoring methods. Concepts of cerebral protection and resuscitation assume unique importance in these patients. This chapter reviews

these issues and also discusses various diseases of the retina and optic nerve.

CEREBRAL BLOOD FLOW, BLOOD VOLUME, AND METABOLISM

Generally, cerebral blood flow (CBF) is governed by cerebral metabolic rate, cerebral perfusion pressure (CPP, defined as the difference between the mean arterial pressure [MAP] and intracranial pressure [ICP]), arterial blood carbon dioxide ($Paco_2$) and oxygen (Pao_2) tensions, the influence of various drugs, and intracranial abnormalities. Under normal physiologic conditions, CBF is autoregulated—that is, CBF remains constant (or nearly so) over a range of perfusion pressures. With intact autoregulation, normal CBF in an awake person is approximately 50 mL/100 g brain tissue per minute. In the past, CBF was thought to be autoregulated over a range of CPPs of 50–150 mm Hg in chronically normotensive patients. However, more recent data suggest that the lower limit of autoregulation may be greater than 50 mm Hg (i.e., 60–70 mm Hg) in normotensive individuals. Also, the autoregulatory range may be dynamic, changing in response to physiologic factors (e.g., sleep/wake cycles) and likely varies among individuals. Given that a normal adult brain weighs approximately 1500 g and normal cardiac output is 5 L/min, CBF is therefore 750 mL/min or 15% of cardiac output during the awake state.

Normal cerebral metabolic rate, generally measured as rate of oxygen consumption ($CMRO_2$), is 3.0–3.8 mL O_2/100 g brain tissue per minute. Under awake resting conditions, total body oxygen consumption is approximately 250 mL O_2/min. Therefore total brain oxygen consumption is 45–57 mL O_2/min or 18%–23% of total body oxygen consumption. $CMRO_2$ can be decreased by temperature reductions and various anesthetic agents and increased by temperature increases and seizures.

Anesthetic and intensive care management of neurologically impaired patients relies heavily on manipulation of intracranial volume and pressure. These in turn are influenced by cerebral blood volume (CBV) and CBF. CBF and CBV do not always change in parallel. For example, vasodilatory anesthetics and hypercapnia may produce parallel increases in CBF and CBV. Conversely, moderate systemic hypotension can produce a reduction in CBF but, as a result of compensatory vasodilation, an increase in CBV. Similarly, partial occlusion of an intracranial artery such as occurs in embolic stroke may reduce regional CBF. However, vessel dilation distal to the occlusion, which is an attempt to restore circulation, can produce an increase in CBV.

Arterial Carbon Dioxide Partial Pressure

Variations in $Paco_2$ produce corresponding changes in CBF (Fig. 13.1). As a guideline, CBF (normally ≈50 mL/100 g brain tissue per minute) increases by 1–2 mL/100 g per minute (or ≈15 mL/min for a 1500-g brain) for every 1 mm Hg increase in $Paco_2$. A similar decrease occurs during hypocarbia, so that CBF is decreased by approximately 50% when $Paco_2$ is acutely reduced to 20 mm Hg.

The impact of $Paco_2$ on CBF is mediated by variations in the pH of the cerebrospinal fluid (CSF) around the walls of arterioles. Decreased CSF pH causes cerebral vasodilation, and increased CSF pH results in vasoconstriction. $Paco_2$ can also modulate CBV. The extent of CBV reduction is dependent on the anesthetic being used. In general, vasoconstricting anesthetics tend to attenuate the effects of $Paco_2$ on CBV.

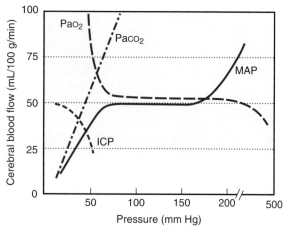

FIG. 13.1 Impact of intracranial pressure (ICP), Pao_2, $Paco_2$, and mean arterial pressure (MAP) on cerebral blood flow.

The ability of hypocapnia to acutely decrease CBF, CBV, and ICP is fundamental to the practice of clinical neuroanesthesia. Concern that cerebral hypoxia due to vasoconstriction can occur when the $Paco_2$ is lowered to less than 20 mm Hg has not been substantiated. The ability of hypocapnia to decrease CBV and thus ICP is attenuated by the return of CSF pH to normal after prolonged periods of hypocapnia. This reduces the effectiveness of induced hypocapnia as a means of long-term control of intracranial hypertension. This adaptive change, which reflects active transport of bicarbonate ions into or out of the CSF, requires approximately 6 hours to return the CSF pH to normal.

Arterial Oxygen Partial Pressure

Decreased Pao_2 does not significantly affect CBF until a threshold value of approximately 50 mm Hg is reached. Below this threshold there is abrupt cerebral vasodilation and CBF increases. Furthermore the combination of arterial hypoxemia and hypercarbia exert synergistic effects on CBF. The effect of isolated hyperoxia (i.e., independent of $Paco_2$) on CBF is less clear, though generally, intense hyperoxia (at normal or supranormal atmospheric pressure) is assumed to produce no meaningful effect or a small reduction (e.g., 10%) in CBF.

Cerebral Perfusion Pressure and Cerebral Autoregulation

The ability of the brain to maintain CBF at constant levels despite changes in CPP is known as *autoregulation* (see Fig. 13.1). Autoregulation is an active vascular response characterized by (1) arterial constriction when CPP is increased and (2) arterial dilation in response to decreases in CPP. For example, in normotensive patients the lower limit of CPP associated with autoregulation is believed to be approximately 50 mm Hg, although the exact value is controversial and may be higher. Below the "lower limit of autoregulation" threshold, cerebral blood vessels are maximally dilated and CBF decreases. CBF then becomes directly related to CPP—that is, it becomes *pressure-dependent blood flow.* Indeed, at a CPP of 30–45 mm Hg, symptoms of cerebral ischemia may appear in the form of nausea, dizziness, and altered consciousness. Autoregulation of CBF also has an upper limit above which the flow becomes more proportional to the CPP. This upper limit of autoregulation in normotensive patients is believed to be a CPP of approximately 150 mm Hg. Above this pressure the cerebral blood vessels are maximally constricted. If CPP increases further, CBF increases and becomes pressure dependent. At even higher pressures, fluid may be forced across blood vessel walls into the brain parenchyma, producing cerebral edema. The risk of cerebral hemorrhage also increases.

Autoregulation of CBF is altered in the presence of chronic hypertension. Specifically the autoregulation curve is displaced to the right, so pressure dependence of CBF occurs at a higher CPP at both the lower and upper thresholds of autoregulation. The adaptation of cerebral blood vessels to increased blood pressure requires some time. The lower limit of autoregulation is shifted upward in chronically hypertensive patients, so decreases in systemic blood pressure that would be tolerated in normotensive patients are not well tolerated in these individuals. Therefore rapid lowering of blood pressure with the use of a vasodilating drug to population-normal values in patients who are chronically hypertensive can result in cerebral ischemia. Gradual decreases in systemic blood pressure over time resulting from antihypertensive drug therapy can improve the tolerance of the brain to hypotension as the autoregulation curve shifts back toward a more normal position. Acute hypertension, as seen in children with acute-onset glomerulonephritis or in patients with short-duration pregnancy-induced hypertension, often produces signs of CNS dysfunction at MAP values that are well tolerated in chronically hypertensive patients. Similarly an acute hypertensive response associated with direct laryngoscopy or surgery may exceed the upper limit of autoregulation in chronically normotensive patients. Autoregulation of CBF may be lost or impaired under a variety of conditions, including the presence of intracranial tumors or head trauma and the administration of volatile anesthetics. Loss of autoregulation in the blood vessels surrounding intracranial tumors reflects acidosis leading to maximum vasodilation, so blood flow becomes pressure dependent in these areas.

Venous Blood Pressure

Increases in the brain's venous blood pressure can influence CBF either directly or indirectly. Directly, increased brain venous pressure contributes to reductions in arterial/venous pressure gradients. Indirectly, increases in brain venous blood pressure increase CBV and ICP (see later discussion), which in turn reduces CPP. If these changes in brain venous blood pressure are not compensated for by an increase in MAP, the CPP reduction will produce the expected effects on CBF.

Venous pressure increases emanating from the central circulation (i.e., central venous pressure [CVP]) are variably transmitted to the brain depending on whether the patient's position is horizontal (maximal CBV increase) or head up (minimal CBV increase). In contrast, venous blood pressure increases emanating from the neck or skull base are more effectively translated to the brain. Regardless of its origin, an increase in brain venous pressure can contribute to increased brain bulk during intracranial surgery and impede the surgeon's access to the target brain areas.

Causes of increased brain venous pressure include venous sinus thrombosis and jugular compression resulting from improper neck positioning, such as extreme flexion or rotation. Superior vena cava syndrome can cause long-term increases in brain venous pressure. With coughing, increases in intrathoracic pressure result in transient increases in CVP. However, if a coughing or bucking patient is tracheally intubated, the glottis is stented open by the endotracheal tube and the effects of a cough or buck on CVP will be different from those in a nonintubated patient. CVP in the tracheally intubated patient will transiently increase during forced exhalation but transiently decrease during forced inhalation, which results in no meaningful change in CVP over an entire coughing or bucking cycle. In such a setting, ICP can still increase, but this increase would be due to increases in CBF and CBV resulting from muscle afferent-mediated stimulation of the brain, a mechanism shared by succinylcholine-induced increases in ICP.

Anesthetic Drugs

Under normal physiologic conditions, changes in $CMRO_2$ usually lead to concomitant same-direction changes in CBF, a phenomenon known as *CBF-CMRO$_2$ coupling.* In contrast, volatile anesthetics such as isoflurane, sevoflurane, and desflurane, particularly when administered in concentrations greater than 0.6–1.0 minimum alveolar concentration (MAC), are potent direct cerebral vasodilators that produce dose-dependent increases in CBF despite concomitant decreases in cerebral metabolic oxygen requirements. Below 1 MAC, volatile anesthetics alter CBF minimally, in part because any direct effects of the anesthetics are counterbalanced by CBF-CMRO$_2$ coupling. When volatile anesthetic–induced $CMRO_2$ depression is maximized concomitant with maximal depression of cerebral electrical activity, larger dosages of volatile anesthetic will dilate cerebral blood vessels. This can lead to increases in CBF, CBV, and possibly ICP. At equi-MAC doses, desflurane causes greater increases in ICP than isoflurane. With halothane, which at clinically relevant dosages does not induce the extent of $CMRO_2$ depression seen with other volatile anesthetics (isoflurane, sevoflurane, desflurane), direct vasodilatory effects predominate, which results in greater increases in CBF at equipotent doses compared with other commonly used volatile agents. This can lead to increased ICP, which makes halothane a less-than-ideal volatile anesthetic agent for neurosurgical procedures in which CBV and ICP management are critical. With all volatile anesthetics, arterial hypocapnia helps to minimize increases in CBV that might accompany administration of these drugs at normocarbia. These same CBV- and ICP-attenuating effects can also be achieved by administration of supplemental cerebral vasoconstricting anesthetics such as thiopental or propofol.

Nitrous oxide also causes an increase in CBF, but in contrast to volatile anesthetics it does not appear to interfere with autoregulation. The exact effects of nitrous oxide on human cerebral hemodynamics remain elusive, probably because of a wide range of interspecies differences in the MAC of nitrous oxide (as determined in laboratory experiments), as well as the invariable presence of other drugs used to maintain general anesthesia. Initiation of nitrous oxide administration after closure of the dura may contribute to the development of a tension pneumocephalus, since there is likely to be air in the intracranial vault following dural closure, and nitrous oxide has greater solubility in air than nitrogen. This leads to an increase in the size and pressure of the air pocket. Clinically, tension pneumocephalus usually presents as delayed emergence from general anesthesia after craniotomy.

Like the volatile anesthetics, ketamine is considered a cerebral vasodilator. Propofol and barbiturates such as thiopental are potent cerebral vasoconstrictors capable of decreasing CBF, CBV, and ICP. Opioids are also cerebral vasoconstrictors, assuming opioid-induced ventilatory depression is controlled and no increase in $Paco_2$ is allowed. Drugs that produce cerebral vasoconstriction predictably decrease CBV and ICP.

Administration of nondepolarizing neuromuscular blocking drugs does not meaningfully alter ICP. However, muscle relaxation may help prevent acute increases in ICP resulting from movement or coughing during direct laryngoscopy. Neuromuscular blocker–induced histamine release, as occurs with atracurium, D-tubocurarine, and metocurine, could theoretically produce cerebral vasodilation and an associated increase in CBV and ICP, particularly if large doses of these drugs are administered rapidly. The use of succinylcholine in the setting of increased ICP may temporarily raise ICP. The mechanism for this effect is most likely increases in muscle afferent activity, a process somewhat independent of visible muscle fasciculations. This can lead to cerebral arousal (which can be seen on electroencephalography [EEG]) and corresponding increases in CBF and CBV. These cerebral effects of succinylcholine can be attenuated or prevented by prior induction of deep anesthesia with a cerebral vasoconstricting anesthetic.

INCREASED INTRACRANIAL PRESSURE

The intracranial and spinal vault contains neural tissue (brain and spinal cord), blood, and CSF and is enclosed by the dura mater and bone. The pressure within this space is referred to as the *intracranial pressure* (ICP). Under normal conditions, brain tissue, intracranial CSF, and intracranial blood have a combined volume of approximately 1200–1500 mL, and normal ICP is usually 5–15 mm Hg (or 7–20 cm H_2O). Any increase in one component of intracranial volume will initially fill a small potential space of only a few milliliters in volume but later must be offset by a decrease in the volume of another intracranial component to prevent an increase in ICP. Under normal

physiologic conditions, changes in one component are well compensated by the potential space or changes in other components, but eventually a point can be reached at which even a small change in intracranial contents results in a large change in ICP (Fig. 13.2). Since ICP is one of the determinants of CPP, homeostatic mechanisms work to increase MAP to help support CPP despite increases in ICP, but eventually compensatory mechanisms can fail and cerebral ischemia will result.

Factors leading to alterations in CSF flow or its absorption into the vasculature can often lead to increased ICP. CSF is produced by two mechanisms: (1) ultrafiltration and secretion by the cells of the choroid plexus and (2) the passage of water, electrolytes, and other substances across the blood-brain barrier. CSF is therefore a direct extension of the extracellular fluid compartment of the CNS. CSF is produced at a constant rate of 500–600 mL/day in adults and is contained within the ventricular system of the brain, the central canal of the spinal cord, and the subarachnoid space, as well as the extracellular compartment of the CNS. CSF is absorbed from microscopic arachnoid villi and macroscopic arachnoid granulations within the dura mater and bordering venous sinusoids and sinuses.

It is important to note that the intracranial vault is considered to be compartmentalized. Specifically there are various meningeal barriers within the intracranial vault that functionally separate the contents: the falx cerebri (a reflection of dura mater that separates the two cerebral hemispheres) and the tentorium cerebelli (a reflection of dura mater that lies rostral to the cerebellum and marks the border between the supratentorial and infratentorial spaces). Increases in the contents of one region of brain may cause regional increases in ICP, and in extreme instances the contents of that compartment can move, or herniate, into a different compartment.

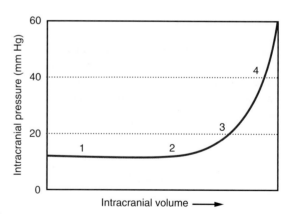

FIG. 13.2 Intracranial elastance curve depicting the impact of increasing intracranial volume on intracranial pressure (ICP). As intracranial volume increases from point 1 to point 2, ICP does not increase because of compensatory mechanisms. Patients on the rising portion of the curve (point 3) can no longer compensate for increases in intracranial volume; the ICP begins to increase and is likely to be associated with clinical symptoms. Additional increases in intracranial volume at this point (point 3), as produced by anesthetic drug–induced increases in cerebral blood volume, can precipitate abrupt increases in ICP (point 4).

Various types of herniation syndromes are categorized based on the region of brain affected (Fig. 13.3). Herniation of cerebral hemispheric contents under the falx cerebri is referred to as *subfalcine herniation*. Typically this condition leads to compression of branches of the anterior cerebral artery and is evident on radiographic imaging as midline shift. Herniation of the supratentorial contents past the tentorium cerebelli is referred to as *transtentorial herniation*, in which evidence of brainstem compression occurs in a rostral-to-caudal manner, resulting in altered consciousness, defects in gaze and afferent ocular reflexes, and finally hemodynamic and respiratory compromise followed by death. The uncus (i.e., the medial portion of the temporal lobe) may herniate over the tentorium cerebelli, which results in a subtype of transtentorial herniation referred to as *uncal herniation*. A specific sign is ipsilateral oculomotor nerve dysfunction because the oculomotor nerve is compressed against the brainstem; this results in pupillary dilatation, ptosis, and lateral deviation of the affected eye, which occurs before evidence of brainstem compression and death. Herniation of the cerebellar tonsils can occur in the setting of elevated infratentorial pressure, which leads to extension of these cerebellar structures through the foramen magnum. Typical signs are those indicating medullary dysfunction, including cardiorespiratory instability and death.

Nonspecific signs and symptoms of increased ICP include headache, nausea, vomiting, and papilledema. As ICP further increases and cerebral perfusion becomes limited, decreased levels of consciousness and possibly coma can be observed. Acute increases in ICP may not be tolerated as well as chronic intracranial hypertension.

Increased ICP is often diagnosed clinically based on the symptoms described earlier, by radiographic means, and by direct measurement of ICP. Typically, computed tomography (CT) or magnetic resonance imaging (MRI) will help identify the cause of an increase in ICP. For example, a large mass or hematoma may be evident. If aqueductal stenosis is present, the third but not fourth ventricle is enlarged.

Several methods are currently available to measure and monitor ICP. The choice of technique depends on the clinical situation. Pressure can be measured in the subdural space, brain parenchyma, or ventricle. The advantage of this last technique, known as a *ventriculostomy,* is that in addition to pressure monitoring it allows for withdrawal of CSF; it is currently considered the gold standard for ICP measurement. This is a major benefit, since the drainage system can be organized so that CSF will only drain if the ICP exceeds a selected value. Such an approach allows some control over ICP. A second advantage of ventriculostomy is that CSF can be easily obtained for laboratory analysis. A lumbar subarachnoid catheter is another available modality. It offers advantages similar to those of ventriculostomy in that CSF can be withdrawn or allowed to passively drain if the ICP increases above a set value. The disadvantage of a lumbar subarachnoid catheter compared with ventriculostomy is that because of compartmentalization of the intracranial contents, lumbar CSF pressure may not accurately reflect ICP in all circumstances. In certain clinical settings (e.g., brain tumor) there is also a risk of herniation of the cerebellar tonsils when CSF is drained using the lumbar subarachnoid approach. Other techniques, such as measurement of optic nerve sheath diameter via ultrasonography, may provide a noninvasive way to assess ICP.

A normal ICP waveform is pulsatile and varies with the cardiac impulse and spontaneous breathing. An ICP remaining below 15 mm Hg is normal. In patients with *increased intracranial elastance* (i.e., dramatic increases in ICP in response to small increases in intracranial volume), not only may ICP be above 15 mm Hg, but abnormal waveforms may appear. There are three types of Lundberg waves that may appear on an ICP waveform tracing. Lundberg A waves (or "plateau waves") are abrupt increases in ICP from 20–100 mm Hg that can last for up to 20 minutes. Lundberg A waves occur in the setting of increased intracranial elastance with impaired oxygen and substrate delivery that results in abrupt vasodilation and an increase in ICP. During these dramatic increases in ICP, patients may become symptomatic and manifest evidence of inadequate cerebral perfusion. Spontaneous hyperventilation or changes in mental status may occur. Anxiety and painful stimulation can initiate abrupt increases in ICP. Lundberg A waves are related to a poor outcome. Lundberg B waves are sharp, brief spikes in ICP to 20–50 mm Hg occurring approximately every 0.5–2 minutes. They also indicate increased intracranial elastance but to a lesser degree than Lundberg A

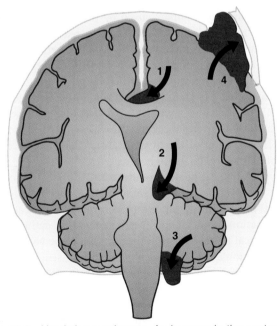

FIG. 13.3 Herniation syndromes. An increase in the contents of the supratentorial space caused by masses, edema, or hematoma can lead to (1) herniation of the cingulate gyrus under the falx (i.e., subfalcine herniation); (2) herniation of contents over the tentorium cerebelli (i.e., transtentorial herniation); (3) herniation of the cerebellar tonsils out through the foramen magnum; and (4) herniation of brain contents out of a traumatic defect in the cranial cavity. (Adapted from Fishman RA. Brain edema. *N Engl J Med.* 1975;293:706-711.)

waves. Lundberg C waves are rhythmic, very-short-duration spikes in ICP up to 20 mm Hg of unknown etiology. Lundberg C waves are considered benign.

Methods to Decrease Intracranial Pressure

Methods to decrease ICP include elevation of the head, hyperventilation, CSF drainage, surgical decompression, and administration of hyperosmotic drugs, diuretics, corticosteroids (but only in very specific conditions), and cerebral vasoconstricting anesthetics such as barbiturates and propofol. It is not possible to reliably identify the level of ICP that will interfere with regional CBF or alter cerebral function and well-being in individual patients. Therefore a frequent recommendation is to treat any sustained increase in ICP that exceeds 20 mm Hg. Treatment may be indicated even when the ICP is less than 20 mm Hg if the appearance of occasional plateau waves suggests the presence of increased intracranial elastance.

Posture is important for ensuring optimal venous drainage from the brain. For example, elevating the patient's head to approximately 30 degrees above heart level encourages venous outflow from the brain and lowers ICP. Extreme flexion or rotation of the head can obstruct the jugular veins and restrict venous outflow from the brain. The head-down position must be used with caution, since this position can increase ICP.

Hyperventilation, and hence lowering of $Paco_2$, is an effective method for rapidly reducing ICP. In adults a frequent recommendation is to maintain $Paco_2$ near 30–35 mm Hg. Lowering the $Paco_2$ more than this may not meaningfully decrease ICP further but may result in adverse changes in systemic physiology. The optimal $Paco_2$-related reduction in ICP is influenced by whether or not the patient is receiving a vasodilating or vasoconstricting anesthetic. However, regardless of the anesthetic used, the effects of hyperventilation will diminish with time and wane after 6 hours. When prolonged hyperventilation is discontinued, rebound increases in ICP are a potential problem, especially if normocapnia is rapidly restored.

Draining CSF from the lateral cerebral ventricles or the lumbar subarachnoid space decreases intracranial volume and ICP. Lumbar CSF drainage via a catheter is usually reserved for operations in which surgical exposure is difficult, such as surgery on the pituitary gland or an intracranial aneurysm. Lumbar CSF drainage is not routinely used for the treatment of intracranial hypertension, particularly that related to mass lesions, because of the fear that pressure gradients induced by drainage could result in cerebral herniation. If the cause of increased ICP is chronic, shunting of CSF from an intracranial ventricle is preferred. For long-term treatment, CSF is typically drained to the right atrium (ventriculoatrial shunt) or the peritoneal cavity (ventriculoperitoneal shunt).

Intravenous (IV) infusion of drugs and fluids such as mannitol and hypertonic saline are effective at decreasing ICP. These drugs produce transient increases in the osmolarity of plasma, which act to draw water from tissues, including the brain. With osmotic diuretics, diuresis and a reduction in systemic blood volume, similar to that occurring with loop diuretics, are important secondary effects. When mannitol or any other diuretic is administered, care should be taken to avoid significant hypovolemia. Excessive fluid losses can result in hypotension and jeopardize maintenance of adequate CPP. In addition, urinary losses of electrolytes, particularly potassium, may occur, and thus careful monitoring and replacement are required. Moreover, an intact blood-brain barrier is necessary so that mannitol can exert maximum beneficial effects on brain size. If the blood-brain barrier is disrupted, these drugs may cross into the brain, causing cerebral edema and increases in brain size. The brain eventually adapts to sustained increases in plasma osmolarity, so long-term use of hyperosmotic drugs results in reduced effectiveness.

Mannitol is ideally administered in doses of 0.25–0.5 g/kg IV. Larger initial doses have little incremental effect on ICP but may predispose the patient to rebound increases in ICP. Hence it is better to give an initial dose of 0.25–0.5 g/kg IV and if the desired effect is not achieved, either administer another dose or switch to another type of therapy. Also, no further mannitol should be administered if serum osmolarity is above 320 mOsm/L. Under ideal conditions, treatment with mannitol results in removal of approximately 100 mL of water from the brain. After mannitol administration, decreases in ICP are seen within 30 minutes, with maximum effects occurring within 1–2 hours. Urine output can reach 1–2 L within an hour after administration of mannitol. Appropriate infusion of crystalloid and colloid solutions may be necessary to prevent adverse changes in plasma electrolyte concentrations and intravascular fluid volume caused by the brisk diuresis. On the other hand, mannitol can initially increase intravascular fluid volume, which emphasizes the need to carefully monitor patients who have limited cardiac reserve or congestive heart failure. Mannitol has direct vasodilating properties. Interestingly, mannitol can transiently contribute to increased CBV and ICP in individuals with normal ICP, but in those with intracranial hypertension, mannitol will *not* further increase ICP. The duration of the hyperosmotic effects produced by mannitol is approximately 6 hours.

Hypertonic saline is an alternate option to increase serum osmolarity and decrease ICP. Hypertonic saline should be administered via a central venous catheter; extravasation from an infiltrated peripheral catheter can lead to local tissue irritation that can be worse with higher concentrations. For an adult patient, administration of 1–2 mL/kg of 3% sodium chloride over 5 minutes can be considered. Additional drug can be administered to obtain a target serum sodium concentration of 145–155 mEq/L and a serum osmolarity below 320 mOsm/L if the initial dose fails to reduce ICP. Serum sodium concentrations greater than 160 mEq/L can lead to renal injury, pulmonary edema, cardiac dysfunction, and seizures. As such, serum sodium should be checked frequently until target serum sodium and osmolarity are obtained and then at least every 6 hours for the duration of the infusion. Hypertonic saline has greater overall risk than mannitol.

Loop diuretics, particularly furosemide, have been used to decrease ICP, although their efficacy is significantly less than that of mannitol or hypertonic saline. Furosemide may be useful in patients with evidence of increased intravascular fluid volume and pulmonary edema and in patients who, because of various co-existing diseases such as congestive heart failure or nephrotic syndrome, would not tolerate the initial increase in intravascular volume associated with mannitol or hypertonic saline infusion. In these patients, furosemide will promote diuresis and systemic dehydration and improve arterial oxygenation along with causing a concomitant decrease in ICP.

Corticosteroids (e.g., dexamethasone, methylprednisolone) are effective in lowering ICP caused by the development of localized vasogenic cerebral edema. This is due in part to a steroid-induced upregulation of the expression of proteins responsible for the integrity of the tight junctions between endothelial cells constituting a major component of the blood-brain barrier. Patients with brain tumors often exhibit improved neurologic status and disappearance of headache within 12–36 hours after initiation of corticosteroid therapy. Corticosteroids are also effective in treating increased ICP in patients with pseudotumor cerebri (benign intracranial hypertension). Corticosteroids are *not* effective in reducing ICP in some other forms of intracranial hypertension such as closed head injury. Corticosteroids can increase blood glucose concentration, which may adversely affect outcome if ongoing cerebral ischemia is present. Because of this, corticosteroids should not be administered for the nonspecific treatment of increased ICP.

Barbiturates in high dosages are particularly effective in treating increased ICP that develops after an acute head injury. Propofol may also be useful in this situation. However, patients receiving prolonged propofol infusions, particularly pediatric patients, should be monitored for drug-associated high-anion-gap metabolic acidosis (propofol infusion syndrome), which can herald multiorgan dysfunction and can be fatal.

Specific Causes of Increased Intracranial Pressure

Increased ICP is typically a sign of an underlying intracranial pathologic process. Therefore one should seek the cause of increased ICP in addition to instituting treatment. Causes of increased ICP are many. Tumors can lead to increased ICP (1) directly because of their size, (2) indirectly by causing edema in normal surrounding brain tissue, or (3) by causing obstruction of CSF flow, as is commonly seen with tumors involving the third ventricle. Intracranial hematomas can cause increased ICP in a manner similar to mass lesions. Blood in the CSF, as is seen in subarachnoid hemorrhage, may lead to obstruction of CSF reabsorption at the arachnoid villi and granulations and may further exacerbate increased ICP. Infection (e.g., meningitis, encephalitis) can lead to edema or obstruction of CSF reabsorption. Some causes of intracranial hypertension not discussed elsewhere in this chapter are described in the following sections.

Aqueductal Stenosis

Stenosis of major CSF flow channels may impede CSF flow and can lead to increased ICP. Aqueductal stenosis, one of the more common causes of obstructive hydrocephalus, results from congenital narrowing of the cerebral aqueduct that connects the third and fourth ventricles. Obstructive hydrocephalus can present during infancy when the narrowing is severe. Lesser obstruction results in slowly progressive hydrocephalus, which may not be evident until adulthood. Symptoms of aqueductal stenosis are the same as those seen with other forms of intracranial hypertension. Seizure disorders are present in approximately one-third of these patients. CT is useful to confirm the presence of obstructive hydrocephalus. Symptomatic aqueductal stenosis is treated by ventricular shunting. Management of anesthesia for ventricular shunt placement must focus on managing intracranial hypertension.

Benign Intracranial Hypertension

Benign intracranial hypertension (pseudotumor cerebri) is a syndrome characterized by an ICP above 20 mm Hg, normal CSF composition, normal sensorium, and absence of intracranial lesions. This disorder typically occurs in obese women and is observed more commonly in patients with polycystic ovary syndrome, systemic lupus erythematosus, Addison's disease, and hypoparathyroidism. It is also associated with hypervitaminosis A. CT scan indicates a normal or even small cerebral ventricular system. Headaches and bilateral visual disturbances typically occur. Of note, symptoms may be exaggerated during pregnancy. Interestingly, no identifiable cause of increased ICP is found in most patients. The prognosis is usually excellent.

Acute treatment of benign intracranial hypertension includes removal of 20–40 mL of CSF from the lumbar subarachnoid space, as well as the administration of acetazolamide to decrease CSF formation. Patients also respond to treatment with corticosteroids. Treatment of a contributing factor (i.e., vitamin A restriction for those with hypervitaminosis A) should be considered early. Further therapy may involve repeated lumbar punctures to remove CSF, which also facilitates measurement of ICP. Interestingly, continued leakage of CSF through the dural puncture site may be therapeutic. Long-term administration of acetazolamide can result in acidemia, which presumably reflects inhibition of hydrogen ion secretion by renal tubules. Surgical therapy, most often insertion of a lumboperitoneal shunt, is indicated only after medical therapy has failed and the patient's vision has begun to deteriorate. Optic nerve sheath fenestration is another surgical alternative to CSF shunting. If untreated, visual function may be threatened.

Anesthesia management for lumboperitoneal shunt placement involves avoiding exacerbation of intracranial hypertension and ensuring an adequate CPP. Hypoxia and hypercarbia must be avoided.

Spinal anesthesia may be used in selected parturients with mildly increased ICP so long as the patient has no significant neurologic deficits or alterations in consciousness. In patients with elevated ICP, epidural analgesia should be avoided in most cases, since the volume of drug required may exacerbate the elevated ICP. In the presence of a *lumboperitoneal shunt,* there is a possibility that local anesthetic solution injected into the subarachnoid space could escape into the peritoneal cavity, decreasing anesthesia density and clinical effect. In parturients with a functioning *ventriculoperitoneal shunt,* spinal and epidural analgesia and anesthesia can be used safely and effectively.

Normal Pressure Hydrocephalus

Normal pressure hydrocephalus usually presents as the triad of dementia, gait changes, and urinary incontinence that develops over a period of weeks to months. The mechanism is thought to be related to compensated but impaired CSF absorption from a previous insult to the brain, such as subarachnoid hemorrhage, meningitis, or head trauma. In most cases, however, the cause is never identified. Lumbar puncture usually reveals normal or low CSF pressure, yet CT or MRI will often demonstrate large ventricles. Treatment typically involves drainage of CSF via ventriculoperitoneal shunting.

INTRACRANIAL TUMORS

Intracranial tumors may be classified as primary (those arising from the brain and its coverings) or metastatic. Tumors can originate from virtually any cell type within the CNS. Supratentorial tumors are more common in adults and often present with headache, seizures, or new neurologic deficits, whereas infratentorial tumors are more common in children and often present with obstructive hydrocephalus and ataxia. Treatment and prognosis depend on both the tumor type and location. Treatment may consist of surgical resection or debulking, chemotherapy, or radiation. Gamma knife irradiation differs from traditional radiation therapy in that multiple radiation sources are used, and because the tumor is addressed from multiple angles, radiation to the tumor can be maximized while the radiation dose to any single area of surrounding brain tissue can be minimized. Such treatment can also be accomplished with the use of x-ray as well as particle-based modalities such as proton beam therapy. Emerging therapies include immunotherapy and oncolytic virotherapy, the latter employing viruses specifically programmed to kill neoplastic cells.

Tumor Types

Astrocytoma

Astrocytes are the most prevalent neuroglial cells in the CNS and give rise to many types of infratentorial and supratentorial tumors. Well-differentiated (low-grade) gliomas are the least aggressive class of astrocyte-derived tumors. They often are found in young adults and generally present as new-onset seizures. Imaging generally shows minimal enhancement with contrast. Surgical or radiation treatment of low-grade gliomas usually results in symptom-free long-term survival.

Pilocytic astrocytomas usually affect children and young adults. They often arise in the cerebellum (cerebellar astrocytoma), cerebral hemispheres, hypothalamus, or optic pathways (optic glioma). The tumor usually appears as a contrast-enhancing, well-demarcated lesion with minimal to no surrounding edema. Because of its benign pathologic characteristics, prognosis following surgical resection is generally very good. However, the location of the lesion, such as within the brainstem, may preclude resection.

Anaplastic astrocytomas are poorly differentiated, usually appear as contrast-enhancing lesions on imaging because of disruption of the blood-brain barrier, and generally evolve into glioblastoma multiforme. Treatment involves resection, radiation, or chemotherapy. Prognosis is intermediate between that for low-grade gliomas and glioblastoma multiforme.

Glioblastoma multiforme (grade IV glioma) accounts for 30% of all primary brain tumors in adults. Imaging usually reveals a ring-enhancing lesion reflecting central necrosis and surrounding edema. Because of microscopic infiltration of normal brain by tumor cells, resection alone is typically inadequate. Instead, treatment usually consists of surgical debulking combined with chemotherapy and radiation and is aimed at palliation, not cure. Despite treatment, life expectancy may be measured in weeks.

Oligodendroglioma

Oligodendrogliomas arise from myelin-producing cells within the CNS and account for only 6% of primary intracranial tumors. Classically, seizures predate the appearance of the tumor on imaging, often by many years. Calcifications within the tumor are common and are visualized on CT imaging. The tumor usually consists of a mixture of both oligodendrocytic and astrocytic cells. Treatment and prognosis depend on the pathologic features. Initial treatment involves resection, since early in the course the tumor consists of primarily oligodendrocytic cells, which are radioresistant. Because of the presence of astrocytic cells, these tumors commonly behave more like anaplastic astrocytomas or glioblastoma multiforme later in their course.

Ependymoma

Arising from cells lining the ventricles and central canal of the spinal cord, ependymomas commonly present in childhood and young adulthood. Their most common location is the floor of the fourth ventricle. Symptoms include obstructive hydrocephalus, headache, nausea, vomiting, and ataxia. Treatment consists of resection and radiation. Tumor infiltration into surrounding tissues may preclude complete resection. Prognosis depends on the completeness of resection.

Primitive Neuroectodermal Tumor

Primitive neuroectodermal tumor represents a diverse class of tumors including retinoblastoma, medulloblastoma, pineoblastoma, and neuroblastoma, all believed to arise from primitive neuroectodermal cells. Medulloblastoma is the most common pediatric primary malignant brain tumor and may disseminate via CSF to the spinal cord. The presentation of medulloblastoma is similar to that of ependymoma. Treatment usually involves a combination of resection, radiation, and possibly intrathecal instillation of chemotherapeutic drugs. Prognosis is very good in children if treatment leads to disappearance of both tumor on MRI and tumor cells within the CSF. Prognosis is less optimistic if there is evidence of tumor dissemination within the CNS.

Meningioma

Meningiomas are usually extraaxial (arising outside of the brain proper), slow-growing, well-circumscribed, benign tumors arising from arachnoid cap cells, not the dura mater. Because of their slow growth, they can be very large at the time of diagnosis. They can occur anywhere arachnoid cap cells exist but are most common near the sagittal sinus, falx cerebri, and cerebral convexity. Tumors are usually apparent on plain radiographs and CT scans as a result of the presence of calcifications. On MRI and conventional angiography, these tumors are often seen to receive their blood supply from the *external carotid artery*. Surgical resection is the mainstay of treatment. Prognosis is usually excellent. However, some tumors may be recurrent and require additional resection. Malignant meningiomas are rare.

Pituitary Tumor

Pituitary adenomas usually arise from cells of the anterior pituitary gland. They may occur along with tumors of the parathyroid glands and pancreatic islet cells as part of multiple endocrine neoplasia (MEN) type I. These tumors are usually divided into functional (i.e., hormone-secreting) and nonfunctional types. The former usually present as an endocrinologic disturbance related to the hormone secreted by the tumor. Functional tumors are usually smaller (<1 cm in diameter) at the time of diagnosis; hence they are often called *microadenomas*. Macroadenomas are usually nonfunctional, present with symptoms related to their mass (i.e., headache or visual changes resulting from compression of the optic chiasm), and are larger at the time of diagnosis (usually >1 cm in diameter). Panhypopituitarism may be caused by either tumor type because of compression of normally functioning pituitary gland tissue. Pituitary tumors may also present as *pituitary apoplexy*, which is characterized by the abrupt onset of headache, visual changes, ophthalmoplegia, and altered mental status due to hemorrhage, necrosis, or infarction within the tumor. These tumors can also invade the cavernous sinus or internal carotid artery or compress various cranial nerves, causing an array of symptoms. Treatment depends on tumor type. Prolactinomas may initially be treated medically with bromocriptine. Surgical resection via the transsphenoidal approach or open craniotomy can be curative for most pituitary tumors.

Corticosteroids, such as dexamethasone for nausea and vomiting prophylaxis, should *not* be administered during pituitary tumor resection. Dexamethasone is a potent suppressor of the hypothalamic-pituitary-adrenal axis. Often, serum cortisol is assessed on the day following surgery to screen for postoperative hypopituitarism, and dexamethasone use may result in a false diagnosis of hypopituitarism.

Acoustic Neuroma

The term "acoustic neuroma" is a misnomer insofar as the tumor is usually a benign schwannoma involving the *vestibular* (not auditory) component of cranial nerve VIII within the internal auditory canal. However, bilateral tumors may occur as part of neurofibromatosis type 2 (NF2). Common presenting symptoms include hearing loss, tinnitus, and disequilibrium. Larger tumors that grow out of the internal auditory canal and into the cerebellopontine angle may cause symptoms related to compression of a cranial nerve, especially the facial nerve, or compression of the brainstem. Treatment usually consists of surgical resection with or without radiation therapy. Surgery generally involves intraoperative cranial nerve monitoring with electromyography or brainstem auditory evoked potentials, because resection carries a high risk for cranial nerve injury. Prognosis is usually very good; however, recurrence of tumor is not uncommon.

Central Nervous System Lymphoma

CNS lymphoma is a rare tumor that can arise as a primary brain tumor, known as a *microglioma*, or via metastatic spread from a systemic lymphoma. Primary CNS lymphoma can occur anywhere within the brain but is most common in supratentorial locations, especially in deep gray matter or the corpus callosum. Primary CNS lymphoma is thought to be associated with a variety of systemic disorders, including systemic lupus erythematosus, Sjögren syndrome, rheumatoid arthritis, immunosuppressed states, and infection with Epstein-Barr virus. Symptoms depend on the location of the tumor. Diagnosis is made by imaging as well as biopsy. During biopsy it may be reasonable to wait to administer corticosteroids such as dexamethasone until after pathologic specimens have been obtained, since these tumors may be very sensitive to steroids. Indeed, steroid-associated tumor lysis before a biopsy is performed may result in failure to obtain an adequate sample to make the diagnosis. The mainstay of treatment is chemotherapy (including *intraventricularly delivered* drugs) and whole-brain radiation. Prognosis is poor despite treatment.

Metastatic Tumor

Metastatic brain tumors originate most often from primary sites in the lung or breast. Malignant melanoma, renal cell cancer, and carcinoma of the colon are also likely to spread to the brain. Metastatic brain tumor is the likely diagnosis when more than one intracranial lesion is present. Because of abnormal angiogenesis in metastatic lesions, these tumors tend to bleed more during resection than other CNS tumors.

Management of Anesthesia

Management of anesthesia during tumor resection procedures can be challenging, since patients may be of any age, and a variety of operative positioning issues may arise. Furthermore, some procedures may be conducted with electrophysiologic monitoring, which may have implications for anesthetic drug choices and the use of muscle relaxants. Some procedures may even be performed in awake patients to facilitate resection of a mass located near an eloquent region of brain, such as the motor cortex. Major goals during anesthesia include (1) maintaining adequate cerebral perfusion and oxygenation of normal brain, (2) optimizing operative conditions to facilitate resection, (3) ensuring rapid emergence from anesthesia at the conclusion of the procedure to facilitate neurologic assessment, and (4) accommodating intraoperative electrophysiologic monitoring if needed.

Preoperative Management

Preoperative evaluation of a patient with an intracranial tumor is directed toward identifying the presence or absence of increased ICP. Symptoms of increased ICP include nausea and vomiting, altered level of consciousness, decreased reactivity of the pupils to light, papilledema, bradycardia, systemic hypertension, and breathing disturbances. Evidence of midline shifts (>0.5 cm) on CT or MRI suggests the presence of increased ICP.

Patients with an intracranial pathologic process may be extremely sensitive to the CNS depressant effects of opioids and sedatives. Drug-induced hypoventilation can lead to hypercarbia and further increase ICP. Likewise, drug-induced sedation can mask alterations in the level of consciousness that accompany intracranial hypertension. On the other hand, preoperative sedation can unmask subtle neurologic deficits that may not usually be apparent. This is thought to result from increased sensitivity of injured neurons to the depressant effects of various anesthetic and sedative agents. Considering all the potential adverse effects of preoperative medication, it is prudent to use premedication very sparingly, particularly if the patient is not being continually observed. Preoperative administration of depressant drugs should be avoided in patients with diminished levels of consciousness. In alert adult patients with intracranial tumors, benzodiazepines in small doses can provide anxiety relief without meaningfully affecting ventilation. The decision to administer an anticholinergic drug or histamine 2 receptor antagonist is not influenced by the presence or absence of increased ICP.

Induction of Anesthesia

Anesthesia induction is typically achieved with drugs such as barbiturates or propofol that produce a rapid, reliable onset of unconsciousness without increasing ICP. This can be followed by a nondepolarizing muscle relaxant to facilitate endotracheal intubation. Administration of succinylcholine may be associated with a modest transient increase in ICP. Mechanical hyperventilation is initiated with the goal of decreasing $Paco_2$ to approximately 35 mm Hg. Adequate depth of anesthesia and profound skeletal muscle paralysis should be achieved before laryngoscopy to suppress or eliminate the noxious stimulation or patient movement that can abruptly increase CBF, CBV, and ICP.

Direct laryngoscopy should be accomplished during profound skeletal muscle paralysis as confirmed by a nerve stimulator. Additional doses of IV anesthetic drugs, lidocaine 1.5 mg/kg IV, esmolol, or potent short-acting opioids may help blunt the response to laryngoscopy or other forms of intraoperative stimulation such as placement of pinions or skin incision.

Abrupt sustained increases in systemic blood pressure, particularly in areas of impaired cerebral vasomotor tone, may be accompanied by undesirable increases in CBF, CBV, and ICP and precipitate cerebral edema. Sustained hypotension must also be avoided to prevent brain ischemia. Positive end-expiratory pressure has a highly variable effect on ICP. Hence it should be used with caution, and attention must be paid to changes in ICP, MAP, and CPP as a result of this intervention. The efficacy of brain volume management can be assessed after craniotomy by direct visualization and communication with the surgeon.

Maintenance of Anesthesia

Maintenance of anesthesia in patients undergoing surgical resection of supratentorial brain tumors is often achieved by combining drugs of various classes, including nitrous oxide, volatile anesthetics, opioids, barbiturates, and propofol. Although modest cerebrovascular differences can be demonstrated with different combinations of drugs, there is no evidence that any particular combination is significantly different from another or superior in terms of effects on ICP and short-term patient outcome.

Use of nitrous oxide is controversial if there is any potential for venous air embolism (e.g., in operations performed with patients in the sitting position). Despite theoretical concerns, however, the actual incidence of venous air embolism in sitting patients is not influenced by nitrous oxide use. Once a venous air embolism has been detected, nitrous oxide use must be discontinued because of the concern that the embolus volume will expand and exacerbate the physiologic consequences of the embolus. Both nitrous oxide and potent volatile anesthetics have the potential to increase CBV and ICP as a result of direct cerebral vasodilation. However, low concentrations of volatile anesthetics (0.6–1.0 MAC) may be useful for preventing or treating increases in blood pressure related to noxious surgical stimulation. Nitrous oxide should be avoided if there is concern for preexisting air within the CNS, as may occur after prior craniotomy, spine surgery involving durotomy, basilar skull fracture, or percutaneous instrumentation (e.g., insertion of a ventricular shunt, pneumoencephalography). Nitrous oxide has the potential to expand these spaces limited by either a pressure ceiling equal to the partial pressure of nitrous oxide (e.g., the partial pressure of 50% nitrous oxide is in excess of 300 mm Hg) or a volume multiplier effect (e.g., 2-fold for 50% nitrous oxide; 4-fold for 75% nitrous oxide).

Spontaneous movement by patients undergoing surgical resection of brain tumors must be prevented. Such movement could result in an increase in intracranial volume and ICP, increased surgical bleeding (making surgical exposure difficult), or direct injury to the head and brain from pinions or surgical instrumentation. Therefore in addition to adequate depth of anesthesia, skeletal muscle paralysis is typically maintained during intracranial surgery.

Fluid Therapy

Relatively isoosmolar solutions (e.g., 0.9% sodium chloride or lactated Ringer solution) do not adversely affect brain water or edema formation, provided the blood-brain barrier is intact and they are used in modest amounts. In contrast, free water in hypoosmolar solutions, such as 0.45% sodium chloride, is rapidly distributed throughout body water, including brain water, and may adversely affect ICP management. Hyperosmolar solutions, such as hypertonic saline, initially tend to decrease brain water by increasing the osmolarity of plasma. Regardless of the crystalloid solution selected, any solution administered in large amounts can increase CBV and ICP in patients with brain tumors. Therefore the rate of fluid infusion should be titrated to maintain euvolemia, and measures should be taken to avoid hypervolemia. Intravascular fluid volume depletion caused by blood loss during surgery should be corrected with packed red blood cells or colloid solutions supplemented with balanced salt solutions. Glucose-containing solutions should be avoided, since hyperglycemia in the setting of CNS ischemia will exacerbate neuronal injury and worsen outcome.

Monitoring

Insertion of an intraarterial catheter is useful for continuous monitoring of blood pressure and blood sampling as needed. Capnography can facilitate ventilation and $Paco_2$ management as well as detect venous air embolism. Continuous ICP monitoring, although not routine, can be of value. Nasopharyngeal or esophageal temperature is monitored to prevent hyperthermia or uncontrolled hypothermia. A urinary bladder catheter has utility in managing perioperative fluid balance. It is essential if drug-induced diuresis is planned; if the patient has diabetes insipidus, the syndrome of inappropriate secretion of antidiuretic hormone, or other aberration of salt or water physiology; or if a lengthy surgical procedure is anticipated and bladder distention is a concern.

Intravenous access with large-bore catheters should be obtained, given the likelihood of bleeding and the need for transfusion or rapid administration of fluids. Central venous catheterization can be useful for both IV access and monitoring of fluid status. It also has utility as a means to aspirate intracardiac air following venous air embolism, should this occur during surgery performed with the patient in the sitting position. For this latter purpose, the tip of a multiorifice catheter should be placed at the junction of the superior vena cava and right atrium. The impact of central access for air aspiration is controversial; even in the setting of a large air embolism, the volume of air that can be aspirated from the catheter may not be enough to improve clinical outcome. Transesophageal echocardiography (TEE) can also be useful for procedures in the sitting position to identify intravenous air and help assess cardiac function. Pulmonary artery catheterization can be considered in patients with cardiac disease.

A peripheral nerve stimulator is helpful for monitoring the persistence of drug-induced skeletal muscle paralysis. One must be aware that when paresis or paralysis of an extremity is associated with the brain tumor, the paretic extremity will show resistance (decreased sensitivity) to nondepolarizing muscle relaxants compared with a normal extremity (Fig. 13.4). These altered muscle responses to neuromuscular blockers most likely reflect the proliferation of acetylcholine-responsive cholinergic receptors that can occur after muscle denervation. Therefore monitoring of skeletal muscle paralysis on the paretic limb may provide misleading information. For example, the response to nerve stimulation on a paretic limb may be erroneously interpreted as inadequate skeletal muscle paralysis. Likewise, at the conclusion of surgery the nerve stimulator response could be interpreted as indicating better recovery from neuromuscular blockade than actually exists.

Monitoring of electrocardiographic (ECG) activity is necessary to detect responses related to intracranial tumors or surgery. ECG changes can reflect increased ICP or, more importantly, surgical retraction or manipulation of the brainstem or cranial nerves. Indeed, the cardiovascular centers, respiratory control areas, and nuclei of the lower cranial nerves lie in close proximity in the brainstem. Manipulation of the brainstem may produce systemic hypertension and bradycardia or hypotension and tachycardia. Cardiac dysrhythmias range from acute sinus dysrhythmia to ventricular premature beats or ventricular tachycardia.

Postoperative Management

Ideally the effects of anesthetics and muscle relaxants should be dissipated or pharmacologically reversed at the conclusion

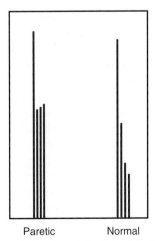

FIG. 13.4 In a surgical patient with mild residual hemiparesis after stroke, the train-of-four ratio recorded from the paretic arm (0.6) is higher than that recorded from the normal arm (0.3), which reflects resistance of the paretic arm to the effects of nondepolarizing muscle relaxants. (Adapted from Moorthy SS, Hilgenberg JC. Resistance to nondepolarizing muscle relaxants in paretic upper extremities of patients with residual hemiplegia. *Anesth Analg.* 1980;59:624-627.)

of surgery. This facilitates immediate assessment of neurologic status and recognition of any adverse events related to the surgery. It is important to have patients awaken with little reaction to the presence of the endotracheal tube. Intraoperative use of opioids may aid in attenuating the patient's response to the endotracheal tube and facilitate optimal timing of extubation. However, it must be appreciated that opioids as well as the local anesthetic lidocaine (which also has general anesthetic properties when given IV or via the trachea) can produce CNS depression. As such, both the dose and timing of these drugs can confound attempts at smooth extubation of the trachea.

In patients in whom consciousness was depressed preoperatively or new neurologic deficits are anticipated as a result of surgery, it may be best to delay tracheal extubation until return of airway reflexes is confirmed and spontaneous ventilation is sufficient to prevent carbon dioxide retention. Hypothermia may be a cause of slow awakening. Other causes of delayed emergence from anesthesia include residual neuromuscular block, residual effects of drugs with sedative effects (i.e., opioids, benzodiazepines, volatile anesthetics), or a primary CNS event such as ischemia, hematoma, or tension pneumocephalus.

Following general anesthesia, a preexisting neurologic deficit may be exacerbated by the sedative effects of anesthetic drugs, which makes a subtle preoperative deficit appear more severe. This *differential awakening* is thought to be due to increased sensitivity of injured neurons to the depressant effects of anesthetic agents. Often these deficits will disappear and neurologic function will return to its baseline state with time. Any persistent new deficit that does not quickly resolve must be further investigated.

Sitting Position and Venous Air Embolism

Craniotomy to remove a supratentorial tumor is usually performed with the patient in the supine position with the head elevated 10–15 degrees to facilitate cerebral venous drainage. Infratentorial tumors have more unusual patient positioning requirements and may be performed with the patient in the lateral, prone, or sitting position.

The sitting position deserves special attention because it has a variety of implications for management of anesthesia. The sitting position is often used for exploration of the posterior cranial fossa, and it may be employed to resect intracranial tumors, clip aneurysms, decompress cranial nerves, or implant electrodes for cerebellar stimulation. In addition, it may be used for surgery on the cervical spine and posterior cervical musculature. Advantages of the sitting position include excellent surgical exposure and enhanced cerebral venous and CSF drainage, which minimizes blood loss and reduces ICP. These advantages are offset by the decreases in systemic blood pressure and cardiac output produced by this position, and the potential hazard of venous air embolism. For these reasons the lateral or prone position is often selected as an alternative. However, so long as no contraindication to the sitting position exists (e.g., a patent foramen ovale), the outcome of patients undergoing surgery in the sitting position is similar or superior to that of patients placed in other positions.

If the sitting position is used, one should account for the effect of hydrostatic pressure gradients on CPP. Specifically, CPP should reflect correction for the hydrostatic pressure difference between the heart and brain. This is generally accomplished by measuring blood pressure via an intraarterial catheter and referencing the pressure transducer to the vertical height of the external auditory meatus, which approximates the position of the circle of Willis. Lack of correction for hydrostatic pressure may put the patient at undue risk of cerebral hypoperfusion, since the measured systemic blood pressure—but not necessarily the true pressure at the level of the brain—will be greater if the transducer is referenced at the level of the heart.

Venous air embolism is a potential hazard whenever the operative site is above the level of the heart, so that pressure in the exposed veins is subatmospheric. Although this complication is most often associated with neurosurgical procedures, venous air embolism may also occur during operations involving the neck, thorax, abdomen, and pelvis and during open heart surgery, repair of liver and vena cava lacerations, obstetric and gynecologic procedures, and total hip replacement. Patients undergoing intracranial surgery are at increased risk not only because the operative site is above the level of the heart but also because veins in the skull and intracranial venous sinuses may not collapse when cut owing to their attachment to bone or dura. Indeed, the cut edge of cranial bone, including that associated with burr holes, is a common site for air entry into veins.

When air enters the right atrium and ventricle, there is interference with right-sided cardiac output and blood flow into the pulmonary artery. Air that eventually enters the pulmonary artery may trigger reflex bronchoconstriction and pulmonary edema. Death is usually secondary to an air lock in the right ventricular outflow tract that causes right-sided cardiac output to severely decrease, acute cor pulmonale to develop, and hypoxemia to occur from the combined cardiac and pulmonary insults.

Small quantities of air can sometimes pass through pulmonary vessels to reach the coronary and cerebral circulations. Large quantities of air can travel directly to the systemic circulation via right-to-left intracardiac shunts created by a patent foramen ovale or septal defects. This passage of air from the right to left circulation is known as *paradoxical air embolism*. Basically a venous embolism becomes an arterial embolism. A known patent foramen ovale or other cardiac defects that could result in a right-to-left shunt are contraindications to use of the sitting position.

Fatal air embolism subsequent to entrainment of systemic venous air has occurred even in the absence of identifiable shunts or intracardiac defects. This may occur because of failure of contrast echocardiography to detect an existing patent foramen ovale or septal defect. There are many theoretical reasons for this failure of detection. One is that Valsalva or other provocative maneuvers are not always successful in mimicking the physiologic changes that occur during general anesthesia and true venous air embolism, and for this reason may underestimate the potential for venous air to pass from the right to the left circulation. Use of the sitting position inherently predisposes neurosurgical patients to paradoxical air embolism because the normal interatrial pressure gradient may become reversed in this position, and the gradients may vary within the cardiac cycle.

When the likelihood of venous air embolism is increased, it is useful but not mandatory to place a right atrial catheter before beginning surgery. Death caused by paradoxical air embolism results from obstruction of the coronary arteries by air, which leads to myocardial ischemia and ventricular fibrillation. Neurologic damage may follow air embolism to the brain.

Early detection of venous air embolism is important for successful treatment. A Doppler ultrasonographic transducer placed over the right cardiac structures is one of the most sensitive detectors of intracardiac air. However, this device cannot provide information regarding the volume of air that has entered the venous circulation, and commonly the transducer detects small amounts of air that are clinically unimportant. TEE by comparison is useful for assessing both the presence and quantity of intracardiac air. A sudden decrease in end-tidal carbon dioxide tension may reflect increased alveolar dead space and/or diminished cardiac output resulting from air embolism. An increase in right atrial and pulmonary artery pressure can reflect acute cor pulmonale and correlates with abrupt decreases in end-tidal carbon dioxide tension. Although end-tidal carbon dioxide tension changes are less sensitive indicators of the presence of air than the findings of Doppler ultrasonography or TEE, they reflect the size of the venous air embolism. Increases in end-tidal nitrogen can identify and partially quantify the presence of venous air embolism. Changes in end-tidal nitrogen tension may precede decreased end-tidal carbon dioxide tension or increased pulmonary artery pressures. During controlled ventilation, sudden attempts by the patient to initiate spontaneous breaths (*gasp reflex*) may be the first indication of venous air embolism. Hypotension, tachycardia, cardiac dysrhythmias, and cyanosis are late signs of venous air embolism. Detection of the characteristic *mill wheel murmur,* as heard through an esophageal stethoscope, is a late sign of catastrophic venous air embolism.

Once a venous air embolism is detected, the surgeon should flood the operative site with fluid, apply occlusive material to all bone edges, and attempt to identify any other sources of air entry such as perforation of a venous sinus. Aspiration of air should be attempted through the right atrial catheter. The ideal location for the tip of the right atrial catheter is controversial, but evidence suggests that the junction of the superior vena cava with the right atrium is preferable. Multiorifice right atrial catheters permit aspiration of larger amounts of air than do single-orifice catheters. Because of its small lumen and slow speed of blood return, a pulmonary artery catheter is not very useful for aspirating air but may provide additional evidence that venous air embolism has occurred. Administration

of nitrous oxide is promptly discontinued to avoid increasing the size of any venous air bubbles. Indeed, elimination of nitrous oxide from the inhaled gases after detection of a venous air embolism often results in decreased pulmonary artery pressures. Pure oxygen is substituted for nitrous oxide. Direct jugular venous compression may increase venous pressure at the surgical site entraining air, but the use of positive end-expiratory pressure to accomplish this same effect has not been shown to be of value.

Extreme hypotension from massive air embolism may require support of the blood pressure using vasoactive drugs with vasoconstrictive and inotropic properties. Bronchospasm is treated with β_2-adrenergic agonists delivered by aerosol. Placing the patient in the supine position in cases of severe air embolism can be useful because it will lead to an increase in venous pressure, decrease further air entrainment, and allow for effective resuscitation. If the patient is to be put in the supine position, the Mayfield head holder should be disengaged from the arch frame so as to not injure the cervical spine during movement. Although the traditional admonition is to treat venous air embolism by placing the patient in the left lateral decubitus position, this is rarely possible or safe during intracranial surgery. It is likely that attempting to attain this patient position would lose valuable time that would be better spent aspirating air and supporting the circulation.

After successful treatment of small or modest venous air embolism, the surgical procedure can be resumed. However, the decision to reinstitute use of nitrous oxide must be individualized. If nitrous oxide is not used, maintenance of an adequate depth of anesthesia requires administration of larger doses of volatile or IV anesthetics. If nitrous oxide is added to the inhaled gases, it is possible residual air in the circulation could again produce symptoms.

Hyperbaric therapy may be useful in the treatment of both severe venous air embolism and paradoxical air embolism. Transfer of patients to a hyperbaric chamber in an attempt to decrease the size of air bubbles and improve blood flow is likely to be helpful only if the transfer can be accomplished within 8 hours.

The postoperative complications that may occur after posterior fossa craniotomy include apnea due to hematoma formation, tension pneumocephalus, and cranial nerve injuries. Macroglossia is also a possibility and is presumably due to impaired venous and lymphatic drainage from the tongue. This is sometimes associated with excessive neck flexion and may be influenced by the simultaneous use of multiple oral instruments (e.g., endotracheal tube, oral airway, esophageal stethoscope, TEE probe).

DISORDERS RELATED TO VEGETATIVE BRAIN FUNCTION

Coma

Coma is a state of profound unconsciousness produced by drugs, disease, or injury affecting the CNS. It is usually caused by dysfunction of regions of the brain that are responsible for maintaining consciousness, such as the pontine reticular activating system, midbrain, or cerebral hemispheres. The causes of coma are many and can be divided into two groups: structural lesions (i.e., tumor, stroke, abscess, intracranial bleeding) and diffuse disorders (i.e., hypothermia, hypoglycemia, hepatic or uremic encephalopathy, postictal state following seizures, encephalitis, drug effects). The most common means used to assess the overall severity of coma is the Glasgow Coma Scale (Table 13.1).

Initial management of any comatose patient involves establishing a patent airway and ensuring adequacy of oxygenation, ventilation, and circulation. One should then attempt to determine the cause of coma. This attempt should begin with obtaining a medical history from family members or caretakers if possible and conducting a physical examination followed by diagnostic studies. Blood pressure and heart rate assessments are important because they might suggest a cause such as hypothermia. Respiratory patterns can also aid in diagnosis. Irregular breathing patterns may reflect an abnormality at a specific site in the CNS (Table 13.2). Ataxic breathing is characterized by a completely random pattern of tidal volumes that results from disruption of medullary neural pathways by trauma, hemorrhage, or compression by tumors. Lesions in the pons may result in apneustic breathing characterized by prolonged *end-inspiratory* pauses maintained for as long as 30 seconds. Occlusion of the basilar artery leading to pontine infarction is a common cause of apneustic breathing. Cheyne-Stokes breathing is characterized by breaths of progressively increasing and then decreasing tidal volume (crescendo-decrescendo pattern) followed by periods of apnea lasting 15–20 seconds. This pattern of breathing may reflect brain injury in the cerebral hemispheres or basal ganglia or may be due to arterial hypoxemia and congestive heart failure. In the presence of congestive heart failure, the delay in circulation from the pulmonary capillaries to the carotid bodies is presumed to be responsible for the Cheyne-Stokes breathing pattern. Central neurogenic hyperventilation is most often due to acute neurologic insults that are associated with cerebral thrombosis, embolism, or closed head injury. Hyperventilation is spontaneous and may be so severe that the $Paco_2$ is decreased to less than 20 mm Hg. The basic neurologic examination can be the key to diagnosis and should, at a minimum, include examination of the pupils and pupillary responses to light, function of the extraocular muscles via reflexes, and gross motor responses in the extremities (Table 13.3).

Under normal conditions, pupils are usually 3–4 mm in diameter, equal bilaterally, and react briskly to light. However,

TABLE 13.1 Glasgow Coma Scale

Response	Score
EYE OPENING	
Spontaneous	4
To speech	3
To pain	2
Nil	1
BEST MOTOR RESPONSE	
Obeys	6
Localizes	5
Withdraws (flexion)	4
Abnormal flexion	3
Extensor response	2
Nil	1
VERBAL RESPONSES	
Oriented	5
Confused conversation	4
Inappropriate words	3
Incomprehensible sounds	2
Nil	1

TABLE 13.2 Abnormal Patterns of Breathing

Abnormality	Pattern	Site of Lesion/Condition
Ataxic (Biot) breathing	Unpredictable sequence of breaths varying in rate and tidal volume	Medulla
Apneustic breathing	Gasps and prolonged pauses at full inspiration	Pons
Cheyne-Stokes breathing	Cyclic crescendo-decrescendo tidal volume pattern interrupted by apnea	Cerebral hemispheres Congestive heart failure
Central neurogenic hyperventilation	Marked hyperventilation	Cerebral thrombosis or embolism
Posthyperventilation apnea	Awake apnea following moderate decreases in $Paco_2$	Frontal lobes

TABLE 13.3 Neurologic Findings Due to Compression of Brainstem During Transtentorial Herniation

Region of Compression	Pupillary Examination	Response to Oculocephalic or Cold Caloric Testing	Gross Motor Findings
Diencephalon	Small pupils (2 mm) reactive to light	Normal	Purposeful, semipurposeful, or decorticate (flexor) posturing
Midbrain	Midsize pupils (5 mm) unreactive to light	May be impaired	Decerebrate (extensor) posturing
Pons or medulla oblongata	Midsize pupils (5 mm) unreactive to light	Absent	No response

Adapted from Aminoff MJ, Greenberg DA, Simon RP. *Clinical Neurology*. 3rd ed. Stamford, CT: Appleton & Lange; 1996:291.

approximately 20% of the general population normally has physiologic anisocoria—that is, a slight (<1 mm) difference in the diameters of the pupils. Compression of the diencephalon (thalamic and hypothalamic structures) leads to small (2 mm) but reactive pupils, probably resulting from interruption of descending sympathetic fibers. Unresponsive midsize pupils (5 mm) usually indicate midbrain compression. A fixed and dilated pupil (>7 mm) usually indicates oculomotor nerve compression and can be seen with brain herniation as well as with anticholinergic or sympathomimetic drug intoxication. Pinpoint pupils (1 mm) usually indicate opioid or organophosphate intoxication, focal pontine lesions, or neurosyphilis.

Evaluation of the function of the extraocular muscles allows assessment of the function of the oculomotor, trochlear, and abducens nerves (cranial nerves III, IV, and VI) and, indirectly, brainstem function. In the comatose patient this testing can be performed by means of passive head rotation (oculocephalic reflex or doll's eye maneuver) or by cold water irrigation of the tympanic membrane (oculovestibular reflex or cold caloric testing). In unresponsive patients with normal brainstem function, oculocephalic maneuvers will produce full conjugate horizontal eye movements. Eliciting the oculovestibular reflex will result in tonic conjugate eye movements toward the side of cold water irrigation of the external auditory canal. Unilateral oculomotor nerve or midbrain lesions will result in failed adduction but intact contralateral abduction. Complete absence of responses can indicate pontine lesions or diffuse disorders.

Evaluation of motor responses to painful stimuli can also be helpful in localizing the cause of coma. Patients with mild to moderate diffuse brain dysfunction above the level of the diencephalon will usually react with purposeful or semipurposeful movements toward the painful stimulus. Unilateral reactions may indicate unilateral lesions such as stroke or tumor. Decorticate responses to pain consist of flexion of the elbow, adduction of the shoulder, and extension of the knee and ankle, and they are usually indicative of diencephalic dysfunction. Decerebrate responses consist of extension of the elbow, internal rotation of the forearm, and leg extension and imply more severe brain dysfunction. Patients with pontine or medullary lesions often exhibit no response to painful stimuli.

In cases in which the cause of coma is unknown, useful discriminatory laboratory tests include measurement of serum electrolytes and blood glucose concentrations to assess for disorders of sodium and glucose as well as the anion gap. Liver and renal function tests help evaluate for hepatic or uremic encephalopathy. Drug and toxicology screens may help identify exogenous intoxicants. A complete blood cell count (CBC) and results of coagulation studies may suggest the risk of intracranial bleeding from thrombocytopenia or coagulopathy. CT or MRI may reveal a structural cause such as tumor or stroke. A lumbar puncture can be performed if meningitis or subarachnoid hemorrhage is suspected.

Outcomes for patients in comatose states depend on many factors but are usually related to the cause and extent of injury to brain tissue.

Management of Anesthesia

Comatose patients may be brought to the operating suite either for treatment of the cause of the coma (e.g., burr hole drainage of an intracranial hematoma) or for treatment of injuries related to the comatose state (e.g., bone fractures caused by a motor vehicle accident in an intoxicated patient).

It is important for the anesthesia provider to be aware of the likely cause of the coma, since anesthetic management will vary depending on the cause as well as the type of planned surgery. Primary overall goals should be to safely establish an airway, provide adequate cerebral perfusion and oxygenation, and optimize operating conditions. Careful attention should be paid to avoiding increases in ICP during stimulating events. Treatments should be instituted to decrease elevations in baseline ICP. Intracranial monitoring may be helpful. Intraarterial catheterization is useful for blood pressure optimization as well as management of hyperventilation if needed. Anesthetic agents that increase ICP (e.g., halothane, ketamine) should be avoided, but other potent volatile agents such as isoflurane and sevoflurane used at low doses (<1 MAC) in combination with IV cerebral vasoconstrictive anesthetics are acceptable. Desflurane should be used with caution because it may increase ICP. Nitrous oxide should be avoided if the patient has known or suspected pneumocephalus (e.g., after recent intracranial surgery or basilar skull fracture). Administration of nondepolarizing muscle relaxants helps facilitate tracheal intubation and patient positioning; however, succinylcholine should be used with caution, since it may transiently increase ICP or potentially cause hyperkalemia in the setting of motor deficits.

Brain Death and Organ Donation

Brain death is defined as the permanent cessation of total brain function. The traditional criteria used to define brain death, which are an adaptation of the original Harvard criteria established in 1968, are as follows:

Coma of an established and irreversible cause. All listed tests and assessments of reflexes should be performed after all possible reversible causes of coma have been ruled out.

1. Lack of spontaneous movement, with the recognition that spinal reflexes may remain intact
2. Lack of all cranial nerve reflexes and function. This includes the failure of heart rate to increase by more than 5 beats per minute in response to intravenously (preferably centrally) administered 0.04 mg/kg atropine, which suggests loss of vagal nuclear, and thus tonic vagal nerve, function.
3. Positive result on an apnea test indicating lack of function of the respiratory control nuclei in the brainstem. The test is performed by initially ensuring a $Paco_2$ of 40 ± 5 mm Hg and an arterial pH of 7.35–7.45. The patient is then ventilated with 100% oxygen for at least 10 minutes. Then while vital signs are monitored and the trachea is insufflated with 100% oxygen, mechanical ventilation is discontinued for 10 minutes. Arterial blood gas values are obtained at 5 and 10

minutes following cessation of mechanical ventilation, and the patient is observed for signs of spontaneous respiration. Given that hypercarbia ($Paco_2 > 60$ mm Hg) is a potent stimulus for ventilation, if no respiratory activity is noted, the result of the apnea test is deemed positive.

Other confirmatory test results include an isoelectric EEG and absence of CBF as demonstrated by various techniques, including transcranial Doppler ultrasonography, cerebral angiography, and MR angiography. Of note, it may be difficult to document an isoelectric EEG if the patient is within an "electrically noisy" environment (e.g., intensive care unit [ICU] or operating room), because it will be difficult to discriminate between extraneous electrical noise and brain electrical activity.

Once the diagnosis of brain death has been established and discussions with the immediate family, legal guardian, or next of kin have taken place, the decision is made either to withdraw artificial means of cardiopulmonary support or to proceed to organ retrieval if that was the wish of the patient or is the desire of the family or legal guardian.

Management of Anesthesia

The major goal when patients diagnosed with brain death undergo surgery for multiorgan retrieval is to optimize oxygenation and perfusion of the organs to be retrieved. It is important to be aware of the various physiologic sequelae of brain death and direct physiologic and pharmacologic management with the needs of the organ recipient, not the donor, in mind. Because of loss of central hemodynamic regulatory mechanisms—that is, the presence of neurogenic shock—brain-dead patients are often hypotensive. Hypovolemia caused by diabetes insipidus, third space losses, or drugs can contribute to hypotension. Aggressive fluid resuscitation should be considered, with efforts made to avoid hypervolemia, which could lead to pulmonary edema, cardiac distention, or hepatic congestion. Vasoconstrictor drugs should be avoided when considering pharmacologic treatment of hypotension. Inotropic agents are preferred for this. Dopamine and dobutamine should be first-line drugs for the treatment of hypotension in euvolemic patients, with low-dose epinephrine as a second-line agent. For those in whom the heart is to be retrieved, catecholamine doses should be minimized because of the theoretical risk of catecholamine-induced cardiomyopathy. ECG abnormalities such as ST-segment and T-wave changes, as well as dysrhythmias, can occur. Causes include electrolyte abnormalities, loss of vagal nerve function, and cardiac contusion (if death was trauma related). Dysrhythmias should be treated pharmacologically or by electrical pacing.

Hypoxemia can occur as a result of diminished cardiac output or multiple pulmonary factors such as aspiration, edema, contusion, or atelectasis. Inspired oxygen concentration and ventilatory parameters should be adjusted in an attempt to maintain normoxia and normocapnia. Excessive positive end-expiratory pressure should be avoided because of its effect on cardiac output as well as the risk of barotrauma in the setting of possible trauma-related lung injury. Oxygen delivery to tissues should be optimized by treating coagulopathy and anemia with blood products.

Diabetes insipidus frequently occurs in brain-dead patients and if not treated can lead to hypovolemia, hyperosmolality, and electrolyte abnormalities that could contribute to hypotension and cardiac dysrhythmias. Treatment should initially include volume replacement with hypotonic solutions titrated to volume status and electrolyte concentrations. In severe cases, patients may need inotropic support and either vasopressin (0.04–0.1 units/h IV) or desmopressin (1–4 µg IV) to treat the diabetes insipidus. Because of its vasoconstrictor properties, vasopressin use should be minimized to avoid end-organ ischemia. A vasodilator such as nitroprusside may be administered with the vasopressin to avoid vasopressin-induced hypertension and vasoconstriction in end organs.

Because of loss of temperature-regulatory mechanisms, brain-dead patients tend to become poikilothermic and will require measures to avoid hypothermia. Although mild hypothermia possibly provides some degree of organ protection, it can also result in cardiac dysrhythmias, coagulopathy, and reduced oxygen delivery to tissue, thus potentially causing harm to the organs to be retrieved. A good rule of thumb for the management of patients for organ donation is the *rule of 100s:* systolic blood pressure greater than 100 mm Hg, urine output greater than 100 mL/h, Pao_2 greater than 100 mm Hg, and hemoglobin level greater than 100 g/L.

CEREBROVASCULAR DISEASE

Stroke is characterized by sudden neurologic deficits resulting from ischemia (88% of cases) or hemorrhage (12% of cases) (Table 13.4). In the United States, stroke is the fourth leading cause of death, and survivors of stroke represent the patient group with the highest rate of major disability. The pathogenesis of stroke differs among ethnic groups. Extracranial carotid artery disease and heart disease–associated embolism more commonly cause ischemic stroke in non-Hispanic whites, whereas intracranial thromboembolic disease is more common in African Americans. Women have lower stroke rates than men at all ages until age 75 years and older. Stroke rates are at their highest after age 75. In developed countries, stroke-related mortality has decreased over the past several decades, probably because of better control of co-existing diseases such as hypertension and diabetes, smoking cessation, and greater awareness of stroke risk factors and the clinical cues of stroke onset (allowing faster initiation of treatment).

Other stroke-related disorders of the cerebrovascular system include atherosclerotic disease of the carotid artery, cerebral aneurysm, arteriovenous malformation (AVM), and Moyamoya disease.

Cerebrovascular Anatomy

Blood supply to the brain is via two pairs of arteries: the internal carotid arteries and the vertebral arteries (Fig. 13.5). These

TABLE 13.4	Characteristics of Stroke Subtypes				
Parameter	Systemic Hypoperfusion	Embolism	Thrombosis	Subarachnoid Hemorrhage	Intracerebral Hemorrhage
Risk factors	Hypotension Hemorrhage Cardiac arrest	Smoking Ischemic heart disease Peripheral vascular disease Diabetes mellitus White race and male gender	Smoking Ischemic heart disease Peripheral vascular disease Diabetes mellitus White race and male gender	Often none Hypertension Coagulopathy Drugs Trauma	Hypertension Coagulopathy Drugs Trauma
Onset	Parallels risk factors	Sudden	Often preceded by transient ischemic attack	Sudden, often during exertion	Gradually progressive
Signs and symptoms	Pallor Diaphoresis Hypotension	Headache	Headache	Headache Vomiting Transient loss of consciousness	Headache Vomiting Decreased level of consciousness Seizures
Imaging	CT (hypodensity) MRI	CT (hypodensity) MRI	CT (hypodensity) MRI	CT (hyperdensity) MRI	CT (hyperdensity) MRI

Adapted from Caplan LR. Diagnosis and treatment of ischemic stroke. *JAMA*. 1991;266:2413-2418.

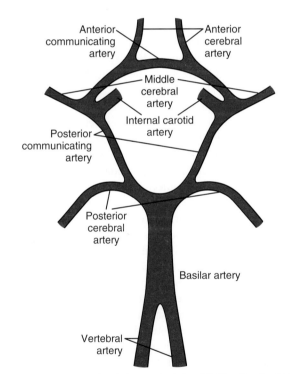

FIG. 13.5 Cerebral circulation and circle of Willis. Cerebral blood supply is from the vertebral arteries (arising from the subclavian arteries) and the internal carotid arteries (arising from the common carotid arteries).

blood vessels join on the inferior surface of the brain to form the circle of Willis, which under ideal circumstances provides collateral circulation to multiple areas of the brain. Unfortunately all the elements of an intact circle of Willis are present and functional in only about one-third of people; some segments may be hypoplastic or absent in the rest. Each internal

carotid artery gives rise to an anterior cerebral artery and continues on to become a middle cerebral artery. These vessels arising from the carotid arteries comprise the *anterior circulation* and ultimately supply the frontal, parietal, and lateral temporal lobes, the basal ganglia, and most of the internal capsule. The vertebral arteries each give rise to a posterior-inferior cerebellar artery before converging at the level of the pons to form the basilar artery. The basilar artery generally gives rise to two anterior-inferior and two superior cerebellar arteries before dividing to become the paired posterior cerebral arteries. Vessels that receive their predominant blood supply from this vertebral-basilar system comprise the *posterior circulation* and typically supply the brainstem, occipital lobes, cerebellum, medial portions of the temporal lobes, and most of the thalamus. The anterior and posterior circulations communicate via the posterior communicating artery, and the left and right anterior cerebral arteries communicate via the anterior communicating artery. Occlusion of specific arteries distal to the circle of Willis results in predictable clinical neurologic deficits (Table 13.5).

Acute Ischemic Stroke

Patients who experience the sudden onset of neurologic dysfunction or describe neurologic signs and symptoms evolving over minutes to hours are most likely experiencing a stroke. A *transient ischemic attack* (TIA) is a sudden vascular-related focal neurologic deficit that resolves promptly (within 24 hours). A TIA is not considered a separate entity but rather evidence of an impending ischemic stroke. Stroke represents a medical emergency, and the prognosis depends on the time elapsed from the onset of symptoms to thrombolytic intervention if thrombosis is the cause of the symptoms. Patients who

TABLE 13.5	Clinical Features of Cerebrovascular Occlusive Syndromes
Occluded Artery	**Clinical Features**
Anterior cerebral artery	Contralateral leg weakness
Middle cerebral artery	Contralateral hemiparesis and hemisensory deficit (face and arm more than leg)
	Aphasia (dominant hemisphere)
	Contralateral visual field defect
Posterior cerebral artery	Contralateral visual field defect
	Contralateral hemiparesis
Penetrating arteries	Contralateral hemiparesis
	Contralateral hemisensory deficits
Basilar artery	Oculomotor deficits and/or ataxia with crossed sensory and motor deficits
Vertebral artery	Lower cranial nerve deficits and/or ataxia with crossed sensory deficits

Adapted from Morgenstern LB, Kasner SE. Cerebrovascular disorders. *Sci Am Med.* 2000:1–15.

receive early treatment to restore cerebral perfusion have better outcomes.

Systemic hypertension is the most significant risk factor for acute ischemic stroke, and long-term treatment of systolic or diastolic hypertension dramatically reduces the risk of a first stroke. Cigarette smoking, hyperlipidemia, diabetes mellitus, excessive alcohol consumption, and increased serum homocysteine concentrations are also associated with increased risk of acute ischemic stroke.

In patients with suspected stroke the brain should be imaged using noncontrast CT, which reliably distinguishes acute intracerebral hemorrhage from ischemia. This distinction is important because treatment of hemorrhagic stroke is substantially different from treatment of ischemic stroke. CT is relatively insensitive to ischemic changes during the first few hours after a stroke but is very sensitive for detection of intracranial bleeding.

Conventional angiography is useful for demonstrating arterial occlusion. The vasculature can also be visualized noninvasively using CT or MR angiography. Alternatively, transcranial Doppler ultrasonography can provide indirect evidence of major vascular occlusion and offers the advantage of real-time bedside monitoring in patients undergoing thrombolytic therapy.

The etiologies of acute ischemic stroke are categorized according to the TOAST classification (*Trial of Org 10172 in Acute Stroke Treatment*) into 5 groups:
1. large-artery atherosclerosis
2. cardioembolism
3. small-vessel occlusion (e.g., lacunar stroke)
4. stroke of other determined etiology (e.g., stroke due to hypercoagulable states or vasculopathy)
5. stroke of undetermined etiology

Management of Acute Ischemic Stroke

Aspirin by mouth is often recommended as initial therapy in patients with an acute ischemic stroke and for prevention of recurrent stroke. Intravenous recombinant tissue plasminogen activator (tPA) is used in patients who meet specific eligibility requirements and in whom treatment can be initiated within a limited time window from the onset of acute symptoms (due to concern for hemorrhagic transformation). Direct infusion of thrombolytic drugs (prourokinase or recombinant tPA) into occluded blood vessels is a potential alternative or adjunctive therapy to IV administration of recombinant tPA. Despite advances in the treatment of acute ischemic stroke, most patients will have residual neurologic dysfunction. The initial stroke severity is a strong predictor of outcome, and early evidence of recovery is a good prognostic sign.

Management of the airway, oxygenation, ventilation, systemic blood pressure, blood glucose concentration, and body temperature are part of the overall medical management of acute ischemic stroke. In the most critically ill stroke patients, cerebral edema and increased ICP may complicate the clinical course. Expanding cerebral infarction may cause focal or diffuse mass effects that typically peak 2–5 days following stroke onset. Large hemispheric strokes may be characterized by *malignant middle cerebral artery syndrome,* in which the edematous infarcted tissue causes compression of the anterior and posterior cerebral arteries and results in secondary infarctions. Similarly, infarction of the cerebellum may result in basilar artery compression and brainstem ischemia. Mortality rates for both middle cerebral artery syndrome and infarction of the cerebellum approach 80%.

Surgical decompression has a role in a small number of stroke patients. Craniotomy with cerebellar resection is a lifesaving intervention for acute cerebellar stroke, because it prevents secondary brainstem and vascular compression. Malignant middle cerebral artery syndrome may be amenable to treatment with hemicraniectomy.

Respiratory function must be evaluated promptly in all stroke patients. Ventilatory drive is usually intact except after massive hemispheric infarction or infarction of the medulla. The ability to protect the lungs from aspiration may be impaired in the acute setting, so tracheal intubation may be necessary. In most patients, however, supplemental oxygen administration without endotracheal intubation is sufficient to maintain arterial oxygen saturation above 95%.

Maintenance of adequate blood pressure is critically important because blood flow to ischemic regions is dependent on CPP. Systemic hypertension is common at the time of initial stroke presentation, and rapid lowering of blood pressure can impair CBF and worsen the ischemic injury. Hypertension often gradually decreases during the first few days following an acute stroke. Antihypertensive drug therapy, such as small IV doses of labetalol, may be used when necessary to maintain the systemic blood pressure below 220/120 mm Hg. Following revascularization, blood pressure targets should be lower to minimize risk for hemorrhagic transformation. A blood pressure below 180/105 mm Hg is recommended during this time. Appropriate intravascular volume replacement in patients with acute stroke improves cardiac output and cerebral perfusion. Hypervolemic hemodilution may be considered in an attempt to increase CBF while decreasing blood viscosity without causing a significant decrease in oxygen delivery.

Hyperglycemia appears to parallel poor outcomes in patients experiencing acute ischemic stroke. During periods of cellular hypoxia or anoxia, as occur with stroke, glucose is metabolized to lactic acid, which results in tissue acidosis and increased tissue injury. Normalization of blood glucose concentration is recommended, using insulin when appropriate. Parenteral administration of glucose should be avoided.

Based on animal data, hypothermia may improve outcomes following acute ischemic stroke, owing to its ability to decrease neuronal oxygen demands, cerebral edema, and neurotransmitter-associated toxicity. However, there are few human studies evaluating the effectiveness of hypothermia for reduction of morbidity and mortality from acute stroke; use of hypothermia in this setting continues to be controversial. It *is* certain that fever must be avoided in patients with acute stroke. Even a mild increase in body temperature can be deleterious. Normothermia should be maintained in acute ischemic stroke patients using antipyretics or cooling blankets as necessary.

Prophylaxis to prevent deep vein thrombosis is initiated early in the treatment of patients experiencing acute ischemic stroke. Heparin 5000 units subcutaneously every 12 hours is the most common intervention. Patients with acute hemorrhage who cannot be given heparin are treated with pneumatic compression stockings.

Patients undergoing radiologic-guided revascularization procedures for acute ischemic stroke may require sedation or general anesthesia to facilitate the procedure. The decision to provide sedation or general anesthesia mostly depends on the severity of stroke. Patients with greater neurologic deficits may be unable to remain motionless. They may also be more likely to require airway management owing to the inability to protect their airway, thus necessitating a general anesthetic. However, general anesthesia in this setting is associated with greater morbidity and mortality than sedation. This outcome difference is likely due to multiple factors, including a selection bias in which patients with greater stroke severity are more likely to require general anesthesia to facilitate the procedure, as well as potentially injurious lower blood pressures that are more likely to occur with general anesthesia.

Perioperative and Periprocedural Stroke

Most perioperative strokes are ischemic, and patients undergoing cardiac, neurologic, and major vascular surgery are at greatest risk for stroke. Invasive radiologic procedures to the heart and major arteries also carry a risk for periprocedural stroke. The higher incidence of stroke in these patient populations is related to (1) a higher incidence of baseline stroke risk factors (e.g., hypertension, atherosclerosis, diabetes mellitus) in these patients, (2) risks of perioperative cerebral embolism

(e.g., open cardiac procedures, invasive radiologic procedures to the cerebrovasculature), and (3) acute alterations in systemic physiology, including systemic or regional hypotension resulting in impairment of blood flow.

Patients having noncardiovascular and nonneurologic surgery or procedures are still at risk for perioperative stroke ($\approx$0.1% for adults). Patients having amputations, abdominal exploration, or small bowel resection are at greatest risk. Other risk factors include increasing age, myocardial infarction within 6 months, renal dysfunction, history of stroke or TIA, hypertension, chronic obstructive pulmonary disease, smoking, and preoperative or intraoperative metoprolol use. β-Blockers, especially metoprolol, should be used with caution in the perioperative period and titrated carefully to avoid hypotension.

Patients who suffer a perioperative stroke have an 8-fold increased risk for death within 30 days of surgery compared to those who do not suffer a stroke. Elective surgery should be delayed following a stroke for up to 9 months to allow for return of cerebral autoregulation, risk factor reduction, and treatment of a cause if one can be identified.

If perioperative stroke occurs, it should be recognized as soon as possible. This can be difficult in the perioperative period because patients may have residual effects from general anesthetics, sedatives, or analgesics. There should be an index of suspicion for stroke if a patient's mental status does not improve as expected, a relationship between opioid administration and fluctuations in consciousness can be ruled out, or there is evidence of a focal neurologic deficit. If one has a high suspicion for stroke, a gross neurologic examination should be conducted and documented to establish a baseline and note focal deficits. Then the patient should undergo a noncontrast CT of the head to rule out other causes such as intracranial hemorrhage. If suspicions for ischemic stroke are confirmed, a neurologist should be consulted to determine whether the patient is a candidate for thrombolytic therapy despite recent surgery. Meanwhile, oxygen delivery to the brain should be optimized.

Acute Hemorrhagic Stroke

Acute hemorrhagic stroke results from extravasation of blood in the cranial vault that in turn impairs perfusion of normal brain tissue. Hemorrhagic stroke is four times more likely than ischemic stroke to cause death. Acute hemorrhagic stroke cannot be reliably distinguished from ischemic stroke based on clinical criteria. A noncontrast CT evaluation is needed to detect the presence of bleeding. The estimated volume of extravasated blood and the level of consciousness are the two best predictors of outcome.

Subtypes of hemorrhagic strokes are defined based on the location of blood. Blood located within the brain proper is called an *intraparenchymal hemorrhage.* Blood located in the epidural, subdural, or subarachnoid spaces is referred to as *epidural hematoma, subdural hematoma,* or *subarachnoid hemorrhage,* respectively. Blood located in the ventricular system is an *intraventricular hemorrhage.* This last form of hemorrhagic stroke is usually not an isolated event but instead occurs in the setting of other types of hemorrhagic stroke.

Intraparenchymal Hemorrhage

Intraparenchymal hemorrhage, also known as *intracerebral hemorrhage,* refers to a collection of blood in the brain parenchyma. A *primary* intraparenchymal hemorrhage occurs in the absence of an obvious anatomic source (e.g., AVM) for the hemorrhage. It occurs at a higher rate in African Americans and those with poorly controlled hypertension. *Secondary* causes of intraparenchymal hemorrhage include rupture of an AVM, trauma, or bleeding from a brain tumor. (This is in contrast to *aneurysm rupture,* which results in *subarachnoid hemorrhage.*) Patients with intracerebral hemorrhage often deteriorate clinically as a result of hematoma expansion or cerebral edema that worsens during the first 24–48 hours following the acute bleed. Late hematoma evacuation is ineffective in decreasing mortality. The efficacy of early surgical evacuation of a hematoma to decrease ischemic injury and edema to the surrounding tissue remains unclear. Intravenous administration of recombinant activated factor VII has minimal effect on the hematoma expansion rate, no significant effect on overall outcome, and may increase the risk for arterial thrombosis.

Intraventricular hemorrhage is a particularly ominous form of intracranial hemorrhage because the blood will occlude CSF drainage. Prompt ventricular drainage should be performed to treat any signs of hydrocephalus. Sedation (with propofol infusion, barbiturates, or benzodiazepines), with or without drug-induced skeletal muscle paralysis, is often helpful in managing patients who require prolonged tracheal intubation to protect the airway and manage ventilation and oxygenation.

The goal of blood pressure management involves balancing the need to maintain cerebral perfusion while decreasing risk for rebleeding or hematoma expansion. Blood pressure should be decreased in patients with a systolic blood pressure above 200 mm Hg or MAP above 150 mm Hg. In patients with systolic blood pressure above 180 mm Hg or MAP above 130 mm Hg and evidence of increased ICP, an ICP monitor should be considered and blood pressure should be lowered to maintain a CPP of 61–80 mm Hg. In patients with systolic blood pressure above 180 mm Hg or MAP above 130 mm Hg and no evidence of increased ICP, blood pressure should be decreased to a systolic blood pressure of approximately 140 mm Hg or a MAP of approximately 110 mm Hg.

Epidural Hematoma

Epidural hematoma most commonly occurs in the setting of trauma. The arteries that supply the dura mater are located between the dura mater and the periosteum of the cranial bones, and epidural hematoma is generally due to traumatic rupture of a meningeal artery. Generally patients have a lucid interval following trauma, but as blood accumulates in the epidural space, hematoma volume can compress the brain and decrease perfusion. This results in progressive deterioration in consciousness as ICP increases and CPP decreases. The prognosis following early hematoma evacuation is excellent.

Subdural Hematoma

Subdural hematoma occurs when blood accumulates between the dura mater and arachnoid layer. Most commonly, subdural hematoma occurs in the setting of trauma. This can occur following either major or minor trauma, with the latter often occurring in older patients with cerebral atrophy, a condition that lends itself to stretching and rupture of bridging veins that run in the subdural space. Patients taking anticoagulants and antiplatelet drugs are at greatest risk. As with epidural hematomas, early evacuation of the hematoma is associated with better outcome.

Signs and symptoms of a subdural hematoma may evolve gradually over several days (in contrast to epidural hematomas) because the hematoma is due to slow venous bleeding. Headache is a universal complaint. Drowsiness and obtundation are characteristic findings, but the magnitude of these changes may fluctuate from hour to hour. Lateralizing neurologic signs eventually occur, manifesting as hemiparesis, hemianopsia, or language disturbances. Elderly patients may have unexplained signs of progressive cognitive decline or dementia.

Conservative medical management of subdural hematomas may be acceptable for patients whose condition stabilizes, but surgical evacuation of the clot is desirable in most patients. Most subdural hematomas can be drained via burr holes; the procedure can be performed under general anesthesia, local anesthesia, or monitored anesthesia care. If the subdural hematoma is particularly large, is chronic, or consists of clotted blood, removal may require craniotomy. Because a subdural hematoma is usually caused by venous bleeding, normocapnia is desirable following evacuation of the hematoma to allow for a larger brain volume, which may help tamponade any sites of venous bleeding.

Subarachnoid Hemorrhage and Intracranial Aneurysms

Spontaneous subarachnoid hemorrhage most commonly results from rupture of an intracranial aneurysm. Various pathologic conditions such as hypertension, coarctation of the aorta, polycystic kidney disease, fibromuscular dysplasia, and the occurrence of cerebral aneurysms in first-degree relatives are associated with the presence of cerebral aneurysms. Larger aneurysms are more likely to rupture. Other risk factors for rupture include hypertension, cigarette smoking, cocaine abuse, female sex, and use of oral contraceptives.

Patients may also present clinically with unruptured aneurysms. A common presentation of an unruptured aneurysm is the development of a new focal neurologic deficit. The cause of this new deficit may be either a mass effect from an expanding aneurysm that compresses normal neurologic structures, or small emboli to the distal cerebral circulation from a thrombus contained within the aneurysm. Headache caused by mass effect can occur. New-onset seizures can indicate an unruptured aneurysm and are thought to result from the formation of a glial scar (gliosis) in brain parenchyma adjacent to the aneurysm. Unruptured aneurysms may also be identified incidentally on cerebral imaging performed for unrelated reasons. Aneurysm diameter is not static. Thus although smaller aneurysms may be followed with serial imaging, larger aneurysms are often considered for surgery because of their increased risk for spontaneous rupture.

The diagnosis of subarachnoid hemorrhage is based on clinical symptoms ("worst headache of my life") and CT demonstration of subarachnoid blood. MRI is not as sensitive as CT for detecting acute hemorrhage, especially with thin layers of subarachnoid blood, although MRI may be useful for demonstrating subacute or chronic subarachnoid hemorrhage or infarction after CT findings have returned to normal. In addition to severe headache, the rapid onset of photophobia, stiff neck, decreased level of consciousness, and focal neurologic changes suggest subarachnoid hemorrhage. Prompt establishment of the diagnosis followed by treatment of the aneurysm can decrease morbidity and mortality. Two of the most common methods used to grade the severity of subarachnoid hemorrhage are the Hunt and Hess classification and the World Federation of Neurologic Surgeons grading system (Table 13.6). These grading systems are useful because their stratification of severity helps with prognosis and with measurement of the efficacy of various therapies.

Changes in the ECG often follow subarachnoid hemorrhage, with ST-segment depression and T-wave inversion being most common. These changes are most often noted within the first 48 hours after hemorrhage and have been attributed to catecholamine release. This same catecholamine release may result in cardiac dysrhythmias and may also be responsible for producing pulmonary edema. Echocardiography has demonstrated temporary depression of myocardial contractility unrelated to coronary artery disease in patients with subarachnoid hemorrhage. Of note, apical cardiac function may be preserved, a phenomenon attributed to the paucity of sympathetic innervation at the cardiac apex.

Treatment of subarachnoid hemorrhage involves localizing the aneurysm with conventional or MR angiography and then excluding the aneurysmal sac from the intracranial circulation while preserving its parent artery. Depending on the location and characteristics of the aneurysm, and the volume and placement of associated bleeding, this can be accomplished by craniotomy and surgery or via percutaneous radiology techniques (e.g., aneurysm coiling). Outcome is optimal when treatment is performed within the first 72 hours after bleeding. Placing a clip across the neck of the intracranial aneurysm is the most definitive surgical treatment. For larger or fusiform aneurysms that lack a definitive neck, surgical options include wrapping the exterior of the aneurysm or aneurysm trapping. In *aneurysm trapping* a clip is placed on the artery both proximal and distal to the aneurysm after the artery distal to the aneurysm has been bypassed, usually by means of the superficial temporal artery. Endovascular techniques that involve placing soft metallic coils in the dome of an aneurysm may be an alternative to surgical therapy but may not be an option for the treatment of all aneurysms, specifically those with a large neck or those that lack a neck. Because of the extremely high morbidity and mortality associated with surgical treatment of basilar tip aneurysms, endovascular treatment is preferred in this situation.

Surgery is often delayed in patients with severe symptoms such as coma. In these patients, other options, including interventional radiographic procedures, may be used. Anticonvulsants are administered should seizure activity occur. Systemic blood pressure is controlled because hypertension increases the risk of rebleeding. Hydrocephalus is

TABLE 13.6	Common Grading Systems for Subarachnoid Hemorrhage

HUNT & HESS CLASSIFICATION

Score	Neurologic Finding	Mortality
0	Unruptured aneurysm	0%–2%
1	Ruptured aneurysm with minimal headache and no neurologic deficits	2%–5%
2	Moderate to severe headache, no deficit other than cranial nerve palsy	5%–10%
3	Drowsiness, confusion, or mild focal motor deficit	5%–10%
4	Stupor, significant hemiparesis, early decerebration	25%–30%
5	Deep coma, decerebrate rigidity	40%–50%

WORLD FEDERATION OF NEUROLOGIC SURGEONS GRADING SYSTEM

Score	Glasgow Coma Scale Score	Presence of Major Focal Deficit
0		Intact unruptured aneurysm
1	15	No
2	13 or 14	No
3	13 or 14	Yes
4	7–12	Yes or no
5	3–6	Yes or no

Adapted from Lam AM. Cerebral aneurysms: anesthetic considerations. In: Cottrell JE, Smith DS, eds. *Anesthesia and Neurosurgery*. 4th ed. St Louis, MO: Mosby; 2001.

common after subarachnoid hemorrhage and is treated with ventricular drainage. Any change in mental status must be promptly evaluated by CT to look for signs of rebleeding or hydrocephalus.

Following subarachnoid hemorrhage, with or without surgical or endovascular treatment of the aneurysm, an important goal is prevention of cerebral vasospasm (intracranial arterial narrowing) and its consequences. Development of vasospasm can be triggered by many mechanisms, the most important of which is the contact of free hemoglobin with the abluminal surface of cerebral arteries. Not surprisingly the incidence and severity of vasospasm correlate with the amount of subarachnoid blood seen on CT. Vasospasm typically occurs 3–15 days after subarachnoid hemorrhage. For this reason, daily transcranial Doppler ultrasonographic examinations may be performed to detect vasospasm. If vasospasm is identified, *triple-H therapy* (*h*ypertension, *h*ypervolemia, *h*emodilution) is initiated. Colloids and crystalloids can be used, and pressor support may be needed. Administration of nimodipine, a calcium channel blocker, has been shown to improve outcome when initiated on the first day and continued for 21 days after subarachnoid hemorrhage. Improvement in clinical outcome with nimodipine occurs without angiographic evidence of vessel luminal enlargement to nimodipine infusion, suggesting that the beneficial effects of nimodipine in this situation may be due to direct neuronal protection. Cerebral angiographic techniques can also be employed to dilate vasospastic arteries mechanically (e.g., via balloons) or chemically (e.g., via intraarterial administration of papaverine or related vasodilating drugs).

Management of Anesthesia

The goals of anesthesia during intracranial aneurysm clipping surgery are to reduce the risk of aneurysm rupture, prevent cerebral ischemia, and facilitate surgical exposure.

The goal during induction of anesthesia is to prevent any increase (particularly a sudden increase) in the transmural pressure of the aneurysmal sac, which could increase the risk of aneurysm rupture. Therefore significant increases in systemic blood pressure must be avoided. In those patients with cerebral aneurysms *without* increased ICP and in those with unruptured aneurysms, it is reasonable to avoid excessive *decreases* in ICP before dural opening so as not to diminish the tamponading forces on the external surface of the aneurysm. Profound hyperventilation then should be avoided. Patients who have increased ICP before surgery present a challenge because they may not tolerate a decrease in MAP to protect against aneurysm rupture without developing cerebral ischemia. Patients with vasospasm also present a quandary because systemic hypertension may improve flow through vasospastic vessels but may increase the risk of aneurysm rebleeding. Aneurysm clipping during the period in which the patient is at high risk of vasospasm is associated with increased mortality. Therefore in patients with vasospasm who require anesthetic care, CPP should be kept elevated to maintain blood flow through vasospastic arteries.

Monitoring of the blood pressure via an intraarterial catheter is desirable to ensure the adequacy of blood pressure control during direct laryngoscopy and at other times of noxious stimulation. Prophylaxis against significant hypertension during direct laryngoscopy may be accomplished by administration of esmolol, lidocaine, propofol, barbiturates, or short-acting opioids. Loss of consciousness is achieved with IV administration of thiopental, propofol, or etomidate. Nondepolarizing neuromuscular blocking drugs are most often selected to facilitate tracheal intubation.

Placement of a CVP catheter may be useful because of large intraoperative fluid shifts associated with osmotic and loop diuretics, intraoperative aneurysm rupture, and the need for fluid resuscitation. A pulmonary artery catheter or TEE may be considered when patients have known cardiac disease. Electrophysiologic monitoring (EEG, somatosensory or motor evoked potentials) may be helpful to identify intraoperative cerebral ischemia.

The goals of anesthetic management include providing a depth of anesthesia appropriate to the level of surgical stimulation, facilitating surgical exposure through optimal brain relaxation, maintaining CPP, reducing transmural pressure in the aneurysm during aneurysm clip placement (and the last portions of surgical exposure to facilitate clip placement), and prompt awakening of the patient at the end of the procedure to permit immediate neurologic assessment. Drugs, fluids, and blood must be immediately available should the aneurysm rupture. The risk of intraoperative rupture is approximately 7%, and rupture most commonly occurs during the late stages of surgical dissection. Management of rupture consists of aggressive volume resuscitation to maintain normovolemia combined with controlled hypotension (e.g., with nitroprusside) to temporarily limit hemorrhage and permit the neurosurgeon to gain control of the aneurysm.

If temporary clipping of the feeding vessel is used to gain control of a ruptured aneurysm, or alternatively to surgically manage a difficult-to-access aneurysm, the systemic blood pressure can be returned to the patient's normal (or even slightly elevated) levels to improve collateral blood flow while that vessel is obstructed by the occlusion clip.

Anesthesia is typically maintained with volatile anesthetics (isoflurane, desflurane, sevoflurane) with or without the addition of nitrous oxide, and also may be supplemented with intermittent (fentanyl) or continuous (remifentanil) infusion of opioids. Alternatively a total IV anesthetic technique (e.g., propofol and short-acting opioid) can be used. Cerebral vasoconstricting anesthetics such as barbiturates and propofol help reduce brain volume and, in the case of barbiturates and possibly propofol, may provide some degree of neuronal protection against ischemia. Muscle paralysis is critical to prevent movement during aneurysm clipping. Also, electrophysiologic monitoring, such as somatosensory or motor evoked potential monitoring, may be employed and may require changes in anesthetic plan to facilitate this monitoring.

Patients may have hydrocephalus as a result of hematoma volume, brain edema, or obstruction of arachnoid granulations by blood, thus impairing CSF reabsorption. Therefore optimization of brain relaxation is important, and combinations of lumbar CSF drainage, mild hyperventilation, administration of loop and/or osmotic diuretics, and proper positioning to facilitate cerebral venous drainage can help optimize surgical exposure. The timing and extent of these interventions is critical in achieving overall management goals. Intraoperative fluid administration is guided by blood loss, urine output, and measurement of cardiac filling pressures. Normovolemia is the goal, which is best achieved by IV administration of balanced salt solutions. Intravenous solutions containing glucose are *not* recommended; hyperglycemia may exacerbate neuronal injury. Current best evidence suggests no benefit to intraoperative hypothermia in patients undergoing aneurysm clipping. However, hyperthermia must be avoided because it increases $CMRO_2$ and CBV.

Traditionally, drug-induced controlled hypotension has been used to decrease transmural pressure in the aneurysm and thereby decrease the risk of aneurysm rupture during microscopic isolation and clipping. Controlled hypotension is used less often today because of concerns about the impairment of autoregulation that follows subarachnoid hemorrhage, unpredictable cerebrovascular responses to drug-induced hypotension, and the risk of global ischemia. As an alternative to drug-induced hypotension, *regional controlled hypotension* produced by placing a vascular clamp on the parent artery supplying the aneurysm provides protection against aneurysm rupture without incurring the risk of global cerebral ischemia. Ideally, temporary occlusion of the parent artery does not exceed 10 minutes. If longer periods of occlusion are needed, the administration of anesthetics that decrease $CMRO_2$, particularly barbiturates, might provide protection against regional cerebral ischemia and infarction. However, the utility and efficacy of this intervention remains controversial. During temporary clamping of the feeding vessel, systemic blood pressure should be maintained toward the higher end of the patient's normal blood pressure range to encourage collateral circulation.

At the conclusion of the surgical procedure, prompt emergence from anesthesia is desirable to facilitate immediate neurologic evaluation of the patient. Use of short-acting inhaled and IV anesthetic drugs make prompt awakening more likely. However, incremental doses of antihypertensive drugs such as labetalol or esmolol may be needed to control the blood pressure as the patient emerges from anesthesia. Lidocaine may be administered intravenously to suppress airway reflexes and the response to the presence of the endotracheal tube; however, this lidocaine may also contribute to some degree of reanesthetizing the patient, since IV lidocaine has general anesthetic properties. Tracheal extubation immediately after surgery is acceptable and encouraged in patients who are awake with adequate spontaneous ventilation and protective upper airway reflexes. Patients who were obtunded preoperatively are likely to require continued mechanical ventilation during the postoperative period. Patients who experience intraoperative rupture of an intracranial aneurysm may recover slowly and benefit from postoperative airway and ventilatory support.

Neurologic status is assessed at frequent intervals in the ICU. Patients may manifest delayed emergence from anesthesia or focal neurologic deficits after intracranial aneurysm surgery, and it may be difficult to distinguish between drug-induced causes (e.g., differential awakening, generalized cerebral depression) and surgical causes (e.g., ischemic or mechanical brain injury). The appearance of a *new focal deficit* should raise suspicion of a surgical cause, since—in all instances other than differential awakening—anesthetic drugs would be expected to cause primarily global effects. Inequality of pupils that was not present preoperatively is also likely to reflect a surgical event. CT or angiography may be necessary if the patient does not awaken promptly. Successful surgical therapy may be followed by delayed neurologic deficits (hours to days later) resulting from cerebral vasospasm. This in turn requires aggressive triple-H therapy or invasive radiologic interventions.

Anesthetic goals for patients undergoing angiographically guided cerebral aneurysm coil placement are similar to those for patients undergoing aneurysm clip placement. Typically, coil placement procedures can be performed using sedation or general anesthesia. The principal advantage of sedation is that intraprocedural neurologic assessment can be performed. However, patient movement during the procedure poses the risk of aneurysm rupture or coil dislodgment resulting in coil embolization. For this reason, general anesthesia is preferred during coil placement. Anesthetic management includes ICP control, maintenance of adequate cerebral perfusion without excessive hypertension, and facilitation of a rapid postprocedural assessment of neurologic function.

Arteriovenous Malformation

AVMs are abnormal collections of blood vessels in which multiple direct arterial-to-venous connections exist without intervening capillaries. There is no neural tissue within the nidus of this malformation. AVMs typically represent high-flow, low-resistance shunts, with vascular intramural pressure being less than systemic arterial pressure. Thus rupture does not appear to be clinically associated with acute or chronic hypertension. These malformations are believed to be congenital and commonly present in adulthood as either hemorrhage or new-onset seizures. The exact cause of AVM-associated seizures is unknown but has been attributed to either a steal phenomenon (e.g., shunting of blood away from normal brain tissue toward the low-resistance AVM) or gliosis due to hemosiderin deposits from previous hemorrhage. Most AVMs are supratentorial. AVMs are associated with a 4%–10% incidence of cerebral aneurysm. AVMs presenting in the neonatal or childhood period usually involve the vein of Galen, and presenting symptoms include hydrocephalus or macrocephaly and prominence of forehead veins, as well as evidence of a high-output cardiac state or heart failure. Diagnosis is made by either MRI or angiography.

Before the advent of focused high-dose radiation and selective cerebral angiography-based treatment regimens, primary surgical treatment of AVMs was associated with a high morbidity and mortality. Currently, treatment may involve a combination of highly focused (Gamma Knife) radiation, angiographically guided embolization, and/or surgical resection. With smaller AVMs, patients may respond completely to radiation or embolization therapy. With larger AVMs, however, these techniques are typically used as adjunctive therapy *before* surgery to decrease the size of the AVM nidus and reduce both the complexity and risks of surgery. Prognosis and perioperative outcome can be estimated using the Spetzler-Martin AVM grading system, which classifies the AVM based on three features (Table 13.7).

Other types of intracranial AVMs include venous angiomas, cavernous angiomas, capillary telangiectasias, and AV fistulas.

Venous Angioma

Venous angiomas or malformations consist of tufts of veins. Often they are occult lesions found during cerebral angiography or MRI performed to evaluate other disease states. Rarely will a venous angioma present as either hemorrhage or new-onset seizures. These are low-flow, low-pressure lesions and usually contain brain parenchyma within the nidus; they are treated only if bleeding or intractable seizures occur.

Cavernous Angioma

Cavernous angiomas, also known as *cavernous hemangiomas* or *cavernomas,* are typically benign lesions consisting of vascular channels without large feeding arteries or large veins. Brain parenchyma is not found within the nidus of the lesion. These low-flow, well-circumscribed lesions often present as new-onset seizures but occasionally manifest as hemorrhage. They may be seen on CT or MRI and typically appear as a flow void on cerebral angiography. Treatment involves surgical resection of symptomatic lesions. They do not respond to radiation, nor are they amenable to embolization, since they are angiographically silent.

Capillary Telangiectasia

Capillary telangiectasias are low-flow, enlarged capillaries and probably one of the least understood vascular lesions in the CNS. They are angiographically silent and difficult to diagnose antemortem. The risk of hemorrhage is low except for lesions occurring in the brainstem. They are often found incidentally at autopsy and are often associated with other disorders, including Osler-Weber-Rendu and Sturge-Weber syndromes. These lesions are not treatable.

Arteriovenous Fistula

AV fistulas are direct communications between arteries and veins without an intervening nidus of smaller blood vessels. They commonly occur between meningeal vessels within the dura mater or between the carotid artery and venous sinuses within the cavernous sinus. Some AV fistulas are thought to occur spontaneously. Many others are associated with a previous traumatic injury or, in the case of carotid cavernous fistulas, with previous (presumably silent) rupture of an intracavernous carotid artery aneurysm. Dural AV fistulas commonly present with pulsatile tinnitus or headache. An occipital bruit can be appreciated in 24% of these cases, since the occipital artery is a common arterial feeder of an AV fistula. Treatment options include angiographically guided embolization or surgical ligation. Surgical treatment is associated with the risk of rapid and significant blood loss.

Patients with carotid cavernous AV fistulas often have orbital or retroorbital pain, arterialization of the conjunctiva, or visual changes. Diagnosis is made by MR or conventional angiography. Embolization is usually an effective treatment option.

Management of Anesthesia

Surgical resection of low-flow vascular malformations such as cavernous angiomas is generally associated with fewer intraoperative and postoperative complications than resection of high-flow vascular lesions such as AVMs and AV fistulas. AVMs often involve multiple feeding and draining vessels, whereas AV fistulas involve a single feeding and a single

TABLE 13.7	Spetzler-Martin Arteriovenous Malformation (AVM) Grading System
Graded Feature	Points Assigned
Nidus size	
Small (<3 cm)	1
Medium (3–6 cm)	2
Large (>6 cm)	3
Eloquence of adjacent brain[a]	
Noneloquent	0
Eloquent	1
Pattern of venous drainage	
Superficial only	0
Deep only or deep and superficial	1

SURGICAL OUTCOME BASED ON SPETZLER-MARTIN AVM GRADE

Grade	Percent of Patients With No Postoperative Neurologic Deficit
1	100
2	95
3	84
4	73
5	69

[a]Eloquent brain includes the sensory, motor, language, and visual areas as well as the hypothalamus, thalamus, internal capsule, brainstem cerebellar peduncles, and deep nuclei.
Adapted from Spetzler RF, Martin NA. A proposed grading system for arteriovenous malformations. *J Neurosurg.* 1986;65:476-483.

draining vessel. As such, surgical resection of AVMs can pose greater clinical challenges during resection and postoperative care.

Preoperatively a patient with an intracranial vascular malformation should be evaluated for evidence of cerebral ischemia or increased ICP. The nature of the malformation—including size, location, mechanism of venous drainage, presence of associated aneurysms, and any prior treatment—should be elicited, since these factors may help in anticipating perioperative complications. Medications, including antiepileptic drugs if the patient has a concurrent seizure disorder, should be administered preoperatively.

In addition to standard monitoring, an intraarterial catheter may be placed before induction of anesthesia. Blood pressure control throughout anesthesia, surgery, and the postoperative period is critical, since hypotension may result in ischemia in hypoperfused areas and hypertension may increase the risk of rupture of an associated aneurysm, exacerbate intraoperative bleeding, or worsen intracranial hypertension. For embolization or surgical resection of a vascular malformation in an eloquent region of brain, monitored anesthesia care with an "awake craniotomy" is an attractive option. In cases requiring general anesthesia, a hemodynamically stable induction is desirable, although AVMs—unlike cerebral aneurysms—are unlikely to hemorrhage during anesthesia induction, even with moderate increases in blood pressure. Barbiturates, propofol, and etomidate are all effective and safe induction agents. Muscle relaxation should be accomplished with a nondepolarizing neuromuscular blocking agent, since succinylcholine may induce further increases in ICP as well as cause hyperkalemia if motor deficits are present. Techniques to blunt hemodynamic responses to stimulating events such as laryngoscopy, pinion placement, and incision should be used as needed. These may include administration of lidocaine (IV or locally), esmolol, or nitroprusside or deepening the anesthetic state with higher concentrations of volatile anesthetics, small doses of IV anesthetics, short-acting opioids, or IV lidocaine.

Given the risk of severe and rapid *intraoperative hemorrhage,* especially with AVMs and AV fistulas, adequate IV access is essential. Further, central venous access may be useful in some cases to monitor volume status or allow rapid administration of large volumes of fluids or blood products. Monitoring via a pulmonary artery catheter or TEE can be useful in patients with cardiac disease.

In cases of large or high-flow vascular malformations, frequent communication with the surgeon is of paramount importance because impressions of the lesions and the surgical and anesthetic requirements for safe resection may change during the operation. This is due in part to changing surgical requirements during various stages of resection of a large complex lesion. Hemodynamic stability, optimal surgical conditions, and rapid emergence from anesthesia at the conclusion of surgery are appropriate goals. Both IV and volatile anesthetic–based techniques are appropriate.

Hypotonic and glucose-containing solutions should be avoided, since the former can exacerbate cerebral edema and the latter can worsen outcome following neurologic ischemia. Mild hyperventilation ($Paco_2$ 30–35 mm Hg) will help facilitate surgical exposure. Lumbar CSF drainage may also help decrease intracranial volume and improve exposure. Cerebral edema of surrounding brain tissue can be a significant problem during and following AVM resection. Since this edema often develops despite normal systemic blood pressure, the etiology is referred to as *normal perfusion pressure breakthrough.* The exact mechanism leading to this is not clear but has been attributed to two possible causes. First, because AVMs represent high-flow, low-resistance vascular lesions, as arterial feeders are ligated during resection or embolization, blood flow is directed toward the surrounding brain tissue. These surrounding blood vessels may have experienced a chronic reduction in vascular resistance to compete with the AVM, so development of cerebral edema is quite possible. Alternatively, stasis of blood and development of microthrombi in the recently ligated feeder arterioles and draining veins can perturb the local microcirculation, leading to cerebral edema. Treatment of cerebral edema may include moderate hyperventilation, administration of mannitol, and blood pressure reduction. In extreme cases, high-dose barbiturate or propofol anesthesia or temporary craniectomy with postoperative ventilatory support may be useful.

Most patients respond quite well to surgical resection, and emergence from anesthesia should be rapid and smooth. Drugs such as β-adrenergic antagonists as well as lidocaine or nitroprusside can be used to control short-term hypertension during emergence. Prompt neurologic assessment should follow emergence.

Moyamoya Disease

Progressive stenosis of intracranial blood vessels with secondary development of an anastomotic capillary network is the hallmark of moyamoya disease. *Moyamoya* is the Japanese term for "puff of smoke" and refers to the angiographic finding of a cluster of small abnormal blood vessels. There seems to be a familial tendency toward the development of this disease, but it may be seen following head trauma or in association with other disorders such as neurofibromatosis, tuberous sclerosis, and fibromuscular dysplasia. Affected arteries have a thickened intima and a thin media. Since similar pathologic findings may be found in other organs, CNS abnormalities may be manifestations of a systemic disease. Intracranial aneurysms occur with increased frequency in those with moyamoya disease. Symptoms of ischemia (e.g., TIAs, cerebral infarcts) are common initial findings in children, whereas hemorrhagic complications are usually the presenting symptoms in adults. The diagnosis is typically made by conventional or MR angiography, which demonstrates a cluster of small abnormal blood vessels. Conventional MRI and CT imaging will show a tissue void or hemorrhage.

Medical treatment is aimed at decreasing ischemic symptoms and usually consists of a combination of vasodilators and anticoagulants. Surgical options include direct anastomosis of the superficial temporal artery to the middle cerebral artery (also known as an *extracranial-intracranial bypass*) or other indirect revascularization procedures, which may be combined with an extracranial-intracranial bypass. These techniques include laying the temporalis muscle directly on the brain surface and suturing the superficial temporal artery to the dura mater. Even with treatment, the overall prognosis is not good. Only about 58% of patients ever attain normal neurologic function.

Management of Anesthesia

Preoperative assessment of the patient with moyamoya disease should involve documentation of preexisting neurologic deficits, a history of hemorrhage, or the concurrent presence of an intracranial aneurysm. Anticoagulant or antiplatelet drug therapy should be discontinued if possible to avoid bleeding complications intraoperatively.

The goals of induction and maintenance of anesthesia include (1) ensuring hemodynamic stability, because hypotension could lead to ischemia in the distribution of the abnormal vessels and hypertension may cause hemorrhagic complications; (2) avoiding factors that lead to cerebral or peripheral vasoconstriction, such as hypocapnia or phenylephrine, which can compromise blood flow in the feeding or recipient vessels; and (3) facilitating rapid emergence from anesthesia so that neurologic function can be assessed. In addition to standard monitoring, intraarterial catheterization is essential to rapidly assess changes in blood pressure. If possible, this should be done before induction of anesthesia to help ensure a hemodynamically stable induction sequence. Central venous catheterization is not essential but can be useful to guide fluid management and can also provide access for administering vasoactive agents or blood products. Any IV induction agent can be used safely. Inhalational induction with sevoflurane is an option for children. Succinylcholine should be used with caution in patients with preexisting neurologic deficits because of the potential risk of hyperkalemia. Hemodynamic responses to stimulating events should be blunted. A volatile anesthetic–based technique may have the theoretical advantage of enhancing cerebral vasodilation. Excessive hyperventilation should be avoided because of its cerebral vasoconstrictive effect. Hypovolemia should be treated with colloid or crystalloid solutions. Dopamine and ephedrine are reasonable options for pharmacologic treatment of hypotension, because they will avoid the adverse effects on the cerebral vasculature that can result from use of a pure vasoconstrictor. Anemia should be avoided to prevent ischemia in already compromised brain regions.

Postoperative complications include stroke, seizure, and hemorrhage. Any of these may present as delayed awakening or a new neurologic deficit.

TRAUMATIC BRAIN INJURY

Traumatic brain injury (TBI) is the leading cause of disability and death in young adults in the United States. Brain injury may result from both closed head injury and penetrating injuries caused by bullets or other foreign objects. Other injuries, including cervical spine injury and thoracoabdominal trauma, frequently accompany acute head injury. Brain injury can be further exacerbated by systemic conditions related to trauma, including hypotension and hypoxia related to excessive bleeding, pulmonary contusion, pulmonary aspiration, or adult respiratory distress syndrome.

Initial management of patients with acute head injury includes immobilizing the cervical spine, establishing a patent airway, protecting the lungs from aspiration of gastric contents, and maintaining brain perfusion by treatment of hypotension. The most useful diagnostic procedure in terms of simplicity and rapidity is CT, which should be performed as soon as possible. CT has greatly facilitated identification of epidural or subdural hematomas. CT may not be needed in patients with minor head trauma who meet the following criteria: no headache or vomiting, younger than age 60, no intoxication, no deficits in short-term memory, no physical evidence of trauma above the clavicles, and no seizures.

It is not unusual for patients with TBI who initially are in stable condition and awake or in light coma to deteriorate suddenly. Delayed hematoma formation or cerebral edema is often responsible for these changes. Uncontrolled brain swelling that is not responding to conventional management may also cause sudden neurologic deterioration. Delayed secondary injury at the cellular level is an important contributor to brain swelling and subsequent irreversible brain damage.

The Glasgow Coma Scale (GCS) provides a reproducible method for assessing the seriousness of brain injury and for following neurologic status (see Table 13.1). *Severe head injury is defined as a GCS score of less than 8.* The type of head injury and patient age are important determinants of outcome when GCS scores are low. For example, patients with acute subdural hematoma have a poorer prognosis than do patients with diffuse brain contusion injury. Mortality in children with severe head injury is lower than that in adults.

Management of Anesthesia

Perioperative management of patients with acute head trauma must consider the risks of ongoing injury to the brain as well as co-existing injuries affecting organs and structures other than the brain. Initially, CBF is usually reduced and then gradually increases with time. Factors contributing to poor outcome in head injury patients are increased ICP and MAPs of less than 70 mm Hg. Normal autoregulation of CBF is often impaired in patients with acute head injury, but carbon dioxide reactivity is usually preserved. Control of increased ICP with mannitol or furosemide is indicated, and in some patients therapeutic craniectomy may be necessary. However, blood-brain barrier disruption may lead to either an attenuated or even paradoxical effect (i.e., increased ICP) with mannitol. Therefore it should be used with caution and with an ICP monitor in place. Hyperventilation, although effective in controlling ICP, may contribute to cerebral ischemia in patients with head injury, and for this reason the current recommendation is to *avoid hyperventilation* as a routine treatment. Barbiturate coma may be useful in some patients to control intracranial hypertension when other measures have failed. Induced mild hypothermia in adult patients with acute head injury does *not* improve outcome. Administration of hypertonic saline and mannitol may decrease brain volume. Associated lung injuries may impair oxygenation and ventilation and necessitate mechanical ventilation. *Neurogenic pulmonary edema* may also contribute to acute pulmonary dysfunction. The exact mechanism of neurogenic pulmonary edema is unknown, but it may be related to hyperactivity of the sympathetic nervous system, resulting in pathogenic alterations in Starling forces in the lung. Coagulopathy occurs in head injury patients and may be exacerbated by hypothermia as well as by massive blood loss and blood transfusion. Disseminated intravascular coagulation can occur following severe head injury and is perhaps related to the release of brain thromboplastin, a brain tissue extract known to activate the coagulation cascade. Replacement of clotting factors may be necessary.

Patients with TBI may require anesthesia for neurosurgical interventions such as hematoma drainage, decompressive craniectomy for cerebral edema, or spinal stabilization. Anesthesia may also be required for the treatment of a variety of nonneurologic problems related to the initial trauma, such as the repair of limb fractures and intraabdominal injuries. Management of anesthesia must include efforts to optimize CPP, minimize the occurrence and severity of cerebral ischemia, and avoid drugs and techniques that could increase ICP. CPP should be maintained in the range of 50–70 mm Hg if possible, and hyperventilation should *not* be used unless it is needed as a temporizing measure to control ICP. During surgical evacuation of acute epidural or subdural hematomas, systemic blood pressure may decrease precipitously at the time of surgical decompression and require aggressive management. Patients with severe head injury may experience impaired oxygenation and ventilation that complicates management during the intraoperative period. In these instances, treatment of hypoxia should be a primary therapeutic concern. Adequate fluid resuscitation is important. Hypertonic sodium chloride solution increases the plasma osmotic pressure and thus removes water from the brain's interstitial space. Hypotonic crystalloid solutions should be avoided because they decrease plasma osmotic pressure and increase cerebral edema. Glucose-containing solutions must be avoided unless specifically indicated, such as for the treatment of laboratory-diagnosed hypoglycemia. Consistent with recent guidelines, the upper limit of blood glucose concentration should be no greater than 180 mg/dL, and further glucose reduction is likely warranted. Corticosteroids are not indicated as a primary treatment of TBI.

Induction and Maintenance of Anesthesia
In patients in hemodynamically stable condition, induction of anesthesia with IV induction drugs and nondepolarizing muscle relaxants is acceptable. Fiberoptically guided endotracheal intubation or tracheostomy should be considered in patients for whom there is concern either that tracheal intubation via direct laryngoscopy cannot be performed easily or that a neurologic deficit may be further exacerbated, such as in cases of cervical spine fracture. These forms of airway management are also appropriate for patients who already show evidence of airway compromise. In moribund patients, establishing a safe and effective airway takes priority over concerns about anesthetic drug selection, since anesthetic drugs may not be needed. One must be aware of the possibility of hidden extracranial injuries (e.g., bone fractures, pneumothorax) that may lead to problems such as extensive blood loss or perturbations in ventilation and circulation. Maintenance of anesthesia often includes continuous infusions of IV anesthetic or analgesic drugs or low doses of a volatile anesthetic, with the goal of optimizing CPP and preventing increases in ICP. Nitrous oxide should be avoided because of the risk of pneumocephalus and concern for nonneurologic injuries such as pneumothorax. Low-dose sevoflurane may be desirable because of its relatively minimal impairment of cerebral autoregulation, although low-dose isoflurane is also a good choice. If acute brain swelling develops, correctable causes such as hypercapnia, arterial hypoxemia, hypertension, and venous obstruction must be considered and corrected if present. Intraarterial monitoring of blood pressure is very useful, but time constraints may limit the use of CVP or pulmonary artery catheter monitoring.

During the postoperative period, it is common to maintain skeletal muscle paralysis, typically in combination with infused sedative and hypnotic drugs, to facilitate mechanical ventilation. Continuous monitoring of ICP is useful in many patients.

CONGENITAL ANOMALIES OF THE BRAIN

Congenital anomalies of the CNS result from defects in the development or architecture of the nervous system. Often these are hereditary conditions. Pathologic processes may be diffuse or involve only those structures and neurons that are anatomically and functionally related.

Chiari Malformation

Chiari malformation refers to a group of disorders consisting of congenital displacement of the cerebellum. Chiari I malformation consists of downward displacement of the cerebellar tonsils over the cervical spinal cord, whereas Chiari II malformation is downward displacement of the cerebellar vermis. This is often associated with a meningomyelocele. Chiari III malformations are extremely rare and represent displacement of the cerebellum into an occipital encephalocele. Chiari IV malformations consist of cerebellar hypoplasia and do not involve displacement of posterior fossa contents.

Signs and symptoms of Chiari I malformation can appear at any age. The most common complaint is occipital headache, often extending into the shoulders and arms, with corresponding cutaneous dysesthesias. Pain is aggravated by coughing or moving the head. Visual disturbances, intermittent vertigo, and ataxia are prominent symptoms. Signs of syringomyelia are present in approximately 50% of patients with this disorder. Chiari II malformations usually present in infancy with obstructive hydrocephalus plus lower brainstem and cranial nerve dysfunction.

Treatment of Chiari malformation consists of surgical decompression by freeing adhesions and enlarging the foramen magnum. Management of anesthesia must consider the possibility of increases in ICP as well as significant intraoperative blood loss, especially in the case of Chiari II malformations.

Tuberous Sclerosis

Tuberous sclerosis (Bourneville disease) is an autosomal dominant disease characterized by intellectual disability, seizures, and facial angiofibromas. Pathologically, tuberous sclerosis can be viewed as a condition in which a constellation of benign hamartomatous lesions and malformations may occur in any organ of the body. Brain lesions include cortical tubers and giant cell astrocytomas. Cardiac rhabdomyoma, although rare, is the most common benign cardiac tumor associated with tuberous sclerosis. Both echocardiography and MRI are useful for detecting cardiac tumors. Wolff-Parkinson-White syndrome can be associated with tuberous sclerosis. Co-existing angiomyolipomas and cysts of the kidney may result in renal failure. Oral lesions such as nodular tumors, fibromas, or papillomas may be present on the tongue, palate, pharynx, and larynx. The clinical spectrum for patients with tuberous sclerosis depends on the organ systems involved and ranges from no symptoms to life-threatening complications.

Anesthesia management must consider the likely presence of intellectual disability and a seizure disorder requiring antiepileptic drugs. Upper airway abnormalities must be identified preoperatively. Cardiac involvement may be associated with intraoperative cardiac dysrhythmias. Impaired renal function may have implications when selecting drugs that depend on renal clearance mechanisms. Although experience is limited, these patients seem to respond normally to inhaled and IV anesthetic drugs, including opioids.

Von Hippel-Lindau Disease

Von Hippel-Lindau disease is a familial disease transmitted by an autosomal dominant gene with variable penetrance. It is characterized by retinal angiomas, hemangioblastomas, visceral tumors and CNS (typically cerebellar) tumors. Although these tumors are benign, they can cause symptoms resulting from pressure on surrounding structures or bleeding. The incidence of pheochromocytoma, renal cysts, and renal cell carcinoma is increased in this syndrome. These patients may require intracranial surgery for resection of hemangioblastomas.

Management of anesthesia in patients with von Hippel-Lindau disease must consider the possibility of pheochromocytoma. Preoperative treatment with antihypertensive drugs and vascular volume reexpansion is indicated if a pheochromocytoma is identified. The possibility of spinal cord hemangioblastomas may limit use of spinal anesthesia, although epidural anesthesia has been described for cesarean section. Exaggerated hypertension, especially during direct laryngoscopy or sudden changes in the intensity of surgical stimulation, may require intervention with esmolol, labetalol, sodium nitroprusside, anesthetic drugs, or a combination of these drugs.

Neurofibromatosis

Neurofibromatosis is due to an autosomal dominant mutation. Both sexes are equally affected. Expressivity is variable, but penetrance of the trait is virtually 100%. The disorder is characterized by tumors that grow in the nervous system. There are three types of neurofibromatosis: NF1, NF2, and schwannomatosis. Each has distinctly different genetic mutations.

NF1 occurs in 1 of 3000–4000 persons. The diagnosis of NF1 is based on the National Institutes of Health criteria. Patients must have at least two of the following:

- at least six café au lait spots
- two or more neurofibromas or one plexiform neuroma
- freckling in the axilla or inguinal areas
- at least two Lisch nodules (hamartomas of the iris)
- optic glioma
- osseous lesions such as sphenoid dysplasia or thinning of long bone cortex, with or without pseudarthrosis
- first-degree relative with NF1

Although both neurofibromas (observed in NF1) and schwannomas (observed in NF2 and schwannomatosis) consist predominantly of Schwann cells, there are differences in their characteristics. Neurofibromas consist of Schwann cells intermixed with other components such as fibroblasts, neurons, and collagen strands, whereas schwannomas consist almost entirely of Schwann cells. In addition, neurofibromas tend to *encase* the parent nerve, often requiring either debulking or en bloc resection of the nerve and tumor. However, schwannomas tend to *displace* the parent nerve, allowing for possible resection with sparing of the parent nerve.

In addition to abnormalities in the diagnostic criteria, patients with NF1 may have macrocephaly, short stature, obstructive hydrocephalus, epilepsy, hypertension, congenital heart defects, and both learning and behavioral disorders. There is an increased incidence of cancer in patients with neurofibromatosis. Commonly associated cancers include neurofibrosarcoma, malignant schwannoma, Wilms tumor, rhabdomyosarcoma, and leukemia. There is an association between NF1 and MEN type IIb that consists of mucocutaneous tumors, medullary thyroid cancer, and pheochromocytoma. Generally, neurofibromas are removed if they become symptomatic, painful, or cancerous. They may also be removed for cosmetic reasons.

NF2 is much rarer than NF1. It is diagnosed by the presence of at least one of the following:

- bilateral vestibular schwannomas
- family history of NF2 or unilateral vestibular schwannoma before age 30

- any two of glioma, meningioma, peripheral nerve schwannoma, or juvenile cataracts (Patients may undergo surgery for resection of tumors associated with this condition or removal of cataracts.)

Schwannomatosis is the rarest variant of neurofibromatosis. It consists of diffuse schwannomas but the absence of a schwannoma of the vestibular nerve.

Management of Anesthesia

Management of anesthesia in patients with neurofibromatosis includes consideration of the many clinical presentations of this disease. The possible presence of a pheochromocytoma should be considered during the preoperative evaluation. Signs of increased ICP may reflect expanding intracranial tumors. Expanding laryngeal neurofibromas may jeopardize airway patency. Patients with neurofibromatosis and scoliosis are likely to have cervical spine defects that could influence positioning for direct laryngoscopy and the subsequent surgical procedure. Responses to muscle relaxants are variable. These patients have been described as both sensitive and resistant to succinylcholine and sensitive to nondepolarizing muscle relaxants. Neuraxial anesthesia should be avoided in patients with tumors involving the proximal peripheral nerves (i.e., tumors near the spine or within the spinal canal). In the absence of such tumors, epidural analgesia is an effective method for producing analgesia during labor and delivery.

DEGENERATIVE DISEASES OF THE BRAIN

Degenerative diseases of the CNS usually involve neuronal malfunction or loss within specific anatomic regions, and as such they represent a diverse group of disease states.

Alzheimer's Disease

Alzheimer's disease is a chronic neurodegenerative disorder. It is the most common cause of dementia in patients older than 65 years and the fourth most common cause of disease-related death in patients older than age 65. Diffuse amyloid-rich senile plaques and neurofibrillary tangles are the hallmark pathologic findings. There are also changes in synapses and in the activity of several major neurotransmitters, especially synapses involving acetylcholine and CNS nicotinic receptors. Two types of Alzheimer's disease have been described: early onset and late onset. Early-onset Alzheimer's disease usually presents before age 60 and appears to be due to missense mutations in several genes. These mutations have an autosomal dominant mode of transmission. Late-onset Alzheimer's disease usually develops after age 60, and genetic factors appear to play a relatively minor role in the risk of developing this disorder. In both forms of the disease, patients typically develop progressive cognitive impairment that can consist of problems with memory as well as apraxia, aphasia, and agnosia. Definitive diagnosis is usually made on postmortem examination. The antemortem diagnosis of Alzheimer's disease is one of exclusion. There is currently no cure for Alzheimer's disease, and treatment focuses on control of symptoms. Pharmacologic options include *cholinesterase inhibitors* such as tacrine, donepezil, rivastigmine, and galantamine. Memantine, an *N*-methyl-D-aspartate (NMDA) receptor antagonist, has also been shown to improve cognitive function, although the mechanism for this effect is not well understood. Drug therapy should be combined with nonpharmacologic therapy, including caregiver education and family support. Even with treatment, the prognosis for patients with Alzheimer's disease is poor.

Patients with Alzheimer's disease may come for a variety of surgical interventions that are common in the elderly population. Patients are often confused and sometimes uncooperative, which makes monitored anesthesia care or regional anesthesia challenging. There is no one single anesthetic technique or drug that is ideal in this group of patients. Shorter-acting sedative-hypnotic drugs, anesthetics, and opioids are preferred, since they allow a more rapid return to baseline mental status. One should be aware of potential drug interactions, especially prolongation of the effect of succinylcholine and relative resistance to nondepolarizing muscle relaxants resulting from the use of cholinesterase inhibitors.

Parkinson's Disease

Parkinson's disease is a neurodegenerative disorder of unknown cause. Increasing age is the single most important risk factor in the development of this disease. There is a characteristic loss of dopaminergic fibers normally present in the basal ganglia, and as a result, regional dopamine concentrations are depleted. Dopamine is presumed to inhibit the rate of firing of the neurons that control the extrapyramidal motor system. Depletion of dopamine results in diminished inhibition of these neurons and unopposed stimulation by acetylcholine.

The classic triad of major signs of Parkinson's disease consists of skeletal muscle tremor, rigidity, and akinesia. Skeletal muscle rigidity first appears in the proximal muscles of the neck. The earliest manifestations may be loss of arm swings when walking and absence of head rotation when turning the body. There is facial immobility manifested by infrequent blinking and by a paucity of emotional expressions. Tremors are characterized as rhythmic alternating flexion and extension of the thumbs and other digits (pill-rolling tremor). Tremors are more prominent during rest and tend to disappear during voluntary movement. Seborrhea, oily skin, diaphragmatic spasms, and oculogyric crises are frequent. Dementia and depression are often present.

Treatment of Parkinson's disease is designed to increase the concentration of dopamine in the basal ganglia or decrease the neuronal effects of acetylcholine. Replacement therapy with the dopamine precursor levodopa combined with administration of a decarboxylase inhibitor such as carbidopa, which prevents peripheral conversion of levodopa to dopamine and optimizes the amount of levodopa available to enter the CNS, is the standard medical treatment. Indeed, levodopa is the most effective treatment for Parkinson's disease, and early treatment with this drug prolongs life. Levodopa is associated with a number of side effects, including dyskinesias and psychiatric disturbances. The increased myocardial contractility and heart rate seen in treated patients may reflect increased levels of circulating dopamine converted from levodopa. Orthostatic hypotension may be prominent in treated patients. Gastrointestinal side effects of levodopa therapy include nausea and vomiting, most likely caused by stimulation of the medullary chemoreceptor trigger zone.

Amantadine, an antiviral agent, is reported to help control the symptoms of Parkinson's disease. The mechanism for its effect is not fully understood. The type B monoamine oxidase inhibitors (MAOIs) selegiline and rasagiline can also help control the symptoms of Parkinson's disease by inhibiting catabolism of dopamine in the CNS. They have an advantage over nonspecific MAOIs because they are not associated with the occurrence of tyramine-related hypertensive crises. They do, however, have a significant reaction with meperidine.

Surgical treatment of Parkinson's disease is reserved for patients with disabling and medically refractory symptoms. Stimulation of the various nuclei within the basal ganglia via an implanted *deep brain stimulating device* can relieve or help control tremors. Fetal tissue transplantation for treatment of Parkinson's disease is based on the demonstration that implanted embryonic dopaminergic neurons can survive in recipients. The effectiveness of this treatment is not currently known.

Deep brain stimulator placement is typically performed on an awake patient. However, in certain circumstances, such as in patients with developmental delay or those with severe claustrophobia, the procedure is performed under general anesthesia. The procedure begins with placement of a rigid head frame, followed by MRI to allow for coordinate determination relative to fiduciary markers on the head frame. The deep brain electrode is then advanced through a burr hole, often with microelectrode recordings taken while the electrode is being advanced, since specific nuclei differ in their spontaneous firing patterns. Following successful brain lead placement, a generator pack is implanted below the clavicle or in the abdomen. Of note, deep brain stimulation is currently also used for treatment of a variety of other disorders, such as essential tremor, dystonia, multiple sclerosis with a significant tremor, and some psychiatric disorders.

Management of Anesthesia

Management of anesthesia in patients with Parkinson's disease requires an understanding of how this disease is treated. The elimination half-life of levodopa and the dopamine it produces is brief, so interruption of drug therapy for more than 6–12 hours can result in an abrupt loss of therapeutic effects. Abrupt drug withdrawal can also lead to skeletal muscle rigidity, which can interfere with ventilation. Therefore levodopa therapy, including the usual morning dose on the day of surgery, must be continued throughout the perioperative period. Oral levodopa can be administered approximately 20 minutes before induction of anesthesia, and the dose may be repeated intraoperatively and postoperatively via an orogastric or nasogastric tube as needed.

The possibility of hypotension and cardiac dysrhythmias must be considered, and butyrophenones (e.g., droperidol, haloperidol) must be available to antagonize the effects of dopamine in the basal ganglia. Acute dystonic reactions following administration of alfentanil might indicate an opioid-induced decrease in central dopaminergic transmission. The use of ketamine is controversial because exaggerated sympathetic nervous system responses might be provoked, but ketamine has been administered safely to patients treated with levodopa. The choice of a muscle relaxant is not influenced by the presence of Parkinson's disease.

Patients undergoing deep brain stimulator implantation may have been told by the surgeon to refrain from taking the usual morning dose of levodopa to facilitate the return of tremors and enhance sensitivity in detecting the efficacy of deep brain stimulation during the procedure. If that is the case, establishing IV access may prove challenging in an extremity with a significant tremor. Patients should receive minimal sedation during lead placement to prevent interference with microelectrode recordings and clinical assessment. Since γ-aminobutyric acid (GABA) is a common neurotransmitter involved in the normal circuitry of the basal ganglia, anesthetic drugs with significant effects on GABA (e.g., propofol, benzodiazepines) can alter the characteristic microelectrode recordings of specific nuclei and should be avoided. Sedative drugs such as opioids and dexmedetomidine are more satisfactory alternatives. Excessive sedation should be avoided not only to minimize difficulty obtaining neurologic assessments, but more importantly to avoid respiratory depression in a patient in whom there is little access to the airway because of the presence of a head frame. A variety of airway management devices (e.g., fiberoptic bronchoscope, laryngeal mask airway) should be readily available should airway compromise become an issue intraoperatively. In patients having general anesthesia for lead implantation, microelectrode recordings cannot be used to facilitate placement of the lead, so choice of anesthetic drugs is not limited. During general anesthesia, lead localization is performed solely by stereotaxis to reach anatomic landmarks.

Lead placement can be a long procedure, so care should be taken to position the patient properly and comfortably. Proper padding should be placed at sites that may be prone to pressure injury.

The procedure is performed with the patient in the sitting position, so there is a risk of air embolism. Precordial Doppler monitoring can help identify air entrainment. If venous air embolism and oxygen desaturation occur, the patient should *not* be encouraged to take a deep breath; this can lower intrathoracic pressure and cause entrainment of even more air. Instead the surgeon should flood the field with saline and attempt to identify and treat the site of air entrainment. In more severe cases the patient should be placed supine and hemodynamic support instituted as required.

Other potential complications of deep brain stimulator placement include hypertension, seizures, and bleeding.

Hypertension should be treated to avoid increasing the risk of intracranial hemorrhage. Seizures often spontaneously abate, but very small doses of a barbiturate, propofol, or a benzodiazepine may be required to terminate their activity despite the potentially suppressive effect of administration of these drugs on microelectrode recordings. The effect of these drugs on ventilatory drive must also be appreciated and minimized. A sudden alteration of consciousness could indicate intracranial hemorrhage. Hemorrhage would require aggressive management, such as emergent removal of the head frame, endotracheal intubation, and craniotomy after imaging.

Hallervorden-Spatz Disease

Hallervorden-Spatz disease is a rare autosomal recessive disorder of the basal ganglia. Although the term *Hallervorden-Spatz disease* is still in use, the more modern terms for this disease include *pantothenate kinase–associated neurodegeneration* (PKAN) and *neurodegeneration with brain iron accumulation* (NBIA). This disease follows a slowly progressive course from its onset during late childhood to death within about 10 years. As the new names suggest, there is a defect in the gene encoding the enzyme pantothenate kinase, and there is accumulation of iron in the brain. Laboratory testing can detect the enzyme defect, and there is a characteristic finding on MRI called the "eye-of-the-tiger" sign in the globus pallidi. There is no effective treatment for this disease. Dementia, dystonia with torticollis, and scoliosis are commonly present. Dystonic posturing often disappears with the induction of general anesthesia. However, skeletal muscle contractures and bony changes that accompany this chronic disease can cause immobility of the temporomandibular joint and cervical spine even in the presence of deep general anesthesia or drug-induced skeletal muscle paralysis.

Management of anesthesia must consider the possibility that these patients may not be able to be positioned optimally for tracheal intubation. Noxious stimulation caused by attempted awake tracheal intubation can intensify dystonia, so an inhalation induction with maintenance of spontaneous ventilation is a common choice. Administration of succinylcholine is potentially dangerous, since skeletal muscle wasting and diffuse axonal changes in the brain that involve upper motor neurons could accentuate the release of potassium. However, safe use of succinylcholine has been reported. Required skeletal muscle relaxation is best provided by deep general anesthesia or administration of nondepolarizing neuromuscular blockers. Emergence from anesthesia is predictably accompanied by return of dystonic posturing.

Huntington's Disease

Huntington's disease is a degenerative disease of the CNS characterized by marked atrophy of the caudate nucleus and to a lesser degree the putamen and globus pallidus. Biochemical abnormalities include deficiencies of acetylcholine (and its synthesizing enzyme choline acetyltransferase) and GABA in the basal ganglia. Selective loss of GABA can decrease inhibition of the dopamine nigrostriatal system. Huntington's disease is transmitted as an autosomal dominant trait. It has a delayed appearance at age 35–40. Identification of the genetic defect may be useful for disease risk prediction in those who have inherited the defective gene.

Manifestations of Huntington's disease consist of progressive dementia combined with choreoathetosis. Chorea is usually considered the first sign of Huntington's disease. This is the reason for the former designation of this disease as *Huntington's chorea*. Behavioral changes such as depression, aggressive outbursts, and mood swings may precede the onset of involuntary movements by several years. Involvement of the pharyngeal muscles makes these patients susceptible to pulmonary aspiration as well as significant weight loss. The disease progresses over several years, and accompanying mental depression makes suicide a frequent cause of death. The duration of Huntington's disease from clinical onset to death averages 17 years.

Treatment of Huntington's disease is symptomatic and directed at decreasing the choreiform movements. Haloperidol and other butyrophenones may be administered to control the chorea and emotional lability associated with the disease. Involuntary movements are best controlled by drugs that interfere with the neurotransmitter effects of dopamine, either by antagonizing dopamine (haloperidol, fluphenazine) or depleting dopamine stores (reserpine, tetrabenazine).

Experience in anesthesia management in patients with Huntington's chorea is too limited to allow recommendation of specific anesthetic drugs or techniques. Preoperative sedation using butyrophenones (e.g., droperidol, haloperidol) may be helpful in controlling choreiform movements. The increased likelihood of pulmonary aspiration must be considered. Use of nitrous oxide and volatile anesthetics is acceptable. Propofol and succinylcholine have been administered without adverse effects, but decreased plasma cholinesterase activity with prolonged responses to succinylcholine has been observed. It has been suggested that these patients may be sensitive to the effects of nondepolarizing muscle relaxants.

Torticollis

Torticollis (also called *cervical dystonia*) is thought to result from disturbances in basal ganglia function. The most common mode of presentation is spasmodic contraction of neck muscles, which may progress to involvement of limb and girdle muscles. Hypertrophy of the sternocleidomastoid muscles may be present. Spasm may involve the muscles of the vertebral column, leading to lordosis, scoliosis, and impaired ventilation. Treatment may include injection of botulinum toxin. Selective peripheral denervation of the affected cervical musculature is currently the favored surgical option to treat severe cervical dystonia. There are no known problems influencing the selection of anesthetic drugs for this procedure, but spasm of nuchal muscles can interfere with maintenance of a patent upper airway before institution of skeletal muscle paralysis. Awake endotracheal intubation may be necessary if chronic skeletal muscle spasm has led to fixation of the cervical vertebrae. Surgery may be performed with the patient in the sitting position. If so, anesthetic considerations related to use of the sitting position and the potential for venous air embolism will come into play.

The sudden appearance of torticollis after administration of anesthetic drugs has been reported. Administration of diphenhydramine 25–50 mg IV produces dramatic reversal of this drug-induced torticollis.

Transmissible Spongiform Encephalopathies

The human transmissible spongiform encephalopathies are Creutzfeldt-Jakob disease (CJD), kuru, Gerstmann-Sträussler-Scheinker syndrome, and fatal familial insomnia. These noninflammatory diseases of the CNS are caused by transmissible slow-acting infectious protein pathogens known as *prions.* Prions differ from viruses in that they lack RNA and DNA and fail to produce a detectable immune reaction. Transmissible spongiform encephalopathies are diagnosed on the basis of clinical and neuropathologic findings, including the presence of diffuse or focal clustered small round vacuoles that may become confluent. Familial progressive subcortical gliosis and some inherited thalamic dementias may also be spongiform encephalopathies. Bovine spongiform encephalopathy (mad cow disease) is a transmissible spongiform encephalopathy that occurs in animals. Infectivity of skeletal muscles, milk, and blood has not been detected.

CJD is the most common transmissible spongiform encephalopathy, with an estimated incidence of one case per million worldwide. Transmission of the prion and the development of clinical disease are still poorly understood. In fact a significant proportion of the population probably carries the CJD prion, but most do not develop clinical disease. Approximately 10%–15% of patients with CJD have a family history of the disease, so both infectious and genetic factors probably play a role in disease development. The time interval between infection and development of symptoms is measured in months to years. The disease develops by accumulation of an abnormal protein thought to act as a neurotransmitter in the CNS. This prion protein is encoded by a specific gene, and random mutations result in variants of CJD. Rapidly progressive dementia with ataxia and myoclonus suggests the diagnosis, although confirmation currently requires brain biopsy. Reliable noninvasive tests are under development. Alzheimer's disease poses the most difficult differential diagnosis. Unlike toxic and metabolic disorders, myoclonus is rarely present at the onset of CJD, and seizures, when they occur, are a late phenomenon. There may also be characteristic EEG abnormalities associated with CJD, but the sensitivity and specificity are not known. No vaccines or treatments are effective.

Universal infection precautions are necessary when caring for patients with CJD. In addition, handling of CSF calls for special precautions (use of double gloves and protective glasses, specimen labeling as "infectious"), since CSF has been the only body fluid shown to result in experimental transmission to primates. Performance of biopsies and autopsies requires similar precautions. The main risk of transmitting CJD is during brain biopsy for diagnostic confirmation of the disease. Instruments used should be disposable or should be decontaminated by soaking in sodium hypochlorite. Alternatively, instruments used for the surgical biopsy can be stored in a freezer and sterilized normally if the biopsy is negative or discarded if the biopsy results are positive.

Human-to-human CJD transmission has occurred inadvertently in association with surgical procedures such as corneal transplantation, stereotactic procedures with previously used electrodes, procedures with contaminated neurosurgical instruments, and human cadaveric dura mater transplantation. Transmission has also been attributed to treatment with human-derived growth hormone and gonadotropic hormones. Although injection or transplantation of human tissues may result in transmission of infectious prions, the hazards of transmission through human blood are debatable, since this disease is not observed more frequently in individuals with hemophilia than in the general population. Nevertheless, transfusion of blood from individuals known to be infected is not recommended.

Management of anesthesia includes use of universal infection precautions, disposable equipment, and sterilization of any reusable equipment using sodium hypochlorite. Surgery in patients known or suspected to be infected might be better performed at the end of the day to allow thorough cleansing of equipment and the operating room before the next use. The number of personnel participating in anesthesia and surgery should be kept to a minimum, and all should wear protective gowns, gloves, and face masks with transparent visors to protect the eyes. Since a proportion of the general population are probably carriers of the prion thought to cause CJD, and both infectious and genetic factors play a role in the development of clinical symptoms, the likelihood of developing CJD after coming in contact with a CJD prion is probably very low. However, this fact does not obviate the need for precautionary measures.

Multiple Sclerosis

Multiple sclerosis is an autoimmune disease affecting the CNS and appears to occur in genetically susceptible persons. There is a high rate of concordance among twins and an increased risk in individuals who have a first-degree relative with the disease. There are also geographic associations with this disease, which reaches its highest incidence in northern Europe, southern Australia, and North America. However, no clear genetic, environmental, or infectious causes have yet been identified. There is also no clear understanding of the immunopathogenic processes that determine the sites of tissue damage in the CNS, the variations in natural history, and the severity of disability caused by this disease.

Pathologically, multiple sclerosis is characterized by diverse combinations of inflammation, demyelination, and axonal damage in the CNS. The loss of myelin covering axons is followed by formation of demyelinative plaques. Peripheral nerves are not affected by multiple sclerosis.

Clinical manifestations of multiple sclerosis reflect its multifocal involvement and are always progressive. Manifestations reflect the sites of demyelination in the CNS and spinal cord. For example, inflammation of the optic nerves (optic neuritis) causes visual disturbances, involvement of the cerebellum leads to gait disturbances, and lesions of the spinal cord cause limb paresthesias and weakness as well as urinary incontinence and impotence. Optic neuritis is characterized by diminished visual acuity and defective pupillary reaction to light. Ascending spastic paresis of skeletal muscles can occur. Intramedullary disease of the cervical cord is suggested by an electrical sensation that runs down the back into the legs in response to flexion of the neck (Lhermitte sign). Typically symptoms develop over the course of a few days, remain stable for a few weeks, and then improve. Because remyelination probably does not occur in the CNS, remission of symptoms most likely results from correction of transient chemical and physiologic disturbances that have interfered with nerve conduction in the areas of demyelination. Increases in body temperature can also cause exacerbation of symptoms, owing to further alterations in nerve conduction in regions of demyelination. There is an increased incidence of seizure disorders in patients with multiple sclerosis.

The course of multiple sclerosis is characterized by exacerbations and remissions at unpredictable intervals over a period of several years. Symptoms eventually persist, leading to severe disability from visual failure, ataxia, spastic skeletal muscle weakness, and urinary incontinence. However, in some patients the disease remains benign, with infrequent mild episodes of demyelination followed by prolonged remissions. The onset of multiple sclerosis after age 35 is typically associated with slow disease progression.

The diagnosis of multiple sclerosis can be established with varying degrees of confidence (i.e., probable or definite) on the basis of clinical features alone or clinical features in combination with oligoclonal immunoglobulin abnormalities in the CSF; prolonged latency of evoked potentials, reflecting slowing of nerve conduction resulting from demyelination; and signal changes in white matter seen on cranial MRI.

No treatment is curative for multiple sclerosis, so treatment is directed at symptom control and slowing disease progression. Corticosteroids, the principal treatment for acute relapses of multiple sclerosis, have immunomodulatory and antiinflammatory effects that restore the blood-brain barrier, decrease edema, and possibly improve axonal conduction. Treatment with corticosteroids shortens the duration of a relapse and accelerates recovery, but whether the overall degree of recovery or progression of the disease

is altered is not known. Interferon beta is the treatment of choice for patients with relapsing-remitting multiple sclerosis. The most common side effect of interferon beta therapy is transient flulike symptoms for 24–48 hours after injection. Slight increases in serum aminotransferase concentrations, leukopenia, or anemia may be present, and co-existing depression may be exaggerated. Glatiramer acetate is a mixture of random synthetic polypeptides synthesized to mimic myelin basic protein. This drug is an alternative to interferon beta and is most useful in patients who become resistant to interferon beta treatment because of serum interferon beta–neutralizing activity. Mitoxantrone is an immunosuppressive drug that functions by inhibiting lymphocyte proliferation. Because of severe cardiac toxicity, its use is limited to patients with rapidly progressive multiple sclerosis. Azathioprine is a purine analogue that depresses both cell-mediated and humoral immunity. Treatment with this drug may decrease the rate of relapses in multiple sclerosis but has no effect on the progression of disability. Azathioprine is considered when patients show no response to therapy with interferon beta or glatiramer acetate. Other immune modulators include natalizumab and fingolimod. Low-dose methotrexate is relatively nontoxic and inhibits both cell-mediated and humoral immunity because of its antiinflammatory effects. Patients with secondary progressive multiple sclerosis may benefit from treatment with this drug.

Management of Anesthesia

Management of anesthesia in patients with multiple sclerosis must consider the impact of surgical stress on the natural progression of the disease. Regardless of the anesthetic technique or drugs selected for use during the perioperative period, it is possible that symptoms and signs of multiple sclerosis will be exacerbated postoperatively. This may be due to factors such as infection and fever. Any increase in body temperature, even as little as 1°C, can cause an exacerbation of multiple sclerosis. It is possible that increased body temperature results in complete block of conduction in demyelinated nerves. The unpredictable cycle of clinical exacerbations and remissions inherent in multiple sclerosis might lead to erroneous conclusions that there are cause-and-effect relationships between disease severity and drugs or events occurring during the perioperative period.

The changing and unpredictable neurologic presentation of patients with multiple sclerosis during the perioperative period must be appreciated when regional anesthetic techniques are selected. Indeed, spinal anesthesia has been implicated in postoperative exacerbations of multiple sclerosis, whereas there is currently no convincing evidence of exacerbations of the disease after epidural anesthesia or peripheral nerve block. The mechanism by which spinal anesthesia might differ in this regard from epidural anesthesia is unknown, but it might involve local anesthetic neurotoxicity. Specifically it is speculated that the demyelination associated with multiple sclerosis renders the spinal cord more susceptible to the neurotoxic effects of local anesthetics. Epidural anesthesia may carry less risk than spinal anesthesia because the concentration of local anesthetics in the white matter of the spinal cord is lower than after spinal anesthesia. Nevertheless, both epidural anesthesia and spinal anesthesia have been used in parturient women with multiple sclerosis.

General anesthesia is the most frequently used technique in patients with multiple sclerosis. There are no unique interactions between multiple sclerosis and the drugs used to provide general anesthesia, and there is no evidence to support the use of one inhaled or injected anesthetic drug over another. In patients with motor weakness, use of succinylcholine can result in exaggerated potassium release and should be avoided. Prolonged responses to the paralyzing effects of nondepolarizing muscle relaxants would be consistent with co-existing skeletal muscle weakness and decreased skeletal muscle mass. However, resistance to the effects of nondepolarizing muscle relaxants has been observed, which perhaps reflects the proliferation of extrajunctional cholinergic receptors characteristic of upper motor neuron lesions.

Corticosteroid supplementation during the perioperative period may be indicated in patients being treated long term with these drugs. Efforts must be made to recognize and prevent even a modest increase in body temperature, since this change may exacerbate symptoms. Periodic neurologic evaluation during the postoperative period is useful for detection of disease exacerbation.

Postpolio Syndrome

Poliomyelitis is caused by an enterovirus that initially infects the reticuloendothelial system. In a minority of patients the virus enters the CNS and preferentially targets motor neurons in the brainstem and anterior horn of the spinal cord. The worldwide incidence of poliomyelitis has significantly decreased since the development of vaccines against this disease. Because poliomyelitis is so rare at this time in the United States, a clinician will see patients with postpolio syndrome (also called *postpolio sequelae*) much more commonly than those with acute polio. Postpolio syndrome manifests as fatigue, skeletal muscle weakness, joint pain, cold intolerance, dysphagia, and sleep and breathing problems (e.g., obstructive sleep apnea), which presumably reflect neurologic damage from the original poliovirus infection. Poliovirus may damage the reticular activating system; this accounts for the fact that these individuals may exhibit exquisite sensitivity to the sedative effects of anesthetics as well as delayed awakening from general anesthesia. Sensitivity to nondepolarizing muscle relaxants is common. Severe back pain following surgery may be due to co-existing skeletal muscle atrophy and scoliosis. Postoperative shivering may be profound, since these individuals are very sensitive to cold. Postoperative pain perception may be abnormal, possibly because of poliovirus damage to endogenous opioid-secreting cells in the brain and spinal cord. Outpatient surgery may not be appropriate for many postpolio patients, since they are at increased risk of

complications, especially those related to respiratory muscle weakness and dysphagia.

SEIZURE DISORDERS

Seizures are caused by transient, paroxysmal, and synchronous discharge of groups of neurons in the brain. Seizure is one of the most common neurologic disorders and may occur at any age. Approximately 5% of the population will experience a seizure at some time during their lives. Clinical manifestations depend on the location and number of neurons involved in the seizure discharge and its duration. Transient abnormalities of brain function, such as occur with hypoglycemia, hyponatremia, hyperthermia, and drug toxicity, typically result in a single seizure. Treatment of the underlying disorder is usually curative. *Epilepsy* is defined as *recurrent seizures* resulting from congenital or acquired factors (e.g., cerebral scarring) and affects approximately 0.6% of the population.

Seizures are grossly classified based on two factors: loss of consciousness and regions of brain affected by the seizure. *Simple seizures* involve no loss of consciousness, whereas altered levels of consciousness are seen in *complex seizures*. *Partial seizures* appear to originate from a limited population of neurons in a single hemisphere, whereas *generalized seizures* appear to involve diffuse activation of neurons in both cerebral hemispheres. A partial seizure may initially be evident in one region of the body and may subsequently become generalized, involving both hemispheres, a process known as *jacksonian march*.

MRI is the preferred method for studying brain structure in patients with epilepsy. Standard EEG is used to identify the location(s) of seizure foci as well as to characterize their electrical properties. The use of videography in addition to EEG allows simultaneous documentation of electrical and clinical seizure activity. Electrocorticography, in which electrodes are surgically placed directly on the cerebral cortex, not only permits more accurate focus identification but also allows mapping of electrical events in relation to identifiable brain surface anatomy, a feature that is valuable during surgical resection of seizure foci. Stimulation of various electrocorticographic electrodes can also help identify eloquent brain areas before seizure focus resection so that those areas can be avoided during surgery.

Pharmacologic Treatment

Seizures are treated with antiepileptic drugs, starting with a single drug and achieving seizure control by increasing the dosage as necessary. Drug combinations may be considered when monotherapy fails. Changes in drug dosage are guided by clinical response (antiseizure effects vs. side effects) rather than by serum drug concentrations. Monitoring of serum drug levels is usually not necessary for patients who are experiencing adequate seizure control without evidence of toxicity. Effective antiepileptic drugs appear to decrease neuronal excitability or enhance neuronal inhibition. Drugs effective for the treatment of partial seizures include carbamazepine, phenytoin, eslicarbazepine, vigabatrin, lacosamide, ezogabine, and valproate. Generalized seizure disorders can be managed with carbamazepine, phenytoin, valproate, barbiturates, gabapentin, levetiracetam, rufinamide, clobazam, or lamotrigine. Except for gabapentin, all of the useful antiepileptic drugs are metabolized in the liver before undergoing renal excretion. Gabapentin appears to undergo no metabolism and is excreted unchanged by the kidneys. Carbamazepine, phenytoin, and barbiturates cause enzyme induction, and long-term treatment with these drugs can alter the rate of their own metabolism as well as that of other drugs. Pharmacokinetic and pharmacodynamic drug interactions are considerations in patients being treated with antiepileptic drugs.

Dose-dependent neurotoxic effects are the most common adverse effects of antiepileptic drugs. All antiepileptic drugs can cause depression of cerebral function with symptoms of sedation.

Phenytoin has many side effects, including hypotension, cardiac dysrhythmias, gingival hyperplasia, and aplastic anemia. It is associated with various cutaneous manifestations, including erythema multiforme and Stevens-Johnson syndrome. Extravasation or intraarterial injection of phenytoin can induce significant vasoconstriction resulting in *purple glove syndrome,* which can lead to skin necrosis, compartment syndrome, and gangrene. These side effects make fosphenytoin, a phosphorylated prodrug that does not share the same toxicity profile as phenytoin, a more attractive option for IV antiepileptic administration.

Valproate produces hepatic failure in approximately 1 in every 10,000 recipients. The mechanism of this hepatotoxicity is unknown, but it may represent an idiosyncratic hypersensitivity reaction. Pancreatitis has also been observed during valproate therapy. Long-term use of valproate is associated with increased surgical bleeding, especially in children. The mechanism is currently unknown but might involve a combination of thrombocytopenia and valproate-induced decreases in von Willebrand factor and factor VIII.

Carbamazepine can cause diplopia, dose-related leukopenia, and hyponatremia (which is usually clinically unimportant) as well as alterations in the hepatic metabolism of various drugs.

Adverse hematologic reactions associated with antiepileptic drugs range from mild anemia to aplastic anemia and are most commonly associated with the use of carbamazepine, phenytoin, and valproate.

Surgical treatment of seizure disorders is considered in patients whose seizures do not respond to antiepileptic drugs or who cannot tolerate the side effects of pharmacologic therapy. Surgery is now being performed much earlier than in the past, particularly in young patients, to avoid social isolation resulting from medication side effects and/or persistent seizures. Partial seizures may respond to resection of a pathologic region within the brain such as a tumor, hamartoma, or scar tissue. Corpus callosotomy may help prevent the generalization of partial seizures to the opposite hemisphere. Finally, hemispherectomy is sometimes needed for persistent catastrophic seizures.

In preparation for surgery the seizure focus is located by imaging and functional studies. MRI is the imaging modality of choice, especially for detection of *mesial temporal sclerosis,* a common cause of complex partial seizures. Nuclear medicine–based modalities such as positron emission tomography (PET) and single-photon emission computed tomography (SPECT) may demonstrate alterations in metabolism or abnormal blood flow in regions of the brain. Video-EEG monitoring can assist in correlating electrical activity and clinical manifestations of seizures.

Electrocorticography, as mentioned earlier, involves placement of electrodes either as a grid directly on the brain surface or deeper within the brain. Electrocorticography offers many advantages over surface EEG recordings, such as increased precision in seizure focus determination, the ability to monitor deep regions of cortex, and the ability to stimulate regions of brain to map eloquent cortex. Electrocorticography can be performed during the same surgical procedure as cortical resection, or electrodes can be placed during one procedure and the patient allowed to return on a different day for seizure focus resection. In the latter case, video monitoring and mapping with grids in place can increase the accuracy of identifying the specific seizure focus for resection.

A more conservative surgical approach to medically intractable seizures involves implantation of a left vagal nerve stimulator. The left side is chosen because the right vagal nerve usually has significant cardiac innervation, which could lead to severe bradydysrhythmias. The mechanism by which vagal nerve stimulation produces its effects is unclear. Patients tolerate this treatment well except for the occurrence of hoarseness in some cases, which reflects the vagal innervation of the larynx.

Status Epilepticus

Status epilepticus is a life-threatening condition that manifests as continuous seizure activity or two or more seizures occurring in sequence without recovery of consciousness between them.

The goal of treatment of status epilepticus is prompt pharmacologic suppression of seizure activity combined with support of the airway, ventilation, and circulation. Hypoglycemia can be ruled out as a cause within minutes, using rapid bedside glucose assessment techniques. If hypoglycemia is present, it can be corrected by IV administration of 50 mL of 50% glucose solution. Routine glucose administration before confirmation of hypoglycemia is potentially dangerous, since hyperglycemia can exacerbate brain injury. Tracheal intubation may be needed to protect the airway and/or optimize oxygen delivery and ventilation. Muscle relaxants should be avoided if muscle movement rather than electrophysiologic monitoring is the principal method of assessing the effectiveness of antiepileptic medications. Administration of an antiepileptic anesthetic (e.g., propofol, thiopental) will temporarily halt seizure activity during tracheal intubation. Monitoring of arterial blood gas levels and pH may be useful for confirming adequacy of oxygenation and ventilation. Metabolic acidosis is a common sequela of ongoing seizure activity. Intravenous administration of sodium bicarbonate may be needed to treat extreme acid-base abnormalities. Hyperthermia occurs frequently during status epilepticus and necessitates active cooling.

Management of Anesthesia

Management of anesthesia in patients with seizure disorders includes considering the impact of antiepileptic drugs on organ function and the effect of anesthetic drugs on seizures. Sedation produced by antiepileptic drugs may have additive effects with that produced by anesthetic drugs, and enzyme induction by antiepileptic drugs may alter the pharmacokinetics and pharmacodynamics of anesthetic drugs.

When selecting anesthetic induction and maintenance drugs, one must consider their effects on CNS electrical activity. Methohexital administration can activate epileptic foci and has been recommended as a method for delineating these foci during electrocorticography in patients undergoing surgical treatment of epilepsy. Alfentanil, ketamine, enflurane, isoflurane, and sevoflurane can cause epileptiform spike-and-wave EEG activity in patients without a history of seizures, but they are also known to suppress epileptiform and epileptic activity. Seizures and opisthotonos have been observed in rare cases after propofol anesthesia, which suggests caution when administering this drug to patients with known seizure disorders. In selection of muscle relaxants, the CNS-stimulating effects of laudanosine, a proconvulsant metabolite of atracurium and cisatracurium, may merit consideration. Various antiepileptic drugs, specifically phenytoin and carbamazepine, shorten the duration of action of nondepolarizing muscle relaxants through both pharmacokinetic and pharmacodynamic means. Topiramate may be the cause of unexplained metabolic acidosis, given its ability to inhibit carbonic anhydrase.

It seems reasonable to avoid administering potentially epileptogenic drugs to patients with epilepsy. Instead, thiobarbiturates, opioids, and benzodiazepines are preferred. Isoflurane, desflurane, and sevoflurane seem to be acceptable choices in patients with seizure disorders. Regardless of the anesthetic drugs used, it is important to maintain treatment with the preoperative antiepileptic drugs throughout the perioperative period.

During intraoperative electrocorticography, monitoring is aimed at identifying *interictal epileptiform activity*, the characteristic patterns of electrical activity that occur in the time between seizures. Many anesthetic agents, such as benzodiazepines, volatile anesthetics, and anesthetic doses of barbiturates and propofol, can significantly suppress epileptiform activity, which renders electrocorticographic monitoring difficult or impossible. During the monitoring period, anesthesia should be managed with agents such as opioids, nitrous oxide, droperidol, diphenhydramine, and possibly dexmedetomidine. If epileptiform activity remains suppressed or is inadequate for analysis, high-dose short-acting opioids (e.g., alfentanil 50 μg/kg as an IV bolus), or small IV boluses of methohexital (0.3 mg/kg) or etomidate (0.05–0.1 mg/kg) can serve to enhance epileptiform activity. Careful attention to maintaining muscle paralysis during this part of the procedure is important. During the preoperative discussion, the patient should be made aware that anesthetic techniques used to improve the quality of electrophysiologic recordings may also increase the risk of awareness during anesthesia.

Despite general anesthesia and muscle relaxation, patients may still exhibit seizure activity. This may manifest as unexplained abrupt changes in heart rate and blood pressure with or without overt clonic movement, depending on the degree of muscle paralysis. Increases in carbon dioxide production from increased brain and muscle metabolism will be reflected in an increased end-tidal carbon dioxide concentration and may result in patient respiratory efforts. Seizures can be terminated by administration of a barbiturate, propofol, or a benzodiazepine that is titrated to seizure cessation. Seizures can also be rapidly terminated by direct application of cold saline to the brain surface. This is a very useful technique in procedures performed in awake patients, because it avoids the use of drugs that could potentially produce somnolence, hypoventilation, airway obstruction, or apnea.

NEUROOCULAR DISORDERS

Disorders involving the visual system discussed in this section are limited to those affecting the retina, optic nerve, and intracranial optic system. Degenerative diseases involving this part of the visual system include Leber optic atrophy, retinitis pigmentosa, and Kearns-Sayre syndrome. The most common cause of new-onset blindness during the perioperative period is ischemic optic neuropathy. Other causes of postoperative visual defects are cortical blindness, retinal artery occlusion, and ophthalmic vein obstruction.

Leber Optic Atrophy

Leber optic atrophy, or Leber hereditary optic neuropathy, is characterized by degeneration of the retina and atrophy of the optic nerves culminating in blindness. This disorder was the first human disorder for which a mitochondrial pattern of inheritance was definitively described. This rare disorder usually presents as loss of central vision in adolescence or early adulthood and is often associated with other neuropathologic conditions, including multiple sclerosis and dystonia.

Retinitis Pigmentosa

Retinitis pigmentosa refers to a genetically and clinically heterogeneous group of inherited retinopathies characterized by degeneration of the retina. These debilitating disorders collectively represent a common form of human visual handicap, with an estimated prevalence of approximately 1 in 3000. Examination of the retina shows areas of pigmentation, particularly in the peripheral regions. Vision is lost first in the periphery of the retina and then moves toward the center until total blindness occurs.

Kearns-Sayre Syndrome

Kearns-Sayre syndrome, a mitochondrial myopathy, is characterized by retinitis pigmentosa associated with progressive external ophthalmoplegia, typically occurring before age 20. Cardiac conduction abnormalities ranging from bundle branch block to complete atrioventricular heart block are common. Complete heart block can occur abruptly, leading to sudden death. Generalized degeneration of the CNS has been observed. Although Kearns-Sayre syndrome is rare, it is possible that patients with this disorder will require anesthesia for insertion of cardiac pacemakers.

Management of anesthesia requires a high index of suspicion for, and preparation to treat, third-degree atrioventricular heart block. Transthoracic pacing capability must be available. Experience is too limited to recommend specific drugs for induction and maintenance of anesthesia. Presumably the response to succinylcholine and nondepolarizing muscle relaxants is not altered, since this disease does not involve motor neurons or the neuromuscular junction.

Ischemic Optic Neuropathy

Ischemic optic neuropathy should be suspected in patients who complain of visual loss during the first week following surgery of any type. Ischemic injury to the optic nerve can result in loss of both central and peripheral vision.

The optic nerve can be functionally divided into an anterior and a posterior segment based on differences in blood supply (Fig. 13.6). Blood supply to the anterior portion is derived from both the central retinal artery and small branches of the ciliary artery. In contrast, blood supply to the posterior segment of the optic nerve is derived from small branches of the ophthalmic and central retinal arteries. Baseline blood flow to the posterior segment of the optic nerve is significantly less than that to the anterior segment. Because of this difference, ischemic events in the anterior and posterior segments of the optic nerve are associated with different risk factors and physical findings. However, the prognosis in terms of improvement of vision is poor in either case. If ischemic optic neuropathy is suspected, urgent ophthalmologic consultation should be obtained so that other treatable causes of perioperative blindness can be excluded.

Anterior Ischemic Optic Neuropathy

The visual loss associated with anterior ischemic optic neuropathy is due to infarction within the watershed perfusion zones between the small branches of the short posterior ciliary arteries. The usual presentation is a sudden, painless, monocular visual deficit varying in severity from a slight decrease in visual acuity to blindness. Asymptomatic optic disk swelling may be the earliest sign. A congenitally small optic disk is often present. The prognosis varies, but the most common outcome is minimal recovery of visual function.

The *nonarteritic form* of anterior ischemic optic neuropathy is more likely than the arteritic form to manifest during the postoperative period. It is usually attributed to decreased oxygen delivery to the optic disk in association with hypotension and/or anemia. This form of visual loss has been associated with hemorrhagic hypotension, anemia, cardiac surgery, head and neck surgery, cardiac arrest, and hemodialysis. It may also occur spontaneously. *Arteritic* anterior ischemic optic neuropathy, which is less common than the nonarteritic form, is associated with inflammation and thrombosis of the short posterior

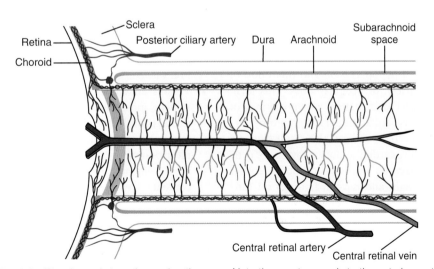

FIG. 13.6 Blood supply to retina and optic nerve. Note the greater supply to the anterior portion of the optic nerve via the central retinal artery. Blood flow to the posterior portion of the optic nerve is supplied by pial perforators and is much less than blood flow to the anterior segment. (Adapted from Hayreh SS. Anatomy and physiology of the optic nerve head. *Trans Am Acad Ophthalmol Otolaryngol.* 1974;78:240-254.)

ciliary arteries. The diagnosis is confirmed by demonstration of giant cell arteritis on a biopsy sample from the temporal artery. High-dose corticosteroids are used to treat arteritic anterior ischemic optic neuropathy and to provide prophylaxis against disease manifestation in the contralateral eye.

Posterior Ischemic Optic Neuropathy

Posterior ischemic optic neuropathy presents as acute loss of vision and visual field defects similar to those in anterior ischemic optic neuropathy. It is presumed to be caused by decreased oxygen delivery to the posterior portion of the optic nerve between the optic foramen and the point of entry of the central retinal artery. However, recent data suggest that impedance of venous outflow from the optic nerve may contribute. Spontaneous occurrence is less frequent than with anterior ischemic optic neuropathy. However, posterior ischemic optic neuropathy is more common than anterior ischemic optic neuropathy as a cause of visual loss in the perioperative period. There may be no abnormal ophthalmoscopic findings initially, which reflects retrobulbar involvement of the optic nerve. Mild disk edema is present after a few days, and CT of the orbits may reveal enlargement of the intraorbital optic nerve.

Posterior ischemic optic neuropathy has been described following prolonged spine surgery performed in the prone position, cardiac surgery, radical neck dissection, hip arthroplasty, and robotic prostatectomy. The etiology of posterior ischemic optic neuropathy appears to be multifactorial. Factors associated with increased risk for posterior ischemic optic neuropathy include male sex, obesity, use of the Wilson frame, long-duration procedures, and increased blood loss during surgery. Other associations such as anemia, hypotension, excessive fluid administration, and excessive use of vasopressors are speculative, with no formal data to support an association.

Cortical Blindness

Cortical blindness may follow profound hypotension or cardiac arrest as a result of hypoperfusion and infarction of watershed areas in the parietal or occipital lobes. This form of blindness has been observed after many different kinds of surgical procedures, such as cardiac surgery, craniotomy, laryngectomy, and cesarean section, and can also result from air or particulate emboli during cardiopulmonary bypass. Cortical blindness is characterized by loss of vision but retention of pupillary reactions to light and normal findings on funduscopic examination. Patients may not be aware of focal vision loss, which usually improves with time. The presence of abnormalities in the parietal or occipital lobes on CT or MRI scans confirms the diagnosis.

Retinal Artery Occlusion

Central retinal artery occlusion presents as painless monocular blindness. It is due to occlusion of a branch of the retinal artery. Visual field defects are often severe initially but improve with time. Ophthalmoscopic examination reveals a pale edematous retina. Unlike ischemic optic neuropathy, central retinal artery occlusion is often caused by emboli from an ulcerated atherosclerotic plaque in the ipsilateral carotid artery. Many retinal artery occlusions are due to emboli during open heart surgery, and these typically resolve promptly. Vasospasm or thrombosis may also cause central retinal artery occlusion following radical neck surgery complicated by hemorrhage and hypotension. The condition can also occur following intranasal injection of α-adrenergic agonists. Stellate ganglion block improves vision in some patients.

Ophthalmic Venous Obstruction

Obstruction of venous drainage from the eyes may occur intraoperatively when patient positioning results in external pressure on the orbits. Placement in the prone position and use of headrests during neurosurgical procedures require careful attention to ensure that the eyeballs and orbits are free from external compression. Ophthalmoscopic examination reveals engorgement of the veins and edema of the macula if obstruction to venous drainage is present.

KEY POINTS

- Major goals when providing anesthesia care for patients undergoing neurologic surgery include maintenance of adequate cerebral oxygen delivery, optimization of operative conditions, and facilitation of a rapid, smooth emergence from anesthesia to allow for immediate assessment of neurologic function.
- In the perioperative period, factors affecting CBF include Pao_2 and $Paco_2$, systemic blood pressure, ICP, cerebral autoregulation, and various drugs.
- Major techniques to decrease ICP include head elevation, hyperventilation, CSF drainage, and administration of hyperosmotic drugs, diuretics, corticosteroids, and cerebral vasoconstrictors.
- Venous air embolism can occur in a variety of circumstances, most commonly in patients who are placed in the sitting (or other head-up) position. Techniques available to monitor for entrainment of air include precordial Doppler ultrasonography, transesophageal echocardiography, and measurement of end-expired carbon dioxide and nitrogen content. Treatment includes discontinuation of nitrous oxide administration, flooding of the surgical field with fluid, aspiration of air via a central venous catheter, and hemodynamic support.
- Succinylcholine should be used with caution in patients with neurologic diseases because of its potential to produce a transient increase in ICP and because of the risk of hyperkalemia in the setting of denervating diseases that cause an upregulation of acetylcholine receptors at the neuromuscular junction.

RESOURCES

American Society of Anesthesiologists Task Force on Perioperative Visual Loss. Practice advisory for perioperative visual loss associated with spine surgery: an updated report by the American Society of Anesthesiologists Task Force on Perioperative Visual Loss. *Anesthesiology*. 2012;116:274-285.

Brott TG, Hobson RW, Howard G, et al. Stenting versus endarterectomy for treatment of carotid artery stenosis. *N Engl J Med*. 2010;363:11-23.

Browne TR, Holmes GL. Epilepsy. *N Engl J Med*. 2001;344:1145-1151.

Connolly Jr ES, Rabinstein AA, Carhuapoma JR, et al. Guidelines for the management of aneurysmal subarachnoid hemorrhage: a guideline for healthcare professionals from the American Heart Association/American Stroke Association. *Stroke*. 2012;43:1711-1737.

Hemphill III JC, Greenberg SM, Anderson CS, et al. Guidelines for the management of spontaneous intracerebral hemorrhage: a guideline for healthcare professionals from the American Heart Association/American Stroke Association. *Stroke*. 2015;46:2032-2060.

Jauch EC, Saver JL, Adams Jr HP, et al. Guidelines for the early management of patients with acute ischemic stroke: a guideline for healthcare professionals from the American Heart Association and American Stroke Association. *Stroke*. 2013;44:870-947.

Leipzig TJ, Morgan J, Horner TG, et al. Analysis of intraoperative rupture in the surgical treatment of 1694 saccular aneurysms. *Neurosurgery*. 2005;56:455-468.

Lukovits TG, Goddeau Jr RP. Critical care of patients with acute ischemic and hemorrhagic stroke: update on recent evidence and international guidelines. *Chest*. 2011;139:694-700.

Mashour GA, Shanks AM, Keterphal S. Perioperative stroke and associated mortality after noncardiac, nonneurologic surgery. *Anesthesiology*. 2011;114:1289-1296.

Mendelow AD, Gregson BA, Fernandes HM, et al. Early surgery versus initial conservative treatment in patients with spontaneous supratentorial intracerebral haematomas in the International Surgical Trial in Intracerebral Haemorrhage (STICH): a randomised trial. *Lancet*. 2005;365:387-397.

Sirven JI, Noe K, Hoerth M, Drazkowski J. Antiepileptic drugs 2012: recent advances and trends. *Mayo Clin Proc*. 2012;87:879-889.

Todd MM, Hindman BJ, Clarke WR, et al. Mild intraoperative hypothermia during surgery for intracranial aneurysm. *N Engl J Med*. 2005;352:135-145.

Wass CT, Lanier WL. Glucose modulation of ischemic brain injury: review and clinical recommendations. *Mayo Clin Proc*. 1996;71:801-812.

Spinal Cord Disorders

JEFFREY J. PASTERNAK, WILLIAM L. LANIER, JR.

The most common cause of acute spinal cord injury is trauma. However, various disease processes, including tumors and congenital and degenerative diseases of the spinal cord and vertebral column, can also cause spinal cord injury.

ACUTE SPINAL CORD INJURY

The mobility of the cervical spine makes it vulnerable to injury, especially *hyperextension* injury. It is estimated that cervical spine injury occurs in 1.5%–3.0% of all major trauma victims. Approximately 4%–5% of patients with traumatic head injury have a concurrent injury to the spine, typically occurring in the upper cervical spine at C1–C3. Trauma can also injure the thoracic and lumbar spinal cord segments.

The clinical manifestations of acute spinal cord injury depend on both the extent and the site of injury. Acute spinal cord injury initially produces a state of spinal shock that is characterized by flaccid muscle paralysis with loss of sensation below the level of injury. *Spinal shock*—that is, loss of neurologic function—is differentiated from *neurogenic shock,* which is a reduction in blood pressure. The extent of injury is commonly described in terms of the International Standards for Neurological Classification of Spinal Cord Injury (ISNCSCI) system (Table 14.1), which characterizes the injury in terms of both motor and sensory impairment. This scale is based on testing 28 dermatomes bilaterally for the response to pinprick and light touch sensation. In addition, 10 key muscle groups are assessed bilaterally with manual muscle testing (Table 14.2). Muscle function is considered to be grade 3 if there is active movement and full range of motion against gravity. Lesser function or total paralysis are noted in grades less than 3. Better function is noted in grades 3 or higher. Evaluation of anal sensory and motor function is also added to the injury classification.

A score of A indicates a "complete" injury in which all motor and sensory function is lost below the level of the lesion, including function at the lower sacral segments of S4 and S5. Lower sacral neurologic function is determined by assessing rectal tone and sensation. Scores of B through D are assigned to "incomplete" lesions in which some degree of spinal cord integrity is maintained below the level of injury. A score of E indicates normal spinal cord function.

The extent of physiologic effects from spinal cord injury depends on the level and degree of injury, with the most severe physiologic derangements occurring with complete injury to the cervical cord and lesser perturbations occurring with less complete injury and more caudal cord injuries. Reductions in blood pressure are common, especially with cervical cord injury, and are influenced by (1) loss of sympathetic nervous system activity and a decrease in systemic vascular resistance and (2) bradycardia resulting from loss of the T1–T4 sympathetic innervation to the heart (i.e., loss of *cardiac accelerator* innervation). Hypotension can also occur with thoracic and lumbar cord injuries, although typically it is less severe than with cervical injuries. *Neurogenic shock,* a condition in which untreated hemodynamic abnormalities are severe enough to impair organ perfusion, typically lasts from 1–3 weeks before compensatory physiologic mechanisms are fully in place.

TABLE 14.1	International Standards for Neurological Classification of Spinal Cord Injury (ISNCSCI)	
Category	Description	Definition
A	Complete	*No sensory or motor* function below level of lesion or in sacral segments S4 and S5
B	Incomplete	Sensory but not motor function is preserved below neurologic level and includes S4–S5 segments
C	Incomplete	Motor function is preserved below level of injury and more than half of key muscles below neurologic level have a grade less than 3
D	Incomplete	Motor function is preserved below level of injury and more than half of key muscles below neurologic level have a grade of 3 or more
E	Normal	Sensory and motor function intact

From Kirshblum SC, Burns SP, Biering-Sorensen F, et al: International standards for neurological classification of spinal cord injury (revised 2011). *J Spinal Cord Med.* 2011;34:535-546.

TABLE 14.2	Key Muscle Groups Tested in ISNCSCI Impairment Evaluation of Acute Spinal Cord Injury
Muscle(s) Tested	Nerve Root Evaluated
Elbow flexors	C5
Wrist extensors	C6
Elbow extensors	C7
Finger flexors	C8
Finger abductors (little finger)	T1
Hip flexors	L2
Knee extensors	L3
Ankle dorsiflexors	L4
Long toe extensors	L5
Ankle plantar flexors	S1

ISNCSCI, International Standards for Neurological Classification of Spinal Cord Injury.

With cervical and upper thoracic cord injury, the major cause of morbidity and mortality is alveolar hypoventilation combined with an inability to clear bronchial secretions. Respiratory muscles are not affected with lumbar and low thoracic injuries, so minimal respiratory impairment can be expected with these injuries. Aspiration of gastric contents, pneumonia, and pulmonary embolism can occur.

Cervical spine radiographs are obtained for a large percentage of patients who come for treatment of various forms of trauma and are intended to identify suspected or occult cervical spine injuries. However, the probability of cervical spine injury is minimal in patients who meet the following five criteria: (1) no midline cervical spine tenderness, (2) no focal neurologic deficits, (3) normal sensorium, (4) no intoxication, and (5) no painful distracting injury. Patients who meet these criteria *do not* require routine imaging studies to rule out occult cervical spine injury.

An estimated two-thirds of trauma patients have multiple injuries that can interfere with cervical spine evaluation. Evaluation ideally includes computed tomography (CT) or magnetic resonance imaging (MRI), but imaging may not be practical in some cases because of the risk of transporting patients in unstable condition. For this reason, standard radiographic views of the cervical spine, often taken with a portable x-ray machine, are relied upon to evaluate for the presence of cervical spine injury and associated instability. For cervical spine imaging to have greatest utility, the entire cervical spine (including the body of the first thoracic vertebra) must be visible. Images are analyzed for alignment of the vertebrae (lateral view), presence of fractures (all views), and the condition of disk and soft tissue spaces. The sensitivity of plain radiographs for detecting cervical spine injury is not 100%, so the likelihood of cervical spine injury must be interpreted in conjunction with other clinical signs, symptoms, and risk factors. If there is any doubt, it is prudent to treat all acute cervical spine injuries as potentially unstable until proven otherwise.

Treatment of a cervical fracture or dislocation entails immediate immobilization to limit neck motion. Soft neck collars have little effect in limiting movement of the neck. Hard neck collars limit neck flexion and extension by only about 25%. Immobilization and traction provided by halothoracic devices are most effective in preventing cervical spine movement. During direct laryngoscopy, *manual in-line stabilization* (in which an assistant's hands are placed on each side of the patient's face, the head is grasped with fingertips resting on the mastoid process, and downward pressure is applied against a firm table surface to hold the head immobile in a neutral position) is recommended to help minimize cervical spine flexion and extension. Cervical spine movement during direct laryngoscopy is likely to be concentrated in the occipito-atlanto-axial area, which suggests an increased risk of spinal cord injury at this level in vulnerable patients, even with the use of in-line stabilization.

Not only can movement of the neck in the presence of cervical spine injury cause mechanical deformation of the spinal cord, but there is an even greater risk that neck motion that elongates the cord will compromise spinal cord blood supply as a result of narrowing the longitudinal blood vessels. In fact, maintenance of spinal cord perfusion pressure may be of more importance than positioning for prevention of spinal cord injury in the presence of cervical spine injury.

Management of Anesthesia

Acute spinal cord injury at the cervical level is accompanied by a marked decrease in vital capacity. Arterial hypoxemia is a consistent early finding following cervical spinal cord injury. Tracheobronchial suctioning has been associated with bradycardia and even cardiac arrest in these patients, so it is important to optimize arterial oxygenation before suctioning the airway.

Patients with acute spinal cord injury often require special precautions during airway management. When laryngoscopy is performed, neck movement must be minimized and hypotension must be avoided so that spinal cord perfusion pressure can be maintained. However, fear of possible spinal cord compression must not prevent necessary airway interventions. Extensive clinical experience supports the use of direct laryngoscopy for orotracheal intubation provided that (1) maneuvers are taken to stabilize the head during the procedure and thus avoid hyperextension of the neck, (2) prior evaluation of the airway did not suggest the likelihood of any technical difficulties, and (3) adequate blood pressure and oxygenation are maintained during airway management. Otherwise, videolaryngoscopes that allow visualization of the larynx with virtually no cervical spine movement are reasonable alternatives to direct laryngoscopy for intubation in patients with known or possible cervical spine trauma. Awake fiberoptic laryngoscopy under topical anesthesia is another alternative to direct laryngoscopy if the patient is cooperative and airway trauma (with associated blood, secretions, and anatomic deformities) does not preclude visualization with the fiberscope. It is important to remember that coughing during topical anesthetization of the airway and fiberoptic intubation may result in cervical spine movement. It is reasonable to have an assistant maintain manual in-line stabilization of the cervical spine during *all* airway manipulations. There is no evidence of increased neurologic morbidity after elective or emergency orotracheal intubation of anesthetized or awake patients with an unstable cervical spine if appropriate steps are taken to minimize neck movement. Awake tracheostomy is reserved for the most challenging airway conditions, in which neck injury, combined with facial fractures or other severe abnormalities of airway anatomy, makes securing the airway by nonsurgical means difficult or unsafe. Airway management in the presence of cervical spine injury should be dictated by common sense, not dogmatic approaches. Certainly, clinical experience supports the safety of a variety of airway management techniques.

The absence of compensatory sympathetic nervous system responses in patients with cervical or high thoracic spinal cord injury makes these patients particularly vulnerable to dramatic decreases in blood pressure following changes in body position, blood loss, or positive pressure ventilation. To minimize these effects, liberal intravenous infusion of crystalloid solutions may be necessary to maintain intravascular volume that has been compromised by vasodilation. Acute blood loss should be treated promptly. Electrocardiographic abnormalities are common during the acute phase of spinal cord injury, especially with cervical cord injuries. Breathing is best managed by mechanical ventilation, since abdominal and intercostal muscle weakness or paralysis is exacerbated by general anesthesia and increases the likelihood of respiratory failure with ensuing hypoxemia and hypercapnia. Body temperature should be monitored and manipulated because patients tend to become poikilothermic in dermatomes below the level of the spinal cord lesion. Maintenance of anesthesia is targeted at ensuring physiologic stability and facilitating tolerance of

TABLE 14.3	Early and Late Complications in Patients With Spinal Cord Injury
Complication	Incidence (%)
2 YEARS AFTER INJURY	
Urinary tract infection	59
Skeletal muscle spasticity	38
Chills and fever	19
Decubitus ulcer	16
Autonomic hyperreflexia	8
Skeletal muscle contractures	6
Heterotopic ossification	3
Pneumonia	3
Renal dysfunction	2
Postoperative wound infection	2
30 YEARS AFTER INJURY	
Decubitus ulcers	17
Skeletal muscle or joint pain	16
Gastrointestinal dysfunction	14
Cardiovascular dysfunction	14
Urinary tract infection	14
Infectious disease or cancer	11
Visual or hearing disorders	10
Urinary retention	8
Male genitourinary dysfunction	7
Renal calculi	6

the endotracheal tube. Volatile and intravenous anesthetics are both satisfactory in this situation. Nitrous oxide should be used with great caution, if at all, given concerns for co-existing trauma and air entrainment in closed spaces, as can occur with basilar skull fracture or rib fracture. Nitrous oxide would then contribute to expansion of pneumocephalus or pneumothorax. Arterial hypoxemia is common following spinal cord injury, which emphasizes the need for continuous pulse oximetry and oxygen supplementation.

Muscle relaxant use should be based on the operative site and the level of spinal cord injury. Succinylcholine does not provoke excessive release of potassium during the first few hours after spinal cord injury. The benefits of succinylcholine, which include rapid onset of action and short duration of paralysis must, as always, be weighed against potential side effects. Use of a nondepolarizing relaxant, with mask ventilation while cricoid pressure is employed, is another alternative to airway management during anesthetic induction and before laryngoscopy. A nondepolarizing relaxant may also facilitate patient positioning.

CHRONIC SPINAL CORD INJURY

Sequelae of chronic spinal cord injury include impaired alveolar ventilation, autonomic hyperreflexia, chronic pulmonary and genitourinary tract infections, renal stones and possible renal dysfunction, anemia, and altered thermoregulation (Table 14.3). Injuries that occur more rostrally along the spinal cord tend to have more significant systemic effects. Chronic urinary tract infection reflects the inability to empty the bladder completely and predisposes to calculus formation. As a result, renal failure may occur and is a common cause of death in patients with chronic spinal cord injury. Prolonged immobility leads to osteoporosis, skeletal muscle atrophy, and decubitus ulcers. Immobility can also predispose patients to deep vein thrombosis, so prophylactic measures such as use of compression stockings, low-dose anticoagulant therapy, or insertion of an inferior vena cava filter may be indicated. Pathologic fractures can occur when these patients are moved. Pressure points should be well protected and padded to minimize the likelihood of trauma to the skin and development of decubitus ulcers.

Depression and chronic pain are common problems following spinal cord injury. Nerve root pain is localized at or near the level of injury. Visceral pain is produced by distention of the bladder or bowel. Phantom body pain can occur in areas of complete sensory loss. As a result of such pain and/or depression, these patients are often treated with analgesics (including opioids) and antidepressants that require attention when anesthetic management is planned.

Several weeks after acute spinal cord injury, spinal cord reflexes gradually return and patients enter a more chronic stage characterized by overactivity of the sympathetic nervous system and involuntary skeletal muscle spasms. Baclofen, which potentiates the inhibitory effects of γ-aminobutyric acid (GABA), is useful for treating spasticity. Abrupt cessation of baclofen therapy, as might occur with hospitalization for an unrelated problem, may result in withdrawal reactions that can include seizures. Diazepam and other benzodiazepines also facilitate the inhibitory effects of GABA and may have specific utility in the management of patients receiving baclofen. Spasticity refractory to pharmacologic suppression may require surgical treatment via dorsal rhizotomy or myelotomy, but typically implantation of a spinal cord stimulator or subarachnoid baclofen pump will be undertaken before rhizotomy is even considered.

Spinal cord injury at or above the fifth cervical vertebra may result in apnea caused by denervation of the diaphragm, which has innervation from C3–C5. When function of the diaphragm is intact, the tidal volume is likely to remain adequate, but the ability to cough and clear secretions from the airway is often impaired because of a decreased expiratory reserve volume resulting from denervation of intercostal and abdominal muscles.

Management of Anesthesia

Anesthetic management in patients with chronic spinal cord injury should focus on preventing autonomic hyperreflexia. When general anesthesia is selected, administration of muscle relaxants is useful to facilitate tracheal intubation and prevent reflex skeletal muscle spasms in response to surgical stimulation. Nondepolarizing muscle relaxants are the primary choice in this circumstance, since succinylcholine may provoke hyperkalemia, most commonly during the initial 6 months after spinal cord injury. Indeed, it seems reasonable to avoid

use of succinylcholine in patients with a spinal cord injury of longer than 24 hours' duration.

The anesthesiologist must be aware of the potential for altered hemodynamics, especially with cervical and high thoracic cord lesions. These can manifest as wide alterations in both blood pressure and heart rate. In chronically immobile patients, the index of suspicion for pulmonary thromboembolism, which can manifest as alterations in hemodynamics and oxygenation, must be high. If intercostal muscle function is impaired, patients may be at high risk of postoperative hypoventilation and may have an impaired cough and a corresponding accumulation of secretions. Baclofen and benzodiazepines should be continued throughout the perioperative period to avoid withdrawal symptoms. Patients with impaired renal function may require close attention to fluid administration, serum electrolyte concentrations, and potential altered pharmacology of drugs eliminated by the kidney. Prophylaxis against deep venous thrombosis should be continued.

AUTONOMIC HYPERREFLEXIA

Autonomic hyperreflexia appears following spinal shock and in association with return of spinal cord reflexes. This reflex response can be initiated by cutaneous or visceral stimulation below the level of spinal cord injury. Surgery and distention of a hollow viscus such as the bladder or rectum are common stimuli.

Stimulation *below* the level of spinal cord injury initiates afferent impulses that enter the spinal cord (Fig. 14.1). Because of reflexes entirely within the spinal cord itself, these impulses elicit an increase in sympathetic nervous system activity along the splanchnic outflow tract. In neurologically intact individuals, this outflow would be modulated by inhibitory impulses from higher centers in the central nervous system, but in the presence of a spinal cord lesion, this outflow is isolated from

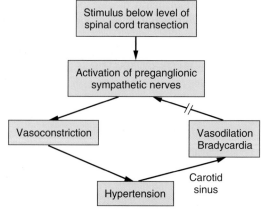

FIG. 14.1 Sequence of events associated with clinical manifestations of autonomic hyperreflexia. Because the efferent impulses from the brain that produce compensatory vasodilation (in response to increased baroreceptor activity) cannot reach the neurologically isolated portion of the spinal cord, unmodulated vasoconstriction develops below the level of the spinal cord injury, resulting in systemic hypertension.

inhibitory impulses from above, so generalized *vasoconstriction* occurs *below* the level of the spinal cord injury.

Hypertension and reflex bradycardia are the hallmarks of autonomic hyperreflexia—severe systemic hypertension causes reflex bradycardia. Reflex cutaneous *vasodilation* occurs *above* the level of the spinal cord injury. Nasal stuffiness reflects this vasodilation. Patients may complain of headache and blurred vision, which indicate severe hypertension. This increase in blood pressure can result in cerebral, retinal, or subarachnoid hemorrhage as well as increased operative blood loss. Loss of consciousness and seizures may also occur, and cardiac dysrhythmias are often present. Pulmonary edema reflects acute left ventricular failure resulting from dramatically increased afterload.

The incidence of autonomic hyperreflexia depends on the level of spinal cord injury. Approximately 85% of patients with lesions above T6 exhibit this reflex. It is unlikely to be associated with spinal cord lesions below T10 (Fig. 14.2). Also, in patients with cervical or high thoracic spinal cord lesions, those with complete lesions are more likely to exhibit autonomic hyperreflexia than those with incomplete lesions.

Management of patients at risk of this phenomenon should begin with efforts to *prevent* the development of autonomic hyperreflexia. Patients who have no history of this reflex are still at risk of its occurrence during surgery, simply because of the intense stimuli surgery can produce. Before surgical or other stimulation is initiated in locations that lack sensory innervation, general, neuraxial, or regional anesthesia should be instituted. Epidural anesthesia has been described for the treatment of autonomic hyperreflexia provoked by uterine contractions during labor. However, epidural anesthesia may be less effective than spinal anesthesia in preventing autonomic hyperreflexia because of its relative sparing of the sacral segments and lesser block density. Blocking afferent

pathways with topical local anesthetics applied to the urethra for a cystoscopic procedure does not prevent autonomic hyperreflexia, because this form of anesthesia does not block the bladder muscle proprioceptors that are stimulated by bladder distention.

Regardless of the anesthesia technique selected, vasodilator drugs having a short half-life (e.g., sodium nitroprusside) should be readily available to treat sudden-onset severe hypertension. Persistence of hypertension may require continuous infusion of vasodilators, perhaps supplemented with longer-acting drugs such as hydralazine. It is important to note that autonomic hyperreflexia may first manifest *postoperatively* when the effects of the anesthetic drugs begin to wane.

SPINAL CORD TUMORS

Spinal cord tumors can be divided into two broad categories. *Intramedullary* tumors are located within the spinal cord and account for approximately 10% of tumors affecting the spinal column. Gliomas and ependymomas account for the vast majority of these intramedullary tumors. *Extramedullary* tumors can be either intradural or extradural. Neurofibromas and meningiomas account for most of the intradural tumors. Metastatic lesions, usually from lung, breast, or prostate cancer or myeloma, are the most common extradural lesions. Other mass lesions of the spinal cord, including abscesses and hematomas, share many of the clinical signs and symptoms of tumors.

Spinal cord tumors typically present with symptoms of cord compression. Pain is a common finding and is usually aggravated by coughing or straining. Motor symptoms and sphincter disturbances may occur. Sometimes spinal tenderness may be present. Diagnosis is usually based on symptoms and imaging of the spinal cord. MRI is the technique of choice. Treatment and prognosis depend on the nature of the lesion, and treatment may include corticosteroids, radiation therapy, chemotherapy, or surgical decompression or excision.

Management of Anesthesia

Management of anesthesia involves ensuring adequate spinal cord oxygenation and perfusion. This is achieved by maintaining PaO_2 at sufficient levels and avoiding hypotension and anemia. Specifics of management will depend on the level of the lesion, the extent of neurologic impairment, and whether or not evoked potential monitoring will be used during surgery.

Tumors involving the cervical spinal cord may influence the approach used to secure the airway. Significant motion of the cervical spine could lead to further cord compromise via compression and a decrease in cord perfusion. With any form of disease that places the cervical spine at risk of new injury, airway management should be similar to that discussed for the management of acute spinal cord injury. This may include in-line stabilization during either standard laryngoscopy,

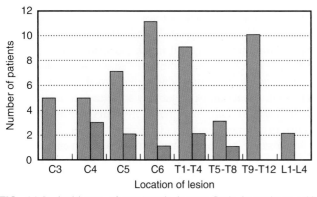

FIG. 14.2 Incidence of autonomic hyperreflexia in patients with spinal cord injury undergoing extracorporeal shock wave lithotripsy. This reflex did not occur in any patient with an injury below T9. Blue bars show the distribution of lesion sites in all patients with spinal cord injury (n = 52); orange bars show the lesion sites in the subset of patients developing autonomic hyperreflexia (n = 9). (Adapted from Stowe DF, Bernstein JS, Madsen KE, et al. Autonomic hyperreflexia in spinal cord injured patients during extracorporeal shock wave lithotripsy. *Anesth Analg.* 1989;68:788-791.)

videolaryngoscopy, or awake fiberoptic tracheal intubation. If the approach to patient management is uncertain, it is useful—*before* administering sedatives or opioids—to have the patient placed in position for airway management and then to move carefully through the anticipated variations of head and neck movements before actual airway manipulation or induction of anesthesia is carried out. Eliciting or exacerbating symptoms upon movement should tip the clinician toward fiberoptic laryngoscopy (with the head held in neutral position) or other options that are less likely to cause movement with its potential for harm to the spinal cord. Use of a light wand or videolaryngoscope may facilitate intubation of the trachea without significant neck extension.

Safe resection of a tumor may require use of intraoperative electrophysiologic monitoring of neurologic function. Electromyography, somatosensory evoked potential monitoring, and motor evoked potential monitoring have a variety of anesthetic implications. The preferred approach may vary from institution to institution.

Succinylcholine should be used with caution in patients with spinal cord tumors, given the risk of associated hyperkalemia. Neuromuscular monitoring with train-of-four stimulation should be performed on a neurologically intact extremity. Upper motor neuron impairment may lead to upregulation of acetylcholine receptors, which makes an affected extremity more resistant to nondepolarizing blockade. If there are significant concerns regarding the possibility of altered responsiveness to neuromuscular block because of tumor-induced spinal cord dysfunction, train-of-four monitoring on the facial nerve may be a reasonable option. One should be careful, however, to monitor evoked muscle twitches, not direct muscle stimulation.

INTERVERTEBRAL DISK DISEASE

Low back pain ranks second only to upper respiratory tract disease as the most common reason for office visits to physicians. An estimated 70% of adults experience low back pain at some time in their lives. Among chronic conditions, low back pain is the most common cause of limitation of activity in patients younger than 45 years. Primary or metastatic cancer is the most common systemic disease affecting vertebral bodies, but it accounts for fewer than 1% of all episodes of low back pain.

One of the most common causes of back pain is intervertebral disk disease. The intervertebral disk is composed of a compressible nucleus pulposus surrounded by a fibrocartilaginous annulus fibrosis. The disk acts as a shock absorber between vertebral bodies. Trauma or degenerative processes lead to changes in the intervertebral disk. Nerve root or spinal cord compression results when the nucleus pulposus protrudes through the annulus fibrosis. With compression of a single nerve root (i.e., a radiculopathy), patients usually complain of pain in a single dermatomal distribution or localized muscle weakness. Spinal cord compression can lead to complex sensory, motor, and autonomic symptoms at and below

the level of the insult. CT or MRI confirms the diagnosis and the location of intervertebral disk herniation.

Cervical Disk Disease

Lateral protrusion of a cervical disk usually occurs at the C5–6 or C6–7 intervertebral spaces. Protrusion can be secondary to trauma or can occur spontaneously. Symptoms are commonly aggravated by coughing. The same symptoms can be due to osteophytes that compress nerve roots in the intervertebral foramina. It is important to note that many people have vertebral osteophytes, but treatment should be dictated based on symptoms and not simply the presence of an osteophyte.

Initial treatment of cervical disk protrusion is typically conservative and includes rest, pain control, and possibly epidural administration of steroids. Surgical decompression is necessary if symptoms do not abate with conservative treatment or if there is significant motor involvement.

Management of Anesthesia

The primary initial concern in the perioperative care of patients with cervical spine disease is airway management. The clinician should base the approach to airway management on the medical history, physical examination findings, review of radiologic studies, and discussion with the surgeon. Direct laryngoscopy can be considered if the patient shows no significant exacerbation of neurologic symptoms with neck movement (especially neck extension), no spinal instability, and no other airway abnormalities. Use of a videolaryngoscope or an assistant to manually maintain neck neutrality during airway management can be considered. If there is any significant concern that laryngoscopy may induce spinal cord compromise, awake fiberoptic intubation followed by a brief neurologic examination after successful tube placement should be considered. For patients with an unstable cervical spine who may be at risk for exacerbation of their injury during positioning for surgery, evoked potential monitoring (especially use of motor evoked potentials) can be conducted before and after positioning to assess for changes. If this is performed, an anesthetic technique that facilitates monitoring should be employed.

In cervical spine procedures performed via an anterior approach, retraction of the airway structures to attain access to the cervical spine may result in injury to the ipsilateral recurrent laryngeal nerve. Many cases of nerve injury are asymptomatic, but injury may manifest as hoarseness, stridor, or (less frequently) frank airway compromise postoperatively. Injury may be due either to direct compression of or traction on the recurrent laryngeal nerve, or compression of nerve fibers within the airway. Such compression of nerve fibers may be caused by the endotracheal tube shaft—rigidly tethered at the mouth and anchored at the distal end by the inflated cuff—during airway retraction, or by direct pressure effects of the inflated cuff. Because of these issues, it is common practice following airway retraction to let air out of the endotracheal tube cuff and then reinflate it to the point at which no air leak is noted.

Lumbar Disk Disease

The most common sites for lumbar disk protrusion are the L4–5 and L5–S1 intervertebral spaces. Disk protrusion at both sites produces low back pain that radiates down the posterior and lateral aspect of the thighs and calves (sciatica). The exact pattern and distribution of symptoms depend on the spinal level and nerve roots affected. A history of trauma, often viewed as trivial by the patient, is commonly associated with the sudden onset of back pain and signals disk protrusion. Alternatively a similar constellation of symptoms can occur as a result of disk degeneration, where loss of disk height leads to compression of nerve roots due to stenosis of the nerve root foramina. Back pain is aggravated by coughing or stretching of the sciatic nerve as, for example, by straight-leg raising. These mechanical signs help distinguish disk protrusion from peripheral nerve disorders. For example, diabetes mellitus–associated peripheral neuropathy may share the symptoms but not the signs of a ruptured lumbar disk.

Treatment of acute lumbar disk protrusion has historically included bed rest, analgesics, and centrally acting "muscle relaxants." Patients with acute low back pain who continue ordinary activities within the limits permitted by the pain have a more rapid recovery than those who stay on bed rest or perform back-mobilizing exercises. When neurologic symptoms persist despite conservative medical management, surgical laminectomy or microdiskectomy can be considered to decompress the affected nerve roots. Epidural steroids (e.g., triamcinolone, methylprednisolone) are an alternative to surgery in certain patients. These drugs act by decreasing inflammation and edema around the nerve roots. Suppression of the hypothalamic-pituitary-adrenal axis is a consideration in patients treated with oral steroids and may have implications for anesthetic management. Although epidural steroid injections may provide short-term alleviation of symptoms caused by sciatica, this treatment offers no significant functional benefit, nor does it decrease the need for surgery.

CONGENITAL AND DEGENERATIVE DISEASES OF THE VERTEBRAL COLUMN AND SPINAL CORD

Spina Bifida Occulta

Spina bifida occulta (incomplete formation of a single lamina in the lumbosacral spine without other abnormalities) is a congenital defect that is present in an estimated 5% of individuals. It usually produces no symptoms and is often discovered as an incidental finding on radiographic examination during evaluation of some other unrelated disease process. Because there are no associated abnormalities, an increased risk with spinal anesthesia is not expected, and large numbers of these patients have undergone spinal anesthesia safely.

Meningocele and Myelomeningocele

During fetal development, closure of the neural tube is required for normal formation of the brain, spinal cord, and their enclosing structures, the cranium and vertebral canal. Failure of the neural tube to appropriately close in the caudal segments results in neural tube defects. Herniation of contents of the spinal canal result in meningocele and myelomeningocele if the herniated contents contain only meninges and cerebrospinal fluid (CSF) versus meninges, CSF, *and* neural elements, respectively. This is opposed to a pseudomeningocele, which is a collection of CSF that does not contain meninges or neural elements and usually results from trauma or surgery. Meningocele is relatively rare and usually associated with a lower incidence and severity of neurologic deficits. Myelomeningocele is the most common severe congenital anomaly of the spine. Although it usually occurs in the lumbosacral region, myelomeningocele can also occur in cervical or thoracic regions of the vertebral column and cord. Increased risk for this defect is associated with maternal folate deficiency and can occur in the setting of other congenital anomalies such as trisomy 13, trisomy 18, and type II Chiari malformations. Hydrocephalus can also occur, especially in the presence of a type II Chiari malformation. A myelomeningocele often results in sensory and motor deficits that can be severe. Patients often have bowel and bladder dysfunction as well. In utero surgical repair of a myelomeningocele may reduce the incidence of associated hydrocephalus and improve overall neurologic function.

Owing to frequent and multiple exposures to latex-containing products from a very early age, patients with myelomeningocele often develop latex sensitivity, so perioperative exposure to latex should be avoided. Perioperative management should include avoidance of succinylcholine because of increased risk for hyperkalemia in the setting of motor deficits. Resistance to nondepolarizing muscle relaxants can occur in weak extremities, so titration of muscle relaxant dose should not be based on monitoring of the lower extremities. The clinician should also be aware of other neurologic deficits that may be related to hydrocephalus, such as the presence of a CSF-diverting shunt or Chiari malformation.

Tethered Spinal Cord Syndrome

During fetal development the vertebral column develops and elongates faster than the spinal cord. Abnormal attachments of the spinal cord to the vertebral column can result in stretching of the spinal cord and development of tethered spinal cord syndrome. These abnormal attachments can occur in the setting of myelomeningocele, dermal sinus tracts, lipomatous tissue in the spinal canal, diastematomyelia (a bifurcated spinal cord), or a filum terminale of reduced elasticity. Also, trauma or injury to the spinal cord and vertebral column can cause scar formation that can lead to cord tethering. Spinal cord stretch leads to dysfunction. Depending on the cause and severity, tethered spinal cord syndrome can present at any stage of life from early childhood through adulthood. Many individuals with a tethered spinal cord have cutaneous manifestations overlying the anomaly, including tufts of hair, hyperpigmented areas, cutaneous lipomas, and skin dimples. Scoliosis and foot deformities such as clubfoot may also occur.

Spinal anesthesia in patients with a tethered spinal cord may increase the risk of cord injury. Normally the conus medullaris lies at the level of L1–L2 in adults. Patients with tethered spinal cord syndrome often have a conus medullaris that lies below the L2 level. There may also be stretch of the cord *without* a low conus medullaris, or there can be a functional cord stretch that may occur only with changes in position. Patients may present with motor and sensory deficits and bladder and bowel incontinence. Surgical management often involves release of tethering if possible. Spinal anesthesia should be avoided in these patients to reduce risk of exacerbation of neurologic deficits. In patients with motor deficits, succinylcholine should be avoided owing to risk for hyperkalemia. Resistance to nondepolarizing muscle relaxants can also occur.

Syringomyelia

Syringomyelia, also known as *syrinx,* is a disorder in which there is cystic cavitation of the spinal cord. The condition is often congenital, but it can also occur following spinal cord trauma or in association with various neoplastic conditions such as gliomas. Rostral extension into the brainstem is called *syringobulbia.* Two main forms of syringomyelia occur, depending on whether there is communication of the cystic region with the subarachnoid space or central canal. There may be only dilation of the central canal of the cord, known as *hydromyelia.* In another form of communicating syringomyelia, there is a communication between the abnormal cystic lesions in the spinal cord proper and the CSF spaces. Communicating syringomyelia is usually associated with a history of basilar arachnoiditis or Chiari I malformation. In contrast the presence of cysts that have no connection to the CSF spaces is called *noncommunicating syringomyelia* and is often associated with a history of trauma, neoplasm, or arachnoiditis.

Signs and symptoms of congenital syringomyelia usually begin during the third or fourth decade of life. Early complaints are those of sensory impairment involving pain and temperature sensation in the upper extremities. This reflects destruction of pain and temperature neuronal pathways that cross within the spinal cord near the central canal. As cavitation of the spinal cord progresses, destruction of lower motor neurons ensues, with development of skeletal muscle weakness and wasting and loss of reflexes. Thoracic scoliosis may result from weakness of paravertebral muscles. Syringobulbia is characterized by paralysis of the palate, tongue, and vocal cords and loss of sensation over the face. MRI is the preferred procedure to diagnose syringomyelia.

There is no known treatment that is effective in arresting the progressive degeneration of the spinal cord or medulla. Surgical procedures designed to restore normal CSF flow have not been predictably effective.

Management of anesthesia in patients with syringomyelia or syringobulbia should consider the neurologic deficits associated with this disease. Thoracic scoliosis can contribute to pulmonary ventilation/perfusion mismatching. Lower motor neuron disease with skeletal muscle wasting suggests that hyperkalemia can develop after administration of succinylcholine. Altered responses to nondepolarizing muscle relaxants can be observed. Thermal regulation may be impaired. Selection of drugs for induction and maintenance of anesthesia is not influenced by this disease. With syringobulbia, any decrease in or absence of protective airway reflexes may influence the timing of endotracheal tube removal postoperatively.

Spondylosis and Spondylolisthesis

Spondylosis is a common acquired degenerative disorder that leads to osteophyte formation and degenerative disk disease. The term *spondylosis* is used synonymously with *spinal stenosis.* There is narrowing of the spinal canal and compression of the spinal cord by transverse osteophytes or nerve root compression by bony spurs in the intervertebral foramina. Spinal cord dysfunction can also result from ischemia of the spinal cord caused by bony compression of the spinal arteries. Symptoms typically develop insidiously after age 50. With cervical spondylosis, neck pain and radicular pain in the arms and shoulders are accompanied by sensory loss and skeletal muscle atrophy. Later, sensory and motor signs may appear in the legs, producing an unsteady gait. Lumbar spondylosis usually leads to radicular pain and muscle atrophy in the lower extremities. Sphincter disturbances are uncommon regardless of the location of spondylosis. Radiographs of the spine often demonstrate osteoarthritic changes, but these changes correlate poorly with neurologic symptoms. Surgery may be necessary to arrest progression of the symptoms, especially if there is evidence of motor loss.

Spondylolisthesis refers to anterior subluxation of one vertebral body on another. This most commonly occurs at the lumbosacral junction. Radicular symptoms usually involve the nerve root inferior to the pedicle of the anteriorly subluxed vertebra. Treatment includes analgesics, antiinflammatory medications, and physical therapy if low back pain is the only symptom. Surgery is reserved for patients who have myelopathy, radiculopathy, or neurogenic claudication.

Amyotrophic Lateral Sclerosis

Amyotrophic lateral sclerosis (ALS) is a degenerative disease involving (1) the lower motor neurons in the anterior horn gray matter of the spinal cord and (2) the corticospinal tracts (i.e., the primary descending upper motor neurons). Therefore this disease process produces both upper and lower motor neuron degeneration. It most commonly affects men aged 40–60 years. When the degenerative process is limited to the motor cortex of the brain, the disease is called *primary lateral sclerosis;* limitation to the brainstem nuclei is known as *pseudobulbar palsy.* Werdnig-Hoffmann disease resembles ALS except that it occurs during the first 3 years of life. Although the cause of ALS is unknown, a genetic pattern is occasionally present, with defects in the gene for the enzyme superoxide dismutase occurring in up to 20% of patients.

Signs and symptoms of ALS reflect upper and lower motor neuron dysfunction. Initial manifestations include skeletal muscle atrophy, weakness, and fasciculations, frequently beginning in the intrinsic muscles of the hands. With time, atrophy and weakness involve most of the skeletal muscles, including the tongue, pharynx, larynx, and chest wall. Early symptoms of bulbar involvement include fasciculations of the tongue plus dysphagia, which leads to pulmonary aspiration. The ocular muscles are generally spared. Autonomic nervous system dysfunction can be manifested as orthostatic hypotension and resting tachycardia. Complaints of cramping and aching sensations, particularly in the legs, are common. Plasma creatine kinase concentrations are normal, which distinguishes this disease from chronic polymyositis. Carcinoma of the lung has been associated with ALS. ALS has no known treatment, and death from respiratory failure is likely within 6 years after the onset of symptoms.

General anesthesia in patients with ALS may be associated with exaggerated respiratory depression. ALS patients are also vulnerable to hyperkalemia following administration of succinylcholine as a result of lower motor neuron disease, and these patients may show prolonged responses to nondepolarizing muscle relaxants. Bulbar involvement with dysfunction of pharyngeal muscles may predispose to pulmonary aspiration. There is no evidence that any specific anesthetic drug or combination of drugs is ideal in these patients. Epidural anesthesia has been used successfully in patients with ALS without neurologic exacerbation or impairment of pulmonary function.

Friedreich's Ataxia

Friedreich's ataxia is an autosomal recessive condition characterized by degeneration of the spinocerebellar and pyramidal tracts. Cardiomyopathy is present in 10%–50% of patients with this disease. Kyphoscoliosis, producing a progressive deterioration in pulmonary function, is seen in nearly 80% of affected individuals. Ataxia is the typical presenting symptom. Dysarthria, nystagmus, skeletal muscle weakness and spasticity, and diabetes mellitus may be present. Friedreich's ataxia is usually fatal by early adulthood, most often because of heart failure.

Management of anesthesia in patients with Friedreich's ataxia is similar to that described for patients with ALS. If cardiomyopathy is present, the negative inotropic effects of anesthetic drugs must be considered when selecting a technique. Kyphoscoliosis may make epidural anesthesia technically difficult. Spinal anesthesia has been used successfully. The likelihood of postoperative ventilatory failure may be increased, especially in the presence of kyphoscoliosis.

KEY POINTS

- The physiologic effects of a spinal cord injury depend on the level of injury, with the most severe physiologic derangements occurring with injury to the cervical cord.

Hypotension is a result of (1) loss of sympathetic nervous system activity and a decrease in systemic vascular resistance and (2) bradycardia resulting from loss of the T1–T4 sympathetic innervation to the heart. These hemodynamic changes are collectively known as neurogenic shock and typically last 1–3 weeks.

- Major goals in caring for patients who have spinal cord disease or are undergoing surgical procedures involving the spinal cord or vertebral column are maintenance of adequate blood flow and oxygen delivery to vulnerable neurologic tissues, optimization of operative conditions, and facilitation of a rapid, smooth emergence from anesthesia to allow immediate assessment of neurologic function.
- Succinylcholine should be used with caution in patients with motor deficits because of the risk of hyperkalemia.
- In acute spinal cord injury, care must be taken during airway manipulation to avoid excessive neck movement. Succinylcholine can be used without a significant risk of hyperkalemia in the first few hours following spinal cord injury.
- Sequelae of chronic spinal cord injury may include impaired alveolar ventilation, cardiovascular instability manifested as autonomic hyperreflexia, chronic pulmonary and genitourinary tract infections, anemia, and altered thermoregulation.
- Patients with cervical and thoracic spinal cord injuries are at risk of developing autonomic hyperreflexia in response to various stimuli, including surgery, bowel distention, and bladder distention. Autonomic hyperreflexia can be prevented by either general or spinal anesthesia, since both methods are effective in blocking the afferent limb of the pathway. Use of topical anesthesia for cystoscopic procedures does not prevent autonomic hyperreflexia, and epidural anesthesia is not reliably effective in preventing autonomic hyperreflexia.
- Spinal cord tumors can be divided into two broad categories. Intramedullary tumors are located within the spinal cord and account for approximately 10% of tumors affecting the spinal column. Gliomas and ependymomas account for the vast majority of intramedullary tumors. Extramedullary tumors can be either intradural or extradural. Neurofibromas and meningiomas account for most of the intradural tumors. Metastatic lesions, usually from lung, breast, or prostate cancer or myeloma, are the most common forms of extradural lesions.
- Low back pain ranks second only to upper respiratory tract disease as the most common reason for office visits to physicians. An estimated 70% of adults experience low back pain at some time in their lives.

RESOURCES

Adzick NS, Thom EA, Spong CY, et al. A randomized trial of prenatal versus postnatal repair of myelomeningocele. N Engl J Med. 2011;364:993-1004.
Hindman BJ, Palecek JP, Posner KL, et al. Cervical spinal cord, root, and bony spine injuries: a closed claims analysis. Anesthesiology. 2011;114:782-795.
Hoffman JR, Mower WR, Wolfson AB, et al. Validity of a set of clinical criteria to rule out injury to the cervical spine in patients with blunt trauma.

National Emergency X-Radiography Utilization Study Group. *N Engl J Med*. 2000;343:94-99.

Jung A, Schramm J. How to reduce recurrent laryngeal nerve palsy in anterior cervical spine surgery: a prospective observational study. *Neurosurgery*. 2010;67:10-15.

Kirshblum SC, Burns SP, Biering-Sorensen F, et al. International standards for neurological classification of spinal cord injury (revised 2011). *J Spinal Cord Med*. 2011;34:535-546.

Lennarson PJ, Smith D, Todd MM, et al. Segmental cervical spine motion during orotracheal intubation of the intact and injured spine with and without external stabilization. *J Neurosurg*. 2000;92:201-206.

Loftus RW, Yeager MP, Clark JA, et al. Intraoperative ketamine reduces perioperative opiate consumption in opiate-dependent patients with chronic back pain undergoing back surgery. *Anesthesiology*. 2010;113:639-646.

Lotto ML, Banoub M, Schubert A. Effects of anesthetic agents and physiologic changes on intraoperative motor evoked potentials. *J Neurosurg Anesthesiol*. 2004;16:32-42.

Diseases of the Autonomic and Peripheral Nervous Systems

JEFFREY J. PASTERNAK, WILLIAM L. LANIER, JR.

The *peripheral nervous system* comprises nerve elements outside the brain and spinal cord. It contains both peripheral nerves and elements of the autonomic nervous system (ANS). Disorders of the ANS can result in significant hemodynamic changes as well as abnormal responses to drugs that work via adrenergic receptors. Diseases affecting peripheral nerves often have implications for perioperative patient management, including the choice of muscle relaxants and control of neuropathic pain.

AUTONOMIC DISORDERS

Multiple System Atrophy

Multiple system atrophy (MSA) involves degeneration and dysfunction of diverse central nervous system structures such as the basal ganglia, cerebellar cortex, locus ceruleus, pyramidal tracts, inferior olivary nuclei, vagal motor nuclei, and spinocerebellar tracts. The extent of degeneration of these structures, individually or in aggregate, results in different clinical manifestations that in the past were considered different disease states. Examples include *striatonigral degeneration, olivopontocerebellar atrophy,* and *Shy-Drager syndrome* when, respectively, parkinsonian features, cerebellar dysfunction, and autonomic dysfunction predominated. Now these disease states are all categorized as *multiple system atrophy.*

MSA with autonomic dysfunction predominating results from degeneration of the locus ceruleus, intermediolateral column of the spinal cord, and peripheral autonomic neurons and manifests as orthostatic hypotension. Other regions of the nervous system may also be affected but to a lesser degree. *Idiopathic orthostatic hypotension,* in contrast to MSA with autonomic dysfunction predominating, is a diagnosis of exclusion when ANS dysfunction occurs in the absence of central nervous system degeneration. In addition to orthostatic hypotension, signs and symptoms of MSA with autonomic dysfunction include urinary retention, bowel dysfunction, and impotence. Postural hypotension, when severe, can produce syncope. Plasma norepinephrine concentrations fail to increase after standing or with exercise. Pupillary reflexes may be sluggish and control of breathing abnormal. Further evidence of ANS dysfunction is failure of baroreceptor reflexes to produce an increase in heart rate or vasoconstriction in response to hypotension.

Treatment includes use of compression stockings, consumption of a high-sodium diet to expand plasma volume, and administration of vasoconstricting α_1-*adrenergic agonist* drugs such as midodrine or α_2-*adrenergic antagonists* such as yohimbine. These drugs facilitate continued release of norepinephrine from postganglionic adrenergic neurons. If symptoms of parkinsonism are present, they can be treated with drugs used to treat Parkinson's disease (e.g., levodopa, anticholinergics). Patients with MSA have an ominous prognosis, with death usually occurring within 8 years of diagnosis. Death is generally a result of cerebral ischemia associated with prolonged hypotension.

Management of Anesthesia

Management of anesthesia for MSA should focus on the decreased ANS activity and hemodynamic aberrations that occur in response to changes in body position, positive airway pressure, and acute blood loss. The negative inotropic effects of anesthetic drugs should also be considered.

The keys to management include continuous monitoring of the systemic blood pressure and prompt correction of hypotension. Crystalloid or colloid solutions can be infused to treat hypotension. If vasopressors are needed, a direct-acting vasopressor such as phenylephrine is preferred. Small doses of phenylephrine should be used initially until the response can be assessed, because the upregulated expression of α-adrenergic receptors in this disease of chronic relative autonomic denervation can produce an exaggerated response to even a small dose of this drug. Spinal or epidural anesthesia can be considered, although the risk of hypotension demands diligence and caution. Autonomic dysfunction in patients with MSA can prevent physiologic compensation for the vasodilation and tachycardia that can result from the use of volatile anesthetics, thus resulting in exaggerated hypotension. Bradycardia that contributes to hypotension is best treated with atropine or glycopyrrolate. Signs of light anesthesia may be less apparent in these patients because the sympathetic nervous system is less responsive to noxious stimulation. Administration of a muscle relaxant that has little or no effect on hemodynamics (e.g., vecuronium, cisatracurium) is preferred. Intravenous ketamine could potentially accentuate blood pressure increases. In contrast, other intravenous anesthesia induction drugs should have their dosage and rate of administration adjusted to lessen the risk of hypotension. Any antiparkinsonian medications should be continued in the perioperative period.

Orthostatic Intolerance Syndrome

Orthostatic intolerance syndrome is a chronic idiopathic disorder of primary autonomic system dysfunction characterized by episodic and position-related hypotension. Orthostatic intolerance syndrome is most often observed in young women. Symptoms include palpitations, tremulousness, light-headedness, fatigue, and syncope. The pathophysiology is unclear, although possible explanations include enhanced sensitivity of β_1-adrenergic receptors, hypovolemia, excessive venous pooling during standing, primary dysautonomia, and lower extremity sympathetic denervation.

Medical treatment of patients with orthostatic intolerance syndrome includes increasing intravascular fluid volume (increased sodium and water intake, administration of mineralocorticoids) to increase venous return. Long-term administration of α_1-adrenergic agonists such as midodrine or other vasoconstrictors may compensate for the decreased sympathetic activity in the legs and blunt heart rate responses to standing.

Management of Anesthesia

Management of anesthesia in patients with orthostatic intolerance syndrome includes preoperative administration of crystalloid or colloid solution to expand intravascular volume. Low-dose phenylephrine infusion may be cautiously administered, with recognition that lower extremity sympathetic nervous system denervation may cause upregulation of α_1-adrenergic receptors and contribute to *receptor hypersensitivity*. The combination of volume expansion and low-dose phenylephrine infusion should be sufficient to augment venous return, maintain blood pressure, and decrease ANS lability in the presence of vasodilating anesthetic drugs or techniques. β-Adrenergic blocking drugs may be used to blunt tachycardia if needed, but care must be taken to avoid excessive hypotension.

Paraganglioma

Paragangliomas are neuroendocrine tumors that arise from neural crest cells. In rare instances they are hormonally active (e.g., secreting norepinephrine), and when this occurs they function as a component of the ANS. These tumors have an origin similar to pheochromocytoma except that paragangliomas exist in extraadrenal locations. They can develop within neuroendocrine tissues surrounding the aorta or within the lung, as well as in the head and neck in proximity to the carotid artery, glossopharyngeal nerve, jugular vein, and middle ear. Distinct terminology based on tumor location, such as carotid body tumor and glomus jugulare, although employed extensively in the past, is currently falling out of favor. Instead these individual tumors are now classified simply as paragangliomas, with the involved location noted (e.g., paraganglioma of the middle ear). Tumor location determines signs and symptoms. For example, paragangliomas in the middle ear can lead to unilateral pulsatile tinnitus, conductive hearing loss, and a bluish red mass behind the tympanic membrane.

Paragangliomas rarely secrete vasoactive substances, but when they do, norepinephrine secretion is the most common (thus mimicking a pheochromocytoma). Paragangliomas typically lack the enzyme that converts norepinephrine to epinephrine, thus epinephrine secretion is even less common than norepinephrine secretion. Other hormones can be produced, including cholecystokinin, thought to play a role in the high incidence of postoperative ileus following tumor resection. Release of serotonin or kallikrein can cause carcinoid-like symptoms such as bronchoconstriction, diarrhea, headache, flushing, and hypertension. Release of histamine or bradykinin can cause bronchoconstriction and hypotension.

Small tumors are most often treated with radiation or embolization, either as a primary treatment or as adjunctive treatment before surgery. Surgery may be required for large or invasive tumors. Preoperative determination of serum concentrations of norepinephrine and catecholamine metabolites may be useful to determine if the tumor is secreting norepinephrine. Phenoxybenzamine or prazosin may be administered preoperatively to lower blood pressure and facilitate volume expansion in patients with increased serum norepinephrine concentrations. Patients with increased serum 5-hydroxyindoleacetic acid (5-HIAA) concentration, especially those with symptoms resembling those of carcinoid syndrome, should receive octreotide preoperatively.

Management of Anesthesia

Anesthetic management can be a challenge in these patients if the tumor is secreting a vasoactive substance prior to surgery. Risks include catecholamine secretion producing exaggerated hemodynamic changes and serotonin secretion producing signs of carcinoid syndrome. Histamine and bradykinin released during surgical manipulation can cause profound hypotension. With paragangliomas in the head and neck, cranial nerve deficits (vagus, glossopharyngeal, hypoglossal nerves) may be present preoperatively or may occur as a result of tumor resection. Airway obstruction resulting from unilateral vocal cord paralysis is a risk after cranial nerve injury. In adults this does not usually result in complete airway obstruction by itself but could produce airway obstruction in combination with airway edema or laryngeal distortion. Other complications can include impaired gastric emptying as a consequence of vagal nerve dysfunction, pulmonary aspiration resulting from cranial nerve dysfunction, and venous air embolism.

Invasive arterial monitoring should be considered, especially in patients with vasoactive substance–secreting tumors. Given the risk of pheochromocytoma-like and carcinoid-like signs occurring intraoperatively, drugs used to treat both hypertension (e.g., sodium nitroprusside, phentolamine, nicardipine) and carcinoid-like signs (e.g., octreotide) should be immediately available.

Venous air embolism is a risk in head and neck surgery, especially if the internal jugular vein is opened to remove tumor. Appropriate monitoring to detect venous air is indicated in this situation. Sudden unexplained cardiovascular collapse and death during resection of these tumors may reflect the presence of a venous air or tumor embolism. If the surgeon finds it necessary to identify the facial nerve, skeletal muscle paralysis should be avoided to allow for monitoring of nerve integrity during surgery. The choice of anesthetic drugs is not uniquely influenced by the presence of paragangliomas, although the potential adverse effects of nitrous oxide have implications if venous air embolism occurs.

Carotid Sinus Hypersensitivity

Carotid sinus hypersensitivity is an uncommon entity caused by exaggeration of normal activity of the baroreceptors in response to mechanical stimulation. For example, stimulation of the carotid sinus by external massage, which in normal individuals produces modest decreases in heart rate and systemic blood pressure, can produce syncope in those with carotid sinus hyperactivity. Affected individuals have an increased incidence of peripheral vascular disease. Carotid sinus hypersensitivity is a recognized albeit transient complication following carotid endarterectomy.

Two distinct cardiovascular responses may be noted in the presence of carotid sinus hypersensitivity. In approximately 80% of affected individuals, a cardioinhibitory reflex mediated by the vagus nerve produces profound bradycardia. In approximately 10% of affected individuals, a vasodepressor reflex mediated by inhibition of vasomotor tone produces decreases in systemic vascular resistance and profound hypotension. The remaining 10% of patients exhibit components of both reflexes.

Carotid sinus hypersensitivity may be treated with drugs, implantation of a cardiac pacemaker, or ablation of the carotid sinus. Use of anticholinergic and vasopressor drugs is limited by their adverse effects, and they are rarely effective in patients with vasodepressor or mixed forms of carotid sinus hypersensitivity. Denervation of the carotid sinus may be attempted in patients in whom the vasodepressor reflex response is refractory to cardiac pacing.

Management of Anesthesia

Anesthetic management in patients with carotid sinus hypersensitivity is often complicated by hypotension, bradycardia, and cardiac dysrhythmias. Continuous invasive monitoring of arterial blood pressure can be valuable. Drugs to treat hypotension and bradycardia should be available. External cardiac pacing may also be useful to treat bradycardia that is unresponsive to pharmacologic therapy.

Hyperhidrosis

Hyperhidrosis is a rare disorder in which an individual produces an excessive amount of sweat. The disorder can be either primary (idiopathic) or secondary to other conditions such as hyperthyroidism, pheochromocytoma, hypothalamic disorders (including that following central nervous system trauma), spinal cord injury, parkinsonism, or menopause. The disorder results from overactivity of sudomotor nerve fibers innervating eccrine sweat glands. The location of excess sweat production in secondary hyperhidrosis depends on the specific cause. Patients with primary hyperhidrosis often complain of excess sweat production in the palms of the hands and axillae, which often leads to social embarrassment. Conservative treatments include topical astringents such as potassium permanganate or tannic acid, or antiperspirants. Although these sudomotor nerve fibers belong to the sympathetic nervous system, the primary neurotransmitter in sweat glands is acetylcholine. Patients may respond to anticholinergic agents or botulinum toxin injections. Botulinum toxin temporarily blocks the nerves that stimulate sweating. Severe cases may require surgical sympathectomy.

Management of Anesthesia

The sympathetic chain is most commonly accessed in the thoracic cavity via video-assisted thoracoscopy. Bilateral hyperhidrosis will require bilateral sympathectomy that can be performed during two separate operations but more commonly is done during a single procedure. Each thoracic cavity will need to be accessed, so one-lung ventilation will be required and is facilitated by placement of a double-lumen endotracheal tube. Successful sympathectomy will produce vasodilation in the ipsilateral upper extremity, documented by an immediate increase in temperature of 1°C or more in that extremity. Therefore continuous cutaneous temperature monitoring on a finger or palm can assess baseline and postlesional temperatures. Laser Doppler measurement of cutaneous blood flow could also be used. The probe is placed on the hands, and sympathectomy results in an immediate and significant increase in blood flow. In otherwise healthy patients this surgery can be performed as an outpatient procedure. Patients often have minimal pain postoperatively, which responds well to opioids and nonsteroidal antiinflammatory drugs (NSAIDs). Common surgical complications include infection, Horner syndrome (resulting from injury to the stellate ganglion during the ablative procedure), and a compensatory hyperhidrosis elsewhere (e.g., trunk or lower extremity).

DISEASES OF THE PERIPHERAL NERVOUS SYSTEM

Idiopathic Facial Paralysis (Bell's Palsy)

Idiopathic facial paralysis is characterized by rapid onset of motor weakness or paralysis of the muscles innervated by the facial nerve. Additional symptoms can include loss of taste sensation over the anterior two-thirds of the tongue, as well as hyperacusis and diminished salivation and lacrimation. There is no cutaneous sensory loss because the trigeminal nerve, not the facial nerve, supplies sensory innervation to the face. The cause of idiopathic facial paralysis is presumed to be inflammation and edema of the facial nerve, most often in the facial nerve canal within the temporal bone. A virus, perhaps herpes simplex virus, may be the cause. During pregnancy there is an increased incidence of idiopathic facial paralysis. The presence of idiopathic facial paralysis does not influence the choice of anesthetic technique.

Spontaneous recovery usually occurs in about 3 months. If no recovery is seen in 4–5 months, the clinical signs and symptoms are probably *not* due to idiopathic facial paralysis. Prednisone (1 mg/kg orally daily for 5–10 days, depending on the extent of facial nerve paralysis) can dramatically relieve pain and decrease the likelihood of complete denervation of the facial nerve. If blinking is not possible, the patient's affected eye should be covered to prevent corneal dehydration.

Surgical decompression of the facial nerve may be needed for persistent or severe cases of idiopathic facial paralysis or for facial paralysis due to trauma. Uveoparotid fever (Heerfordt syndrome) is a rare manifestation of sarcoidosis characterized by bilateral anterior uveitis, parotitis, and low-grade fever as well as the presence of facial nerve paralysis in 50%–70% of patients. Facial nerve paralysis associated with postoperative uveoparotid fever may be erroneously attributed to mechanical pressure over the nerve during general anesthesia.

Trigeminal Neuralgia (Tic Douloureux)

Trigeminal neuralgia is characterized by brief but intense episodes of unilateral facial pain. These events can occur spontaneously or be triggered by local sensory stimuli to the affected side

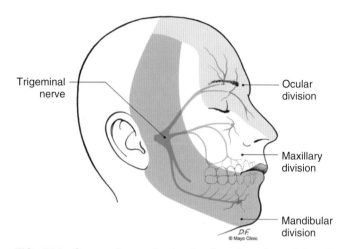

FIG. 15.1   Sensory innervation by the three branches of the trigeminal nerve. (By permission of the Mayo Foundation for Medical Education and Research. All rights reserved.)

of the face. Trigeminal neuralgia can be diagnosed purely on the basis of clinical signs and symptoms. Patients report brief stabbing pain or clusters of stabbing pain in the face or mouth that are restricted to one or more divisions of the trigeminal nerve, most often the mandibular division (Fig. 15.1). Trigeminal neuralgia most often develops in otherwise healthy individuals during late middle age. The appearance of this neuralgia at an earlier age should arouse suspicion of multiple sclerosis. The pathophysiology of the pain associated with trigeminal neuralgia is uncertain. However, compression of the nerve root by a blood vessel is sometimes the cause. The most common blood vessel causing such compression is a branch of the superior cerebellar artery. Antiepileptic drugs are useful for treating trigeminal neuralgia. The anticonvulsant carbamazepine is the drug of choice, but baclofen and lamotrigine are also effective. Surgical therapy (selective radiofrequency destruction of trigeminal nerve fibers, transection of the sensory root of the trigeminal nerve, microsurgical decompression of the trigeminal nerve root) is recommended for individuals who develop pain refractory to drug therapy.

Patients undergoing surgery may experience bradycardia caused by activation of the trigeminocardiac reflex. In patients having microsurgical decompression, placement of a retractor to gain access to the root of the trigeminal nerve can stretch the vestibulocochlear nerve (cranial nerve VIII) and potentially result in hearing loss. Therefore intraoperative monitoring of brainstem auditory evoked potentials may be used to assess the integrity of cranial nerve VIII. The potential enzyme-inducing effects of anticonvulsant drugs must be considered when predicting drug effects. Carbamazepine can also alter hepatic function and produce leukopenia and thrombocytopenia.

Glossopharyngeal Neuralgia

Glossopharyngeal neuralgia is characterized by episodes of intense pain in the throat, neck, tongue, and ear. Swallowing, chewing, coughing, or talking can trigger the pain. This neuralgia may also be associated with severe bradycardia and syncope, presumably because of the close association of the glossopharyngeal and vagus nerves, especially the branch of the glossopharyngeal nerve carrying afferent impulses from the carotid sinus (Hering's nerve).

Glossopharyngeal neuralgia is usually idiopathic but has been described in patients with cerebellopontine angle vascular anomalies and tumors, vertebral and carotid artery occlusive disease, arachnoiditis, and extracranial tumors arising in the area of the pharynx, larynx, and tonsils. The diagnosis of glossopharyngeal neuralgia is supported by pain in the distribution of the glossopharyngeal nerve and relief of this pain by topical anesthesia of the oropharynx at the tonsillar pillar.

In the absence of pain, cardiac symptoms associated with glossopharyngeal neuralgia may be confused with the cardiac conduction disease sick sinus syndrome or carotid sinus hyperactivity. Failure of carotid sinus massage to produce cardiac symptoms rules out carotid sinus hypersensitivity. Glossopharyngeal nerve block is useful for differentiating glossopharyngeal neuralgia from atypical trigeminal neuralgia or sick sinus syndrome. This nerve block does not, however, differentiate glossopharyngeal neuralgia from carotid sinus hyperactivity, because afferent pathways of both syndromes are mediated by the glossopharyngeal nerve.

Glossopharyngeal neuralgia–associated cardiac symptoms should be treated aggressively. Cardiovascular symptoms can be treated acutely with atropine, isoproterenol, a cardiac pacemaker, or a combination of these modalities. Pain associated with this syndrome is managed by administration of anticonvulsant drugs such as carbamazepine or phenytoin. Prevention of cardiovascular symptoms and predictable pain relief can be achieved by intracranial transection of the glossopharyngeal nerve and the upper two roots of the vagus nerve. Although permanent pain relief is possible after repeated glossopharyngeal nerve block, this neuralgia is sufficiently life-threatening to justify intracranial transection of the nerve in patients who do not respond to medical therapy.

Management of Anesthesia

Preoperative evaluation of patients with glossopharyngeal neuralgia is directed at assessing cardiac status and intravascular fluid volume. Hypovolemia may be present, since these patients avoid oral intake and its associated pharyngeal stimulation in an attempt to avoid triggering the pain attacks. In addition, drooling can contribute to fluid losses. A preoperative history of syncope or documented bradycardia concurrent with an episode of pain introduces the possible need for transcutaneous cardiac pacing or placement of a transvenous cardiac pacemaker before induction of anesthesia. Continuous monitoring of blood pressure via an intraarterial catheter is useful. Topical anesthesia of the oropharynx with lidocaine is helpful to prevent bradycardia and hypotension that may occur in response to pharyngeal stimulation during direct laryngoscopy.

Cardiovascular changes should be expected in response to surgical manipulation during intracranial transection of the glossopharyngeal and vagus nerve roots. Bradycardia and hypotension are likely during manipulation of the vagus nerve. Anticholinergic drugs should be immediately available to treat these vagally mediated responses. Hypertension, tachycardia, and ventricular premature beats may occur after surgical transection of the glossopharyngeal nerve and the upper two roots of the vagus nerve because of the sudden loss of sensory input from the carotid sinus. Hypertension is usually transient but can persist into the postoperative period. In this setting, hydralazine may be useful. Experience is too limited to permit recommendations for specific anesthetic drugs or muscle relaxants. The possible development of vocal cord paralysis after vagal nerve transection should be considered and may manifest as airway obstruction following tracheal extubation.

Charcot-Marie-Tooth Disease

Charcot-Marie-Tooth disease (CMT) is the most common inherited cause of chronic motor and sensory peripheral neuropathy. It has an estimated incidence of 1 in 2500 individuals. CMT is the clinical manifestation of a heterogeneous group of genetic mutations that lead to alterations in peripheral nerve function. Details of the more common forms of CMT are outlined in Table 15.1. CMT is stratified into a variety of subtypes: type 1 subtypes are characterized by autosomal dominant or X-linked inheritance and demyelination, type 2 subtypes by autosomal dominant inheritance and axonal dysfunction, type 3 by autosomal dominant or recessive inheritance, and type 4 by autosomal recessive inheritance. The mechanisms and manifestations of type 3 and type 4 CMT are broad and not as well defined as type 1 and 2 forms of CMT. Type 3 and 4 forms of CMT are quite rare.

The more common forms of CMT, especially type 1A, present as distal skeletal muscle weakness, muscle wasting, and loss of tendon reflexes that become evident by the middle teenage years. Classically this neuropathy is described as being restricted to the lower third of the legs, producing foot deformities (high pedal arches and talipes) and peroneal muscle atrophy ("stork-leg" appearance). The disease may slowly progress to include wasting of the quadriceps muscles as well as the muscles of the hands and forearms. Mild to moderate stocking-glove sensory loss occurs in many patients. Pregnancy may precipitate exacerbations of CMT.

Treatment of mild forms of CMT is limited to supportive measures, including splinting, tendon transfers, and various arthrodeses. Many individuals with mild forms of CMT experience long-term disability, but their lifespan is not decreased. Severe forms of CMT, especially those that present earlier in life, are associated with significant disability and reduced lifespan.

Management of Anesthesia

Management of anesthesia in patients with CMT should focus on the response to neuromuscular blocking drugs and the possibility of postoperative respiratory failure resulting from weakness of the respiratory muscles. Cardiac manifestations

TABLE 15.1 | **Characteristics of More Common Genotypes of Charcot-Marie-Tooth Disease**

Type	Subtype	Inheritance Pattern	Chromosome	Mutation	Clinical Comments
1					**All type 1 variants of CMT are predominantly demyelinating.**
	1A	AD	11	Duplication of peripheral myelin protein 22 gene	Most common form of CMT
	1B	AD	1	Myelin protein zero gene	Phenotype typical of CMT-1A, with varying wide range of severity
	1C	AD	16	Lipopolysaccharide TNF-α factor gene	
	1D	AD	10	Early growth response protein gene	Usually severe phenotype
	1E	AD	17	Point mutation of peripheral myelin protein 22 gene	Earlier onset and more severe phenotype than type 1A
	1F	AD	8	Neurofilament light chain protein gene	
	1X	XL	X	Gap junction beta protein gene	Second most common form of CMT
2					**All type 2 variants of CMT are predominantly characterized by axonal dysfunction.**
	2A	AD	1	Mitofusin 2 gene	Fusion of mitochondria is a notable finding.
	2B	AD	3	Ras-related protein 7A gene	Predominantly a sensory neuropathy
	2C	AD	12	Unknown gene	Diaphragm and vocal cord paresis are characteristic
	2D	AD	7	Glycyl tRNA synthetase gene	Can be a sensory/motor or purely motor neuropathy
	2E	AD	8	Neurofilament light gene	
3	Dejerine-Sottas syndrome	AD or AR	Multiple	Many mutations can lead to Dejerine-Sottas syndrome.	Final common pathway of a group of mutations
					Severe symptoms before age 3 and poor prognosis
4	4A	AR	8	Ganglioside-induced differentiation-associated protein 1 gene	Primarily demyelinating
					Vocal cord paresis can be present.
	4B1	AR	11	Myotubularin-related protein 2 gene	
	4B2	AR	11	Myotubularin-related protein 13 gene	Onset in infancy
					Notable for both proximal and distal neurologic deficits
	4B3	AR	22	Myotubularin-related protein 5 gene	
	4C	AR	5	Defect in SH3 domain and tetratricopeptide repeats 2 gene	Most common autosomal recessive form of CMT
	4D	AR	8	Unknown gene	Deafness is characteristic of CMT-4D
	4E	AR	1 or 10	Defect in myelin protein zero gene or early growth response protein 2 gene	Also known as *congenital hypomyelination syndrome*
	4F	AR	19	Periaxin gene	
	4G	AR	10	Unknown gene	
	4H	AR	12	Actin filament–binding protein frabin gene	
	4J	AR	6	Factor-induced gene 4	

AD, Autosomal dominant; *AR,* autosomal recessive; *CMT,* Charcot-Marie-Tooth disease; *RNA,* ribonucleic acid; *TNF-α,* tumor necrosis factor α; *XL,* X-linked.

attributed to this neuropathy, including conduction disturbances, atrial flutter, and cardiomyopathy, are seen occasionally. Drugs known to trigger malignant hyperthermia have been used safely in patients with CMT. The response to neuromuscular blocking drugs seems to be normal in patients with mild forms of CMT. It may be reasonable to avoid succinylcholine because of theoretical concerns about exaggerated potassium release in individuals with neuromuscular diseases. However, succinylcholine has been used safely in some patients with mild forms of CMT, without producing hyperkalemia or triggering malignant hyperthermia. Safe use of succinylcholine has not yet been described in patients with rarer forms of CMT and should be used with caution or avoided in this subset of patients. Use of epidural anesthesia for labor and delivery has been described.

Brachial Plexus Neuropathy

Primary brachial plexus neuropathy, otherwise known as *idiopathic brachial neuritis, Parsonage-Turner syndrome,* or *shoulder-girdle syndrome,* is characterized by acute onset of severe pain in the upper arm. The pathophysiology of primary brachial plexus neuropathy is currently unknown. The pain is typically most severe at the onset of the neuropathy. As the pain diminishes, patchy paresis or paralysis of the skeletal muscles innervated by branches of the brachial plexus appears. Skeletal muscle wasting, particularly involving the shoulder girdle and arm, is common. *Secondary* causes of brachial plexus neuropathy include trauma to the neck or upper limb. In neonates, shoulder dystocia during delivery is another cause of brachial plexus neuropathy.

Electrophysiologic studies are valuable in diagnosing brachial plexus neuropathy and demonstrating the multifocal pattern of denervation. Muscle fibrillations and slowing of nerve conduction velocity are observed. The diaphragm may also be affected. Sensory disturbances occur in most patients but tend to be minimal and generally disappear over time.

Nerve biopsy findings in individuals with hereditary brachial plexus neuropathy and Parsonage-Turner syndrome suggest an inflammatory-immune pathogenesis. Autoimmune neuropathies may also occur during the postoperative period independent of the site of surgery. It is possible that the stress of surgery activates an unidentified dormant virus in the nerve roots, a circumstance that would be similar to the onset of herpes zoster after surgery. In addition, strenuous exercise or pregnancy may be inciting events for brachial plexus neuropathy.

Guillain-Barré Syndrome (Acute Idiopathic Polyneuritis)

Guillain-Barré syndrome is characterized by sudden onset of skeletal muscle weakness or paralysis that typically begins in the legs and spreads cephalad over the ensuing days to involve the arms, trunk, and face. Since the virtual elimination of poliomyelitis, this syndrome has become the most common cause of acute generalized paralysis, with an annual incidence of 1–2 cases per 100,000. Bulbar involvement typically manifests as bilateral facial paralysis. Difficulty swallowing due to pharyngeal muscle weakness and impaired ventilation due to intercostal muscle paralysis are the most serious signs of this process. Because of lower motor neuron involvement, paralysis is flaccid and corresponding tendon reflexes are diminished. Sensory disturbances (e.g., paresthesias) generally precede the onset of paralysis and are most prominent in the distal extremities. Pain is often present.

TABLE 15.2	Diagnostic Criteria for Guillain-Barré Syndrome

FEATURES REQUIRED FOR DIAGNOSIS
Progressive bilateral weakness in arms and legs
Areflexia

FEATURES STRONGLY SUPPORTING THE DIAGNOSIS
Progression of symptoms over 2–4 weeks
Symmetry of symptoms
Mild sensory symptoms or signs
Cranial nerve involvement (especially bilateral facial nerve weakness)
Decreased nerve conduction velocity
Autonomic nervous system dysfunction
No fever at onset
Elevated concentration of protein in CSF with a cell count <10/mm^3
Spontaneous recovery starting 2–4 weeks after progression halts

FEATURES MAKING THE DIAGNOSIS UNLIKELY
Definite sensory level
Marked persistent asymmetry of the weakness
Severe and persistent bowel and bladder dysfunction
>50 white cells/mm^3 in CSF

CSF, Cerebrospinal fluid.

ANS dysfunction is a prominent finding in patients with Guillain-Barré syndrome and is usually manifested as fluctuations in blood pressure, sudden profuse diaphoresis, peripheral vasoconstriction, resting tachycardia, and cardiac conduction abnormalities. Orthostatic hypotension may be so severe that elevating the patient's head onto a pillow may lead to syncope. Thromboembolism may occur secondary to immobility. Sudden death associated with this disease is most likely caused by ANS dysfunction.

Complete spontaneous recovery from acute idiopathic polyneuritis can occur within a few weeks if segmental demyelination is the predominant pathologic process. However, axonal degeneration (as detected by electromyographic screening) may result in slower recovery that takes several months and leaves some residual weakness. The mortality rate associated with Guillain-Barré syndrome is 3%–8%, and death is most often a result of sepsis, acute respiratory failure, pulmonary embolism, or cardiac arrest.

The diagnosis of Guillain-Barré syndrome is based on clinical signs and symptoms (Table 15.2) supported by finding an increased protein concentration in the cerebrospinal fluid. Cerebrospinal fluid cell counts typically remain within the normal range. In approximately half of patients, this syndrome develops after respiratory or gastrointestinal infection, which suggests that the cause may be related to either viral or mycoplasma infection.

Treatment of Guillain-Barré syndrome is symptomatic. Vital capacity is monitored, and when it decreases to less than 15 mL/kg, mechanical support of ventilation is initiated. Arterial blood gas measurements help in assessing the adequacy of ventilation and oxygenation. Pharyngeal muscle weakness, even in the absence of ventilatory failure, may require insertion of a cuffed endotracheal tube or tracheostomy to protect the lungs from aspiration of secretions or gastric fluid. ANS dysfunction may require treatment of hypertension or hypotension. Corticosteroids are *not* useful. Plasma exchange or infusion of gamma globulin may benefit some patients but does not affect overall outcome.

Management of Anesthesia

Abnormal ANS function and the presence of lower motor neuron lesions are the major factors to consider in developing an anesthetic plan for patients with Guillain-Barré syndrome. Compensatory cardiovascular responses may be absent, so profound hypotension occurs in response to changes in posture, blood loss, or positive airway pressure. Conversely, noxious stimulation such as direct laryngoscopy can cause exaggerated increases in blood pressure. Because of these unpredictable changes in blood pressure, it may be prudent to monitor blood pressure continuously with an intraarterial catheter. Patients may also exhibit exaggerated responses to indirect-acting vasopressors, probably as a result of upregulation of postsynaptic receptors.

Succinylcholine should *not* be administered; there is a risk of excessive potassium release from denervated skeletal muscles. A nondepolarizing muscle relaxant with minimal circulatory effects (e.g., vecuronium, cisatracurium) may be used if needed. Even if a patient is breathing spontaneously before surgery, mechanical ventilation may be required during the postoperative period.

Entrapment Neuropathies

Entrapment neuropathies occur at anatomic sites where peripheral nerves pass through narrow passages, an anatomic arrangement that makes compression a possibility. Examples include the median nerve passing through the carpal tunnel at the wrist and the ulnar nerve passing through the cubital tunnel at the elbow. Peripheral nerves are probably more sensitive to compressive (ischemic) injury in patients who have generalized polyneuropathies such as those that occur with diabetes mellitus or hereditary peripheral neuropathies. A peripheral nerve may also be more susceptible to compression if the same fibers have been partially damaged proximal to the site of compression *(double crush hypothesis)*. For example, spinal nerve root compression (cervical radiculopathy) may increase the vulnerability of nerve fibers to injury at distal entrapment sites, such as the carpal tunnel at the wrist. Peripheral nerve damage resulting from compression depends on the severity of the compression and the anatomy of the nerve. The outermost nerve fibers—that is, those that innervate more proximal tissues—are more vulnerable to ischemia from compression than the fibers lying more deeply in the nerve bundle. Focal demyelination of nerve fibers causes slowing or blocking of nerve impulse conduction through the damaged area. Electromyographic studies are adjuncts to nerve conduction studies and can show patterns characteristic of denervation and subsequent reinnervation of muscle fibers by surviving axons.

Carpal Tunnel Syndrome

Carpal tunnel syndrome is the most common entrapment neuropathy. It results from compression of the median nerve between the transverse carpal ligament and the carpal bones at the wrist. This neuropathy most often occurs in otherwise healthy women (three times more frequently than in men) and is often bilateral, although the dominant hand is typically involved first. Patients describe repeated episodes of pain and paresthesias in the wrist and hand following the distribution of the median nerve. The exact cause of carpal tunnel syndrome is unknown, but affected individuals often engage in occupations that require repetitive movements of the hands and fingers. Nerve conduction studies are the definitive method for confirming the diagnosis and demonstrate reduced conduction velocity in the median nerve at the wrist. In previously asymptomatic patients who acquire symptoms of carpal tunnel syndrome shortly after an unrelated surgery, it is likely that accumulation of third space fluid resulted in an increase in tissue pressure and contributed to compression of the nerve. Pregnancy with peripheral edema may also precipitate the initial manifestations of carpal tunnel syndrome. Cervical radiculopathy may produce similar symptoms unilaterally but rarely bilaterally.

Immobilizing the wrist with a splint is a common treatment for carpal tunnel syndrome that is expected to be transient (pregnancy) or caused by a medically treatable disease (hypothyroidism, acromegaly). Injection of corticosteroids into the carpal tunnel may relieve symptoms but is seldom curative. Definitive treatment of carpal tunnel syndrome is decompression of the median nerve by surgical division of the transverse carpal ligament.

Ulnar Neuropathy

Compression of the ulnar nerve after it passes through the condylar groove and enters the cubital tunnel results in clinical symptoms typical of ulnar nerve neuropathy. These often include numbness and tingling in the ring and little fingers. It may be difficult to differentiate clinical symptoms of ulnar nerve neuropathy caused by compression in the condylar groove from symptoms related to entrapment in the cubital tunnel. Surgical treatment of cubital tunnel entrapment syndrome (by tunnel decompression and transposition of the nerve) may be helpful in relieving symptoms, but sometimes it may make symptoms worse, perhaps by interfering with the nerve's blood supply.

Meralgia Paresthetica

The *lateral femoral cutaneous nerve,* a pure sensory nerve, can become entrapped as it crosses under the inguinal ligament near the attachment of the ligament to the anterior superior iliac spine. Patients complain of burning pain down the lateral portion of the thigh, but they may also experience sensory loss in that region and possibly point tenderness at the site of entrapment. Meralgia paresthetica often occurs in overweight individuals and is exacerbated by wearing tight-fitting garments such as belts. It may also occur following abdominal surgery or iliac crest bone graft harvesting, during pregnancy, or in conditions involving fluid overload (e.g., ascites, congestive heart failure). Treatment is usually conservative, since meralgia paresthetica tends to regress spontaneously. Treatment options include weight loss, removal of offending garments, elimination of activities involving hip flexion, topical cooling, and administration of analgesics. Refractory cases may require local anesthetic and corticosteroid injections at the site of entrapment and possible surgical decompression.

Complex Regional Pain Syndrome

Complex regional pain syndrome (CRPS), formerly known as *reflex sympathetic dystrophy* or *causalgia,* is a disorder that may occur following an injury or surgery in a region of the body, most frequently a limb. However, CRPS can also develop in the absence of an identifiable inciting injury. CRPS is more common in women, especially postmenopausal women. Although the exact etiology of CRPS is unknown, inappropriate activation of the inflammatory cascade, dysregulation of pain-mediating neuropeptides (i.e., substance P, neuropeptide Y, calcitonin gene-related peptide), central nervous system sensitization to pain stimuli, dysregulation of the sympathetic nervous system, and a possible genetic predisposition may all play a role. Symptoms include pain, swelling, decreased hair growth, skin changes, and bone demineralization. Pain is often the most debilitating symptom of CRPS. Pain is described as burning, stinging, or tearing, and its distribution is often inconsistent with the anatomic distribution of known nervous system structures (i.e., nerve, dermatome, plexus). Patients may also have motor and autonomic dysfunction, with the latter manifesting as changes in skin temperature, color, and sweat production. In the past, CRPS was often considered to evolve through three stages, although this notion has widely been abandoned by most clinicians. However, because these stages may still be encountered in clinical practice, they are worth mentioning:

stage 1: development of throbbing, burning pain in a limb, not corresponding to an anatomic distribution; may have allodynia and vasomotor disturbances

stage 2: development of soft tissue edema, muscle atrophy, and skin changes lasting 3–6 months

stage 3: limitation in range of motion, contractures, skin atrophy and fragility, nail changes, lack of hair growth, and bone demineralization

The diagnosis of CRPS is based on the Budapest Criteria as outlined in Table 15.3. Other tests such as bone scintigraphy, autonomic testing, and magnetic resonance imaging can help support the diagnosis of CRPS.

Management of CRPS should ideally start with prevention. There is some evidence that vitamin C supplementation in the setting of an injury may reduce the risk for CRPS. Management should be multidisciplinary and include pain control combined with physical therapy, psychological support, and patient education. Pain management may involve the use of NSAIDs, antiepileptic drugs (i.e., gabapentin, pregabalin),

TABLE 15.3	Budapest Clinical Criteria for Diagnosis of Complex Regional Pain Syndrome

The patient must have *all* the following:
1. Continued pain that is disproportionate to the inciting event
2. Report at least one *symptom* in three of the categories
3. Demonstrate at least one *sign* in two of the categories at the time of evaluation
4. No other diagnosis that better explains the signs and symptoms

Sensory: allodynia or hyperesthesia
Vasomotor: temperature asymmetry and/or skin color changes and/or skin color asymmetry
Sudomotor/edema: edema and/or sweating changes and/or sweating asymmetry
Motor/trophic: decreased range of motion and/or motor dysfunction (weakness, tremor, dystonia) and/or trophic changes of hair, nails, or skin

From the findings of the International Association for the Study of Pain (IASP) conference in Budapest, Hungary 2007.

tricyclic antidepressants, bisphosphonates, ketamine, opioids, and topical lidocaine or capsaicin. For refractory pain a pain management specialist may consider trigger point injections, sympathetic nerve blocks, spinal cord stimulation, or epidural clonidine. The prognosis of CRPS is highly variable, but 60% of patients still have symptoms 6 years after the onset of this syndrome.

Management of Anesthesia

Elective surgery on a limb with CRPS should be delayed if possible until pain and control of other symptoms has been optimized. Great care must be taken in positioning. Given the limitation in range of motion and the fragile skin in patients with CRPS, there should be extra padding of pressure points, and the extremities should not be positioned in a manner that would exceed the tolerable range of motion noted by the patient in the awake state. Increased analgesic requirements are typical following surgery, even if the procedure was not performed on the affected limb, since most patients with CRPS have been taking analgesics chronically. One should expect an increase in pain due to concomitant *hyperalgesia* if the procedure is performed on the affected limb. A multimodal approach to postoperative pain management should be considered. This can include parenteral and oral opioid and nonopioid analgesics and adjuvant drugs such as gabapentin, pregabalin, and tricyclic antidepressants. Regional anesthesia should also be considered if possible. Consultation with a pain management specialist in the perioperative period can be beneficial.

Diseases Associated With Peripheral Neuropathies

Diabetes Mellitus

Diabetes mellitus is commonly associated with peripheral polyneuropathy. The incidence of this problem increases with the duration of the diabetes and decreases with better glycemic control. The etiology of diabetic neuropathy is multifactorial and may include microvascular damage resulting in neuronal ischemia, formation of glycosylated intraneuronal proteins, activation of protein kinase C, inhibition of glutathione (which increases reactive oxygen species), and activation of the sorbitol–aldose reductase pathway. Neurons that utilize this last pathway (e.g., retinal and renal cells) do not require insulin to facilitate intracellular entry of glucose. The increased intracellular glucose is converted to sorbitol via aldose reductase, and since sorbitol cannot cross cell membranes, this results in increased intracellular osmolarity, cellular osmotic stress, and subsequent neuronal dysfunction.

Electrophysiologic studies show evidence of denervation and reduced nerve conduction velocity. The most common neuropathy is distal, symmetrical, and predominantly sensory. The principal manifestations are an unpleasant tingling, numbness, burning, and aching in the lower extremities, along with skeletal muscle weakness and distal sensory loss. Discomfort is prominent at night and often relieved by walking. Symptoms often progress and may extend to the upper extremities. Impotence, urinary retention, gastroparesis, resting tachycardia, and postural hypotension are common and reflect ANS dysfunction. For reasons that are not understood the peripheral nerves of patients with diabetes mellitus are more vulnerable to injury resulting from nerve compression or stretch, as may occur during intraoperative and postoperative positioning.

Alcohol Abuse

Polyneuropathy of chronic alcoholism is nearly always associated with nutritional and vitamin deficiencies. Symptoms characteristically begin in the lower extremities, with pain and numbness in the feet. Weakness and tenderness of the intrinsic muscles of the feet, loss of the Achilles tendon reflex, and hyperalgesia in a stocking-glove distribution are early manifestations. Restoration of a proper diet, abstinence from alcohol, and multivitamin therapy promote slow but predictable resolution of the neuropathy.

Vitamin B_{12} Deficiency

The earliest neurologic symptoms of vitamin B_{12} deficiency resemble the neuropathy typically seen in patients who abuse alcohol. Paresthesias in the legs, with sensory loss in a stocking distribution plus absent Achilles tendon reflexes are characteristic findings. Similar neurologic findings have been reported in dentists who experience long-term exposure to nitrous oxide and in individuals who habitually inhale nitrous oxide for nonmedical purposes. Nitrous oxide is known to inactivate certain vitamin B_{12}–dependent enzymes that in turn could lead to symptoms of neuropathy.

Uremia

Distal polyneuropathy with sensory and motor components often occurs in the extremities of patients with chronic renal failure. Symptoms tend to be more prominent in the legs than in the arms. Presumably, metabolic abnormalities are responsible for the axonal degeneration and segmental demyelination that accompany this neuropathy. Slowing of nerve conduction has been correlated with increased plasma concentrations of parathyroid hormone and myoinositol, a component of myelin. Improved nerve conduction velocity often occurs within a few days after renal transplantation. However, hemodialysis is ineffective in reversing this polyneuropathy.

Cancer

Peripheral sensory and motor neuropathies occur in patients with a variety of malignancies, especially those involving the lung, ovary, and breast. Polyneuropathy that develops in elderly patients should always arouse suspicion of undiagnosed cancer. Myasthenic (Eaton-Lambert) syndrome may be observed in patients with carcinoma of the lung. This paraneoplastic syndrome results from the abnormal production of an antibody against presynaptic calcium channels located on cholinergic neurons. As a result of calcium channel blockade, decreased quantities of acetylcholine are released from nerve terminals at the neuromuscular junction, and this results in weakness. Myasthenic syndrome is associated with an increased sensitivity to both depolarizing and nondepolarizing neuromuscular blocking drugs. Invasion of the lower trunks of the brachial plexus by a tumor in the lung apex (Pancoast syndrome) produces arm pain, paresthesias, and weakness of the hands and arms.

Collagen Vascular Diseases

Collagen vascular diseases are commonly associated with peripheral neuropathies. These occur most often in systemic lupus erythematosus, polyarteritis nodosa, rheumatoid arthritis, and scleroderma. Detection of multiple mononeuropathies suggests a vasculitis of nerve trunks and should stimulate a search for the presence of a collagen vascular disease.

Sarcoidosis

Sarcoidosis is a disorder of unknown etiology in which noncaseating granulomas occur in multiple organ systems, most commonly the lungs, lymphatics, bone, liver, and nervous system. Polyneuropathy resulting from the presence of granulomatous lesions in peripheral nerves is a frequent finding. Unilateral or bilateral facial nerve paralysis may result from sarcoid involvement of this nerve in the parotid gland(s) and is often one of the first manifestations of sarcoidosis.

AIDS-Associated Neuropathy

Peripheral neuropathy is common in patients with acquired immunodeficiency syndrome (AIDS) but not in patients with human immunodeficiency virus (HIV) infection *without* AIDS. AIDS-associated neuropathy is typically a distal symmetric polyneuropathy, and patients complain of numbness, tingling, and sometimes pain in their feet. There may be loss of vibratory sensation and light touch. Although the exact cause is unclear, infection with cytomegalovirus or *Mycobacterium avium-intracellulare*, lymphomatous invasion of peripheral nerves, or adverse effects of antiretroviral medication may be responsible.

Perioperative Peripheral Neuropathies

Perioperative neuropathies have been described following a variety of surgical procedures and affecting a multitude of nerves. Although such neuropathies were originally thought to be primarily the result of errors in patient positioning during surgery, epidemiologic data suggest that in most circumstances, preexisting aberrations of patient anatomy and physiology predispose the patient to this kind of injury. These include obesity, bony abnormalities, edema formation, metabolic derangements, and preexisting nerve abnormalities manifested as conduction delays. The failure of sedated pain-free patients to frequently reposition themselves in bed postoperatively (and hence a failure to relieve pressure on individual nerves) may also be involved. *Ulnar neuropathy* is the most common perioperative neuropathy, typically affecting obese males who undergo abdominal or pelvic surgical procedures. Symptoms of ulnar neuropathy do not typically present until at least 48 hours after surgery, and patients are often found to have *contralateral* nerve conduction dysfunction as well as the new ulnar neuropathy. This indicates a predisposition to this injury. Postoperative *brachial plexus neuropathy* may initially be mistaken for ulnar neuropathy, and it appears to be associated with brachial plexus stretch resulting from sternal retraction during median sternotomy, placement in steep Trendelenburg position, and prone positioning with shoulder abduction and contralateral head rotation. Lower extremity neuropathies are associated with procedures performed in the lithotomy position and usually affect the *common peroneal nerve*. It is theorized that the risk of common peroneal nerve damage is increased if the nerve becomes compressed by leg-holder hardware as the nerve crosses over the fibular head. Sciatic and femoral neuropathy may also be associated with lithotomy positioning, but these are seen much less often than peroneal neuropathy.

Management of patients who develop perioperative peripheral neuropathies begins with (1) taking a history and performing a physical examination, which should focus on identifying risk factors for or a history of neuropathy; (2) determining whether the deficit is sensory, motor, or mixed;

and (3) documenting the distribution of the deficit. Most sensory deficits resolve within 5 days, so if the deficit is purely sensory, expectant management is usually adequate. Since motor fibers tend to be located deeper within nerves, the presence of a motor deficit suggests a more extensive injury. In this situation a neurology consultation is warranted.

KEY POINTS

- When caring for patients with diseases affecting the autonomic nervous system, one must carefully monitor for and be prepared to treat significant changes in heart rate and blood pressure.
- In the setting of autonomic disorders, changes in catecholamine release and adrenergic receptor density may occur. Therefore one should titrate the dosage of direct-acting adrenergic agonists and avoid the use of indirect-acting adrenergic agonists.
- Succinylcholine should be used with caution in patients with neurologic diseases affecting the peripheral nervous system because of the risk of hyperkalemia resulting from upregulation of acetylcholine receptors at the neuromuscular junction.
- Diseases affecting the peripheral nervous system may be associated with significant neuropathic pain. Both opioid and nonopioid analgesics should be considered for management of this pain.

RESOURCES

Apfelbaum JL. Practice advisory for the prevention of perioperative peripheral neuropathies. *Anesthesiology.* 2011;114:1-14.

Baets J, De Jonghe P, Timmerman V. Recent advances in Charcot-Marie-Tooth disease. *Curr Opinion Neurol.* 2014;27:532-540.

de Mos M, Huygen FJ, van der Hoeven-Borgman M, et al. Outcome of the complex regional pain syndrome. *Clin J Pain.* 2009;25:590-597.

Harden RN, Bruehl S, Stanton-Hicks M, Wilson PR. Proposed new diagnostic criteria for complex regional pain syndrome. *Pain Med.* 2007;8:326-331.

Harden RN, Oaklander AL, Burton AW, et al. Complex regional pain syndrome: practical diagnostic and treatment guidelines, 4th edition. *Pain Med.* 2013;14:180-229.

Scrivani SJ, Mathews ES, Maciewicz RJ. Trigeminal neuralgia. *Oral Surg Oral Med Oral Pathol Oral Radiol Endod.* 2005;100:527-538.

Diseases of Aging

SHAMSUDDIN AKHTAR

INTRODUCTION

Compared to 100 years ago, people are living much longer. The US life expectancy for men in 1900 was 48 years and for women, 51 years. Currently the average life expectancy in the United States exceeds 75 years. The *elderly,* defined as those older than 65 years, constitute one of the fastest growing segments of the population. In 2010 the US elderly population numbered 47 million, representing 17% of the total population, and by 2030 there will be approximately 80 million

elderly (Fig. 16.1). This is a worldwide phenomenon. In the United States alone, by the year 2025 there are expected to be 15 million individuals aged 85 years. The social, economic, and political costs of these demographic changes is enormous.

Surgeries that were considered prohibitively high risk and rare in octogenarians 2 decades ago are now being performed routinely. Many elderly patients and octogenarians now undergo complex major cardiac, orthopedic, and other noncardiac surgery. With the changing demographics and advancement in surgical techniques, this trend is likely to grow.

Elderly patients utilize disproportionately more medical care than younger people. By some estimates, 35% of total US medical costs are spent on patients older than 65 years. Per capita healthcare costs are three times higher in patients older than 85 years versus those younger than 65. About 40% of all surgery and inpatient procedures are performed on elderly patients.

Though the impact of aging and its associated diseases has been recognized for a long time, optimal care of the elderly continues to evolve. Most providers of anesthesia for adults are now involved in the care of geriatric patients and so can be considered "geriatric anesthesiologists." Thus it is imperative that an anesthesiologist know the impact of aging on physiology and pharmacology, the impact of comorbidities, and the composite effect of all these changes on perioperative outcomes. Elderly patients are not only "old" or "very old"; they are a unique phenotype comprising an aged biological system, multiple comorbid diseases, and a spectrum of geriatric syndromes. Preoperative assessment of the elderly patient must involve assessment of geriatric syndromes, functional status, frailty, cognition, nutritional status, and goals of care.

BIOLOGY OF AGING

In the past few decades there has been significant research on the process of aging, the mechanisms that underlie aging, and potential interventions that could delay aging. Aging appears to be driven by progressive accumulation of a variety of random molecular defects that build up in cells and tissues. Aging is thus a continuous process, starting early and developing

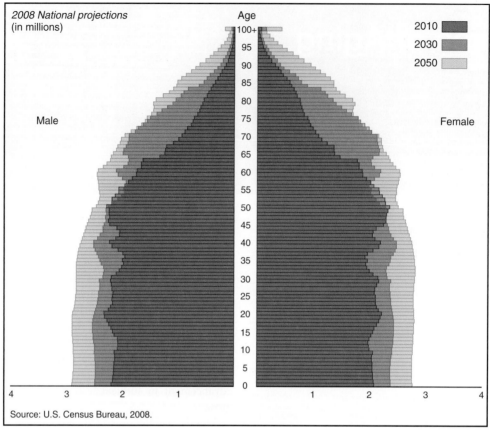

FIG. 16.1   Age and sex structure of the US population for 2010, 2030, and 2050 (2008 national projections in millions). (Source: US Census Bureau, 2008.)

gradually, instead of being a distinct phase that begins in middle to later life. It is well recognized that all individuals do not age at the same rate. Five key elements seem to contribute to the individuality of the human aging process: *genes, nutrition, lifestyle, environment,* and *chance.*

Aging and longevity are clearly influenced by genes. Although genes influence longevity, they appear to account for only about 25% of the variance in the human lifespan. Multiple genes contribute to the aging phenotype, but there are no specific genes for aging. Mutations that extend lifespan make creatures resistant to multiple forms of lethal injuries due to oxidative agents, heat, heavy metals, radiation, and so forth. However, genes that allow the organism to survive in youth may have deleterious effects at an older age. And a variety of gene mutations with late deleterious effects may exist, giving rise to the senescent phenotype.

There are many mechanisms that can lead to defects and aging, and it is highly likely that no single process is responsible for aging. The following mechanisms are considered to be the most important and may work synergistically:

Oxidative damage: Free radicals—that is, reactive oxygen species—are byproducts of oxygen use and energy metabolism. These free radicals can cause damage to chromosomal DNA and subsequently impair gene function, damage mitochondrial DNA, and damage telomeres.

DNA damage and repair: Age-related increases in somatic mutations and other forms of DNA damage are well recognized. They can produce permanent alterations of DNA sequences and hence function. A key enzyme involved in the repair of damaged DNA is poly(ADP-ribose) polymerase 1 (PARP-1), and its levels correlate positively to lifespan. Centenarians who have maintained generally good health have higher levels of PARP-1 than the general population. *Telomeres* are regions of repetitive nucleotide sequences found at the end of each chromosome. They protect the ends of the chromosome from deterioration and from fusion with nearby chromosomes. A growing body of evidence links telomere length to aging and mortality. With normal aging, telomeres shorten in several tissues, thus limiting the ability of these tissues to regenerate over time, ultimately leading to loss of function and cell death. However, premature shortening of telomeres can occur and has been associated with certain diseases such as vascular dementia, psychological and physiologic stress, and others. Telomere shortening is potentially one way by which environmental factors contribute to premature aging.

Mitochondrial senescence: Mitochondria are intricately involved in energy metabolism and generation of oxygen radicals. Just like somatic DNA, mitochondrial DNA also develops point mutations and deletions over time. An increased incidence of mutated mitochondrial DNA has been noted in aging brain tissue, muscle cells, and gut epithelium.

Malfunction of proteins: Damaged, misfolded, or malfunctioning proteins also accumulate over time and are seen in many age-related diseases such as Parkinson's disease, Alzheimer's disease, and senile cataracts. Though these faulty proteins *should* be cleared rapidly, their accumulation and aggregation over time becomes less efficient. Malfunctioning or accumulated proteins lead to loss of particular functions and ultimately to dysfunction of the entire cell.

Environmental factors: Aging is affected by environmental factors that interact with the genome in various ways. It has been recognized that a low-calorie diet leads to a longer lifespan. This phenomenon is explained by the *"disposable soma theory,"* which postulates that natural selection has led to those pathways that optimize utilization of metabolic resources (energy) among competing physiologic demands (growth, maintenance, reproduction). Insulin and insulin-like growth factor gene systems seem to play a crucial role in these processes. Activation of these genes alters the function of a variety of downstream stress response genes, genes encoding for a variety of antimicrobial proteins, and pathways involved in protein turnover.

The boundary between aging and disease pathogenesis is somewhat arbitrary. The same cellular and molecular functions that contribute to improved lifespan are also responsible for degenerative diseases like osteoporosis, osteoarthritis, and dementia.

PHYSIOLOGIC EFFECTS OF AGING

Central Nervous System

Aging affects the brain, and cognitive decline with aging has been taken for granted. It is considered an unavoidable consequence of brain senescence. Though there are changes with aging, new evidence suggests that part of these changes are due to aging-related medical conditions. Brain function associated with the normal process of aging should be differentiated from specific changes due to neurodegenerative diseases.

All major cell types in the brain undergo structural changes with aging. These changes include neuronal cell death, dendritic retraction and expansion, synaptic loss and remodeling, and changes in glial cell (astrocyte and microglia) reactivity. There is an overall reduction in neuronal regenerative capacity. The mass of the brain decreases by approximately 15% with aging. This decrease is due to cell loss and shrinkage of cell volume. There is a compensatory increase in cerebrospinal fluid volume. However, all areas of the brain do not shrink at the same rate. Some areas (e.g., pons) are not affected by aging, whereas there is a significant decline in thalamic and cortical gray matter size. Cells in the hippocampus continue to regenerate. White matter does not decrease with aging.

Changes in brain structure are not limited only to cell volume but also to synaptic connections. Neural connections play a critical role in brain function and are responsible for the *neural plasticity* of the brain. With aging, neural plasticity decreases, yet neuronal connectivity may increase.

Cellular signaling transduction pathways, cytokines, and growth factors that are involved in neuronal excitability and plasticity are also affected by aging. There are significant changes in neurotransmitter signaling. Cholinergic signaling, which plays a crucial role in learning and memory, can be especially impaired in patients with Alzheimer's disease. Presynaptic and postsynaptic dopaminergic neurotransmission can also be significantly affected by aging. In conjunction with thalamic contraction there is impairment of dopamine signal transduction pathways. These pathways play a significant role in age-related deficits in motor control and may explain the susceptibility of the elderly to the extrapyramidal side effects of dopamine receptor antagonist drugs. Norepinephrine levels are increased in some parts of the aging brain, while levels of α_2-agonist receptors may decrease. Levels of ionic glutamate receptors and γ-aminobutyric acid $(GABA)_A$ binding sites decrease with age. Neurovascular, endocrine, and immunologic changes are also noted in the brain with aging (Fig. 16.2). Aging brain has decreased cerebral blood flow due to a reduction in cerebral metabolic rate and is more susceptible to metabolic stress.

Significant cognitive dysfunction is related to aging and age-related diseases. The incidence of many chronic diseases increases proportionally with age, so it can be difficult to differentiate age-related cognitive dysfunction from disease-related cognitive dysfunction in any particular patient. Hypertension, diabetes mellitus, nutritional deficiency, chronic obstructive pulmonary disease, obstructive sleep apnea, thyroid dysfunction, alcoholism, depression, and medications (opioids, benzodiazepines, anticonvulsants, antipsychotics, antidepressants, antihistamines, decongestants, and central nervous system stimulants) can also affect cognitive function. General intellectual functioning, attention, memory, and psychomotor function decline with age, but language and executive function remain more or less intact.

Cardiovascular System

Tissue elasticity decreases with age, whereas the proportion of collagen increases. Elastin becomes fragmented because of increased activity of matrix metalloproteinases, and collagen becomes increasingly cross-linked. These changes produce *increased stiffness* in tissues, causing significant structural and physiologic changes in the cardiovascular system.

Two major structural effects occur in blood vessels: stiffening and atherosclerosis. The first is a natural change in the composition of blood vessel walls, with decreasing amounts of elastin and increasing amounts of collagen. The cumulative effects of free radicals and glycosylation of proteins add to the progressive stiffness and thickening of arteries, but the aortic lumen actually *increases* in diameter despite the arterial stiffness/thickening. Atherosclerosis and arterial stiffening due to elastin/collagen changes occur simultaneously, but

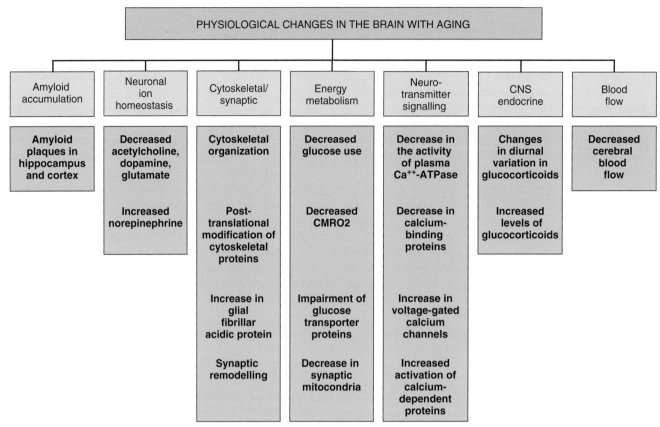

FIG. 16.2   Central nervous system changes with aging. *CMRO2,* Cerebral metabolic rate; *CNS,* central nervous system.

these processes are quite different. Atherosclerosis is a heterogeneous process that happens quite uniformly throughout the conduit arteries. The severity of blood turbulence and shear stress provide a nidus for the atherosclerotic process. *Inflammation* is the hallmark of atherosclerosis, with increased cholesterol as a cofactor. Atherosclerosis causes *occlusion* of arteries, whereas age-related changes typically cause *dilatation.* Functionally the arteries become less responsive to both vasoconstrictors and vasodilators owing to changes in the endothelium. Though levels of endothelin 1 (a potent vasoconstrictor) are increased, the effect of other vasoconstrictor chemicals such as norepinephrine, ephedrine, and phenylephrine is attenuated.

The consequence of stiff arteries is that the pulse wave of the ejected blood travels faster. Velocity increases twofold between the ages of 20 and 80, independent of blood pressure. Stiffer arteries also allow pressure to reflect from the periphery back to the heart quicker while the aortic valve is still open and the heart is ejecting, effectively increasing the afterload on the heart (Fig. 16.3). Thus systolic blood pressure is augmented. Data from the Framingham Heart Study show that systolic blood pressure increases by about 5 mm Hg per decade until the age of 60 and thereafter increases by 10 mm Hg per decade. Diastolic pressure remains unchanged. The net effect is an increase in the systolic blood pressure without a change in diastolic blood pressure.

These changes lead to alterations in *ventricular-vascular coupling.* The heart responds to the increased impedance by developing left ventricular hypertrophy. Left ventricular mass increases by 15% between age 30 and 70, with subsequent effects on systolic and diastolic function (Fig. 16.4). These chronic changes make the myocardium more prone to ischemia. Decreased oxygen supply due to an increase in left ventricular end-diastolic pressure and decreased aortic diastolic pressure occurs at the same time as oxygen demand increases owing to ventricular hypertrophy, increased left ventricular end-systolic pressure, increased aortic pressure, and increased duration of systole (Fig. 16.5).

The incidence of diastolic dysfunction increases with age, and this has been proven by detailed echocardiographic studies. Any systolic dysfunction in the elderly should be considered abnormal, especially if it is accompanied by a wall motion abnormality. Though the cardiac myocytes continue to multiply during life, their ability to keep pace with apoptosis decreases. Consequently there is a net loss of about half of cardiac myocytes during life. Older myocytes are stiffer and lack the ability for ischemic preconditioning. The incidence of heart failure increases significantly with age. With heart failure the ratio of β_1- to β_2-adrenergic receptors also changes. In persons without heart failure the left ventricle has 80% β_1-adrenergic receptors and 20% β_2-adrenergic receptors. In heart failure the ratio changes to 60% β_1 receptors and 40% β_2

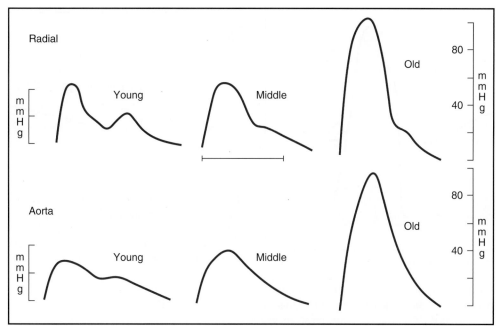

FIG. 16.3   Impact of vascular changes with aging on pulse waveforms of the ascending aorta and radial artery. Pulse pressure is increased almost fourfold in the ascending aorta and twofold in the upper limb. (Adapted from O'Rourke MF, Hashimoto J. Mechanical factors in arterial aging: a clinical perspective. *J Am Coll Cardiol.* 2007;50:1-13.)

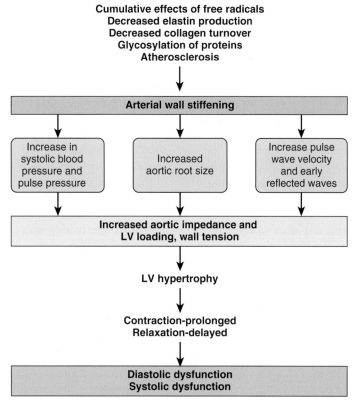

FIG. 16.4   Impact of vascular changes on myocardial function with aging. *LV,* Left ventricular.

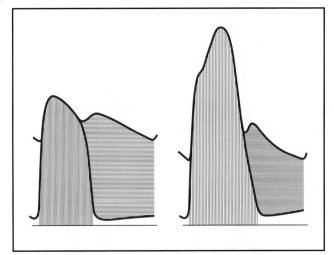

FIG. 16.5 Ascending aortic (*horizontally lined area*) and left ventricular (*vertically lined area*) pressure waves in young and old subjects, with the young subject on the left and the old subject on the right. In the older person, myocardial oxygen demands are increased by the increase in left ventricular (LV) and aortic systolic pressure and by the increased duration of systole. Myocardial oxygen supply is reduced by a shorter duration of diastole, lower aortic pressure during diastole, and increased LV pressure during diastole caused by LV dysfunction. (Adapted from O'Rourke MF, Hashimoto J. Mechanical factors in arterial aging: a clinical perspective. *J Am Coll Cardiol.* 2007;50:1-13.)

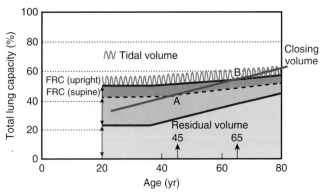

FIG. 16.6 Changes in lung volumes and capacities with aging. Residual volume and functional residual capacity (FRC) increase with age, whereas total lung capacity remains the same. Closing volume increases with age and exceeds FRC in the supine position at about age 45 and exceeds FRC in the upright position at about age 65. (Adapted from Corcoran TB, Hillyard S. Cardiopulmonary aspects of anaesthesia for the elderly. *Best Pract Res Clin Anaesthesiol.* 2011;25:329-354.)

receptors. This can have a significant impact on how adrenergic agonists and blockers impact ventricular function.

Ventricular septal thickness increases with age, as does thickness of the aortic and mitral valve leaflets. Annular dilatation is very common, and 90% of healthy octogenarians demonstrate some form of mild multivalvular regurgitation, which is typically central and associated with normal-appearing valve leaflets. Left atrial chamber size also increases. The incidence of aortic sclerosis and stenosis increases with age.

The electrical system of the heart also declines with age. The number of pacemaker cells is reduced by about 90% by age 70. Prolongation of the PR interval, QRS duration, and QT interval is noted. The incidence of dysrhythmias, especially atrial fibrillation, increases significantly. The *resting heart rate* slows, and there is a marked decrease in *maximum heart rate* in response to exercise. The response to atropine administration is half that of younger individuals. Decreased chronotropic, inotropic, and lusitropic responses to dobutamine have been noted in the elderly. Heart rate variability (i.e., variation in instantaneous heart rate and the R-R interval), which is considered a marker of physiologic reserve, is also decreased.

Normal age-related changes in cardiovascular physiology include a decrease in peak heart rate, peak cardiac output, and peak ejection fraction. In addition, there are changes in autonomic tone and baroreceptor reflex activity. There is overall dampening of autonomic and baroreceptor activity with aging. This results in a slower resting heart rate and decreased ability to increase cardiac output by a change in heart rate. Compared to younger

individuals, increases in cardiac output in the elderly are achieved by increasing end-diastolic volume rather than by increasing heart rate. This results in an increased reliance on atrial contraction for maintenance of cardiac output. Overall the ability of the cardiovascular system to withstand stress is significantly decreased.

Respiratory System

Age-related physiologic changes in the respiratory system can be grouped into three broad categories: (1) mechanical changes, (2) changes in gas exchange, and (3) changes in sensing mechanisms. A progressive decrease in elasticity changes respiratory mechanics and alveolar architecture. The chest wall becomes stiffer as lung tissue loses its intrinsic elastic recoil. Thus chest wall compliance decreases while lung compliance increases. Total lung capacity remains the same, residual volume increases, and vital capacity decreases. Mechanical changes lead to increased work of breathing and make the elderly more prone to respiratory failure. Owing to a progressive decline in diaphragmatic strength and changes in the airway, expiratory flows such as FEV_1 (forced expiratory volume in the first second of expiration) and $FEF_{75\%}$ (forced expiratory flow at 75% of forced vital capacity) decrease (Fig. 16.6).

Complex changes at the alveolar level cause a reduction in arterial oxygen tension with age. It is estimated that the arterial partial pressure of oxygen (Pao_2) decreases at an average rate of 0.35 mm Hg per year. Mean arterial oxygen tension *on room air* decreases from 95 mm Hg at age 20 to less than 70 mm Hg at age 80. These changes in arterial oxygenation are caused by an increase in ventilation/perfusion mismatching and to a lesser extent by intrapulmonary shunting. The reduction in elastic tissue in the lung interstitium results in emphysematous changes in lung/airway architecture. Therefore there is an increased tendency of airways to close (i.e., closing volume increases). Closing volume approaches tidal volume, so the elderly are more prone to atelectasis. Residual volume also increases as a proportion of total lung capacity. It is 20% at age 20 and 40% at age 70. Protective cough mechanisms may become attenuated and both decrease the ability to clear secretions and increase the risk of aspiration. The endurance of the respiratory muscles also decreases. Functionally there is reduced respiratory drive in response to hypoxia, hypercarbia, and a resistive load. Increased airway reactivity is also seen.

Renal System, Fluids, and Electrolytes

Various aspects of renal function decline with normal aging. The salient changes in renal function that accompany normal aging are as follows:

Renal vascular dysautonomy: This term is used to indicate the attenuation of autonomic renal vascular reflexes that are present to protect the kidney from hypotensive and hypertensive states.

Senile hypofiltration: This describes the progressive decline in the glomerular filtration rate (GFR) of about 1 mL/year after age 30 that is seen in about two-thirds of the elderly.

Tubular dysfunction: This leads to reduction in the maximal tubular capacity to reabsorb and excrete solutes, especially sodium.

Medullary hypotonicity: This phenomenon describes the reduction in tonicity of the renal medulla, which causes a reduced antidiuretic hormone effect and thereby a reduction in water absorption. Elderly patients are unable to maximally concentrate or dilute urine.

Tubular frailty: This term refers to renal tubular cells being more susceptible to hypoxic or nephrotoxicity injury and taking longer to recover from acute tubular necrosis.

The clinical consequences of all of these changes can be profound. The aging kidney is more susceptible to injury, less able to accommodate hemodynamic changes, and not able to handle water and salt perturbations. A low GFR and diminished tubular function lead to reduced ability to concentrate urine, which means that the obligatory urinary volume to excrete waste products has to increase. However, also owing to decreased GFR, the ability to excrete excess free water is diminished, making the elderly more prone to fluid overload, pulmonary edema, and development of hypoosmolar states (e.g., hyponatremia) if large amounts of hypoosmolar fluids are administered.

Aging also causes decreased sensitivity of volume and osmoreceptors, so the thirst response may be diminished and drinking behavior altered. Bladder dysfunction or incontinence can also alter drinking behavior to avoid embarrassing situations. Since many elderly patients have mobility problems or difficulties with the activities of daily living (ADLs), inability to reach fluids or difficult access to fluids further predisposes them to dehydration.

Gastrointestinal System

Aging significantly affects the motility of the oropharyngeal/upper esophageal area, colonic function, gastrointestinal immunity and gastrointestinal drug metabolism. Liver size, blood flow, and perfusion normally decline by 30%–40% between the 3rd and 10th decades. However, these changes do *not* have a significant impact on liver function. Liver function has to decrease by 70% to have clinically relevant effects. No significant abnormalities are noted on conventional liver function tests in the elderly.

Immune System

Significant changes in the immune system include both changes in the innate immune system (macrophages, neutrophils, natural killer cells, etc.) and in the adaptive immune systems. The bactericidal activity of immune cells is decreased. Increased levels of cytokines and chemokines have been noted, which is consistent with a low-grade chronic inflammatory process in the elderly. Age-related functional changes have also been noticed in T-cell and B-cell functions. These changes are thought to impact the ability of the elderly to fight infection and control cancers.

Endocrine Function Changes

The endocrine glands tend to atrophy in the elderly and reduce hormone production. This frequently leads to impaired endocrine function, such as impaired glucose homeostasis. Deficiencies of insulin, thyroxine, growth hormone, renin, aldosterone, and testosterone are often present. Chronic electrolyte abnormalities, diabetes mellitus, hypothyroidism, impotence, and osteoporosis are common.

The resting metabolic rate declines approximately 1% per year after age 30, and total energy expenditure also goes down, probably secondary to a decline in lean body mass. However, in elderly persons with multiple morbidities and those affected by chronic illness, total energy expenditure *increases*. Sick individuals often expend most of their energy performing simple ADLs. Longitudinal studies have demonstrated that peak oxygen consumption declines progressively with aging, so the elderly are unable to cope with high oxygen demands.

Sarcopenia and Body Composition

There is a 10%–15% decrease in intracellular fluid owing to loss of muscle mass. Total fat content decreases, but the percentage of fat per total body weight increases. Weight tends to decline with aging because of a significant reduction in lean body mass, which is predominantly composed of muscle and visceral organs. Muscle atrophy is greater in fast-twitch than in slow-twitch muscle fibers, presumably secondary to loss of motor neurons. Waist circumference increases throughout one's lifespan are due to increasing visceral fat. In some individuals, fat can also accumulate inside muscle tissue, affecting muscle quality and function. Fibroconnective tissue also builds up with aging, and it too can affect muscle quality and function. This loss of muscle mass and quality results in reduced muscle strength that ultimately affects functioning and mobility. The elderly become progressively frail.

TABLE 16.1	Comparison of Different Central Nervous System Disorders		
Diagnosis	Distinguishing Features	Symptoms	Course
Dementia	Memory impairment	Disorientation, agitation	Slow onset, progressive, chronic
Delirium	Fluctuating level of consciousness, decreased attention	Disorientation, visual hallucinations, agitation, apathy, withdrawal, memory and attention impairment	Acute; most cases remit with correction of underlying medical condition
Psychotic disorders	Deficit in reality testing	Social withdrawal, apathy	Slow onset with prodromal syndrome; chronic with exacerbations
Depression	Sadness, loss of interest and pleasure in usual activities	Disturbances of sleep, appetite, concentration; low energy; feelings of hopelessness and worthlessness; suicidal ideation	Single episode or recurrent episodes; may be chronic

FRAILTY

Frailty is defined as a state of reduced physiologic reserve that is associated with increased susceptibility to disability. It is related to normal changes of aging, chronic disease, and inflammation and is characterized by failure of the body to respond to additional stresses such as surgery or infection. There is no universally accepted definition or assessment tool for frailty. A proposed phenotype definition of frailty is characterized by weight loss, fatigue, impaired grip strength, low physical activity, and slow gait speed and in some patients, cognitive decline. All these changes lead to a decreased reserve. Compared to their younger counterparts, elderly patients are likely to decompensate more quickly and recover more slowly from physiologic or pathologic insults. Frailty is an independent predictor of in-hospital mortality.

GERIATRIC SYNDROMES

Geriatric syndromes encompass clinical conditions that are frequently encountered in older people. The pathophysiology of geriatric syndromes is multifactorial and can involve multiple unrelated organ systems. These syndromes have deleterious effects on independent functioning and quality of life. The list of geriatric syndromes includes incontinence, delirium, falls, pressure ulcers, sleep disorders, problems with eating or feeding, pain, and depressed mood. In addition, dementia and physical disability can also be considered geriatric syndromes. Geriatric syndromes are the phenotypic consequences of frailty. Virtually all geriatric syndromes are characterized by changes in four domains: (1) alteration in body composition, (2) gaps in energy supply and demand, (3) signaling disequilibrium, and (4) neurodegeneration. Only dementia and falls will be discussed here.

Dementia

Intellectual decline is one of the early hallmarks of dementia. Major differences are seen in the elderly in terms of intellectual function compared to themselves in early adulthood. In any patient with a slowly progressive dementia, sudden changes in cognitive, behavioral, or health status may occur. Mental status is often a barometer of health in these patients, and abrupt changes necessitate a search for any additional problem that may be occurring (Table 16.1). Numerous population-based studies report decreased longevity in elderly individuals who experience cognitive decline. *Diminishing cognitive performance over any time interval is predictive of an earlier death.* Perhaps the most important challenge in treating dementia is identifying cases of *reversible dementia,* such as chronic drug intoxication, vitamin deficiencies, subdural hematoma, major depression, normal-pressure hydrocephalus, and hypothyroidism.

Unfortunately, most causes of dementia, including degenerative brain diseases such as Alzheimer's disease and other common multiinfarct states are incurable. This does not mean, however, that symptoms cannot be treated and ameliorated. Pharmacotherapy for dementia is tailored to control behavioral problems and sleep disorders that may be present and to prevent further intellectual decline and neurodegeneration. These treatments include vitamin E, nonsteroidal antiinflammatory drugs, estrogen replacement therapy, and centrally acting acetylcholinesterase inhibitors.

For the anesthesiologist the challenges in caring for elderly patients with declining mental capacity are many. Perioperative interactions with the patient and family must take into account the patient's compromised ability to process general and medical information and capability to provide truly informed consent. Documentation of baseline cognitive and neurologic function may become significant if postoperative alterations in mental function are encountered. If acute deterioration is suspected, a neurologic consultation is advised.

Falls and Balance Disorders

Unstable gait and falls are a serious concern in older patients. Problems with balance and falls tend to be multifactorial. Poor muscle strength, neural damage in the basal ganglia and cerebellum, and peripheral neuropathy are all recognized risk factors for falls. The American Geriatric Society recommends asking all older adults about falls and gait instability. Patients with a history of multiple falls should undergo an evaluation of gait and balance to determine the precipitating factors.

PHARMACOKINETIC AND PHARMACODYNAMIC CHANGES WITH AGING

Elderly patients often suffer from multiple morbidities and are taking multiple medications. *Polypharmacy is the norm in the elderly.* The effects of drug interactions are substantially increased with advanced age. Older, sicker patients require less anesthesia. Their increased sensitivity to anesthetics has been attributed to loss of neuronal tissue or poorly defined changes in receptor functions. Progressive changes in functional connectivity in the aging brain and the varying effects of anesthetics provide other possible explanations for this increased sensitivity. This sensitivity may explain both anesthetic "toxicity" and the cognitive dysfunction associated with anesthesia in the elderly.

Management of Anesthesia

The pharmacokinetics of anesthetic drugs are affected by progressive physiologic changes that occur with aging. Total body water decreases by 10%–15%, and this decrease causes a decrease in the measured central compartment volume. This can lead to an increase in initial plasma concentration following rapid intravenous (IV) administration of an anesthetic drug. Body fat increases as muscle mass decreases, so lipid-soluble drugs (most IV anesthetics) have a large volume of distribution with the potential for prolonged clinical effects.

Changes in serum proteins include a decrease in plasma albumin and a slight increase in α_1-acid glycoprotein. These changes could theoretically affect circulating free drug concentrations and the concentration of drug at the effect site. In practice, however, these protein changes do *not* appear to have a significant impact on geriatric anesthetic pharmacology. A greater concern is the need for *adjustment of drug dosages* based on a smaller lean body mass and weight in the elderly.

Drugs that are metabolized by microsomal cytochrome P450 enzymes may be affected. These changes result in a reduction in clearance of about 30%–40%, which corresponds to the degree hepatic blood flow is reduced in the elderly. As renal function declines, drugs that are cleared by the kidneys should be administered judiciously. In particular, neuromuscular blockers that are excreted by the kidneys must be very carefully dosed.

Inhalational Anesthetics

The minimum alveolar concentration (MAC) required to achieve adequate anesthetic depth progressively decreases with age. By some estimates, MAC values decrease by about 6% per decade after age 40 for volatile anesthetics and about 8% per decade for nitrous oxide. The exact mechanism for this is unknown. The effects of volatile anesthetics and nitrous oxide are additive. Thus an 80-year-old patient who gets 66% nitrous oxide will require only 0.3% sevoflurane to achieve 1 MAC anesthetic concentration (Fig. 16.7) The hemodynamic impact of excessive anesthetic administration is well recognized.

Propofol

The pharmacodynamics and pharmacokinetics of propofol are significantly altered with aging. Age-related changes have been found for both induction drug doses and infusion doses. This dosing adjustment may be nearly a 50% decrease. Elderly patients develop deeper anesthetic stages (as evidenced by electroencephalography [EEG]), need more time to reach deeper anesthetic stages, and require more time for recovery. They need less propofol for steady-state maintenance of a defined stage of hypnosis. The hemodynamic effects of propofol are much greater in the elderly.

Interestingly there are gender differences in propofol pharmacokinetics. Propofol clearance is decreased much more in women than in men. Propofol infusion rates to achieve a persistent level of moderate sedation are lower in the elderly. Current literature suggests at least a 20% reduction in the induction dose of propofol. Though the drug has been extensively studied, investigations have been limited to relatively healthy older patients. Current practice for anesthetic care of the *very elderly* is based on extrapolation of these data.

Etomidate

Etomidate is an anesthetic and amnestic but not an analgesic. It is often considered an ideal drug for the elderly because it causes less hemodynamic instability than propofol or thiopental. However, it has a smaller initial volume of distribution and reduced clearance in the elderly. A significant increase in sensitivity to this drug has also been shown. Like propofol, *much lower induction doses* are recommended in the elderly.

Thiopental

The central volume of distribution for thiopental decreases in the elderly, and the total dose of this drug will need to be reduced. An optimal dose in an 80-year-old patient is suggested to be 50%–80% of the dose needed for an adult patient. Recovery after a bolus dose of thiopental is delayed in older patients because of the decreased central volume of distribution.

Midazolam

Elderly patients are significantly more sensitive to midazolam than younger patients, primarily because of *pharmacodynamic* differences. However, the exact mechanism of this pharmacodynamic difference is unknown. The duration of effect of midazolam may be much longer and could potentially contribute to postoperative delirium. Furthermore, midazolam is metabolized to the pharmacologically active metabolite *hydroxymidazolam,* which is excreted by the kidneys and may accumulate in patients with diminished renal function. A 75% reduction in dose from a 20-year-old to a 90-year-old has been recommended.

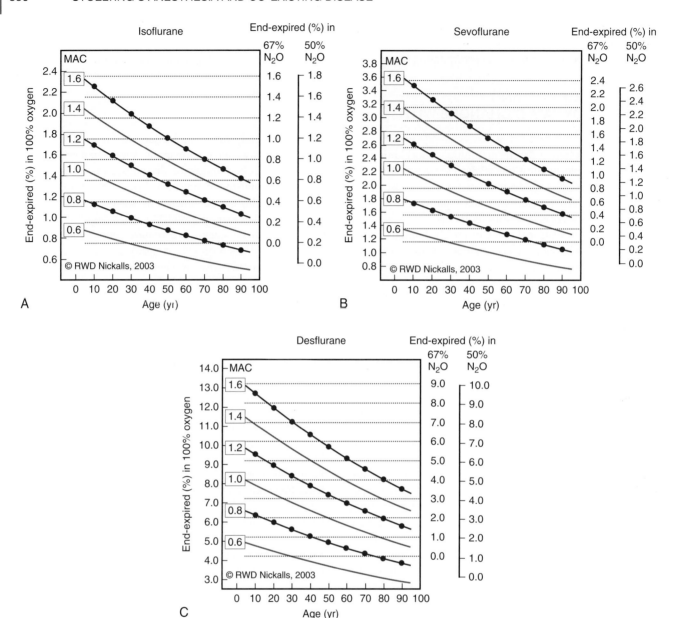

FIG. 16.7 Iso-MAC charts for isoflurane (A), sevoflurane (B), and desflurane (C) (age > 1 year). (Adapted from Nickalls RW, Mapleson WW. Age-related iso-MAC charts for isoflurane, sevoflurane and desflurane in man. *Br J Anaesth.* 2003;91:170-174.)

Opioids

Pharmacodynamic changes within the opioid receptor system have been noted with aging. Receptor density, receptor affinity, and binding may change. Though increased sensitivity to opioids is attributed to *pharmacodynamic* changes, age-related *pharmacokinetic* changes, especially on opioid metabolism, affect the choice of opioids to be used in the elderly. The liver metabolizes the opioids, and the kidneys excrete the metabolites. Metabolites of some opioids, including codeine, morphine, and meperidine, are pharmacologically active and contribute to both analgesia and many side effects. The primary risk of opioids is respiratory depression, the incidence of which is *markedly increased* with age.

Fentanyl

Fentanyl is a highly selective μ-receptor agonist. Age has a greater effect on fentanyl pharmacodynamics than on its pharmacokinetics. A 50% increase in the potency of fentanyl has been reported in octogenarians. Since elderly patients are much more sensitive to fentanyl, they should receive reduced IV doses.

Remifentanil

Remifentanil is an ultrashort-acting synthetic opioid and is metabolized by nonspecific tissue and plasma esterases. This makes it an ideal drug for use in the elderly because it has a very short half-life and is not dependent on liver and renal function for clearance. However, elderly patients are quite sensitive to remifentanil. The equilibrium constant is decreased by approximately 50% over the age range of 20–85 years. The onset and offset of remifentanil effect is also slower in elderly individuals. Elderly patients need only about half the bolus dose of younger patients to achieve the same effect. This is because of increased pharmacodynamic sensitivity rather than pharmacokinetic changes. Elderly patients require an infusion rate about *one-third* that of younger patients because of the combined impact of increased sensitivity and decreased clearance.

Meperidine

Meperidine is a relatively weak μ-agonist with about 10% of the potency of morphine. It is metabolized to an active metabolite, normeperidine, which is excreted by the kidneys and has a very long half-life of 15–30 hours. Use of meperidine has been associated with development of postoperative delirium in elderly patients, so its use is *not* recommended in older adults except in the very small doses needed to manage postoperative shivering.

Neuromuscular Blocking Drugs

The pharmacodynamics of neuromuscular blocking drugs are not significantly altered by age. The ED_{95} of neuromuscular blockers is essentially the same for young and old patients. In contrast *the pharmacokinetics of neuromuscular drugs are significantly altered with age.* The onset to maximal block may be delayed, and metabolism by the liver and excretion by the kidneys can be significantly prolonged in elderly patients with hepatic and/or renal dysfunction. Recovery time from neuromuscular blockade could be increased by as much as 50%, and the impact of residual neuromuscular blockade on pharyngeal function can be very significant in the elderly. Since cisatracurium is not dependent on hepatic or renal function for clearance, it may be considered a neuromuscular blocker of choice for the elderly.

PERIOPERATIVE OUTCOMES AFTER CARDIAC AND NONCARDIAC SURGERY

Perioperative outcomes are dependent on many factors, the two most important of which are the surgical risk of the procedure and the number of defined clinical risk factors in the patient. As the number of clinical risk factors increases and the risk of the surgical procedure increases, the overall risk of a poor outcome also increases. Surgery performed in high-volume centers with specialized staff and extra resources may have better outcomes.

Based on their physiologic changes, it is expected that outcomes in the elderly would be worse than in their younger counterparts. However, this has not been clearly shown. One reason for this unexpected observation is that the rate of decline of function varies significantly among individuals. The rate of decline is dependent on genetic factors, co-existing diseases, and environmental insults. Thus a "healthy" 80-year-old may be more physiologically robust than a 70-year-old with

several comorbidities. Complicated surgery or procedures cannot be denied to elderly patients solely on the basis of age and the presence of any comorbidities. The functional level of the patient must also be considered.

The probability that an octogenarian will be *completely healthy* is remote. According to 2011 American Heart Association statistics, the prevalence of cardiovascular disease in patients older than 80 years is 78%–85%. The incidence of hypertension (>65%), coronary artery disease (23%–37%), and congestive heart failure (13%–15%) are all higher (Fig. 16.8). Furthermore the incidence of diabetes mellitus, renal insufficiency, atrial fibrillation, and chronic obstructive pulmonary disease increases significantly with aging.

Elderly patients do have significantly worse outcomes than their younger counterparts. This has been shown in national databases and individual studies. The operative mortality of octogenarians undergoing cardiac surgery is reported to be 6%–11%, compared with 3%–4% in younger patients. Octogenarians have a significantly higher risk for *any complication* with cardiac surgery, including neurologic events, pneumonia, dysrhythmias, and wound infection (Fig. 16.9). Operative mortality is two to five times higher in octogenarians than in younger patients. This is also true for noncardiac surgery (Fig. 16.10).

A high rate of postoperative complications—as high as 60%—has been reported. Pulmonary insufficiency or infection was one of the leading causes of postoperative morbidity. One-fifth of patients required prolonged (>24 hours) mechanical ventilation. Atrial fibrillation and surgical wound infection are more frequent. The stroke rate is about twice that of younger patients. *Neurocognitive dysfunction* is very common after both cardiac and noncardiac surgery in the elderly. *Delirium* is very common after major surgery, and the incidence of a long-term decline in cognitive function is also very common. This has been most clearly demonstrated after coronary artery bypass surgery. The incidence of cognitive dysfunction after noncardiac surgery is three to nine times more frequent than in the elderly who do *not* undergo surgery. Many of these complications account for increased hospital length of stay and increases in cost.

Functional recovery after cardiac and noncardiac surgery is *not* the norm. Some studies report that fewer than 50% of elderly patients are discharged back to their homes. Instead, many patients are discharged to long-term rehabilitation facilities or nursing homes.

PERIOPERATIVE CARE OF ELDERLY PATIENTS

Preoperative Assessment

It is well recognized that elderly patients have a decreased reserve and hence are more prone to major adverse events. Comprehensive preoperative assessment is crucial in determining perioperative risk and optimizing care. Because of the complexity of geriatric patients, it is not uncommon that

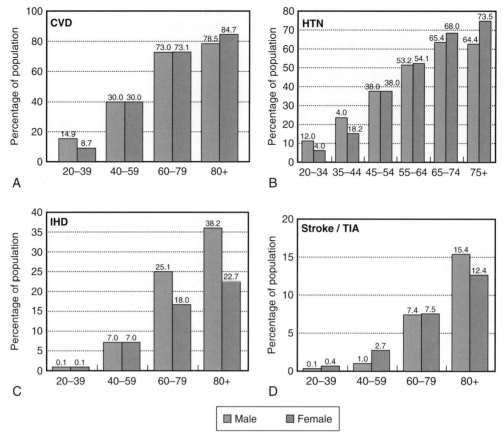

FIG. 16.8   Incidence of cardiovascular disease based on age and gender. A, Cardiovascular disease (CVD). B, Hypertension (HTN). C, Ischemic heart disease (IHD). D, Stroke/transient ischemic attack (TIA). (Data from Lloyd-Jones D, Adams RJ, Brown TM, et al. on behalf of the American Heart Association Statistics Committee and Stroke Statistics Subcommittee. Heart disease and stroke statistics—2010 update: a report from the American Heart Association. *Circulation.* 2010;121:e46-e215.)

COMPLICATIONS AND OUTCOMES FOR OCTOGENARIANS
UNDERGOING CARDIAC SURGERY

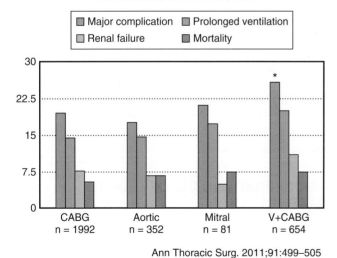

Ann Thoracic Surg. 2011;91:499–505

FIG. 16.9   Morbidity after cardiac surgery in octogenarians. *CABG,* Coronary artery bypass grafting; *V+CABG,* valve surgery in addition to CABG. (Data from Bhamidipati CM, LaPar DJ, Fonner E Jr, et al. Outcomes and cost of cardiac surgery in octogenarians is related to type of operation: a multi-institutional analysis. *Ann Thorac Surg.* 2011;91:499-505.)

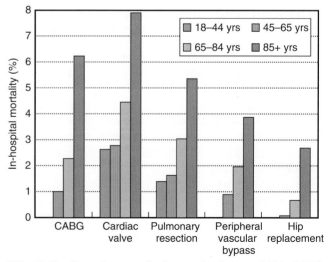

FIG. 16.10   Operative mortality by age for the year 2009. *CABG,* Coronary artery bypass grafting. (Data from Healthcare cost and utilization project [HCUP]. Nationwide inpatient sample 2009. www.hcup-us.ahrq.gov.)

geriatric consultation is obtained preoperatively or that an elderly patient is comanaged with a geriatrician.

Traditional risk indices cannot predict outcomes in octogenarians. They do not take into account frailty, which has been difficult to define but signifies decreased functional capacity in an elderly individual. The *Frailty Index* is able to predict outcomes in the nonsurgical elderly population and may have a role in perioperative risk assessment. Adding the Frailty Index to the established Revised Cardiac Risk Index can improve risk prediction by 8%–10% and can be of incremental value in cardiovascular risk assessment. Geriatric preoperative assessment must include review of geriatric syndromes, evaluation of frailty, nutritional status, assessment of functional status, baseline cognitive status, review of medications, and goals of care.

Nutrition and Anorexia

Normal aging is associated with a decline in food intake, which is more marked in men than in women. This is partly a result of a low level of physical activity, a decline in lean body mass, and a slow rate of protein turnover. Loss of taste sensation, reduced stomach compliance, and high levels of certain hormones also lead to a decrease in appetite. About a quarter of elderly individuals meet the criteria for malnutrition. *Malnutrition* or *undernutrition* is associated with multiple adverse health consequences, such as impaired muscle function, decreased bone mass, immune dysfunction, anemia, reduced cognitive function, poor wound healing, delayed recovery from surgery, and increased risk of falling. If there is a concern regarding malnutrition due to

alcohol consumption, vitamin B_{12} and folate levels should be measured. Patients with an unintentional weight loss of more than 10%–15% over the last 6 months, a body mass index (BMI) below 18.5, or a serum albumin below 3 g/dL are considered to be at *severe nutritional risk. Preoperative nutritional support* should be provided to these patients. Though there is consensus that nutritional assessment is important, nutritional supplementation in the perioperative period has not been shown to improve outcome.

Functional Status

Poor functional status has been identified as a risk factor for surgical site infection and postoperative complications. About one-fourth of patients older than age 65 have impairment in their *basic* ADLs: bathing, dressing, eating, transferring from bed to chair, continence, toileting; or their *instrumental (I)ADLs:* transportation, shopping, cooking, using the telephone, managing money, taking medications, housecleaning, laundry. Half of persons older than 85 years have impairment in their ADLs. Functional status can be assessed by performance times in up-and-go mobility tests and a review of ADLs and IADLs. Some tests require special training and performance by specific healthcare professionals, whereas others can be easily performed in a preoperative clinic—for example, walking speed over a 4-meter distance (Table 16.2). Elderly patients with impaired mobility and increased dependency are at increased risk of postoperative complications. Common serious impairments in hearing and vision should also be elicited.

TABLE 16.2	**Tools for Functional Assessment in Older Patients**	
Measurement Instrument	Evaluation	Activities/Reference
Index of Independence in ADLs	Self-reported	Difficulty/need for help in bathing, dressing, toileting, transferring, continence, feeding
Instrumental ADLs	Self-reported	Difficulty using the telephone, using a car/public transportation, shopping, preparing meals, housework, managing medications, financial management
Functional Independence Measure	Consensus by multidisciplinary team	Motor (eating, grooming, bathing, dressing, toileting, managing bladder/bowels, transferring, walking, climbing stairs); cognitive (auditory comprehension, verbal expression, social interaction, problem solving, memory)
Barthel Index	Professionally evaluated	Independence or need for help in feeding, transferring from bed to chair and back, grooming, transferring to and from toilet, bathing, walking, climbing stairs, dressing, continence
Mobility Questionnaire	Self-reported	Severe difficulty walking ¼ mile and/or climbing stairs
Short Physical Performance Battery	Objective performance based	Time required to walk 4 meters, rise from a chair 5 times, maintain balance
Berg Balance Scale	Objective and professionally evaluated	Performance in 14 tasks related to balance
Walking Speed	Objective performance	Measure walking speed over a 4-meter course
6-Minute Walk	Objective performance based	Distance covered in 6 minutes
Long-Distance Corridor Walk (400 meters)	Objective performance based	Time to fast-walk 400 meters

ADLs, Activities of daily living.
From Ferrucci L, Studenski S. Clinical problems of aging. In: Kasper DL, Fauci AS, Hauser SL, et al., eds. *Harrison's Principles of Internal Medicine.* 19th ed. New York: McGraw-Hill Education; 2015.

Cognition

An older individual's cognitive capacity, decision-making capacity, and risk for postoperative delirium should be assessed. For patients without a known history of dementia, a cognitive assessment tool such as the Mini-Cog test should be performed. The Mini-Cog is a 3-item recall and clock drawing test that efficiently screens for cognitive impairment; 1 point is awarded for each item recalled and 2 points for a normal-appearing clock. A score of 0–2 points indicates a positive screen for dementia. This screening is the initial step in identifying patients who may lack the capacity to make medical decisions and are at high risk for delirium. For patients lacking capacity, advance directives or a surrogate decision maker should be used.

Medication Review

As noted earlier, polypharmacy is the norm in the elderly. Over half of these patients take more than 5 medications weekly, and a fifth take more than 10. The risk of adverse events during a hospitalization increases significantly with the number of medications a patient is taking. Preoperative evaluation is an ideal opportunity to review medications. Anticholinergic medications such as diphenhydramine, promethazine, metoclopramide, and paroxetine should be discontinued if possible. They are associated with delirium and gait instability. Up to 25% of elderly patients may be using benzodiazepines chronically and may be at risk of a withdrawal syndrome in the postoperative period. It is prudent to taper off these drugs prior to surgery so they cannot contribute to postoperative confusion, gait instability, and delirium. By some estimates, over half of elderly patients also take over-the-counter herbal products. The American Society of Anesthesiologists (ASA) recommends that whenever possible, herbal products be discontinued at least 1–2 weeks prior to surgery. Garlic extract and ginkgo biloba increase the risk of perioperative bleeding.

Goals of Care

Preoperative assessment of an elderly patient is an excellent opportunity to discuss goals of care. This time provides the family and patient the opportunity to make important decisions, formalize decisions, express their wishes, and complete legal paperwork.

Preoperative Assessment of Patients Undergoing Urgent or Emergent Surgery

Many elderly patients present for urgent or emergent surgery after trauma, falls, hip fractures, intracranial bleeding, or intraabdominal/vascular emergencies. The urgency of the surgery may preclude detailed preoperative evaluation and optimization. Decisions need to be made regarding the value of waiting for medical problems to be optimized versus proceeding promptly to surgery. Basic evaluation of the cardiorespiratory system, looking for signs of acute heart failure, fat embolism, acute lung injury, and signs of dehydration, should be done. Increased oxygen requirements and low oxygen saturation may denote worsening left ventricular function, acute

lung injury, aspiration, and/or pneumonia. Acute delirium may be evident even before the surgery and should be investigated (if possible) prior to surgery to rule out a new intracranial process. Patients coming for urgent or emergent surgery have worse outcomes than patients who come for elective surgery. Patients and their caregivers should be given realistic information regarding intraoperative risk and potential postoperative outcomes, including the need for mechanical ventilation, intensive care unit (ICU) admission, and a prolonged hospital stay.

Intraoperative Management

Monitoring

Age alone is not an indication for invasive monitoring. The impact of transesophageal echocardiography, pulmonary artery catheterization, or noninvasive cardiac output monitors is yet to be defined in the elderly population, but the decision to use these monitors should be based on their potential benefits and risks, the potential for considerable blood loss or large fluid shifts during surgery, the patient's ASA physical status, the presence of concurrent illnesses, and the planned surgery.

Anesthetic Management

Choosing an anesthetic plan for an elderly patient requires consideration of many details. Several retrospective and prospective studies have failed to show a difference in outcome or a clear benefit for regional or neuraxial anesthesia versus general anesthesia. These studies could not identify any meaningful difference in mortality and morbidity except for a clearly reduced incidence of deep vein thrombosis with regional anesthesia. There is some evidence that use of regional anesthesia may decrease intraoperative blood loss in certain subsets of surgical patients. However, regional anesthesia is not suitable for all surgery.

Anesthetic requirements are reduced significantly in the elderly. The MAC of sevoflurane in an octogenarian is 30% lower than that of a younger person (see Fig. 16.7). IV anesthetics have more pronounced hemodynamic effects, and smaller doses are required to achieve the same anesthetic depth. Dose of an induction drug and opioids should be decreased by at least 25%. *Benzodiazepines should be avoided* whenever possible. Meperidine should *not* be used in the elderly. It is prudent to use cisatracurium in patients with renal and/or liver dysfunction.

The elderly have decreased skin elasticity and reduced skin and soft tissue perfusion, which increases the risk of skin breakdown or ulcerations. The presence of osteoarthritis and osteoporosis also poses a risk of injury. Bony prominences must be protected and padded.

Elderly patients are often dehydrated. Because of decreased left ventricular compliance and limited β-adrenergic receptor responsiveness, these patients are more prone to develop hypotension when hypovolemic, and congestive heart failure when hypervolemic. A thorough assessment of intravascular volume status is essential *before* induction of anesthesia.

Measures to conserve body heat and decrease the risk of hypothermia should be implemented. Prolonged elimination of anesthetic drugs and slower postoperative awakening can occur as a result of intraoperative heat loss. Elderly patients can respond to hypothermia by shivering during the early postoperative period. Shivering results in a greatly increased oxygen demand, which is a special concern in patients with coronary disease or in those with compromised cardiovascular reserve.

Fluid Therapy/Blood Transfusion

Fluid therapy should not be considered routine. It should be given as much importance as administration of any drug. Owing to atherosclerosis, stiff ventricles, diastolic dysfunction, and coronary artery disease, elderly patients do not tolerate hypovolemia or hypervolemia. Inappropriate fluid administration can have dire consequences. *Hypovolemia* leads to severe hypotension and organ hypoperfusion; *overhydration* can lead to congestive heart failure.

Blood component therapy should also be used judiciously. There is some evidence suggesting that higher hemoglobin and hematocrit values may be more desirable in elderly patients.

Postoperative Management

Postoperative Delirium and Cognitive Dysfunction

Neurocognitive dysfunction is very common in the elderly after both cardiac and noncardiac surgery. Delirium affects 15%–55% of hospitalized older patients. It is characterized by (1) a rapid decline in the level of consciousness, with difficulty focusing, shifting, or sustaining attention; and (2) a cognitive change (e.g., incoherent speech, memory gaps, disorientation, hallucination) not explained by preexisting dementia and/or a medical history suggestive of preexisting cognitive impairment, frailty, and comorbidity. The mechanism of postoperative delirium remains elusive, but it has been hypothesized that the stress of surgery and its associated inflammatory response result in leukocyte migration into the central nervous system, where leukocytes play an active role in the pathophysiology of postoperative delirium. Most patients with postoperative delirium experience a complete recovery, but this disorder is far from benign. Hospitalized patients with delirium have up to a 10-fold higher risk of developing other medical complications and have longer hospital stays, increased medical costs, an increased need for long-term care, and a higher 1-year mortality rate.

The strongest predisposing factor for postoperative delirium is preexisting dementia. Other factors that can contribute to delirium include dehydration, alcohol consumption (or withdrawal), psychoactive drugs, visual impairment, and hearing deprivation. Stressful conditions that can precipitate delirium include surgery, anesthesia, persistent pain, sleep deprivation, immobilization, hypoxia, malnutrition, metabolic and electrolyte derangements, and treatment with opioids and anticholinergic agents. Even though it is a common condition, there are *no known substantive prevention measures.* Early identification,

supportive measures, and symptomatic treatment are the rule. Short-term use of haloperidol can be considered to control symptoms of agitation, paranoia, fear, and delirium. However, prophylactic use of antipsychotic medications has *not* been shown to improve outcomes and is not recommended. Use of antipsychotic medications in patients with dementia is associated with increased mortality.

Postoperative Pain Control

Management of acute postoperative pain is challenging in the elderly, especially in patients with baseline cognitive dysfunction. The American Geriatric Society has developed comprehensive guidelines for the management of acute postoperative pain. Though not based on strong levels of evidence, they provide an adequate framework for pain management in the elderly. Many elderly patients may also suffer from chronic pain. Acute procedural pain should be differentiated from chronic pain or pain due to complications of a procedure (e.g., new pain, increased intensity of pain, pain not relieved by previously effective strategies), and treatment should be directed accordingly. Conducting a pain history before a procedure can help discriminate procedural from chronic pain.

The principles of pain management in the elderly are the same as for a younger population, but the tools for assessing pain have to be adapted to compensate for the cognitive and sensory impairments in the elderly. Adaptations for auditory impairments include positioning oneself clearly in view of the patient, speaking in a slow, normal tone of voice, reducing extraneous noise, and (if appropriate) making sure the patient has a functioning hearing aid. Adequate time to process information and respond to questions must be allowed. Adaptations for visual impairment include using simple lettering (at least 14-point font size), adequate line spacing, and nonglare paper and making sure the patient has his/her eyeglasses.

The cognitive status of the older adult impacts the approach to pain assessment, patient and family education, and pain treatment options. A baseline assessment of cognitive status provides the basis for evaluating changes in cognitive status throughout an episode of illness. Older adults with mild to moderate cognitive impairment are often able to rate pain using self-reporting instruments, and an individual patient's ability to do so should be assessed. It may be necessary to try several assessment tools to evaluate which one can be used most easily by the cognitively impaired individual. Even many severely impaired persons can respond to simple questioning about the presence of pain and may be able to use a simple rating scale to assess it. Scales that are the simplest and most usable for cognitively impaired older adults include verbal descriptor scales, pain thermometers, and pain scales with faces.

Elderly adults who cannot report pain must be assessed for the presence of factors that cause pain. Whenever an older adult with cognitive impairment shows a change in mental status, pain should be considered a potential etiology. Potential sources of pain include a distended bladder, the incision, infection, inflammation, fracture, positioning, urinary tract infection, and constipation. Treating the underlying cause of pain using etiology-specific interventions is important. Observing behavior when the patient is engaged in activity (e.g., transfers, ambulation, repositioning) can provide clues to the level of pain the patient may be experiencing. Assessing pain by only observing a patient at rest can be misleading. Nonverbal cognitively impaired patients need to be observed closely for essential information on which to make a judgment regarding the presence of pain. Failure to assess and treat pain in the elderly, and specifically in cognitively impaired individuals, is often due to the mistaken belief by healthcare providers that the perception of pain is decreased in individuals with cognitive impairment.

Some drugs should be avoided in the elderly. *Beer's criteria,* which lists drugs potentially harmful to the elderly, should be referenced. The use of *meperidine* is *not* recommended in older individuals. The use of *transdermal fentanyl* is *not* recommended for acute pain management in opioid-naïve older adults because of its potential for delirium and respiratory depression. *Agonist-antagonist opioids* should be *avoided* in older adults, since their side effects can be pronounced. *Butorphanol* and *pentazocine* produce psychotomimetic effects and may lead to delirium. Pentazocine causes hallucinations, dysphoria, delirium, and agitation in older adults and has been shown to be no more effective in controlling pain than aspirin or acetaminophen. Analgesics with a long, highly variable half-life (e.g., opioids such as *methadone* and *levorphanol*) should also be *avoided.* Drugs with a long half-life can readily accumulate in older adults and result in toxicity (i.e., respiratory depression, sedation).

Care of the Elderly in the ICU

It is not uncommon to have elderly patients transferred to the ICU because of the need for mechanical ventilation or postoperative hemodynamic monitoring after major surgery. Postoperative care of elderly patients is governed by the same goals as their intraoperative care. The presence of comorbidities and the patient's tolerance of the intraoperative course help determine the intensity of postoperative monitoring. For sedation, dexmedetomidine is a better drug than benzodiazepines because it is associated with less delirium and earlier recovery.

The care of a geriatric patient in the ICU can be very challenging. Dealing with social, ethical, and end-of-life issues can be particularly daunting. To achieve the best possible outcomes, physicians need to be mindful of the sensitivities and wishes of the patient and provide a realistic prognosis to family members and caregivers.

KEY POINTS

- Aging appears to be driven by progressive accumulation of a variety of random molecular defects that build up in cells and tissues. Aging is a continuous process, starting early and developing gradually, rather than a distinct phase that begins in middle to later life. It is well recognized that individuals

do not all age at the same rate. Five key elements seem to contribute to the individuality of the human aging process: genes, nutrition, lifestyle, environment, and chance.

- The boundary between aging and disease pathogenesis is somewhat arbitrary. The same cellular and molecular functions that contribute to improved lifespan are also responsible for degenerative diseases like osteoporosis, osteoarthritis, and dementia.

- All major cell types in the brain undergo structural changes with aging. These changes include neuronal cell death, dendritic retraction and expansion, synaptic loss and remodeling, and changes in glial cell (astrocyte and microglia) reactivity. The mass of the brain decreases by about 15% with aging. This decrease is due to cell loss and shrinkage of cell volume. There is a compensatory increase in cerebrospinal fluid volume.

- The incidence of many chronic diseases increases proportionally with age, so it can be difficult to differentiate age-related cognitive dysfunction from disease-related cognitive dysfunction in any particular patient. Hypertension, diabetes mellitus, nutritional deficiency, chronic obstructive pulmonary disease, obstructive sleep apnea, thyroid dysfunction, alcoholism, depression, and medications (opioids, benzodiazepines, anticonvulsants, antipsychotics, antidepressants, antihistamines, decongestants, central nervous system stimulants) can also affect cognitive function.

- Two major structural effects occur in blood vessels. The first is the natural change in the composition of blood vessel walls, with decreasing amounts of elastin and increasing amounts of collagen; the vessels become stiff and thickened. The second is the effect of atherosclerosis.

- The incidence of diastolic dysfunction increases with age, and this has been proven by detailed echocardiographic studies. Any systolic dysfunction in the elderly should be considered abnormal, especially if it is accompanied by a wall motion abnormality.

- Closing volume approaches tidal volume in the elderly, so they are more prone to atelectasis.

- The aging kidney is more susceptible to injury, less able to accommodate hemodynamic changes, and not able to handle significant changes in water and salt balance.

- *Frailty* is defined as a state of reduced physiologic reserve associated with an increased susceptibility to disability. It is related to normal changes of aging, chronic disease, and inflammation and is characterized by failure of the body to respond to additional stresses such as surgery or infection.

- The list of geriatric syndromes includes incontinence, delirium, falls, pressure ulcers, sleep disorders, problems with eating or feeding, pain, and depressed mood.

- Perioperative outcomes are dependent on many factors, the two most important of which are the surgical risk of the procedure and the number of defined clinical risk factors in a patient. As the number of clinical risk factors increases and the risk of the surgical procedure increases, the overall risk of a poor outcome also increases.

- Neurocognitive dysfunction is very common after both cardiac and noncardiac surgery in the elderly. Delirium is very common after major surgery, and a long-term decline in cognitive function is also very common after surgery.
- Anesthetic requirements are reduced significantly in the elderly.
- Elderly adults who cannot report pain must be assessed for the presence of factors that cause pain. Whenever an older adult with cognitive impairment shows a change in mental status, pain should be considered a potential etiology.

RESOURCES

Akhtar S, Ramani R. Geriatric pharmacology. *Anesthesiol Clin.* 2015;33:457-469.

American Geriatrics Society 2015 Beers Criteria Update Expert Panel. American Geriatrics Society 2015 Updated Beers Criteria for Potentially Inappropriate Medication Use in Older Adults. *J Am Geriatr Soc.* 2015;63:2227-2246.

American Geriatrics Society Expert Panel on Postoperative Delirium in Older Adults. Postoperative delirium in older adults: best practice statement from the American Geriatrics Society. *J Am Coll Surg.* 2015;220:136-148.

Bhamidipati CM, LaPar DJ, Fonner E, et al. Outcomes and cost of cardiac surgery in octogenarians is related to type of operation: a multi-institutional analysis. *Ann Thorac Surg.* 2011;91:499-505.

Catic AG. The perioperative geriatric consultation. In: Barnet SR, ed. *Manual of Geriatric Anesthesia.* New York: Springer; 2013:43-62.

Ferrucci L, Studenski S. Clinical problems of aging. In: Kasper DL, Fauci AS, Hauser SL, et al., eds. *Harrison's Principles of Internal Medicine.* 19th ed. New York: McGraw-Hill Education; 2015.

Hubbard RE, Story DA. Patient frailty: the elephant in the operating room. *Anaesthesia.* 2014;69(suppl 1):26-34.

Neufeld KJ, Yue J, Robinson TN, et al. Antipsychotic medication for prevention and treatment of delirium in hospitalized adults: a systematic review and meta-analysis. *J Am Geriatr Soc.* 2016;64:705-714.

Nickalls RW, Mapleson WW. Age-related iso-MAC charts for isoflurane, sevoflurane and desflurane in man. *Br J Anaesth.* 2003;91:170-174.

O'Rourke MF, Hashimoto J. Mechanical factors in arterial aging: a clinical perspective. *J Am Coll Cardiol.* 2007;50:1-13.

Partridge JS, Harari D, Martin FC, et al. The impact of pre-operative comprehensive geriatric assessment on postoperative outcomes in older patients undergoing scheduled surgery: a systematic review. *Anaesthesia.* 2014;69(suppl 1):8-16.

Sadean MR, Glass PS. Pharmacokinetics in the elderly. *Best Pract Res Clin Anaesthesiol.* 2003;17:191-205.

Diseases of the Liver and Biliary Tract

TRICIA BRENTJENS, PAUL DAVID WEYKER, CHRISTOPHER A.J. WEBB

EPIDEMIOLOGY OF LIVER DISEASE

The liver is one of the most metabolically active organs in the body and is responsible for numerous homeostatic and synthetic processes that are vital for survival. Not surprisingly, liver dysfunction and ultimately liver failure are poorly tolerated. Therefore liver disease is a leading cause of death and a major cause for morbidity in the United States, where an estimated two million deaths are caused by liver disease annually. Although there are many causes for liver disease, the underlying pathophysiology of liver failure in various diseases is similar and ranges from hepatic inflammation and fibrosis to cirrhosis and finally hepatic failure. In the United States, viral hepatitis and alcoholic liver disease (ALD) are the most common causes of chronic liver disease. However, nonalcoholic steatohepatitis (NASH) is becoming an ever-more-common indication for liver transplantation.

FUNCTION OF THE LIVER

Although medical science has found ways to replace the function of some important organs (heart, lungs, kidneys, digestive system), there is as yet no reliable means of replacing many of the critical functions of the liver. Broadly speaking, the functions of the liver can be broken down into five major categories; metabolic, synthetic, immunologic, regenerative, and homeostatic.

Some of the blood supply to the liver arises from the portal vein, which carries blood from the digestive system. This blood contains nutrients, cytokines, and bacteria absorbed from the gut. From a metabolic standpoint, the liver plays an important role in drug, protein, lipid, and glucose metabolism. It is responsible for the synthesis of procoagulants and anticoagulants, albumin, cholesterol, thrombopoietin, angiotensinogen, and insulinlike growth factor (IGF)-1. It plays an important role in *innate* and *adaptive immunity*. It is notable that approximately 10% of the cells in the liver are macrophages, natural killer (NK) cells, T lymphocytes, and B lymphocytes. The liver, unlike other organs, is *able to regenerate* after trauma or partial hepatectomy. It aids in *homeostasis* of intravascular volume by storage of blood during hypervolemic states and by production of renin and angiotensinogen. It also helps maintain glucose homeostasis via gluconeogenesis and glycogenolysis.

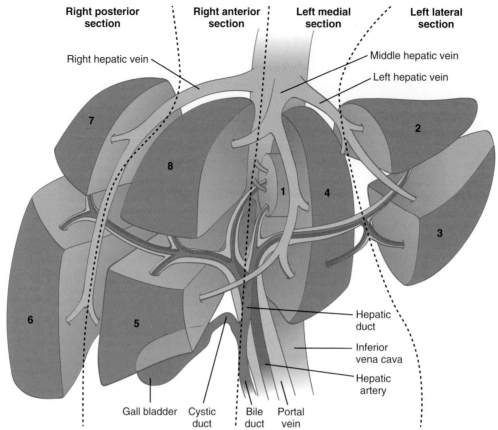

FIG. 17.1 Anatomic and functional subdivisions of the liver. The eight functional anatomic segments of the liver are demonstrated in this drawing. Each segment has its own blood supply and biliary drainage. (From Siriwardena AK, et al. Management of colorectal cancer presenting with synchronous liver metastases. *Nat Rev Clin Oncol.* 2014;11:446-459.)

Liver Anatomy and Physiology

Liver anatomy is important for both the anesthesiologist and the surgeon involved in the treatment of patients with liver disease. Fig. 17.1 illustrates the liver segments, blood supply, and biliary anatomy. The most important aspect of liver anatomy for the anesthesiologist is its blood supply. The liver derives its blood supply from the hepatic artery and portal vein. These two blood vessels receive about 20%–25% (≈1500 mL/min) of cardiac output. The hepatic artery provides approximately 25% of the blood flow to the liver, with the portal vein providing the remaining 75% (Fig. 17.2). Owing to the difference in oxygen content of portal venous blood compared to hepatic artery blood, about half of the liver's oxygen supply is derived from the portal vein and half from the hepatic artery. When portal vein blood flow decreases, there is a corresponding increase in hepatic artery blood flow. It is thought that this effect is due to locally produced adenosine that accumulates in low-flow states, causing arterial vasodilation and thus increasing hepatic artery blood flow. This physiologic response is critical in maintaining relatively constant blood flow and satisfactory oxygen supply to the liver. Blood exits the liver from the hepatic veins.

Normally blood travels from the portal vein through the low-resistance hepatic sinusoids into the hepatic veins then

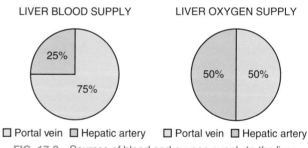

LIVER BLOOD SUPPLY   LIVER OXYGEN SUPPLY

☐ Portal vein ☐ Hepatic artery   ☐ Portal vein ☐ Hepatic artery

FIG. 17.2 Sources of blood and oxygen supply to the liver.

into the vena cava and finally into the right atrium. In a healthy liver the portal venous pressure is generally only 1–5 mm Hg higher than that of the hepatic veins. This pressure difference is the driving force of blood flow through the liver. In cirrhosis, fibrosis causes an increase in intrahepatic vascular resistance and thus impedes blood flow through the liver. This creates higher portal pressures (i.e., portal hypertension). Directly measuring portal venous pressure is not easily accomplished, so instead a *wedged hepatic venous pressure* (WHVP) is used as a surrogate measure of portal venous pressure, much like using pulmonary capillary wedge pressure as a surrogate measurement of left atrial pressure. The *hepatic venous pressure gradient* (HVPG) is the difference between the portal vein

TABLE 17.1	Causes of Hepatic Function Based on Liver Function Test Results			
Hepatic Dysfunction	Bilirubin	Aminotransferase Enzymes	Alkaline Phosphatase	Causes
Prehepatic	Increased unconjugated fraction	Normal	Normal	Hemolysis Hematoma resorption Bilirubin overload from blood transfusion
Intrahepatic (hepatocellular)	Increased conjugated fraction	Markedly increased	Normal to slightly increased	Viral infection Drugs Alcohol Sepsis Hypoxemia Cirrhosis
Posthepatic (cholestatic)	Increased conjugated fraction	Normal to slightly increased	Markedly increased	Biliary tract stones or tumors Sepsis

TABLE 17.2	Liver Function Test Abnormalities in Liver Disease				
Liver Disease	Aminotransferases	Alkaline Phosphatase	Bilirubin	International Normalized Ratio	Albumin
Chronic alcoholic liver disease	AST:ALT ratio, 2:1; AST and ALT levels normal to <8× upper limit of normal	Normal to elevated in decompensated or late-stage disease	Normal to elevated in decompensated or late-stage disease	Normal to elevated in decompensated or late-stage disease	Normal to decreased in decompensated or late-stage disease
Nonalcoholic fatty liver disease	AST:ALT ratio, <1; AST and ALT levels normal to <5× upper limit of normal	Normal to 2–3× upper limit of normal	Normal to elevated in decompensated or late-stage disease	Normal to elevated in decompensated or late-stage disease	Normal to decreased in decompensated or late-stage disease
Chronic viral hepatitis	AST and ALT levels normal to 10× upper limit of normal	Normal to slightly elevated	Normal to elevated in decompensated or late-stage disease	Normal to elevated in decompensated or late-stage disease	Normal to decreased in decompensated or late-stage disease
Acute viral hepatitis	AST and ALT > 25× upper limits of normal	Normal to elevated	Normal to elevated in decompensated or late-stage disease	Normal to elevated in decompensated or late-stage disease	Normal to decreased in decompensated or late-stage disease
Shock liver	AST:ALT ratio, 1:1; AST and ALT > 50× upper limit of normal	Normal to elevated	Normal to elevated in decompensated or late-stage disease	Normal to elevated in decompensated or late-stage disease	Normal to decreased in decompensated or late-stage disease

and hepatic vein pressure. *Portal hypertension* is defined as a gradient of more than 6 mm Hg, with the condition becoming clinically significant at gradients in excess of 10 mm Hg.

Assessment of Liver Function

Assessment of liver function should begin with a thorough history and physical exam. The history should include questions about known liver disease as well as identification of potential risk factors for liver disease, such as excessive alcohol use, intravenous (IV) drug use, or use of medication that may be hepatotoxic.

Physical examination clues to underlying liver disease include hepatomegaly, splenomegaly, spider nevi, gynecomastia, jaundice, ascites, or caput medusa. Patients with advanced liver disease may have alterations in mental status and asterixis as manifestations of hepatic encephalopathy.

Laboratory assessment of liver function usually falls into two major categories: (1) measurement of dysfunction of the hepatocytes or biliary system, which manifests as alterations in levels of hepatic transaminases and bilirubin, and (2) assessment of the liver's synthetic function, which is assessed via alterations in levels of albumin and coagulation factors. Traditional liver function tests (LFTs) include the serum aminotransferases (alanine aminotransferase [ALT] and aspartate aminotransferase [AST]), alkaline phosphatase, lactate dehydrogenase (LDH), and bilirubin (Table 17.1).

Specific patterns of LFT abnormalities provide clues as to the underlying liver disease (Table 17.2). Hepatocellular disease typically manifests as elevations in AST and ALT out of proportion to alkaline phosphatase changes. Cholestatic disease produces alkaline phosphatase levels out of proportion to changes in AST and ALT. Other clues can be found in the relative concentrations of liver enzymes. For example, an AST:ALT ratio of 2:1 is commonly seen in patients with ALD, but a ratio of less than 1 is more common in NASH. *Chronic viral hepatitis* often presents with mildly elevated (<10 times normal values) AST and ALT levels, whereas *acute viral hepatitis* is often associated with levels more than 25 times normal. *Shock liver* can be associated with the highest levels of liver enzymes (i.e., levels > 50 times normal).

Bilirubin is the breakdown product of hemoglobin and myoglobin. *Unconjugated bilirubin* is transported to the liver, where it is conjugated into a more water-soluble form and excreted in the bile, a process that is energy dependent. Laboratory tests can differentiate direct (conjugated) and indirect (unconjugated) bilirubin. Higher concentrations of *indirect bilirubin* are most commonly due to a hemolytic process, breakdown of a hematoma, portal hypertension, and more rarely to inborn errors of metabolism. Increases in *direct bilirubin* are due to hepatic dysfunction, biliary obstruction, or impaired hepatic excretion of bilirubin, which is particularly common in sepsis.

The *international normalized ratio* (INR) is a laboratory test that evaluates the extrinsic pathway of coagulation. It is greatly dependent on factor VII, a vitamin K–dependent clotting factor produced in the liver and having a relatively short half-life. The INR can be used as a test of the synthetic function of the liver. Indeed, INR prolongation has been shown to be an independent risk factor for mortality in patients with liver disease. For this reason the INR is part of the calculation in the Model for End-Stage Liver Disease (MELD) equation.

Albumin, the most abundant plasma protein, is produced exclusively by the liver. It plays a vital role in maintaining colloid osmotic pressure and binds cations, fatty acids, and bilirubin. Low plasma albumin can be caused by hepatic dysfunction, decreased protein intake, loss of albumin in the kidneys, and catabolic states.

DISEASES OF THE BILIARY TRACT

Biliary Tract Anatomy

The biliary tract is the pathway along which bile is secreted from the liver, stored, and transported to the first part of the duodenum, where it aids in digestion of fats. The biliary tract includes bile ducts of various sizes (which make, store, and secrete bile) and the gallbladder. Bile flows out of the liver via the left and right hepatic ducts, which then combine to form the common hepatic duct, which then joins with the cystic duct to form the common bile duct. Half of the bile secreted between meals goes directly to the common bile duct and half is diverted via the cystic duct to the gallbladder for storage.

Cholelithiasis

Inflammatory biliary tract disease and gallstones are common in the United States. Approximately 30 million Americans have gallstones. The prevalence is significantly greater in females than males and increases with age, obesity, rapid weight loss, and pregnancy. Gallstone formation is most likely related to abnormalities in the physiochemical characteristics of bile. About 90% of gallstones in countries consuming a Western diet high in protein and fat are radiolucent and composed primarily of cholesterol. Most of the remaining gallstones are radiopaque and composed of calcium bilirubinate. Patients who have gallbladder stones are often asymptomatic, but obstruction of the cystic duct or the common bile duct by a gallstone causes acute inflammation.

Signs and symptoms of *acute cholecystitis* include abdominal pain with right upper quadrant tenderness, nausea, vomiting, and fever. Patients with acute cholecystitis are treated with IV fluids, antibiotics, and opioids for pain relief. Surgery is typically performed once the patient's condition has stabilized. Laparoscopic cholecystectomy is the procedure of choice. Fewer than 5% of patients will require conversion to open cholecystectomy. Common duct stones can be removed intraoperatively or subsequently by endoscopic retrograde cholangiopancreatography (ERCP). Patients with septic shock who are considered too ill to undergo surgery require a *percutaneous cholecystostomy*.

Anesthetic considerations for laparoscopic cholecystectomy are similar to those for other kinds of laparoscopic surgery. However, the use of opioids during this surgery is controversial because opioids might cause spasm of the sphincter of Oddi. The incidence of opioid-induced sphincter spasm is quite low (<3%), and it is possible to antagonize this spasm by administration of glucagon, naloxone, or nitroglycerin.

Choledocholithiasis

The term *choledocholithiasis* indicates that a gallstone is lodged in the common bile duct. Patients with choledocholithiasis typically present with signs of *cholangitis* if the stone is obstructing the common bile duct. Fever, rigors, jaundice, and right upper quadrant pain will be present. The often severe pain caused by a stone lodged in a duct is termed *biliary colic*. This pain can be extraordinarily intense. Some stones pass into the duodenum or a pancreatic duct and can result in acute pancreatitis. Serum bilirubin and alkaline phosphatase levels typically increase abruptly and markedly when a stone obstructs the common bile duct.

Endoscopic sphincterotomy is the initial treatment for patients with suspected choledocholithiasis. ERCP can be used to identify the cause of common bile duct obstruction, as well as to remove a stone or place a biliary stent if needed.

HYPERBILIRUBINEMIA

Gilbert Syndrome

The most common example of a *hereditary hyperbilirubinemia* is Gilbert syndrome. It is inherited as an autosomal dominant

TABLE 17.3 | Characteristic Features of Viral Hepatitis

Parameter	Type A	Type B	Type C	Type D
Mode of transmission	Fecal-oral Sewage-contaminated shellfish	Percutaneous Sexual	Percutaneous	Percutaneous
Incubation period	20–37 days	60–110 days	35–70 days	60–110 days
Results of serum antigen and antibody tests	IgM early, IgG appears during convalescence	HBsAg and anti-HBcAg early and persist in carriers	Anti-HCV in 6 weeks to 9 months	Anti-HDV late; may be short-lived
Immunity	Antibodies in 45%	Antibodies in 5%–15%	Unknown	Protected if immune to type B
Course	Does not progress to chronic liver disease	Chronic liver disease develops in 1%–5% of adults and 80%–90% of children	Chronic liver disease develops in up to 75%	Coinfection with type B
Prevention after exposure	Pooled gamma globulin Hepatitis A vaccine	Hepatitis B immunoglobulin Hepatitis B vaccine	Interferon plus ribavirin	Unknown
Mortality	<0.2%	0.3%–1.5%	Unknown	Acute icteric hepatitis: 2%–20%

HBcAg, Hepatitis B core antigen; *HBsAg,* hepatitis B surface antigen; *HCV,* hepatitis C virus; *HDV,* hepatitis D virus; *IgG,* immunoglobulin G; *IgM,* immunoglobulin M.
Adapted from Keefe EB. Acute hepatitis. *Sci Am Med.* 1999:1-9.

trait with variable penetrance. The primary defect is a mutation in the glucuronosyltransferase enzyme. Plasma bilirubin concentrations rarely exceed 5 mg/dL but can increase twofold to threefold with fasting, illness, or stress.

Crigler-Najjar Syndrome

Crigler-Najjar syndrome is a rare hereditary form of *severe unconjugated hyperbilirubinemia* that is inherited as an autosomal recessive trait and results from a mutation in the glucuronosyltransferase enzyme, which is typically reduced to below 10% of normal. Severe jaundice appears in the first days of life and can lead to brain damage in infants. Treatment includes daily exchange transfusions in the neonatal period and daily phototherapy (12 hours/day) as well as oral calcium treatment to bind bile in the gut. Long-term phenobarbital therapy may decrease jaundice by stimulating activity of glucuronosyltransferase. Definitive treatment is liver transplantation before significant brain damage develops.

Benign Postoperative Intrahepatic Cholestasis

Benign postoperative intrahepatic cholestasis occurs most often when surgery has been complicated by hypotension, hypoxemia, or the need for blood transfusion. This hyperbilirubinemia may be caused by an increase in bilirubin production from breakdown of transfused red blood cells or resorption of a hematoma and/or decreased hepatic clearance of bilirubin. An increase in conjugated bilirubin and alkaline phosphatase are seen. This condition typically resolves in tandem with improvement in the underlying surgical or medical condition.

HEPATITIDES

Viral Hepatitis

Chronic viral hepatitis is a leading cause of liver disease worldwide and is caused primarily by hepatitis A, B, and C viruses. Less common causes include hepatitis D and E viruses. An extensive review of viral hepatitis is beyond the scope of this chapter, so this section will focus on chronic hepatitis B and C, since these viruses are most commonly associated with chronic viral hepatitis and its complications (Table 17.3).

Hepatitis B virus (HBV) continues to be one of the most common chronic viral infections affecting developing countries. Global reporting suggests that up to 400 million people are chronically infected. In developed countries, however, vaccination has dramatically decreased the incidence of chronic hepatitis B infection. Transmission of hepatitis B is primarily via vertical transmission (mother to fetus) in developing countries where hepatitis B is endemic. In areas where this virus is not endemic, infection occurs primarily via sexual or hematogenous spread. For unclear reasons, men are more likely than women to develop chronic hepatitis B infection. Clinical manifestations may vary between acute and chronic infections, but both stages can present as subclinical infection, fulminant hepatitis, or end-stage liver disease. During acute hepatitis B infection, most patients (70%) will present with subclinical (anicteric) disease, whereas the other 30% will present with icterus. During the acute phase, hepatic function tests may show markedly elevated ALT and AST levels (up to 2000 IU/L), and ALT levels tend to be higher than AST levels. The transaminase levels usually normalize within 4 months. Persistently elevated levels (>6 months) correlate with progression to chronic viral hepatitis. Fulminant hepatic failure due to acute hepatitis B infection is relatively rare and affects fewer than 0.5% of patients. Immune-mediated hepatocyte destruction appears to be the primary mechanism of this form of hepatic failure.

HBV is detectable in the blood via polymerase chain reaction (PCR) assay for many years after the initial acute infection. Cytotoxic T cells specific for hepatitis B antigens mitigate reactivation of hepatitis B in immunocompetent individuals. The risk of progression to chronic hepatitis B infection is determined mostly by age at the time of initial infection. Almost all neonatal hepatitis B infections become chronic, but fewer than 5% of acute hepatitis B infections in adults progress to a chronic form. Extrahepatic manifestations of hepatitis B infection (polyarteritis nodosa, membranous nephropathy, aplastic anemia) occur in about 20% of individuals with chronic hepatitis B. These are related to circulating immune complexes. Treatment for *acute* hepatitis B is supportive. *Prophylactic use of antiviral medication is not recommended.* However, patients with preexisting liver disease, those with fulminant hepatic failure, immunocompromised individuals, patients who develop a coagulopathy (INR > 1.5), or those with persistent hyperbilirubinemia for more than 4 weeks *should be treated* with antiviral therapy. Use of interferon is *contraindicated* because of the risk of hepatic inflammation and necrosis.

Hepatitis C virus (HCV) is the most common cause of end-stage liver disease in the United States and thus the most frequent disease necessitating liver transplantation. Unlike HBV, the majority of those who become infected with HCV progress to chronic infection. However, only 5%–30% of these chronically infected patients will actually develop cirrhosis. Clinically the majority of patients with acute HCV infection present with malaise, anorexia, arthralgias, and weakness. Common extrahepatic manifestations include hematologic diseases (cryoglobulinemia, lymphoma), renal diseases (membranous nephropathy, membranoproliferative glomerulonephritis), and several dermatologic diseases. Initial diagnostic tests involve detection of HCV antibodies. Patients who often have false-negative test results, such as the immunocompromised, should undergo additional testing to confirm the presence of HCV RNA.

Treatment of HCV infection involves a combination of antiviral medications with or without interferon. The HCV genotype, side-effect profile, prior treatment, severity of the liver disease, and risk of drug-drug interactions help determine the optimal combination therapy. One particular drug regimen that combines the use of daclatasvir with sofosbuvir has demonstrated a 98% response rate, as evidenced by the absence of HCV RNA after only 12 weeks of treatment in patients with HCV genotype 1. Patients with HCV genotype 3, which has been the most aggressive genotype in terms of rapidly developing liver dysfunction and the development of liver cancer, as well as a very resistant genotype to antiviral therapy, show a 90% response rate to this same combination therapy.

Nonalcoholic Fatty Liver Disease

Nonalcoholic fatty liver disease (NAFLD) is the accumulation of hepatic fat that is not due to heavy alcohol use. It is one of the most common causes of liver disease worldwide and the most common cause of liver disease in developed countries. In the United States, reports show a prevalence of NAFLD that ranges from 10%–46%, with the highest prevalence in the Hispanic population.

Histologically there are two main types of NAFLD: nonalcoholic fatty liver (NAFL) and NASH. In the latter, liver biopsies show significant liver inflammation that in many cases mimics the histopathology of alcoholic steatohepatitis. Risk factors for NAFLD include the metabolic syndrome, diabetes mellitus type 2, total parenteral nutrition, patients who have had jejunal-ileal bypass weight loss surgery, and certain medications (amiodarone, calcium channel blockers, glucocorticoids, etc.). Although the etiology of hepatic fat accumulation is not fully understood, potential mechanisms include excessive lipogenesis, inappropriate movement of free fatty acids from adipose tissue, impaired utilization of free fatty acids, and small intestinal bacterial overgrowth. Common to all these mechanisms is the overproduction of oxygen free radicals, which leads to hepatocellular injury. Microbial overgrowth has also been associated with endotoxin-induced hepatic injury. Management of patients with NAFLD involves treatment of the primary medical problems: weight loss, diabetes management, treatment of hyperlipidemia, avoidance of alcohol, and vaccination against hepatitis A and B.

Alcoholic Liver Disease

ALD is one of the most common causes of cirrhosis and the second leading cause of end-stage liver disease requiring liver transplantation. Worldwide, ALD accounts for nearly 500,000 deaths every year. Similar to other causes of liver disease, ALD includes a spectrum of disease ranging from *alcoholic steatosis* and *alcoholic steatohepatitis* to cirrhosis and hepatocellular carcinoma. Alcoholic steatosis develops in about 20% of heavy drinkers and can be reversed if alcohol intake is stopped. Progression from steatosis to cirrhosis will occur in up to a fifth of patients. Alcoholic steatohepatitis as diagnosed on liver biopsy shows signs similar to NASH: inflammation, hepatocyte degeneration, and fibrosis. However, what is unique about alcoholic steatohepatitis on biopsy is the infiltration of neutrophils in the liver. Patients with *alcoholic steatohepatitis* have rates of progression to cirrhosis that are twice those of patients with only *steatosis*. Alcoholic cirrhosis is the most serious form of alcohol-related liver disease and demonstrates extensive hepatic fibrosis and loss of normal hepatic function.

Clinically the signs and symptoms of ALD will vary depending on the degree of hepatic impairment. Patients with alcoholic steatosis or steatohepatitis may be clinically asymptomatic but on physical exam demonstrate *hepatomegaly*. Patients who progress to cirrhosis may present with the classic stigmata of chronic liver disease: spider angiomata, jaundice, icterus, palmar erythema, and gynecomastia. Alcoholic cirrhosis leading to end-stage liver disease can manifest as multiorgan failure marked by worsening ascites, peripheral edema, neuropathy, pancreatic dysfunction, platypnea/orthodeoxia, renal failure, or hepatic encephalopathy with or without asterixis.

LFTs will correlate with disease progression. Classically the AST:ALT ratio is greater than 2. The specific diagnosis of ALD requires a history of alcohol abuse combined with clinical signs and symptoms of liver disease. However, other common etiologies of liver disease should also be considered. Treatment for ALD involves a multidisciplinary approach that includes alcohol cessation, nutritional therapy/supplementation, and management of any co-existing medical problems. For patients who have progressed to hepatic failure, management includes supportive care and evaluation for liver transplantation.

Inborn Errors of Metabolism

Some inborn errors of metabolism involve inherited abnormal biochemical pathways that can lead to the accumulation of hepatotoxic substances that can cause liver disease and even liver failure. Although more commonly diagnosed in the pediatric population, age of onset can be variable.

Wilson Disease

Wilson disease (see also Chapter 19, "Inborn Errors of Metabolism") is an autosomal recessive disease that involves impaired copper metabolism, which leads to copper deposition in the liver as well as in extrahepatic tissues, including the basal ganglia and cornea (Kayser-Fleischer ring). The incidence ranges from 1/30,000 to 1/100,000. Diagnosis combines histopathology with molecular genetic testing. Clinically, patients with Wilson disease can present with a self-limited hepatitis or even chronic active hepatitis. Aminotransferases will be elevated, but levels tend to be lower than those seen with viral or autoimmune hepatitis. Acute fulminant hepatic failure could be the initial presentation, but this occurs in fewer than 3% of cases. If left untreated, Wilson disease patients can develop cirrhosis. Rarely, chronic liver inflammation or cirrhosis can lead to hepatocellular carcinoma. Common extrahepatic manifestations of copper deposition include joint pain/arthritis, cardiomyopathy, nonimmune hemolytic anemia, and renal failure. Treatment of Wilson disease includes administration of zinc with or without the chelating drug trientine. Zinc prevents gastrointestinal absorption of copper.

α_1-Antitrypsin Deficiency

α_1-Antitrypsin (A1AT) deficiency is an autosomal codominant genetic disease transmitted with variable expression. It affects up to 1 in 3000 live births. Normally, A1AT counteracts the proteolytic effects of neutrophil elastase and other neutrophil proteases. Clinically, deficiency in A1AT results in early onset of emphysematous lung disease and in adult-onset liver disease. The pathophysiology of the liver disease may be abnormal accumulation of polymerized A1AT in hepatocytes. This polymerization is inappropriate and results in folding of the molecule, which then cannot exit the hepatocyte. Patients with A1AT deficiency–related liver disease present with elevated aminotransferases in addition to a hepatitis-like syndrome that may or may not involve cholestasis and jaundice. The incidence of progression of the liver disease is extremely variable. The pediatric literature suggests that 2%–3% of patients will progress to cirrhosis and end-stage liver disease requiring transplantation. Treatment of A1AT deficiency–related liver disease differs from the treatment of the A1AT deficiency lung disease. Intravenous A1AT augmentation with protein concentrates containing this enzyme can restore both blood and alveolar epithelial cell A1AT levels to normal and *improve* the lung disease. However, such infusions do *not* correct the underlying problem of abnormal polymerized A1AT in the liver. A1AT deficiency is not a common indication for liver transplantation in adults. However, in children it is the main metabolic liver disease that can lead to liver transplantation.

Hemochromatosis

Hemochromatosis is an autosomal recessive inborn error of metabolism that primarily affects Caucasians of Northern European descent (see Chapter 19, "Inborn Errors of Metabolism"). It is characterized by a genetic mutation and deficiency in the *HFE* gene, the result of which is excessive iron storage in the body that ultimately leads to cellular dysfunction and organ damage. Onset occurs in the fourth decade or later. Men show an earlier onset than women (who lose iron with menstruation). Patients can present with the classic triad of cirrhosis, diabetes mellitus (due to destruction of pancreatic beta cells), and bronzing of the skin. However, patients often present earlier with nonspecific symptoms such as arthralgias, lethargy, and muscle weakness. Hepatic involvement in this disease is common, since the liver is one of the major sites for iron storage. Elevated levels of iron within hepatocytes ultimately lead to elevated aminotransferase levels and hepatocellular destruction. Cardiac involvement can range from dysrhythmias to dilated cardiomyopathy. An elevated serum transferrin saturation (>45%) and serum ferritin levels (>300 ng/mL in men and >200 ng/mL in women) are indicative of hemochromatosis. Definitive diagnosis involves molecular genetic testing. Biopsy of the liver may be done to evaluate for the presence of cirrhosis. Treatment involves therapeutic phlebotomy to physically remove iron from the body. Patients with hemochromatosis who have end-stage liver disease may require liver transplantation.

Autoimmune Hepatitis

Autoimmune hepatitis (AIH) is an inflammatory liver disease that is characterized by both T-cell and autoantibody-mediated destruction of hepatocytes. Several genes are believed to be involved in its pathogenesis, with most of these localized to the human leukocyte antigen (HLA) region. Although patients affected by AIH can present in early childhood or at an advanced age, most present around the fifth decade of life. Up to 25% of patients will have subclinical disease with an incidental finding of elevated transaminases. Almost 40% will present with an acute hepatitis. Diagnostic workup includes liver function panels, autoantibody testing and liver biopsy. As in other autoimmune disorders, treatment centers on immunomodulation with corticosteroids. Azathioprine may be added to a corticosteroid regimen to reduce steroid-induced side effects. Therapeutic response is guided by resolution of symptoms in addition to normalization of transaminase levels, improvement in immunoglobulin levels (specifically IgG), and confirmation with a liver biopsy to show that there has been no progression and perhaps even some resolution of hepatic inflammation.

Primary Biliary Cirrhosis

Primary biliary cirrhosis (PBC) is an autoimmune cholestatic form of liver disease that is due to destruction of *small* intrahepatic bile ducts by T cells. PBC primarily occurs in women (female-to-male ratio is 10:1). Both genetic and environmental risk factors appear to play a role in the pathogenesis of this disorder. Population studies have demonstrated a link between primary biliary cirrhosis and certain HLA alleles. Additionally, certain hair dyes, nail polishes, and exposure to certain bacteria (*Escherichia coli, Mycobacterium gordonae*) have been correlated with the development of PBC. Clinical manifestations of PBC are similar to those of other forms of liver disease and include pruritus, jaundice, fatigue, hyperpigmented skin, and hepatosplenomegaly. Other autoimmune diseases may also be present. The diagnostic workup involves LFTs, with results showing an elevated alkaline phosphatase level (typically 1.5 times normal) and elevated aminotransferase levels, in addition to serologic markers such as antimitochondrial antibodies and antinuclear antibodies. Liver biopsy will reveal chronic inflammation and destruction of interlobular bile ducts.

Treatment of PBC involves the use of ursodeoxycholic acid (UDCA), which has been shown to delay the progression of this disease as well as improve overall transplant-free survival. Since the diagnosis is often made earlier than in the past, and since UDCA has been so successful in treatment, liver transplantation for patients with PBC is quite uncommon today.

Primary Sclerosing Cholangitis

Primary sclerosing cholangitis (PSC) is a chronic inflammatory liver disease characterized by inflammatory scarring and ultimately areas of severe narrowing in *medium and large* bile ducts. PSC results in cholestasis and if left untreated can progress to liver failure. The pathogenesis of PSC is not fully understood but is likely to be multifactorial, with factors such as ischemic ductal injury, bacterial infection, mutations within the HLA allele, and the presence of autoantibodies causing immune-mediated destruction of the bile ducts. Similar to primary biliary cirrhosis, patients with this disease can be asymptomatic or have another autoimmune disease. Classically PSC is associated with ulcerative colitis, with some reports suggesting 75%–90% of patients with PSC also have ulcerative colitis,

based on rectal and sigmoid colon biopsies. Because of the cholestasis, patients typically present with pruritus, jaundice, and hepatosplenomegaly. Workup includes LFTs and serologies (gamma globulins, IgM, perinuclear antineutrophil cytoplasmic antibodies, and HLA-DRw52a). Cholangiography will demonstrate multifocal stricturing and dilatation of intrahepatic and extrahepatic bile ducts. Liver biopsy is not a useful tool to diagnose this disease because the findings are very nonspecific and mirror those seen with primary biliary cirrhosis. Unlike treatment of primary biliary cirrhosis, medical management of PSC has proven to be difficult. Various immunomodulators including UDCA, corticosteroids, cyclosporine, methotrexate, tacrolimus, azathioprine, penicillamine, and etanercept have been tried with conflicting results. Antibiotic therapy with vancomycin or metronidazole for 12 weeks has been shown to decrease transaminase levels but not affect overall disease progression.

Minimally invasive interventions such as balloon dilation or stent placement for management of strictures have also demonstrated conflicting results, and it is still unclear whether or not dilation of a stricture improves outcome. Surgical interventions other than liver transplantation include biliary reconstruction, as well as proctocolectomy for patients with ulcerative colitis. With biliary reconstruction there seems to be a decrease in progression of the PSC that can persist for several years after surgery. In patients who undergo liver transplantation, the risk of PSC *recurrence* can be as high as 20%. Interestingly, recurrent PSC and the need for retransplantation are much more common in patients with ulcerative colitis who have *not* undergone a proctocolectomy. Therefore it is not uncommon to perform a proctocolectomy either before or during liver transplantation to mitigate this problem.

Drug/Toxin-Induced Liver Disease

Accidental or intentional overdose of acetaminophen is the most common drug-induced liver disease that causes fulminant hepatic failure. Many other drugs can also cause hepatic dysfunction. Antituberculosis medications, antibiotics, antifungals, and antiepileptic medications are the drug classes most often associated with liver dysfunction. Halothane, which is no longer used in the United States, was known to cause liver injury in 1 in 10,000 anesthetics in adults. Recreational drugs such as cocaine and amphetamines have also been associated with hepatic necrosis (Table 17.4).

Cardiac Causes of Liver Disease

The liver receives about 25% of cardiac output under normal conditions. The hepatic veins drain directly into the inferior vena cava within centimeters of the right atrium. Owing to this unique anatomy, cardiac pathology can lead to acute and chronic liver disease. Right ventricular failure leads to elevated central venous pressure and thus to elevated hepatic venous and sinusoidal pressures. Chronically elevated hepatic sinusoidal pressure leads to progressive fibrosis and then cirrhosis

TABLE 17.4	Common Drugs Associated With Liver Disease

ANALGESIC
Acetaminophen
Nonsteroidal antiinflammatory drugs

CARDIOVASCULAR
Statins
Amiodarone
Methyldopa
Angiotensin-converting enzyme inhibitors

ANTIMICROBIAL
Isoniazid
Rifampicin
Pyrazinamide
Tetracycline
Macrolides
Sulfonamides
Azole antifungals
Fluoroquinolones
β-Lactams

NEUROLOGIC/ANTIEPILEPTIC
Phenobarbital
Phenytoin
Carbamazepine
Lamotrigine
Felbamate
Valproate
Chlorpromazine
Tricyclic antidepressants
Selective serotonin reuptake inhibitors
Norepinephrine reuptake inhibitors

RECREATIONAL
Amphetamines
Cocaine
Ecstasy
Ethanol

and portal hypertension. Other cardiac conditions that cause chronically elevated central venous pressure (e.g., constrictive pericarditis, tricuspid valve disease, congenital heart disease palliated with a Fontan procedure) can cause what is called *cardiac cirrhosis.*

Any process that leads to decreased cardiac output, such as acute myocardial infarction, dysrhythmia, or severe hypovolemia, could lead to *shock liver.*

ACUTE LIVER FAILURE

Acute liver failure is defined as rapid development of severe liver damage, with impaired hepatic synthetic function and encephalopathy, in someone who previously had normal liver function or compensated liver disease. Acute liver failure develops in less than 4 weeks. This time measurement begins at the first appearance of physical findings (e.g., jaundice) to the loss of 80%–90% of liver function. Acute liver failure includes fulminant hepatic failure, which is liver failure that

develops within 8 days of the onset of symptoms and signs of liver failure. The underlying cause of the liver failure and the grade of encephalopathy at the time of presentation are critical determinants of outcome. In the United States the most common cause of acute liver failure is acetaminophen overdose. Other causes include idiosyncratic drug reactions, viral hepatitis, alcoholic hepatitis, acute fatty liver of pregnancy, Budd-Chiari syndrome, and Reye syndrome. Acute liver failure has a very high mortality rate. Death is often due to cerebral edema leading to increased intracranial pressure and coma. Patients with acute liver failure should ideally receive intensive care in a hospital with a liver transplantation program.

There is ongoing research involving *extracorporeal hepatic support therapy.* These are treatment options that could function either as treatment for an episode of liver failure or as a bridge to liver transplantation. In general these therapies are categorized as nonbiological or biological systems. *Nonbiological hepatic support systems* are similar to hemodialysis for renal failure. They rely on semipermeable membranes and various absorbents, most notably albumin, to remove bound toxins. This is also called *albumin dialysis,* and there are US Food and Drug Administration (FDA)-approved devices in use at this time. *Biological hepatic support systems* would do blood purification via a dialysis-like system, but they would also contain active hepatocytes. So theoretically, these systems could metabolize small molecules such as ammonia and synthesize various proteins. Such biological systems are under development but are not close to clinical availability.

CIRRHOSIS

Cirrhosis is the manifestation of liver disease that results from chronic liver inflammation that produces scarring. Histologically, cirrhosis is characterized by fibrous deposition that causes distortion of normal hepatic architecture. There can be areas of regenerative growth of hepatocytes between the areas of fibrous tissue. The fibrosis disrupts the sinusoids and other vascular structures, causing an increase in resistance to intrahepatic blood flow. This increased flow resistance causes *portal hypertension.* In the United States the most common causes of cirrhosis are hepatitis C, ALD, and NASH. Less common causes include autoimmune hepatitis, primary biliary cirrhosis, PSC, hepatitis B, and α_1-antitrypsin disease.

Cirrhosis has many systemic manifestations, including a hyperdynamic circulation, decreased systemic vascular resistance, and a compensatory increase in cardiac output. Cirrhosis is also associated with development of hepatocellular carcinoma. The systemic effects of cirrhosis are illustrated in Table 17.5. The severity of cirrhosis has been classified using the Child-Pugh scoring system (Table 17.6). However, the MELD score is now used more often because it is not only an index of disease severity but also a reliable measure of 3-month mortality risk. The MELD equation takes into account the patient's creatinine, bilirubin, and INR. The higher the MELD score, the more severe the liver disease and the higher the near-term mortality.

TABLE 17.5	Systemic Effects of Cirrhosis	
Organ System	Effects of Cirrhosis	Anesthetic Considerations
Neurologic	Hepatic encephalopathy	Decreased anesthetic and analgesic requirements, intubation to protect airway
Cardiac	Portopulmonary hypertension, hyperdynamic circulation	Right ventricular failure, cardiogenic shock, vasodilatory shock
Respiratory	Hepatopulmonary syndrome, decreased functional residual capacity	Hypoxemia refractory to oxygen therapy, PEEP
Renal	Hepatorenal syndrome, hyponatremia	Maintenance of renal perfusion, caution with drugs eliminated by kidney, avoidance of nephrotoxic drugs
Gastrointestinal	Portal hypertension, varices/variceal bleeding, ascites, malnutrition	Risk of gastrointestinal bleeding, "full stomach" precautions, hypoalbuminemia, changes in drug binding
Hematologic	Coagulopathy, anemia, thrombocytopenia, neutropenia	Risk of hemorrhage; vitamin K administration, blood component transfusion as needed
Immunologic	Compromised immune system	Risk of infection; *very careful sterile technique*
Endocrine	Less glucose production and storage, decreased metabolism of insulin, hypogonadism	Hypoglycemia

TABLE 17.6	Child-Pugh Scoring System to Assess Severity of Liver Disease		
Sign of Hepatic Dysfunction	1 Point	2 Points	3 Points
Encephalopathy (grade)	None	Grade I-II	Grade III-IV
Ascites	Absent	Mild	Severe
Bilirubin (mg/dL)	<2	2–3	>3
Albumin (g/dL)	>3.5	2.8–3.5	<2.8
International normalized ratio	<1.7	1.7–2.2	>2.2

Portal Hypertension

Portal hypertension is most commonly caused by increased resistance to blood flow within the liver in a patient with cirrhosis. However, other causes such as portal vein thrombosis and Budd-Chiari syndrome can also cause portal hypertension. An HVPG above 6 mm Hg defines the presence of portal hypertension (normal gradient < 5 mm Hg). Portal hypertension produces splenomegaly, formation of varices, ascites, gastropathy, and hepatorenal syndrome. When the HVPG exceeds 12 mm Hg, the patient is at high risk of variceal bleeding. Portal hypertension produces splanchnic vasodilation due to local release of nitric oxide and vascular endothelial growth factor. This splanchnic vasodilation can cause relative renal hypoperfusion and thus activation of the renin-angiotensin-aldosterone system. This leads to salt and water retention.

Ascites and Spontaneous Bacterial Peritonitis

Portal hypertension, hypoalbuminemia, and salt and water retention contribute to progressive accumulation of fluid within the peritoneal cavity (i.e., *ascites*) (Fig. 17.3). A threshold HVPG of 12 mm Hg is needed for the formation of ascites. Progressive ascites can worsen renal perfusion and decrease pulmonary compliance. Medical treatment includes sodium restriction and diuresis with spironolactone. Recurrent paracentesis or insertion of a *transjugular intrahepatic portosystemic shunt* (TIPS) can be used to manage refractory ascites. Patients with ascites are at high risk of developing *spontaneous bacterial peritonitis,* which is peritonitis that develops despite the absence of an obvious source of infection. Gram-negative bacteria are usually cultured from the ascites; early diagnosis and antibiotic therapy are essential. This entity has a very high morbidity and mortality even with timely initiation of antibiotic therapy.

Varices

Varices are formed when there is development of portal-systemic collaterals. The most common sites for these are in the lower esophagus and stomach. Portal hypertension causes these veins to dilate to accommodate the increase in collateral blood flow. The threshold HVPG necessary to develop varices is 10–12 mm Hg. The elevated pressure within these thin-walled blood vessels increases the risk of spontaneous rupture and thus variceal bleeding. Variceal bleeding can be massive and lead to death if not promptly treated.

Endoscopic treatments of variceal bleeding include ligation and sclerotherapy. Both methods are effective at controlling esophageal variceal bleeding. Endoscopic treatment plus administration of a vasoconstrictor such as octreotide provides the best therapy for an episode of acute variceal bleeding. Antibiotic therapy is also administered. Recurrent bleeding can be prevented by either TIPS insertion or a surgically created portosystemic shunt. Nonselective β-blockers (e.g., nadolol, propranolol) are used to chronically reduce portal pressure and help prevent rebleeding.

Hepatic Encephalopathy

Hepatic encephalopathy is defined as the neuropsychiatric dysfunction found in patients with significant liver disease. It is graded on a scale of I to IV based on severity. Grade I encephalopathy manifests as only mild changes in behavior, with

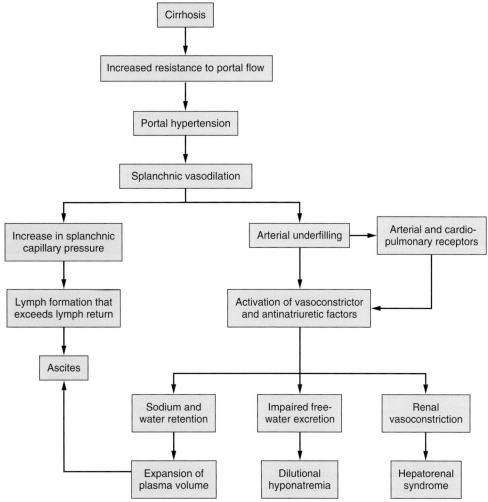

FIG. 17.3   Pathogenesis of ascites. (From Gines P, Cardenas A, Arroyo V, et al. Management of cirrhosis and ascites. *N Engl J Med.* 2004;350:1646-1654. Copyright 2004 Massachusetts Medical Society. All rights reserved.)

minimal change in the level of consciousness. Grade IV is the most severe grade and represents coma and unresponsiveness to painful stimuli. Patients with hepatic encephalopathy may have *asterixis,* a flapping tremor of the hands when the wrist is extended. Hepatic encephalopathy is often precipitated by gastrointestinal bleeding or infection. Portosystemic shunts can also cause or worsen hepatic encephalopathy, since ammonia and other metabolites are allowed to bypass the liver. Treatment of hepatic encephalopathy involves (1) treatment of the underlying cause, (2) restriction of protein intake. (3) oral administration of lactulose or rifaximin to decrease ammonia absorption, (4) correction of electrolyte abnormalities, and (5) avoidance of sedatives, opioids, and anesthetic drugs if possible.

Hepatorenal Syndrome

Hepatorenal syndrome is a form of *functional renal failure* (i.e., there is no visible renal pathology) that can occur in patients with acute liver failure or cirrhosis. Portal hypertension causes splanchnic and systemic arterial vasodilation, likely due to

overproduction of nitric oxide and prostaglandins. This arterial vasodilation leads to *relative renal hypoperfusion* and activation of the renin-angiotensin-aldosterone system. This produces renal vasoconstriction and a decreased glomerular filtration rate.

There are two types of hepatorenal syndrome described: type 1, with a rapid onset (considerable renal dysfunction in 1–2 weeks) and a very poor prognosis; and type 2, with a more gradual onset and an association with a better outcome than type 1. Both types can be seen with diuretic-resistant ascites. Treatment may involve diuretic withdrawal, administration of albumin, and use of midodrine and octreotide to treat splanchnic vasodilation. Definitive treatment may require liver transplantation.

Hepatopulmonary Syndrome

Hepatopulmonary syndrome (HPS) is a triad consisting of liver disease, hypoxemia, and intrapulmonary vascular shunting. The intrapulmonary shunting causes ventilation/perfusion

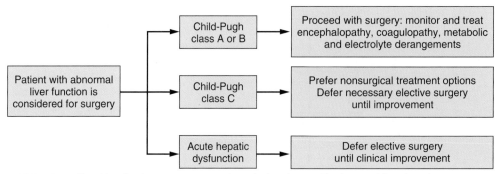

FIG. 17.4 Algorithm for the management of surgical patients with abnormal liver function.

mismatch and an increased alveolar-arterial oxygen gradient. Classically these patients may have platypnea and orthodeoxia. *Platypnea* is shortness of breath that is relieved by lying down and worsens when sitting or standing up. *Orthodeoxia* is hypoxemia that is worse in an upright position and gets better when lying down. The exact mechanism of these unusual pulmonary signs is unknown.

If a patient is suspected of having HPS, diagnosis can be confirmed by echocardiography. With HPS, injected agitated saline will appear as air bubbles on the *left* side of the heart three to four beats after the original appearance of the agitated saline in the *right* atrium. The only definitive treatment for HPS is liver transplantation.

Portopulmonary Hypertension

Portopulmonary hypertension is defined as a mean pulmonary artery pressure greater than 25 mm Hg (i.e., pulmonary arterial hypertension) in a patient with known liver disease and portal hypertension. The exact etiology is unknown, but histologically there is pulmonary endothelial smooth muscle proliferation and often thrombus in situ. There does not seem to be a correlation between the severity of the liver disease and the severity of the portopulmonary hypertension. Diagnosis is often made during a pretransplant echocardiogram. A mean pulmonary arterial pressure above 45 mm Hg is considered an absolute contraindication to liver transplantation.

ANESTHESIA FOR PATIENTS WITH LIVER DISEASE

Given the large population of patients with some degree of chronic liver disease, many elective surgeries are performed every day on patients with liver dysfunction. Routine liver function testing on every patient who presents for elective surgery is not indicated. However, patients with known or suspected liver disease should have this form of testing. Careful assessment of a patient's level of hepatic dysfunction must be performed. Patients with acute hepatitis, fulminant hepatic failure, or late-stage cirrhosis (Child class C) have an unacceptably high perioperative mortality (>80%) and thus should not undergo elective surgery. Patients with less severe hepatic

TABLE 17.7	Survival Statistics According to Child-Pugh Class		
Points	Class	1-Year Survival	2-Year Survival
5–6	A	100%	85%
7–9	B	81%	57%
10–15	C	45%	35%

dysfunction (Child class A and B cirrhosis) can generally undergo anesthesia safely when they are medically optimized (Fig. 17.4 and Table 17.7).

Induction of anesthesia can be accomplished with propofol or etomidate. However, a smaller induction dose of drug may be needed compared to that for patients without liver disease. The one exception is the dosing of patients whose liver disease is related to active substance abuse. Patients with a large amount of ascites likely have a significant aspiration risk, and positioning and a rapid-sequence induction may mitigate that risk. Cisatracurium and succinylcholine are probably the safest neuromuscular blockers, since they undergo *no* hepatic metabolism. Maintenance of anesthesia can be performed with any inhalation anesthetic. Patients with hepatic dysfunction may require lower doses of opioids for perioperative pain management, owing to decreased hepatic clearance of opioids. These patients have diminished physiologic reserves and consequently are at an increased perioperative risk of bleeding, infection, deterioration in liver function, and death compared to those without liver disease.

PROCEDURES AND OPERATIONS FOR LIVER DISEASE

Transjugular Intrahepatic Portosystemic Shunt

TIPS is a procedure performed in interventional radiology in which a shunt is placed between the hepatic and portal veins. Indications include refractory ascites and reducing the risk for variceal rebleeding in patients with a prior variceal hemorrhage. Thorough cardiac evaluation prior to performance of a TIPS procedure is very important, since heart failure, pulmonary hypertension, and severe tricuspid regurgitation are considered contraindications to this procedure. Anesthetic

TABLE 17.8	Special Considerations in Liver Transplantation	
Surgical Phase	Surgical Considerations	Anesthetic Considerations
Preoperative	Transplantation evaluation (including psychological evaluation, MELD score, UNOS listing	Preoperative evaluation, vascular access, blood product availability
Dissection	Surgical incision, mobilization of liver and vascular structures, isolation of bile duct	Hemodynamic compromise from loss of ascites, hemorrhage during dissection, decreased venous return
Anhepatic	Clamping of hepatic artery and portal vein, removal of diseased liver, anastomosis of IVC and portal vein of donor liver	Hemodynamic compromise from clamping IVC, metabolic (lactic) acidosis, hypocalcemia from citrate intoxication, hyperkalemia, hypothermia, hypoglycemia
Reperfusion	Anastomosis of hepatic artery and biliary system, reperfusion of transplanted liver	Hemodynamic instability, dysrhythmias, hyperkalemia, acidosis, cardiac arrest
Posttransplantation	Hemostasis, evaluation of graft function, ultrasound for vascular patency	ICU admission, early or late extubation, hemodynamic management

ICU, Intensive care unit; *IVC,* inferior vena cava; *MELD,* Model for End-Stage Liver Disease; *UNOS,* United Network for Organ Sharing.

considerations include adequate IV access and the immediate availability of properly matched blood, since there is a risk of hemorrhage during this vascular procedure.

Partial Hepatectomy

Partial hepatectomy is often performed in patients with resectable liver tumors. Extensive preoperative evaluation must be undertaken to determine whether the patient has significant cirrhosis and also to know the tumor size. It is important that the surgeon leaves a sufficient remnant of liver tissue to provide adequate liver function while the liver regenerates after the surgery. About 25%–30% of liver tissue is needed for this. Important anesthetic considerations include adequate IV access, availability of blood products, drugs to control hemodynamics during the procedure, and of course a safe anesthetic. Depending on the location of the tumor(s), the portal vein or inferior vena cava may need to be clamped to provide surgical exposure and/or prevent serious blood loss. This can lead to hemodynamic compromise/hypotension.

Minimizing fluid administration prior to resection of the tumor specimen can help keep the venous pressure low, mitigate bleeding, and improve surgical exposure. Patients are often treated in an intensive care unit after a partial hepatectomy because of concerns about further bleeding. Pain management can be accomplished with patient-controlled analgesia. Epidural catheters are used in some institutions for a significant part of the anesthetic as well as for postoperative analgesia. Care must be taken to check coagulation studies prior to epidural catheter removal, since coagulation is often abnormal for several days after liver resection.

Liver Transplantation

Liver transplantation is the only effective long-term treatment for end-stage liver disease. The first human liver transplantation was performed in 1963, but it was not until the development of effective immunosuppressive drugs (e.g., cyclosporine) that liver transplantation became a viable treatment for hepatic

failure. Today there are over 6700 liver transplants performed in the United States annually. The list of people waiting for a liver transplant has more than 12,000 patients actively listed. Cirrhosis due to HCV is the most common indication for liver transplantation in the United States at the present time. Other common indications include alcoholic cirrhosis and hepatocellular carcinoma. Current 5-year survival is better than 70%, and there are more than 56,000 people living with a transplanted liver in the United States.

Organ allocation is complex, but in general, priority is given to patients with more severe disease, such as those requiring admission to an intensive care unit. The MELD score is used to predict mortality due to liver disease and help allocate organs.

The surgical technique of a liver transplantation is often described as having three main phases: the dissection/mobilization phase, the anhepatic phase, and the reperfusion phase. Specific anesthetic concerns for each phase are illustrated in Table 17.8.

Postoperative care of a liver transplant recipient involves intensive care. Most cases will require several hours of mechanical ventilation while the metabolic acidosis clears and graft function improves. Right upper quadrant ultrasound is performed to assess vascular patency. After extubation, pain management is often achieved with intermittent boluses of an IV opioid such as fentanyl or hydromorphone or by patient-controlled analgesia.

KEY POINTS

- The function of the liver can be broken down into five major categories: metabolic, synthetic, immunologic, regenerative, and homeostatic.
- The liver gets its blood supply from the portal vein and hepatic artery, which together receive about 20%–25% of cardiac output. The hepatic artery provides approximately 25% of the liver blood flow while the portal vein provides the remaining 75%. Each of these blood vessels provides roughly half of the liver's oxygen supply.
- Assessment of liver function via laboratory testing falls into two major categories: dysfunction of hepatocytes/biliary

system, which can be seen as alterations in levels of liver enzymes and bilirubin; and assessment of synthetic function, which is measured by alterations in albumin levels and the INR.

- Bilirubin is the breakdown product of hemoglobin and myoglobin. Increases in *indirect bilirubin* are most commonly due to a hemolytic process, breakdown of a hematoma, portal hypertension, and inborn errors of metabolism. Increases in *direct bilirubin* are due to hepatic dysfunction, biliary obstruction, or impaired hepatic bilirubin excretion, which is commonly seen in sepsis.

- Hepatitis C virus (HCV) is the most common cause of end-stage liver disease in the United States and thus is the most frequent disease for which liver transplantation is required.

- Acute liver failure is the rapid development of severe liver injury that presents with impaired synthetic function (INR > 1.5) and hepatic encephalopathy in a patient without underlying liver disease or in one with *stable* chronic liver disease.

- Cirrhosis is the common end stage of liver disease that can result from many different kinds of chronic liver diseases. Histologically, cirrhosis is characterized by formation of fibrous deposits that cause distortion of normal hepatic anatomy. This fibrosis disrupts the sinusoids and other vascular structures in the liver, leading to an increased resistance to blood flow. This increased resistance to flow is the cause of portal hypertension.

- Portal hypertension is a hepatic venous pressure gradient (HVPG) above 6 mm Hg (normal gradient < 5 mm Hg). Portal hypertension produces splenomegaly, formation of esophageal and gastric varices, and gastropathy. When the HVPG exceeds 12 mm Hg, the patient is likely to develop ascites and variceal bleeding.

- *Hepatic encephalopathy* is defined as the neuropsychiatric dysfunction found in patients with liver dysfunction. It is graded on a severity scale of I to IV, with grade I manifesting as only mild changes in behavior. Grade IV is the most severe and manifests as coma and unresponsiveness to painful stimuli.

- Patients with acute hepatitis, fulminant hepatic failure, or late-stage cirrhosis (Child class C disease) have an unacceptably high perioperative mortality (>80%) and thus should *not* undergo elective surgery. Patients with less severe hepatic dysfunction (Child class A and B cirrhosis) can generally undergo anesthesia safely if they are medically optimized.

- Transjugular intrahepatic portosystemic shunt (TIPS) is a procedure whereby a shunt is placed between the hepatic vein and the portal vein. It reduces the degree of portal hypertension.

- Liver transplantation is the only effective long-term treatment for end-stage liver disease. Cirrhosis due to HCV is the most common indication for liver transplantation in the United States. Current 5-year survival after liver transplantation is better than 70%. There are now more than 56,000 people living with a transplanted liver in the United States.

- The surgical technique of liver transplantation has three main phases: the dissection/mobilization phase, the anhepatic phase, and the reperfusion phase.

RESOURCES

del Olmo JA, Flor-Lorente B, Flor-Civera B, et al. Risk factors for nonhepatic surgery in patients with cirrhosis. *World J Surg*. Jun 2003;27:647-652.

Faust TW, Reddy KR. Postoperative jaundice. *Clin Liver Dis*. 2004;8:151-166.

Friedman LS. The risk of surgery in patients with liver disease. *Hepatology*. 1999;29:1617-1623.

Hannaman MJ, Hevesi ZG. Anesthesia care for liver transplantation. *Transplant Rev*. 2011;25:36-43.

Keegan MT, Plevak DJ. Preoperative assessment of the patient with liver disease. *Am J Gastroenterol*. 2005;100:2116-2127.

Mandell MS, Lockrem J, Kelley SD. Immediate tracheal extubation after liver transplantation: experience of two transplant centers. *Anesth Analg*. 1997;84:249-253.

Millwala F, Nguyen GC, Thuluvath PJ. Outcomes of patients with cirrhosis undergoing non-hepatic surgery: risk assessment and management. *World J Gastroenterol*. 2007;13:4056-4063.

O'Leary JG, Friedman LS. Predicting surgical risk in patients with cirrhosis: from art to science. *Gastroenterology*. 2007;132:1609-1611.

Rizvon MK, Chou CL. Surgery in the patient with liver disease. *Med Clin North Am*. 2003;87:211-227.

Teh SH, Nagorney DM, Stevens SR, et al. Risk factors for mortality after surgery in patients with cirrhosis. *Gastroenterology*. 2007;132:1261-1269.

Wagener G. *Liver Anesthesiology and Critical Care Medicine*. New York: Springer; 2012.

Diseases of the Gastrointestinal System

HOSSAM TANTAWY, TORI MYSLAJEK

The principal function of the gastrointestinal (GI) tract is to provide the body with a supply of water, nutrients, and electrolytes. Each division of the GI tract—esophagus, stomach, small and large intestines—is adapted for specific functions such as passage, storage, digestion, and absorption of food. Impairment of any part of the GI tract may have significant effects on a patient coming for surgery.

PROCEDURES TO EVALUATE AND TREAT DISEASES OF THE GASTROINTESTINAL SYSTEM

Upper Gastrointestinal Endoscopy

Upper GI endoscopy, or *esophagogastroduodenoscopy* (EGD), can be done for diagnostic and/or therapeutic purposes and is usually performed in the left lateral decubitus position. It involves placement of a fiberoptic endoscope into the esophagus and through the stomach into the pylorus. EGD is a relatively safe procedure with a mortality rate ranging from 0.01–0.4 per 1000 and an overall complication range of 0.6–5.4 per 1000. Most complications are cardiopulmonary in nature. EGD may be performed with or without sedation/anesthesia. If deep sedation/general anesthesia is chosen, the anesthesiologist shares the upper airway with the gastroenterologist, which introduces a unique challenge. In addition, these procedures are frequently performed outside of the main operating room suite, challenging anesthesiologists to provide a high level of patient safety with little or no immediate backup while simultaneously meeting the efficiency demands of the endoscopy center. Currently there is no consensus on which anesthetic drugs or technique is best for minimizing complications and maximizing efficiency.

Respiratory complications of EGD include desaturation, airway obstruction, laryngospasm, and aspiration. Studies suggest that the incidence of respiratory complications in nonintubated patients is higher than in intubated patients and that there is no decrement in efficiency because of endotracheal intubation.

Because there is no consensus for the best anesthetic technique for upper GI endoscopy, and because the expectations vary between gastroenterologists and anesthesiologists, the anesthesiologist must have a thorough understanding of both diagnostic and therapeutic EGD procedures and patient comorbidities to formulate an appropriate anesthetic plan. Many relatively healthy patients for diagnostic endoscopy can be managed without the assistance of an anesthesiologist. Typically an anesthesia team is involved if a patient is not a good candidate for conscious sedation or there are other comorbid conditions that pose challenges to nonanesthesiologists, such as the need for endotracheal intubation. Patients with a difficult airway or at risk of airway obstruction (e.g., patients with sleep apnea) require an endotracheal tube, especially if prone positioning will be used. Patients at risk for aspiration, such as those with a full stomach, gastroparesis, achalasia, and morbid obesity, may also require endotracheal intubation.

Endoscopic procedures that may be technically challenging or unusually stimulating (e.g., stent changes, dilations, per oral endoscopic myotomy) may require general anesthesia to ensure control of noxious stimuli. Patients with complex medical conditions should have their procedures done in an operating room suite or in a hospital setting with ready access to appropriate extra equipment and personnel and to have a higher level of postoperative care.

Colonoscopy

Like EGD, colonoscopy can be done for diagnostic or therapeutic purposes and with or without deep sedation/anesthesia. There is no consensus on the anesthetic technique that best maximizes safety and efficiency.

A major concern prior to colonoscopy is bowel preparation, with its high risk of dehydration and the required period of fasting necessary to provide a safe anesthetic. Most bowel preps are completed the evening prior to the procedure, and a traditional 6- to 8-hour nothing-by-mouth period is requested by the anesthesiologist to decrease the risk of pulmonary aspiration of gastric contents. Recent prep protocols may call for some of the bowel prep to be done the day before the colonoscopy and some on the morning of the procedure. This method, known as the *split-dose bowel prep*, may provide a superior prep and has greater patient tolerance. It has been shown that gastric residual volume is the same after a split-prep with 2 hours of fasting in the morning as when there is an overnight fast with the traditional prep. This suggests that the risk of aspiration may be similar for these two preps. However, a consensus has not yet been reached in this regard.

Other Diagnostic Tools

High-resolution manometry (HRM) should be done if a motility disorder is suspected. HRM uses a catheter that can detect pressures at 1-cm or smaller intervals along the length and circumference of the catheter. Thus it allows pressure readings to be made simultaneously along the entire length of the esophagus, including at the upper and lower esophageal sphincters. The patient is given small aliquots of fluid to swallow after the catheter has been placed through the esophagus and into the proximal stomach. The catheter passes through the gastroesophageal (GE) junction. Measurements are made in a three-dimensional display of time, distance down the esophagus, and pressure at all points along the esophagus. This creates a test result called *esophageal pressure topography*.

A *barium contrast study* is a noninvasive study that remains useful, especially for patients who are poor candidates for endoscopy. It can demonstrate esophageal reflux, hiatal hernias, ulcerations, erosions, and strictures.

Reflux testing can be done via ambulatory esophageal pH recordings over a 24- to 48-hour time period using a transmitter anchored to the esophageal mucosa or a transnasal wire electrode.

DISEASES OF THE ESOPHAGUS

Symptoms of Esophageal Disease

To evaluate esophageal symptoms, a thorough clinical history can provide some clues and help focus the evaluation. The most common symptoms of esophageal disease are dysphagia, heartburn, and regurgitation. Others include chest pain, odynophagia, and globus sensation.

Dysphagia is a symptom referring to difficulty swallowing. Patients typically describe a sensation of food getting stuck in the chest or throat. Dysphagia can be classified based on its anatomic origin (i.e., oropharyngeal or esophageal).

TABLE 18.1	Etiologies of Dysphagia

MECHANICAL DISORDERS

Benign Strictures
- Peptic stricture
- Schatzki ring
- Esophageal webs
- Anastomotic stricture
- Eosinophilic esophagitis
- Post fundoplication
- Radiation-induced strictures
- Post endoscopic mucosal resection
- Extrinsic compression from vascular structures
- Extrinsic compression from benign lymph nodes or an enlarged left atrium

Malignant Strictures
- Esophageal adenocarcinoma
- Squamous cell cancer
- Extrinsic compression from malignant lymph nodes

MOTILITY DISORDERS
- Achalasia
- Hypotensive peristalsis
- Hypertensive peristalsis
- Nutcracker esophagus
- Distal/diffuse esophageal spasm
- Functional obstruction
- GERD
- Other diseases: pseudoachalasia, Chagas disease, scleroderma

Oropharyngeal dysphagia is commonly seen after head and neck surgery and with certain neurologic conditions such as stroke and Parkinson's disease. *Esophageal dysphagia* is classified based on its physiology (i.e., mechanical or due to dysmotility) (Table 18.1). The clinical history of the dysphagia—better or worse with solids or liquids, episodic or constant, or progressive in character—helps guide the diagnostic workup. Dysphagia only for solid food usually indicates a structural disorder, and dysphagia for both liquids and solids suggests a motility disorder.

Heartburn is a symptom described as burning or discomfort behind the sternum, possibly radiating to the neck. The association between heartburn and gastroesophageal reflux disease (GERD) is so strong that current management of heartburn includes empirical treatment for GERD, realizing that in a few patients the "heartburn" could have a cardiac cause. *Regurgitation* refers to the effortless return of gastric contents into the pharynx without the nausea or retching that would be experienced with vomiting.

Chest pain caused by esophageal disease is often difficult to distinguish from chest pain due to a cardiac origin. The description of heartburn in addition to the pain may be helpful to clarify that the discomfort is caused by gastroesophageal reflux. *Odynophagia* is pain with swallowing. This symptom is often described with esophagitis of infectious origin and with esophageal ulcers. *Globus sensation* is the feeling of "a lump in the throat." Patients with this sensation are often referred for a dysphagia evaluation.

EGD permits direct visualization of esophageal abnormalities as well as collection of biopsy and cytology specimens. It is the best form of evaluation when mechanical causes of dysphagia are suspected. This modality can also detect mucosal lesions and the presence of Barrett's esophagus. It allows for dilation of strictures during the examination.

Esophageal Motility Disorders

Esophageal motility disorders frequently present with dysphagia, heartburn, or chest pain. The most common disorders are achalasia, diffuse esophageal spasm, and GERD.

The Chicago Classification
Using HRM, the Chicago Classification of esophageal motility assesses 10 swallows and can classify patients as having (1) normal esophageal motility, (2) abnormal GE junction relaxation, (3) a major motility disorder with normal GE junction relaxation, or (4) borderline peristalsis.

Achalasia
Achalasia is a neuromuscular disorder of the esophagus with an incidence of 1 per 100,000 persons per year. It consists of esophageal outflow obstruction caused by inadequate relaxation of the lower esophageal sphincter (LES) and a dilated hypomotile esophagus. It is theorized that there is loss of ganglion cells in the myenteric plexus in the esophageal wall, either as a result of a degenerative neuronal disease or as a result of infection. This is followed by absence of the inhibitory neurotransmitters nitric oxide and vasoactive intestinal polypeptide on the LES. Thus there is unopposed cholinergic stimulation of the LES, and it consequently fails to relax. The end result is hypertension of the LES, reduced peristalsis, and esophageal dilatation with impaired emptying of food into the stomach and thus food stasis in the esophagus.

Symptoms include dysphagia with both liquids and solids (95%), regurgitation (60%), heartburn (40%), and chest pain (40%). In the long term, this disease is associated with an increased risk of esophageal cancer. Pulmonary aspiration is common, with resultant pneumonia, lung abscess, and/or bronchiectasis. The diagnosis of achalasia can be made by esophagram, which reveals the classic "bird's beak" appearance. EGD can exclude other structural issues, but esophageal manometry is the standard for definitive diagnosis. With HRM and the Chicago Classification, achalasia can be classified into three distinct patterns. Type I (classic) involves minimal esophageal pressurization and has a better outcome, with myotomy as the initial treatment rather than dilation or botulinum toxin injection. Type II shows pressurization of the entire esophagus and has the best outcome regardless of the initial treatment. Type III involves esophageal spasm with premature contractions and has the worst outcome.

Treatment
All treatments for achalasia are palliative. They *can* relieve the obstruction caused by the LES but *cannot* correct the peristaltic

deficiency of the esophagus. Medications, including nitrates and calcium channel blockers, can be used to try to relax the LES. Invasive measures include endoscopic botulinum toxin injection, pneumatic dilation, laparoscopic Heller myotomy, and *per oral endoscopic myotomy* (POEM). The POEM procedure involves endoscopically dividing the circular muscular layer of the LES but leaving the longitudinal muscular layer intact. Therefore it may offer the efficacy of surgery with the morbidity of an endoscopic procedure. However, the procedure is not without risk. Up to 40% of patients will develop a pneumothorax or pneumoperitoneum, and half of these will require a chest tube or peritoneal drain. Dilation is the most effective nonsurgical treatment, and laparoscopic Heller myotomy remains the best surgical treatment of achalasia. Esophagectomy can be considered in very advanced disease and would eliminate the risk of esophageal cancer as well as mitigate symptoms.

Anesthetic Concerns

Patients with achalasia are at high risk of perioperative aspiration and must be treated using full-stomach precautions. The dilated esophagus may retain food for many days after ingestion, so the duration of fasting is meaningless in terms of aspiration risk. A large-bore nasogastric tube can be inserted to decompress and empty the esophagus prior to induction, or a large-channel endoscope can be passed to evacuate most of the esophageal contents. Rapid-sequence induction/endotracheal intubation or awake intubation is required in all patients.

Patients presenting for repair via POEM require general anesthesia and mechanical ventilation. Prior to the procedure, patients may fast for up to 48 hours. The procedure is performed in the supine position, and the esophagus is insufflated with carbon dioxide. During insufflation, patients may have an increase in $ETCO_2$ that can be managed with controlled mechanical ventilation.

Distal Esophageal Spasm

Distal esophageal spasm (DES) is now the preferred term for describing *diffuse esophageal spasm* because it is typically the distal portion of the esophagus that is spastic. DES typically occurs in elderly patients and is most likely due to autonomic nervous system dysfunction. An esophagram may show a "corkscrew esophagus" or a "rosary bead esophagus." Pain produced by esophageal spasm may mimic angina pectoris and does frequently respond favorably to treatment with nitroglycerin, which can confuse the clinical picture. The antidepressants trazodone and imipramine can decrease chest pain due to distal esophageal spasm. The phosphodiesterase inhibitor sildenafil can also reduce this pain.

Esophageal Structural Disorders

Esophageal Diverticula

Esophageal diverticula are outpouchings of the wall of the esophagus. The most common locations for these are pharyngoesophageal (Zenker's diverticulum), midesophageal, and epiphrenic (supradiaphragmatic diverticulum).

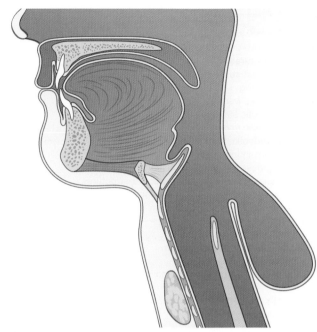

FIG. 18.1 Lateral view of neck showing the location of a Zenker's diverticulum in relationship to the cricoid cartilage. Note that it is directly behind the cricoid cartilage. (From Law R, Katzka DA, Baron TH. Zenker's diverticulum. *Clin Gastroenterol Hepatol.* 2014;12:1773-1782, with permission.)

Zenker's diverticulum (Fig. 18.1) appears in a natural zone of weakness in the posterior hypopharyngeal wall (Killian's triangle) and can cause significant bad breath from retention of food particles consumed up to several days previously. A midesophageal diverticulum may be caused by traction from old adhesions or inflamed lymph nodes or by propulsion associated with esophageal motility abnormalities. An epiphrenic diverticulum may be associated with achalasia. Large symptomatic esophageal diverticula are removed surgically.

Small or medium-sized Zenker's diverticula are usually asymptomatic. If they become large and filled with food, they can compress the esophagus and cause dysphagia. Regurgitation of food contents and the risk of aspiration of this material from a diverticulum can occur at any time during anesthesia—during induction, during endotracheal intubation, after intubation, or with surgical manipulation—and there can be leakage around the endotracheal tube cuff. Various anesthetic regimens are acceptable during surgical repair of a Zenker's diverticulum, with a top priority given to efforts to prevent aspiration. The effectiveness of cricoid pressure in reducing the risk of aspiration during rapid-sequence induction/intubation is doubtful in this situation. A preoperative barium swallow analyzed by an expert in this technique could help determine whether cricoid pressure will be useful or not. If the diverticular sac is immediately behind the cricoid cartilage, cricoid pressure might force the contents of the sac into the pharynx rather than protect the patient from regurgitation. Most often, general anesthesia is induced in the head-up position *without* cricoid pressure.

Regardless of anesthetic technique, the pouch may be emptied prior to anesthetic induction by the patient exerting external pressure. Insertion of a nasogastric tube should be avoided because it can perforate the diverticulum. For echocardiography the probe needs to be inserted very carefully to prevent perforation of the diverticulum.

Hiatal Hernia

A *hiatal hernia* is a herniation of part of the stomach into the thoracic cavity through the esophageal hiatus in the diaphragm. A *sliding hiatal hernia* is one in which the GE junction and fundus of the stomach slide upward. This type of hernia is seen in about 30% of patients having upper GI tract radiographic examinations. Many of these patients are asymptomatic (i.e., no symptoms of reflux). This hernia may result from weakening of the anchors of the GE junction to the diaphragm, from longitudinal contraction/shortening of the esophagus, or from increased intraabdominal pressure. A *paraesophageal hernia* is one in which the GE junction stays in its normal location and a pouch of stomach is herniated *next to* the GE junction through the esophageal hiatus. Hiatal hernias are very infrequently repaired. The fact that most patients with hiatal hernias do not have symptoms of reflux esophagitis emphasizes the importance of the integrity of the LES.

Esophageal Tumors

Esophageal cancer occurs in 4–5 per 100,000 people in the United States. It usually presents with progressive dysphagia to solid food and weight loss. Esophageal cancer has a poor survival rate because abundant esophageal lymphatics lead to early lymph node metastases. Esophageal cancer can be a squamous cell cancer or an adenocarcinoma. Formerly, most esophageal cancers were of the squamous cell type and situated about midesophagus. Today most esophageal cancers are adenocarcinomas and are located at the lower end of the esophagus. It is postulated that adenocarcinomas are linked to the dramatic increase in GERD, Barrett's esophagus, and obesity.

Esophagectomy

Esophagectomy can be a curative or palliative option for malignant esophageal lesions. It can also be considered when benign obstructive conditions are not responsive to conservative management. There are several surgical approaches to esophagectomy, including transthoracic, transhiatal, and minimally invasive. Minimally invasive esophagectomy combines a laparoscopic resection of the GE junction and the proximal stomach with a thoracoscopic resection of the esophagus. Survival rates at 5 years with any of these surgical approaches ranges from 12%–60%.

Morbidity and Mortality. The morbidity and mortality of esophagectomy are quite high. Morbidity rates are almost 50% in specialized high-volume centers, and mortality rates approach 5%. Most major postoperative complications are respiratory, and these contribute to poor outcomes. Acute lung injury and/or acute respiratory distress syndrome (ARDS)

occur in up to 10%–20% of esophagectomies. Mortality approaches 50% if ARDS occurs.

The cause of ARDS in the setting of esophagectomy is not completely understood, but it may be that inflammatory mediators and gut-related endotoxins trigger the pulmonary dysfunction. Another contributing factor may be the use of prolonged one-lung ventilation. The current practice of protective lung ventilation (limiting the tidal volume during mechanical ventilation to 5 mL/kg plus PEEP) likely decreases ventilator-associated trauma. A history of smoking, low body mass index, long duration of surgery, cardiopulmonary instability, and the occurrence of a postoperative anastomotic leak also increase the risk of ARDS.

Other common postoperative complications include anastomotic leaks, dumping syndrome and esophageal stricture.

Anesthetic Implications. Patients are often malnourished (protein-calorie malnutrition) before esophagectomy and for many months afterward. Fortunately over the past decade, regular surveillance of patients with Barrett's esophagus has lead to the diagnosis of some esophageal cancers in very early stages, so these patients typically arrive for surgery in good nutritional balance. Some patients presenting for esophagectomy have had chemotherapy and/or radiation therapy, so pancytopenia, dehydration, and lung injury can be present.

In the postoperative period, patients may need to return to the operating room for correction of an anastomotic leak. They may have acute lung injury, sepsis, or shock. *There is a very significant risk of aspiration in all patients who have had an esophagectomy, a risk that persists for life.*

Recurrent laryngeal nerve injury has been described in patients after esophagectomy, likely related to the cervical portion of the surgery. A vocal cord palsy can lead to airway compromise during extubation and postoperatively and does increase the risk of aspiration. Spontaneous resolution of recurrent laryngeal nerve palsy has been described in about 40% of patients.

Thoracic epidural analgesia for perioperative pain management has been shown to reduce the incidence of pulmonary complications and promote earlier return of bowel function. The latter facilitates expeditious resumption of enteric feeding. The best analgesic drugs for thoracic epidural analgesia are uncertain. Local anesthetics, local anesthetics combined with opioids, and opioids alone can be used. Hemodynamic variables and fluid management will be affected by the choice of the epidural analgesic medication(s).

Gastroesophageal Reflux Disease

GERD is defined as gastroesophageal reflux that causes bothersome symptoms, mucosal injury in the esophagus or at extraesophageal sites, or a combination of both. It is a common problem, with approximately 15% of adults in the United States being affected based on self-reporting of chronic heartburn. The most common symptoms are heartburn and regurgitation. Dysphagia and chest pain are less commonly noted.

Pathophysiology of GERD

Natural antireflux mechanisms consist of the LES, the crural diaphragm, and the anatomic location of the GE junction below the diaphragmatic hiatus. The LES opens with swallowing and closes afterward to prevent gastric acid in the stomach from refluxing into the esophagus. At rest the LES exerts a pressure high enough to prevent gastric contents from entering the esophagus.

With GE junction incompetence, gastric contents can reenter the esophagus, causing symptoms and/or mucosal damage. Three common mechanisms of incompetence are (1) transient LES relaxation (elicited by gastric distention); (2) LES hypotension (average resting tone, 13 mm Hg in patients with GERD vs. 29 mm Hg in patients without GERD); and (3) anatomic distortion of the GE junction, such as with a hiatal hernia. The reflux contents may include hydrochloric acid, pepsin, pancreatic enzymes, and bile. Bile is a cofactor in the development of Barrett's metaplasia and adenocarcinoma.

Complications of GERD

Chronic peptic esophagitis is caused by reflux of acidic gastric fluid into the esophagus, producing retrosternal discomfort (i.e., "heartburn"). Local complications include esophagitis, strictures, ulcers, Barrett's metaplasia, and its associated risk of adenocarcinoma. With the laryngopharyngeal reflux variant of GERD, gastric contents reflux into the pharynx, larynx, and tracheobronchial tree, resulting in chronic cough, bronchoconstriction, pharyngitis, laryngitis, bronchitis, or pneumonia. Recurrent pulmonary aspiration can lead to progressive pulmonary fibrosis or chronic asthma. It is notable that up to 50% of patients with asthma have either endoscopic evidence of esophagitis or an increased esophageal acid exposure on 24-hour ambulatory pH monitoring.

Treatment

Therapy for GERD includes lifestyle modification, including avoidance of foods that reduce LES tone (e.g., fatty and fried foods, alcohol, peppermint, chocolate) and avoidance of acidic foods (e.g., citrus and tomato products). Pharmacologic measures aim to inhibit gastric acid secretion, with proton pump inhibitors being more effective than histamine (H_2) receptor antagonists. These drugs do not prevent reflux but increase the pH of the reflux, which allows esophagitis to heal. Surgical options for severe symptoms include laparoscopic Nissen fundoplication, in which an antireflux barrier is created by wrapping the proximal stomach around the distal esophagus.

Perioperative Management and Anesthetic Considerations

Depending on the planned surgery and anesthetic, medications to treat GERD may be given preoperatively. Cimetidine and ranitidine decrease gastric acid secretion and increase gastric pH. Cimetidine's effect begins in 1–1.5 hours and lasts for about 3 hours. Ranitidine is 4–6 times more potent than cimetidine and has fewer side effects. Famotidine and nizatidine can be given intravenously and are similar in effect to ranitidine but have a longer duration of action. Proton pump inhibitors are generally given orally the night before surgery and again on the morning of surgery.

Sodium citrate is an oral nonparticulate antacid that increases gastric pH. It can be given with a gastrokinetic agent (e.g., metoclopramide) shortly prior to induction of anesthesia. It is generally used in those who are diabetic, morbidly obese, or pregnant.

In terms of anesthetic management, GERD represents an *aspiration risk*. For pulmonary aspiration to occur, gastric contents must flow to the esophagus (GE reflux), contents must reach the pharynx (esophagopharyngeal reflux), and laryngeal reflexes must be obtunded (as with sedation or general anesthesia). For this aspirated material to cause an aspiration pneumonitis, it is believed there must be a volume of at least 0.4 mL/kg (≈30 mL in a 70-kg person) of gastric contents aspirated, and the pH of the gastric contents must be below 2.5.

Other factors that contribute to the likelihood of intraoperative aspiration of gastric contents include urgent or emergent surgery, a full stomach, a difficult airway, inadequate anesthetic depth, use of the lithotomy position, autonomic neuropathy, insulin-dependent diabetes mellitus, gastroparesis, pregnancy, increased intraabdominal pressure, severe illness, and morbid obesity.

Patients with GERD may have certain complications of their GERD that can affect anesthetic management. *Mucosal complications* (e.g., esophagitis, esophageal stricture) can result in esophageal dilatation and compound the risk for aspiration. *Extraesophageal* or *respiratory complications* (e.g., laryngitis, bronchitis, bronchospasm, recurrent pneumonia, progressive pulmonary fibrosis) can also have anesthetic implications.

Rapid-sequence induction with immediate endotracheal intubation is typically used in patients with GERD. Cricoid pressure is also applied to assist in reducing the risk of aspiration. Cricoid pressure compresses the lumen of the pharynx between the cricoid cartilage and the cervical vertebrae. The force applied to the cricoid cartilage should be sufficient to prevent aspiration but not so great as to cause possible airway obstruction or to permit esophageal rupture in the event of vomiting. Succinylcholine increases LES pressure and intragastric pressure, but the barrier pressure (LES pressure minus intragastric pressure) is unchanged.

Endotracheal intubation is essential for protecting the airway in anesthetized patients when aspiration is considered a risk. The endotracheal tube is superior to all other airway devices in reducing the risk of aspiration.

PEPTIC ULCER DISEASE

Burning epigastric pain exacerbated by fasting and improved with meal consumption is the typical symptom complex associated with *peptic ulcer disease,* ulcers in the mucosal lining of the stomach or duodenum. The lifetime prevalence of peptic ulcer disease in the United States is about 12% in men and 10% in women. Interestingly an estimated 15,000 deaths per year occur as a consequence of complicated peptic ulcer disease. Bleeding, peritonitis, dehydration, perforation, and sepsis, especially in elderly debilitated or malnourished patients, are risk factors for death caused by peptic ulcer disease.

Helicobacter pylori

Barry Marshall and Robin Warren received the Nobel Prize for their work in establishing the link between *Helicobacter pylori* and peptic ulcer disease, one of the great advances in medicine in the past 50 years. *H. pylori* infection is virtually *always* associated with chronic active gastritis, but only 10%–15% of infected individuals actually develop a peptic ulceration. Ironically the earliest stages of *H. pylori* infection are accompanied by a marked *decrease* in gastric acid secretion. Then this organism induces increased acid secretion through both direct and indirect actions of the organism and proinflammatory cytokines. These actions affect the function of G, D, and parietal cells in the stomach and also reduce duodenal mucosal bicarbonate production.

Complications

Bleeding

Peptic ulcer disease is the most common cause of nonvariceal upper GI bleeding, and *hemorrhage* is the leading cause of death associated with peptic ulcer disease. The lifetime risk of hemorrhage in patients with a duodenal ulcer who have not had surgery and do not receive maintenance drug therapy is approximately 35%. The current risk of mortality from bleeding is between 10% and 20%. Significant risk factors for rebleeding or in-hospital mortality include a systolic blood pressure below 100 mm Hg, heart rate above 100 beats per minute, the presence of melena, syncope or altered mentation, concomitant renal, liver, or cardiac disease, and the findings at endoscopy.

Perforation

The lifetime risk of perforation in patients with duodenal ulceration who do not receive treatment is approximately 10%. Perforation is usually accompanied by sudden and severe epigastric pain caused by spillage of highly acidic gastric secretions into the peritoneum. The mortality of emergency ulcer surgery is correlated with the presence of preoperative shock, significant co-existing medical illnesses, and perforation longer than 48 hours before surgery.

Obstruction

Gastric outlet obstruction can occur acutely or slowly. These patients should be considered to have a full stomach when they come for surgery. Acute obstruction is caused by edema and inflammation in the pyloric channel and the first portion of the duodenum. Pyloric obstruction is suggested by recurrent vomiting, dehydration, and hypochloremic alkalosis resulting from loss of acidic gastric secretions. Treatment consists of nasogastric suction, hydration, and intravenous administration of antisecretory drugs (i.e., proton pump inhibitors). In most instances, acute obstruction resolves within 72 hours

TABLE 18.2	Classification of Gastric Ulcers
Type of Gastric Ulcer	Location
Type I	Along the lesser curvature close to incisura; no acid hypersecretion
Type II	Two ulcers, first on gastric body, second duodenal; usually acid hypersecretion
Type III	Prepyloric with acid hypersecretion
Type IV	At lesser curvature near gastroesophageal junction; no acid hypersecretion
Type V	Anywhere in stomach, usually seen with NSAID use

with these supportive measures. However, repeated episodes of ulceration and healing can lead to pyloric scarring and a subsequent fixed stenosis and chronic gastric outlet obstruction.

Gastric Ulcer

Benign *gastric ulcers* are a form of peptic ulcer disease occurring with one-third the frequency of benign duodenal ulcers. There are five types of gastric ulcers, as described in Table 18.2. Use of nonsteroidal antiinflammatory drugs (NSAIDs) is the other common cause of gastroduodenal ulcer disease. If *H. pylori* is also present, the risk of NSAID-induced ulcers is significantly increased.

Stress Gastritis

Major trauma accompanied by shock, sepsis, respiratory failure, burns, hemorrhage, massive transfusion, or head injury is often associated with the development of *acute stress gastritis*. Acute stress gastritis is particularly prevalent after central nervous system injury, intracranial hypertension, and thermal injury involving more than 35% of body surface area. The major complication of stress gastritis is gastric hemorrhage. The incidence of gastric bleeding is significantly associated with a coagulopathy, thrombocytopenia, an international normalized ratio (INR) higher than 1.5, and an activated partial thromboplastin time (aPTT) greater than twice normal.

Treatment

Antacids

Antacids are rarely used by clinicians as a primary therapy for gastritis. However, patients often use them for symptomatic relief of dyspepsia. The most commonly used antacids are aluminum hydroxide and magnesium hydroxide, and many over-the-counter brands (e.g., Maalox, Mylanta) contain a combination of both aluminum and magnesium hydroxide to avoid the side effects of constipation or diarrhea. Neither magnesium nor aluminum-containing preparations should be used in patients with chronic renal failure. The former can cause hypermagnesemia and the latter can cause neurotoxicity. Other potent antacids include calcium carbonate (Tums) and sodium bicarbonate. Long-term use of calcium carbonate can lead to milk-alkali syndrome (hypercalcemia and hyperphosphatemia) with possible development of renal stones and progression to renal insufficiency. Sodium bicarbonate use may induce metabolic alkalosis.

H₂-Receptor Antagonists

Four H$_2$-receptor antagonists—cimetidine, ranitidine, famotidine, and nizatidine—are currently available, and their structures share homology with histamine. All will significantly inhibit basal and stimulated gastric acid secretion. This class of drugs is effective for the treatment of active ulcer disease (4–6 weeks of treatment) and as adjuvant therapy (with antibiotics) for the management of *H. pylori* infection. Cimetidine was the first H$_2$-receptor antagonist used for the treatment of acid peptic disorders, with healing rates approaching 80% at 1 month. Ranitidine, famotidine, and nizatidine are all more potent H$_2$-receptor antagonists than cimetidine. Cimetidine and ranitidine, but not famotidine and nizatidine, bind to hepatic cytochrome P450. Therefore, careful monitoring of treatment with drugs such as warfarin, phenytoin, and theophylline that also use cytochrome P450 for metabolism is indicated.

Proton Pump Inhibitors

Omeprazole, esomeprazole, lansoprazole, rabeprazole, and pantoprazole are substituted benzimidazole derivatives that covalently bind and irreversibly inhibit hydrogen-potassium–adenosine triphosphatase (H$^+$,K$^+$-ATPase). These are the most potent acid-inhibitory drugs available. Proton pump inhibitors inhibit all phases of gastric acid secretion. Onset of action is rapid, with a maximum effect achieved within 2–6 hours and a duration of action of up to 72 hours. As with any drug that leads to a significant reduction in gastric hydrochloric acid production, proton pump inhibitors may interfere with absorption of drugs such as ketoconazole, ampicillin, iron, digoxin, and diazepam. Their absorption may be either increased or decreased depending on the characteristics of the particular drug. Hepatic cytochrome P450 may also be inhibited by some proton pump inhibitors (omeprazole, lansoprazole).

Prostaglandin Analogues

Because of their central role in maintaining mucosal integrity and repair, prostaglandin analogues were developed for the treatment of peptic ulcer disease. At present the prostaglandin E$_1$ derivative *misoprostol* is the only drug in this class approved by the U.S. Food and Drug Administration for clinical use in the prevention of gastroduodenal mucosal injury induced by NSAIDs. Prostaglandin analogues enhance mucosal bicarbonate secretion, stimulate mucosal blood flow, and decrease mucosal cell turnover. The most common side effect is diarrhea. Other toxicities include uterine contractions and uterine bleeding. Thus misoprostol is contraindicated in women who may be pregnant.

Cytoprotective Agents

Sucralfate is a complex sucrose salt in which the hydroxyl groups have been substituted by aluminum hydroxide and sulfate. It can act by several mechanisms. In the gastric environment, aluminum hydroxide dissociates from the sulfate anion, which can then bind to positively charged tissue proteins found within the ulcer bed. This process provides a physicochemical barrier, impeding further tissue injury by either acid or pepsin. Sucralfate may also induce a trophic effect by binding growth factors (e.g., endothelial growth factor), enhance prostaglandin synthesis, stimulate mucus and bicarbonate secretion, and enhance mucosal defense and repair. Toxicity from sucralfate is rare, and constipation is the most common side effect. Sucralfate should be avoided in patients with chronic renal insufficiency to prevent aluminum-induced neurotoxicity.

Colloidal bismuth subcitrate and bismuth subsalicylate (Pepto-Bismol) are the most widely used bismuth-containing antacids and antiulcer drugs. The mechanism by which these agents induce ulcer healing is unclear. Potential mechanisms include ulcer coating, prevention of further pepsin and hydrochloric acid–induced damage, binding of pepsin, and stimulation of prostaglandins, bicarbonate, and mucus secretion. Long-term use of high dosages, especially of colloidal bismuth subcitrate, could lead to neurotoxicity.

Miscellaneous Drugs

Anticholinergic drugs designed to inhibit activation of the muscarinic receptor in parietal cells have limited success in ulcer healing because of their relatively weak acid-inhibiting effect and significant side effects (dry eyes, dry mouth, urinary retention).

Treatment of *Helicobacter pylori* Infection

The National Institutes of Health, American Digestive Health Foundation, and European Maastricht and Asia Pacific consensus conferences recommend that *H. pylori* be eradicated in patients with peptic ulcer disease. Eradication of this organism is associated with a dramatic decrease in ulcer recurrence. However, no single drug is effective in eradicating *H. pylori*. Combination triple therapy for 14 days provides the greatest efficacy and consists of a proton pump inhibitor (at about double the usual dose) and two antibiotics. The antibiotics used with the greatest frequency are amoxicillin, metronidazole, tetracycline, and clarithromycin, but an increase in antimicrobial resistance will cause changes in antibiotic therapy as needed.

Surgical Treatment

Operative intervention is reserved for the treatment of complicated ulcer disease. The most common complications requiring surgery are hemorrhage, perforation, and obstruction, as well as failure of a recurrent ulcer to respond to medical therapy and/or the inability to exclude malignant disease. The first goal of any surgical treatment should be removal of the source of the ulcer so that ulcer healing can be achieved and the risk of recurrence minimized. The second goal is treatment of co-existing anatomic complications such as pyloric stenosis or perforation. The third major goal should be prevention of undesirable long-term side effects from the surgery.

Three procedures—truncal vagotomy and drainage, truncal vagotomy and antrectomy, and proximal gastric vagotomy—have traditionally been used for surgical treatment of peptic ulcer disease. Surgical treatment now, however, is often directed exclusively at correcting the immediate problem (e.g., closure of a duodenal perforation *without gastric denervation*). Division of both vagal trunks at the esophageal hiatus (truncal vagotomy) denervates the acid-producing fundal mucosa as well as the remainder of the viscera supplied by the vagus nerve. Because denervation results in impairment of gastric emptying, truncal vagotomy must be combined with a procedure to eliminate pyloric sphincter dysfunction, usually a pyloroplasty.

ZOLLINGER-ELLISON SYNDROME

In 1955 Zollinger and Ellison described two patients with gastroduodenal and intestinal ulceration together with gastrin hypersecretion and a non–beta islet cell tumor of the pancreas (gastrinoma). The incidence of Zollinger-Ellison syndrome varies from 0.1%–1% of individuals with peptic ulcer disease. Men are affected more often than women, and in the majority of cases the disorder is identified in patients between the ages of 30 and 50.

Pathophysiology

Gastrin stimulates acid secretion through gastrin receptors on parietal cells and via histamine release. It also exerts a trophic effect on gastric epithelial cells. Long-standing hypergastrinemia causes markedly increased gastric acid secretion by both parietal cell stimulation and increased parietal cell mass. This increased gastric acid output leads to peptic ulcer disease, erosive esophagitis, and diarrhea.

Abdominal pain and peptic ulceration are seen in up to 90% of patients with Zollinger-Ellison syndrome; diarrhea is seen in 50%, and 10% have diarrhea as their only symptom. Gastroesophageal reflux is seen in about half of patients. Initial presentation and ulcer location in the duodenal bulb may be indistinguishable from that in ordinary peptic ulcer disease. Ulcers in unusual locations (second part of the duodenum and beyond), ulcers refractory to standard medical therapy, and ulcer recurrence after acid-reducing surgery or ulcers presenting with complications (bleeding, obstruction, and perforation) should create suspicion of a gastrinoma. Gastrinomas can develop in the presence of multiple endocrine neoplasia (MEN) type I, a disorder involving primarily three organ sites: the parathyroid glands, pancreas, and pituitary gland. In view of the stimulatory effect of calcium on gastric secretion, the hyperparathyroidism and hypercalcemia seen in MEN I patients may have a direct effect on ulcer disease. Resolution of hypercalcemia by parathyroidectomy will reduce gastrin and gastric acid output in gastrinoma patients.

Treatment

The first step in the evaluation of a patient with suspected Zollinger-Ellison syndrome is obtaining a fasting gastrin level

TABLE 18.3	Causes of Increased Fasting Serum Gastrin Level
Hypochlorhydria and achlorhydria (± pernicious anemia)	Retained gastric antrum
G-cell hyperplasia	Gastric outlet obstruction
Renal insufficiency	Massive small bowel obstruction
Rheumatoid arthritis	Vitiligo
Pheochromocytomas	Diabetes mellitus
Helicobacter pylori infection	Use of antisecretory drugs

(Table 18.3). Gastric acid induces feedback inhibition of gastrin release. Such feedback is *absent* in Zollinger-Ellison syndrome. Unfortunately up to 50% of patients with gastrinomas have metastatic disease at the time of diagnosis.

Patients with duodenal ulcers as part of Zollinger-Ellison syndrome are treated initially with proton pump inhibitors at doses higher than those used to treat GERD and peptic ulcer disease, and then the doses of these drugs are guided by gastric acid measurements. A potentially curative surgical resection of a gastrinoma is indicated in the absence of evidence of MEN I syndrome and the absence of an unresectable liver metastasis or co-existing significant medical disorders that are likely to limit life expectancy.

Management of Anesthesia

Management of anesthesia for gastrinoma excision must consider the presence of gastric hypersecretion as well as the likely presence of a large gastric fluid volume. Esophageal reflux is common in these patients despite the ability of gastrin to increase LES tone. Depletion of intravascular fluid volume and electrolyte imbalances (hypokalemia, metabolic alkalosis) may accompany profuse watery diarrhea. The associated endocrine abnormalities (MEN I syndrome) can also influence the management of anesthesia. Antacid prophylaxis with proton pump inhibitors and H_2-receptor antagonists is maintained up to the time of surgery. A preoperative coagulation screen and liver function tests are recommended, since alterations in fat absorption can influence production of clotting factors. Administration of a proton pump inhibitor or ranitidine or octreotide is useful for preventing gastric acid hypersecretion during surgery.

POSTGASTRECTOMY SYNDROMES

A number of syndromes have been described following gastric operations performed for peptic ulcer disease or gastric neoplasm. The overall occurrence of severe postoperative symptoms is low, perhaps 1%–3% of cases, but the symptoms can be rather disabling. The two most common postgastrectomy syndromes are dumping and alkaline reflux gastritis.

Dumping

Dumping syndrome consists of a series of vasomotor and GI symptoms and signs. There may be two phases to dumping:

early and late. Dumping is caused by the entry of hyperosmolar gastric contents into the proximal small bowel, which results in a shift of fluid into the small bowel lumen, plasma volume contraction, and acute intestinal distention. Release of vasoactive GI hormones may also play a role. Early dumping symptoms occur 15–30 minutes after a meal and include nausea, epigastric discomfort, diaphoresis, crampy abdominal pain, diarrhea, tachycardia, palpitations, and in extreme cases, dizziness or even syncope. The late phase of dumping follows a meal by 1–3 hours and can include vasomotor symptoms thought to be secondary to hypoglycemia, which occurs as a result of excessive insulin release. Dietary modifications—consumption of frequent small meals with a few simple sugars and a reduction in the amount of fluid ingested with a meal—can be very helpful.

Octreotide therapy has been reported to improve dumping symptoms in diet-refractory cases. The drug is administered subcutaneously before a meal or by depot injection monthly. Somatostatin analogues have beneficial effects on the vasomotor symptoms of dumping, probably as a result of the pressor effects of the somatostatin analogues on splanchnic blood vessels. In addition, somatostatin analogues inhibit the release of vasoactive peptides from the gut, decrease peak plasma insulin levels, and slow intestinal transit. Acarbose (an α-glucosidase inhibitor that delays the digestion of carbohydrates) is often beneficial in late dumping.

Alkaline Reflux Gastritis

Alkaline reflux gastritis is identified by the occurrence of the clinical triad of (1) postprandial epigastric pain often associated with nausea and vomiting, (2) evidence of reflux of bile into the stomach, and (3) histologic evidence of gastritis. There is no pharmacologic treatment for alkaline reflux gastritis. The only proven treatment is operative diversion of intestinal contents from contact with the gastric mucosa. The most common surgical procedure for this purpose is a Roux-en-Y gastrojejunostomy.

INFLAMMATORY BOWEL DISEASE

Inflammatory bowel diseases are the second most common chronic inflammatory disorders (after rheumatoid arthritis). The diagnosis of ulcerative colitis and Crohn's disease, and the differentiation between these disorders, is based on nonspecific clinical and histologic patterns that are often obscured by intercurrent infection, iatrogenic events, medication, or surgery. The incidence of inflammatory bowel disease in the United States is approximately 18 per 100,000.

Ulcerative Colitis

Ulcerative colitis is a mucosal disease involving the rectum and extending proximally to involve part or all of the colon. Approximately 40%–50% of patients have disease limited to the rectum and rectosigmoid, 30%–40% have disease extending beyond the sigmoid but not involving the entire colon, and 20% have a pancolitis. Proximal spread occurs in continuity without areas of spared mucosa. In severe disease the mucosa is hemorrhagic, edematous, and ulcerated. The major symptoms and signs of ulcerative colitis are diarrhea, rectal bleeding, tenesmus, passage of mucus, and crampy abdominal pain. Symptoms in moderate to severe disease may also include anorexia, nausea, vomiting, fever, and weight loss. Active disease can be associated with an *increase* in levels of acute-phase reactants, platelet count, and erythrocyte sedimentation rate and a *decrease* in hematocrit. In severely ill patients the serum albumin level is low and leukocytosis may be present.

Complications

Catastrophic illness is an initial presentation in only 15% of patients with ulcerative colitis. In 1% of patients a severe episode may be accompanied by massive hemorrhage, which usually stops with treatment of the underlying disease. However, if the patient requires 6–8 units of blood within 24–48 hours, colectomy is frequently performed. *Toxic megacolon* is defined as a dilated transverse colon with loss of haustrations. It occurs in approximately 5% of episodes and can be triggered by electrolyte abnormalities or narcotics. Toxic megacolon will resolve about half of the time with medical therapy, but urgent colectomy may be required in those who do not experience improvement with conservative treatment. Perforation of the colon is the most dangerous complication of ulcerative colitis, and the physical signs of peritonitis may not be obvious, especially if the patient is receiving glucocorticoids. The mortality rate associated with perforation of the colon is approximately 15%. Some patients can develop toxic colitis and such severe ulcerations that the bowel may perforate without dilating. Obstruction caused by benign stricture formation occurs in 10% of patients.

Crohn's Disease

Although Crohn's disease usually presents as acute or chronic bowel inflammation, the inflammatory process typically evolves into one of two patterns of disease, a penetrating-fistulous pattern or an obstructing pattern, each with different treatments and prognoses.

The most common site of inflammation is the terminal ileum. Therefore the usual presentation is ileocolitis with a history of recurrent episodes of right lower quadrant pain and diarrhea. A spiking fever suggests intraabdominal abscess formation. Weight loss, often 10%–20% of body weight, is common and a consequence of fear of eating, anorexia, and diarrhea. An inflammatory mass may be palpated in the right lower quadrant of the abdomen and mimic acute appendicitis. Local extension of the mass can cause obstruction of the right ureter or inflammation of the bladder, manifested as dysuria and fever. Bowel obstruction may take several forms. In the early stages, bowel wall edema and spasm produce intermittent obstruction and increasing postprandial pain. Over the course of years, persistent inflammation gradually progresses

TABLE 18.4	Extraintestinal Manifestations of Inflammatory Bowel Disease
Dermatologic	Erythema nodosum, pyoderma gangrenosum
Rheumatologic	Peripheral arthritis
Ocular	Conjunctivitis, anterior uveitis/iritis, episcleritis
Hepatobiliary	Hepatomegaly, fatty liver, biliary cirrhosis, cholelithiasis, primary sclerosing cholangitis
Urologic	Renal calculi, ureteral obstruction
Coagulation disorders	Thromboembolic disease (pulmonary embolism, cerebrovascular accidents, arterial emboli) with increased levels of fibrinopeptide A, factor V, factor VIII and fibrinogen, accelerated thromboplastin generation, antithrombin III deficiency, protein S deficiency
Other	Endocarditis, myocarditis, and pleuropericarditis Interstitial lung disease Secondary/reactive amyloidosis

TABLE 18.5	Indications for Surgery in Inflammatory Bowel Disease

ULCERATIVE COLITIS

Massive hemorrhage, perforation, toxic megacolon, obstruction, intractable and fulminant disease, cancer

CROHN'S DISEASE

Stricture, obstruction, hemorrhage, abscess, fistulas, intractable and fulminant disease, cancer, unresponsive perianal disease

to fibrous narrowing and stricture formation. Diarrhea decreases and is replaced by chronic bowel obstruction. Severe inflammation of the ileocecal region may lead to localized wall thinning, with microperforation and formation of fistulas to the adjacent bowel, skin, urinary bladder, or mesentery.

Extensive inflammatory disease is associated with a loss of digestive and absorptive surfaces, which results in malabsorption and steatorrhea. Nutritional deficiencies can also result from poor intake and enteric losses of protein and other nutrients, causing hypoalbuminemia, hypocalcemia, hypomagnesemia, coagulopathy, and hyperoxaluria with nephrolithiasis. Vertebral fractures are caused by a combination of vitamin D deficiency, hypocalcemia, and prolonged glucocorticoid use. Pellagra from niacin deficiency can occur in extensive small bowel disease, and malabsorption of vitamin B_{12} can lead to a megaloblastic anemia and neurologic symptoms.

Diarrhea is a sign of active disease caused by bacterial overgrowth in obstructed areas, fistulization, bile acid malabsorption resulting from a diseased or resected terminal ileum, and intestinal inflammation with decreased water absorption and increased secretion of electrolytes.

Stricture formation can produce symptoms of bowel obstruction. Colonic disease may fistulize into the stomach or duodenum, causing feculent vomitus, or into the proximal or middle small bowel.

Up to one-third of patients with Crohn's disease have at least one extraintestinal manifestation of the disease, such as arthritis, a dermatologic condition, uveitis, or renal calculi. Patients with perianal Crohn's disease are at an even higher risk of developing extraintestinal manifestations (Table 18.4).

Treatment of Inflammatory Bowel Disease

Surgical Treatment

Crohn's disease is a recurring disorder that cannot be cured by surgical resection. However, some of the complications of Crohn's disease may require surgery. Patients with extensive

colonic disease may require a total proctocolectomy and end ileostomy. The most common surgery is resection of an area of small intestine involved in a fistula or obstruction. Resection of half of the small bowel comes close to the upper limit of resection, because removal of more than two-thirds of the small intestine results in *short bowel syndrome* and the need for parenteral nutrition.

Nearly half of patients with extensive chronic ulcerative colitis undergo surgery within the first 10 years of their illness; indications for surgery are listed in Table 18.5. The complication rate is approximately 20% in elective, 30% in urgent, and 40% in emergent proctocolectomy. The complications are primarily hemorrhage, sepsis, and neural injury. In contrast to Crohn's disease, a total proctocolectomy can be a curative procedure in ulcerative colitis. Newer versions of this surgery can maintain continence while surgically removing the involved rectal mucosa.

Medical Treatment

5-Acetylsalicylic acid (5-ASA) is the mainstay of therapy for mild to moderate inflammatory bowel disease. It was originally developed to deliver both antibacterial (sulfapyridine) and topical antiinflammatory (5-acetylsalicylic acid) therapy into the lumen of the small intestine and colon. 5-ASA is effective in inducing remission in both ulcerative colitis and Crohn's disease and in maintaining remission in ulcerative colitis. Adverse reactions to 5-ASA are uncommon. Sulfa-free aminosalicylate preparations such as mesalamine can deliver a larger amount of the pharmacologically active ingredient 5-acetylsalicylic acid to the site of active bowel disease while limiting systemic toxicity. There are many preparations of mesalamine available. Different tablet coatings can deliver the drug to different areas of the intestines and/or prolong drug effect.

The majority of patients with moderate to severe ulcerative colitis benefit from oral or parenteral glucocorticoids. Prednisone is usually started at dosages of 40–60 mg/day for active ulcerative colitis that is unresponsive to 5-ASA therapy. Topically applied glucocorticoids are beneficial for distal colitis and may serve as an adjunct in those who have rectal involvement. These glucocorticoids are absorbed from the rectum in significant amounts and can lead to adrenal suppression after prolonged use.

Glucocorticoids are also effective for treatment of moderate to severe Crohn's disease. Controlled-ileal-release budesonide is nearly equipotent to prednisone in treating ileocolonic Crohn's disease and has fewer glucocorticoid side effects. Steroids play no role in maintenance therapy in either ulcerative colitis or Crohn's disease. Once clinical remission has been induced, corticosteroids should be tapered and discontinued.

Antibiotics have no role in the treatment of active or quiescent ulcerative colitis. However, "pouchitis," which occurs in approximately one-third of ulcerative colitis patients after colectomy, usually responds to treatment with metronidazole or ciprofloxacin. These two antibiotics should be used as first-line drugs in perianal and fistulous Crohn's disease and as second-line therapy in active Crohn's disease after 5-acetylsalicylic acid drugs become ineffective.

Azathioprine and 6-mercaptopurine are purine analogues commonly used in the management of glucocorticoid-dependent inflammatory bowel syndromes. Azathioprine is readily absorbed and then converted to 6-mercaptopurine, which is then metabolized to an active end product. Efficacy is seen within 3–4 weeks. Pancreatitis occurs in 3%–4% of patients, generally within the first few weeks of therapy, and is completely reversible when these immunomodulatory drugs are discontinued.

Methotrexate inhibits dihydrofolate reductase, which results in impaired DNA synthesis. Additional antiinflammatory properties may be related to a decrease in interleukin (IL)-1 production.

Cyclosporine alters the immune response by acting as a potent inhibitor of T cell–mediated responses. Although cyclosporine acts primarily via inhibition of IL-2 production by helper T cells, it also decreases recruitment of cytotoxic T cells and blocks other cytokines, interferon-γ, and tumor necrosis factor. It has a more rapid onset of action than 6-mercaptopurine and azathioprine. Renal function should be monitored frequently. An increase in creatinine requires a dosage reduction or discontinuation of the drug.

Tacrolimus is a macrolide antibiotic with immunomodulatory properties similar to cyclosporine. A particular advantage of its use in inflammatory bowel disease is its excellent absorption in the small bowel even if bile is not present or the mucosa is not intact. Thus it can be taken orally with good effect.

Other biologic therapies are being used with Crohn's disease and ulcerative colitis. These include anti–tumor necrosis factor antibodies such as infliximab. Both of these diseases respond well to infliximab, but difficulties with this therapy include development of antibodies to infliximab and a significantly increased risk of development of certain forms of leukemia and lymphoma.

Natalizumab is an immunoglobulin antibody against α-integrin indicated for treatment of Crohn's disease refractory to or intolerant of anti–tumor necrosis factor therapy. It causes remission in about 40% of patients with advanced Crohn's disease. Its major adverse effect is the potential for development of progressive multifocal leukoencephalopathy (PML) associated with the Creutzfeldt-Jakob virus. The risk of developing PML with natalizumab therapy is about 1:1000.

TABLE 18.6	Secretory Characteristics of Carcinoid Tumors in Various Sites		
	Foregut	Midgut	Hindgut
Serotonin secretion	Low	High	Rare
Other substances secreted	ACTH, 5-HTP, GRF	Tachykinins; rarely 5-HTP, ACTH	Rarely 5-HTP, ACTH; other peptides
Carcinoid syndrome	Atypical	Typical	Rare

ACTH, Corticotropin; GRF, growth hormone–releasing factor; 5HTP, 5-hydroxytryptophan.

TABLE 18.7	Location and Presentation of Carcinoid Tumors
Carcinoid Location	Presentation
Small intestine	Abdominal pain (51%), intestinal obstruction (31%), tumor (17%), gastrointestinal bleeding (11%)
Rectum	Bleeding (39%), constipation (17%), diarrhea (17%)
Bronchus	Asymptomatic (31%)
Thymus	Anterior mediastinal mass
Ovary and testicle	Mass discovered on physical examination or ultrasonography
Metastases	In the liver; frequently presents as hepatomegaly

CARCINOID TUMORS

Carcinoid tumors originate from the GI tract most of the time. They can occur in almost any GI tissue. Less than a quarter of carcinoid tumors are first found in the lung. These tumors typically secrete GI peptides and/or vasoactive substances (Table 18.6).

Carcinoid Tumors Without Carcinoid Syndrome

Carcinoid tumors (Table 18.7) are often found incidentally during surgery for suspected appendicitis. Symptoms are often vague, so the diagnosis is often delayed.

Carcinoid Tumors With Systemic Symptoms Due to Secreted Products

Carcinoid tumors can contain GI peptides such as gastrin, insulin, somatostatin, motilin, neurotensin, tachykinins (substance K, substance P, neuropeptide K), glucagon, gastrin-releasing peptide, vasoactive intestinal peptide, pancreatic peptide, other biologically active peptides (corticotropin, calcitonin, growth hormone), prostaglandins, and bioactive amines (serotonin). These substances may or may not be released by the tumor in sufficient amounts to cause symptoms. Midgut carcinoids are more likely to produce various peptides than foregut carcinoids. Only 25% of carcinoids are capable of producing mediators; carcinoids that do not often present as a mass and/or bowel obstruction.

Carcinoid Syndrome

Carcinoid syndrome occurs in approximately 10% of patients with carcinoid tumors and is a result of the large amounts of serotonin and vasoactive substances reaching the systemic circulation. The two most common signs are flushing and diarrhea (with the associated dehydration and electrolyte abnormalities). The characteristic flush is of sudden onset. Physically it appears as a deep red blush, especially in the neck and face, often associated with a feeling of warmth and occasionally associated with pruritus, tearing, diarrhea, or facial edema. Hypotension and hypertension can occur, as well as bronchoconstriction. Flushes may be precipitated by stress, alcohol, exercise, certain foods, and drugs such as catecholamines, pentagastrin, and serotonin reuptake inhibitors. Carcinoid tumors may have cardiac manifestations resulting from endocardial fibrosis, primarily on the chambers of the right side of the heart and on the tricuspid and pulmonic valves. Usually the left side of the heart is protected from this disease because of the ability of the lung to clear the vasoactive substances secreted by the carcinoid tumor. But left-sided lesions can occur if there is pulmonary involvement or via a right-to-left intracardiac shunt. Other clinical manifestations include wheezing and pellagra-like skin lesions. Retroperitoneal fibrosis can cause ureteral obstruction.

Most patients with carcinoid syndrome overproduce serotonin, which is responsible for the diarrhea through its effects on gut motility and intestinal secretion. Serotonin receptor antagonists relieve the diarrhea in most patients. Serotonin does not, however, appear to be involved in the flushing. In patients with gastric carcinoid tumors the red, patchy, pruritic flush is likely due to histamine release and can be prevented by H_1- and H_2-receptor blockers. Both histamine and serotonin may be responsible for bronchoconstriction.

A potentially life-threatening complication of carcinoid syndrome is development of a *carcinoid crisis*. Clinically this manifests as intense flushing, diarrhea, abdominal pain, and cardiovascular signs, including tachycardia, hypertension, or hypotension. If not adequately treated, it can be fatal. The crisis may occur spontaneously or be provoked by stress, chemotherapy, or biopsy. Anesthetic drugs that can precipitate a carcinoid crisis are noted in Table 18.8.

The diagnosis of carcinoid syndrome relies on measurement of urinary or plasma serotonin concentrations or measurement of serotonin metabolites in the urine. The measurement of 5-hydroxyindoleacetic acid (5-HIAA) is performed most frequently. False-positive test results may occur if the patient is eating serotonin-rich foods.

TABLE 18.8	Drugs Associated With Carcinoid Crisis

DRUGS THAT MAY PROVOKE MEDIATOR RELEASE
Succinylcholine, mivacurium, atracurium, tubocurarine
Epinephrine, norepinephrine, dopamine, isoproterenol, thiopental

DRUGS NOT KNOWN TO RELEASE MEDIATORS
Propofol, etomidate, vecuronium, cisatracurium, rocuronium, sufentanil, alfentanil, fentanyl, remifentanil
All inhalation agents; desflurane may be the better choice in patients with liver metastasis because of its low rate of metabolism.

Treatment

Therapy for carcinoid tumors includes avoiding conditions that precipitate flushing, treating heart failure and/or wheezing, providing dietary supplementation with nicotinamide, and controlling diarrhea. If the patient continues to have symptoms, serotonin receptor antagonists or somatostatin analogues are useful. Many of these drugs have very short half-lives and must be given as continuous infusions. The 5-HT_1 and 5-HT_2 receptor antagonists can control the diarrhea but usually do not decrease flushing. The 5-HT_3 receptor antagonists (e.g., ondansetron, tropisetron, alosetron) can control diarrhea and nausea in the majority of patients and even occasionally ameliorate the flushing. A combination of H_1- and H_2-receptor antagonists may be useful in controlling flushing.

Most neuroendocrine tumors have somatostatin receptors on their cells, so somatostatin can bind to these receptors and prevent symptoms, including flushing. Synthetic analogues of somatostatin such as octreotide control symptoms in more than 80% of patients with a carcinoid tumor. Lanreotide is the most widely used drug in this class. It is given in a depot form by subcutaneous injection every 4 weeks. Somatostatin analogues are effective in both relieving symptoms and decreasing urinary 5-HIAA levels. They can also prevent development of a carcinoid crisis during known precipitating events such as surgery, anesthesia, chemotherapy, and stress. Octreotide should be administered 24–48 hours before surgery and then continued throughout the procedure.

The bronchoconstriction of carcinoid tumors is typically resistant to treatment, and β-agonists may exacerbate the problem owing to mediator release. Octreotide and histamine blockers combined with ipratropium have been used with good results.

Transarterial chemoembolization (TACE) with or without chemotherapy can reduce tumor size in most patients, but surgery is the only potentially curative therapy for nonmetastatic carcinoid tumors.

Management of Anesthesia

General anesthesia is required for carcinoid tumor resection surgery. No single anesthetic medication has been associated with worse outcomes during this kind of surgery, but it is suggested to avoid histamine-releasing medications. Invasive arterial blood pressure monitoring is necessary for intraoperative management because of the potential for rapid changes in hemodynamic variables. Administration of octreotide preoperatively and before manipulation of the tumor will attenuate most adverse hemodynamic responses. Ondansetron, a serotonin antagonist, is a good antiemetic for these patients. Delayed awakening in this patient population has been described, and patients may need to be admitted to the intensive care unit for postoperative monitoring. Symptoms may persist postoperatively if the surgery was palliative, there is known metastatic disease, or there are undiagnosed metastases.

Use of epidural analgesia in patients who have been adequately treated with octreotide is a safe technique, provided the local anesthetic is administered in a gradual manner accompanied by careful hemodynamic monitoring.

ACUTE PANCREATITIS

Acute pancreatitis is an acute inflammatory disorder of the pancreas. The incidence has increased 10-fold since the 1960s, which could reflect increased alcohol use and/or improved diagnostic techniques.

Pathogenesis

The pancreas contains numerous digestive enzymes (proteases). Autodigestion of the pancreas is normally prevented by packaging of the proteases in precursor form, synthesis of protease inhibitors, and the low intrapancreatic concentration of calcium, which decreases trypsin activity. Loss of any of these protective mechanisms leads to enzyme activation, autodigestion, and acute pancreatitis.

Gallstones and alcohol abuse are the causative factors in 60%–80% of patients with acute pancreatitis. Gallstones are believed to cause pancreatitis by transiently obstructing the ampulla of Vater, which causes pancreatic ductal hypertension. Acute pancreatitis is also common in patients with acquired immunodeficiency syndrome and those with hyperparathyroidism and its associated hypercalcemia. Trauma-induced acute pancreatitis is generally associated with blunt trauma rather than penetrating injury. Blunt trauma may compress the pancreas against the spine. Postoperative pancreatitis can occur after abdominal and other noncardiac surgery and after cardiac surgery, especially procedures that require cardiopulmonary bypass. Clinical pancreatitis develops in 1%–2% of patients following endoscopic retrograde cholangiopancreatography (ERCP).

Excruciating, unrelenting midepigastric pain that radiates to the back occurs in almost every patient with acute pancreatitis. Sitting and leaning forward may decrease the pain. Nausea and vomiting can occur at the peak of the pain. Abdominal distention with ileus often develops. Dyspnea may reflect the presence of pleural effusions or ascites. Low-grade fever, tachycardia, and hypotension are fairly common. Shock may

occur as a result of (1) hypovolemia from exudation of blood and plasma into the retroperitoneal space, (2) release of kinins that cause vasodilation and increase capillary permeability, and (3) systemic effects of pancreatic enzymes released into the general circulation.

Obtundation and psychosis may reflect alcohol withdrawal. Tetany may occur as a result of hypocalcemia, since in this situation calcium binds to free fatty acids and forms soaps.

The hallmark of acute pancreatitis is an increase in serum amylase and lipase concentration. Contrast-enhanced computed tomography is the best noninvasive test for documenting the morphologic changes associated with acute pancreatitis. ERCP can be useful for evaluating and treating certain forms of pancreatitis such as traumatic pancreatitis (localization of injury) and severe gallstone pancreatitis (papillotomy, stone removal, and drainage).

The differential diagnosis of acute pancreatitis includes a perforated duodenal ulcer, acute cholecystitis, mesenteric ischemia, and bowel obstruction. Acute myocardial infarction may cause severe abdominal pain, but the serum amylase concentration is not increased. Patients with pneumonia may also have significant epigastric pain and fever.

Multifactor scoring systems have been devised to help identify high-risk patients. One such system is the Ranson criteria. These criteria include (1) age older than 55 years, (2) white blood cell count above 16,000 cells/mm^3, (3) blood urea nitrogen concentration above 16 mmol/L, (4) aspartate transaminase level above 250 units/L, (5) arterial Pao$_2$ below 60 mm Hg, (6) fluid deficit greater than 6 L, (7) blood glucose level above 200 mg/dL in a person without a history of diabetes mellitus, (8) lactate dehydrogenase level above 350 IU/L, (9) corrected calcium concentration less than 8 mg/dL, (10) a decrease in hematocrit of more than 10, and (11) metabolic acidosis with a base deficit greater than 4 mmol/L. It is noteworthy that the serum amylase concentration is not one of the criteria.

In the Ranson scoring system, mortality is related to the number of criteria present. Patients with 0–2 criteria have a mortality rate below 5%. Patients meeting 3 or 4 criteria have a 20% mortality rate; those with 5 or 6 criteria have a 40% mortality rate. The presence of 7 or 8 criteria is associated with nearly 100% mortality.

Complications

About 25% of patients who develop acute pancreatitis experience significant complications. Shock can develop early in the course and is a major risk factor for death. Sequestration of large volumes of fluid in the peripancreatic space, hemorrhage, and systemic vasodilation contribute to hypotension. Arterial hypoxemia is often present early in the course of the disease. ARDS is seen in 20% of patients. Renal failure occurs in 25% of patients and is associated with a poor prognosis. GI hemorrhage and coagulation defects from disseminated intravascular coagulation may occur. Infection of necrotic pancreatic material or abscess formation is a serious complication associated with a mortality rate higher than 50%.

Treatment

Aggressive intravenous fluid administration is necessary to treat the significant hypovolemia that occurs in all patients, even those with mild pancreatitis. Colloid replacement may be necessary. Traditionally, oral intake is stopped to rest the pancreas and prevent aggravation of the accompanying ileus. Some data suggest that feeding patients via a postpyloric route such as a nasojejunal tube or feeding jejunostomy may be helpful, especially in patients who are intubated and mechanically ventilated as a result of ARDS or renal failure. Parenteral feeding is indicated if patients do not tolerate enteral feeding. Nasogastric suction may be needed to treat persistent vomiting or ileus. Opioids are administered to manage the severe pain. Endoscopic removal of obstructing gallstones is indicated early after the onset of symptoms to decrease the risk of cholangitis. Drainage of intraabdominal collections of fluids or necrotic material can now be accomplished without surgery.

ERCP is a fluoroscopic examination of the biliary or pancreatic ducts by endoscopically guided injection of contrast through the duodenal papilla. Interventions via ERCP include drainage through tubes of various sizes that can be changed (upsized) if needed. Other interventions include stent placement, sphincterotomy, stone extraction, and hemostasis.

Chronic Pancreatitis

The incidence of chronic pancreatitis is difficult to determine, since the disease may be asymptomatic or abdominal pain may be attributed to other causes. The persistent inflammation characteristic of chronic pancreatitis leads to irreversible damage to the pancreas. There is loss of both exocrine and endocrine function.

Chronic pancreatitis is most often due to chronic alcohol abuse. Alcohol may have a direct toxic effect on the pancreas. Diets high in protein seem to predispose alcoholic patients to the development of chronic pancreatitis. Up to 25% of adults in the United States with chronic pancreatitis are diagnosed with *idiopathic chronic pancreatitis;* it has been suggested that a significant number of these cases could be related to genetic defects. Chronic pancreatitis also occurs in association with cystic fibrosis and hyperparathyroidism.

Chronic pancreatitis is often characterized as epigastric pain that radiates to the back and is frequently postprandial. However, up to one-third of patients have painless chronic pancreatitis. Steatorrhea is present when at least 90% of pancreatic exocrine function is lost. Diabetes mellitus is the end result of loss of endocrine function. Pancreatic calcifications develop in most patients with alcohol-induced chronic pancreatitis.

The diagnosis of chronic pancreatitis may be based on a history of chronic alcohol abuse and demonstration of pancreatic calcifications. Patients who have chronic pancreatitis are often thin or even emaciated. This is due to maldigestion of proteins and fats because the amount of pancreatic enzymes entering the duodenum is reduced to less than 20% of normal. Serum amylase concentrations are usually normal. Ultrasonography is useful for documenting the presence of an enlarged pancreas or identifying a pseudocyst. Computed tomography in patients with chronic pancreatitis demonstrates dilated pancreatic ducts and changes in the size of the pancreas. ERCP is the most sensitive imaging test for detecting early changes in the pancreatic ducts caused by chronic pancreatitis.

Treatment of chronic pancreatitis includes management of pain, malabsorption, and diabetes mellitus. Opioids are often required for adequate pain control, and in some patients, celiac plexus blockade may be considered. An internal surgical drainage procedure (pancreaticojejunostomy) or endoscopic placement of stents and/or extraction of stones may be helpful in patients whose pain is resistant to medical management. Enzyme supplements are administered to facilitate fat and protein absorption. Insulin is administered as needed.

GASTROINTESTINAL BLEEDING

GI bleeding (Table 18.9) most often originates in the upper GI tract (from peptic ulcer disease). Bleeding in the lower GI tract from diverticulosis or tumor accounts for about 10%–20% of cases of GI bleeding and commonly affects older patients.

Upper Gastrointestinal Tract Bleeding

Patients with acute upper GI tract bleeding may experience hypotension and tachycardia if blood loss exceeds 25% of total blood volume. Patients with *orthostatic hypotension* generally have a hematocrit below 30%. The hematocrit may be normal early in the course of acute hemorrhage because there has been insufficient time for equilibration of plasma volume. After fluid resuscitation, anemia becomes more overt. Melena indicates that bleeding has occurred at a site above the

TABLE 18.9	Common Causes of Upper and Lower Gastrointestinal Tract Bleeding
Cause	Incidence (%)
UPPER GASTROINTESTINAL TRACT BLEEDING	
Peptic ulcer	
Duodenal ulcer	36
Gastric ulcer	24
Mucosal erosive disease	
Gastritis	6
Esophagitis	6
Esophageal varices	6
Mallory-Weiss tear	3
Malignancy	2
LOWER GASTROINTESTINAL TRACT BLEEDING	
Colonic diverticulosis	42
Colorectal malignancy	9
Ischemic colitis	9
Acute colitis of unknown cause	5
Hemorrhoids	5

Adapted from Young HS. Gastrointestinal bleeding. *Sci Am Med.* 1998:1-10.

cecum. Blood urea nitrogen levels are typically above 40 mg/dL because of absorbed nitrogen from the blood in the small intestine. Elderly individuals, those with esophageal variceal bleeding, those with malignancy, and those who develop bleeding during hospitalization for other medical conditions have a mortality rate exceeding 30%. Multiple organ system failure rather than hemorrhage is the usual cause of death in such patients. Upper endoscopy after hemodynamic stabilization is the diagnostic/therapeutic procedure of choice in patients with acute upper GI bleeding.

For patients with bleeding peptic ulcers, endoscopic coagulation (thermotherapy or injection with epinephrine or a sclerosing material) is indicated when active bleeding is visible. Even patients receiving anticoagulants can be safely treated with endoscopic coagulation of a peptic ulcer. Perforation occurs in approximately 0.5% of patients undergoing endoscopic coagulation. With bleeding esophageal varices, endoscopic ligation of the bleeding varices is as effective as sclerotherapy. A transjugular intrahepatic portosystemic shunt (TIPS) may be used in patients with esophageal variceal bleeding resistant to control by endoscopic coagulation or sclerotherapy. However, insertion of such a shunt can lead to worsening encephalopathy. Mechanical balloon tamponade of bleeding varices can be accomplished with a Blakemore-Sengstaken tube. However, such a device is rarely used now that endoscopic therapy for bleeding varices is so successful. Surgical treatment of nonvariceal upper GI tract bleeding may be undertaken to oversew an ulcer or perform gastrectomy for diffuse hemorrhagic gastritis in patients who continue to bleed despite optimal supportive therapy and in whom endoscopic coagulation is unsuccessful.

EGD is overall quite safe for evaluation of upper GI bleeding. However, cardiopulmonary complications remain a concern because of the potential for aspiration of blood and/or gastric contents and the presence of other medical conditions. Endotracheal intubation is the preferred method for airway protection for upper GI bleeding severe enough to require endoscopy.

Lower Gastrointestinal Tract Bleeding

Lower GI tract (colonic) bleeding usually occurs in older patients and typically presents as abrupt passage of bright red blood and clots via the rectum. Causes include diverticulosis, tumors, ischemic colitis, and certain forms of infectious colitis. Sigmoidoscopy to exclude anorectal lesions is indicated as soon as a patient is hemodynamically stable. Colonoscopy can be performed after the bowel has been cleansed. If bleeding is persistent and brisk, angiography and embolic therapy may be attempted. Up to 15% of patients with lower GI tract bleeding require surgical intervention to control it.

ADYNAMIC ILEUS

Adynamic ileus, formerly known as *acute colonic pseudo-obstruction,* is a form of colonic ileus characterized by massive dilatation of the colon in the absence of a mechanical obstruction. The disorder is characterized by loss of effective colonic peristalsis and subsequent distention of the colon. This syndrome generally develops in seriously ill patients hospitalized for major medical problems. These patients have electrolyte disorders, are immobile, or have received narcotic or anticholinergic medications. The disorder can also be observed in surgical patients after a variety of non-GI operations. If left untreated, the colonic dilatation could result in ischemia of the right colon and cecum and, if the ileocecal valve is competent, in perforation. One hypothesis as to the etiology of colonic pseudo-obstruction invokes an imbalance in neural input to the colon distal to the splenic flexure. It suggests an *excess of sympathetic stimulation* and a *paucity of parasympathetic input.* This can result in spastic contraction of the distal colon and functional obstruction. Plain radiographs of the abdomen reveal dilatation of the proximal colon and a decompressed distal colon, with some air in the rectosigmoid region. Patients in whom the cecal diameter is less than 12 cm (risk of perforation is much greater if cecal diameter exceeds 12 cm) can undergo an initial trial of conservative therapy. This would include correction of electrolyte abnormalities, avoidance of narcotic and anticholinergic drugs, hydration, mobilization, tap water enemas, and nasogastric suction. The majority of patients who will have resolution of this problem with conservative therapy will have this happen within 2 days. This suggests that a 48-hour trial of conservative management is warranted in patients in stable condition. Patients for whom conservative therapy fails should be considered for an active intervention. This could include repetitive colonoscopy or administration of neostigmine. Intravenous neostigmine at a dose of 2–2.5 mg given over 3–5 minutes results in immediate colonic decompression in 80%–90% of patients, presumably by improving parasympathetic tone in the bowel. Because symptomatic bradycardia is an expected side effect of neostigmine administration, all patients undergoing this treatment require cardiac monitoring. Placement of a cecostomy is another active intervention that may be needed.

KEY POINTS

- Natural antireflux mechanisms consist of the lower esophageal sphincter, the crural diaphragm, and the anatomic location of the gastroesophageal junction below the diaphragmatic hiatus.
- Factors that contribute to the likelihood of aspiration during anesthesia and surgery include the urgency of surgery, the presence of a difficult airway, inadequate anesthetic depth, lithotomy position, increased intraabdominal pressure, insulin-dependent diabetes mellitus, autonomic neuropathy, pregnancy, severe illness, and obesity.
- Patients with silent aspiration may present with symptoms and signs of bronchial asthma.
- All patients who have undergone esophagectomy have a lifelong very high risk of aspiration.

- Major trauma accompanied by shock, sepsis, respiratory failure, hemorrhage, massive transfusion, burns, head injury, or multiorgan injury is often associated with development of acute stress gastritis.
- Following gastric surgery for peptic ulcer disease or gastric neoplasm, patients may develop dumping syndrome or alkaline reflux gastritis.
- Inflammatory bowel diseases are the second most common chronic inflammatory diseases (after rheumatoid arthritis). Ulcerative colitis and Crohn's disease are associated with abdominal pain, fluid and electrolyte disturbances, bleeding, bowel perforation, peritonitis, fistula formation, GI tract obstruction, cancer, and numerous extraintestinal manifestations of the diseases.
- Carcinoid tumors may be associated with carcinoid syndrome due to release of large amounts of serotonin and other vasoactive substances into the systemic circulation, causing flushing, diarrhea, tachycardia, hypertension, or hypotension.
- Gallstones and alcohol abuse cause the majority of cases of acute pancreatitis. Chronic pancreatitis is usually caused by chronic alcohol abuse, but up to 25% of cases are labeled as idiopathic in origin.
- Gastrointestinal bleeding most often originates in the upper GI tract and is often due to peptic ulcer disease. About 20% of GI bleeding originates in the lower GI tract and can be due to diverticulosis, tumors, ischemic colitis, or certain forms of infectious colitis.

RESOURCES

Agrawal D, Elsbernd B, Singal A, Rockey D. Gastric residual volume after split-dose compared with evening-before polyethylene glycol bowel preparation. *Gastrointest Endosc*. 2015;83:574-580.

Aitkenhead AR. Anaesthesia and bowel surgery. *Br J Anaesth*. 1984;56:95-101.

Bowers SP. Esophageal motility disorders. *Surg Clin North Am*. 2015;95:467-482.

Cortinez FLI. Refractory hypotension during carcinoid resection surgery. *Anaesthesia*. 2000;55:505-506.

Cooper GS, Kou TD, Rex DK. Complications following colonoscopy with anesthesia assistance: a population-based analysis. *JAMA Intern Med*. 2013;173:551-556.

Dantoc MM, Cox MR, Eslick GD. Does minimally invasive esophagectomy (MIE) provide for comparable oncologic outcomes to open techniques? *J Gastrointest Surg*. 2012;16:486-494.

Dierdorf SF. Carcinoid tumor and carcinoid syndrome. *Curr Opin Anaesthesiol*. 2003;16:343-347.

Hunter AR. Colorectal surgery for cancer: the anaesthetist's contribution. *Br J Anaesth*. 1986;58:825-826.

Lohse N, Lundstrom LH, Vestergaard TR, et al. Anaesthesia care with and without tracheal intubation during emergency endoscopy for peptic ulcer bleeding: a population-based cohort study. *Br J Anaesth*. 2015;114:901-908.

Longo DL, Fauci AS, Kasper DL, et al., eds. Disorders of the gastrointestinal system. In: *Harrison's Principles of Internal Medicine*. 18th ed. New York: McGraw-Hill; 2012:2402.

Mulholland MW, Lillemoe KD, Doherty GM. *Greenfield's Surgery: Scientific Principles and Practice*. Philadelphia: Lippincott Williams & Wilkins; 2006.

Navaneethan U, Eubanks S. Approach to patients with esophageal dysphagia. *Surg Clin North Am*. 2015;95:483-489.

Ng A, Smith G. Gastroesophageal reflux and aspiration of gastric contents in anesthetic practice. *Anesth Analg*. 2001;93:494-513.

Patino M, Glynn S, Soberano M, et al. Comparison of different anesthesia techniques during esophagogastroduodenoscopy in children: a randomized trial. *Ped Anesth*. 2015;25:1013-1019.

Redmond MC. Perianesthesia care of the patient with gastroesophageal reflux disease. *J Perianesthesia Nurs*. 2003;18:535-544.

Rudolph SJ, Landsverk BK, Freeman ML. Endotracheal intubation for airway protection during endoscopy for severe upper GI hemorrhage. *Gastrointest Endosc*. 2003;57:58-61.

Salem MR, Khoransani A, Saatee S, et al. Gastric tubes and airway management in patients at risk of aspiration: History, current concepts, and proposal of an algorithm. *Anesth Analg*. 2014;118:569-579.

Sanghera SS, Nurkin SJ, Demmy TL. Quality of life after an esophagectomy. *Surg Clin North Am*. 2012;92:1315-1535.

Sontag SJ, O'Connell S, Khandewal S, et al. Most asthmatics have gastroesophageal reflux with or without bronchodilator therapy. *Gastroenterology*. 1990;99:613-620.

Steinberg W, Tenner S. Acute pancreatitis. *N Engl J Med*. 1994;330:1198-1210.

Young HS. Diseases of the pancreas. *Sci Am Med*. 1997:1-16.

Young HS. Gastrointestinal bleeding. *Sci Am Med*. 1998:1-10.

Inborn Errors of Metabolism

HOSSAM TANTAWY, JING TAO

Inborn errors of metabolism manifest as a variety of metabolic defects that may complicate the management of anesthesia (Table 19.1). In some instances these defects are clinically asymptomatic and become manifest only in response to specific triggering events, such as ingestion of certain foods or administration of certain drugs, including some anesthetic drugs.

PORPHYRIAS

Porphyrias are a group of metabolic disorders, each of which results from deficiency of a specific enzyme in the heme synthetic pathway. The synthetic pathway of porphyrins is determined by a sequence of enzymes. A defect in any of these enzymes results in accumulation of the preceding intermediate form of porphyrin and produces a form of *porphyria* (Fig. 19.1). In human physiology, heme is the most important porphyrin and is bound to proteins to form hemoproteins that include hemoglobin and cytochrome P450 isoenzymes. Production of heme is regulated by the activity of aminolevulinic acid (ALA) synthase, which is present in mitochondria. The formation of ALA synthase is controlled by endogenous concentrations of heme in a feedback loop that ensures that the

level of heme production parallels requirements. ALA synthase is readily inducible, and therefore its supply can respond rapidly to increased heme requirements such as those resulting from administration of drugs that need cytochrome P450 isoenzymes for their metabolism. In the presence of porphyria, any increase in heme requirements results in accumulation of pathway intermediates.

Classification

Porphyrias are classified as either *hepatic* or *erythropoietic* depending on the primary site of overproduction or accumulation of the precursor porphyrin (Table 19.2). However, for anesthesiologists, the more functional classification of *acute* versus *nonacute* porphyrias may be more important, since only acute forms of porphyria are relevant to the management of anesthesia (Table 19.3). They are the only forms of porphyria that can result in life-threatening reactions in response to drugs often used in the perioperative period.

Acute Porphyrias

Acute porphyrias are inherited autosomal dominant disorders with variable expression. The enzyme defects in these forms of porphyria are deficiencies rather than absolute deficits of heme pathway enzymes. Although there is no direct influence of gender on the pattern of inheritance, attacks occur more frequently in women and are most frequent during the third and fourth decades of life. Attacks are rare before puberty or following the onset of menopause. Acute attacks of porphyria are most commonly precipitated by events that *decrease* heme concentrations and thus *increase* the activity of ALA synthase and stimulate production of porphyrinogens. Enzyme-inducing drugs are the

TABLE 19.1	Selected Inborn Errors of Metabolism

Porphyria
Purine metabolism disorders
Carbohydrate metabolism disorders
Hemochromatosis
Wilson disease

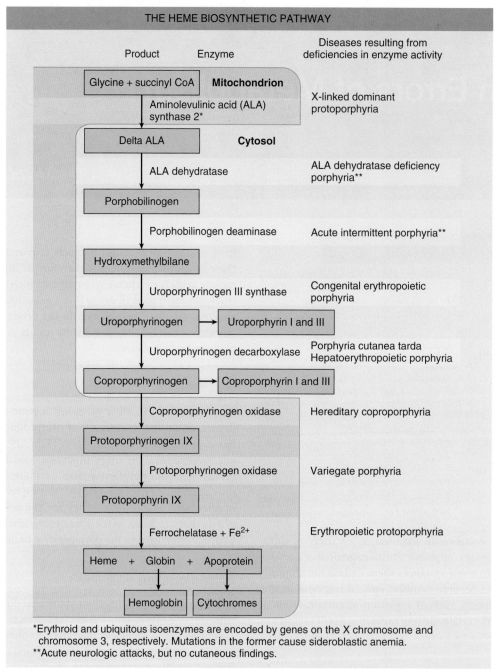

THE HEME BIOSYNTHETIC PATHWAY

Product   Enzyme   Diseases resulting from
                                              deficiencies in enzyme activity

Glycine + succinyl CoA   **Mitochondrion**

    Aminolevulinic acid (ALA)   X-linked dominant
    synthase 2*   protoporphyria

Delta ALA   **Cytosol**

    ALA dehydratase   ALA dehydratase deficiency
                                             porphyria**

Porphobilinogen

    Porphobilinogen deaminase   Acute intermittent porphyria**

Hydroxymethylbilane

    Uroporphyrinogen III synthase   Congenital erythropoietic
                                             porphyria

Uroporphyrinogen → Uroporphyrin I and III

    Uroporphyrinogen decarboxylase   Porphyria cutanea tarda
                                             Hepatoerythropoietic porphyria

Coproporphyrinogen → Coproporphyrin I and III

    Coproporphyrinogen oxidase   Hereditary coproporphyria

Protoporphyrinogen IX

    Protoporphyrinogen oxidase   Variegate porphyria

Protoporphyrin IX

    Ferrochelatase + Fe^{2+} Erythropoietic protoporphyria

Heme + Globin + Apoprotein

Hemoglobin   Cytochromes

*Erythroid and ubiquitous isoenzymes are encoded by genes on the X chromosome and
chromosome 3, respectively. Mutations in the former cause sideroblastic anemia.
**Acute neurologic attacks, but no cutaneous findings.

FIG. 19.1   The heme biosynthetic pathway. The enzyme facilitating each step in this pathway is noted, as well as the type of porphyria created by that particular enzyme deficiency. (From Bolognia JL, Schaffer JV, Duncan KO, Ko, CJ. *Dermatology Essentials.* Philadelphia: Elsevier; 2014, Fig. 41.1.)

most important triggers in the development of acute porphyria. However, these acute attacks may also be precipitated by physiologic hormonal fluctuations such as those that accompany menstruation, fasting (e.g., before elective surgery), dehydration, stress (e.g., associated with anesthesia and surgery), and infection. Pregnancy in patients with acute porphyria is often associated with spontaneous abortion. Furthermore, pregnancy may be complicated by systemic hypertension and an increased incidence of low-birth-weight infants.

Acute Intermittent Porphyria

Of all the acute porphyrias, acute intermittent porphyria affecting the central and peripheral nervous systems produces the most serious symptoms and signs and is the one most likely to be life threatening. The defective enzyme is porphobilinogen deaminase, and the gene encoding this enzyme is located on chromosome 11. Since the enzyme block is early in the heme synthetic pathway, an excess of these early precursors of heme can cause development of an acute attack but not skin disease.

TABLE 19.2	Traditional Classification of Porphyrias

HEPATIC
Acute intermittent porphyria
Variegate porphyria
Hereditary coproporphyria
Aminolevulinic acid dehydratase porphyria
Porphyria cutanea tarda

ERYTHROPOIETIC
Congenital erythropoietic protoporphyria
Erythropoietic protoporphyria
X-linked protoporphyria

TABLE 19.3	Acute and Nonacute Porphyrias

ACUTE PORPHYRIAS
Acute intermittent porphyria
Variegate porphyria
Hereditary coproporphyria
Aminolevulinic acid dehydratase porphyria

NONACUTE PORPHYRIAS
Porphyria cutanea tarda
Congenital erythropoietic protoporphyria
Erythropoietic protoporphyria
X-linked protoporphyria

Variegate Porphyria

Variegate porphyria is characterized by neurotoxicity *and* cutaneous photosensitivity. The skin lesions are bullous eruptions that occur on exposure to sunlight as a result of conversion of porphyrinogens to porphyrins. This photosensitivity can be attributed to increases in light-absorbing porphyrin intermediates and their metabolites. The enzyme defect is late in the heme synthetic pathway at the level of protoporphyrinogen oxidase, and the gene encoding this enzyme is on chromosome 1.

Hereditary Coproporphyria

Acute attacks of hereditary coproporphyria are less common and less severe than attacks of acute intermittent porphyria or variegate porphyria. These patients typically experience neurotoxicity and cutaneous hypersensitivity, although these signs tend to be less severe than is seen in variegate porphyria. The defective enzyme is coproporphyrinogen oxidase, encoded by a gene on chromosome 9.

ALA Dehydratase Porphyria

ALA dehydratase (ALAD) porphyria is a rare autosomal recessive disorder. The gene encoding ALAD is on chromosome 9.

Nonacute Porphyrias

Porphyria Cutanea Tarda

Porphyria cutanea tarda is due to an enzymatic defect (decreased hepatic activity of uroporphyrinogen decarboxylase) transmitted as an autosomal dominant trait. ALA synthase activity is unimportant in this form of porphyria, and drugs capable of precipitating attacks in other forms of porphyria *do not* provoke acute attacks in this porphyria. Likewise, neurotoxicity does not accompany this form of porphyria. Signs and symptoms of porphyria cutanea tarda appear as photosensitivity reactions, especially in men older than 35 years. Porphyrin accumulation in the liver can be associated with hepatocellular necrosis. Anesthetic drugs are not hazardous in affected patients, although the choice of drugs should take into consideration the likely presence of liver disease.

Congenital Erythropoietic Protoporphyria

Erythropoietic porphyrias are forms of porphyria that, in contrast to porphyrin synthesis in the liver, have porphyrin synthesis in the red blood cells in bone marrow. Congenital erythropoietic protoporphyria (CEP) is a rare form of porphyria transmitted as an autosomal recessive trait. Hemolytic anemia, bone marrow hyperplasia, and splenomegaly are often present. Infections are common, and photosensitivity can be severe. Of note, the urine of affected patients turns red when exposed to light. Neurotoxicity and abdominal pain *do not* occur, and administration of barbiturates does not adversely affect this disease. Death often occurs during childhood.

Erythropoietic Protoporphyria

Erythropoietic protoporphyria (EPP) is a much more common and less debilitating form of erythropoietic porphyria. Signs and symptoms include photosensitivity, vesicular cutaneous eruptions, and edema. In occasional patients, cholelithiasis develops secondary to increased excretion of protoporphyrin. Administration of barbiturates does not adversely affect the course of the disease, and survival to adulthood is common.

X-Linked Protoporphyria

This form of erythropoietic porphyria has only recently been identified. Its clinical manifestation is very similar to that of EPP except for its mode of inheritance and the degree of zinc binding to red blood cell protoporphyrins.

Acute Attacks of Porphyria

Acute attacks of porphyria are characterized by severe abdominal pain, autonomic nervous system instability, electrolyte disturbances, and neuropsychiatric manifestations ranging from mild to life-threatening events. Skeletal muscle weakness that may progress to quadriparesis and respiratory failure is a potentially lethal neurologic manifestation of an acute attack of porphyria. Central nervous system involvement is likely the result of increased concentrations of ALA in the brain. This chemical appears to be toxic to the brain. Central nervous system manifestations of acute porphyria include upper motor neuron lesions and cranial nerve palsies, with abnormalities of the cerebellum and basal ganglia seen less frequently. These neurologic lesions in combination with autonomic neuropathy and hypovolemia can cause significant cardiovascular instability. Seizures may occur during an attack of acute porphyria. Psychiatric disturbances may develop, but despite classic tales of so-called werewolf behavior and other bizarre psychiatric problems, mental disorders are not very common.

Gastrointestinal symptoms of acute porphyria include abdominal pain, vomiting, and diarrhea. However, despite severe abdominal pain that may mimic acute appendicitis, acute cholecystitis, or renal colic, clinical examination of the abdomen is typically normal. Abdominal pain is thought to be related to autonomic neuropathy. Dehydration and electrolyte disturbances involving sodium, potassium, and magnesium may be prominent. Tachycardia and hypertension or, less commonly, hypotension are manifestations of cardiovascular instability.

Complete and prolonged remissions are likely between episodes, and many individuals with the genetic defect of a porphyria never develop symptoms. It is important to note, however, that patients at known risk of porphyria but previously asymptomatic (silent or latent porphyria) may experience their first symptoms in response to administration of triggering drugs during the perioperative period. ALA synthase concentrations are increased during all acute attacks of porphyria.

Triggering Drugs

Drugs may trigger an acute attack of porphyria by inducing the activity of ALA synthase or interfering with the negative feedback control at the final common pathway of heme synthesis. It is not possible to predict which drugs will be porphyrinogenic, although chemical groupings such as the allyl groups present on barbiturates and certain steroid structures have been incriminated in the induction of porphyria. *Only the acute forms of porphyria are affected by drug-induced enzyme induction.* It is not clear why the manifestations of nonacute porphyrias are apparently unaffected by enzyme-inducing drugs.

Labeling drugs as safe or unsafe for patients with porphyria is often based on anecdotal experience with the use of particular drugs in porphyric patients and reports of induction of acute attacks. Drugs may be tested in cell culture models for their ability to induce ALA synthase activity or for their effects on porphyrin synthesis. Alternatively, the action of drugs on the porphyrin synthetic pathway can be investigated in animal models. Both cell culture and animal models tend to *overestimate* the ability of drugs to induce excess porphyrin intermediates.

It is difficult to assess the porphyrinogenic potential of anesthetic drugs, since other factors such as sepsis or stress may also precipitate a porphyric crisis in the perioperative period. Any classification of anesthetic drugs with regard to their ability to precipitate a porphyric crisis is likely to be imperfect (Table 19.4). Particular care is needed when selecting drugs for patients with acute intermittent porphyria or clinically active forms of porphyria and when prescribing drugs in combination; exacerbation of porphyria is more likely under these circumstances.

Management of Anesthesia

The principles of safe anesthetic management of patients with the potential for an acute attack of porphyria include identification of susceptible individuals and determination of potentially porphyrinogenic drugs. Laboratory identification of porphyric individuals is not easy, since many show only subtle or even no biochemical abnormalities during an asymptomatic phase. In the presence of a suggestive family history, determination of erythrocyte porphobilinogen activity is the most appropriate screening test for patients suspected of having acute intermittent porphyria. A careful family history should be obtained and a thorough physical examination performed (although there is often no physical evidence of a porphyria or only subtle skin lesions), and the presence or absence of peripheral neuropathy and autonomic nervous system instability should be noted.

Guidelines for drug selection include the following: (1) There is evidence that a single exposure to a potent inducer might be well tolerated, but *not* during an acute attack. (2) Exposure to multiple potential inducers is more dangerous than exposure to any single drug. (3) Lists of "safe" and "unsafe" anesthetic drugs and adjuncts may be based on animal or cell culture experiments, so the actual clinical effects of these agents may be unknown. Note that the American Porphyria Foundation maintains up-to-date information on all aspects of porphyrias, and they maintain an up-to-date drug database for healthcare professionals that contains expert assessments of the potential of drugs to provoke attacks of acute porphyria (see Table 19.4).

If an acute exacerbation of porphyria is suspected during the perioperative period, particular attention must be given to skeletal muscle strength and cranial nerve function, since these signs may predict impending respiratory failure and an increased risk of pulmonary aspiration. Cardiovascular examination may reveal systemic hypertension and tachycardia that necessitate treatment. Postoperative mechanical ventilation may be required. During an acute exacerbation, severe abdominal pain may mimic a surgical abdomen. Patients experiencing an acute porphyric crisis must be assessed carefully for fluid balance and electrolyte status.

Preoperative starvation should be minimized, but if a prolonged fast is unavoidable, preoperative administration of a glucose-containing infusion is prudent, since caloric restriction has been linked to precipitation of attacks of acute porphyria.

Based on current evidence, patients can receive benzodiazepines for preoperative anxiolysis. Aspiration prophylaxis may include proton pump inhibitors and/or histamine-2 receptor blockers.

Regional Anesthesia

There is no contraindication to the use of regional anesthesia in patients with porphyria. However, if a regional anesthetic is being considered, it is essential to perform a neurologic examination before initiating the blockade to minimize the likelihood that worsening of any preexisting neuropathy would be erroneously attributed to the regional anesthetic. Autonomic

TABLE 19.4	Potential of Drugs to Provoke Acute Porphyria Attacks[a]
Anesthetic Medications	**Recommendation**
INHALATION ANESTHETICS	
Nitrous oxide, isoflurane, sevoflurane, desflurane	All OK
INTRAVENOUS ANESTHETICS	
Propofol, dexmedetomidine	OK
Thiopental, thiamylal, methohexital, etomidate, ketamine	All BAD
NARCOTIC OPIOIDS FOR INTRAVENOUS ADMINISTRATION	
Morphine, meperidine, hydromorphone, methadone	All OK
Fentanyl, alfentanil, sufentanil	All OK
Remifentanil, tramadol	No Data
NARCOTIC OPIOIDS FOR ORAL ADMINISTRATION	
Codeine, hydrocodone, oxycodone	All OK
NONNARCOTIC ANALGESICS	
Aspirin, acetaminophen, some NSAIDs	OK
Ketorolac	BAD
NEUROMUSCULAR BLOCKERS	
Succinylcholine, pancuronium, vecuronium	All OK
REVERSAL DRUGS FOR NEUROMUSCULAR BLOCKERS	
Atropine, glycopyrrolate	OK
Edrophonium, neostigmine, pyridostigmine, physostigmine	All OK
LOCAL ANESTHETICS	
Lidocaine, tetracaine, bupivacaine, mepivacaine, ropivacaine	All OK
Benzocaine	No data
SEDATIVES	
Midazolam, diazepam, lorazepam	All OK
ANTIEMETICS	
Ondansetron, scopolamine, metoclopramide	All OK
Famotidine, ranitidine, cimetidine	All OK
CARDIOVASCULAR MEDICATIONS	
Esmolol, propranolol, labetalol, metoprolol, atenolol	All OK
Epinephrine, dopamine, dobutamine	All OK
Adenosine	OK
Amiodarone	BAD
Calcium channel blockers	Many are BAD. *Check each calcium channel blocker before administration!*
NARCOTIC ANTAGONIST	
Naloxone	OK

[a]Expert assessments.

BAD, Probably unsafe or very likely to be unsafe for prolonged use; *No data,* insufficient data available to make a recommendation about its use; *NSAIDs,* nonsteroidal antiinflammatory drugs; *OK,* very likely or probably likely to be safe for prolonged use.

Adapted from the American Porphyria Foundation Drug Database posted at www.porphyriafoundation.org.

nervous system blockade induced by the regional anesthetic could unmask cardiovascular instability, especially in the presence of autonomic neuropathy, hypovolemia, or both. There is no evidence that any local anesthetic has ever induced an acute attack of porphyria or neurologic damage in porphyric individuals. Regional anesthesia *has* been safely used in parturient women with acute intermittent porphyria. However, regional anesthesia is used very infrequently in patients experiencing an attack of acute intermittent porphyria, owing to concerns about hemodynamic instability, mental confusion, and porphyria-related neuropathy.

General Anesthesia

Perioperative monitoring should consider the frequent presence of autonomic dysfunction and the possibility of blood pressure lability.

Intravenous induction drugs include some of the most dangerous medications for patients at risk for acute porphyria. Specifically, *any barbiturate,* etomidate, and ketamine are contraindicated. Fortunately, propofol is well tolerated, either in a bolus dose or by continuous infusion. Propofol could be given with or without midazolam, a narcotic, or dexmedetomidine.

Nitrous oxide is well established as a safe inhaled anesthetic in patients with porphyria. Safe use of isoflurane, sevoflurane, and desflurane is also established. Virtually all opioids for intravenous administration have been administered safely, though there are no specific data available about the safety of remifentanil. Naloxone is also a safe drug in these patients. Neither depolarizing nor nondepolarizing neuromuscular blocking drugs introduce any predictable risk when administered to these patients, nor do their reversal drugs.

Prophylaxis for postoperative nausea and vomiting can be safely accomplished with ondansetron and/or scopolamine. Safe oral analgesics for control of postoperative pain include codeine, oxycodone, hydrocodone, acetaminophen, and many nonsteroidal antiinflammatory drugs (NSAIDs). However, *ketorolac is not safe.* There is insufficient evidence to recommend the use of tramadol.

It is important to remember that many drugs other than anesthetic or analgesic drugs might be administered intraoperatively or postoperatively: antibiotics, bronchodilators, antihypertensives, drugs for heart rate control, anticoagulants and their reversals, antidysrhythmics, glucagon, octreotide, and others. The "safe" members of each drug class likely to be needed perioperatively should be determined *preoperatively* so timely administration of these drugs can occur whenever necessary.

Treatment of a Porphyric Crisis

The first step in treating an acute porphyric crisis is removal of any known triggering factors. Adequate hydration and carbohydrate loading are necessary. Sedation using a phenothiazine or benzodiazepine can be useful. Pain often necessitates administration of opioids. Nausea and vomiting are treated with conventional antiemetics. β-Blockers can be administered to control tachycardia and hypertension. Since many traditional anticonvulsants are regarded as unsafe, seizures may be treated with a benzodiazepine or propofol. Electrolyte disturbances, including hypomagnesemia, must be treated aggressively.

Because intravenous heme is more effective and its response rate quicker if heme treatment is given early in the course of an acute attack, it is no longer recommended that heme therapy for a severe attack be delayed pending a trial of glucose therapy. Now *all* patients with severe attacks should get heme therapy initially. Those with only a mild attack can be treated first with glucose. Heme is administered as hematin, heme albumin, or heme arginine. It is presumed that these forms of heme supplement the intracellular pool of heme and thus suppress ALA synthase activity via the negative feedback loop. Heme arginine and heme albumin lack the potential adverse effects associated with hematin (coagulopathy, thrombophlebitis). Recovery after an acute attack of porphyria depends on the degree of neuronal damage and usually is rapid if treatment is started early.

DISORDERS OF PURINE METABOLISM

Gout

Gout is a disorder of purine metabolism and may be classified as primary or secondary. *Primary gout* is due to an inherited metabolic defect that leads to overproduction of uric acid. *Secondary gout* is hyperuricemia resulting from an identifiable cause, such as administration of chemotherapeutic drugs that cause rapid lysis of purine-containing cells. Gout is characterized by hyperuricemia with recurrent episodes of acute arthritis caused by deposition of urate crystals in joints. Deposition of urate crystals typically initiates an inflammatory response that causes pain and limited motion of the joint. At least half of the initial attacks of gout are confined to the first metatarsophalangeal joint—that is, the joint at the base of the great toe. Persistent hyperuricemia can also result in deposition of urate crystals in extraarticular locations, manifested most often as nephrolithiasis. Urate crystal deposition can also occur in the myocardium, aortic valve, and extradural spinal regions. The incidence of systemic hypertension, ischemic heart disease, and diabetes mellitus is increased in patients with gout.

Treatment

Treatment of gout is designed to decrease plasma concentrations of uric acid by administration of uricosuric drugs (e.g., probenecid) or drugs that inhibit conversion of purines to uric acid by xanthine oxidase (e.g., allopurinol). Colchicine, which lacks any effect on purine metabolism, is considered the drug of choice for management of acute gouty arthritis. It relieves joint pain presumably by modifying leukocyte migration and phagocytosis. Side effects of colchicine include vomiting and diarrhea. Large doses of colchicine can produce hepatorenal dysfunction and agranulocytosis.

Management of Anesthesia

Management of anesthesia in the presence of gout focuses on prehydration to facilitate continued renal elimination of uric acid. Administration of sodium bicarbonate to alkalinize the urine also facilitates excretion of uric acid. Even with appropriate precautions, acute attacks of gout often follow surgical procedures in patients with a history of gout.

Extraarticular manifestations of gout and side effects of drugs used to control the disease deserve consideration when formulating a plan for anesthetic management. Renal function must be evaluated, since clinical manifestations of gout usually increase with deteriorating renal function. The increased incidence of systemic hypertension, ischemic heart disease, and diabetes mellitus in patients with gout must be considered. Although rare, adverse renal and hepatic effects may be associated with use of probenecid and colchicine. Limited temporomandibular joint motion from gouty arthritis, if present, can make direct laryngoscopy difficult.

Lesch-Nyhan Syndrome

Lesch-Nyhan syndrome is a genetic disorder of purine metabolism that occurs exclusively in males. Biochemically the defect is characterized by decreased or absent activity of hypoxanthine-guanine phosphoribosyltransferase, which leads to excessive purine production and increased uric acid concentrations throughout the body. It has been called *juvenile gout*. Clinically, patients are often intellectually disabled and exhibit characteristic spasticity and self-mutilation. Self-mutilation often involves trauma to perioral tissues. Subsequent scarification around the mouth may cause difficulty with direct laryngoscopy for tracheal intubation. Seizures are associated with this syndrome. Spasticity of skeletal muscles can be significant. Athetoid dysphagia makes swallowing very difficult, and co-existing malnutrition is typically present. This dysphagia can also increase the likelihood of aspiration if vomiting occurs. Sympathetic nervous system responses to stress are often enhanced. Hyperuricemia is associated with nephropathy, urinary tract calculi, and arthritis. Death is often due to renal failure.

Management of anesthesia is influenced principally by potential airway difficulties and by the neurologic and renal dysfunction that is present.

DISORDERS OF CARBOHYDRATE METABOLISM

Disorders of carbohydrate metabolism typically reflect genetically determined enzyme defects (Table 19.5). Glycogen storage disease (GSD) type IA is the more severe form. It involves deficiency of the enzyme glucose-6-phosphatase itself. Death usually occurs in early childhood. GSD type IB is caused by an inability to translocate glucose-6-phosphatase across microsomal membranes.

Hypoglycemia and lactic acidosis are the most common signs of both type I GSDs and can result from even short periods of fasting. There may also be coagulation difficulties due to poor platelet adhesiveness. Long-term complications include gout due to hyperuricemia, hyperlipidemia leading to pancreatitis, ischemic heart disease, hepatic adenoma, renal dysfunction, and osteoporosis.

Management of anesthesia in patients with type I GSDs should include evaluation for the existence of disease complications such as renal dysfunction and heart disease. Arterial

TABLE 19.5	Disorders of Carbohydrate Metabolism
GSD type Ia (von Gierke disease)	
GSD type Ib	
GSD type II (Pompe disease)	
GSD type V (McArdle disease)	
Galactosemia	
Fructose 1,6-diphosphate deficiency	
Pyruvate dehydrogenase deficiency	

GSD, Glycogen storage disease.

pH should be monitored perioperatively. Because even a short fast can induce hypoglycemia and metabolic acidosis, preoperative fasting must be minimized and glucose-containing infusions should be administered.

HEMOCHROMATOSIS

Hemochromatosis is an autosomal recessive disease that is one of the most common genetic diseases in the United States. It is characterized by an excess in total body iron. This iron is then deposited in parenchymal cells, especially in the liver, pancreas, and heart. Most patients are asymptomatic until about age 40, when the tissue damage from excessive iron becomes manifest, often as hepatomegaly/cirrhosis, diabetes mellitus, and/or congestive heart failure. Less commonly, bronzing of the skin and arthropathy develop.

The primary defect in this disease is a genetic mutation in the *HFE* gene involved in iron metabolism. This *HFE* gene controls the link between body iron stores and intestinal absorption of iron. Normally, intestinal iron absorption is equal to body iron losses. In hemochromatosis, intestinal iron absorption *exceeds* the body's requirement for iron.

The mainstay of treatment of hemochromatosis is phlebotomy to physically remove iron from the body. Phlebotomy may be done once or twice a week at first then tapered to less frequent treatment as the goal ferritin level is reached. Chelating agents such as deferoxamine remove less iron than phlebotomy and are used only when phlebotomy is not feasible. Certain complications of the iron deposition of hemochromatosis, such as skin pigmentation, hepatomegaly, and heart failure, can be improved with treatment, but diabetes and established cirrhosis cannot be reversed.

Anesthetic management should focus on preoperative assessment of any liver disease, diabetes mellitus, and the presence of cardiac dysfunction. Monitoring methods and anesthetic technique and drugs should be tailored to the severity of liver and cardiac involvement. In addition, transfusion of packed red blood cells should be avoided if at all possible because this will add to the iron overload problem.

WILSON DISEASE

Wilson disease is a rare autosomal recessive disease of copper metabolism caused by a mutation in a gene necessary for copper transport. This defect in copper transport impairs biliary copper excretion and results in accumulation of copper, most prominently in the liver. As the disease progresses there can be copper buildup in other organs, especially the brain.

Presentation of Wilson disease is often in the teenage years, and signs can range from abdominal pain and hepatitis to acute liver failure or cirrhosis. Neurologic and psychiatric signs and symptoms are seen later in the course of this disease. Movement disorders such as dystonia, tremors, and a Parkinson-like syndrome are often seen. Dysarthria and dysphagia are also common, as is autonomic neuropathy.

The diagnosis of Wilson disease is best made by liver biopsy. Serum ceruloplasmin levels may be reduced, and urinary copper levels can be increased in heterozygotes. Kayser-Fleischer rings (brown rings around the rim of the cornea) are seen on slit lamp examination in virtually all patients with neuropsychiatric manifestations of Wilson disease but in fewer than 50% of patients who have not yet developed symptoms of the disease or those with only liver involvement.

The traditional anticopper treatment of Wilson disease was the chelator penicillamine, which has significant toxicity, especially the potential to worsen neurologic disease. Currently if a chelator is chosen for therapy, it is trientine, which is much less toxic. However, for most patients with Wilson disease, especially those without severe liver or neuropsychiatric disease, zinc is now the preferred treatment, and it is nontoxic. Zinc blocks intestinal absorption of copper and induces production of a liver protein that sequesters excess copper. Patients with more advanced disease (e.g., hepatic failure, neurologic signs) are treated with both zinc and a copper-chelating drug.

Anesthetic management includes preoperative evaluation of the length and severity of the Wilson disease and current treatment. Examination for signs of significant liver disease and neuropsychiatric disease and appropriate laboratory investigations are undertaken.

A principal goal of anesthetic management should focus on avoiding techniques and drugs that could worsen affected organs. Care should be taken when giving anxiolytics, narcotics, or sedating medications; their sedative effects may be exaggerated in patients who are already experiencing some of the neurodepressive effects of Wilson disease. Drugs metabolized by the liver may have sustained effects secondary to liver dysfunction.

Although theoretically, general anesthesia may increase the risk of further liver damage by causing vasodilation, hypotension, and decreased liver perfusion, it can be safely performed in patients with Wilson disease. Regional and neuraxial anesthesia are also safe. Regional anesthesia can be performed even in advanced stages of Wilson disease, because peripheral nerves are *not* affected by the copper overload.

KEY POINTS

- Acute attacks of porphyria are characterized by severe abdominal pain, autonomic nervous system instability, electrolyte disturbances, and neuropsychiatric manifestations. These can range from mild disturbances to life-threatening events.
- Skeletal muscle weakness that may progress to quadriparesis and respiratory failure is the most dangerous neurologic manifestation of an acute attack of porphyria. Seizures may also occur.
- Because carbohydrate administration can suppress porphyrin synthesis, carbohydrate supplementation preoperatively is recommended to reduce the risk of an attack of acute porphyria.
- Initial treatment of a severe acute porphyric crisis should include administration of heme. This will stop production of ALA synthase and production of the problematic porphyrin intermediate.
- Anesthetic management of a patient with hemochromatosis must focus on the severity of hepatic disease, diabetes mellitus, and congestive heart failure, which are the most common and important clinical features of the hereditary form of this disease. Red blood cell transfusion should be avoided if possible.
- Anesthetic management of a patient with Wilson disease must include careful consideration of the hepatic and neuropsychiatric dysfunction often present in untreated disease. Dysphagia may increase the risk of pulmonary aspiration of gastric contents. Severe dystonia may make the physical tasks of administering general anesthesia quite difficult. Positioning may be complicated by orthostatic hypotension.

RESOURCES

American Porphyria Foundation. www.porphyriafoundation.com.

Anderson KE, Bloomer JR, Bonkovsky HL, et al. Recommendations for the diagnosis and treatment of the acute porphyrias. *Ann Intern Med.* 2005;142:439-450.

Bacon RB, Adams PC, Kowdley KV, et al. Diagnosis and management of hemochromatosis: 2011 practice guidelines by the American Association for the Study of Liver Diseases. *Hepatology.* 2011;54:328-343.

Gorcheln A. Drug treatment in acute porphyria. *Br J Clin Pharmacol.* 1997;44:427-434.

James MF, Hift RJ. Porphyrias. *Br J Anaesth.* 2000;85:143-153.

Jensen NF, Fiddler DS, Striepe V. Anesthetic considerations in porphyrias. *Anesth Analg.* 1995;80:591-599.

Roberts EA, Schilsky ML. Diagnosis and treatment of Wilson disease: an update. *Hepatology.* 2008;47:2089-2111.

Nutritional Diseases: Obesity and Malnutrition

VERONICA MATEI, WANDA M. POPESCU

Nutritional diseases can be caused by either an underconsumption of essential nutrients or an overconsumption of poor nutrients. Both result in forms of abnormal nutrition (i.e., malnutrition). Currently the most prevalent nutritional disease worldwide is obesity. Because of its detrimental impact on overall health and functional status, obesity is considered by the World Health Organization (WHO) to be one of the eight significant causes of chronic illness and the leading preventable cause of medical illness in the world. About two-thirds of the world's population lives in countries where being overweight and obese kills more people than being underweight. In the United States, obesity is considered a national epidemic and a serious public health threat. The rise in obesity rates has begun to plateau, but the prevalence of severe obesity remains substantial, with estimates indicating that 14.5% of the US population has a body mass index (BMI) of 35 or higher.

Most evidence suggests that obesity is due to a combination of elements, including genetic, environmental, psychological, and socioeconomic factors. Controlling the obesity epidemic will depend on a better understanding of its causes as well as a systems-based approach to its medical management.

OBESITY

Definition

Obesity is defined as an abnormally high amount of adipose tissue compared with lean muscle mass ($\geq$20% over ideal body weight). It is associated with increased morbidity and mortality due to a wide spectrum of medical and surgical diseases (Table 20.1). BMI is the most commonly used quantifier of obesity despite the fact that it does not measure adipose tissue directly. BMI is calculated as weight in kilograms divided by the square of the height in meters (BMI = kg/m^2). This BMI ratio is used because of its simplicity. However, there are flaws in the formula that should be taken into consideration when using the BMI clinically. For example, persons with an unusually high percentage of lean muscle mass (e.g., body builders) may have a high BMI that does not correlate with a high ratio of adipose tissue. In general, calculation of BMI provides a useful indicator of weight categories that may lead to health problems (Table 20.2). It should be noted that the weight term *morbid obesity* has been replaced with the term *clinically severe obesity*.

Epidemiology

Over the past 20 years, obesity has increased dramatically. Currently a third of the American adult population is obese, defined as having a BMI of 30 or higher. Prevalence rates vary by ethnicity and race, with African American women having the highest prevalence (82%). The prevalence of childhood obesity has nearly tripled and is currently estimated to be about 25%.

As the prevalence of obesity increases, so do its associated healthcare costs. On average the annual healthcare costs for an obese patient are approximately 42% more than for a normal-weight patient. In addition to being associated with major comorbid conditions, including diabetes mellitus, hypertension, and cardiovascular disease, obesity is also associated with a decrease in life expectancy. The risk of premature death is doubled in the obese population, and the risk of death resulting from cardiovascular disease is increased fivefold in the obese compared with the nonobese.

TABLE 20.1	Medical and Surgical Conditions Associated With Obesity
Organ System	Comorbid Conditions
Respiratory system	Obstructive sleep apnea
	Obesity hypoventilation syndrome
	Restrictive lung disease
Cardiovascular system	Systemic hypertension
	Coronary artery disease
	Congestive heart failure
	Cerebrovascular disease, stroke
	Peripheral vascular disease
	Pulmonary hypertension
	Hypercoagulable syndromes
	Hypercholesterolemia
	Hypertriglyceridemia
	Sudden death
Endocrine system	Metabolic syndrome
	Diabetes mellitus
	Cushing syndrome
	Hypothyroidism
Gastrointestinal system	Nonalcoholic steatohepatitis
	Hiatal hernia
	Gallstones
	Fatty liver infiltration
	Gastroesophageal reflux disease
	Delayed gastric emptying
Musculoskeletal system	Osteoarthritis of weight-bearing joints
	Back pain
	Inguinal hernia
	Joint pain
Malignancy	Pancreatic
	Kidney
	Breast
	Prostate
	Cervical, uterine, endometrial
	Colorectal
Other	Kidney failure
	Depression
	Overall shorter life expectancy

Modified from Adams JP, Murphy PG. Obesity in anaesthesia and intensive care. *Br J Anaesth*. 2000;85:91-108.

TABLE 20.2	Body Mass Index (BMI) Weight Categories
Category	BMI Range (kg/m^2)
ADULTS	
Underweight	<18.5
Normal	18.5–24.9
Overweight	25–29.9
Obese class I	30–34.9
Obese class II	35–39.9
Obese class III (severe)	≥40
CHILDREN (2–18 yr)	
Overweight	85th–94th percentile
Obese	95th percentile or ≥ 30
Severely obese	99th percentile

Pathophysiology

Weight gain results when caloric intake exceeds energy expenditure. Energy expenditure is primarily determined by basal metabolic rate, which is responsible for maintaining homeostasis of bodily functions. Most metabolic activity occurs within lean tissue and involves small sources of energy expenditure, including the thermal effect of physical activity and the heat produced by food digestion, absorption, and storage. Exercise can increase energy consumption not only during exercise but also for up to 18 hours afterward. It does so by increasing the thermal effects of physical activity and, *with regular exercise over time, the body's basal metabolic rate increases.* Caloric restriction (i.e., fasting) *without exercise,* on the other hand, *leads to a reduction in basal metabolic rate* due to promotion of the body's efforts to conserve energy. This reduction in basal metabolic rate leads to slow weight loss during the dieting phase but rapid weight gain when normal caloric intake is resumed.

Fat Storage

A positive caloric balance is stored by the body as fat in adipocytes. This fat is primarily in the form of triglycerides. Triglycerides serve as an efficient form of energy storage because of their high caloric density and hydrophobic nature. Adipocytes are able to increase to a maximum size, and then they begin dividing. It is believed that at BMIs up to 40 kg/m^2, adipocytes are only increased in size, whereas in clinically severe obesity, there exists an absolute increase in the total number of fat cells. The storage of triglycerides is regulated by lipoprotein lipase. The activity of this enzyme varies in different parts of the body. For example, it is more active in abdominal fat than in hip fat. The increase in metabolic activity of abdominal fat may contribute to the higher incidence of metabolic disturbances associated with *central (abdominal) obesity.* Abdominal obesity is more common in men and is therefore known as *android fat distribution.* Peripheral fat around the hips and buttocks is more common in women and is known as *gynecoid fat distribution.* It is currently accepted that a *waist-to-hip ratio* of more than 1.0 in men and more than 0.8 in women is a strong predictor of ischemic heart disease, stroke, diabetes mellitus, and death, independent of the total amount of body fat. Environmental factors such as stress and cigarette smoking stimulate cortisol production, which may facilitate further deposition of extra calories as abdominal fat.

Cellular Disturbances

Obesity leads to severe metabolic derangements, mainly because of disturbances in insulin regulation. At a cellular level, fatty infiltration of the pancreas leads to decreased secretion of insulin while at the same time, engorgement of adipocytes promotes insulin resistance. In addition the engorged adipocytes are capable of secreting various cytokines, including interleukin (IL)-1, IL-6, and tumor necrosis factor (TNF)-α. These cytokines worsen glucose intolerance by decreasing the secretion of adiponectin, a powerful insulin sensitizer. Leptin, another hormone secreted by adipose tissue, travels centrally to the ventromedial hypothalamus and modulates secretion of neuropeptides that regulate energy expenditure and food intake. *Leptin induces satiety* when present in high concentrations. Leptin secretion accelerates inflammatory changes by activating monocytes and decreasing the capacity of neutrophils to activate and migrate. Acting in opposition to leptin, the hormone *ghrelin increases appetite.* Ghrelin appears to modulate appetite both peripherally and centrally by affecting the mechanosensitivity of gastric vagal afferents, making them less sensitive to distention and thus facilitating overeating. With central obesity the high level of fatty infiltration of omental adipocytes (usually devoid of fat) leads to an increased influx of fatty acids, hormones, and cytokines. All these substances eventually stimulate the liver to produce increased levels of very low-density lipoproteins and apolipoprotein B. As a result the pancreas is stimulated to secrete more insulin and more pancreatic polypeptides. This results in diffuse intracellular inflammatory changes.

Genetic Factors

From a Darwinian perspective the ability of the body to conserve and store energy probably conferred a survival advantage. However, in affluent societies where food is very calorie dense and serving sizes are abnormally large, this ability to conserve and store energy likely proves deleterious to survival. For this reason, scientists are looking for specific genes that may favor energy storage and diminish energy expenditure as possible explanations for the current obesity epidemic. Discovery of the various hormones responsible for signaling satiety in the brain and thus maintaining a normal body weight has led scientists to believe that overeating resulting in obesity may be due to genetic mutations. In fact, research suggests that many forms of severe obesity may be related to a combination of inherited gene mutations. Genetic factors have been shown to influence the degree of weight gain and predict which individuals are most likely to gain weight. Statistical analyses suggest that more than half of the variations in individual BMIs are genetically influenced. For example, mutations in the gene that controls the hypothalamic melanocortin receptor, which is involved in appetite suppression, helps explain about 5% of severe early childhood obesity. Homozygous mutations in genes responsible for leptin and ghrelin secretion and receptor activity are also associated with extreme childhood obesity. However, it is clear that the metabolic consequences of inheriting maladaptive genes do not fully explain and are not entirely responsible for the current obesity epidemic.

Environmental Factors

Environmental factors, consumption of high-calorie foods, decreased physical activity, and aging are all important in the development of obesity. The technologic developments of the past 50 years have contributed significantly to decreased physical activity and sedentary lifestyles. There has also been a change in our food habits, with the development of "fast food" and intense food marketing and industry competition. These new food habits amplify the obesity problem.

Some people try to solve their weight problem by following popular fad diets that claim to aid in weight loss. Although these "lose-weight-quick" diets appear to work initially, it is unlikely that they contribute to sustained weight loss. Both proteins and carbohydrates can be metabolically converted into fat. Evidence is lacking to prove that changing the relative proportions of protein, carbohydrates, and fat in the diet without reducing overall caloric intake will promote weight loss. The bottom line is quite simple: *if an individual is to lose weight and keep the weight off, daily energy expenditure must exceed daily caloric intake.* If daily caloric (energy) intake exceeds energy expenditure by only 2%, the cumulative effect after 1 year is approximately a 5-lb increase in body weight. The critical elements of weight loss are both diet and exercise. Even slight exertion has been shown to provide some benefit to a highly sedentary adult, and the benefit is not exclusively related to weight loss. Exercise has a positive impact on cardiovascular health and glucose control. It limits the progressive decline in lean body tissue with age, decreases the risk of developing osteoporosis, and improves overall psychological well-being.

Psychological and Socioeconomic Factors

Often throughout history, obesity was viewed as a sign of wealth and elite socioeconomic status. Today, however, much more emphasis is placed on appearing slim and fit. Media and marketing pressures can lead overweight individuals, particularly women, to experiment with quick-weight-loss schemes and to develop obsessive, unhealthy eating disorders to avoid discrimination. Nearly 37% of women in the United States are at risk of developing major depression related to obesity. Eating disorders linked to both depression and obesity include binge eating disorder and night-eating syndrome (Table 20.3). These eating disorders are seen in a large proportion of patients attending obesity clinics. It is important to recognize the characteristics of eating disorders, as well as signs of depression and anxiety, because psychological assessment and counseling are essential for treatment of these conditions. Use of antidepressants to treat depression related to obesity can be risky because many of these drugs are associated with weight gain (Table 20.4).

In the past, US Food and Drug Administration (FDA) nutrition labeling policies allowed the food industry to sell packaged foods prepared with potentially harmful chemicals that prolonged shelf life, and to add ingredients that increased the caloric density of the food without increasing its macronutrient content. In 2016 the FDA updated its requirements for nutrition facts labeling to support better-informed food choices by consumers.

Fast food restaurants have made huge profits by attracting consumers with sugary and salty foods rich in fats, extracted sugars, and refined starches. All of these may taste good but when eaten in large quantities are toxic to the body. Clever

TABLE 20.3	Criteria for Common Eating Disorders

BINGE EATING DISORDER

Consumption of large meals rapidly and without control
Three or more of the following: rapid eating, solitary or secretive eating, eating despite fullness, eating without hunger, self-disgust, guilt, depression
Striking distress while eating
No compensatory features (i.e., no excess exercise, purging, or fasting)
Persistence for >2 days/wk for 6 mo
If vomiting is part of the disorder, it is classified as *bulimia*.

NIGHT-EATING SYNDROME

Evening hyperphagia (>50% of daily intake occurs after evening meal)
Guilt, tension, and anxiety while eating
Frequent waking with more eating
Morning anorexia
Consumption of sugars and other carbohydrates at inappropriate times
Persistence for >2 mo

Adapted from Stunkard AJ. Binge-eating disorder and the night-eating syndrome. In: Wadden TA, Stunkard AJ, eds. *Handbook of Obesity Treatment*. New York: Guilford Press; 2002:107-121.

TABLE 20.4	Drugs Causing Weight Gain

Anticonvulsants: phenytoin, sodium valproate
Antidepressants: tricyclics, selective serotonin reuptake inhibitors, monoamine oxidase inhibitors, mirtazapine, lithium
Antihistamines
Antipsychotics, especially olanzapine
Corticosteroids
Insulin
Oral contraceptive and progestogenic compounds and blockers
Oral hypoglycemic agents: glitazones (peripheral rather than visceral gain), sulfonylureas

Adapted from Haslam DW, James WPT. Obesity. *Lancet*. 2005;366:1197-1209.

marketing trends to "supersize" meal portions to fool consumers into believing they are getting more value for their dollar have also led to an unhealthy and unnecessary increase in calorie consumption.

Diseases Associated With Obesity

Obesity can have detrimental effects on many organ systems. The most profound effects are on the endocrine, cardiovascular, respiratory, gastrointestinal (GI), immune, musculoskeletal, and nervous systems. Individuals with clinically severe obesity have limited mobility and may therefore appear to be asymptomatic even in the presence of significant respiratory and cardiovascular impairment.

Endocrine Disorders

Many of the comorbid conditions caused by obesity are related to the *metabolic syndrome,* also known as *syndrome X*. This syndrome has been defined in a number of ways. The most accepted definition requires the presence of at least three of the following signs: large waist circumference, high triglyceride levels, low levels of high-density lipoprotein (HDL) cholesterol, glucose intolerance, and hypertension.

Glucose Intolerance and Diabetes Mellitus Type 2

Obesity is an important risk factor for the development of non–insulin-dependent (type 2) diabetes mellitus. Increased adipose tissue leads to increased resistance of peripheral tissues to the effects of insulin, which ultimately results in glucose intolerance and overt diabetes mellitus. Events that increase stress levels in these patients (e.g., surgery) may necessitate the use of exogenous insulin. *Resolution of type 2 diabetes* can be achieved in more than 75% of obese patients simply by weight loss.

Endocrinopathies Causing Obesity

Certain diseases of the endocrine system may promote the development of obesity. Examples are hypothyroidism and Cushing disease. It is important to consider the possibility of an endocrine disorder when evaluating an obese patient.

Cardiovascular Disorders

Cardiovascular disease is a major cause of morbidity and mortality in obese individuals and may manifest as systemic hypertension, coronary artery diseases, or heart failure. In patients with clinically severe obesity, cardiac function is best at rest and exercise is poorly tolerated. Physical activity may cause exertional dyspnea and/or angina pectoris. Any increase in cardiac output is achieved by an increase in heart rate without an increase in stroke volume or ejection fraction. Changing position from sitting to supine is associated with an increase in pulmonary capillary wedge pressure and mean pulmonary artery pressure, as well as a decrease in heart rate and systemic vascular resistance. Obese individuals with cardiac dysfunction may choose to sleep sitting up in a chair to avoid symptoms of orthopnea and paroxysmal nocturnal dyspnea.

Systemic Hypertension

Mild to moderate systemic hypertension is 3–6 times more frequent in obese than in lean patients and is seen in approximately 50%–60% of obese patients. The mechanism of hypertension in obesity is multifactorial (Fig. 20.1). Obesity-induced hypertension is related to insulin effects on the sympathetic nervous system and extracellular fluid volume. Hyperinsulinemia appears to increase circulating levels of norepinephrine, which has direct pressor activity and increases renal tubular reabsorption of sodium, which results in hypervolemia. Cardiac output increases by an estimated 100 mL/min for each kilogram of adipose tissue weight gain. At the cellular level, insulin activates adipocytes to release angiotensinogen, which activates the renin-angiotensin-aldosterone pathway; this in turn leads to sodium retention and development of hypertension. An increase in circulating cytokines is seen in obesity, and this may cause damage to and fibrosis of the arterial wall, thereby increasing arterial stiffness. If hypertension is not well controlled, a mixed eccentric and concentric left ventricular hypertrophy can develop that eventually leads to heart failure

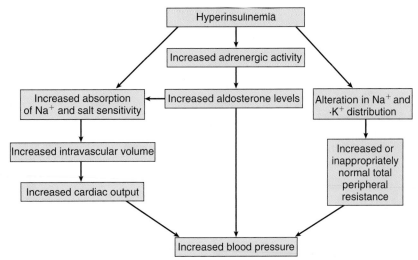

FIG. 20.1 Development of hypertension in obesity. (Adapted from Thakur V, Richards R, Reisin E. Obesity, hypertension, and the heart. *Am J Med Sci.* 2001;321:242-248.)

and pulmonary hypertension. *Weight loss can significantly improve or even completely resolve this hypertension.* In general a decrease of 1% in body weight can decrease systolic blood pressure by 1 mm Hg and diastolic blood pressure by 2 mm Hg.

Cardiac Disease

Coronary Artery Disease. Obesity seems to be an independent risk factor for the development of ischemic heart disease, and this coronary artery disease is more common in obese individuals with central obesity. This risk is compounded by the presence of dyslipidemia, a chronic inflammatory state, hypertension, and diabetes mellitus. Insulin resistance and abnormal glucose tolerance are associated with progression of atherosclerosis. Young obese patients are showing a significant incidence of single-vessel coronary artery disease, particularly in the right coronary artery. Obese men seem to be affected 10–20 years before women, which may reflect a protective effect from estrogen that dissipates after menopause.

Heart Failure. Obesity is an independent risk factor for heart failure. In its staging of heart failure, the American College of Cardiology and the American Heart Association lists metabolic syndrome and obesity as stage A of heart failure. This means that they have heart failure risk factors but that no symptoms or overt evidence of heart failure has yet developed. Possible mechanisms for the development of heart failure are structural and functional modifications of the heart resulting from volume overload and vascular stiffness. These changes cause pressure overload that leads to concentric left ventricular hypertrophy, a progressively less compliant left ventricle that develops diastolic dysfunction, and finally a left ventricle with systolic dysfunction. Increased metabolic demands and a larger circulating blood volume result in a hyperdynamic circulation. Right ventricular afterload may be increased because of associated sleep-disordered breathing and changes in left ventricular function (Fig. 20.2). Insulin resistance also appears to play a significant role in the development of heart failure. Car-

diac steatosis, lipoapoptosis, and activation of specific cardiac genes that promote left ventricular remodeling and cardiomyopathy may contribute to obesity-related cardiomyopathy. The increased demands placed on the cardiovascular system by obesity decrease cardiovascular reserve and limit exercise tolerance. Cardiac dysrhythmias in obese individuals may be precipitated by arterial hypoxemia, hypercarbia, ischemic heart disease, obesity hypoventilation syndrome, or fatty infiltration of the cardiac conduction system. It is important to note that ventricular hypertrophy and dysfunction worsen with the duration of obesity. However, *some of these structural and functional changes can be reversed with significant weight loss.*

Respiratory Disorders

Respiratory derangements associated with obesity are related to the presence of redundant tissue in the upper airway, thorax, and abdomen that affects lung volumes, gas exchange, lung compliance, and work of breathing.

Lung Volumes

Obesity can produce a restrictive pattern of ventilation resulting from the added weight of the thoracic cage, chest wall, and abdomen. The added weight impedes motion of the diaphragm, especially in the supine position, which results in an overall decrease in functional residual capacity (FRC), expiratory reserve volume, and total lung capacity. FRC declines exponentially with increasing BMI and may decrease to the point that small airway closure occurs (i.e., closing volume becomes greater than FRC). This results in ventilation/perfusion mismatching, right-to-left intrapulmonary shunting, and arterial hypoxemia. General anesthesia accentuates these changes. A 50% decrease in FRC occurs in anesthetized patients who are obese compared with a 20% decrease in nonobese individuals. Application of positive end-expiratory pressure (PEEP) can improve FRC and arterial oxygenation but at the potential expense of reducing cardiac output and oxygen delivery.

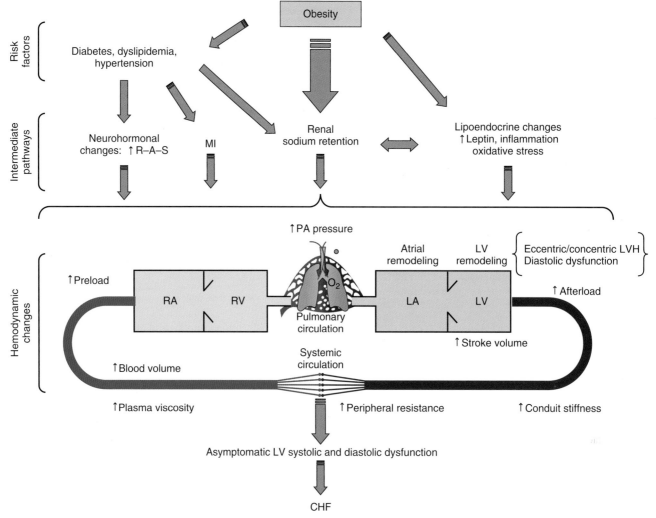

FIG. 20.2 Cardiac changes in obesity leading to heart failure. ↑, Increased; *CHF,* congestive heart failure; *LA,* left atrium; *LV,* left ventricle; *LVH,* left ventricular hypertrophy; *MI,* myocardial infarction; *PA,* pulmonary artery; *RA,* right atrium; *RAS,* renin-angiotensin system; *RV,* right ventricle. (Adapted from Vasan RS. Editorial: cardiac function and obesity. *Heart.* 2003;89:1127-1129.)

This decrease in FRC impairs the ability of obese patients to tolerate periods of apnea, such as during direct laryngoscopy for endotracheal intubation. They are likely to experience oxygen desaturation following induction of anesthesia despite adequate preoxygenation. This phenomenon reflects a *decreased* oxygen reserve due to the reduced FRC and an *increased* oxygen consumption resulting from the increased metabolic activity of excess adipose tissue.

Gas Exchange and Work of Breathing
Because of the obese patient's increased body mass, oxygen consumption and carbon dioxide (CO_2) production are increased. To maintain normocapnia, obese patients must increase minute ventilation, which also increases their work of breathing. Obese patients typically increase their minute ventilation by rapid, shallow breathing because this pattern uses the least amount of energy and helps prevent fatigue from the increased work of breathing. Individuals with clinically severe obesity may exhibit only modest decreases

in arterial oxygenation and modest increases in the alveolar-arterial oxygen difference. The $Paco_2$ and ventilatory response to CO_2 remain within the normal range in obese patients, which reflects the high diffusing capacity and favorable characteristics of the CO_2 dissociation curve. However, arterial oxygenation may deteriorate markedly during induction of anesthesia (a period of increased oxygen consumption and decreased oxygen reserves) so that a higher fraction of inspired oxygen (Fio_2) is required to maintain an acceptable level of oxygen saturation.

Lung Compliance and Airway Resistance
Increased BMI is associated with decreased lung compliance and increased airway resistance. Accumulation of fat tissue in and around the chest wall and abdomen and the added effect of an increased pulmonary blood volume cause this decrease in lung compliance, which is associated with a decrease in FRC and impaired gas exchange. These changes are most evident when obese individuals assume the supine position.

Obstructive Sleep Apnea

Obstructive sleep apnea (OSA) is defined as cessation of breathing for periods lasting longer than 10 seconds during sleep. There may be frequent episodes of apnea and hypopnea during sleep. *Hypopnea* is a reduction in the size or number of breaths compared with normal ventilation and is associated with some degree of arterial desaturation. Apnea occurs when the pharyngeal tissues collapse. Pharyngeal patency depends on the action of dilator muscles that prevent upper airway collapse. Pharyngeal muscle tone is decreased during sleep, and in many individuals this reduced tone leads to significant narrowing of the upper airway, resulting in turbulent airflow and snoring. In susceptible individuals this may progress to severe snoring and ultimately to sleep apnea. Sleep fragmentation is the most likely explanation for daytime somnolence, which is associated with impaired concentration, memory problems, and even motor vehicle accidents. Airway obstruction may induce physiologic changes that include arterial hypoxemia and hypercarbia, polycythemia, systemic hypertension, pulmonary hypertension, and right ventricular failure. In addition, patients may complain of morning headaches caused by nocturnal CO_2 retention and cerebral vasodilation. OSA is diagnosed using polysomnography in a sleep laboratory, where episodes of apnea during sleep can be observed and quantified. The average number of incidents per hour measures the severity of OSA. More than five incidents per hour is considered evidence of *sleep apnea syndrome.* The main predisposing factors for development of OSA are male gender, middle age, and obesity (BMI > 30 kg/m^2). Additional factors such as evening alcohol consumption or use of pharmacologic sleep aids can worsen the problem. Treatment of OSA is aimed at applying enough positive airway pressure through a nasal mask to sustain patency of the upper airway during sleep. Patients treated with positive airway pressure demonstrate improved neuropsychiatric function and reduced daytime somnolence. Patients with mild OSA who do not tolerate positive airway pressure may benefit from nighttime application of oral appliances designed to enlarge the airway by keeping the tongue in an anterior position or by displacing the mandible forward. Nocturnal oxygen therapy is another possibility for individuals who experience significant oxygen desaturation. In severe cases of sleep apnea, surgical treatment including uvulopalatopharyngoplasty, tracheostomy, or maxillofacial surgery (i.e., genioglossal advancement) may be performed. In many instances, *weight loss results in a significant improvement in or even complete resolution of OSA symptoms.*

Obesity Hypoventilation Syndrome

Obesity hypoventilation syndrome (OHS) is the long-term consequence of OSA. It is characterized by nocturnal episodes of *central apnea* (apnea without respiratory efforts), reflecting progressive desensitization of the respiratory center to nocturnal hypercarbia. At its extreme, OHS culminates in Pickwickian syndrome, which is characterized by obesity, daytime hypersomnolence, hypoxemia, hypercarbia, polycythemia, respiratory acidosis, pulmonary hypertension, and right ventricular failure. Even light sedation can cause complete airway collapse and/or respiratory arrest in a Pickwickian patient. All patients with a history of OSA or OHS must be thoroughly evaluated preoperatively. Obese patients *without* a documented history of sleep apnea should be screened preoperatively with a tool such as the STOP-BANG questionnaire.

Gastrointestinal Disorders

Nonalcoholic Fatty Liver Disease/Nonalcoholic Steatohepatitis

Obesity is the most important risk factor associated with *nonalcoholic fatty liver disease* (NAFLD) and *nonalcoholic steatohepatitis* (NASH) (see Chapter 17, "Diseases of the Liver and Biliary Tract"). Obesity causes an excess of intrahepatic triglycerides, impaired insulin activity, and additional release of inflammatory cytokines. These factors can lead to destruction of hepatocytes and disruption of hepatic physiology and architecture. Because of the increasing prevalence of obesity, NASH has become one of the most common causes of end-stage liver disease in the United States. Approximately one-third of overweight children, adolescents, and adults have NASH. About 85% of *severely obese adults* have NASH. In most cases this form of hepatitis follows a benign course. However, in severe cases it may progress to cirrhosis, portal hypertension, and/or hepatocellular carcinoma requiring liver transplantation. Most patients are asymptomatic, but some may experience fatigue and abdominal discomfort. Liver function test results may be abnormal. Among patients with NASH, 22% also develop diabetes mellitus, 22% develop systemic hypertension, and 25% die of coronary heart disease within 5–7 years. *Weight reduction,* especially bariatric surgery–induced weight loss, *has been shown to significantly improve the metabolic abnormalities associated with fatty liver disease or even cure this form of hepatic inflammation.*

Gallbladder Disease

Gallbladder disease is closely associated with obesity. Most commonly, obese patients have cholelithiasis resulting from supersaturation of bile with cholesterol resulting from abnormal cholesterol metabolism. Women with a BMI of more than 32 kg/m^2 have a three times higher risk of developing gallstones, and those with a BMI of more than 45 kg/m^2 have a seven times higher risk of gallstones than lean people. Paradoxically, rapid weight loss, especially after bariatric surgery, *increases* the risk of gallstones.

Gastric Emptying and Gastroesophageal Reflux Disease

Obesity per se is not a risk factor for delayed gastric emptying or gastroesophageal reflux disease (GERD). Indeed, many obese patients may actually have increased gastric emptying, although they have greater gastric fluid volumes.

Inflammatory Syndrome of Obesity

A higher rate of perioperative infection is seen in the obese population. This phenomenon may be due to the inability of neutrophils to activate, migrate, and adhere at sites of inflammation as a result of adipose tissue secretion of various proinflammatory cytokines or "adipokines." Markers of inflammation such as C-reactive protein, interleukins (IL-1,

IL-6), and tumor necrosis factor are released by adipocytes. Elevated concentrations of these inflammatory markers consistently decrease after weight-loss surgery. In addition, adiponectin, an adipose tissue–derived cytokine associated with insulin sensitivity, decreases in obese states and increases with weight loss.

Cancer

The depressed immune function of the obese patient significantly increases the risk of development of certain cancers. The WHO International Agency for Research on Cancer estimates that obesity and lack of physical activity are responsible for 25%–33% of breast, colon, endometrial, renal, and esophageal cancers. Prostate and uterine cancer are also seen in a higher percentage of overweight patients. Peripheral conversion of sex hormones in adipose tissue by aromatase, together with decreased concentrations of plasma steroid-binding globulin, may be responsible for the increased incidence of some of these cancers.

Thromboembolic Disorders

The risk of deep vein thrombosis in obese patients undergoing surgery is approximately double that of nonobese individuals. This increased risk presumably reflects the compounded effects of polycythemia, increased intraabdominal pressure, increased fibrinogen levels associated with a chronic inflammatory state, and immobilization leading to venostasis. At a cellular level, adipocytes produce excessive plasminogen activator inhibitor, and tissues have a decreased capacity for synthesis of tissue plasminogen activator. As a result there is a decrease in fibrinolysis that renders the obese patient susceptible to development of deep vein thrombosis or fatal pulmonary embolism. This phenomenon is worsened in the perioperative period. The use of low-molecular-weight heparin perioperatively can decrease thromboembolic complications during this time. In calculating the dosing for heparin, it is suggested that the dose be based on total body weight, since this correlates with drug clearance. Perioperative use of sequential compression stockings is also indicated.

The risk of stroke is increased in obese patients. Studies report an association between stroke and an increased waist/hip ratio and BMI. For every 1 unit increase above a normal BMI, there is a 4% increase in the risk of ischemic stroke and a 6% increase in the risk of hemorrhagic stroke. This increased stroke risk may be related to the prothrombotic and chronic inflammatory state that accompanies excess adipose tissue accumulation.

Musculoskeletal Disorders
Degenerative Joint Disease

Osteoarthritis and degenerative joint disease are being seen more frequently in men and women 40–60 years of age, a trend that closely parallels the incidence of obesity. Obesity leads to joint pain and arthritis of the hips, knees, and carpometacarpal joints of the hands, not only because of mechanical loading of weight-bearing joints but also because of the accompanying inflammatory and metabolic effects of increased adipose tissue. Co-existing disorders of glucose intolerance, lipid metabolism, hyperuricemia, gout, and vitamin D deficiency may further contribute to the problem of osteoarthritis in obese patients. Extra care must be taken in the positioning of patients with arthritis or degenerative joint disease.

Nervous System

Obese patients, especially those affected by diabetes, may have symptoms of autonomic nervous system dysfunction and peripheral neuropathy. Deficiencies of essential micronutrients such as vitamin B_{12}, thiamine, folate, trace minerals, iron, and calcium, in combination with hyperglycemia, can lead to autonomic nervous system dysfunction. Weight loss in severely obese patients is associated with significant improvement in autonomic cardiac modulation. Because pressure sores and nerve injuries are more common in the superobese and diabetic populations, particular attention must be given to padding the extremities and protecting pressure-prone areas during surgery.

Treatment of Obesity

Successful treatment of obesity requires a significant degree of patient motivation. It is estimated that fewer than 20% of obese patients are sufficiently motivated to accept treatment. Only after patients have acknowledged their weight problem and shown themselves capable of complying with a weight-loss program (even if unsuccessful) should pharmacologic or surgical treatment be considered. Patient motivation is required to achieve sustained positive results; ultimately the treatment of obesity requires a lifelong commitment to lifestyle modifications in the form of increased physical activity and decreased caloric intake. The benefits of weight loss in obesity are well documented. Medical and surgical weight-loss plans should be aimed at decreasing the severity of obesity rather than meeting a cosmetic standard of thinness. A weight loss of only 5–20 kg can be associated with a decrease in systemic blood pressure and plasma lipid concentrations and better control of diabetes mellitus.

Nonpharmacologic Therapy

The first step in any weight-loss program is dieting. Caloric restriction to 500–1000 kcal/day less than a regular diet promotes weight loss. Restricting caloric intake beyond this amount may initially help the patient lose weight faster, but the likelihood of long-term adherence to such a restricted diet is very low. Behavior modification therapy may be required to help patients stay motivated and adhere to lifestyle changes. The addition of exercise programs to dieting programs helps in maintaining successful long-term weight loss. Unfortunately, most patients with severe obesity do not maintain weight loss over time without pharmacologic or surgical intervention.

Medical Therapy

Current National Institutes of Health (NIH) and European Union recommendations suggest adding pharmacotherapy to weight-management programs in patients with a BMI of 27 kg/m^2 or higher and a persistent comorbid condition such as hypertension or glucose intolerance, and in patients with a BMI of more than 30 kg/m^2 with no comorbidities. When used properly, weight-loss drugs increase by threefold to fourfold the proportion of patients achieving at least a 5% weight loss at 1 year.

Prescription drugs designed to control caloric intake may produce their effects in several ways. All the currently available drugs approved for *short-term treatment* of obesity (no longer than 12 weeks) do so by producing amphetamine-like effects that decrease appetite by suppressing the hypothalamic appetite regulatory center. These drugs include phentermine (Adipex-P, Suprenza), benzphetamine (Didrex), diethylpropion (Tenuate), phentermine with topiramate (Qsymia), and phendimetrazine (Bontril).

Several drugs are currently available for *long-term treatment* of obesity and work via several different mechanisms. One class treats obesity by affecting GI lipase inhibitor, which then blocks fat absorption. Orlistat (Xenical) is in this class, as is Alli, which is a reduced-dosage form of orlistat available over the counter. Another drug in the long-term treatment class is lorcaserin (Belviq), a serotonergic drug with a high affinity for the 5-hydroxytryptamine 2C receptor that targets the receptor subtype affecting appetite. A somewhat similar drug is Contrave, which is a combination of naltrexone, a pure opioid antagonist, and bupropion, a dopamine reuptake inhibitor. It is postulated that this drug regulates food intake and body weight via the hypothalamic melanocortin system and the mesolimbic reward system.

Another weight loss drug is liraglutide (Saxenda, Victoza), an acylated glucagon-like peptide 1 (GLP-1) analogue. GLP-1 is a physiologic regulator of appetite and caloric intake via GLP-1 receptors that are present in several areas of the brain involved in appetite regulation, including the hypothalamus. Additional effects of liraglutide include a concurrent reduction in glycemic variables, since this drug is the active ingredient in Victoza, an injectable treatment for diabetes mellitus. The principal adverse effect of liraglutide is the risk of developing thyroid tumors.

Several efforts are underway to develop an *obesity vaccine*. One research effort is directed against the hormone ghrelin, which stimulates appetite. The goal of this vaccine is to inactivate ghrelin by producing an antibody response against it, decreasing the amount of hormone available to enter the central nervous system and stimulate the appetite. This research is in phase II trials. Other obesity vaccine research is directed against somatostatin. Somatostatin has many effects in the body, including its ability to suppress pancreatic release of several hormones (insulin, glucagon). Very early trials showed that this "flab jab" vaccine caused loss of 10% of body weight in the 4 days after its injection in mice. However, most of the weight was regained over time.

Surgical Therapy

Adult bariatric surgery results in significant sustained weight loss in patients who are severely obese. Bariatric surgery also improves obesity-related comorbid conditions, especially hypertension and diabetes. Such surgery is currently the most cost-effective treatment for patients with a BMI over 40 kg/m^2 or for patients with a BMI over 35 kg/m^2 if significant comorbid conditions are present. With recognition of the long-term benefits of this surgery for patients with clinically severe obesity, bariatric surgery is performed much more often now than previously. In the United States, bariatric surgery is being performed as frequently as cholecystectomy. It appears that the mean percentage of excess weight loss after Roux-en-Y gastric bypass is 68%, whereas for gastric banding it is 62%. Patients have a 77% likelihood of resolution of diabetes mellitus and a 62% likelihood of resolution of hypertension with weight-loss surgery.

Current strategies for surgically assisted weight loss fall into one of three categories: gastric restriction, intestinal malabsorption, or combined restrictive-malabsorptive bariatric surgery (Fig. 20.3 and Table 20.5). Most often these surgeries are performed via laparoscopic techniques, which have the advantages of decreased pain, decreased rates of complication (i.e., pulmonary complications, thromboembolism, wound infection, hernia development), and shorter recovery times.

Types of Bariatric Surgery

Restrictive Bariatric Procedures. Laparoscopic adjustable gastric banding, sleeve gastrectomy, and vertical banded gastroplasty are examples of restrictive weight loss procedures in which a small gastric pouch with a small outlet is created. The mechanism of weight loss may be related to appetite suppression and early satiety or to vagal nerve compression or reduced secretion of gastric hormones such as ghrelin. Adjustable gastric banding is the most commonly performed bariatric procedure in Europe, Latin America, and Australia. It has been used in the United States since 2001. The surgery entails placement of an adjustable silicone band around the upper end of the stomach, which creates a small pouch and restrictive stoma that slows the passage of food into the small intestine. This procedure requires no cutting of, or entry into, the stomach or small intestine and should therefore be associated with a low complication rate. The gastric band is adjusted after surgery by injection of saline into a subcutaneous port (placed at the time of surgery) to adjust the stoma size. Sleeve gastrectomy involves resection of the greater curvature of the stomach, which compromises about 75% of the stomach. The smaller gastric reservoir produces early satiety, and the remnant stomach secretes decreased levels of gastric hormones. The normal absorptive physiology of the entire small intestine is left intact in all of these restrictive procedures. Therefore specific nutrient deficiencies are rare unless there is a significant change in eating habits or surgical complications occur.

Malabsorptive Bariatric Procedures. Malabsorptive procedures include distal gastric or jejunoileal bypass, biliopancreatic diversion (BPD), and duodenal switch. These operations typically combine gastric volume reduction with a bypass of various

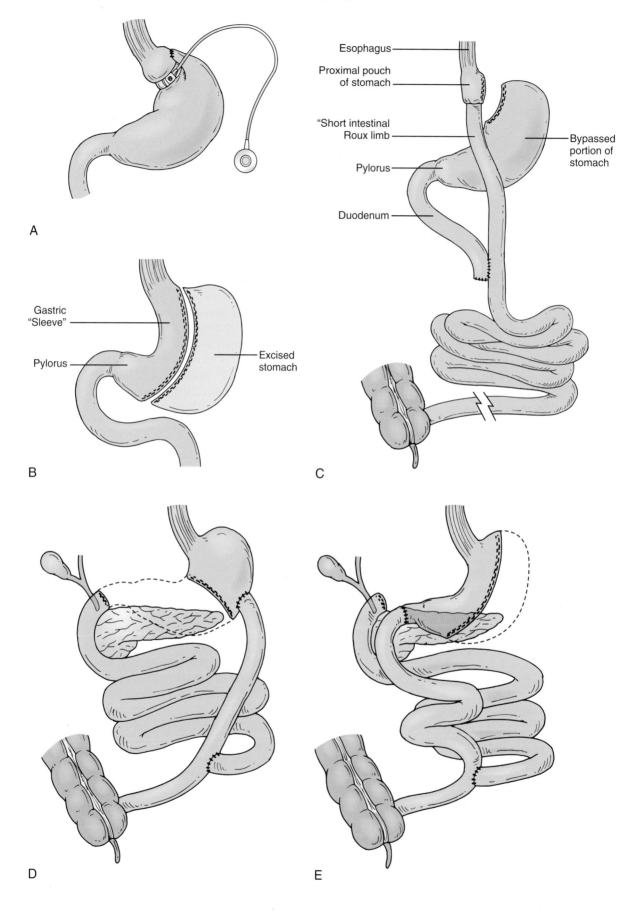

A

B

Gastric
"Sleeve"

Pylorus

Excised
stomach

C

Esophagus

Proximal pouch
of stomach

"Short intestinal
Roux limb

Pylorus

Duodenum

Bypassed
portion of
stomach

D

E

FIG. 20.3   A, Adjustable gastric band (AGB). A silicone band is looped around the proximal stomach to create a 15- to 20-mL pouch with an adjustable outlet. The stomach is wrapped around
the band anteriorly to prevent the band from slipping out of position. The band consists of a rigid
outer ring and an inner inflatable balloon reservoir connected by tubing to a subcutaneous port
that can be accessed through the skin to adjust the tightness. B, Sleeve gastrectomy. A narrow
gastric sleeve is created by stapling the stomach vertically. The fundus and greater curve of the
stomach are removed from the abdomen. C, Roux-en-Y gastric bypass (RYGB). A small gastric
pouch (15–30 mL) is created by division of the upper stomach, connected to a 100- to 150-cm
limb of jejunum called the *Roux limb*. The small gastric pouch results in restriction of food intake.
D, Biliopancreatic diversion (BPD). Most of the small bowel is bypassed, and only 50–100 cm of a
common channel remains for absorption of calories and nutrients. The upper pouch is larger than
that of the RYGB to allow for ingestion of larger amounts of protein to prevent malnutrition. E, Biliopancreatic diversion with duodenal switch (BPD-DS). To avoid dumping syndrome and maintain the
pylorus, the procedure was modified with the pouch based on the lesser curve of the stomach and
an anastomosis at the first portion of the duodenum. (From Ding S, McKenzie T, Vernon A, Goldfine
A. Bariatric surgery. In: Jameson JL, De Groot LJ, de Kretser DM, eds. *Endocrinology: Adult and
Pediatric.* 7th ed. Philadelphia: Elsevier; 2015:479.)

TABLE 20.5   Most Common Bariatric Surgeries

	Combined Restrictive-Malabsorptive	Restrictive	Malabsorptive
Name	Roux-en-Y gastric bypass	Adjustable gastric banding (Lap-Band surgery) Laparoscopic sleeve gastrectomy	Jejunoileal bypass or biliopancreatic diversion
How stomach is made smaller	Upper portion of stomach is stapled to lower part of intestines, leaving only a small gastric pouch	*Gastric banding:* silicone band is placed around top portion of stomach and adjusted until desired size of stomach is achieved. *Sleeve gastrectomy:* greater curvature of stomach is resected, with ≈25% of stomach remaining	80% of stomach is removed, along with a significant portion of small intestine, which leaves behind a smaller absorptive area
Hospital stay	2–3 days	Overnight	1–2 days
Operating time	2 hr	1 hr	1.5 hr
Advantages	Greatest weight loss of all types of surgery, with improvement in obesity-related health issues	Lower mortality and morbidity with banding because band is adjustable and placement does not require cutting, stapling, or rerouting stomach. Nutritional deficiencies usually not an issue, since intestines left intact	Significant weight loss
Disadvantages	Need for continuous lifelong nutritional surveillance and supplementation	Need for more frequent outpatient visits and longest time to achieve weight loss	Malabsorption of essential vitamins and nutrients like B_{12}, folic acid, and iron, as well as protein-calorie malnutrition

lengths of small intestine. After creation of a small gastric pouch, the small bowel is divided proximal to the ileocecal valve and connected directly to the gastric pouch, which produces a *gastroileostomy*. The remaining proximal limb of small intestine (biliopancreatic conduit) is anastomosed end-to-side to the distal ileum, proximal to the ileocecal valve. This provides a common channel that allows for mixture of nutrients with digestive enzymes in the ileum. The length of the common channel determines the degree of malabsorption. Because these procedures induce weight loss by extensively bypassing the small intestine and promoting malabsorption, they are associated with a high incidence of anemia, deficiency of fat-soluble vitamins, and protein-calorie malnutrition in the first year after surgery. Because of these risks of nutritional and metabolic complications, these operations are not performed as frequently as restrictive procedures.

Combined Bariatric Procedure. The combined bariatric procedure called *Roux-en-Y gastric bypass* (RYGB) includes both gastric restriction and some degree of malabsorption. It is the preferred surgical approach for clinically severe obesity. In the RYGB procedure, the surgeon creates a very small proximal gastric pouch that is connected to a Roux limb via an enteroenterostomy to the jejunum near the ligament of Treitz. The procedure bypasses the distal stomach, duodenum, and proximal jejunum, so there is a marked loss of absorptive surface area for nutrients, electrolytes, and bile salts. The RYGB procedure requires the longest operating time and postoperative hospital stay compared with other forms of bariatric surgery. However, it results in the greatest weight loss and improvement in obesity-related health issues.

Surgical Complications

Complications and mortality rates for bariatric surgery depend on several factors: age, gender, BMI, existing comorbid conditions, procedure type and complexity, and experience of the surgeon and surgical center. Higher mortality rates have been associated with abdominal obesity, male gender, BMI of 50 kg/m^2 or more, diabetes mellitus, sleep apnea, older age, and performance of the surgery at a lower-volume bariatric surgery center. Recent improvements in mortality rates are likely due to better perioperative care. Overall 30-day mortality for bariatric surgery ranges from 0.1%–2%. Gastric banding has the lowest mortality rate. Mortality for gastric bypass and sleeve gastrectomy is 0.5%. Malabsorptive operations are associated with a higher mortality rate. The mortality of RYGB ranges from 0.5%–1.5%. The most severe complications of bariatric surgery include anastomotic leaks, stricture formation, pulmonary embolism, sepsis, gastric prolapse, and bleeding. Less common complications include wound dehiscence, hernia or seroma formation, lymphocele, lymphorrhea, and suture extrusion.

Nutritional complications are seen after malabsorptive and combined bariatric procedures. These complications are a result of the marked reduction in vitamin and mineral uptake. The majority of patients can maintain a relatively normal nutritional status after RYGB, but deficiencies of iron, vitamin B_{12}, vitamin K, and folate are common. Some patients develop subclinical micronutrient deficiency. Taking multivitamins with mineral supplements reduces but does not totally prevent development of vitamin or mineral deficiencies. Chronic vitamin K deficiency can lead to an abnormal prothrombin time with a normal partial thromboplastin time. Patients who come for elective surgery with vitamin K deficiency and coagulopathy respond to administration of a vitamin K analogue such as phytonadione within 6–24 hours. Fresh frozen plasma or prothrombin complex concentrates may be required for prothrombin time correction for emergency surgery or active bleeding.

Additional complications of bariatric surgery include occurrence of an undesirable *dumping syndrome* in some patients. Other patients experience major nutritional complications. Three of the most clinically significant nutritional complications are protein-calorie malnutrition, Wernicke encephalopathy, and peripheral neuropathy. In the long term, patients are also at risk for metabolic bone disease. Pregnant women and adolescents are at higher risk for nutritional complications after RYGB because of their higher physiologic nutritional needs. Long-term nutritional follow-up is essential to promote a healthy life after weight-loss surgery. Even when surgery-related mortality is taken into account, several studies have shown a significant survival benefit in patients who underwent bariatric surgery compared with those who did not. The survival benefit is specifically due to a decrease in the rate of myocardial infarction, resolution of diabetes mellitus, and fewer cancer-related deaths.

Protein-Calorie Malnutrition. Severe malnutrition is the most serious metabolic complication of bariatric surgery. Red meat is poorly tolerated after bariatric surgery because it is much harder to break down and pass through the small stomach outlet. If the outlet becomes plugged, vomiting will result.

If the patient does not consume enough alternative protein sources, such as milk, yogurt, eggs, fish, and poultry, protein malnutrition can develop. Protein-calorie malnutrition is generally more common with a biliopancreatic diversion (BPD) and very rare with vertical banded gastroplasty. Protein-calorie malnutrition has a reported incidence of 7%–12% in patients who have undergone BPD. Hypoalbuminemia has been reported as early as 1 year after BPD. In the United States today the common channel is typically 75–150 cm in length. In cases of severe malnutrition, enteral or parenteral nutritional therapy may be necessary. Mild to moderate cases usually respond to dietary counseling. More frequent monitoring may be necessary for patients prone to protein-calorie malnutrition.

Fat Malabsorption. Fat-soluble vitamin malabsorption and fat malabsorption (evidenced by steatorrhea) are common with RYGB and BPD. Indeed, this phenomenon is the principal means by which BPD promotes weight loss. The length of the common channel in BPD regulates the degree of fat absorption and determines the severity of malabsorption. Evidence has shown that a 100-cm common channel is better tolerated than a 50-cm channel and is associated with less diarrhea and steatorrhea and improved protein metabolism. Problems with fat-soluble vitamin imbalances and fat malabsorption are rarely seen with vertical banded gastroplasty.

Consideration of Bariatric Surgery in Pediatric and Adolescent Patients

With over 10% of children now classified as overweight or obese, bariatric surgery in adolescents is becoming more prevalent. Nevertheless, in severely obese children and adolescents, first-line therapy should be noninvasive. This includes family-based behavioral techniques that support changes in diet, promote reduced caloric intake and healthy nutrition, and increase exercise levels.

An NIH consensus statement indicated that bariatric surgery in adolescents is safe and effective for long-term sustained weight loss and resolution of comorbid conditions. The American Society for Metabolic and Bariatric Surgery (ASMBS) has expanded the patient population suitable for bariatric surgery to include adolescents and possibly individuals with a BMI of 30–34.9 kg/m^2 who have associated comorbid conditions. The 2012 ASMBS Pediatric Best Practice Guidelines recommend that bariatric surgery be performed in adolescents with a BMI above 35 kg/m^2 and a severe comorbidity such as severe OSA, moderate to severe NASH, diabetes mellitus type 2, pseudotumor cerebri, or adolescents with a BMI above 40 kg/m^2. The most common weight loss operations in adolescents are sleeve gastrectomy and RYGB. Despite the lower complication rate seen with adjustable gastric banding, the FDA has approved this device for *adults only*. One of the side effects seen after weight loss surgery in female adolescents is an *increase in fertility*.

Management of Anesthesia in Obese Patients

Preoperative Evaluation

A thorough preoperative evaluation is necessary for all patients with clinically severe obesity coming for surgery. The focus of the history and physical examination should be on the cardiovascular and respiratory systems and on airway evaluation. Many of these patients lead sedentary lives, so eliciting symptoms associated with cardiorespiratory disease may be difficult. Even a thorough history and physical examination combined with an electrocardiogram (ECG) may underestimate the extent of cardiovascular disease in these patients. In some cases, more extensive preoperative diagnostic testing may include chest radiography, a sleep study, cardiac stress testing, transthoracic echocardiography, and room air arterial blood gas sampling. These may be necessary to fully evaluate the health status of an obese patient.

The anesthesiologist should inquire about the presence of chest pain, shortness of breath at rest or with minimal exertion, and palpitations, and the position in which the patient sleeps. The most common symptoms of pulmonary hypertension are exertional dyspnea, fatigue, and syncope, which reflect an inability to increase cardiac output during activity. If pulmonary hypertension is suspected, avoidance of nitrous oxide and other drugs that may further worsen pulmonary vasoconstriction is essential. Intraoperatively, inhaled anesthetics may be beneficial because they cause bronchodilation and decrease hypoxic pulmonary vasoconstriction.

Symptoms of OSA such as snoring, apneic episodes during sleep, daytime somnolence, morning headaches, and frequent sleep arousal should be sought. If a diagnosis of severe OSA or OHS is suspected, further evaluation is required. Symptoms of acid reflux, coughing, inability to lie flat without coughing, or heartburn may indicate GERD or delayed gastric emptying. If these symptoms are not already controlled with proton pump inhibitors, it may be necessary to start these medications preoperatively. Prolonging the period of preoperative fasting from the standard 8 hours to 12 hours and prohibiting the intake of clear liquids starting at 8 hours preoperatively may be prudent. In patients with a history of hypertension, eliciting symptoms such as frequent headaches and changes in vision can indicate whether the blood pressure is well controlled. In those with uncontrolled hypertension, referral to an internist for optimization should be considered. In diabetic patients, symptoms of claudication, peripheral neuropathy, renal dysfunction, retinopathy, or an elevated hemoglobin A_{1c} level should signal the possibility of advanced diabetes mellitus, poorly controlled blood glucose levels, and microvascular and/or macrovascular disease.

Obese patients have unique issues that may contribute to cardiovascular, pulmonary, and thromboembolic complications. High-risk patients should be identified early to ensure optimal management of co-existing diseases before surgery. A look at prior anesthetic records, with special attention to induction and intubation, may help identify problems with airway management and indicate the weight of the patient at the time of the previous surgery.

Physical Examination and Airway Examination
The physical examination should attempt to identify signs suggestive of cardiac and respiratory disease. Signs of left or right ventricular failure (e.g., increased jugular venous pressure, extra heart sounds, rales, hepatomegaly, peripheral edema) may be very difficult to elicit in the severely obese patient because of body habitus. Pedal edema is a very common finding in obese patients and may be due to right-sided heart failure, varicose veins, or simply extravasation of intravascular fluid associated with decreased mobility.

A detailed assessment of the upper airway must be performed to look for the following anatomic features: fat face and cheeks, short neck, large tongue, large tonsillar size, excessive palatal and pharyngeal soft tissue, limited cervical and/or mandibular mobility, large breasts, increased neck circumference at the level of the thyroid cartilage, or a Mallampati score of 3 or higher.

A history of sleep apnea should raise the possibility of upper airway abnormalities that may predispose to difficulties with mask ventilation and exposure of the glottic opening during direct laryngoscopy, such as decreased anatomic space to accommodate anterior displacement of the tongue. When awake, these patients may compensate for their compromised airway anatomy by increasing the craniocervical angulation, which increases the space between the mandible and cervical spine and elongates the tongue and soft tissues of the neck. This compensation is lost when these patients become unconscious.

Studies have not shown a statistically significant link between obesity per se and the likelihood of difficult intubation. Rather, physical examination findings such as a very thick neck or a Mallampati score higher than 3 more reliably predict the possibility of a difficult intubation. In selected patients, awake endotracheal intubation using fiberoptic laryngoscopy may be the most appropriate method for securing the airway, but it is important to remember that neither clinically severe obesity nor a high BMI are absolute indications for awake intubation. The obese patient should also be evaluated for ease of peripheral intravenous (IV) catheter placement. If severe difficulty with IV access is anticipated, the patient should be informed of the possibility of placement of a central venous catheter before induction. If a patient is found to be at very high risk of intraoperative or postoperative deep vein thrombosis, placement of an inferior vena cava filter before surgery should be considered.

Preoperative Diagnostic Tests
ECG examination may demonstrate findings suggestive of right ventricular hypertrophy, left ventricular hypertrophy, cardiac dysrhythmias, or myocardial ischemia or infarction. It is important to keep in mind that the ECG may not always be reliable in the patient with clinically severe obesity because of morphologic features such as (1) displacement of the heart by an elevated diaphragm, (2) increased cardiac workload with associated cardiac hypertrophy, (3) increased distance between the heart and the recording electrodes caused by excess adipose tissue in the chest wall and possibly increased epicardial fat, and (4) the potential for associated chronic lung disease to alter the ECG. Chest radiographic examination may show signs of heart failure,

increased vascular markings, pulmonary congestion, pulmonary hypertension, hyperinflated lungs, or other pulmonary disease. Transthoracic echocardiography is useful to evaluate left and right ventricular systolic and diastolic function as well as to identify pulmonary hypertension. In cases of severe OSA, results of arterial blood gas analysis on a sample drawn with the patient breathing room air may be helpful in guiding intraoperative and postoperative ventilatory management and oxygen supplementation.

Home Medications

Most home medications should be continued preoperatively, with the exception of oral hypoglycemics, anticoagulants (e.g., warfarin, aspirin, clopidogrel), and nonsteroidal antiinflammatory drugs (NSAIDs). Patients taking histamine-2 receptor blockers such as famotidine, *nonparticulate* antacids, or proton pump inhibitors should be counseled to take these medications on the morning of surgery. Obese patients are at high risk of acute postoperative pulmonary embolism because of their chronic inflammatory state, so perioperative deep vein thrombosis prophylaxis with either unfractionated or low-molecular-weight heparin is indicated.

If continuous positive airway pressure (CPAP) or bilevel positive airway pressure (BiPAP) is used at home, the patient should be advised to bring the mask on the day of surgery so that this therapy can be continued in the postoperative period. Currently, no data exist to support preoperative initiation of CPAP or BiPAP to improve postoperative outcomes in patients with sleep apnea.

Intraoperative Management
Positioning

Specially designed operating tables (or two regular tables joined together) may be required for bariatric surgery. Regular operating room tables have a maximum weight limit of approximately 205 kg, but operating tables capable of holding up to 455 kg, with a little extra width to accommodate the extra girth, are now available. To transfer the patient from the stretcher to the operating table, an air transfer mattress device (e.g., HoverMatt) can be used to laterally transfer and reposition patients and minimize injury to staff. Some severely obese patients will require "ramping," which is a means of positioning the patient using a ramp that extends from behind the lumbar area to the neck and allows the head to be positioned above the chest in a horizontal plane formed between the sternal notch and the external auditory meatus. This position allows better ventilatory mechanics and facilitates intubation (Fig. 20.4). Particular care should be paid to protecting pressure areas because pressure sores and nerve injuries are more common in the superobese and in obese patients with diabetes mellitus. Brachial plexus, sciatic, and ulnar nerve palsies have been reported in patients with increased BMI. Upper and lower limbs, because of their increased weight, have a higher likelihood of sliding off the operating table, which can produce peripheral nerve injuries. It is desirable to keep the arms in neutral position on the arm boards so their position can be monitored and excess pressure from tight tucking and draping can be avoided.

Laparoscopic Surgery

The degree of intraabdominal pressure determines the effects of pneumoperitoneum on venous return, myocardial performance, and ventilatory status. There is a biphasic cardiovascular response to increases in intraabdominal pressure. At an intraabdominal pressure of approximately 10 mm Hg, there is an *increase* in venous return, probably from a reduction in splanchnic sequestration of blood. This is associated with an increase in cardiac output and arterial pressure. Hypovolemia, however, blunts this response. Compression of the inferior vena cava occurs at intraabdominal pressures of approximately 20 mm Hg, and this results in *decreased* venous return from the lower body, increased renal vascular resistance, decreased renal blood flow, and decreased glomerular filtration. Concomitantly, obese patients manifest a disproportionate increase in systemic vascular resistance caused not only by aortic compression but also by increased secretion of vasopressin. These patients have higher left ventricular end-systolic wall stress *before* pneumoperitoneum (caused by increased end-systolic left ventricular dimensions) and *during* pneumoperitoneum. Since higher left ventricular end-systolic wall stress is a determinant of myocardial oxygen demand, more aggressive control of blood pressure (ventricular afterload) may be needed in patients with clinically severe obesity to optimize myocardial oxygen supply and demand. Both pneumoperitoneum and Trendelenburg positioning can reduce femoral venous blood

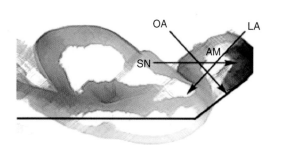 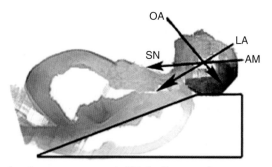

FIG. 20.4   "Ramping" to achieve proper positioning for airway management. *AM,* Auditory meatus; *LA,* laryngeal axis; *OA,* oral axis; *SN,* sternal notch. (Illustration by Brooke E. Albright, MD.)

flow, increasing the risk of lower extremity thrombosis. High intraabdominal pressure in conjunction with placement in Trendelenburg position increases intrathoracic pressure and may impede adequate ventilation. Moreover, absorption of CO_2 can worsen hypercarbia and induce respiratory acidosis, thereby increasing pulmonary hypertension.

Choice of Anesthesia

According to the American Society of Anesthesiologists (ASA) Practice Guidelines, local or regional anesthesia should be the primary anesthetic choice for obese patients undergoing surgery, with general anesthesia used only when necessary. Placement of an epidural or peripheral nerve block can significantly aid in managing postoperative pain and reduce the need for narcotics, which decreases the incidence of postoperative respiratory depression.

Regional Anesthesia. Regional anesthesia—spinal anesthesia, epidural anesthesia, and peripheral nerve block—may be technically difficult in obese patients, since landmarks are obscured by excess adipose tissue. It is estimated that the risk of a failed block is about 1.5 times higher in patients with a BMI above 30 kg/m^2 than in patients with a low BMI. There is also a higher likelihood of block-related complications. The success rate for blocks is significantly higher when ultrasonographic guidance is used to assist in needle placement. A distinct advantage of regional anesthesia in the obese patient is the ability to limit the amount of intraoperative and postoperative opioid use, which thereby limits the risk of respiratory depression and improves patient safety and satisfaction. Interestingly, obese patients require as much as 20% *less* local anesthetic for spinal or epidural anesthesia than nonobese patients, presumably because of fatty infiltration and vascular engorgement from increased intraabdominal pressure, which decreases the volume of the epidural space. It is difficult to reliably predict the sensory level of anesthesia that will be achieved by neuraxial blockade in these patients.

General Anesthesia. Induction of general anesthesia in the obese patient is not without risks. The anesthetic plan, including all risks, benefits, and alternatives to general anesthesia, should be discussed thoroughly with the patient and surgeon before the operation. The possible need for postoperative respiratory support via CPAP, BiPAP, or mechanical ventilation should also be discussed.

Airway Management

Management of the airway is one of the great challenges associated with general anesthesia in the obese patient. An emergency airway cart that provides access to rescue intubating devices such as supraglottic devices, a flexible bronchoscope, a light wand, and resuscitation drugs should be immediately available. Use of an intubating laryngeal mask airway has been shown to be successful for tracheal *intubation* in 96% of obese patients and for successful *ventilation* in 100% of obese patients. Use of a videolaryngoscope may facilitate tracheal intubation. Since the introduction of videolaryngoscopy, awake fiberoptic tracheal intubation is used less frequently, but it remains an option

for airway management in certain patients. For very high-risk patients with extremely limited pulmonary reserve or abnormal airway anatomy, a surgeon with considerable experience in performing tracheostomy should be immediately available to perform an emergency tracheostomy if needed.

Before intubation, there must be adequate time for positioning and preoxygenation. Proper patient positioning is essential to successful intubation of the trachea. Often the large body habitus, particularly a large chest, short neck, or excess neck soft tissue, limits placement of the laryngoscope and glottic exposure. Successful intubation is contingent upon adequate alignment of the oral, pharyngeal, and laryngeal axes, also known as the *sniffing position*. To achieve this position, the obese patient may require ramping, in which a wedge-shaped device is placed behind the torso and a pillow is placed behind the head to slightly extend the neck so that the sternal notch is in line horizontally with the auditory meatus (see Fig. 20.4). Adequate preoxygenation is critically important in obese patients, since they have a decreased FRC and higher oxygen consumption. Therefore they experience desaturation much faster than nonobese patients when they are apneic. Studies have shown that when patients undergo 5 minutes of preoxygenation with an FIO_2 of 100% via CPAP at a pressure of 10 cm H_2O, the time that apnea can be tolerated without oxygen desaturation increases by 50%, allowing more time for direct laryngoscopy and tracheal intubation.

The decision to perform a rapid-sequence induction should be made on a case-by-case basis. Multiple risk factors for pulmonary aspiration may be present in the obese population: higher gastric residual volume, lower pH of gastric contents, higher intraabdominal pressure, and higher incidence of GERD and diabetes.

Management of Ventilation

In the obese population, several factors make controlled mechanical ventilation problematic. Obese patients have a decreased FRC and decreased lung oxygen reserves and experience desaturation faster during periods of hypoventilation or apnea than do normal-weight individuals. Positioning for adequate surgical exposure (prone or Trendelenburg position) can worsen ventilation problems by decreasing chest wall compliance. If pneumoperitoneum is required for surgical exposure (laparoscopic or robotic surgery), ventilation may be impaired by the increased abdominal pressure, which worsens lung compliance. Recruitment maneuvers (e.g., Valsalva maneuver) can be used to prevent atelectasis. PEEP improves ventilation/perfusion matching and arterial oxygenation in obese patients, but at high levels (PEEP of 15–20 cm H_2O) adverse effects on cardiac output and oxygen delivery may offset these benefits. Using pressure-controlled ventilation and changing the inspiratory/expiratory ratio can help limit peak airway pressure. When spontaneous ventilation is resumed at the conclusion of surgery, it is best to maintain the patient in a semi-upright position and apply pressure-support ventilation with PEEP to help reduce the risk of atelectasis. In a spontaneously breathing obese patient, the supine position is often associated with hypoxemia. Currently there are no data to indicate which mode of mechanical ventilation is best for obese patients.

Induction and Maintenance of Anesthesia

Any combination of drugs can be used for induction and maintenance of general anesthesia in patients with clinically severe obesity, but some drugs appear to have a better pharmacokinetic profile than others.

Pharmacokinetics of Anesthetic Drugs

The physiologic changes associated with obesity may lead to alterations in distribution, binding, and elimination of many drugs. The volume of distribution in obese individuals may be influenced by a variety of factors, including increased blood volume and cardiac output, decreased total body water (fat contains less water than other tissues), altered protein binding of drugs, and the lipid solubility of the drug being administered. The effect of obesity on protein binding is variable. Despite the occasional presence of liver dysfunction, hepatic clearance of drugs is usually not altered. Heart failure and decreased liver blood flow could slow elimination of drugs that are highly dependent on hepatic clearance. Renal clearance of drugs may increase in obese individuals because of increased renal blood flow and glomerular filtration rate.

The impact of obesity on dosing of injected drugs is difficult to predict. Total blood volume is likely to be increased, which would tend to decrease the plasma concentration achieved following IV injection of a drug. However, *fat has relatively low blood flow, so an increased dose of drug calculated based on total body weight could result in an excessive plasma concentration.* Cardiac output is increased in the obese patient, which affects drug distribution and dilution in the first minute after administration. Because both cardiac output and plasma volume are increased, an initially higher dose of a drug may be required for loading to attain peak plasma concentration. *The most clinically useful approach is to calculate the initial dose of drug to be injected into an obese patient based on lean body weight rather than total body weight.* Lean body weight is total body weight minus fat weight (Fig. 20.5). In clinically severe obesity, lean body weight is increased and accounts for 20%–40% of excess body weight. Ideal body weight does not take into account the increase in lean body weight in severely obese patients. Therefore lean body weight is more highly correlated with cardiac output and drug clearance and should be used for initial dosing. Subsequent doses of drugs should be based on the pharmacologic response to the initial dose. Repeated injections of a drug, however, can result in cumulative drug effects and prolonged responses, reflecting storage of drugs in fat and subsequent release from this inactive depot into the systemic circulation as the plasma concentration of drug declines. It is important to note that *oral absorption of drugs is not influenced by obesity.*

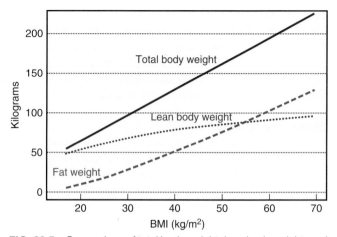

FIG. 20.5 Comparison of total body weight, lean body weight, and fat weight with increasing body mass index (BMI) in a male of standard height. (Adapted from Lemmens H. Perioperative pharmacology in morbid obesity. *Curr Opin Anaesthesiol.* 2010;23:485-491.)

An increased incidence of NASH in obese patients warrants caution when selecting drugs that have been associated with postoperative liver dysfunction. Awakening of obese patients is more prompt after exposure to desflurane or sevoflurane than after administration of either isoflurane or propofol. The rapid elimination of nitrous oxide is useful, but the frequent need for increased supplemental oxygen limits the usefulness of nitrous oxide in obese patients.

Maintenance of anesthesia is best managed with drugs with minimal potential for accumulation in adipose tissue. Propofol, benzodiazepines, atracurium, cisatracurium, and narcotics such as sufentanil and fentanyl are highly lipophilic and accumulate in fatty tissue when administered by infusion over a long period. Usually, highly lipophilic drugs show a significant increase in volume of distribution in obese patients, and it would seem that dosing of these should be based on total body weight. However, because the majority of these drugs have the potential to accumulate in adipose tissue over time, a prolonged effect can be seen. An exception is remifentanil. This drug is also highly lipophilic; however, because it is rapidly metabolized by plasma esterases, it has limited potential for accumulation in fat tissue. It is therefore favored over other narcotics for intraoperative analgesia. Ketamine and dexmedetomidine may also be useful anesthetic adjuncts in patients who are susceptible to narcotic-induced respiratory depression. For common anesthetic drug dosing recommendations, refer to Table 20.6.

Administration of hydrophilic substances such as muscle relaxants should be based on lean body weight, because their peak plasma concentrations are *independent* of the volume of distribution, which is greatly increased in obese patients. The large volume of distribution is due to the high ratio of extracellular to intracellular fluid, since the water content of adipose tissue is almost completely extracellular. Because the effect of this increased extracellular fluid on neuromuscular blockade is unclear, it is *recommended that neuromuscular blockers be dosed based on lean body weight* and that the degree of blockade be carefully monitored with a peripheral nerve stimulator.

TABLE 20.6	Recommended Weight Basis for Dosing of Common Anesthetic Drugs in Obese Patients	
Total Body Weight	**Lean Body Weight**
Propofol: loading	Propofol: maintenance
Midazolam	Thiopental
Succinylcholine	Vecuronium
Cisatracurium and atracurium: loading	Cisatracurium and atracurium: maintenance
Pancuronium[a]	Rocuronium
	Remifentanil
	Fentanyl
	Sufentanil

[a]Pancuronium requires higher dosing to maintain 90% depression of twitch height in obese patients but will also have a longer duration of action at higher dosages.

The pharmacokinetics of succinylcholine are unique. Because the level of plasma pseudocholinesterase and the volume of distribution are increased, patients with clinically severe obesity have larger absolute succinylcholine requirements than normal-weight patients. Therefore to achieve profound neuromuscular blockade and facilitate intubation, administration of *succinylcholine should be based on total body weight* rather than lean body weight.

Recent studies suggest sugammadex (Bridion) may be a better agent than neostigmine in reversing neuromuscular blockade in obese patients, since it has an improved ability to prevent postoperative recurarization in comparison to neostigmine. Sugammadex should be given at a dose of 2 mg/kg based on lean body weight and administered after recovery of neuromuscular blockade has reached the second twitch in response to train of four stimulation.

Monitoring

The extent of surgery and concomitant comorbid conditions should be the primary factors that determine the need for and extent of monitoring beyond routine monitoring. For surgery performed under local or regional anesthesia with moderate sedation, the ASA Practice Guidelines recommend continuous capnography monitoring to decrease the risk of undetected airway obstruction, which is especially prevalent in the obese population. For surgery performed under general anesthesia, hemodynamic monitoring may be needed in selected patients. The technical difficulty of placing invasive hemodynamic monitors may be increased in this patient population. If noninvasive blood pressure cuffs are used, it is important to fit a correctly sized cuff. If the cuff is too small, blood pressure measurements may be falsely elevated. Alternatives to standard blood pressure cuffs include noninvasive blood pressure monitoring systems that detect blood pressure in the radial artery or finger. An intraarterial catheter should be inserted if noninvasive monitoring is inadequate or if the obese patient has severe cardiopulmonary disease. When IV access is problematic, use of ultrasonography to guide the placement of peripheral and/or central lines may increase the success rate and decrease the complication rate associated with these

procedures. Transesophageal echocardiography (TEE) and pulmonary artery catheterization can be performed intraoperatively in patients with heart failure, pulmonary hypertension, or other medical conditions that make continuous assessment of volume status or cardiac function necessary. Continuous TEE monitoring allows immediate detection of alterations in cardiac function as well as accurate assessment of volume status to guide fluid management. However, TEE monitoring requires expensive equipment and trained personnel and may not be readily available in all operative settings.

Fluid Management

Calculation of *fluid requirements* in the obese patient *should be based on lean body weight,* with a goal of euvolemia. Achieving this goal may be very difficult because there is a high association between severe obesity and diastolic dysfunction. In patients with preexisting cardiac disease, large fluid loads may not be tolerated well, and development of pulmonary edema is more likely. During laparoscopic surgery, decreased urinary output does not necessarily reflect hypovolemia, and liberal fluid administration may have a negative impact on overall outcome.

Emergence

Tracheal extubation is considered when obese patients are fully awake and alert and have recovered from the depressant effects of the anesthetics. Although there are no specific studies to guide the practice of tracheal extubation in obese patients, certain maneuvers can facilitate better respiratory mechanics before extubation. These include placement in the semi-upright position (>30 degrees head up), provision of pressure-support ventilation with PEEP or CPAP until extubation, oxygen supplementation, and placement of a nasopharyngeal airway to help maintain airway patency. A history of OSA or OHS mandates intense postoperative respiratory monitoring to ensure a patent upper airway and acceptable oxygenation and ventilation. In certain high-risk patients, placement of a tube exchanger before extubation may be prudent and is usually well tolerated even if left in place for several hours.

The notion that patients with clinically severe obesity emerge slowly from the effects of general anesthesia owing to delayed release of volatile anesthetics from fat stores is *not* accurate. Poor total fat blood flow limits delivery of volatile anesthetics for storage. Overall, recovery times are comparable in obese and lean individuals undergoing surgery that requires anesthesia for less than 4 hours.

Postoperative Management

Although episodic arterial hypoxemia may occur at any time from the immediate postoperative period to as late as 2–5 days after surgery, no data support routine intensive care unit admission to decrease morbidity and mortality. Early episodic arterial hypoxemia may be due to perioperative opioid use. The patients at highest risk for developing postoperative hypoxemia are those with a history of OSA. The sitting position is a useful posture to improve arterial oxygenation. Routine administration of oxygen during the postoperative period is controversial because oxygen administration can increase the duration of apnea by delaying the arousal effect produced by arterial hypoxemia. Therefore it is preferable to provide supplemental oxygen *only* if arterial oxygen desaturation occurs. Once the patient's saturation can be maintained at baseline levels or above 90% on room air with good pain control, pulse oximetry may be discontinued.

Transport

Before transport from the operating room to the recovery room, the obese patient should be fully awake and alert, sitting in a semi-upright position, receiving supplemental oxygen, and monitored by pulse oximetry. Verbal contact should be maintained throughout transport to assess wakefulness and adequacy of respiratory effort.

Postoperative Analgesia

Because opioid-induced ventilatory depression is a concern, a multimodal approach to postoperative pain control is usually employed. This includes use of techniques that decrease narcotic requirements. Peripheral and central nerve block with continuous infusion of local anesthetic with or without small doses of opioids is an effective method for postoperative analgesia in obese patients. Supplementation with NSAIDs, α_2-receptor agonists, *N*-methyl-D-aspartate (NMDA) receptor antagonists, sodium channel blockers, or other nonopioid analgesics is highly recommended, since these drugs do not contribute to postoperative respiratory depression. Ketorolac is an NSAID that has been used successfully to reduce pain in the postoperative period. The principal side effects are GI discomfort and the potential for increased operative site bleeding. Ketorolac is *not suitable* for use in patients who have undergone bariatric surgery, because these patients are at especially high risk for development of GI bleeding. IV acetaminophen can serve as a great adjunct to multimodal analgesia in obese patients. Dosing of IV acetaminophen for patients who weigh more than 50 kg should be 1 g IV every 6 hours as needed, not to exceed 4 g in 24 hours. Because acetaminophen is metabolized by the liver and excreted in the urine, dosage should be decreased in patients with liver or kidney disease. Both dexmedetomidine, a selective α_2-receptor agonist, and clonidine, a less selective α_2-receptor agonist, have been shown to reduce opioid requirements if administered by continuous infusion in the perioperative period. Ketamine has been shown to enhance the analgesic effects of morphine by inhibiting opioid activation of NMDA receptors. Given in small doses postoperatively, ketamine can decrease pain and increase wakefulness and oxygen saturation. If opioids are eventually required to control postoperative pain, patient-controlled analgesia is a good option. *Dosages of opioids should be based on lean body weight.*

In addition, local anesthetic wound infiltration or ultrasound-guided transversus abdominis plane (TAP) blocks after laparoscopic bariatric surgery and other abdominal surgery can be used as part of multimodal pain control therapy.

Respiratory and Cardiovascular Monitoring and Management

Adequacy of ventilation should be assessed and monitored for at least 24–48 hours postoperatively. If the patient was on CPAP or BiPAP at home, this should be resumed postoperatively. If the patient had not been diagnosed with sleep apnea preoperatively but experiences frequent airway obstruction and hypoxemic episodes in the recovery room, CPAP or BiPAP can be initiated. These noninvasive ventilatory modes should be used very cautiously in the period immediately after gastric bypass surgery, however, because there is some risk of stomal dehiscence associated with their use. Respiratory monitoring in the first few postoperative hours should be intensive. Any sign suggestive of respiratory fatigue or cardiovascular instability should be evaluated and treated immediately. If obese patients require reintubation, it is best performed in a controlled fashion rather than under emergency conditions.

Discharge to an Unmonitored Setting

The decision about when to discharge patients to a regular hospital room or to home can be difficult in some obese patients, but it is generally considered safe to discharge a patient to an unmonitored setting (regular hospital bed or home) when pain is adequately controlled and the patient is no longer at significant risk of postoperative respiratory depression.

Postoperative Complications

Postoperative morbidity and mortality rates are higher in obese patients than in nonobese patients. This is due primarily to the presence of preexisting medical illnesses and the risk of aspiration during endotracheal intubation. Wound infection is twice as common in obese patients. Postoperative mechanical ventilation is often needed in obese patients who have a history of CO_2 retention and have undergone prolonged surgery. The hazards of OSA and OHS may extend several days into the postoperative period. The maximum decrease in Pao_2 typically occurs 2–3 days postoperatively. Weaning from mechanical ventilation may be difficult because of increased work of breathing, decreased lung volumes, and ventilation/perfusion mismatching. The likelihood of deep vein thrombosis and pulmonary embolism is increased, which emphasizes the importance of early postoperative ambulation and the need for prophylactic anticoagulation. Obese patients tend *not to be able* to mobilize their fat stores during critical illness and need to rely on carbohydrates for energy. This increased carbohydrate metabolism raises the respiratory quotient and accelerates protein catabolism. If these patients take nothing by mouth for a prolonged period, a protein malnutrition syndrome may develop.

Enhanced Recovery After Surgery (ERAS) protocols, also known as *fast-track protocols,* are designed to reduce morbidity after surgery and to decrease hospital stay. These protocols were initially introduced in the setting of elective colorectal surgery. They are currently being adapted for other types of abdominal surgery, including bariatric procedures. Bariatric ERAS protocols consist of several evidence-based perioperative care interventions, such as using laparoscopic techniques, avoiding prophylactic nasogastric tubes and abdominal drains, early postoperative feeding and ambulation, implementation of multimodal analgesia and antiemetic therapy, and thromboprophylaxis. The effectiveness of bariatric ERAS protocols is not well defined at this time.

MALNUTRITION AND VITAMIN DEFICIENCIES

Malnutrition

Nutrients are essential for the maintenance of biochemical pathways that control cardiac function, respiration, immune responses, and cognition. Proteins are especially important for muscle and tissue synthesis, and their component amino acids have a wide range of biological roles. Malnutrition results from an imbalance in nutritional intake or inadequate caloric support. It can be due to loss of appetite, underconsumption of nutrients in the diet, or malabsorption. Estimates suggest that malnourished patients have hospital stays 50% longer than well-nourished patients and are at higher risk of wound infection, immunosuppression, renal dysfunction, and other complications. Anemia and vitamin B_{12} deficiency further impair recovery. To minimize the risk of malnutrition, it is recommended that *all* patients admitted to a hospital be screened and monitored for signs of malnutrition. Biological markers suggestive of malnutrition include a serum albumin concentration below 3 g/dL, a transferrin level below 200 mg/dL, and a prealbumin level below 15 mg/dL. Cholesterol, zinc, iron, vitamin B_{12}, and folic acid levels may also be significantly reduced in malnourished patients. Of all these markers, prealbumin may be the most useful because its half-life is only 2 days, and therefore changes in nutritional status can be detected quite early. However, prealbumin levels should always be measured in conjunction with C-reactive protein levels, since inflammation can raise the level of prealbumin and affect interpretation of results. In the presence of low levels of *both* prealbumin and C-reactive protein, it is likely the patient is malnourished. Treatment of malnutrition is aimed at balancing nutritional intake with energy needs. If nutritional therapy is necessary, enteral feeding or parenteral nutrition can be initiated.

Enteral Nutrition

When the GI tract is functioning, enteral nutrition can be provided by means of nasogastric or gastrostomy tube feedings or by postpyloric methods such as nasojejunal tubes or feeding jejunostomy tubes. Continuous infusion is the usual method for administering enteral feedings. The rate, composition, and volume of the feeding solution is individualized based on laboratory data.

The question of when to stop postpyloric feedings in patients with upcoming surgery is unclear. However, *nasogastric and orogastric feedings should be stopped 8 hours before surgery,* and the stomach should be suctioned before the patient is taken to the operating room. Complications of

TABLE 20.7	Complications of Total and Peripheral Parenteral Nutrition

Hypokalemia
Hypophosphatemia
Bacterial translocation from the gastrointestinal tract
Renal dysfunction
Nonketotic hyperosmolar hyperglycemic coma
Hypomagnesemia
Venous thrombosis
Osteopenia
Hyperchloremic metabolic acidosis
Hypocalcemia
Infection, sepsis
Elevated liver enzyme levels
Fluid overload
Refeeding syndrome

enteral feedings are infrequent but include hyperglycemia, causing osmotic diuresis and hypovolemia. Exogenous insulin administration may be a consideration if blood glucose concentrations are elevated. The osmolarity of elemental diets (i.e., tube feedings) is high at 550–850 mOsm/L; they often cause diarrhea.

Parenteral Nutrition

Parenteral nutrition is indicated when the GI tract is not functioning. *Peripheral parenteral nutrition* using an isotonic solution delivered through a peripheral vein is limited by osmolality and volume constraints. It may be useful as a supplement to oral intake or when the anticipated need for nutritional support is less than 14 days. *Total parenteral nutrition* (TPN) is used when the daily caloric requirements exceed 2000 kcal or prolonged nutritional support is required. In such cases a catheter is inserted into a central vein to permit infusion of hypertonic solutions in a daily volume of approximately 40 mL/kg.

Potential complications of TPN are numerous (Table 20.7). Blood glucose concentrations must be monitored because hyperglycemia is very common and may require treatment with *exogenous* insulin. Hypoglycemia may occur if the TPN infusion is abruptly discontinued, since increased circulating *endogenous* concentrations of insulin will persist. Hyperchloremic metabolic acidosis may occur because of the liberation of hydrochloric acid during the metabolism of amino acids present in most parenteral nutrition solutions. Parenteral feeding of patients with compromised cardiac function is associated with the risk of congestive heart failure from fluid overload. Increased production of CO_2 resulting from metabolism of large amounts of glucose may result in the need to initiate mechanical ventilation or failure to wean from mechanical ventilation.

Vitamin Deficiencies

Table 20.8 lists the more common vitamin deficiencies.

TABLE 20.8	Vitamin Deficiencies	
Vitamin Deficiency	Causes of Deficiency	Signs of Deficiency
Thiamine (B$_1$) (beriberi)	Chronic alcoholism, which results in decreased intake of thiamine	Low systemic vascular resistance; high cardiac output; polyneuropathy (demyelination, sensory deficit, paresthesia); exaggerated blood pressure response to hemorrhage, change in body position, positive pressure ventilation
Riboflavin (B$_2$)	Almost always caused by dietary deficiency, photodegradation of milk or other dairy products	Magenta tongue, angular stomatitis, seborrhea, cheilosis
Niacin (B$_3$)	Carcinoid tumor; niacin (nicotinic acid) is synthesized from tryptophan; in carcinoid tumor, tryptophan is used to form serotonin instead of niacin, which makes patients with these tumors more susceptible to deficiency.	Mental confusion, irritability, peripheral neuropathy, achlorhydria, diarrhea, vesicular dermatitis, stomatitis, glossitis, urethritis, excessive salivation
Pyridoxine (B$_6$)	Alcoholism, isoniazid therapy	Seborrhea, glossitis, convulsions, neuropathy, depression, confusion, microcytic anemia
Folate (B$_9$)	Alcoholism; therapy with sulfasalazine, pyrimethamine, or triamterene	Megaloblastic anemia, atrophic glossitis, depression, increased homocysteine level
Cyanocobalamin (B$_{12}$)	Gastric atrophy (pernicious anemia), terminal ileal disease, strict vegetarianism	Megaloblastic anemia, loss of vibratory and positional sense, abnormal gait, dementia, impotence, loss of bladder and bowel control, increased levels of homocysteine and methylmalonic acid
Biotin	Ingestion of raw egg whites (contain the protein avidin, which strongly binds the vitamin and reduces its bioavailability)	Mental changes (depression, hallucinations); paresthesias; a scaling rash around the eyes, nose, and mouth; alopecia
Ascorbic acid (C)	Smoking, alcoholism	Capillary fragility, petechial hemorrhage, joint and skeletal muscle hemorrhage, poor wound healing, catabolic state, loosened teeth and gangrenous alveolar margins, low potassium and iron levels
A	Dietary lack of leafy vegetables and animal liver, malabsorption	Loss of night vision, conjunctival drying, corneal destruction, anemia
D (rickets)	Limited sun exposure, inflammatory bowel disease and other fat malabsorption syndromes	Thoracic kyphosis, which can lead to hypoventilation; parathyroid hormone activity, which leads to increased osteoclastic activity and bone resorption
E	Occurs only with fat malabsorption or genetic abnormalities of vitamin E metabolism or transport	Peripheral neuropathy, spinocerebellar ataxia, skeletal muscle atrophy, retinopathy
K	Prolonged antibiotic therapy that eliminates the intestinal bacteria that form the vitamin; failure of fat absorption	Bleeding

KEY POINTS

- Obesity is the most prevalent nutritional disease and is considered one of the most preventable causes of illness worldwide.
- Obesity leads to an increased incidence of glucose intolerance, diabetes mellitus, systemic hypertension, coronary artery diseases, heart failure, cancer, and thromboembolic events. A waist/hip ratio higher than 1.0 in men and 0.8 in women is a strong predictor of ischemic heart disease, stroke, diabetes, and death independent of total body fat.
- Compared with the normal-weight population, the risk of premature death is doubled and the risk of death resulting from cardiovascular disease is increased fivefold in the obese population.
- Bariatric surgery results in significant and sustained weight loss as well as a diminution in obesity-related comorbid conditions. It is associated with a survival benefit.

- Regional anesthesia is the preferred method of primary anesthesia in the severely obese patient. Use of ultrasonography significantly increases the success rate of regional anesthesia in this population.
- Airway management is one of the greatest challenges associated with general anesthesia in obese patients. Mask ventilation can be difficult owing to the presence of increased soft tissues in the head, neck, and chest. Videolaryngoscopy has improved the safety and efficacy of tracheal intubation after induction of anesthesia. Awake intubations are now less often required.
- In the obese population, pneumoperitoneum during laparoscopic surgery may have significant deleterious effects on cardiopulmonary performance, including decreased cardiac output and stroke volume, increased systemic vascular resistance, and decreased functional residual capacity.
- The impact of obesity on appropriate dosing of intravenous anesthetic drugs is difficult to predict. A useful clinical

approach is to calculate the initial dose of injected drug based on lean body weight rather than total body weight.

- A multimodal approach to postoperative pain control is usually employed to decrease the risk of opioid-induced respiratory depression in the obese patient.
- Current guidelines recommend screening and monitoring for signs of malnutrition in all patients admitted to the hospital. In situations in which oral intake is prohibited and treatment of malnutrition is needed, supplementation can be provided by initiating enteral or parenteral nutrition.

RESOURCES

Bergland A, Gislason H, Raeder J. Fast-track surgery for bariatric laparoscopic gastric bypass with focus on anaesthesia and peri-operative care. Experience with 500 cases. *Acta Anaesthesiol Scand.* 2008;52:1394-1399.

Buchwald H. Consensus Conference Panel. Bariatric surgery for morbid obesity: health implications for patients, health professionals, and third-party payers. *J Am Coll Surg.* 2005;200:593-604.

Gonzalez H, Minville V, Delanoue K, et al. The importance of increased neck circumference to intubation difficulties in obese patients. *Anesth Analg.* 2008;106:1132-1136.

Lemmens H. Perioperative pharmacology in morbid obesity. *Curr Opin Anaesthesiol.* 2010;23:485-491.

Michalsky M, Reichard K, Inge T, et al. American Society for Metabolic and Bariatric Surgery. ASMBS pediatric best practices guidelines. *Surg Obes Relat Dis.* 2012;8:1-7.

Ogden CL, Caroll MD, Kit BK, et al. Prevalence of childhood and adult obesity in the United States, 2011-2012. *JAMA.* 2014;311:806-814.

Poirier P, Cornier MA, Mazzone T, et al. Bariatric surgery and cardiovascular risk factors: a scientific statement from the American Heart Association. *Circulation.* 2011;123:1683-1701.

Sinha AC, Singh PM. Controversies in perioperative anesthetic management of the morbidly obese: I am a surgeon, why should I care? *Obes Surg.* 2015;25:879-887.

Schumann R. Anaesthesia for bariatric surgery. *Best Pract Res Clin Anaesthesiol.* 2011;25:83-93.

Terkawi AS, Durieux ME. Perioperative anesthesia care for obese patients. *Anesthesiology News.* 2015:1-11.

Yanovski SZ, Yanovski JA. Long-term drug treatment for obesity: a systematic and clinical review. *JAMA.* 2014;311:74-86.

Fluid, Electrolyte, and Acid-Base Disorders

ROBERT B. SCHONBERGER

Alterations of water, osmolal, and electrolyte content and distribution as well as acid-base disturbances are common in the perioperative period and rarely happen in isolation, because they are inherently interrelated. They both affect and are affected by the function and stability of several organ systems. Central nervous system (CNS) impairment, cardiac dysfunction, and neuromuscular changes are especially common in the presence of water, osmolal, electrolyte, and acid-base disturbances. Several perioperative events can exacerbate such alterations (Table 21.1). Management of patients with these disturbances is based on an assessment of the cause and severity of the condition, an understanding of the interrelationships among these disturbances, and an awareness of the patient's comorbid conditions.

ABNORMALITIES OF WATER, OSMOLALITY, AND ELECTROLYTES

Water and Osmolal Homeostasis

In the nonobese adult, total body water comprises approximately 60% of body weight (obesity decreases this proportion). Body water is divided into intracellular fluid (ICF) and extracellular fluid (ECF) compartments according to the location of the water relative to cell membranes (Fig. 21.1). ECF consists primarily of an *interstitial* compartment (three-fourths of ECF) and an *intravascular* plasma compartment (one-fourth of ECF). Water shifts between compartments according to the balance of hydrostatic and oncotic pressure across membranes, and thus water homeostasis relies on the maintenance of osmolality within a narrow physiologic range. The integrity of living cells depends on preservation of water homeostasis, as well as on the energy-intensive maintenance of intracellular and extracellular concentrations of ions termed *electrolytes*. These electrolytes, in addition to being a major determinant of both osmolality and acid-base balance, are responsible for electrical potentials across cell membranes. Changes in electrolyte homeostasis especially impact excitable cells in the CNS and musculature that rely on action potentials for rapid and organized transfer of information.

Water and osmolal homeostasis are predominantly mediated by osmolality-sensing neurons located in the anterior hypothalamus. In response to osmolal elevations, these neurons stimulate thirst and cause pituitary release of vasopressin (antidiuretic hormone). Vasopressin is stored as granules in the posterior pituitary and acts through G protein–coupled receptors in the collecting ducts of the kidney to cause water retention, which in turn decreases serum osmolality. Vasopressin receptors are also present in other tissues and, most noticeably for the anesthesiologist, are present in high density on vascular smooth muscle cells, where they induce vasoconstriction. As a major site of vasopressin effects, the kidney is responsible for maintaining water homeostasis by excreting urine with large variations in total osmolality. Under normal circumstances, serum osmolality is tightly regulated by thirst and renal control of water excretion. The normal range of serum osmolality is 280–290 mOsm/kg.

TABLE 21.1	Common Causes of Water, Osmolal, Electrolyte, and Acid-Base Disturbances During the Perioperative Period

Disease states
  Endocrinopathies
  Nephropathies
  Gastroenteropathies
Drug therapy
  Diuretics
  Corticosteroids
Nasogastric suction
Surgery
  Transurethral resection of the prostate
  Translocation of body water due to tissue trauma
  Resection of portions of the gastrointestinal tract
Management of anesthesia
  Intravenous fluid administration
  Alveolar ventilation
  Hypothermia

TOTAL BODY WATER = 0.6 × BODY WEIGHT

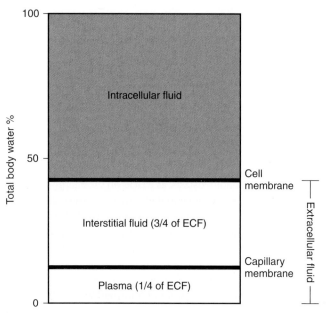

FIG. 21.1   Total body water (≈60% of total body weight) is designated as intracellular fluid (ICF) or extracellular fluid (ECF) depending on the location of the water relative to cell membranes. ECF is further divided into interstitial and plasma compartments depending on its location relative to vascular walls. Two-thirds of total body water is ICF. Of ECF, 75% is interstitial, 25% is intravascular.

The osmolality of serum represents the total number of osmotically active particles (i.e., solutes) per kilogram of solvent. When osmolality is assessed, a shorthand indirect measurement of expected serum osmolality can easily be calculated as 2[Na] + [Glucose]/18 + [Blood urea nitrogen (BUN)]/2.8, and this calculated value should always be compared with direct laboratory-measured actual osmolality. A significant difference in these values (known as an *osmolal gap*) should alert the clinician to the presence of unmeasured osmotically active particles. Increases in serum osmolality

may be encountered as a result of free water depletion (e.g., dehydration or diabetes insipidus) or the presence of additional solutes (most commonly from ingestion of ethanol or other toxins, hyperglycemia, or iatrogenic administration of osmolal loads such as mannitol or glycine). Perioperative attempts to induce fluid shifts by deliberate administration of osmolal loads should take into consideration the patient's preexisting serum osmolality to avoid extreme increases in serum osmolality (>320 mOsm/kg). Mannitol should not be administered to an intoxicated patient with elevated intracranial pressure, for example, without prior consideration of the preexisting effects of ethanol molecules and water diuresis on the osmolal state of the patient.

Although vasopressin is predominantly secreted in response to increased osmolality, its release is also stimulated by large isoosmolar decreases in effective circulating volume. In addition, the pain and stress of the perioperative period are upregulators of vasopressin release, and the stress response to critical illness can include water retention, oliguria, and dilutional hyponatremia (Table 21.2).

In contrast to osmolal homeostasis, the homeostatic response to isotonic changes in total body water relies on juxtaglomerular sensation of changes in effective circulating volume and consequent changes in kidney renin excretion. Renin converts angiotensinogen into angiotensin I, which is converted to angiotensin II in the lung. Angiotensin II induces adrenal release of aldosterone, which promotes sodium reabsorption and potassium loss in the distal tubules and also leads to increases in water resorption. Elevations in circulating volume also cause increased release of natriuretic peptides that promote a return to water homeostasis.

Fluid resuscitation in patients with hypovolemia necessitates consideration of the cause and severity of the hypovolemia and patient comorbid conditions. Crystalloid administration should take into consideration a patient's electrolyte and acid-base balance as well as concerns regarding the acute cardiovascular effects of additional volume and the neurologic effects of changes in volume, osmolality, and glucose levels.

Infusion of colloids, including blood products, should be done in the context of appropriate goals for hemoglobin concentration, platelet numbers, and coagulation factors and must take into consideration the course of any ongoing blood loss and the health status of the patient. Synthetic volume expanders have been advocated to achieve volume expansion with reduced tissue edema compared to crystalloids. However, there is no good evidence that they provide advantages in outcomes in comparison to appropriately balanced crystalloid solutions. Indeed, some have been associated with *increased* bleeding and a *higher* incidence of renal dysfunction in addition to their increased cost in comparison with crystalloids.

DISORDERS OF SODIUM

As the ion with the highest concentration in the ECF, sodium contributes most of the effective osmoles to serum. This underlying connection between serum sodium concentration and

TABLE 21.2	Factors and Drugs Affecting Vasopressin Secretion	
Stimulation of Vasopressin Release	Inhibition of Vasopressin Release	Drugs That Stimulate Vasopressin Release and/or Potentiate Renal Action of Vasopressin
Contracted ECF volume	Expanded ECF volume	Amitriptyline
Hypernatremia	Hyponatremia	Barbiturates
Hypotension	Hypertension	Carbamazepine
Nausea and vomiting		Chlorpropamide
Congestive heart failure		Clofibrate
Cirrhosis		Morphine
Hypothyroidism		Nicotine
Angiotensin II		Phenothiazines
Catecholamines		Selective serotonin reuptake inhibitors
Histamine		
Bradykinin		

ECF, Extracellular fluid.

osmolality is critical for understanding disorders of sodium homeostasis. Under normal circumstances, serum sodium concentration is maintained between 136 and 145 mmol/L, primarily by the action of vasopressin on water and osmolal homeostasis.

Variations in measured sodium concentration frequently occur along with derangements in total body water. Assessment and treatment of changes in sodium concentration must therefore consider osmolality as well as the total body water of the patient. Total body water can be increased, normal, or decreased in the context of derangements in sodium concentration, and the cause and treatment of serum sodium disorders depend on the osmolality and volume status of the patient.

Hyponatremia

Hyponatremia commonly exists in concert with hypoosmolality when water retention or water intake exceeds renal excretion of dilute urine. Hyponatremia exists in approximately 15% of hospitalized patients, most commonly as a dilutional effect in the setting of increased vasopressin release. In the outpatient setting, hyponatremia is more likely to be a result of chronic disease, and in heart failure has been shown to be an independent predictor of 30-day and 1-year mortality.

Signs and Symptoms

The signs and symptoms of hyponatremia depend on the rate at which the hyponatremia has developed and are less pronounced in chronic cases. In addition, younger patients appear to tolerate a decrease in serum sodium better than elderly patients.

Anorexia, nausea, and general malaise may occur early, but CNS signs and symptoms predominate later in the course and in acutely deteriorating cases of hyponatremia (Table 21.3). As mentioned earlier, hyponatremia usually occurs along with extracellular hypotonicity. The associated osmolal gradient allows water to move into brain cells, which results in cerebral edema and increased intracranial pressure. Brain cells may compensate over time by lowering intracellular osmolality by

TABLE 21.3	Symptoms and Signs of Hyponatremia
Symptoms	Signs
Anorexia	Abnormal sensorium
Nausea	Disorientation, agitation
Lethargy	Cheyne-Stokes breathing
Apathy	Hypothermia
Muscle cramps	Pathologic reflexes
	Pseudobulbar palsy
	Seizures
	Coma
	Death

movement of potassium and organic solutes out of brain cells. This reduces water movement into the intracellular space. However, when adaptive mechanisms fail or hyponatremia progresses, CNS dysfunction can manifest as a change in sensorium, seizures, brain herniation, or death.

Diagnosis

Although hyponatremia usually co-exists with hypoosmolality, osmolality should be measured in all cases of hyponatremia, particularly to avoid overlooking a pathologic hyperosmolar state caused by dangerous concentrations of glucose or exogenous toxins, or iatrogenic infusions of osmolal loads.

In such hyperosmolal situations, plasma volume expands as interstitial and intracellular water migrates into the intravascular space, causing a relative dilution of the serum sodium concentration without a reduction in the amount of total body sodium. Total body water may be increased, unchanged, or decreased depending on the competing effects of water administered with the osmolal load and the likely presence of an osmotic diuresis.

In patients with normal osmolality, a *pseudohyponatremia* can be seen as a laboratory artifact in cases of severe hyperlipidemia or hyperproteinemia when plasma volume is increased in the presence of normal serum sodium concentrations. Measuring sodium concentrations in *serum* rather than in plasma avoids this misinterpretation of laboratory data.

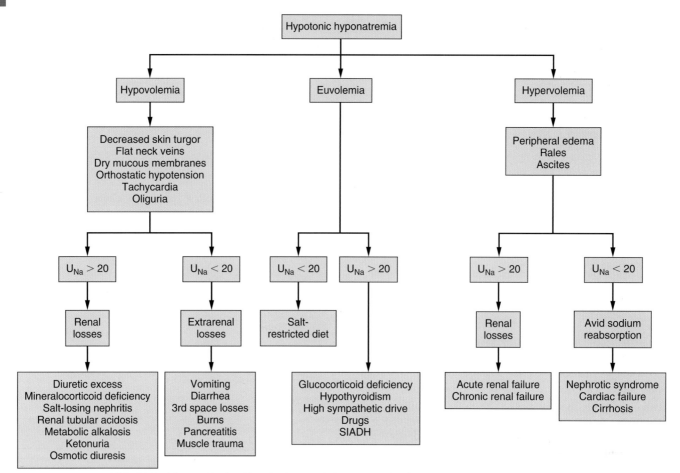

FIG. 21.2 Diagnostic algorithm for hypotonic hyponatremia. *SIADH,* Syndrome of inappropriate antidiuretic hormone secretion; U_{Na}, urinary sodium concentration (mEq/L) in a spot urine sample. (Adapted from Schrier RW. *Manual of Nephrology.* 6th ed. Philadelphia: Lippincott Williams & Wilkins; 2006.)

Once the two situations of hyperosmolality and normal osmolality have been excluded, the approach to the diagnosis of hypoosmolal hyponatremia includes evaluation of the severity of the electrolyte derangement and the underlying volume status of the patient. *Hypervolemic* hyponatremia suggests the possibility of renal failure, congestive heart failure, or a hypoalbuminemic state such as cirrhosis or nephrotic syndrome. *Euvolemic* hyponatremia is commonly seen in the syndrome of inappropriate antidiuretic hormone secretion (SIADH) or in situations of habitual ingestion of hypotonic solutions (e.g., water), as seen in psychogenic polydipsia. *Hypovolemic* hyponatremia should prompt an investigation into the source of free water loss. This free water loss may be from renal losses (e.g., from diuretics, mineralocorticoid deficiency, or other salt-wasting nephropathy) or extrarenal losses (e.g., gastrointestinal [GI] losses or third spacing).

Often the clinical context of hyponatremia offers the principal clue to its cause. For example, massive absorption of irrigating solutions that do not contain sodium, such as during transurethral resection of the prostate, is a relatively common cause of intraoperative hyponatremia. When the clinical context does not lead to a diagnosis, urinary sodium concentration measured from a spot urine sample can help further differentiate among the various causes of hyponatremia (Fig. 21.2).

Treatment

Treatment of *hypotonic* hyponatremia will depend on the volume status of the patient. In hypovolemic hyponatremia, appropriate volume resuscitation should be pursued, usually with normal saline. If renal sodium losses are suspected, mineralocorticoid deficiency and the possibility of adrenal insufficiency should not be overlooked. Cases of massive third spacing, such as often accompany pancreatitis or burns, require tailored resuscitation based on the totality of electrolyte and hematologic derangements.

In *euvolemic* or *hypervolemic* patients, treatment involves withholding free water and encouraging free water excretion with a loop diuretic. Administration of saline is necessary only if significant symptoms are present. In these as in all cases of hyponatremia, the rate of correction depends on whether the development of hyponatremia was acute (i.e., occurred in <48 hours) or was chronic.

TABLE 21.4	Signs and Symptoms of TURP Syndrome	
System	Signs and Symptoms	Cause
Cardiovascular	Hypertension, reflex bradycardia, pulmonary edema, cardiovascular collapse	Rapid fluid absorption (reflex bradycardia may be secondary to hypertension or increased ICP)
	Hypotension	Third spacing secondary to hyponatremia and hypoosmolality; cardiovascular collapse
	ECG changes (wide QRS, elevated ST segments, ventricular dysrhythmias)	Hyponatremia
Respiratory	Tachypnea, oxygen desaturation, Cheyne-Stokes breathing	Pulmonary edema
Neurologic	Nausea, restlessness, visual disturbances, confusion, somnolence, seizures, coma, death	Hyponatremia and hypoosmolality causing cerebral edema and increased ICP, hyperglycinemia, hyperammonemia
Hematologic	Disseminated intravascular hemolysis	Hyponatremia and hypoosmolality
Renal	Renal failure	Hypotension, hyperoxaluria (oxalate is a metabolite of glycine)
Metabolic	Acidosis	Deamination of glycine to glyoxylic acid and ammonia

ECG, Electrocardiogram; *ICP,* intracranial pressure, *TURP,* transurethral resection of the prostate.

Acute symptomatic hyponatremia must be treated promptly. Solute-free fluids are withheld and hypertonic saline (3% NaCl) and furosemide are administered to enhance renal excretion of free water. Serum electrolyte levels should be checked frequently and this treatment continued until symptoms disappear, which will likely occur before the serum sodium concentration returns to normal.

Chronic symptomatic hyponatremia should be corrected slowly to avoid the risk of osmotic demyelination. During the development of chronic hyponatremia, brain cells retain their normal intracellular volume as the serum sodium decreases by exporting "effective osmoles." Approximately half of these effective osmoles are potassium ions and anions, and the remainder are small organic compounds. While hyponatremia is being corrected, brain cells must reaccumulate these effective osmoles or water will move out of the cells into the now relatively hypertonic ECF, causing cell shrinkage. Such shrinkage can trigger central pontine myelinolysis, which can result in quadriplegia, seizures, coma, and death. The risk of osmotic demyelination is higher in patients who are malnourished or potassium depleted. Guidelines for correction of chronic symptomatic hyponatremia call for an initial correction in serum sodium concentration of approximately 10 mEq/L. Thereafter, correction should not exceed 1 to 1.5 mEq/L/hr or a daily maximum increase of 12 mEq/L.

Treatment of *chronic asymptomatic hyponatremia* should consider the underlying cause of the electrolyte disturbance. Appropriate sodium intake and volume restriction are often the cornerstones of treatment. Patients with hypervolemic hyponatremia due to congestive heart failure respond very well to the combination of an angiotensin-converting enzyme inhibitor and a loop diuretic.

Management of Anesthesia

If at all possible, significant hyponatremia, especially if symptomatic, should be corrected before surgery. If the surgery is urgent, appropriate corrective treatment should continue throughout the surgery and into the postoperative period. Frequent measurement of serum sodium concentration is necessary to avoid overly rapid correction of hyponatremia with resultant osmotic demyelination or overcorrection resulting in hypernatremia. If the treatment of hyponatremia includes hypertonic sodium infusion during surgery, it should be infused via a pump while losses caused by the surgery are replaced with standard crystalloid or colloid solutions as required. Treatment of the underlying cause of the hyponatremia should also continue throughout the perioperative period.

Induction and maintenance of anesthesia in patients with hypovolemic hyponatremia are fraught with the risk of hypotension. In addition to fluid therapy, vasopressors and/or inotropes may be required to treat the hypotension, and these should be available before the start of induction. *Hypervolemic hyponatremic* patients, particularly those with heart failure, may benefit from invasive hemodynamic monitoring to assess cardiac function and guide fluid therapy.

Transurethral Resection of the Prostate (TURP) Syndrome

Benign prostatic hyperplasia is often treated surgically by transurethral resection of the prostate (TURP). This procedure involves resection via a cystoscope, with continuous irrigation of the bladder to aid visualization of the surgical field and removal of blood and resected material. The irrigating fluid is usually a nearly isotonic *nonelectrolyte* fluid containing glycine or a mixture of sorbitol and mannitol. This irrigating fluid can be absorbed rapidly via open venous sinuses in the prostate gland and can cause volume overload and hyponatremia. The constellation of findings associated with absorption of bladder irrigation solution is known as *TURP syndrome.* This syndrome is more likely to occur when resection is prolonged (>1 hour), when the irrigating fluid is suspended more than 40 cm above the operative field, when hypotonic irrigation fluid is used, and when the pressure in the bladder is allowed to increase above 15 cm H_2O. TURP syndrome (Table 21.4) manifests principally with cardiovascular signs of fluid overload and neurologic signs and symptoms of hyponatremia. Use of hypotonic irrigating solutions can also induce hemolysis because red blood cells encounter a significant influx of free water from hypotonic ECF. Hypertension and pulmonary edema are common. If a glycine irrigant is used, transient blindness can occur that is thought to result from the inhibitory neurotransmitter effects of glycine on several populations of retinal ganglion cells. Glycine breaks down into glyoxylic acid and ammonia, and excessive ammonia levels are themselves known to cause encephalopathy.

Monitoring for the development of TURP syndrome includes direct neurologic assessment in patients under regional anesthesia and measurement of hemodynamics, serum sodium concentration, and osmolality in patients under general anesthesia. Treatment consists of terminating the surgical procedure so no more fluid is absorbed, administration of loop diuretics if needed for relief of cardiovascular symptoms, and administration of hypertonic saline if severe neurologic symptoms or signs are present or the serum sodium concentration is less than 120 mEq/L.

Hypernatremia

Hypernatremia is defined as a serum sodium concentration above 145 mEq/L. It is much less common than hyponatremia because the vasopressin-driven thirst mechanism is very effective in responding to the hypertonic state of hypernatremia. Even in patients with renal disorders of sodium retention or severe water loss, patients will regulate their serum sodium concentration close to or within the normal range if they have access to water. Therefore hypernatremia is much more likely to be seen in the very young, the elderly, and those people who are debilitated, have altered mental status, or are unconscious.

In the perioperative setting, hypernatremia is most likely a result of iatrogenic overcorrection of hyponatremia or treatment of acidemia with sodium bicarbonate. Free water losses from diabetes insipidus and extrarenal GI losses may also lead to hypernatremia. Because sodium is the major contributor to ECF osmolality, hypernatremia induces the movement of water across cell membranes into the ECF. Hypernatremia and the associated hyperosmolality will always lead to cellular dehydration and shrinkage.

Signs and Symptoms

Signs and symptoms of hypernatremia can vary from mild to life threatening (Table 21.5). The earliest signs and symptoms include restlessness, irritability, and lethargy. As hypernatremia progresses, muscular twitching, hyperreflexia, tremors, and ataxia may develop. The signs and symptoms progress as the osmolality increases above 325 mOsm/kg. Muscle spasticity, seizures, and death may ensue. The very young, the very old, and those with preexisting CNS disease exhibit more severe symptoms at any given serum sodium concentration or degree of hyperosmolality.

The most prominent abnormalities in hypernatremia are neurologic. Dehydration of brain cells occurs as water shifts out of the cells into the hypertonic interstitium. Capillary and venous congestion as well as venous sinus thrombosis have all

TABLE 21.5	Symptoms and Signs of Hypernatremia
Symptoms	Signs
Polyuria	Muscle twitching
Polydipsia	Hyperreflexia
Orthostasis	Tremor
Restlessness	Ataxia
Irritability	Muscle spasticity
Lethargy	Focal and generalized seizures
	Death

been reported. As the brain cells shrink, cerebral blood vessels may stretch and tear, which results in intracranial hemorrhage.

Usually the signs and symptoms are more severe when hypernatremia is *acute* rather than chronic and when excessive elevations in serum sodium levels are present. Mortality rates of up to 75% have been reported in adults with severe acute hypernatremia (serum sodium concentration > 160 mEq/L), and survivors of severe acute hypernatremia often have permanent neurologic deficits. During the development of chronic hypernatremia, brain cells generate "idiogenic osmoles" that restore intracellular water in spite of the ongoing hypernatremia and protect against brain cell dehydration. If chronic hypernatremia is corrected too rapidly, these idiogenic osmoles predispose to the development of cerebral edema.

Diagnosis

The diagnosis and treatment of hypernatremia should focus on the severity of the derangement and the volume status of the patient. The presence of hypervolemia, euvolemia, or hypovolemia dictates the appropriate diagnostic and treatment modalities (Fig. 21.3).

In *hypovolemic hypernatremia* the patient has lost more water than sodium via renal or extrarenal routes. This may occur as a result of excessive diuresis, GI losses, or insensible fluid losses from burns or sweating.

Patients with *hypervolemic hypernatremia* will show signs of ECF volume expansion, such as jugular venous distention, peripheral edema, and pulmonary congestion. The differential diagnosis includes a history of hypertonic fluid administration, oral intake of salt tablets, and endocrine abnormalities marked by excessive aldosterone secretion.

Euvolemic and *hypovolemic hypernatremia* occur secondary to water loss without salt loss and may be seen with either extrarenal pathologic conditions (e.g., GI tract losses or insensible losses from burns or sweating) or from renal losses (e.g., diabetes insipidus, loop diuretics, or osmotic diuresis).

As with hyponatremia, testing of a spot urine sample for sodium concentration and osmolality can help distinguish among the causes of hypernatremia (see Fig. 21.3).

Treatment

Treatment is determined by how severe the hypernatremia is, how rapidly it developed, and whether the ECF volume is increased or decreased.

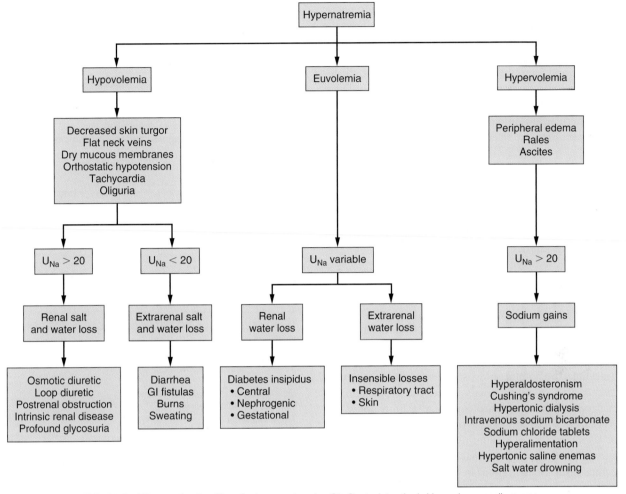

FIG. 21.3 Diagnostic algorithm for hypernatremia. *GI,* Gastrointestinal; U_{Na}, urinary sodium concentration (mEq/L) in a spot urine sample. (Adapted from Schrier RW. *Manual of Nephrology.* 6th ed. Philadelphia: Lippincott Williams & Wilkins; 2006.)

In *hypovolemic hypernatremia* the water deficit is replenished with normal saline or a balanced electrolyte solution until the patient is euvolemic, and then the plasma osmolality is corrected with hypotonic saline or 5% dextrose solution.

In patients with *hypervolemic hypernatremia* the primary treatment is diuresis with a loop diuretic unless the cause is renal failure, in which case hemofiltration or hemodialysis may be needed.

Patients with *euvolemic hypernatremia* require water replacement either orally or with 5% dextrose intravenously. Treatment of diabetes insipidus depends on whether there is a central deficit of vasopressin release or a renal insensitivity to vasopressin's actions.

Acute hypernatremia should be corrected over several hours. However, to avoid cerebral edema, *chronic* hypernatremia should be corrected more slowly over 2–3 days. Ongoing sodium and water losses should also be calculated and replaced.

Management of Anesthesia
If at all possible, surgery should be delayed until the hypernatremia has been corrected and its associated symptoms have

abated. Frequent serum sodium measurement and urine output monitoring will be required perioperatively, and invasive hemodynamic monitoring may be useful to assess volume status. Hypovolemia will be exacerbated by induction and maintenance of anesthesia, and prompt correction of hypotension with fluids, vasopressors, and/or inotropes may be required. The volume of distribution of hydrophilic drugs will be altered in hypovolemia and hypervolemia. However, the accentuated hemodynamic responses to anesthetic drug administration are most likely a consequence of the vasodilation and negative inotropic effects of anesthetic drugs rather than the result of changes in their volume of distribution.

DISORDERS OF POTASSIUM

Potassium is the major intracellular cation. The normal total body potassium content depends on muscle mass; it is maximal in young adults and decreases progressively with age. Less than 1.5% of total body potassium is found in the extracellular space. Therefore serum potassium concentration is more a reflection of factors that regulate transcellular potassium distribution than of total body potassium. Total body potassium is regulated over long periods of time, principally by the distal nephron in the kidneys; the distal nephron secretes potassium in response to aldosterone, which leads to an increase in urine volume and nonresorbable anions and metabolic alkalosis. More than 90% of potassium taken in by diet is excreted in the urine, and most of the remainder is eliminated in the feces. As the glomerular filtration rate decreases in renal failure, the amount of potassium excreted by the GI route increases.

Hypokalemia

Signs and Symptoms

Signs and symptoms of hypokalemia are generally restricted to the cardiac and neuromuscular systems and include dysrhythmias, muscle weakness, cramps, paralysis, and ileus.

Diagnosis

Hypokalemia is diagnosed by the presence of a serum potassium concentration below 3.5 mmol/L and results from decreased net potassium intake, intracellular shifts, or increased potassium losses. The differential diagnosis requires determining whether the hypokalemia is acute and secondary to intracellular potassium shifts, such as might be seen with hyperventilation or alkalosis, or whether the hypokalemia is chronic and associated with depletion of total body potassium stores (Table 21.6). If the hypokalemia is the result of potassium losses, a spot urinary potassium reading will guide the diagnosis to either renal or extrarenal causes. Appropriately low urine potassium concentrations in the setting of hypokalemia point to a normally functioning kidney in the setting of inadequate potassium intake or GI losses. Renal potassium losses are indicated by a spot urinary potassium value of more than 15–20 mEq/L despite the presence of hypokalemia. In cases of renal potassium loss, assessment of the transtubular potassium concentration gradient, hemodynamics, and acid-base status will further help to elucidate the diagnosis. Hypertension with hypokalemia is usually the result of a hyperaldosterone state. Renal losses in the setting of acidemia point to a diagnosis of renal tubular acidosis or diabetic ketoacidosis. Renal losses in the setting of alkalemia can indicate a response to diuretics or can be seen in genetic disorders such as Liddle syndrome (associated with hypertension) or Bartter syndrome (which has tubular effects similar to those of loop diuretics). Hypomagnesemia can also exacerbate renal potassium losses. Hypokalemia without a change in total body potassium stores can be caused by familial hypokalemic periodic paralysis.

Treatment

Treatment of hypokalemia depends on the degree of potassium depletion and the underlying cause. If the hypokalemia is profound or is associated with life-threatening signs, potassium must be administered intravenously. In the presence of paralysis or malignant dysrhythmias, the rate of potassium repletion can be as high as 20 mEq over 30 minutes (via an infusion pump) and repeated as needed. If a malignant

TABLE 21.6	Causes of Hypokalemia

HYPOKALEMIA DUE TO INCREASED RENAL POTASSIUM LOSS
Thiazide diuretics
Loop diuretics
Mineralocorticoids
High-dose glucocorticoids
Antibiotics (penicillin, nafcillin, ampicillin)
Drugs associated with magnesium depletion (aminoglycosides)
Surgical trauma
Hyperglycemia
Hyperaldosteronism

HYPOKALEMIA DUE TO EXCESSIVE GASTROINTESTINAL LOSS OF POTASSIUM
Vomiting and diarrhea
Zollinger-Ellison syndrome
Jejunoileal bypass
Malabsorption
Chemotherapy
Nasogastric suction

HYPOKALEMIA DUE TO TRANSCELLULAR POTASSIUM SHIFT
β-Adrenergic agonists
Tocolytic drugs (ritodrine)
Insulin
Respiratory or metabolic alkalosis
Familial periodic paralysis
Hypercalcemia
Hypomagnesemia

Adapted from Gennari JF. Hypokalemia. *N Engl J Med*. 1998;339:451-458.

dysrhythmia appears during potassium repletion, the rate of potassium administration may be the cause. Therefore electrocardiographic (ECG) monitoring is required whenever rapid potassium repletion is undertaken. In the setting of urgent potassium repletion, potassium solutions *without* dextrose are preferred. Otherwise the insulin secretion stimulated by the glucose will induce intracellular potassium transfer.

The enteral route of potassium repletion is preferred in cases of *nonemergent* potassium repletion to avoid the risks of high-dose intravenous (IV) potassium administration. If IV repletion is chosen in a nonemergency situation, it should proceed at a rate of less than 20 mEq/h. Peripheral infusion of a concentrated potassium solution will result in pain and/or inflammation at the IV site, so administration via a central venous catheter is preferred.

Management of Anesthesia

Whether or not to treat hypokalemia before surgery is an ongoing subject of debate and depends on the chronicity and severity of the deficit. Because of the limitations on the rate of potassium repletion and the large total body potassium deficits that accompany chronic hypokalemia, safe repletion of total body potassium stores often requires days. Although total body depletion is variable in its relationship to serum potassium concentrations, chronic hypokalemia with serum concentrations of less than 3.0 mEq/L may require delivery of 600 mEq or

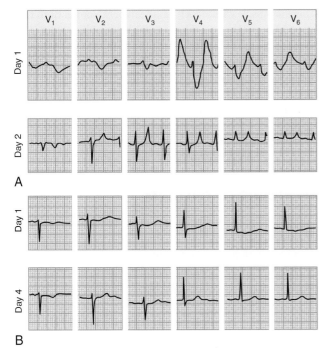

FIG. 21.4 Electrocardiographic changes in hyperkalemia (A) and hypokalemia (B). A, On day 1, at a K⁺ level of 8.6 mEq/L, the P wave is no longer recognizable and the QRS complex is diffusely prolonged. Initial and terminal QRS delays are characteristic of K⁺-induced intraventricular conduction slowing and are best illustrated in leads V_2 and V_6. On day 2, at a K⁺ level of 5.8 mEq/L, the P wave is recognizable, with a PR interval of 0.24 seconds; the duration of the QRS complex is approximately 0.10 seconds, and the T waves are characteristically "tented." B, On day 1, at a K⁺ level of 1.5 mEq/L, the T and U waves are merged. The U wave is prominent and the QU interval is prolonged. On day 4, at a K⁺ level of 3.7 mEq/L, the tracing is normal. (From Bonow R, Mann D, Zipes D, et al., eds. *Braunwald's Heart Disease: A Textbook of Cardiovascular Medicine.* 9th ed. Philadelphia: Saunders; 2011. Courtesy Dr. C. Fisch.)

more of potassium to achieve a normal total body potassium. It is therefore unlikely that administration of small aliquots of potassium immediately before surgery will make any significant difference in potassium balance. Moreover, such interventions carry the risk of inadvertent hyperkalemia that may exacerbate the risk of dysrhythmias in the perioperative period. However, it has been suggested that even small improvements in potassium balance may help normalize transmembrane potentials and reduce the incidence of perioperative dysrhythmias. Recommendations on this controversial issue are based more on expert opinion, clinical judgment, and local practice patterns than on evidence from peer-reviewed studies.

It may be prudent to correct significant hypokalemia in patients with other risk factors for dysrhythmias, such as those with congestive heart failure, those taking digoxin, and those with ECG evidence of hypokalemia. ECG abnormalities associated with potassium derangement are illustrated in (Fig. 21.4). Classically, U waves are seen. Anesthetic management of patients with significant hypokalemia should prevent further decreases in serum potassium concentration by avoiding

TABLE 21.7	Causes of Hyperkalemia

INCREASED TOTAL BODY POTASSIUM CONTENT
Acute oliguric renal failure
Chronic renal disease
Hypoaldosteronism
Drugs that impair potassium excretion
  Triamterene
  Spironolactone
  Nonsteroidal antiinflammatory drugs
Drugs that inhibit the renin-angiotensin-aldosterone system

ALTERED TRANSCELLULAR POTASSIUM SHIFT
Succinylcholine
Respiratory or metabolic acidosis
Lysis of cells resulting from chemotherapy
Iatrogenic bolus

PSEUDOHYPERKALEMIA
Hemolysis of blood specimen
Thrombocytosis/leukocytosis

administration of insulin, glucose, β-adrenergic agonists, bicarbonate, and diuretics, as well as by avoiding hyperventilation and respiratory alkalosis.

Because of the effect of hypokalemia on skeletal muscle, there is the theoretical possibility of prolonged action of muscle relaxants. Doses of neuromuscular blockers should, as always, be guided by nerve stimulator testing.

Potassium levels should be measured frequently if repletion is ongoing or changes resulting from drug administration, surgical progress, or ventilation are expected.

Hyperkalemia

Hyperkalemia is defined as a serum potassium concentration of more than 5.5 mEq/L. As with hypokalemia, hyperkalemia can result from transcellular movement of potassium out of cells or from alterations in potassium intake or excretion. In hospitalized patients, hyperkalemia is frequently the result of iatrogenic potassium loads (Table 21.7).

Signs and Symptoms

Signs and symptoms of hyperkalemia depend on the acuity of the increase. Chronic hyperkalemia is often asymptomatic, and dialysis-dependent patients can withstand considerable variations in serum potassium concentration between dialysis sessions (usually 2–3 days) with remarkably few symptoms. Chronic hyperkalemia may be associated with nonspecific symptoms such as general malaise and mild GI disturbances. More acute or significant increases in serum potassium manifest as complications of a change in membrane depolarization, and neuromuscular and cardiac changes including weakness, paralysis, nausea, vomiting, bradycardia, or asystole may result.

Diagnosis

The first step in the diagnosis of hyperkalemia is to rule out a spuriously high potassium level due to hemolysis of the specimen. A spuriously high potassium level may also occur with thrombocytosis and leukocytosis, because potassium may leak from these cells in vitro. True hyperkalemia can be identified on ECG first as a peaked T wave, followed in more severe cases by disappearance of the P wave and prolongation of the QRS complex, which progresses to sine waves and then eventually to asystole (see Fig. 21.4).

Common causes of hyperkalemia in the perioperative period include acidosis, rhabdomyolysis, and succinylcholine administration. If the increase in serum potassium level is thought to be associated with increased total body potassium, decreased renal excretion or increased potassium intake is likely. Measurement of the urinary potassium excretion rate can aid in the differential diagnosis between cellular potassium shifts and problems with potassium excretion.

Treatment

Immediate treatment of hyperkalemia is required if life-threatening dysrhythmias or ECG signs of severe hyperkalemia are present. This treatment is aimed at antagonizing the effects of a high potassium level on the transmembrane potential and redistributing the potassium intracellularly. Calcium chloride or calcium gluconate is administered intravenously to stabilize cellular membranes. The onset of action is immediate. Potassium can be driven intracellularly by the action of insulin with or without glucose. This measure will be effective within 10–20 minutes. Other adjuvant therapies include sodium bicarbonate administration and hyperventilation to promote alkalosis and movement of potassium intracellularly. Potassium driven intracellularly may eventually move out of the cells again, so therapy may need to continue beyond acute correction of the derangement.

When hyperkalemia is due to increased total body stores of potassium, potassium must be eliminated from the body. This can be achieved by administration of a loop diuretic such as furosemide, infusion of saline to encourage diuresis, or use of an ion exchange resin. The primary potassium exchange resin in use is sodium polystyrene sulfonate (Kayexalate) given either orally or by enema. Dialysis may be required to remove potassium in cases of emergent hyperkalemia or in patients with poor renal function.

Management of Anesthesia

It is recommended that the serum potassium concentration be less than 5.5 mEq/L for elective surgery. Correction of hyperkalemia before surgery is preferable, but if this is not feasible, steps should be taken to lower the potassium level immediately before induction of anesthesia by one or more of the methods indicated previously. Potassium levels may influence selection of drugs for induction and maintenance of anesthesia, because preoperative medications that induce some degree of hypoventilation and respiratory acidosis may cause further transcellular potassium shifts. Also, succinylcholine (which only increases serum potassium concentration by ≈0.5 mEq/L in healthy patients) is best avoided in the absence of an urgent need for it. The effects of muscle relaxants may be exaggerated if there is muscle weakness from the hyperkalemia. Both respiratory and metabolic acidosis must be avoided, since either will exacerbate the hyperkalemia and its effects. Potassium-containing IV fluids such as lactated Ringer solution (which contains 4 mEq/L of potassium) and Normosol (which contains 5 mEq/L of potassium) should be avoided. Dialysis patients who are scheduled for surgery in which intraoperative potassium loads are anticipated can be managed preoperatively by decreasing the potassium content of the dialysate to reduce serum potassium levels in anticipation of surgery.

DISORDERS OF CALCIUM

Only 1% of total body calcium is present in the ECF. The remainder is stored in bone. In the ECF, 60% of calcium is free or coupled with anions and is thus filterable, and the remaining 40% is bound to proteins, mainly albumin. Only the ionized calcium in the extracellular space is physiologically active. Ionized calcium concentrations are affected by both albumin concentration and the pH of plasma. Net calcium balance occurs when absorption from the diet equals losses of calcium in feces and urine. Several hormones regulate calcium metabolism: parathyroid hormone, which increases bone resorption and renal tubular reabsorption of calcium; calcitonin, which inhibits bone resorption; and vitamin D, which augments intestinal absorption of calcium. The activity of these hormones is altered in response to changes in plasma ionized calcium concentration. Other hormones, including thyroid hormone, growth hormone, and adrenal and gonadal steroids, also affect calcium homeostasis, but their secretion is determined by factors other than plasma calcium concentration.

Hypocalcemia

Hypocalcemia is defined as a reduction in serum ionized calcium concentration. It is important to note that many blood chemistry analysis systems measure total calcium rather than ionized calcium. Several formulas exist to convert total calcium to ionized calcium, but none of these is totally reliable.

Binding of calcium to albumin is pH dependent, and acid-base disturbances can change the bound fraction and therefore the concentration of ionized calcium without changing total body calcium. Alkalosis reduces the ionized calcium concentration, so ionized calcium may be significantly reduced after bicarbonate administration or in the setting of hyperventilation. Many hospitalized patients are also hypoalbuminemic, and the reduction in bound calcium will reduce the measured serum calcium level. When serum calcium concentration is interpreted in the setting of a low albumin level, corrected calcium concentration can be calculated as follows: measured calcium (mg/dL) + 0.8 [4 − albumin (mg/dL)].

Signs and Symptoms

The signs and symptoms of hypocalcemia depend on the rapidity and degree of reduction in ionized calcium. Most of these signs and symptoms are evident in the cardiovascular and neuromuscular systems and include paresthesias, irritability, seizures, hypotension, and myocardial depression. ECG changes associated with hypocalcemia are marked by prolongation of the QT interval (Fig. 21.5). In the postoperative period following thyroid or parathyroid resection, hypocalcemia-induced laryngospasm can be life threatening.

Diagnosis

Hypocalcemia is often caused by decreased parathyroid hormone secretion, end-organ resistance to parathyroid hormone, or disorders of vitamin D metabolism. These are usually seen clinically as complications of thyroid or parathyroid surgery, magnesium deficiency, and renal failure. In the operating room, acute hypocalcemia is often encountered as a result of calcium binding to the citrate preservative in blood products during massive transfusion.

Treatment

Acute symptomatic hypocalcemia with seizures, tetany, and/or cardiovascular depression must be treated *immediately* with IV calcium. The duration of treatment will depend on serial calcium measurements. Treatment of hypocalcemia in the presence of hypomagnesemia is ineffective unless magnesium is also replenished. Metabolic or respiratory *alkalosis* should be corrected. If metabolic or respiratory *acidosis* is present with hypocalcemia, the calcium level should be corrected before the acidosis is treated; correcting an acidosis with bicarbonate or hyperventilation will only exacerbate the hypocalcemia.

Less acute and asymptomatic hypocalcemia may be treated with oral calcium and vitamin D supplementation.

Management of Anesthesia

Symptomatic hypocalcemia must be treated before surgery, and every effort must be made to minimize any further decrease in serum calcium level intraoperatively, as might occur with hyperventilation or administration of bicarbonate. A decrease in ionized calcium levels should always be considered during massive transfusion of blood containing citrate. Hypothermia, liver disease, and renal failure impair citrate clearance and further increase the likelihood of significant hypocalcemia in transfusion recipients.

Sudden decreases in ionized calcium levels may be seen in the early postoperative period after thyroidectomy or parathyroidectomy and may precipitate laryngospasm.

Hypercalcemia

Hypercalcemia results from increased calcium absorption from the GI tract (milk-alkali syndrome, vitamin D intoxication, granulomatous diseases such as sarcoidosis), decreased renal calcium excretion in renal insufficiency, and increased bone resorption of calcium (primary or secondary hyperparathyroidism, malignancy, hyperthyroidism, and immobilization).

Signs and Symptoms

Hypercalcemia is associated with neurologic and GI signs and symptoms such as confusion, hypotonia, depressed deep tendon reflexes, lethargy, abdominal pain, and nausea and vomiting, especially if the increase in serum calcium level is relatively acute. A shortened ST segment and QT interval are seen on ECG (see Fig. 21.5). Chronic hypercalcemia is often associated with polyuria, hypercalciuria, and nephrolithiasis.

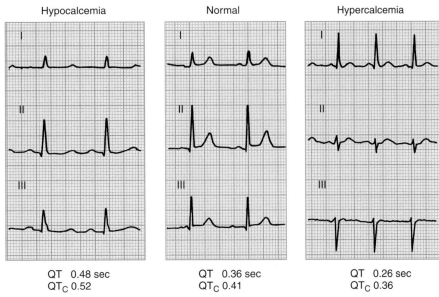

FIG. 21.5 Electrocardiographic changes in calcium disorders. Prolongation of the QT interval (ST-segment portion) is typical of hypocalcemia. Hypercalcemia may cause abbreviation of the ST segment and shortening of the QT interval. *QT$_C$*, Corrected QT interval. (Data from Goldberger AL. *Clinical Electrocardiography: A Simplified Approach.* 6th ed. St Louis, MO: Mosby; 1999.)

Diagnosis

Almost all patients with hypercalcemia have either hyperparathyroidism or cancer. Primary hyperparathyroidism is typically associated with a serum calcium concentration below 11 mEq/L and no symptoms, whereas malignancy often presents with acute symptoms and a serum calcium level higher than 13 mEq/L.

Treatment

Treatment of hypercalcemia is directed toward increasing urinary calcium excretion and inhibiting bone resorption and further GI absorption of calcium.

Since hypercalcemia is frequently associated with hypovolemia secondary to polyuria, volume expansion with saline not only corrects the fluid deficit but also increases urinary excretion of calcium along with the administered sodium. Loop diuretics also enhance urinary excretion of both sodium and calcium but should be used *only after* appropriate volume resuscitation.

Calcitonin, bisphosphonates, or mithramycin may be required in disorders associated with osteoclastic bone resorption. Hydrocortisone may reduce GI absorption of calcium in granulomatous disease, vitamin D intoxication, lymphoma, and myeloma. Oral phosphate may also be given to reduce GI uptake of calcium if renal function is normal. Dialysis may be required for life-threatening hypercalcemia. Surgical removal of the parathyroid glands may be required to treat primary or secondary hyperparathyroidism.

Management of Anesthesia

Management of anesthesia for emergency surgery in a patient with hypercalcemia is aimed at restoring intravascular volume before induction and increasing urinary excretion of calcium with loop diuretics (*thiazide diuretics should be avoided* because they *increase renal tubular reabsorption of calcium*). Ideally, surgery should be postponed until calcium levels have normalized.

Central venous pressure or pulmonary artery pressure monitoring may be advisable in some patients requiring fluid resuscitation and diuresis as part of the perioperative treatment of hypercalcemia. Dosing of muscle relaxants must be guided by neuromuscular monitoring if muscle weakness, hypotonia, or loss of deep tendon reflexes is present.

DISORDERS OF MAGNESIUM

Magnesium is predominantly found intracellularly and in mineralized bone. Between 60% and 70% of serum magnesium is ionized, with 10% complexed to citrate, bicarbonate, or phosphate and approximately 30% bound to protein, mostly albumin. There is little difference between extracellular and intracellular ionized magnesium concentrations, so there is only a small transmembrane gradient for ionized magnesium. It is the ionized fraction of magnesium that is associated with clinical effects.

Magnesium is absorbed from and secreted into the GI tract and filtered, reabsorbed, and excreted by the kidneys. Renal reabsorption and excretion are passive, following sodium and water.

Hypomagnesemia

Some degree of hypomagnesemia occurs in up to 10% of hospitalized patients. An even higher percentage of patients in intensive care units (ICUs), especially those receiving parenteral nutrition or dialysis, have hypomagnesemia. Coronary care unit patients with hypomagnesemia have a higher mortality rate than those with normal serum levels of magnesium.

Signs and Symptoms

Signs and symptoms of hypomagnesemia are similar to those of hypocalcemia and involve mostly the cardiac and neuromuscular systems. Dysrhythmias, weakness, muscle twitching, tetany, apathy, and seizures can be seen. Hypokalemia and/or hypocalcemia that had been refractory to supplementation will respond after correction of hypomagnesemia.

Diagnosis

Hypomagnesemia is most commonly due to reduced GI uptake (reduced dietary intake or reduced absorption from the GI tract) or to renal wasting of magnesium. These entities can be differentiated by measuring the urinary magnesium excretion rate. Much less frequently, hypomagnesemia is due to intracellular shifts of magnesium with no overall change in total body magnesium, to hungry bone syndrome after parathyroidectomy, or to exudative cutaneous losses after burn injury.

Treatment

Treatment of hypomagnesemia depends on the severity of the deficiency and the signs and symptoms that are present. If cardiac dysrhythmias or seizures are present, magnesium is administered intravenously as a bolus (2 g of magnesium sulfate = 8 mEq of magnesium), and the dose is repeated until symptoms abate. After life-threatening signs have resolved, a slower infusion of magnesium sulfate can be continued for several days to allow for equilibration of intracellular and total body magnesium stores. If renal wasting is present, supplementation must be increased to account for the magnesium lost in urine.

Hypermagnesemia is a potential side effect of the treatment of hypomagnesemia, so the patient should be monitored for signs of hypotension, facial flushing, and loss of deep tendon reflexes.

Management of Anesthesia

Management of anesthesia in patients with hypomagnesemia includes attention to the signs of magnesium deficiency, magnesium supplementation, and treatment of refractory hypokalemia or hypocalcemia if needed. If the hypomagnesemia is secondary to malnutrition or alcoholism, the anesthetic implications of these diseases must also be considered. Intraoperative magnesium supplementation to reduce postoperative dysrhythmias has been suggested but was recently found to make no difference in rates of postoperative atrial fibrillation in a randomized trial of cardiac surgery patients.

Ventricular dysrhythmias (typically *polymorphic ventricular tachycardia*) should be anticipated and treated as necessary. Muscle relaxation should be guided by the results of peripheral nerve stimulation, since hypomagnesemia can be associated with both muscle weakness and muscle excitation. Fluid loading (particularly with sodium-containing solutions) and diuretic use should be avoided because renal excretion of magnesium passively follows sodium excretion.

Hypermagnesemia

Hypermagnesemia (i.e., serum magnesium concentration > 2.5 mEq/L) is much less common than hypomagnesemia, because a magnesium load can be briskly excreted if renal function is normal. Even patients with renal failure rarely have symptomatic hypermagnesemia unless there is a significant increase in dietary or IV intake. However, milder elevations in serum magnesium levels are frequently found in ICU and dialysis patient populations. Hypermagnesemia may be a complication of magnesium sulfate administration to treat preeclampsia/eclampsia or to provide perinatal neurologic protection in premature delivery. Magnesium infusion during pheochromocytoma surgery is popular in some centers but may also result in hypermagnesemia.

Signs and Symptoms
Signs and symptoms of hypermagnesemia begin to occur at serum levels of 4–5 mEq/L and include lethargy, nausea and vomiting, and facial flushing. At levels above 6 mEq/L, a loss of deep tendon reflexes and hypotension occur. Paralysis, apnea, heart block, and/or cardiac arrest are likely if the magnesium level exceeds 10 mEq/L.

Diagnosis
Evaluation of hypermagnesemia involves assessing renal function (creatinine clearance) and detecting any source of excess magnesium intake, such as parenteral infusion, oral ingestion of antacids, and administration of magnesium-based enemas or cathartics. Once these have been excluded, less common causes of hypermagnesemia, including hypothyroidism, hyperparathyroidism, Addison's disease, and lithium therapy, can be considered.

Treatment
Life-threatening signs of hypermagnesemia may be temporarily ameliorated with IV calcium administration, but hemodialysis may be required. Lesser degrees of hypermagnesemia can be treated with forced diuresis with saline and loop diuretics to increase renal excretion of magnesium.

Management of Anesthesia
Invasive cardiovascular monitoring may be necessary perioperatively to measure and treat the hypotension and vasodilation associated with hypermagnesemia and to guide fluid resuscitation and ongoing replacement of fluids during forced diuresis. Acidosis exacerbates hypermagnesemia, so careful attention must be paid to ventilation and arterial pH. Initial and subsequent doses of muscle relaxants should be reduced in the presence of muscle weakness and guided by results of peripheral nerve stimulation. Hypermagnesemia and skeletal muscle weakness are not uncommon causes of failure to wean from mechanical ventilation in the ICU setting, especially in patients with renal failure.

ACID-BASE DISORDERS

Arterial acid-base balance is normally tightly regulated within the pH range of 7.35–7.45 to ensure optimal conditions for cellular enzyme function. Values of arterial blood pH less than 7.35 are termed *acidemia*, and values higher than 7.45 are termed *alkalemia*. The related terms *acidosis* and *alkalosis* refer to acid-base derangements that produce either excess H^+ or excess OH^-, respectively, that may be present regardless of arterial pH. Intracellular pH is lower than extracellular pH and is maintained at a closely regulated level of 7.0–7.3. Acid-base regulation in the setting of normal metabolism requires handling of the continuous production of acidic metabolites, totaling approximately 1 mEq/kg body weight per day.

Stability of pH is accomplished by a system of intracellular and extracellular buffers, most importantly the HCO_3/CO_2 buffer pair. Carbon dioxide can enter or leave the body via the lungs, and bicarbonate can enter or leave the body via the kidneys. Maintenance of a normal bicarbonate concentration relative to carbon dioxide tension results in an optimal ratio of approximately 20:1. Maintenance of this ratio of 20:1 allows for a relatively normal pH despite deviations from normal of either bicarbonate concentration or carbon dioxide tension. Other buffers include proteins, bone apatite, and phosphate ions.

The relationship of the CO_2/HCO_3 buffer system to pH is expressed by the Henderson-Hasselbalch equation: $pH = 6.1 + \log (\text{serum bicarbonate concentration}/0.03 \times Paco_2)$.

Changes in respiration regulate carbon dioxide tension, whereas renal regulation adjusts bicarbonate concentration. These changes may be the cause of a primary acid-base disorder or can occur as a compensatory mechanism in response to another underlying disorder. In non–mechanically ventilated, nonsedated patients, compensatory respiratory or renal responses can normalize an altered pH but will not overcompensate and alter the pH to the point of reversing the primary disorder. This is not always true in the operating room, where mechanical ventilation and sedation/unconsciousness allow for potential overcompensation or undercompensation of acid-base disorders. Familiarity with the clinical history is then a key part of understanding the patient's primary acid-base abnormality.

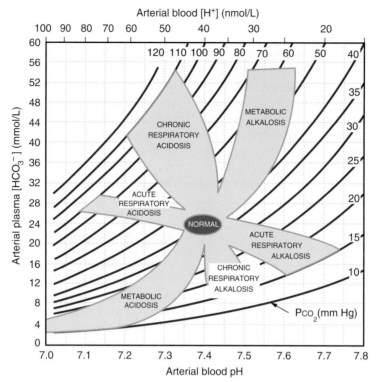

FIG. 21.6   Acid-base nomogram (map). Shaded areas represent the 95% confidence limits of the normal respiratory and metabolic compensations for primary acid-base disturbances. Data falling outside the shaded areas denote a mixed disorder if a laboratory error is not present. (Data from Brenner B, Clarkson M, Oparil S, et al., eds. *Brenner and Rector's The Kidney.* 8th ed. Philadelphia: Saunders; 2007.)

Renal compensation for acid-base derangements may include increases in resorption or secretion of filtered bicarbonate in the proximal tubule. In addition, protons (i.e., hydrogen ions) can be reabsorbed in the distal tubule and collecting duct or excreted into the urine. Hydrogen ion excretion in the urine regenerates the bicarbonate originally consumed by buffering a hydrogen ion in the ECF. The excreted hydrogen ions are themselves buffered by titratable renal buffers (mainly ammonia) and lost in the urine.

Evaluation of acid-base disturbances begins with a determination of the primary pH derangement by measurement of arterial pH, $Paco_2$, and HCO_3. A high or low pH will demonstrate the primary acid-base disorder and allow evaluation of whether there is appropriate compensation. In cases of normal pH, there may still be chronic compensated acidosis or alkalosis that can offer insight into a patient's comorbid condition.

Identification of acid-base disturbance follows a series of steps:

1. Identify whether the pH is increased or decreased. An increase defines alkalemia, and a decrease defines acidemia.
2. Identify the change in $Paco_2$ and bicarbonate from their normal levels of 40 mm Hg and 24 mEq/L, respectively.
3. If both $Paco_2$ and bicarbonate change in the same direction (i.e., both are increased or both are decreased), there is a primary acid-base disorder with a compensatory

secondary disorder that brings the ratio of bicarbonate to carbon dioxide tension back toward 20:1.
4. If bicarbonate and $Paco_2$ change in opposite directions, there is a mixed acid-base disorder.
5. Determine the primary acid-base disorder by comparing the fractional change of the measured bicarbonate or carbon dioxide tension to the normal value.
6. There are equations and nomograms that calculate the expected change in one of the three parameters involved in acid-base determination (pH, bicarbonate, or carbon dioxide tension) for a given change in one of the other two parameters (Fig. 21.6). If the actual change is markedly different from the expected change, there is a mixed acid-base disorder.
7. Finally, calculate the anion gap to determine whether there is an anion gap metabolic acidosis. Elevation in the anion gap requires subsequent identification of the unmeasured anion.

Signs and Symptoms

Major adverse consequences of severe systemic acidosis (pH < 7.2) can occur independently of whether the acidosis is of respiratory, metabolic, or mixed origin (Table 21.8). The effects of acidosis are particularly detrimental to the cardiovascular system. Acidosis decreases myocardial contractility, although clinical effects are minimal until the pH decreases to less than

TABLE 21.8	Adverse Consequences of Severe Acidosis

NERVOUS SYSTEM
Obtundation
Coma

CARDIOVASCULAR SYSTEM
Impaired myocardial contractility
Decreased cardiac output
Decreased arterial blood pressure
Sensitization to reentrant cardiac dysrhythmias
Decreased threshold for ventricular fibrillation
Decreased responsiveness to catecholamines

VENTILATION
Hyperventilation
Dyspnea
Fatigue of respiratory muscles

METABOLISM
Hyperkalemia
Insulin resistance
Inhibition of anaerobic glycolysis

Adapted from Adrogué HJ, Madias NE. Management of life-threatening acid-base disorders. *N Engl J Med*. 1998;338:26-34.

TABLE 21.9	Adverse Consequences of Alkalosis

NERVOUS SYSTEM
Decreased cerebral blood flow
Seizures
Lethargy
Delirium
Tetany

CARDIOVASCULAR SYSTEM
Arteriolar vasoconstriction
Decreased coronary blood flow
Decreased threshold for angina pectoris
Predisposition to refractory dysrhythmias

VENTILATION
Hypoventilation
Hypercarbia
Arterial hypoxemia

METABOLISM
Hypokalemia
Hypocalcemia
Hypomagnesemia
Hypophosphatemia
Stimulation of anaerobic glycolysis

Adapted from Adrogué JH, Madias NE. Management of life-threatening acid-base disorders. *N Engl J Med*. 1998;338:107-111.

TABLE 21.10	Causes of Respiratory Acidosis

Drug-induced ventilatory depression
Permissive hypercapnia
Upper airway obstruction
Status asthmaticus
Restriction of ventilation (rib fractures/flail chest)
Disorders of neuromuscular function
Malignant hyperthermia
Hyperalimentation

7.2, which perhaps reflects the effects of catecholamine release in response to the acidosis. When the pH is less than 7.1, cardiac responsiveness to catecholamines decreases and compensatory inotropic effects are diminished. The detrimental effects of acidosis may be accentuated in those with underlying left ventricular dysfunction or myocardial ischemia and in those in whom sympathetic nervous system activity is impaired, such as by β-adrenergic blockade or general anesthesia.

Major adverse consequences of severe systemic alkalosis (pH > 7.60) reflect impairment of cerebral and coronary blood flow caused by arteriolar vasoconstriction (Table 21.9). Associated decreases in serum ionized calcium concentration probably contribute to the neurologic abnormalities associated with systemic alkalosis. Alkalosis predisposes patients, especially those with co-existing heart disease, to significant and even refractory ventricular dysrhythmias. Alkalosis depresses ventilation and can frustrate efforts to wean patients from mechanical ventilation. Hypokalemia accompanies both metabolic and respiratory alkalosis but is more prominent in the presence of metabolic alkalosis. Alkalosis stimulates anaerobic glycolysis and increases the production of lactic acid and ketoacids. Although alkalosis can decrease the release of oxygen to the tissues by tightening the binding of oxygen to hemoglobin, chronic alkalosis negates this effect by increasing the concentration of 2,3-diphosphoglycerate in erythrocytes.

Respiratory Acidosis

Respiratory acidemia is present when a decrease in alveolar ventilation results in an increase in the $Paco_2$ sufficient to decrease arterial pH to less than 7.35 (Table 21.10). The most likely cause of respiratory acidosis during the perioperative period is drug-induced depression of ventilation by opioids, general anesthetics, or neuromuscular blockers. Respiratory acidosis may be complicated by metabolic acidosis when renal perfusion is decreased to the extent that reabsorption mechanisms in the renal tubules are impaired. For example, cardiac output and renal blood flow may be so decreased in patients with chronic obstructive pulmonary disease and cor pulmonale as to lead to metabolic acidosis.

Respiratory acidosis is treated by correcting the disorder responsible for hypoventilation. Mechanical ventilation is necessary when the increase in $Paco_2$ is marked and carbon dioxide narcosis is present. It must be remembered that rapid lowering of chronically increased $Paco_2$ levels by mechanical ventilation decreases body stores of carbon dioxide much more rapidly than the kidneys can produce a corresponding decrease in serum bicarbonate concentration. The resulting metabolic alkalosis can cause neuromuscular irritability and excitation of the CNS, including seizures. It is best to decrease the $Paco_2$ slowly to permit sufficient time for renal tubular elimination of bicarbonate.

TABLE 21.11	Causes of Respiratory Alkalosis

Iatrogenic (mechanical hyperventilation)
High altitude
Central nervous system injury
Hepatic disease
Pregnancy
Salicylate overdose

TABLE 21.12	Causes of Metabolic Acidosis

Lactic acidosis
Diabetic ketoacidosis
Renal failure
Hepatic failure
Methanol and ethylene glycol intoxication
Aspirin intoxication
Increased skeletal muscle activity
Cyanide poisoning
Carbon monoxide poisoning

Metabolic alkalosis may accompany respiratory acidosis when the body stores of chloride and potassium are decreased. For example, decreased serum chloride concentrations facilitate renal tubular reabsorption of bicarbonate, which leads to metabolic alkalosis. Hypokalemia stimulates renal tubules to excrete hydrogen, which may produce metabolic alkalosis or aggravate a co-existing alkalosis caused by chloride deficiency. Treatment of metabolic alkalosis associated with these electrolyte disturbances requires administration of potassium chloride.

Respiratory Alkalosis

Respiratory alkalosis is present when an increase in alveolar ventilation results in a decrease in $Paco_2$ sufficient to increase the pH to greater than 7.45 (Table 21.11). The most likely cause of acute respiratory alkalosis during the perioperative period is iatrogenic hyperventilation. Respiratory alkalosis occurs normally during pregnancy and is an important adaptive response to high altitude.

Treatment of respiratory alkalosis is directed at correcting the underlying disorder responsible for alveolar hyperventilation. During anesthesia, this is most often accomplished by adjusting the ventilator to decrease alveolar ventilation. The hypokalemia and hypochloremia that may co-exist with respiratory alkalosis may also require treatment.

Metabolic Acidosis

Metabolic acidosis lowers blood pH, which stimulates the respiratory center to hyperventilate and lower carbon dioxide tension. Respiratory compensation does not in general fully counterbalance the increased acid production, but the pH will return *toward* normal.

Acidoses of metabolic origin are typically divided into those with a normal anion gap and those with a high anion gap.

A *high anion gap* occurs when a fixed acid is added to the extracellular space. The acid dissociates, the hydrogen ion combines with bicarbonate forming carbonic acid, and the decreased bicarbonate concentration produces an increased anion gap. Lactic acidosis, ketoacidosis, renal failure, and the acidoses associated with many poisonings are examples of *high–anion gap metabolic acidoses.*

Non–anion gap metabolic acidosis is the result of a net increase in chloride concentration. Bicarbonate loss is counterbalanced by a net gain of chloride ions to maintain electrical neutrality. Therefore a normal anion gap acidosis is often called a *hyperchloremic metabolic acidosis.* The most common causes of a normal–anion gap acidosis are IV infusion of sodium chloride and GI and renal losses of bicarbonate (diarrhea, renal tubular acidosis, early renal failure).

Signs and Symptoms

Since acidosis is secondary to an underlying disorder, the presentation of acidosis is complicated by the signs and symptoms of the causative disorder. Derangements of pH have wide-ranging effects on tissue, organ, and enzyme function, and the signs and symptoms attributable to an acidosis relate to these effects. The clinical features of metabolic acidosis depend also on the rate of development of acidosis and are likely to be more dramatic in rapidly developing acidosis in which compensatory respiratory or renal changes are not able to limit the fall in pH.

Diagnosis

Diagnosis depends on a high index of suspicion and laboratory testing. Most commonly, arterial blood is analyzed for pH, carbon dioxide tension, bicarbonate concentration, and anion gap. Common causes of metabolic acidosis are listed in Table 21.12.

Metabolic acidosis can be of renal or extrarenal origin. Metabolic acidosis of renal origin involves a primary disorder of renal acidification. This occurs when the kidneys are unable to regenerate sufficient bicarbonate to replace that lost by the buffering of normal endogenous acid production (distal renal tubular acidosis) or when an abnormally high fraction of filtered bicarbonate is not reabsorbed in the proximal tubule and is subsequently lost in the urine (proximal renal tubular acidosis or acetazolamide use). Combined defects occur in renal failure. The most common causes of extrarenal sources of metabolic acidosis are GI bicarbonate losses, ketoacidosis, and lactic acidosis.

Treatment

Treatment of metabolic acidosis includes treatment of the cause of the acidosis—for example, insulin and fluids for diabetic ketoacidosis and improvement in tissue perfusion for lactic acidosis. Administration of sodium bicarbonate for acute treatment of metabolic acidosis is very controversial. Many recommend that bicarbonate be given only if the

TABLE 21.13	Causes of Metabolic Alkalosis

Hypovolemia
Vomiting
Nasogastric suction
Diuretic therapy
Bicarbonate administration
Hyperaldosteronism
Chloride-wasting diarrhea

pH is less than 7.1 or the bicarbonate concentration is less than 10 mEq/L. There is concern that the bicarbonate reacts with hydrogen ions, generating carbon dioxide, which diffuses into cells and lowers intracellular pH even more than before the bicarbonate treatment. It is also postulated that administration of bicarbonate to patients with chronic metabolic acidosis may result in transient tissue hypoxia because acute changes in pH toward normal (or alkalosis) may negate the rightward shift of the oxyhemoglobin dissociation curve caused by acidemia (Bohr effect) and result in increased hemoglobin affinity for oxygen, which reduces oxygen delivery at the tissue level.

The 2015 American Heart Association Guidelines Update for Cardiopulmonary Resuscitation and Emergency Cardiovascular Care do *not* recommend administering sodium bicarbonate routinely during cardiac arrest and cardiopulmonary resuscitation. However, sodium bicarbonate may be considered for life-threatening hyperkalemia or cardiac arrest associated with hyperkalemia, or for cardiac arrest associated with a significant prearrest metabolic acidosis.

Management of Anesthesia

Elective surgery should be postponed until an acidosis has been treated. For urgent surgery in a patient with metabolic acidosis, invasive hemodynamic monitoring should be considered to guide fluid resuscitation and monitor cardiac function in marked acidosis. Laboratory measurement of acid-base parameters should be performed frequently throughout the perioperative period because pH can change rapidly and significantly in response to changes in ventilation, volume status, circulation, and drug administration.

Acidosis affects the proportion of drug in the ionized and un-ionized states. Volume of distribution may also be affected in patients who have uncorrected hypovolemia.

Metabolic Alkalosis

Metabolic alkalosis is marked by an increase in plasma bicarbonate concentration and is usually compensated for by an increase in carbon dioxide tension. Common causes of metabolic alkalosis are listed in Table 21.13.

Metabolic alkalosis can be of renal or extrarenal origin and can be caused by either a net loss of hydrogen ions (e.g., loss of hydrochloric acid with vomiting) or a net gain of bicarbonate (e.g., caused by tubular defects of bicarbonate reabsorption). Abnormal losses of chloride with or without hydrogen ion (e.g., in cystic fibrosis or villous adenoma) also induce increased renal bicarbonate reabsorption in an attempt to maintain electroneutrality. Therefore metabolic alkaloses can be characterized as chloride responsive or chloride resistant. Another classification of metabolic alkalosis is *volume-depletion alkalosis* (resulting from vomiting, diarrhea, or chloride losses) and *volume-overload alkalosis* (resulting from primary or secondary mineralocorticoid excess).

Metabolic alkalosis can also occur secondary to renal compensation for chronic respiratory disease with hypercarbia. In these patients, bicarbonate levels may be quite high and associated with urinary losses of chloride along with obligatory losses of sodium and potassium. If the respiratory disorder is treated with mechanical ventilation and the carbon dioxide tension is reduced rapidly, a profound metabolic alkalosis may result.

Signs and Symptoms

Progressively more binding of calcium to albumin occurs as an alkalosis develops, so the signs and symptoms of alkalosis, especially those related to the neuromuscular and central nervous systems, may be very similar to those of hypocalcemia. Metabolic alkalosis may be accompanied by volume contraction, hypochloremia and hypokalemia, or volume overload and sodium retention, depending on the cause.

Diagnosis

As with metabolic acidosis, the diagnosis of metabolic alkalosis is dependent on a high index of suspicion and laboratory testing. Metabolic alkaloses secondary to chloride losses are associated with low urinary chloride levels (typically <10 mEq/L) and volume contraction. In contrast, metabolic alkaloses associated with mineralocorticoid excess are typically associated with volume overload and spot urine chloride values above 20 mEq/L.

Treatment

Volume-depletion metabolic alkalosis is treated by chloride replacement along with fluid resuscitation using saline, which is itself weakly acidic. If the alkalosis has been caused by gastric losses of hydrochloric acid, proton pump inhibitors can be given to stop perpetuation of the alkalosis. Metabolic alkalosis associated with loop diuretics can be improved by adding or substituting potassium-sparing diuretics. In the case of volume-overload metabolic alkalosis due to excess mineralocorticoid concentrations, administration of spironolactone plus potassium chloride may be useful if the source of mineralocorticoid secretion cannot be eliminated.

Management of Anesthesia

Management of anesthesia includes judicious volume replacement and adequate supplementation with chloride, potassium, and magnesium as needed. Invasive monitoring may be helpful in some patients. Care must be taken not to eliminate a compensatory metabolic alkalosis in patients with chronic lung disease and significant carbon dioxide retention, because successful weaning from mechanical ventilation will likely necessitate a return to the chronic respiratory acidosis and metabolic alkalosis the patient had at presentation.

KEY POINTS

- Total body water content is categorized as ICF and ECF, according to the location of the water relative to cell membranes. The distribution and concentration of electrolytes can differ greatly between fluid compartments. The electrophysiology of excitable cells is dependent on the intracellular and extracellular concentrations of sodium, potassium, and calcium.

- Water balance is predominantly mediated by osmolality sensors, neurons located in the anterior hypothalamus that stimulate thirst and cause pituitary release of vasopressin (antidiuretic hormone). Vasopressin is stored as granules in the posterior pituitary and acts through G protein–coupled receptors in the collecting ducts of the kidney, causing water retention that in turn corrects serum osmolality.

- As hyponatremia develops, it is usually associated with extracellular hypotonicity, which results in water movement into cells and can manifest as cerebral edema and increased intracranial pressure. Initial compensation is afforded by the movement of brain extracellular fluid into the cerebrospinal fluid. Later compensation includes the lowering of intracellular osmolality by the movement of potassium and organic solutes out of brain cells. This reduces water movement into the intracellular space. However, when these adaptive mechanisms fail or hyponatremia progresses, CNS manifestations of hyponatremia occur.

- The volume overload, hyponatremia, and hypoosmolality that may accompany transurethral resection of the prostate is known as *TURP syndrome*. This syndrome is more likely to occur when resection is prolonged (>1 hour), when the irrigating fluid is suspended more than 40 cm above the operative field, and when the pressure in the bladder is allowed to increase above 15 cm H_2O. TURP syndrome manifests principally with cardiovascular signs of volume overload and neurologic signs of hyponatremia.

- Hypokalemia is diagnosed by testing the serum potassium concentration. The differential diagnosis requires determining whether the hypokalemia is acute and secondary to intracellular potassium shifts, such as might be seen with hyperventilation or alkalosis, or is chronic and associated with depletion of total body potassium stores.

- Immediate treatment of hyperkalemia is required if life-threatening dysrhythmias or ECG signs of severe hyperkalemia are present. This treatment is aimed at antagonizing the effects of a high potassium on the transmembrane potential and redistributing potassium intracellularly. Calcium chloride or calcium gluconate is administered to stabilize cellular membranes. Hyperventilation, sodium bicarbonate administration, and insulin administration promote movement of potassium intracellularly.

- Binding of calcium to albumin is pH dependent, and acid-base disturbances can change the fraction and therefore the concentration of ionized calcium without changing total body calcium. Alkalosis reduces the ionized calcium concentration, so ionized calcium may be significantly reduced after bicarbonate administration or with hyperventilation.

- Signs and symptoms of hypermagnesemia begin to occur at serum levels of 4–5 mEq/L and include lethargy, nausea and vomiting, and facial flushing. At levels above 6 mEq/L, a loss of deep tendon reflexes and hypotension occur. Paralysis, apnea, and/or cardiac arrest are likely if the magnesium level exceeds 10 mEq/L.

- Major adverse consequences of severe systemic acidosis (pH < 7.2) can occur whether the acidosis is of respiratory, metabolic, or mixed origin. Acidosis decreases myocardial contractility, although clinical effects are minimal until the pH decreases below 7.2, which perhaps reflects the effects of catecholamine release in response to the acidosis. When the pH is less than 7.1, cardiac responsiveness to catecholamines decreases and compensatory inotropic effects are diminished. The detrimental effects of acidosis may be accentuated in those with underlying left ventricular dysfunction or myocardial ischemia and in those in whom sympathetic nervous system activity is impaired, such as by β-adrenergic blockade or general anesthesia.

- Major adverse consequences of severe systemic alkalosis (pH > 7.60) reflect impairment of cerebral and coronary blood flow due to arteriolar vasoconstriction. Associated decreases in serum ionized calcium concentration contribute to the neurologic abnormalities associated with systemic alkalosis. Alkalosis predisposes patients—especially those with coexisting heart disease—to severe, often refractory, ventricular dysrhythmias. Alkalosis also depresses ventilation.

RESOURCES

Adrogué HJ, Madias NE. Management of life-threatening acid-base disorders. *N Engl J Med.* 1998;338:26-34: 107-111.

Berend K, de Vries A, Gans R. Disorders of fluids and electrolytes: physiological approach to assessment of acid-base disturbances. *N Engl J Med.* 2014;371:1434-1445.

Bonow R, Mann D, Zipes D, et al, eds. *Braunwald's Heart Disease: a Textbook of Cardiovascular Medicine.* Philadelphia: Saunders; 2011.

Brenner B, Clarkson M, Oparil S, et al, eds. *Brenner and Rector's The Kidney.* Philadelphia: Saunders; 2007.

Fauci AS, Braunwald E, Hauser SL, et al, eds. *Harrison's Principles of Internal Medicine.* New York: McGraw Hill; 2007.

Gennari FJ. Hypokalemia. *N Engl J Med.* 1998;339:451-458.

Link MS, Berkow LC, Kudenchuk PJ, et al. 2015 American Heart Association guidelines update for cardiopulmonary resuscitation and emergency cardiovascular care. Part 7: adult advanced cardiovascular life support. *Circulation.* 2015;132:S444-S464.

Sterns RH. Disorders of plasma sodium—causes, consequences, and correction. *N Engl J Med.* 2015;372:55-65.

Wahr JA, Parks R, Boisvert D, et al. Preoperative serum potassium levels and perioperative outcomes in cardiac surgical patients. *JAMA.* 1999;281: 2203-2210.

CHAPTER 22

Renal Disease

NATALIE F. HOLT

Medicare spent $87 billion on treatment of all stages of renal disease in 2012. Over 26 million adults in the United States have some form of kidney disease. Many may not even know it because the signs and symptoms may be subtle. It is the ninth leading cause of death in this country. The most important precursors of renal disease are diabetes mellitus, systemic hypertension, a family history of kidney disease, and age older than 65 years. So it is likely that many patients with some degree of renal dysfunction will appear for surgery, or that patients with these precursor medical problems may develop some acute renal injury or worsening of their preexisting renal dysfunction in the perioperative period.

The kidneys are responsible for or contribute to a number of essential functions, including water conservation, electrolyte homeostasis, acid-base balance, and several neurohumoral and hormonal functions. Knowing how the kidneys perform these important functions aids in understanding the clinical presentation, signs and symptoms, and treatment of renal diseases.

The kidneys are the most highly perfused organs in the body, receiving 15%–25% of cardiac output; the majority of blood is distributed to the renal cortex. Each kidney consists of approximately a million nephrons, each of which has distinct anatomic parts: Bowman's capsule, proximal tubule, loop of Henle, distal tubule, and collecting duct (Fig. 22.1).

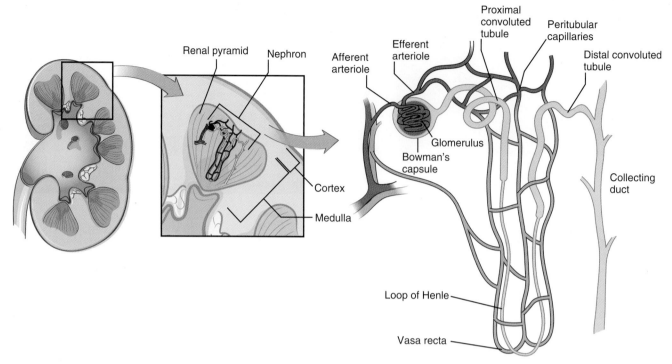

FIG. 22.1 Anatomy of the kidney and glomerulus. The kidneys receive 15%–25% of cardiac output; the majority of blood is distributed to the renal cortex. Each kidney consists of approximately a million nephrons, each of which has distinct anatomic parts: Bowman's capsule, proximal tubule, loop of Henle, distal tubule, and collecting duct. A glomerulus, a tuft of capillaries, is surrounded by Bowman's capsule and is supplied by an afferent arteriole and drained by a slightly smaller efferent arteriole. The juxtaglomerular apparatus is a specialized structure between the afferent arteriole and distal tubule that contributes to the control of renal perfusion and extrarenal hemodynamics. As plasma flows along the nephron, virtually all the fluid and solutes are reabsorbed by a number of active and passive transport systems. The main functions of the kidneys are water and sodium homeostasis, which are intimately linked and regulated by a number of feedback loops and hormonal controls. (From https://www.boundless.com/biology/textbooks/boundless-biology-textbook/osmotic-regulation-and-the-excretory-system-41/human-osmoregulatory-and-excretory-systems-229/kidney-structure-860-12107/.)

Renal blood flow is autoregulated between mean arterial pressures of approximately 50 and 150 mm Hg. A *glomerulus,* which is a tuft of capillaries, is surrounded by Bowman's capsule and supplied by an afferent arteriole and drained by a slightly smaller efferent arteriole. The *juxtaglomerular apparatus* is a specialized structure between the afferent arteriole and distal tubule that contributes to the control of renal perfusion and extrarenal hemodynamics. The glomeruli filter the plasma at a rate of 180 L/day, allowing all but protein and polysaccharides to pass into the nephron. As plasma flows along the nephron, virtually all the fluid and solutes are reabsorbed by a number of active and passive transport systems. The main function of the kidneys is water and sodium homeostasis, which are intimately linked and regulated by a number of feedback loops and hormonal controls.

CLINICAL ASSESSMENT OF RENAL FUNCTION

There are a number of tests that are useful in evaluating renal function and diagnosing disease (Table 22.1).

Glomerular Filtration Rate

The glomerular filtration rate (GFR) is considered the best measure of renal function, because it parallels the various functions of the nephrons. The GFR may be calculated from timed urine volumes plus urinary and plasma creatinine concentrations (creatinine clearance), or from direct measurements of the clearance of either endogenous or exogenous substances (creatinine and inulin, respectively). Alternatively, a number of formulas exist that estimate the GFR from various serum

TABLE 22.1	Tests Used to Evaluate Renal Function
Test	Reference Value
GLOMERULAR FILTRATION RATE	
Blood urea nitrogen concentration	10–20 mg/dL
Serum creatinine concentration	0.6–1.3 mg/dL
Creatinine clearance	110–140 mL/min
Urine protein (albumin) excretion	<150 mg/day
RENAL TUBULAR FUNCTION AND/OR INTEGRITY	
Urine specific gravity	1.003–1.030
Urine osmolality	50–1400 mOsm/L
Urine sodium excretion	<40 mEq/L
Glucosuria	
Enzymuria	
N-Acetyl-β-glucosaminidase	
α-Glutathione S-transferase	
FACTORS THAT INFLUENCE INTERPRETATION	
Dehydration	
Variable protein intake	
Gastrointestinal bleeding	
Catabolism	
Advanced age	
Skeletal muscle mass	
Accurate timing of urine volume measurement	

TABLE 22.2	Calculations Used to Measure or Estimate Glomerular Filtration Rate

CREATININE CLEARANCE

Creatinine clearance = (Urine creatinine × Urine volume) ÷ Serum creatinine × Time

COCKCROFT-GAULT EQUATION

GFR (mL/min) = [(140 − age in years) × Lean body weight (kg)]/ [Serum Cr (mg/dL) × 72] × (0.85 if female)

MODIFICATION OF DIET IN RENAL DISEASE (MDRD) EQUATION

GFR (mL/min/1.73 m^2) = 186.3 × Serum Cr$^{-1.154}$ × Age$^{-0.203}$ × (0.742 if female) × (1.21 if African American)

Cr, Creatinine; *GFR,* glomerular filtration rate.
Adapted from Cockcroft DW, Gault MH. Prediction of creatinine clearance from serum creatinine. *Nephron.* 1976;16:31-41; and Levey AS, Bosch JP, Lewis JB, et al. A more accurate method to estimate glomerular filtration equation from serum creatinine: a new prediction equation. *Ann Intern Med.* 1999;130:461-470.

and urinary indices (Table 22.2). Normal values for GFR are 90 mL/min/1.73 m^2 or better and vary with gender, body weight, and age. GFR decreases by approximately 1% per year after the age of 20. Clinical manifestations of uremia generally appear when the GFR falls below 15 mL/min/1.73 m^2. Alterations in GFR are also associated with predictable changes in erythropoietic activity.

Creatinine Clearance

Creatinine, an endogenous marker of renal filtration, is produced at a relatively constant rate by hepatic conversion of skeletal muscle creatine. Creatinine is freely filtered by the kidney and is not reabsorbed. As a result, creatinine clearance is the most reliable measure of GFR. Creatinine clearance does not depend on corrections for age or the presence of a steady state.

Serum Creatinine

Serum creatinine levels can be used as an estimate of the GFR. Creatinine is generally neither secreted nor reabsorbed in the kidney, so the amount that appears in the urine in a specified time interval reflects the amount that was filtered at the glomerulus during that time interval. Normal serum creatinine concentrations range from 0.6–1.0 mg/dL in women and 0.8–1.3 mg/dL in men, which reflects differences in skeletal muscle mass. Accelerated creatinine production may increase serum creatinine concentrations in the absence of a concomitant decrease in GFR, and small reductions in serum creatinine level may reflect large decreases in GFR. For example, the maintenance of normal serum creatinine concentrations in elderly patients with known decreases in GFR reflects decreased creatinine production owing to the decreased skeletal muscle mass that accompanies aging. Serum creatinine values are also slow to reflect acute changes in renal function. For example, if acute kidney injury occurs and the GFR decreases from 100 mL/min to 10 mL/min, serum creatinine values do not increase correspondingly for about a week.

Blood Urea Nitrogen

Blood urea nitrogen (BUN) concentrations vary with the GFR. However, the influences of dietary intake, co-existing disease, and intravascular fluid volume on BUN concentrations make it potentially misleading as a test of renal function. For example, production of urea is increased by consumption of a high-protein diet or gastrointestinal (GI) bleeding, which results in increased BUN concentrations despite a normal GFR. Other causes of increased BUN concentrations despite a normal GFR include dehydration and increased catabolism, as occurs during a febrile illness. Increased BUN concentrations in the presence of dehydration most likely reflect increased urea absorption due to slow movement of fluid through the renal tubules. When the latter is responsible for increased BUN concentrations, serum creatinine levels remain normal. BUN concentrations can also remain normal with consumption of a low-protein diet (as in hemodialysis patients) despite decreases in GFR. Even given these extraneous influences, BUN concentrations higher than 50 mg/dL *usually* reflect a decreased GFR.

Renal Tubular Function and Integrity

Renal tubular function is most often assessed by measuring the urine concentrating ability. The presence of proteinuria may also reflect renal tubular damage.

Urine Concentrating Ability

The diagnosis of renal tubular dysfunction is established by demonstrating that the kidneys do not produce appropriately concentrated urine in the presence of a physiologic stimulus for the release of antidiuretic hormone. In the absence of diuretic therapy or glucosuria, a urine specific gravity higher than 1.018 suggests that the ability of renal tubules to concentrate urine is adequate. Treatment with diuretics or the presence of hypokalemia or hypercalcemia may interfere with the ability of renal tubules to concentrate urine. The inorganic fluoride resulting from metabolism of sevoflurane is theoretically capable of interfering with the urine concentrating ability of the renal tubules; however, the clinical significance of this observation has yet to be established.

Proteinuria

Proteinuria is relatively common and is present in 5%–10% of adults undergoing screening examinations. Transient proteinuria may be associated with fever, congestive heart failure, seizure activity, pancreatitis, and exercise. This form of proteinuria resolves with treatment of the underlying condition. Orthostatic proteinuria occurs in up to 5% of adolescents while in the upright position and disappears with recumbency. Generally, orthostatic proteinuria resolves spontaneously and is not associated with any deterioration in renal function. Persistent proteinuria generally connotes significant renal disease. Microalbuminuria is the earliest sign of diabetic nephropathy. Severe proteinuria may result in hypoalbuminemia, with an associated decrease in plasma oncotic pressure and increases in unbound drug concentrations.

Fractional Excretion of Sodium

The fractional excretion of sodium (FE_{Na}) is a measure of the percentage of filtered sodium that is excreted in the urine (Table 22.3). It is the filtered sodium divided by the GFR. It is most useful in differentiating between prerenal and renal causes of azotemia. An FE_{Na} higher than 2% (or urinary sodium concentration > 40 mEq/L) reflects decreased ability of the renal tubules to conserve sodium and is consistent with tubular dysfunction. An FE_{Na} of less than 1% (or urinary sodium excretion < 20 mEq/L) occurs when normally functioning renal tubules are conserving sodium.

Urinalysis

Examination of the urine is useful for diagnosing renal and urinary tract disease. Urinalysis is intended to detect the presence of protein, glucose, acetoacetate, blood, and leukocytes. The urine pH and solute concentrations (specific gravity) are determined, and sediment microscopy is used to identify the presence of cells, casts, microorganisms, and crystals. Hematuria may be caused by bleeding anywhere between the glomerulus and urethra. Microhematuria may be benign or may reflect glomerulonephritis, renal calculi, or cancer of the genitourinary tract. Joggers may experience transient hematuria, presumably as a result of trauma to the urinary tract. Sickle cell disease is a consideration in African Americans who exhibit hematuria. In the absence of protein or red blood cell casts in the urine, glomerular disease as a cause of hematuria is unlikely. Red blood cell casts are pathognomonic of acute glomerulonephritis. White blood cell casts are most commonly seen with pyelonephritis.

Other Biomarkers of Renal Function

Cystatin C is a protein produced by all nucleated cells and is freely filtered but not resorbed by the kidneys. Cystatin C–based measures of GFR have been developed and appear to be more accurate than creatinine-based estimates in specific populations such as those with cirrhosis, obesity, malnutrition, or reduced muscle mass. It is a stronger predictor than serum creatinine of the risk of death and cardiovascular events in older patients.

ACUTE KIDNEY INJURY

Acute kidney injury (AKI) is characterized by deterioration of renal function over a period of hours to days, resulting in failure of the kidneys to excrete nitrogenous waste products and to maintain fluid and electrolyte homeostasis. Commonly used definitions of AKI include an increase in serum creatinine concentration of more than 0.3 mg/dL within 48 hours, or more than 50% over a period of 7 days. An acute drop in urine output to less than 0.5 mL/kg/h (*oliguria*) may also be indicative of AKI. Despite major advances in dialysis therapy and critical care, the mortality rate among patients with severe AKI requiring dialysis remains high. When AKI occurs in the setting of multiorgan failure, the mortality rate usually exceeds 50%. The most common causes of death are sepsis, cardiovascular dysfunction, and pulmonary complications.

Etiology

The incidence of AKI depends on the definition used and the patient population studied. Some degree of AKI is thought to affect 5%–7% of all hospitalized patients. AKI is associated with a number of other systemic diseases, acute clinical conditions, drug treatments, and interventional therapies. It almost invariably accompanies multiorgan failure syndromes in the critically ill patient population.

The causes of AKI are classically divided into prerenal, intrarenal (or intrinsic), and postrenal (Table 22.4). *Azotemia* is a condition marked by abnormally high serum concentrations of nitrogen-containing compounds such as BUN and creatinine and is a hallmark of AKI, regardless of cause.

TABLE 22.3	Calculation of Fractional Excretion of Sodium (FE_{Na})

FE_{Na} (%) = [(P_{Cr} × U_{Na})/(P_{Na} × U_{Cr})] × 100

Urine and plasma concentrations of creatinine and sodium are measured in mg/dL. P_{Cr}, Plasma creatinine concentration; P_{Na}, plasma sodium concentration; U_{Cr}, urine creatinine concentration; U_{Na}, urine sodium concentration.

Prerenal Azotemia

Prerenal azotemia accounts for nearly half of hospital-acquired cases of AKI. Prerenal azotemia is rapidly reversible if the underlying cause is corrected. If left untreated, sustained prerenal azotemia is the most common factor that predisposes patients to ischemia-induced acute tubular necrosis. Elderly patients are uniquely susceptible to prerenal azotemia because of their predisposition to hypovolemia (poor fluid intake) and high incidence of renovascular disease. Among hospitalized patients, prerenal azotemia may also be due to congestive heart failure, liver dysfunction, or septic shock. Reduced renal blood flow may be a result of anesthetic drug–induced decreases in perfusion pressure, particularly in the presence of hypovolemia and surgical blood loss.

Assessment of volume status, hemodynamics, and drug therapy is required to identify prerenal causes of acute oliguria. Invasive monitoring (central venous catheter, pulmonary artery catheter) may be helpful to assess intravascular volume status; alternatively, echocardiography may be used for this purpose. Urinary indices are often helpful in distinguishing prerenal from intrinsic AKI (Table 22.5). The use of urinary indices is based on the assumption that the ability of renal tubules to reabsorb sodium and water is maintained in the presence of prerenal causes of AKI, whereas these functions are impaired in the presence of tubulointerstitial disease or acute tubular necrosis. Blood and urine specimens for determination of urinary indices must be obtained before the administration of fluids, dopamine, mannitol, or diuretic drugs.

Renal Azotemia

Intrinsic renal diseases that result in AKI are categorized according to the primary site of injury (glomerulus, renal tubules, interstitium, renal vasculature). Injury to the renal tubules is most often due to ischemia or nephrotoxins (e.g., aminoglycosides, radiographic contrast drugs). Prerenal azotemia and ischemic tubular necrosis are a continuum, with the initial decreases in renal blood flow leading to ischemia of the renal tubular cells. Although some cases of ischemic AKI are reversible if the underlying cause is corrected, irreversible cortical necrosis occurs if the ischemia is severe or prolonged. Injury may also occur during reperfusion because of an influx of inflammatory cells, cytokines, and oxygen free radicals.

Ischemia and toxins often combine to cause AKI in severely ill patients with conditions such as sepsis or acquired immunodeficiency syndrome (AIDS). AKI resulting from acute interstitial nephritis is most often caused by allergic reactions to drugs. Other causes of renal azotemia include glomerulonephritis, pyelonephritis, renal artery emboli, renal vein thrombosis, and vasculitis.

Postrenal Azotemia

AKI occurs when urinary outflow tracts are obstructed, as with prostatic hyperplasia or cancer of the prostate or cervix.

TABLE 22.4 Causes of Acute Kidney Injury

PRERENAL AZOTEMIA
Hemorrhage
Gastrointestinal fluid loss
Trauma
Surgery
Burns
Cardiogenic shock
Sepsis
Hepatic failure
Aortic or renal artery clamping
Thromboembolism

RENAL AZOTEMIA
Acute glomerulonephritis
Vasculitis
Interstitial nephritis (drug allergy, infiltrative diseases)
Acute tubular necrosis
  Ischemia
  Nephrotoxic drugs (aminoglycosides, nonsteroidal antiinflammatory drugs)
  Solvents (carbon tetrachloride, ethylene glycol)
  Heavy metals (mercury, cisplatin)
  Radiographic contrast dyes
  Myoglobinuria
  Intratubular crystals (uric acid, oxalate)

POSTRENAL AZOTEMIA
Nephrolithiasis
Benign prostatic hyperplasia
Clot retention
Bladder carcinoma

Adapted from Klahr S, Miller SB. Acute oliguria. *N Engl J Med*. 1998;338:671-675; and Thadhani R, Pascual M, Bonventre JV. Acute renal failure. *N Engl J Med*. 1996;334:1148-1169.

TABLE 22.5 Characteristic Urinary Indices in Patients With Acute Oliguria Resulting From Prerenal or Renal Causes

Index	Prerenal Causes	Renal Causes
Urinary sodium concentration (mEq/L)	<20	>40
Urine osmolality (mOsm/kg)	>500	<400
Fractional excretion of sodium (%)	<1	>1.1
Fractional excretion of urea (%)	<35	>35
Ratio of urine to plasma creatinine concentration	>40	<20
Ratio of urine to plasma osmolarity	>1.5	<1.0
Sediment	Normal, occasional hyaline casts	Renal tubular epithelial cells, granular casts

Adapted from Schrier RW, Wang W, Poole B, et al. Acute renal failure: definition, diagnosis, pathogenesis, and therapy. *J Clin Invest*. 2004;114:5-14.

TABLE 22.6	Risk Factors for Perioperative Renal Failure

PREOPERATIVE FACTORS
Preexisting renal insufficiency
Advanced age
Heart disease (congestive heart failure, ischemia)
Smoking
Diabetes mellitus
Liver failure
Pregnancy-induced hypertension
ASA physical status 4 or 5

INTRAOPERATIVE FACTORS
Emergency, intraperitoneal, intrathoracic, suprainguinal vascular, transplant surgery
Aortic cross-clamping
Cardiopulmonary bypass
Inotrope use
Erythrocyte transfusion

POSTOPERATIVE FACTORS
Erythrocyte transfusion
Vasoconstrictor use
Diuretic use
Antidysrhythmic use
Sepsis
Nephrotoxins (radiocontrast dyes, nonsteroidal antiinflammatory drugs, aminoglycoside antibiotics)

ASA, American Society of Anesthesiologists.
Adapted from Chenitz KB, Lane-Fall MB. Decreased urine output and acute kidney injury in the postanesthesia care unit. *Anesthesiol Clin.* 2012;30:513-526.

It is important to diagnose postrenal causes of AKI promptly because the potential for recovery is inversely related to the duration of the obstruction. Renal ultrasonography is useful for determining the presence of obstructive nephropathy. Percutaneous nephrostomy can relieve obstruction and improve outcomes.

Risk Factors

Risk factors for the development of AKI include preexisting renal disease, advanced age, congestive heart failure, peripheral vascular disease, diabetes, emergency surgery, and major surgery such as coronary revascularization and aortic aneurysm repair (Table 22.6). Sepsis and multiple organ system dysfunction resulting from trauma introduce the risk of AKI. Iatrogenic components that predispose to AKI include inadequate fluid replacement, hypotension, delayed treatment of sepsis, and administration of nephrotoxic drugs or dyes.

Appropriate hydration and optimal preservation of intravascular fluid volume are essential to maintain renal perfusion. It is also important to maintain adequate systemic blood pressure and cardiac output and to prevent peripheral vasoconstriction. Hypotension may result in inadequate renal perfusion and loss of renal autoregulation. Potentially nephrotoxic substances are logically avoided in patients with prerenal oliguria, and diuretic therapy is contraindicated.

Diagnosis

Signs and symptoms of AKI are often absent in the early stages, and a high degree of suspicion is required to identify subtle changes that accompany the development of AKI. Patients may show generalized malaise or demonstrate evidence of fluid overload such as dyspnea, edema, and hypertension. As protein and amino acid metabolites accumulate, patients become lethargic, nauseated, and confused. Hyperkalemia and acidosis may affect cardiac rhythm and contractility. Encephalopathy, coma, seizures, and death may ensue. Other signs and symptoms of AKI are associated with its specific cause, such as hypotension, jaundice, hematuria, or urinary retention.

The diagnosis of AKI is made based on laboratory data demonstrating an increase in serum creatinine of at least 0.3 mg/dL over 48 hours or more than 50% over 7 days. An acute drop in urine output to less than 0.5 mL/kg/h for more than 6 hours is also suggestive of AKI. *Anuria* is defined as urine output of less than 100 mL/day and is a sign of severe kidney injury. A number of diagnostic biomarkers referred to as the *acute kidney injury biomarker panel* are also useful. These include neutrophil gelatinase–associated lipocalin (NGAL), urinary kidney injury molecule-1, urinary interleukin-18, and urinary liver-type fatty acid–binding protein. Enzymes present in the renal tubular cells (N-acetyl-β-D-glucosaminidase, α-glutathione S-transferase) may be also detectable in the urine. These markers occur very early in AKI, before traditional measurements of creatinine are abnormal. Ideally they may allow earlier physiologic or pharmacologic interventions to prevent more severe acute kidney damage. These enzymes may also be present following sevoflurane anesthesia, which presumably reflects transient drug-induced tubular dysfunction, and in this situation are not accompanied by changes in BUN or serum creatinine concentrations.

Urinalysis is helpful in diagnosing whether the cause of AKI is prerenal, intrarenal, or postrenal.

Complications

Complications of AKI manifest in the central nervous, cardiovascular, hematologic, and GI systems. Metabolic derangements are also common. In addition, infections occur frequently in patients who develop AKI and are leading causes of morbidity and mortality.

Neurologic complications of AKI include confusion, asterixis, somnolence, seizures, and polyneuropathy. These changes appear to be related to the buildup of protein and amino acids in the blood. These symptoms and signs may be ameliorated by dialysis.

Cardiovascular complications include systemic hypertension, congestive heart failure, and pulmonary edema, principally as reflections of sodium and water retention. The presence of congestive heart failure or pulmonary edema suggests the need to decrease the intravascular fluid volume. Cardiac dysrhythmias may develop; peaked T waves and widened QRS complexes are indicative of hyperkalemia. Uremic pericarditis may also occur.

Hematologic complications include anemia and coagulopathy. Hematocrit values between 20% and 30% are common as a result of hemodilution and decreased erythropoietin production. Patients with renal insufficiency are also at increased risk of bleeding complications caused by uremia-induced platelet dysfunction. Preoperative dialysis may be indicated in high-risk patients. Alternatively, desmopressin (DDAVP) can be administered preoperatively to temporarily increase concentrations of von Willebrand factor (vWF) and factor VIII and improve coagulation.

Metabolic derangements include hyperkalemia and metabolic acidosis. Sodium and water retention result in hypertension and edema. Frequent monitoring of arterial blood gas concentrations and electrolyte levels is indicated. Hyperkalemia may be treated with the use of dietary restriction, exchange resins, and insulin. Bicarbonate is useful for the management of acidosis. Hyperphosphatemia and hypocalcemia are common. Treatment depends on whether the patient is symptomatic. Phosphate binders are generally used when the serum phosphate concentration is above 6 mg/dL. Calcium levels often normalize with reduction in phosphate levels.

Gastrointestinal complications include anorexia, nausea, vomiting, and ileus. GI bleeding occurs in as many as one-third of patients who develop AKI and may contribute to anemia. Gastroparesis may occur as a result of uremia. Administration of histamine-2 (H_2) receptor antagonists and/or proton pump inhibitors may decrease the risk of GI bleeding.

Infection commonly affects the respiratory and urinary tracts and sites where breaks in normal anatomic barriers have occurred because of indwelling catheters. Impaired immune responses resulting from uremia may contribute to the increased likelihood of infections in patients with AKI.

Treatment

There are no specific treatment modalities for AKI. Management is aimed at limiting further renal injury and correcting fluid, electrolyte, and acid-base derangements. Underlying causes should be sought and terminated or reversed if possible. Specifically, hypovolemia, hypotension, and low cardiac output should be corrected and sepsis treated. A mean arterial pressure of 65 mm Hg should be maintained, but there is no evidence supporting a better outcome with supraphysiologic values of either systemic blood pressure or cardiac output.

Fluid resuscitation and vasopressor therapy are universally emphasized in the prevention and treatment of AKI. There is no evidence to support the use of colloid over crystalloid. In fact, administration of hydroxyethyl starch has been shown in some studies to exacerbate renal injury. Traditionally, 0.9% saline, which is somewhat hypertonic, was the preferred crystalloid for use in patients with renal dysfunction, because it lacks potassium. However, recent research suggests that it may cause hyperchloremic metabolic acidosis and secondarily lead to hyperkalemia. Therefore *isotonic* saline or other bicarbonate-containing balanced salt solutions may be a better choice.

With regard to the use of vasopressors in the treatment of AKI associated with sepsis, concern has been expressed that renal vasoconstriction may exacerbate tubular injury. It is true that α_1-agonists such as norepinephrine reduce renal blood flow in healthy volunteers. However, in patients with sepsis-related AKI, their effects depend on the balance of a variety of factors. In general it appears that improved systemic pressure is accompanied by reduced renal sympathetic tone and vasodilation. Therefore the overall effect of using norepinephrine in septic patients is to increase GFR and urinary output. Arginine vasopressin is an alternative to traditional vasopressors in the treatment of septic shock and may be effective when other agents have failed. This drug appears to selectively constrict renal efferent arterioles; therefore it may help preserve GFR and urinary output better than α_1-agonists. However, its superiority in the management of septic shock has yet to be demonstrated.

The use of dopamine either to treat or prevent AKI is not supported by the literature; in fact, dopamine use has been associated with a number of undesirable side effects.

The practice of trying to convert oliguric to nonoliguric AKI by using diuretics is not advised and may actually increase mortality risk and permanent renal injury. In severe sepsis, administration of activated protein C and steroid replacement (in those patients who demonstrate adrenal insufficiency) may reduce mortality.

Prophylactic administration of *N*-acetylcysteine, a thio-containing antioxidant that acts as a free radical scavenger, may provide protection against radiographic dye–induced nephropathy. However, because of conflicting data and the risk of complications such as anaphylactoid reactions, it is not universally recommended. Volume loading, preferably with isotonic saline, is the preferred preventive strategy.

Alkalinization of urine with sodium bicarbonate is helpful in the treatment of pigment-induced nephropathy, such as that caused by rhabdomyolysis, because it increases the solubility of myoglobin and prevents formation of tubular precipitates. Prophylactic administration of sodium bicarbonate also appears to reduce the incidence of contrast-induced nephropathy by decreasing the formation of damaging free radicals.

Dialysis (also known as *renal replacement therapy*) is still the mainstay of treatment for severe AKI. There are five main indications for its use: volume overload, hyperkalemia, severe metabolic acidosis, symptomatic uremia, and overdose with a dialyzable drug. Two dialysis methods exist: hemodialysis and peritoneal dialysis. The purpose of both is to remove excess fluid and solutes from the blood and optimize electrolyte balance. Dialysis may be performed as continuous or intermittent therapy, and controversy exists as to whether one or the other method is superior.

Prognosis

The overall prognosis for hospital-acquired AKI is poor. Many AKI study series report mortality rates higher than 20%, and once dialysis is required, mortality rates are invariably in excess of 50%. Those who succumb usually die of failure of other organ systems after prolonged and complex hospital courses. Only about 15% of patients developing AKI will fully recover renal function, 5% will retain a degree of renal insufficiency that remains stable, and another 5% will experience continued deterioration of renal function throughout the remainder of their lives. Fifteen percent will be left with stable renal insufficiency for a period but remain at high risk of developing chronic renal failure later in life.

Drug Dosing in Patients With Renal Impairment

Renal impairment affects most organ systems of the body and consequently the pharmacology of many drugs. Selecting drugs that do not rely on the kidneys for excretion is ideal but not always possible.

The first step in tailoring drug dosing for patients with renal impairment is to estimate the creatinine clearance, since the rate of elimination of drugs excreted by the kidneys is proportional to the GFR. If the patient is oliguric, the creatinine clearance can be approximated by a value of 5 mL/min. If the normal drug regimen starts with a loading dose to rapidly achieve therapeutic levels, the following guidelines may be used:

- If after clinical examination, the extracellular fluid volume appears to be *normal,* use the loading dose suggested for patients with normal renal function.
- If the extracellular fluid is *contracted,* reduce the loading dose.
- If the extracellular fluid is *expanded,* use a higher loading dose.

There are also formulas to calculate loading and maintenance doses based on renal function, depending on either the fraction of drug excreted in the urine or the difference in drug half-life in patients with normal renal function and those with impaired function.

For medications with wide therapeutic ranges or long plasma half-lives, the interval between doses is generally increased. For medications with narrow therapeutic ranges or short plasma half-lives, reduced doses at normal intervals are advised. In reality a combination of the two methods of dosage adjustment is frequently used (Table 22.7).

Management of Anesthesia

Because of the high morbidity and mortality, only lifesaving surgery should be undertaken in patients with AKI. The principles that guide anesthesia management are the same as those that guide supportive treatment of AKI: (1) maintenance of an adequate systemic blood pressure and cardiac output and (2) avoidance of further renal insults, including hypovolemia, hypoxia, and exposure to nephrotoxins. Invasive hemodynamic monitoring is mandatory, as are frequent blood gas analyses and electrolyte measurements.

In general, administration of diuretics to maintain urine output in patients who are not oliguric has *not* been shown to improve either renal outcome or patient survival. However, when a dilutional anemia has been caused by overzealous hydration, use of diuretics may minimize the risk of fluid overload caused by administration of blood or blood products. For patients who meet the criteria, postoperative dialysis should be initiated as soon as the patient is in hemodynamically stable condition.

CHRONIC KIDNEY DISEASE

Chronic kidney disease (CKD) is marked by the presence of kidney damage (usually defined as estimated GFR < 60 mL/min/1.73 m²) for 3 or more months, and it may be caused by a multitude of disease processes (Table 22.8). In the United States, diabetes mellitus and hypertension are responsible for two-thirds of all cases of CKD. The clinical manifestations of CKD reflect the inability of the kidneys to excrete nitrogenous waste products, regulate fluid and electrolyte balance, and secrete hormones. In most patients, regardless of the cause, a decrease in GFR to less than 25 mL/min results in end-stage renal disease (ESRD) requiring dialysis or transplantation (Table 22.9).

TABLE 22.7	Analgesic Dosage Adjustments in Patients With Renal Insufficiency			
Drug	Adjustment Method	GFR > 50 mL/min	GFR 10–50 mL/min	GFR < 10 mL/min
Acetaminophen	↑ Interval	q4h	q6h	q8h
Acetylsalicylic acid	↑ Interval	q4h	q4–6h	Avoid
Alfentanil	↔ Dose	100%	100%	100%
Codeine	↓ Dose	100%	75%	50%
Fentanyl	↓ Dose	100%	75%	50%
Ketorolac	↓ Dose	100%	50%	25%–50%
Meperidine	↓ Dose	100%	Avoid	Avoid
Methadone	↓ Dose	100%	100%	50%–75%
Morphine	↓ Dose	100%	75%	50%
Remifentanil	↔ Dose	100%	100%	100%
Sufentanil	↔ Dose	100%	100%	100%

↑, Increase; ↓, decrease; ↔, no change; *GFR,* glomerular filtration rate.
Adapted from Schrier RW, ed. *Manual of Nephrology.* 8th ed. Philadelphia: Lippincott Williams & Wilkins; 2015.

The best source of data on the incidence and etiology of CKD and ESRD is the United States Renal Data System of the National Institutes of Health. According to these data, in 2012 the prevalence (i.e., number of people) of ESRD reached 1943 per million, or approximately 636,000 individuals. Overall prevalence continues to increase, partly because of aging of the population and partly because patients with ESRD are surviving longer. However, the incidence (i.e., number of new cases) of ESRD—which had been undergoing a year-by-year increase between 1980 and 2010—now seems to have plateaued or even decreased slightly. It was quoted as 353 per million in 2012, or about 115,000 individuals.

There are striking racial and ethnic variations in the incidence and prevalence of ESRD. Based on data from 2012, the incidence of ESRD among African American and Native American populations is 3.3 and 1.5 times greater, respectively, than the rate among whites. The rate of ESRD among Hispanics is 1.5 times higher than among non-Hispanics. Furthermore, African Americans and Hispanics tend to reach ESRD at a younger age than whites. Hypertensive nephropathy accounts for a relatively higher proportion of ESRD cases among African Americans compared with other racial or ethnic groups. A combination of genetic variables and disparities in healthcare access are likely to underlie some of these differences.

Diagnosis

Signs of CKD are often diverse and undetected. When symptoms do appear, complaints are nonspecific, such as fatigue, malaise, and anorexia. In most patients the diagnosis is made during routine testing. In addition to serum creatinine level, urinary sediment analysis is helpful in establishing the diagnosis and possible cause of renal dysfunction.

Progression of Chronic Kidney Disease

Intrarenal hemodynamic changes (glomerular hypertension, glomerular hyperfiltration and permeability changes, glomerulosclerosis) are likely responsible for progression of renal disease. Decreases in both systemic and glomerular hypertension can be achieved with administration of angiotensin-converting enzyme (ACE) inhibitors and/or angiotensin II receptor blockers (ARBs). In addition to having beneficial effects on intraglomerular hemodynamics and systemic pressures, ACE inhibitors and ARBs have renoprotective effects that manifest as reductions in proteinuria and slowing of the progression of glomerulosclerosis in patients with diabetic or nondiabetic nephropathy. These drugs do not appear to be more beneficial than other antihypertensives in treating patients with CKD who do not have proteinuria.

TABLE 22.8	Causes of Chronic Kidney Disease

Glomerulopathies
  Primary glomerular disease
  Focal glomerulosclerosis
  Membranoproliferative glomerulonephritis
  Membranous nephropathy
  Immunoglobulin A nephropathy
  Diabetes mellitus
  Amyloidosis
  Postinfective glomerulonephritis
  Systemic lupus erythematosus
  Wegener granulomatosis
Tubulointerstitial diseases
  Analgesic nephropathy
  Reflux nephropathy with pyelonephritis
  Myeloma kidney
  Sarcoidosis
Hereditary diseases
  Polycystic kidney disease
  Alport syndrome
  Medullary cystic disease
Systemic hypertension
Renal vascular disease
Obstructive uropathy
Human immunodeficiency virus infection

Adapted from Tolkoff-Rubin NE, Pascual M. Chronic renal failure. *Sci Am Med*. 1998:1-12.

TABLE 22.9	Stages of Chronic Kidney Disease	
GFR Stages	GFR (mL/min/1.73 m^2)	Description
G1	≥90	Kidney damage with normal or increased GFR
G2	60–89	Kidney damage with mildly decreased GFR
G3a	45–59	Mildly to moderately decreased GFR
G3b	30–44	Moderately to severely decreased GFR
G4	15–29	Severely decreased GFR
G5	<15 or dialysis	Kidney failure
Albuminuria Stages	Albumin Excretion Rate (mg per 24 hours)	Description
A1	<30 mg	Normal to mildly increased
A2	30–300 mg	Moderately increased
A3	>300 mg	Severely increased

GFR, Glomerular filtration rate.
Adapted from the Kidney Disease: Improving Global Outcomes (KDIGO) 2012 clinical practice guideline for the evaluation and management of chronic kidney disease. Summary of recommendation statements. *Kidney Int*. 2013;3(Suppl):5. Available at http://www.kdigo.org/clinical_practice_guidelines/pdf/CKD/KDIGO_2012_CKD_GL.pdf.

In animal models, protein intake can influence the progression of renal disease, and consequently, moderate protein restriction is recommended for all patients with renal insufficiency. In patients who are diabetic, strict control of blood glucose concentrations can delay the onset of proteinuria and slow the progression of nephropathy, neuropathy, and retinopathy. There is some evidence that hyperlipidemia may accelerate the rate of renal disease; therefore treatment of hyperlipidemia with statin therapy is advised. In addition, smoking cessation is recommended because smoking has been linked to an increased risk of development of kidney disease.

Adaptation to Chronic Kidney Disease

Normally functioning kidneys precisely regulate the concentrations of solutes and water in the extracellular fluid despite large variations in daily dietary intake. Because of substantial renal reserve function, patients with CKD often remain relatively asymptomatic until renal function is less than 10% of normal.

The kidneys demonstrate three stages of adaptation to progressive impairment of renal function. The first stage involves substances such as creatinine and urea, which are dependent largely on glomerular filtration for urinary excretion. As GFR decreases, plasma concentrations of these substances begin to rise, but the increase is not directly proportional to the degree of GFR impairment. For example, serum creatinine concentrations frequently remain within normal limits despite a 50% decrease in GFR. Beyond a certain point, however, when the renal reserve has been exhausted, even minimal further decreases in the GFR can result in significant increases in serum creatinine and urea concentrations.

The second stage of adaptation to progressive renal impairment is seen with solutes such as potassium. Serum potassium concentrations are maintained within normal limits until GFR approaches 10% of normal, at which point hyperkalemia manifests. As nephrons are lost, the remaining nephrons increase their secretion of potassium by increasing blood flow and sodium delivery to the collecting tubules. In addition, because aldosterone secretion increases in patients with renal failure, there is a greater loss of potassium through the GI tract. This system of enhanced GI secretion is an effective compensatory mechanism in the presence of normal dietary intake of potassium but can be easily overwhelmed by an acute *exogenous* potassium load such as administration of potassium or by an acute *endogenous* potassium load such as hemolysis or tissue trauma associated with surgery).

The third stage of adaptation involves sodium homeostasis and regulation of the extracellular fluid compartment volume. In contrast to the levels of other solutes, sodium balance remains intact despite progressive deterioration in renal function and variations in dietary intake. Nevertheless, the system can be overwhelmed by abruptly increased sodium intake (resulting in volume overload) or decreased sodium intake (resulting in volume depletion).

Complications

Uremic Syndrome

Uremic syndrome is a constellation of signs and symptoms (anorexia, nausea, vomiting, pruritus, anemia, fatigue, coagulopathy) that reflect the kidney's progressive inability to perform its excretory, secretory, and regulatory functions. The clinical syndrome is the result of failure of the kidney to excrete a number of uremic toxins that include urea, p-cresol, and β_2-microglobulin. The BUN concentration is a useful clinical indicator of the severity of the uremic syndrome and the patient's response to therapy. This is in contrast to the serum creatinine concentration, which correlates poorly with uremic symptoms. Traditional treatment of uremic syndrome is dietary protein restriction to decrease protein catabolism and urea production combined with dialysis.

Renal Osteodystrophy

Changes in bone structure and mineralization are common in patients with progressive CKD. The most important factors are secondary hyperparathyroidism and decreased vitamin D production by the kidneys. This impairs intestinal absorption of calcium. Hypocalcemia stimulates parathyroid hormone (PTH) secretion, which leads to bone resorption to restore serum calcium concentrations. As GFR decreases, there is a parallel decrease in phosphate clearance and an increase in serum phosphate concentrations. This results in reciprocal decreases in serum calcium concentrations. Radiographs demonstrate evidence of bone demineralization. Further evidence of bone resorption is noted by increased serum alkaline phosphatase concentrations. Treatment of renal osteodystrophy is intended to prevent skeletal complications and includes restriction of dietary phosphate intake plus oral calcium and vitamin D supplementation. Antacids may be administered to bind phosphorus in the GI tract; however, magnesium-containing antacids introduce the risk of hypermagnesemia, and aluminum-containing antacids are equally undesirable. If medical therapies fail to control hypocalcemia resulting from secondary hyperparathyroidism, subtotal parathyroidectomy may be recommended.

Accumulation of aluminum in patients undergoing long-term renal dialysis, although decreasing in frequency, may result in bone pain, fractures, and weakness. Hyperparathyroidism seems to protect against aluminum-induced bone disease. If aluminum toxicity is present, deferoxamine chelation therapy is helpful.

Anemia

Anemia frequently accompanies CKD and is presumed to be responsible for many of the symptoms (fatigue, weakness, decreased exercise tolerance) characteristic of uremic syndrome. This anemia is normochromic and normocytic and is due primarily to decreased erythropoietin production by the kidneys. Excess parathyroid hormone production also contributes to anemia by replacing bone marrow with fibrous tissue.

The anemia of CKD is treated with recombinant human erythropoietin (epoetin) or darbepoetin. Blood transfusions are avoided if possible because the resultant sensitization to antigens of the human leukocyte antigen (HLA) complex makes future kidney transplantation less successful. Intermittent injections of parenteral iron are recommended to maximize the response to erythropoietin. Development or exacerbation of systemic hypertension is a risk of erythropoietin administration.

Uremic Bleeding

Patients with CKD have an increased tendency to bleed despite the presence of a normal platelet count, prothrombin time, and plasma thromboplastin time. The bleeding time is the screening test that best correlates with the tendency to bleed; neither BUN nor creatinine correlates well with bleeding risk. Hemorrhagic episodes (GI bleeding, epistaxis, hemorrhagic pericarditis, subdural hematoma) are significant sources of morbidity in patients with CKD and contribute to persistent anemia.

Desmopressin is used to treat uremic bleeding. An analogue of antidiuretic hormone, desmopressin increases circulating levels of the factor VIII–vWF complex and thereby improves coagulation. In patients with uremia, intravenous (IV) infusion or subcutaneous injection of desmopressin (0.3 µg/kg) is particularly useful for preventing clinical hemorrhage when invasive procedures such as surgery are planned. Desmopressin is fast acting and short-lived. The maximal effect is present within 2–4 hours and lasts for about 6–8 hours. Tachyphylaxis appears to develop with repeat doses and may be related to depletion of endothelial stores of vWF.

Conjugated estrogens have also been shown to improve bleeding times in patients with uremia, an effect that is probably mediated by the action of estradiol via estrogen receptors. The time to onset of action is about 6 hours, but the effects last for 14–21 days. It has also been observed that erythropoietin shortens the bleeding time by enhancing platelet aggregation and increasing platelet counts.

Neurologic Changes

Neurologic changes may be early manifestations of progressive renal insufficiency. Initially, symptoms may be mild (impaired abstract thinking, insomnia, irritability), but as renal disease progresses, more significant changes (seizures, obtundation, uremic encephalopathy, coma) may develop. A disabling complication of advanced renal failure is development of a distal symmetric mixed motor and sensory polyneuropathy marked by paresthesias or hyperesthesias or distal weakness of the lower extremities. The arms may also be affected, but the incidence is less than in the legs. Diabetic neuropathy may be superimposed on uremic neuropathy. Hemodialysis may improve some aspects of uremic encephalopathy and reduce the severity of peripheral neurologic symptoms.

Cardiovascular Changes

Systemic hypertension is the most significant risk factor accompanying CKD and contributes to the congestive heart failure, coronary artery disease, and cerebrovascular disease that occur in these patients. Uncontrolled systemic hypertension also speeds progression of renal dysfunction. The pathogenesis of systemic hypertension in these patients involves intravascular volume expansion resulting from retention of sodium and water and activation of the renin-angiotensin-aldosterone system.

Dyslipidemias are common at all stages of CKD and increase the risk of cardiovascular morbidity and mortality. Along with lifestyle and dietary modifications, therapy is advised when fasting triglyceride levels are above 500 mg/dL and/or low-density lipoprotein levels are above 100 mg/dL.

Silent myocardial ischemia is probably common owing to peripheral neuropathy. Chemical stress testing may be preferred to exercise stress testing, because patients in renal failure are often unable to exercise adequately. However, dipyridamole thallium testing may be less accurate in patients with uremia, as a result of decreased sensitivity of the microvasculature to dipyridamole. The baseline electrocardiogram (ECG) may be altered by metabolic derangements. For unknown reasons, baseline plasma creatine kinase concentrations are often increased in patients with CKD. Because this increase is accounted for principally by the MM isoenzyme of creatine kinase, the value of the MB fraction for diagnosis of an acute myocardial infarction remains intact.

Dialysis is the indicated treatment for patients who are hypertensive because of hypervolemia (volume is removed to attain "dry weight") and those who develop uremic pericarditis. Dialysis is less likely to control systemic hypertension because of activation of the renin-angiotensin-aldosterone system. Increasing dosages of antihypertensive drugs are recommended for these patients. ACE inhibitors are used cautiously in patients in whom GFR is dependent on increased efferent arteriolar vasoconstriction (bilateral renal artery stenosis, transplanted kidney with unilateral stenosis), which is mediated by angiotensin II. Administration of ACE inhibitors to these patients can result in efferent arteriolar dilation and decreased GFR, leading to a sudden deterioration in renal function.

Cardiac tamponade and hemodynamic instability associated with uremic pericarditis is an indication for prompt drainage of the effusion, often via placement of a percutaneous pericardial catheter. In some patients, surgical drainage with creation of a pericardial window or pericardiectomy is necessary. The development of hypotension unresponsive to intravascular fluid volume replacement may be an important clue that cardiac tamponade is present.

Treatment

Management of patients with CKD includes aggressive treatment of the underlying cause, pharmacologic therapy to delay disease progression and prevent complications, and preparation for renal replacement therapy as ESRD ensues.

Blood Pressure

Since hypertension is both a cause and a consequence of CKD and is directly correlated with deterioration of renal function, blood pressure control is imperative. In patients with proteinuric CKD, target blood pressure is less than 130/80 mm Hg. In patients without proteinuria, target blood pressure is less than 140/90 mm Hg. Multimodal drug therapy is usually needed to achieve desired blood pressure control. ACE inhibitors or ARBs are recommended as first-line therapy in patients with proteinuria; these drugs have been shown to slow the rate of progression of CKD. Second-, third-, and fourth-line agents are diuretics, calcium channel blockers, and aldosterone antagonists.

Nutrition

A number of studies involving both diabetic and nondiabetic patients with CKD have demonstrated that modest protein restriction reduces the progression of renal disease. However, an overly restrictive diet places patients at risk for malnutrition and its associated complications. A daily protein intake of approximately 0.6 g/kg is currently advised.

Dietary phosphorus should be restricted to 600–800 mg/day when serum phosphorus or parathyroid hormone levels are elevated. Phosphate binders are used when dietary restriction alone is ineffective. Vitamin D supplementation is also sometimes used to help normalize phosphorus and calcium levels. In patients with advanced disease and chronic metabolic acidosis, administration of alkali salts is advised. Sodium intake should be restricted to less than 1.5–2 g/day to prevent hypertension and fluid overload.

Long-term follow-up of diabetic patients with CKD has shown that euglycemia is associated with a reduction in proteinuria and reversal of the typical lesions seen in diabetic nephropathy. However, this is a long-term change, and the benefits may not manifest for 5–10 years. Current guidelines recommend a glycosylated hemoglobin level below 7%. Metformin is recommended for most patients with type 2 diabetes and stable stage 1, 2, or 3 CKD. However, owing to the risk of lactic acid accumulation, metformin should be discontinued if there are acute changes in renal function or the patient is at risk of such changes, such as during illness or in the perioperative period.

Anemia

Anemia often accompanies CKD and is associated with decreased health-related quality of life. The decision to initiate treatment should be individualized, with consideration of the potential benefits and risks of therapy. Anemia is responsive to treatment with erythropoietin in all stages of CKD. In general the target hemoglobin level should be in the range of 10–11.5 mg/dL.

Renal Replacement Therapy

There is no absolute GFR at which dialysis is required; however, it is generally advised when the GFR reaches 10 mL/min/1.73 m^2 or less. There is clear evidence that effective dialysis is significantly correlated with survival. Since clinical signs and symptoms are not reliable indicators of dialysis adequacy, the response to dialysis should be measured and monitored routinely. The composition of the dialysate solution and the time spent on dialysis can be calculated from a number of different formulas or models. All of them essentially measure the clearance of urea by estimating the difference in predialysis and postdialysis plasma BUN levels. Urea is used in this calculation because it is a small, readily dialyzed molecule that accounts for 90% of the waste nitrogen that accumulates between hemodialysis treatments. Furthermore the fractional clearance of urea has been shown to correlate with morbidity and mortality in dialysis patients.

Hemodialysis and Associated Clinical Challenges

Hemodialysis involves the diffusion of solutes across a semipermeable membrane between the blood and a dialysis solution (Fig. 22.2). This results in removal of metabolic waste products and excess fluid volume, as well as replenishment of body buffers. During the procedure, blood is heparinized and passed through a plastic dialyzer. The dialysate, type of dialysis membrane, and solute clearance are the most important modifiable factors. A typical dialysis session lasts for 3 or 4 hours and results in a 65%–70% reduction in BUN. The annual mortality for patients on hemodialysis is nearly 25% and is most often attributed to cardiovascular causes or infection.

Vascular Access. A surgically created vascular access site is necessary for effective hemodialysis (Fig. 22.3). Native arteriovenous fistulas (e.g., cephalic vein anastomosed to the radial artery) are superior to polytetrafluoroethylene grafts as sites of vascular access because of their longer lifespan and lower incidence of thrombosis and infection. The most common access-related complication is intimal hyperplasia, which results in stenosis proximal to the venous anastomosis. Other complications related to access include thrombosis, infection, aneurysm formation, and limb ischemia. When dialysis is urgently required, vascular access is obtained with a double-lumen dialysis catheter, most often using the jugular or femoral vein.

Complications

Intradialytic Complications. Hypotension is the most common adverse event during hemodialysis and most likely represents osmolar shifts and ultrafiltration-induced volume depletion. Hypotensive episodes may also be due to myocardial ischemia, cardiac dysrhythmias, or pericardial effusion with cardiac tamponade. Changes in potassium concentration may contribute to development of dysrhythmias. Most hypotensive episodes are successfully treated by slowing the rate of ultrafiltration and/or administering IV saline.

Hypersensitivity reactions to the ethylene oxide used to sterilize dialysis machines, as well as adverse reactions to the specific hemodialysis membrane material polyacrylonitrile, may occur. Reactions to polyacrylonitrile are seen most commonly in patients receiving ACE inhibitors. When blood comes in contact with the polyacrylonitrile membrane, the membrane's high negative surface charge stimulates enzymes,

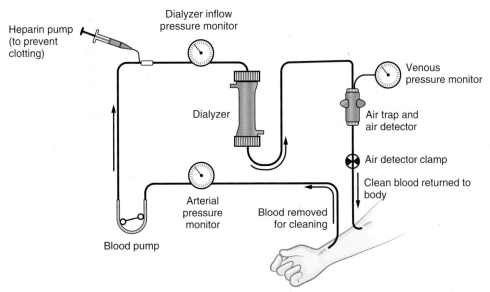

FIG. 22.2   Hemodialysis circuit. Hemodialysis involves the diffusion of solutes across a semipermeable membrane between the blood and a dialysis solution. This results in removal of metabolic waste products and excess fluid volume, as well as replenishment of body buffers. During the procedure, blood is heparinized and passed through a plastic dialyzer. Filtered blood is then returned to circulation after passing through an air detection trap. (From http://www.niddk.nih.gov/health-information/health-topics/kidney-disease/hemodialysis/Pages/facts.aspx.)

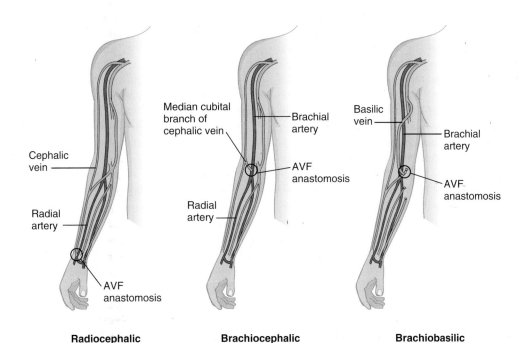

Radiocephalic   **Brachiocephalic**   **Brachiobasilic**

FIG. 22.3   Anatomy of common arteriovenous fistulas (AVFs). Native vessels are preferred for use when vascular access is required for hemodialysis. Both the artery and vein must have lumens of adequate diameter for the procedure to be successful. The radial artery and cephalic vein are the preferred access points when adequate. Alternative access points include the brachial artery and basilic vein. (From Pereira B, Sayegh M, Blake P (eds). *Chronic Kidney Disease, Dialysis, and Transplantation.* 2nd ed. Philadelphia: Saunders; 2005:344.)

which generate bradykinins. Normally bradykinin is degraded by kinases, but ACE inhibitors block this response, and profound peripheral vasodilation and hypotension occurs. Reactions to the cellulose membranes used in some dialyzers can also occur and are believed to be mediated by complement. These reactions are often delayed in onset, and symptoms are generally mild.

Dialysis disequilibrium syndrome is marked by nausea, headaches, and fatigue but may progress to seizures or coma. The condition is thought to result from rapid changes in pH and solute concentrations in the central nervous system (CNS). Management includes reducing the rate of dialysate and blood flow and using dialyzers with smaller surface area.

Muscle cramps are a frequent complaint and most likely reflect changes in potassium concentrations.

Nutrition and Fluid Balance. During progressive renal failure, catabolism and anorexia lead to loss of lean body mass, but concomitant fluid retention masks weight loss and may even lead to weight gain. *Protein-calorie malnutrition is extremely common.* Decreased oral intake, hemodialysis-induced catabolism, and hormonal imbalances are common. Amino acids as well as water-soluble vitamins are removed by dialysis, which contributes to malnutrition. Routine assessment of nutritional status using plasma biomarkers (albumin, prealbumin) is advised, and many patients benefit from oral or parenteral nutritional supplements.

There is no justification for stringent restriction of dietary potassium in patients undergoing hemodialysis. Patients with ESRD have decreased total body potassium stores and an inexplicable tolerance of hyperkalemia. The expected cardiac and neuromuscular responses to hyperkalemia are less pronounced in patients receiving hemodialysis than in those with normal renal function. Clearance of potassium by hemodialysis is efficient, and because most potassium is intracellular, hypokalemia will likely be suggested by a blood sample obtained soon after completion of hemodialysis and before transcellular equilibration has occurred.

Patients should receive counseling with regard to regulation of sodium and fluid intake. Normal weight gain between dialysis treatments is 3%–4% of total body mass.

Decreased catabolism of insulin in many patients receiving hemodialysis may result in decreased insulin requirements compared with needs before the initiation of hemodialysis. The presentation of diabetic ketoacidosis may be atypical, with respiratory alkalosis or acidosis but without metabolic acidosis and hypovolemia.

Infection. Infection is the second leading cause of death in patients with ESRD. Contributing factors include impaired phagocytosis and neutrophil chemotaxis and malnutrition. It is recommended that all patients receiving hemodialysis be immunized against pneumococcus, hepatitis B virus, and influenza virus. Malnutrition or inadequate dialysis may impair antibody responses to vaccines, however, and the diagnosis of infection may be difficult because many patients do not show typical symptoms such as fever.

Tuberculosis in patients receiving hemodialysis is usually extrapulmonary and often presents with atypical symptoms that mimic those of inadequate dialysis. Because anergy in response to skin testing is common, unexplained weight loss and anorexia, with or without persistent fever, should prompt further testing to rule out tuberculosis.

Hepatitis B or C virus infection in patients receiving hemodialysis is often asymptomatic, and liver aminotransferase concentrations may not be increased. A substantial proportion of patients undergoing hemodialysis have antibodies to hepatitis C. Of note, dosage adjustments of drugs used to treat human immunodeficiency virus (HIV) infection are not required during hemodialysis.

Peritoneal Dialysis

Peritoneal dialysis requires placing an anchored plastic catheter in the peritoneal cavity for infusion of a dialysate that remains in place for several hours. During that time, diffusive solute transport occurs across the peritoneal membrane until fresh fluid is exchanged for the old fluid. Automated peritoneal dialysis, in which a mechanized cycler infuses and drains peritoneal dialysate at night, is used by many patients.

Peritoneal dialysis may be desirable for patients with congestive heart failure or unstable angina who may not tolerate the rapid fluid shifts or fluctuations in systemic blood pressure that often accompany hemodialysis. Peritoneal dialysis is also indicated for patients with extensive vascular disease that prevents creation of a vascular access site for hemodialysis.

In patients with diabetes, insulin can be infused with the dialysate to provide precise regulation of blood glucose concentrations.

The presence of abdominal hernias or adhesions may interfere with the ability to use peritoneal dialysis effectively. Peritonitis presenting as abdominal pain and fever is the most common serious complication of peritoneal dialysis. Treatment is with antibiotics, which may include cephalosporins, aminoglycosides, and vancomycin. Survival rates and annual costs are similar with peritoneal dialysis and hemodialysis, but hospitalization rates are higher among patients treated with peritoneal dialysis.

Drug Clearance in Patients Undergoing Dialysis

Patients who are undergoing dialysis require special consideration with respect to drug dosing intervals. Supplemental dosing may be needed for drugs that are cleared by dialysis. When possible, drug doses are best scheduled for administration after completion of a dialysis session.

Drug properties that influence clearance by dialysis include protein binding, water solubility, and molecular weight. Low-molecular-weight (<500 Da), water-soluble, non–protein-bound drugs are readily cleared by dialysis as well as by continuous venovenous hemofiltration and continuous arteriovenous hemofiltration.

Perioperative Hemodialysis

Patients should undergo adequate dialysis within 24 hours of elective surgery to minimize the likelihood of volume

TABLE 22.10	Drugs Used in Anesthesia Practice That Depend Significantly on Renal Elimination
Class	Drugs
Induction agents	Phenobarbital
	Thiopental
Muscle relaxants	Metocurine
	Pancuronium
	Vecuronium
Cholinesterase inhibitors	Edrophonium
	Neostigmine
Cardiovascular drugs	Atropine
	Digoxin
	Glycopyrrolate
	Hydralazine
	Milrinone
Antimicrobials	Aminoglycosides
	Cephalosporins
	Penicillins
	Sulfonamides
	Vancomycin
Analgesics	Codeine
	Meperidine
	Morphine

Adapted from Malhotra V, Sudheendra V, O'Hara J, et al. Anesthesia and the renal and genitourinary systems. In: Miller RD, Cohen N, Eriksson LI, et al., eds. *Miller's Anesthesia*. 8th ed. Philadelphia: Elsevier; 2015.

overload, hyperkalemia, and uremic bleeding. Depending on the planned surgery, the use of heparin may be avoided or minimized during preoperative hemodialysis. Patients on peritoneal dialysis who are undergoing abdominal surgery are generally switched to hemodialysis in the immediately postoperative period.

Urgent hemodialysis is not required after radiocontrast dye studies in those who are undergoing regular hemodialysis. Although these dyes can be removed by hemodialysis, the volume administered in most studies does not result in pulmonary edema in patients maintained on an adequate dialysis regimen, and nephrotoxicity is not a concern in patients with ESRD.

Management of Anesthesia

Management of anesthesia in patients with CKD requires an understanding of the pathologic changes that accompany renal disease, co-existing medical conditions, and the impact of reduced renal function on drug pharmacokinetics (Table 22.10). Optimal management of modifiable risk factors is imperative.

Preoperative Evaluation

Preoperative evaluation of patients with CKD includes consideration of renal function, underlying pathologic processes, and comorbid conditions. In addition to identifying patients with preexisting renal dysfunction, it is important to recognize those who are at high risk of developing perioperative renal failure.

Evaluation of the trend in serum creatinine concentration is useful to determine whether renal function is stable. Blood volume status may be estimated by comparing body weight before and after hemodialysis and measuring vital signs with particular attention to orthostatic hypotension or tachycardia. Because diabetes is often present in these patients, glucose management is of concern. Blood pressure should be well controlled before elective surgery. Antihypertensive therapy is frequently continued; however, ACE inhibitors and ARBs are often withheld on the day of surgery to reduce the risk of intraoperative hypotension. Preoperative medication must be individualized, with recognition that these patients may exhibit unexpected sensitivity to CNS depressant drugs.

A common recommendation is that the serum potassium concentration should not exceed 5.5 mEq/L on the day of surgery. The patient should be evaluated preoperatively for the presence of anemia, but the introduction of recombinant human erythropoietin therapy has decreased the number of patients with renal failure who come for elective surgery with a hematocrit of less than 30%. The preoperative presence of a coagulopathy may be addressed with administration of desmopressin. Gastric aspiration prophylaxis should be considered, especially in diabetic patients. However, all H_2-receptor blockers are excreted renally; therefore dosage adjustment is required. Patients maintained on dialysis should undergo dialysis within the 24 hours preceding elective surgery.

Induction of Anesthesia

Induction of anesthesia and tracheal intubation can be safely accomplished with most IV induction agents (propofol, etomidate, thiopental) in current use. Thiopental has an increased volume of distribution and reduced protein binding in patients with CKD; therefore a dose reduction is advised. Many patients with ESRD respond to induction of anesthesia as if they were hypovolemic. The likelihood of hypotension is increased by uremia as well as by administration of antihypertensives. Exaggerated CNS effects of anesthetic induction drugs may also reflect uremia-induced disruption of the blood-brain barrier.

If indicated, rapid-sequence induction with succinylcholine may be performed if the potassium concentration is less than 5.5 mg/dL. Potassium release following administration of succinylcholine is not exaggerated in patients with CKD. Alternatively a nondepolarizing muscle relaxant with a short onset of action (e.g., rocuronium) may be selected.

Attenuated sympathetic nervous system activity impairs compensatory peripheral vasoconstriction; thus small decreases in blood volume, institution of positive pressure ventilation, abrupt changes in body position, or drug-induced myocardial depression can result in an exaggerated decrease in systemic blood pressure. Patients being treated with ACE inhibitors or ARBs may be at increased risk of experiencing intraoperative hypotension, especially in the setting of acute surgical blood loss or neuraxial anesthesia.

Maintenance of Anesthesia

A balanced anesthetic technique using a volatile agent, muscle relaxant, and opioids is most often employed. Elimination of volatile anesthetics is not dependent on renal function. Sevoflurane may be avoided because of concerns related to fluoride nephrotoxicity or production of compound A, although there is no evidence that patients with co-existing renal disease are at increased risk of renal dysfunction after administration of sevoflurane. Total IV anesthesia is also an option.

Potent volatile anesthetics are useful for controlling intraoperative systemic hypertension and decreasing the doses of muscle relaxants needed for adequate surgical relaxation. Excessive depression of cardiac output is a potential hazard of volatile anesthetics. Decreases in blood flow must be minimized to avoid jeopardizing oxygen delivery to the tissues.

Selection of nondepolarizing muscle relaxants for maintenance of skeletal muscle paralysis during surgery is influenced by the known clearance mechanisms of these drugs. Renal disease may slow excretion of vecuronium and rocuronium, whereas clearance of mivacurium, atracurium, and cisatracurium from plasma is independent of renal function. Renal failure may delay clearance of laudanosine, the principal metabolite of atracurium and cisatracurium. Laudanosine lacks effects at the neuromuscular junction, but at high plasma concentrations, it may stimulate the CNS. Regardless of the drug selected, it is prudent to decrease the initial dose and administer subsequent doses based on the responses observed using a peripheral nerve stimulator.

Opioids are useful because they lack cardiodepressant effects and may help minimize the need for volatile anesthetics. Both morphine and meperidine undergo metabolism to potentially neurotoxic compounds (morphine-3-glucoronide and normeperidine, respectively) that rely on renal clearance. Morphine-6-glucoronide, a morphine metabolite more potent than its parent compound, may also accumulate in patients with CKD and result in profound respiratory depression. Hydromorphone also has an active metabolite, hydromorphone-3-glucoronide, that may accumulate in patients with CKD; however, hydromorphone may be used safely with proper monitoring and dose adjustment. Alfentanil, fentanyl, remifentanil, and sufentanil lack active metabolites. However, the elimination half-life of fentanyl may be prolonged in patients with CKD.

Renal excretion accounts for approximately 50% of the clearance of neostigmine and approximately 75% of the elimination of edrophonium and pyridostigmine. Therefore the risk of recurarization following reversal of muscle relaxant is decreased because the half-lives of these drugs are likely to be prolonged to a greater extent than the half-lives of the nondepolarizing muscle relaxants.

Fluid Management and Urine Output

Patients with severe renal dysfunction who do not require hemodialysis and those without renal disease undergoing operations associated with a high incidence of postoperative renal failure may benefit from preoperative hydration with balanced salt solutions. Indeed, most patients come to the operating room with a contracted extracellular fluid volume. A bolus of balanced salt solution to restore circulating volume (500 mL IV) should increase urine output in the presence of hypovolemia. Lactated Ringer solution (containing 4 mEq/L potassium) or other potassium-containing fluids should be used with caution. Maintaining a urine output of at least 0.5 mL/kg/h is generally reasonable.

Stimulation of urine output with osmotic (mannitol) or tubular (furosemide) diuretics in the absence of adequate intravascular fluid volume replacement is *not* advised. *Intraoperative urine output has not been shown to be predictive of postoperative renal insufficiency.* Indeed, the most likely cause of oliguria is an inadequate circulating fluid volume, and administration of diuretics in this setting may further compromise renal function.

Patients dependent on hemodialysis require special attention with respect to perioperative fluid management. An absence of renal function narrows the margin of safety between insufficient and excessive fluid administration. Noninvasive operations require replacement of only insensible water losses. The small amount of urine output can be replaced with 0.45% sodium chloride. Thoracic or abdominal surgery can be associated with loss of significant intravascular fluid volume to the interstitial spaces. This loss is often replaced with balanced salt solutions or colloid. Blood transfusions are considered if the oxygen-carrying capacity must be increased or if blood loss is excessive. Measuring the central venous pressure is often useful for guiding fluid replacement.

Monitoring

To preserve blood vessels for future dialysis access, venipuncture should be avoided entirely in the nondominant arm as well as in the upper part of the dominant arm. Similarly it is recommended that radial and ulnar artery cannulation be avoided in case these vessels are needed for an arteriovenous fistula in the future. The same may be said of the brachial and even the axillary arteries. Use of the femoral arteries carries the risk of line infection, particularly since these patients may already be immunocompromised. Remaining options include the dorsalis pedis or posterior tibial arteries, which may be inconvenient because of positioning or difficult to access because of edema and tissue induration. Whichever site is chosen, it is important to note that neither the arterial pressure nor the arterial blood gas concentrations will be accurate if the cannula is placed in the same extremity as a functioning or partially patent AV fistula.

Venous pressure monitoring is often extremely helpful, if not necessary, since a volume load is not well tolerated by patients with even modest decreases in renal function. The choice of right atrial or pulmonary artery pressure monitoring is guided by the presence of underlying cardiopulmonary disease. Strict asepsis must be maintained when placing these lines, because patients with CKD are extremely prone to infection. Central venous access may be difficult in patients who have a tunneled venous access device or temporary dialysis catheter in situ or who have had many such catheters previously, since they can develop stenosis of the veins. Transesophageal echocardiography is an additional option for monitoring hemodynamic status.

Although their use is discouraged, temporary dialysis catheters may be used as the venous access for surgery if IV access proves unsuccessful. However, it must be remembered that (1) the catheter must be accessed aseptically, just as it is at the time of dialysis; (2) heparin must be aspirated before connecting to an IV line or pressure transducer; and (3) heparin must be reintroduced and the line aseptically sealed at the time of discontinuation of its use.

Associated Concerns

Attention to patient positioning on the operating room table is important. Poor nutritional status renders the skin particularly prone to bruising and sloughing, and extra padding is required to protect vulnerable nerves around the elbows, knees, and ankles. Fistulas must be protected at all costs and be well padded to prevent pressure injury. Blood pressure cuffs should not be applied to the arm with the fistula. If at all possible, the arm with the fistula should not be tucked but should be positioned so that the fistula thrill can be checked periodically throughout surgery.

Regional Anesthesia

Neuraxial anesthesia may be considered in patients with CKD. A sympathetic blockade of T4–T10 levels may theoretically improve renal perfusion by attenuating catecholamine-induced renal vasoconstriction and suppressing the surgical stress response. However, platelet dysfunction and the effects of residual heparin in patients receiving hemodialysis must also be considered. In addition, adequate intravascular fluid volume must be maintained to minimize hypotension.

Brachial plexus blockade is useful for placing the vascular shunts necessary for long-term hemodialysis. In addition to providing analgesia, this form of regional anesthesia abolishes vasospasm and produces vasodilation that facilitates the surgical procedure. The suggestion that the duration of brachial plexus anesthesia is shortened in patients with CKD has not been confirmed in controlled studies. The presence of uremic neuropathies should be evaluated before induction of regional anesthesia. Co-existing metabolic acidosis may decrease the threshold for seizures in response to local anesthetics.

Postoperative Management

Although residual neuromuscular blockade after apparent reversal of nondepolarizing neuromuscular blockade with anticholinesterase drugs is rare, this diagnosis should be considered in patients with CKD who manifest signs of skeletal muscle weakness during the early postoperative period. Other explanations (antibiotics, acidosis, electrolyte imbalances) should also be considered when muscle weakness persists or reappears in these patients.

Caution should be exercised in the use of parenteral opioids for postoperative analgesia in view of the potential for exaggerated CNS depression and hypoventilation after administration of even small doses of opioids. Administration of naloxone may be necessary if depression of ventilation is severe. Selection of opioids that do not have active metabolites and do not rely on the kidneys for excretion is appropriate. Nonsteroidal antiinflammatory drugs (NSAIDs) are best avoided because they may exacerbate hypertension, precipitate edema, and increase the risk of cardiovascular complications.

Continuous ECG monitoring is helpful for detecting cardiac dysrhythmias, such as those related to hyperkalemia. Continuation of supplemental oxygen into the postoperative period is a consideration, especially if anemia is present. It is prudent to check levels of electrolytes, BUN, and creatinine as well as hematocrit postoperatively. A chest radiograph may be useful if pulmonary edema is a concern. Uremic coagulopathy should be considered in the workup of postoperative bleeding. Controversy exists over the preferred maintenance fluid for patients with CKD. Although 0.9% saline was traditionally favored because it lacks potassium, it may exacerbate preexisting acidosis.

RENAL TRANSPLANTATION

Candidates for renal transplantation are selected from among patients with ESRD who are maintained on established programs of long-term renal replacement therapy. In adults the most common causes of ESRD are systemic hypertension, diabetes mellitus, and glomerulonephritis. Despite concerns regarding renal dysfunction in the donor kidney in the presence of these diseases, such disease generally progresses slowly. A kidney from a cadaver donor can be preserved by perfusion at low temperatures for up to 48 hours, which makes its transplantation a semi-elective surgical procedure. Attempts are made to match HLA antigens and ABO blood groups between donor and recipient. Paradoxically the presence of certain common shared HLA antigens in the blood administered to a potential transplant recipient has been observed to induce tolerance to donor antigens and thus improve graft survival. The donor kidney is placed in the lower abdomen and receives its vascular supply from the iliac vessels. The ureter is anastomosed directly to the bladder. Immunosuppressive therapy is instituted during the perioperative period.

Management of Anesthesia

General Anesthesia

Although both regional and general anesthesia have been successfully used for renal transplantation, general anesthesia is more common. Renal function after kidney transplantation is not predictably influenced by choice of volatile anesthetic. Decreased cardiac output resulting from negative inotropic effects of volatile anesthetics is minimized to avoid jeopardizing the adequacy of tissue oxygen delivery (especially if anemia is present) and to promote renal perfusion. A high-normal systemic blood pressure is required in the presence of euvolemia to maintain adequate urine flow. Selection of muscle relaxants is influenced by their dependence on renal clearance. In this regard, atracurium and cisatracurium are attractive selections because their clearance from plasma is organ independent. A newly transplanted kidney is able to clear neuromuscular blockers and the anticholinesterase drugs used for their reversal at the same rate as healthy native kidneys.

Central venous pressure monitoring is useful for guiding the rate and volume of crystalloid infusions. Optimal hydration during the intraoperative period is intended to maximize renal blood flow and improve early function of the transplanted kidney. Mannitol is often administered to facilitate urine formation by the newly transplanted kidney and to reduce the risk of acute tubular necrosis. Mannitol is an osmotic diuretic that facilitates urine output by decreasing excess tissue and intravascular fluid. In addition, mannitol increases renal blood flow through local release of prostaglandins. To expand intravascular volume and promote urine production, albumin may also be helpful when a cadaveric kidney is transplanted.

When the vascular clamps are released, renal preservative solution from the transplanted kidney and venous drainage from the legs are released into the circulation. Cardiac arrest has been described after completion of the arterial anastomosis to the transplanted kidney and release of the vascular clamp. This event is most likely due to sudden hyperkalemia caused by washout of the potassium-containing preservative solutions from the newly perfused kidney. Unclamping may also be followed by hypotension resulting from the abrupt addition of up to 300 mL to the capacity of the intravascular fluid space and the release of vasodilating chemicals from previously ischemic tissues.

Regional Anesthesia

The advantage of regional anesthesia compared with general anesthesia is avoidance of the need for tracheal intubation and administration of neuromuscular blocking drugs. This advantage is negated, however, if regional anesthesia must be extensively supplemented with injected or inhaled drugs. Furthermore, blockade of the peripheral sympathetic nervous system, as produced by regional anesthesia, can complicate control of systemic blood pressure, especially considering the unpredictable intravascular fluid volume status of many of these patients. Use of regional anesthesia, particularly epidural anesthesia, is controversial in the presence of abnormal coagulation.

Postoperative Complications

The newly transplanted kidney may undergo acute immunologic rejection, which manifests in the vasculature of the transplanted kidney. It can be so rapid that inadequate circulation is evident almost immediately after blood supply to the kidney is established. The only treatment for this acute rejection reaction is removal of the transplanted kidney, especially if the rejection process is accompanied by disseminated intravascular coagulation. A hematoma also may arise in the graft postoperatively, causing vascular or ureteral obstruction.

Delayed signs of graft rejection include fever, local tenderness, and deterioration of urine output. Treatment with high doses of corticosteroids and antilymphocyte globulin may be helpful. Additional therapies used to treat delayed graft rejection include monoclonal antibodies, tacrolimus, and mycophenolate mofetil. Delayed graft function is a relatively common complication of cadaveric kidney transplantation. The most common cause is acute tubular necrosis; precipitating factors include renal ischemia in the donor, use of cyclosporine, and surgical conditions, including prolonged cold and warm ischemia times. Dialysis may be required until kidney function resumes. Ultrasonography and needle biopsy are performed to differentiate between the possible causes of kidney malfunction.

Opportunistic infections resulting from long-term immunosuppression are common after renal transplantation. Long-term survival is unsatisfactory in renal transplant recipients who are immunosuppressed and who also carry hepatitis B surface antigen. The frequency of cancer is 30–100 times higher in transplant recipients than in the general population. Large-cell lymphoma is a well-recognized complication of transplantation; it occurs almost exclusively in patients with evidence of Epstein-Barr virus infection.

Anesthetic Considerations in Renal Transplant Recipients Undergoing Surgery

Renal transplant recipients are often elderly individuals with co-existing cardiovascular disease and diabetes mellitus. The side effects of immunosuppressant drugs (systemic hypertension, lowered seizure threshold, anemia, thrombocytopenia) must be considered when planning the management of anesthesia in these patients. Serum creatinine concentrations are likely to be normal in the presence of normally functioning renal grafts. Nevertheless, GFR and renal blood flow are likely to be lower than in healthy individuals, and the activity of drugs excreted by the kidneys may be prolonged. The presence of azotemia, proteinuria, and systemic hypertension may indicate chronic rejection of the kidney transplant.

Drugs that are potentially nephrotoxic or dependent on renal clearance should be avoided, and diuretics should be administered only after careful evaluation of the patient's intravascular volume status. Decreases in renal blood flow resulting from hypovolemia or other causes should be minimized.

PRIMARY DISEASES OF THE KIDNEYS

A number of pathologic processes can primarily involve the kidneys or occur in association with dysfunction of other organ systems. Knowledge of the associated pathologic features and other characteristics of these diseases is important when managing these patients during the perioperative period.

Glomerulonephritis

Acute glomerulonephritis is usually due to deposition of antigen-antibody complexes in the glomeruli. The source of antigens may be exogenous (after streptococcal infection) or endogenous (collagen vascular diseases). Clinical manifestations of glomerular disease include hematuria, proteinuria, hypertension, edema, and increased serum creatinine concentration. The presence of urinary red blood cell casts is also highly suggestive of renal dysfunction resulting from a glomerular process. Proteinuria reflects an increase in glomerular permeability. Prompt diagnosis is important because treatment with immunosuppressive drugs may help prevent permanent kidney injury.

Two general patterns of glomerular disease exist. A *nephritic pattern* is associated with inflammation and an active urine sediment containing red and white blood cells and a variable amount of proteinuria. A *nephrotic pattern* is characterized by marked proteinuria and a relatively inactive urine sediment.

Nephrotic Syndrome

Nephrotic syndrome is defined as a daily urinary protein excretion exceeding 3.5 g associated with hypoalbuminemia (<3 g/dL) and peripheral edema. Hyperlipidemia, thromboembolism, and infections are frequent complications. Nephrotic syndrome may occur in the context of a systemic disorder (e.g., diabetes, systemic lupus erythematosus), or it may occur as a primary renal disease. In adults the most common cause of nephrotic syndrome is focal segmental glomerulosclerosis. HIV infection may cause nephrotic syndrome and renal insufficiency; in some patients this is the first clinical manifestation of the infection. Pregnancy-induced hypertension may also be associated with nephrotic syndrome. In children, minimal change disease is responsible for the majority of cases of nephrotic syndrome.

Pathophysiology

The primary source of protein loss in nephrotic syndrome is at the glomerulus, and the major protein lost is albumin. Sodium retention and edema formation in patients with nephrotic syndrome have been presumed to reflect decreased plasma oncotic pressure with resultant hypovolemia. Increased tubular reabsorption of sodium was assumed to be a homeostatic response to hypovolemia. More recent evidence suggests that sodium retention is a primary event that precedes the development of proteinuria. Increased sodium reabsorption by the distal renal tubules may be due to an inappropriately low natriuretic response to atrial natriuretic peptide. Hyperlipidemia and hypercholesterolemia accompany nephrotic syndrome and may be associated with an increased risk of vascular disease.

Thromboembolic Complications

Thromboembolic complications such as renal vein thrombosis, pulmonary embolism, and deep vein thrombosis are major risks in patients with nephrotic syndrome, particularly those who have membranous glomerulonephritis. Arterial thromboses are less common than venous thromboses, although the risk of acute myocardial infarction in these patients may be increased. Prophylactic administration of heparin or oral anticoagulants may be considered in patients at high risk.

Infection

Pneumococcal peritonitis has been responsible for fatalities in children with nephrotic syndrome. Viral infections may be more likely in immunosuppressed patients, whereas susceptibility to bacterial infections seems to be related to decreased levels of immunoglobulin (Ig)G.

Protein Binding

Plasma levels of vitamins and hormones may be decreased in patients with nephrotic syndrome as a result of proteinuria. Hypoalbuminemia decreases the available binding sites for many drugs and increases their circulating levels of unbound drug. In this regard, when plasma drug levels are monitored, low levels of highly protein-bound drugs do not necessarily indicate low therapeutic concentrations.

Nephrotic Edema

Generalized edema is a function of an increase in total body sodium content. Potent loop diuretics such as furosemide are needed to offset the kidney's propensity to retain sodium. In addition, thiazide or potassium-sparing diuretics may be added to decrease sodium reabsorption in the distal nephrons. The goal is to reduce edema *slowly;* abrupt natriuresis may cause hypovolemia and even acute kidney injury. It may also produce hemoconcentration, which increases the risk of thromboembolic complications. Albumin solutions are administered to expand the plasma volume only if symptomatic hypovolemia is present. In particularly severe cases, plasma ultrafiltration may be considered.

Goodpasture Syndrome

Goodpasture syndrome, also known as *anti–glomerular basement membrane antibody disease,* is a rare autoimmune disease that manifests as rapidly progressing glomerulonephritis, sometimes in combination with pulmonary hemorrhage. Antibodies are directed against a specific domain in the type IV collagen found in the basement membrane of the glomerulus and alveoli. The syndrome occurs most often in young males. Pulmonary disease occurs in 50%–60% of cases; when present, symptoms may precede clinical evidence of renal disease. Plasmapheresis is the preferred treatment. Corticosteroids are also employed to reduce inflammatory damage and can be combined with cyclophosphamide to suppress the immune response. The prognosis is poor, and most patients develop renal failure within a year of diagnosis. However, those who survive the first year with intact renal function generally do well, and relapses are uncommon.

Acute Interstitial Nephritis

Acute interstitial nephritis has been observed as an allergic reaction to drugs, including penicillin and cephalosporin antibiotics, NSAIDs, proton pump inhibitors, sulfonamides, allopurinol, and diuretics. Other less common causes include autoimmune diseases (systemic lupus erythematosus) and infiltrative diseases (sarcoidosis). Patients exhibit decreased urine concentrating ability, proteinuria, and systemic hypertension. Patients may also have allergic symptoms such as rash or eosinophilia or eosinophiluria. Renal failure caused by acute interstitial nephritis is often reversible after withdrawal of the offending drug or treatment of the underlying disease. Corticosteroid therapy may be beneficial.

Hereditary Nephritis

Hereditary nephritis (Alport syndrome) is a genetic disorder involving a defect in type IV collagen; inheritance is usually X-linked, but autosomal recessive and autosomal dominant forms also exist. As a result, the disorder is more frequent in males than in females. Renal disease is often accompanied by hearing loss and ocular abnormalities, because the type IV collagen affected by the genetic defect is common to these locations. In women the disease is usually mild, but in men the symptoms may be severe and progressive. Drug therapy has not proven successful, although lowering the intraglomerular pressure with ACE inhibitors may slow the progression of renal disease. ESRD is likely before the age of 50. Renal transplantation is the preferred treatment and is associated with good outcomes.

Polycystic Kidney Disease

Polycystic kidney disease is a genetic disorder inherited as an autosomal dominant trait. It is a relatively common condition, affecting 1 in every 400 to 1000 live births; however, approximately half of patients have clinically silent disease. The condition is marked by the development of cysts in the kidney, as well as in other organs such as the liver and pancreas. Intracranial aneurysms and cardiac valve abnormalities may also be present. When symptoms do occur, systemic hypertension, hematuria, kidney stones, and urinary tract infections are common. The disease typically progresses slowly until renal failure occurs during middle age. Hemodialysis or renal transplantation is eventually necessary in most patients.

Renal Tubular Acidosis

Renal tubular acidosis (RTA) is a syndrome that causes metabolic acidosis resulting from inappropriate alkalinization of the urine. Several subtypes of the disorder are recognized. Type 1 RTA is caused by impaired bicarbonate reabsorption in the proximal renal tubule. Type 2 RTA is due to impaired secretion of hydrogen ions in the distal tubule. The result of either defect is a hypokalemic, hyperchloremic metabolic acidosis and inappropriately alkaline urine. These conditions may be hereditary or secondary to an underlying systemic illness (autoimmune disorder, multiple myeloma). Type 4 RTA also causes a metabolic acidosis but is distinct from the other types in that it is associated with hyperkalemia rather than hypokalemia. Type 4 RTA occurs when plasma aldosterone levels are inappropriately low or the kidney fails to respond normally to aldosterone. Type 4 RTA is often seen in patients with CKD.

Fanconi Syndrome

Fanconi syndrome results from inherited or acquired disturbances of proximal renal tubular function. There is renal loss of substances normally conserved by the proximal renal tubules, including potassium, bicarbonate, phosphate, amino acids, glucose, and water. Symptoms include polyuria, polydipsia, metabolic acidosis, and skeletal muscle weakness. Bone pain and osteomalacia (reflecting loss of phosphate) are also common, and patients may have vitamin D–resistant rickets. Management of anesthesia includes attention to fluid and electrolyte abnormalities and the recognition that left ventricular failure due to uremia is often present in advanced stages of the disease.

Bartter and Gitelman Syndromes

Bartter and Gitelman syndromes are inherited renal salt-wasting disorders caused by defects in sodium, chloride, and potassium channels in the thick ascending limb of the distal convoluted tubule. Juxtaglomerular hyperplasia, hyperaldosteronism, and hypokalemic acidosis are pathognomonic of these disorders. Treatment consists of spironolactone and sodium and potassium supplementation. Patients with Bartter syndrome also benefit from treatment with NSAIDs. These syndromes alone do not lead to renal failure. However, if patients develop ESRD for other reasons, transplantation of a kidney from a healthy donor results in normal renal solute handling.

Nephrolithiasis

Although the pathogenesis of nephrolithiasis is poorly understood, several predisposing factors are recognized for the five major types of renal stones that occur (Table 22.11). Most stones are composed of calcium oxalate and result from excess calcium excretion by the kidneys. In these patients, causes of hypercalcemia (hyperparathyroidism, sarcoidosis, cancer) must be considered. Urinary tract infections with urea-splitting organisms that produce ammonia favor the formation of magnesium ammonium phosphate (struvite) stones. Formation of uric acid stones is favored by a persistently acidic urine (pH < 6.0), which decreases the solubility of uric acid. Approximately 50% of patients with uric acid stones have gout.

Stones in the renal pelvis are typically painless unless their presence is complicated by infection or obstruction. By

TABLE 22.11	Composition and Characteristics of Renal Stones			
Type of Stone	Incidence (%)	Radiographic Appearance	Cause	
Calcium oxalate	70	Opaque	Primary hyperparathyroidism Idiopathic hypercalciuria Hyperoxaluria	
Magnesium ammonium phosphate (struvite)	15	Opaque	Alkaline urine (usually resulting from chronic bacterial infection)	
Calcium phosphate	8	Opaque	Renal tubular acidosis	
Uric acid	5	Translucent	Acid urine Gout Hyperuricosuria	
Cystine	2	Opaque	Cystinuria	

contrast, renal stones passing down the ureter can produce intense flank pain, often radiating to the groin, associated with nausea and vomiting, and mimicking an acute abdomen. Hematuria is common during ureteral passage of stones, whereas ureteral obstruction may precipitate renal failure.

Treatment

Treatment of a renal stone depends on identifying the composition of the stone and correcting predisposing factors, such as hyperparathyroidism, urinary tract infection, or gout. High fluid intake sufficient to maintain a daily urine output of 2–3 L is often part of the therapy. Extracorporeal shock wave lithotripsy is a noninvasive treatment for renal stones that uses focused high-intensity acoustic impulses to break up stones into pieces that may be excreted in the urine. The advantages of this approach as an alternative to percutaneous nephrolithotomy are that it is associated with low morbidity and can be performed on an outpatient basis. Cardiac dysrhythmias may occur during extracorporeal shock wave lithotripsy, presumably as a result of premature stimulation of the atria by the electrical discharge that precedes each shock wave. Lithotripsy devices are equipped with ECG gating that helps limit the risk of ventricular fibrillation caused by the "R-on-T" phenomenon.

Renal Hypertension

Renal disease is the most common cause of secondary systemic hypertension. Accelerated or malignant hypertension is likely to be associated with renal disease. Furthermore, the appearance of systemic hypertension in young patients suggests the diagnosis of renal disease rather than essential hypertension. Hypertension due to renal dysfunction reflects parenchymal disease of the kidneys or renovascular disease.

Chronic pyelonephritis and glomerulonephritis are parenchymal diseases often associated with systemic hypertension, particularly in younger patients. Less common forms of renal parenchymal disease that can cause systemic hypertension include diabetic nephropathy, cystic disease of the kidneys, and renal amyloidosis.

Renovascular disease is caused by narrowing of the renal arteries resulting from either fibromuscular dysplasia or atheroma. Sudden onset of a marked increase in systemic blood pressure or the presence of hypertension before the age of 30 years should arouse suspicion of renovascular disease. A bruit may be audible on auscultation of the abdomen over the kidneys. Systemic hypertension due to renovascular disease does not respond well to treatment with antihypertensive drugs. Renovascular hypertension is treated with renal artery angioplasty, stent placement, or endarterectomy or by nephrectomy.

Uric Acid Nephropathy

Acute uric acid nephropathy occurs when uric acid crystals precipitate in the renal collecting tubules or ureters, producing acute oliguric renal failure. This precipitation occurs when uric acid concentrations reach a saturation point in acidic urine. The condition is particularly likely to occur when uric acid production is greatly increased, as in patients with myeloproliferative disorders being treated with chemotherapeutic drugs. These patients are particularly vulnerable to uric acid nephropathy when they become dehydrated or acidotic. Treatment includes IV fluids and allopurinol in an attempt to wash out the uric acid crystals.

Hepatorenal Syndrome

Acute oliguria manifesting in patients with decompensated cirrhosis of the liver is called *hepatorenal syndrome*. Indeed, cirrhosis of the liver is associated with decreased GFR and renal blood flow that precede overt renal dysfunction by several weeks. The typical patient is deeply jaundiced and moribund; ascites, hypoalbuminemia, and hypoprothrombinemia are present. Renal failure in these patients reflects reduction in effective circulating volume, partly as a result of diuretic treatment and partly as a result of splanchnic arteriolar dilatation. Treatment is directed at restoring intravascular fluid volume. Administration of normal saline may aggravate ascites. Therefore whole blood or packed red blood cells may be a more appropriate form of volume replacement. Vasopressin receptor agonists such as ornipressin and terlipressin cause splanchnic vasoconstriction and may help increase renal perfusion and GFR. A peritoneal-venous shunt (LeVeen shunt) for the treatment of ascites may also be associated with improved renal function.

TABLE 22.12	Signs and Symptoms of Transurethral Resection of the Prostate (TURP) Syndrome	
System	Signs and Symptoms	Cause
Cardiovascular	Hypertension, reflex bradycardia, pulmonary edema, cardiovascular collapse, ECG changes (wide QRS, elevated ST segment, ventricular dysrhythmias)	Rapid fluid absorption, reflex bradycardia (secondary to hypertension or increased ICP), third-spacing secondary to hyponatremia and hypoosmolality
Respiratory	Tachypnea, hypoxemia, Cheyne-Stokes breathing	Pulmonary edema
Neurologic	Nausea, restlessness, visual disturbances, confusion, somnolence, seizure, coma, death	Hyponatremia and hypoosmolality causing cerebral edema and increased ICP, hyperglycinemia (glycine is an inhibitory neurotransmitter that potentiates NMDA receptor activity), hyperammonemia
Hematologic	Disseminated intravascular coagulation, hemolysis	Hyponatremia and hypoosmolality
Renal	Renal failure	Hypotension, hyperoxaluria (oxalate is a metabolite of glycine)
Metabolic	Acidosis	Deamination of glycine to glyoxylic acid and ammonia

ECG, Electrocardiogram; *ICP,* intracranial pressure; *NMDA,* N-methyl-ᴅ-aminotransferase.

There is an increased incidence of postoperative AKI in patients with obstructive jaundice who undergo surgery. The cause of renal failure in these patients is unclear, but preoperative administration of mannitol is recommended in the hope of providing some renoprotective effect.

Benign Prostatic Hyperplasia

Benign prostatic hyperplasia (BPH) is a nonmalignant enlargement of the prostate caused by excessive growth of both the glandular and stromal elements of the gland. Symptoms occur as a result of compression of the urethral canal and disruption of the normal flow of urine. BPH is common worldwide in men older than age 40.

Medical Therapy

Prostatic tissue growth is androgen sensitive, so androgen deprivation decreases the size of the prostate and thereby the resistance to outflow through the prostatic urethra. Finasteride, an inhibitor of the 5α-reductase enzyme, reduces both serum and prostatic testosterone levels and is moderately effective for symptomatic treatment of BPH. Side effects are minimal. α-Adrenergic antagonists (terazosin, doxazosin, tamsulosin) are administered to block adrenergic receptors in hyperplastic prostatic tissue, the prostatic capsule, and the bladder neck and thereby decrease smooth muscle tone and resistance to urinary flow. These drugs also have antihypertensive effects and may cause orthostatic hypotension in some patients.

Invasive Treatments

The most commonly used minimally invasive treatments of BPH are transurethral microwave thermotherapy (TUMT) and transurethral needle ablation (TUNA). These procedures rely on the generation of heat to cause tissue necrosis and shrinkage of the prostate.

Surgical treatments include transurethral incision of the prostate (TUIP) and transurethral resection of the prostate (TURP). TUIP is usually effective in patients whose prostates weigh 30 g or less and in whom the primary urinary outlet obstruction is located at the bladder neck. As the incisions are deepened, the bladder neck and prostatic urethra spring open, and the bladder outlet obstruction is relieved. TURP involves resection of prostatic tissue using electrocautery or sharp excision. The procedure is associated with a fair amount of bleeding; patients are admitted postoperatively for continuous bladder irrigation to prevent formation of obstructing blood clots.

Newer procedures using laser therapy to destroy prostate tissue have also been developed. Advantages of laser ablation of the prostate are brief operating time (≤20 minutes) and reduced perioperative bleeding.

Transurethral Resection of the Prostate (TURP) Syndrome

During TURP, an irrigation solution (glycine, sorbitol, mannitol) is used to facilitate surgical visualization and remove blood and resected tissue. The procedure is accompanied by absorption of this irrigation fluid directly through the prostatic venous plexus or more slowly through the retroperitoneal and perivesical spaces. TURP syndrome is characterized by intravascular fluid volume shifts and the effects of plasma solute absorption (Table 22.12). Solute changes such as hyponatremia may alter neurologic function independent of volume-related effects. Although monitoring of serum sodium concentrations during TURP is effective for assessing intravascular fluid absorption, there may be benefit in monitoring serum osmolality as well. Hypoosmolality appears to be the principal factor contributing to the neurologic and hypovolemic changes considered to reflect TURP syndrome. Supportive care remains the most important therapeutic approach for managing cardiovascular, CNS, and renal complications of TURP syndrome.

Neuraxial anesthesia has conventionally been the anesthetic technique of choice for TURP, because it allows for monitoring of TURP syndrome symptoms during the procedure.

Intravascular Volume Expansion. Rapid intravascular fluid volume expansion from systemic absorption of irrigating fluids (absorption rates may reach 200 mL/min) can cause systemic hypertension and reflex bradycardia. Patients with poor left ventricular function may develop pulmonary edema due to acute circulatory volume overload. Factors that influence the amount of irrigating solution absorbed include the intravesicular pressure, which is determined by the height of the irrigation bag above the prostatic sinuses (height should be limited to <40 cm above the prostate) and the number of prostatic sinuses opened (resection time should be limited to 1 hour, and a rim of tissue should be left on the capsule). If intravesical pressures are maintained below 15 cm H_2O, absorption of irrigating fluids is minimal.

The most widely used indicator of intravascular fluid volume absorption is hyponatremia. Before treating TURP syndrome with hypertonic saline, it is important to exclude the presence of hypervolemia with near-normal plasma sodium concentrations. Cardiovascular compromise and impaired arterial oxygenation due to pulmonary edema require aggressive intervention, which may include administration of inotropic drugs or diuretics.

Intravascular Volume Loss. Perioperative hypotension during TURP is sometimes preceded by systemic hypertension. It is conceivable that hyponatremia in association with systemic hypertension can result in water flux along osmotic and hydrostatic pressure gradients out of the intravascular space and into the lungs, with resultant pulmonary edema and hypovolemic shock. Sympathetic nervous system blockade produced by regional anesthesia may compound the hypotension, as may intraoperative endotoxemia, which is common during TURP.

Hyponatremia. Acute hyponatremia due to intravascular absorption of sodium-free irrigating fluids may cause confusion, agitation, visual disturbances, pulmonary edema, cardiovascular collapse, and seizures. ECG changes may accompany progressive decreases in serum sodium concentrations. Spinal anesthesia associated with hypotension may cause nausea and vomiting indistinguishable from that caused by acute hyponatremia. Furthermore, some hyponatremic patients show no signs of water intoxication.

Hypoosmolality. Hypoosmolality rather than hyponatremia may be the crucial physiologic derangement leading to CNS dysfunction in TURP syndrome. This is predictable because the blood-brain barrier is essentially impermeable to sodium but freely permeable to water. Cerebral edema caused by acute hypoosmolality can result in increased intracranial pressure, with resultant bradycardia and hypertension.

Diuretics administered to treat hypervolemia during TURP may accentuate hyponatremia and hypoosmolality. A patient's serum sodium concentration and osmolality may continue to decrease following TURP because of continued absorption of irrigating solutions from the perivesicular and retroperitoneal spaces. If the serum osmolality is near normal, no interventions to correct serum sodium concentrations are recommended for asymptomatic patients even in the presence of hyponatremia. Instituting treatment in the absence of symptoms risks too rapid a correction because the correction rate is difficult to control. The most feared complication of correction of hyponatremia is central pontine myelinolysis (osmotic demyelination syndrome), which has been observed after both rapid and slow correction of serum sodium concentrations in patients undergoing TURP.

Hyperammonemia. Hyperammonemia is a result of the use of glycine-containing irrigation solutions, with subsequent systemic absorption of glycine and its oxidative deamination to glyoxylic acid and ammonia. Alterations in CNS function may accompany hyperammonemia, but its role in TURP syndrome remains unclear. Endogenous arginine in the liver prevents hepatic release of ammonia and facilitates conversion of ammonia to urea. The time necessary to deplete endogenous arginine stores may be as brief as 12 hours, which approximates the preoperative fasting time. Prophylactic administration of IV arginine blunts the increase in serum ammonia concentrations associated with the presence of glycine in the systemic circulation.

Hyperglycinemia. Glycine is an inhibitory neurotransmitter similar to γ-aminobutyric acid in the spinal cord and brain. The use of glycine-containing irrigation solutions during TURP may cause visual disturbances, including transient blindness, which reflects the role of glycine as an inhibitory neurotransmitter in the retina. Therefore glycine likely affects retinal physiology independent of the cerebral edema caused by hyponatremia and hypoosmolality. Vision returns to normal within 24 hours as serum glycine concentrations approach baseline values. Reassurance that unimpaired vision will return is probably the best treatment.

Glycine may also lead to encephalopathy and seizures through its ability to potentiate the effects of N-methyl-D-aspartate (NMDA), an excitatory neurotransmitter. Magnesium exerts a negative control on the NMDA receptor, and hypomagnesemia caused by dilution (resulting from systemic absorption of irrigating solutions during TURP or administration of loop diuretics) may increase the susceptibility to seizures. For this reason a trial of magnesium therapy may be indicated in patients who develop seizures and in whom glycine-containing irrigating solutions have been used.

Glycine may also exert toxic effects on the kidneys. Hyperoxaluria due to metabolism of glycine to oxalate and glyoxylic acid may compromise renal function in patients with preexisting renal disease.

KEY POINTS

- The kidneys receive 15%–25% of total cardiac output, and renal blood flow is autoregulated between mean arterial pressures of approximately 50–150 mm Hg.
- The kidneys are involved in water conservation, electrolyte homeostasis, acid-base balance, and several neurohumoral

and hormonal functions. Some or all of these functions are affected by renal disease. Glomerular filtration rate is the best measure of renal function.

- Patient risk factors for perioperative acute kidney injury (AKI) include advanced age, preexisting renal dysfunction, diabetes, hypertension, and peripheral vascular disease. High-risk surgical procedures include those requiring aortic cross-clamping and cardiopulmonary bypass. Prevention of AKI hinges on maintaining adequate renal perfusion and avoiding nephrotoxins.

- Treatment of AKI is supportive, aimed at limiting further injury by maintaining hemodynamic stability and adequate intravascular fluid volume.

- Preoperative evaluation of patients with chronic kidney disease (CKD) should take into consideration not only baseline renal function but also the high prevalence of comorbid conditions, including cardiovascular disease and diabetes.

- Current guidelines advise that CKD patients with proteinuria should have their blood pressure maintained below 130/80 mm Hg, and those without proteinuria should have their blood pressure maintained below 140/90 mm Hg. ACE inhibitors and/or ARBs are first-line therapies for those with proteinuria, and diuretics are preferred first-line agents for those without proteinuria. However, most patients require treatment with multiple antihypertensive drugs.

- Provision of anesthesia for patients with CKD focuses on meticulous fluid and electrolyte management, acid-base maintenance, and attention to drug pharmacokinetics in renal failure. Vessels of the nondominant forearm should be preserved in anticipation of vascular access requirements for hemodialysis.

- During renal transplantation, hypotension and cardiac dysrhythmias may develop when the vascular clamps are released. This event is likely due to washout of potassium-containing preservative fluid from the newly perfused kidney, abrupt addition of fluid to the intravascular space, and the release of vasodilating chemicals from previously ischemic tissues.

RESOURCES

Chenitz KB, Lane-Fall MB. Decreased urine output and acute kidney injury in the postanesthesia care unit. *Anesthesiol Clin*. 2012;30:513-526.

Gravenstein D. Transurethral resection of the prostate (TURP) syndrome: a review of the pathophysiology and management. *Anesth Analg*. 1997;84:438-446.

Hoste EA, De Corte W. Implementing the Kidney Disease: improving Global Outcomes/acute kidney injury guidelines in ICU patients. *Curr Opin Crit Care*. 2013;19:544-553.

Josephs SA, Thakar CV. Perioperative risk assessment, prevention, and treatment of acute kidney injury. *Int Anesthesiol Clin*. 2009;47:89-105.

Moore EM, Bellomo R, Nichol AD. The meaning of acute kidney injury and its relevance to intensive care and anaesthesia. *Anaesth Intensive Care*. 2012;40:929-948.

Schmid S, Jungwirth B. Anesthesia for renal transplant surgery: an update. *Eur J Anesthesiol*. 2012;29:552-558.

Wagener G, Brentjens TE. Anesthetic concerns in patients presenting with renal failure. *Anesthesiol Clin*. 2010;28:39-54.

Weisbord SD, Gallagher M, Kaufman J, et al. Prevention of contrast-induced AKI: a review of published trials and the design of the Prevention of Serious Adverse Events Following Angiography (PRESERVE) Trial. *Clin J Am Soc Nephrol*. 2013;8:1618-1631.

Zacharias M, Herbison GP, Mugawar M, et al. Interventions for protecting renal function in the perioperative period. *Cochrane Database Syst Rev*. 2013: CD003590.

CHAPTER 23

Endocrine Disease

RUSSELL T. WALL, III

DIABETES MELLITUS

Normal glucose physiology is marked by a balance between glucose utilization and endogenous production or dietary delivery (Fig. 23.1). The liver is the primary source of endogenous glucose production via glycogenolysis and gluconeogenesis. Following a meal, plasma glucose level increases, which stimulates an increase in plasma insulin secretion that promotes glucose utilization. Late in the postprandial period (2–4 hours after eating) when glucose utilization exceeds glucose production, a transition from exogenous glucose delivery to endogenous production becomes necessary to maintain a normal plasma glucose level. Approximately 70%–80% of glucose released by the liver is metabolized by insulin-insensitive tissues such as the brain, gastrointestinal (GI) tract, and red blood cells. During this time, diminished insulin secretion is fundamental to maintenance of a normal plasma glucose concentration. Hyperglycemia-producing hormones (glucagon, epinephrine, growth hormone, cortisol) comprise the glucose counterregulatory system and support glucose production. Glucagon plays a primary role by stimulating glycogenolysis and gluconeogenesis and inhibiting glycolysis.

Diabetes mellitus results from an inadequate supply of insulin and/or an inadequate tissue response to insulin. This leads to increased circulating glucose levels with eventual microvascular and macrovascular complications. Type 1a diabetes is caused by autoimmune destruction of beta cells within

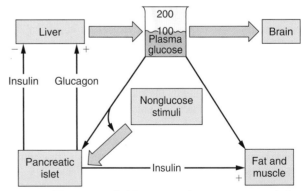

FIG. 23.1 The pancreatic islets act as glucose sensors to balance hepatic glucose release to insulin-insensitive tissues (brain) and insulin-sensitive tissues (fat, muscle). Insulin inhibits glucose release by the liver and stimulates glucose utilization by insulin-sensitive tissues. With hyperglycemia, insulin secretion increases. With hypoglycemia, the reverse occurs. (Adapted from Porte D Jr. Beta-cells in type II diabetes mellitus. *Diabetes.* 1991;40:166-180.)

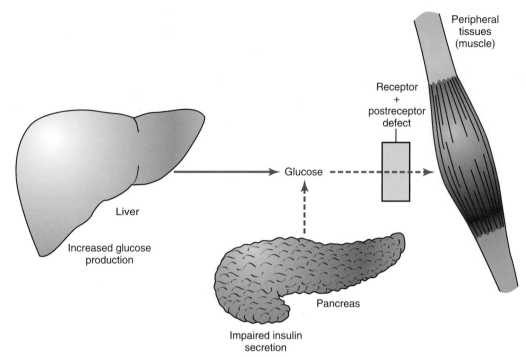

FIG. 23.2 Abnormalities in type 2 diabetes. (Adapted from Inzucchi S, ed. *The Diabetes Mellitus Manual: A Primary Care Companion to Ellenberg and Rifkin's Sixth Edition.* New York: McGraw-Hill; 2005:79.)

pancreatic islets, resulting in complete absence or minimal circulating levels of insulin. Type 1b diabetes is a rare disease of absolute insulin deficiency that is not immune mediated. Type 2 diabetes also is not immune mediated and results from defects in insulin receptors and postreceptor intracellular signaling pathways.

Signs and Symptoms

Type 1 Diabetes

Between 5% and 10% of all cases of diabetes are type 1. There are 1.4 million individuals with type 1 diabetes in the United States and 10–20 million globally. Currently the incidence is increasing by 3%–5% per year. The disorder is usually diagnosed before the age of 40 and is one of the most common chronic childhood illnesses.

Type 1 diabetes is caused by T cell–mediated autoimmune destruction of beta cells in the pancreas. The exact cause is unknown, although environmental triggers such as viruses (especially enteroviruses), dietary proteins, or drugs or chemicals may initiate the autoimmune process in genetically susceptible hosts. At least 80%–90% of beta cell function must be lost before hyperglycemia occurs.

The presentation of clinical disease is often sudden and severe, secondary to loss of a critical mass of beta cells. Patients demonstrate hyperglycemia over several days to weeks associated with fatigue, weight loss, polyuria, polydipsia, blurring of vision, and signs of intravascular volume depletion. The diagnosis is based on the presence of a random blood glucose level higher than 200 mg/dL and a hemoglobin (Hb)A_{1c} level above

7.0%. The presence of ketoacidosis indicates severe insulin deficiency and unrestrained lipolysis.

Type 2 Diabetes

Type 2 diabetes is responsible for 90% of all cases of diabetes mellitus in the world. In 2000 there were approximately 150 million individuals with type 2 diabetes globally, and the number is expected to double by 2025. Patients with type 2 diabetes are typically in the middle to older age group and are overweight, although there has been a significant increase in younger patients and even children with type 2 diabetes over the past decade.

Type 2 diabetes is characterized by relative beta cell insufficiency and insulin resistance. In the initial stages of the disease, an insensitivity to insulin on the part of peripheral tissues leads to an increase in pancreatic insulin secretion to maintain normal plasma glucose levels. As the disease progresses and pancreatic cell function decreases, insulin levels are unable to compensate and hyperglycemia occurs. Three important defects are seen in type 2 diabetes: (1) an increased rate of hepatic glucose release, (2) impaired basal and stimulated insulin secretion, and (3) inefficient use of glucose by peripheral tissues (i.e., insulin resistance) (Fig. 23.2). Although relative beta cell insufficiency is significant, type 2 diabetes is characterized by insulin resistance in skeletal muscle, adipose tissue, and the liver. It appears that insulin resistance is an inherited component of type 2 diabetes, with obesity and a sedentary lifestyle being acquired and contributing factors. Impaired glucose tolerance is associated with an increase in body weight, a decrease in insulin secretion, and a reduction

TABLE 23.1	Diagnostic Features of Metabolic Syndrome

At least three of the following:
    Fasting plasma glucose level ≥ 110 mg/dL
    Abdominal obesity (waist girth > 40 inches in men, >35 inches in women)
    Serum triglyceride level ≥ 150 mg/dL
    Serum high-density lipoprotein cholesterol level < 40 mg/dL in men, <50 mg/dL in women
    Blood pressure ≥ 130/85 mm Hg

Adapted from Expert Panel on Detection, Evaluation, and Treatment of High Blood Cholesterol in Adults: Executive summary of the third report of the National Cholesterol Education Program (NCEP) Expert Panel on Detection, Evaluation, and Treatment of High Blood Cholesterol in Adults (Adult Treatment Panel III). *JAMA.* 2001;285:2486-2497.

TABLE 23.2	Diagnostic Criteria for Diabetes Mellitus

Symptoms of diabetes (polyuria, polydipsia, unexplained weight loss) plus a random plasma glucose concentration ≥ 200 mg/dL
or
Fasting (no caloric intake for ≥ 8 hr) plasma glucose level ≥ 126 mg/dL
or
2-hr plasma glucose level > 200 mg/dL during an oral glucose tolerance test

Adapted from Diagnosis and classification of diabetes mellitus. American Diabetes Association. *Diabetes Care.* 2010;33(Suppl 1):S62.

in peripheral insulin action. The transition to clinical diabetes is characterized by these same factors plus an increase in hepatic glucose production.

The increasing prevalence of type 2 diabetes among children and adolescents appears related to obesity, since 85% of affected children are overweight or obese at the time of diagnosis. Obese patients exhibit a compensatory hyperinsulinemia to maintain normoglycemia. These increased insulin levels may desensitize target tissues, causing a reduced response to insulin. The mechanisms for hyperinsulinemia and insulin resistance from weight gain remain elusive.

Metabolic syndrome, or *insulin-resistance syndrome,* is a constellation of clinical and biochemical characteristics frequently seen in patients who have or are at risk of developing type 2 diabetes (Table 23.1). This syndrome combines insulin resistance with hypertension, dyslipidemia, a procoagulant state, and obesity and is associated with premature atherosclerosis and subsequent cardiovascular disease. This syndrome affects at least 25% of people in the United States.

Diagnosis

The American Diabetes Association (ADA) has established diagnostic criteria for diabetes mellitus (Table 23.2). Measurement of fasting plasma glucose level is the recommended screening test for diabetes mellitus. The upper limit for normal fasting glucose level is 100 mg/dL. Hyperglycemia not sufficient to meet the diagnostic criteria for diabetes is classified as

either impaired fasting glucose or impaired glucose tolerance, depending on whether it is identified through measurement of fasting plasma glucose level or an oral glucose tolerance test. Any fasting glucose level between 101 and 125 mg/dL is categorized as impaired fasting glucose. Glucose levels, especially in type 2 diabetics, usually increase over years to decades, progressing from the normal range to the impaired glucose tolerance range and finally to clinical diabetes.

The HbA_{1c} test provides a valuable measure of long-term glycemic control. Hemoglobin is nonenzymatically glycosylated by glucose, which freely crosses red blood cell membranes. The percentage of hemoglobin molecules participating in this reaction is proportional to the average plasma glucose concentration during the preceding 60–90 days. The normal range for HbA_{1c} is 4%–6%. Increased risk of microvascular and macrovascular disease begins when the HbA_{1c} proportion is 6.5% or higher. Measurement of HbA_{1c} is recommended at least twice a year and more frequently (every 3 months) if glycemic control is inadequate or therapy has changed.

Treatment

The cornerstones of treatment for type 2 diabetes are dietary adjustments along with weight loss, exercise therapy, and oral antidiabetic drugs. Reduction of body weight through diet and exercise is the first therapeutic measure to control type 2 diabetes. The decrease in adiposity improves hepatic and peripheral tissue insulin sensitivity, enhances postreceptor insulin action, and may possibly increase insulin secretion. Nutritional guidelines of the ADA emphasize maintenance of optimal plasma glucose and lipid levels.

Oral Antidiabetic Drugs

The four major classes of oral antidiabetic medications are (1) the secretagogues (sulfonylureas, meglitinides), which increase insulin availability; (2) the biguanides (metformin), which suppress excessive hepatic glucose release; (3) the thiazolidinediones or glitazones (rosiglitazone, pioglitazone), which improve insulin sensitivity; and (4) the α-glucosidase inhibitors (acarbose, miglitol), which delay GI glucose absorption (Fig. 23.3). These agents are used to maintain *glucose control,* which is defined as a fasting glucose level of 90–130 mg/dL, peak postprandial glucose level below 180 mg/dL, and HbA_{1c} level below 7% in the initial stages of the disease.

The sulfonylureas are usually the initial pharmacologic treatment for type 2 diabetes mellitus. They act by stimulating insulin secretion from pancreatic beta cells; they can also enhance insulin-stimulated peripheral tissue utilization of glucose. The second-generation agents (glyburide, glipizide, glimepiride) are more potent and have fewer side effects than their predecessors. Unfortunately, because of the natural history of type 2 diabetes characterized by decreasing beta cell function, these drugs are not effective indefinitely. Hypoglycemia is the most common side effect. Whether or not harmful cardiac effects from sulfonylureas have been demonstrated is controversial. Another class of insulin secretagogues act as

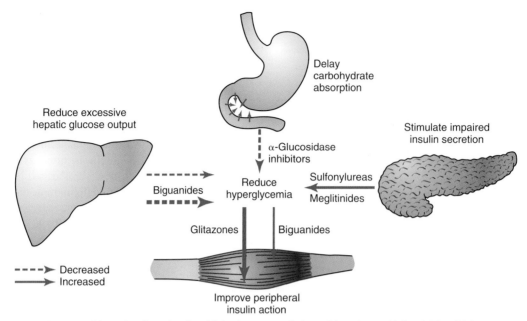

FIG. 23.3 Sites of action of oral antidiabetic agents. (Adapted from Inzucchi S, ed. *The Diabetes Mellitus Manual: A Primary Care Companion to Ellenberg and Rifkin's Sixth Edition.* New York: McGraw-Hill; 2005:168.)

GLP-1 (glucagon-like peptide 1) agonists or enhance endogenous GLP-1 activity in the gut. Exenatide and liraglutide are examples and have been approved for treatment for type 2 diabetes. These agents (incretins) increase glucose-stimulated insulin secretion, suppress glucagon, and slow gastric emptying. Dipeptidyl peptidase-4 inhibitors (saxagliptin, sitagliptin, vildagliptin) inhibit the degradation of native GLP-1 and thus enhance glucose-stimulated insulin secretion.

The biguanides decrease hepatic gluconeogenesis and to a lesser degree enhance utilization of glucose by skeletal muscle and adipose tissue by increasing glucose transport across cell membranes. In addition to lowering glucose levels, they decrease plasma levels of triglycerides and low-density lipoprotein cholesterol and reduce postprandial hyperlipidemia and plasma free fatty acids. The risk of hypoglycemia is less than that with the sulfonylureas. Lactic acidosis is a rare but serious side effect of the biguanides; the risk is particularly high in patients with renal insufficiency. It is much less common with metformin than with its predecessor phenformin.

The thiazolidinediones or glitazones are insulin sensitizers that decrease insulin resistance by binding to peroxisome proliferator–activated receptors located in skeletal muscle, liver, and adipose tissue. These drugs influence the expression of genes encoding proteins for glucose and lipid metabolism, endothelial function, and atherogenesis; as a result, they may influence diabetic dyslipidemia in addition to hyperglycemia.

The α-glucosidase inhibitors inhibit α-glucosidase enzymes in the brush border of enterocytes in the proximal small intestine, which results in a delay in intraluminal production and subsequent absorption of glucose. They are administered before a main meal to ensure their presence at the site of action.

In most patients, therapy is initiated with a sulfonylurea or biguanide and titrated to achieve fasting and peak postprandial glucose levels recommended by the ADA (Fig. 23.4). Combination therapy with oral agents directed at more than one mechanism is often effective. If combination oral therapy is unsuccessful, a bedtime dose of intermediate-acting insulin is added, since hepatic glucose overproduction is typically highest at night. If oral agents plus single-dose insulin therapy is ineffective, type 2 diabetic patients are switched to insulin therapy alone.

Tight control of type 2 diabetes provides significant benefits in preventing and slowing the progression of microvascular disease and possibly macrovascular disease. Not only must hyperglycemia be treated, but all abnormalities of insulin resistance (metabolic syndrome) must be managed, with the goals of therapy including an HbA_{1c} level below 7%, a low-density lipoprotein level below 100 mg/dL, a high-density lipoprotein level higher than 40 mg/dL in men and higher than 50 mg/dL in women, a triglyceride level below 200 mg/dL, and a blood pressure lower than 130/80 mm Hg.

Insulin

Insulin is necessary to manage all cases of type 1 diabetes and many cases of type 2 diabetes (Table 23.3). In the United States, 30% of patients with type 2 diabetes are treated with insulin. Conventional insulin therapy uses twice-daily injections. Intensive insulin therapy requires three or more daily injections or a continuous infusion (Figs. 23.5–23.9).

The various forms of insulin include *basal insulins,* which are intermediate acting (NPH, Lente, lispro protamine, aspart protamine) and administered twice daily or *long acting* (Ultralente, glargine, detemir) and administered once daily; and insulins that are *short acting* (regular) or *rapid acting* (lispro,

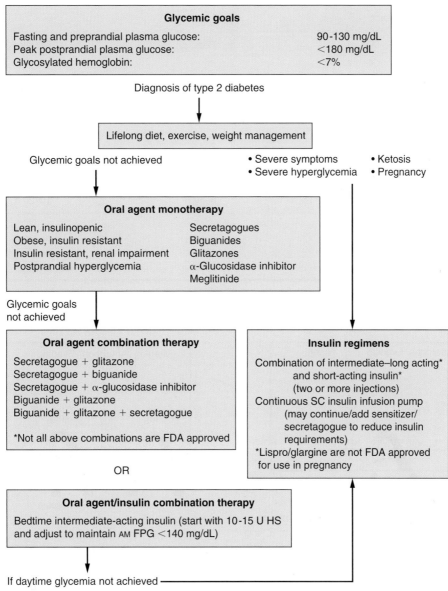

Glycemic goals

Fasting and preprandial plasma glucose:	90-130 mg/dL
Peak postprandial plasma glucose:	<180 mg/dL
Glycosylated hemoglobin:	<7%

Diagnosis of type 2 diabetes

Lifelong diet, exercise, weight management

Glycemic goals not achieved

- Severe symptoms
- Severe hyperglycemia
- Ketosis
- Pregnancy

Oral agent monotherapy

Lean, insulinopenic
Obese, insulin resistant
Insulin resistant, renal impairment
Postprandial hyperglycemia

Secretagogues
Biguanides
Glitazones
α-Glucosidase inhibitor
Meglitinide

Glycemic goals not achieved

Oral agent combination therapy

Secretagogue + glitazone
Secretagogue + biguanide
Secretagogue + α-glucosidase inhibitor
Biguanide + glitazone
Biguanide + glitazone + secretagogue

*Not all above combinations are FDA approved

Insulin regimens

Combination of intermediate–long acting*
and short-acting insulin*
(two or more injections)
Continuous SC insulin infusion pump
(may continue/add sensitizer/
secretagogue to reduce insulin
requirements)
*Lispro/glargine are not FDA approved
for use in pregnancy

OR

Oral agent/insulin combination therapy

Bedtime intermediate-acting insulin (start with 10-15 U HS
and adjust to maintain AM FPG <140 mg/dL)

If daytime glycemia not achieved

FIG. 23.4 Algorithm for treatment of type 2 diabetes. *FDA,* US Food and Drug Administration; *FPG,* fasting plasma glucose level; *HS,* at bedtime; *SC,* subcutaneous. (Adapted from Inzucchi S, ed. *The Diabetes Mellitus Manual: A Primary Care Companion to Ellenberg and Rifkin's Sixth Edition.* New York: McGraw-Hill; 2005:193.)

aspart, glulisine), which provide glycemic control at mealtimes. Rapid-acting insulins are preferred over regular insulin for prandial coverage. Insulin glargine has a later onset of action, longer duration of action, a less pronounced peak of action, and a lower incidence of hypoglycemia, especially at night. A long-acting insulin is usually prescribed with a short-acting insulin to mimic physiologic insulin release with meals. In general, patients with type 1 diabetes require 0.5–1 U/kg/day divided into multiple doses, with approximately 50% given as basal insulin.

Regular insulin is preferred over insulin analogues for intravenous (IV) infusions because it is less expensive and equally effective. Sliding scale short-acting insulin alone is inadequate for inpatient glucose management and should not be used.

Hypoglycemia is the most frequent and dangerous complication of insulin therapy. The hypoglycemic effect can be exacerbated by simultaneous administration of alcohol, sulfonylureas, biguanides, thiazolidinediones, angiotensin-converting enzyme (ACE) inhibitors, monoamine oxidase inhibitors, and nonselective β-blockers.

Repetitive episodes of hypoglycemia, especially at night, can result in *hypoglycemia unawareness,* a condition in which the patient does not respond with the appropriate autonomic warning symptoms before neuroglycopenia. The diagnosis in adults requires a plasma glucose level below 50 mg/dL. Symptoms are adrenergic (sweating, tachycardia, palpitations, restlessness, pallor) and neuroglycopenic (fatigue, confusion, headache, somnolence, convulsions, coma). Treatment

TABLE 23.3	Insulin Preparations			
Insulin	Onset	Peak	Duration
RAPID ACTING			
Lispro (Humalog)	10–15 min	1–2 h	3–6 h
Aspart (NovoLog)	10–15 min	1–2 h	3–6 h
Glulisine (Apidra)	20–30 min	30–90 min	1–2.5 h
SHORT ACTING			
Human regular	30 min	2–4 h	5–8 h
INTERMEDIATE			
Human NPH	1–2 h	6–10 h	10–20 h
Lente	1–2 h	6–10 h	10–20 h
LONG ACTING			
Ultralente	4–6 h	8–20 h	24–48 h
Glargine (Lantus)	1–2 h	—	24 h
Detemir (Levemir)	1–2 h	6–8 h	24 h

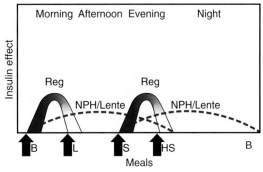

FIG. 23.5 Insulin effect of two daily doses of NPH/Lente plus regular insulin. ↑, Time of insulin injection; *B*, breakfast; *L,* lunch; *S,* supper; *HS,* bedtime. (Adapted from Hirsch IB, Farkas-Hirsch R, Skyler JS. Intensive insulin therapy for treatment of type I diabetes. *Diabetes Care.* 1990;13:1265-1283.)

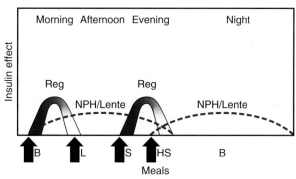

FIG. 23.6 Insulin effect of a regimen of three injections per day: NPH/Lente plus regular insulin in morning, regular insulin before supper, NPH/Lente at bedtime. ↑, Time of insulin injection; *B*, breakfast; *HS*, bedtime; *L,* lunch; *S,* supper.

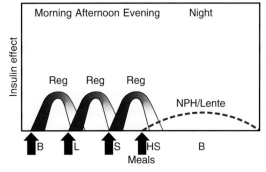

FIG. 23.7 Insulin effect of a regimen of four injections per day: short-acting insulin before each meal and NPH/Lente at bedtime. ↑, Time of insulin injection; *B*, breakfast; *HS*, bedtime; *L,* lunch; *S,* supper.

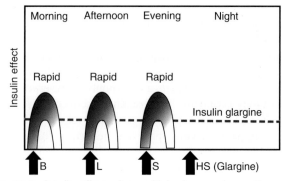

FIG. 23.8 Insulin effect of a multiple-dose regimen: three premeal doses of rapid-acting insulin (lispro/aspart) plus basal insulin (glargine). ↑, Time of insulin injection; *B*, breakfast; *HS*, bedtime; *L,* lunch; *S,* supper.

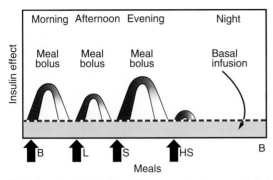

FIG. 23.9 Insulin effect of continuous subcutaneous infusion of short- or rapid-acting insulin before meals and snacks. ↑, Time of insulin injection; *B,* breakfast; *HS,* bedtime; *L,* lunch; *S,* supper.

TABLE 23.4	Diagnostic Features of Diabetic Ketoacidosis
Serum glucose level (mg/dL)	≥300
pH	≤7.3
HCO$_3^-$ (mEq/L)	≤18
Serum osmolarity (mOsm/L)	<320
Serum and urine ketone levels	Moderate to high

TABLE 23.5	Diagnostic Features of Hyperglycemic Hyperosmolar Syndrome
Glucose level (mg/dL)	≥600
pH	≥7.3
HCO$_3^-$ (mEq/L)	≥15
Serum osmolarity (mOsm/L)	≥350

includes administration of sugar in the form of sugar cubes, glucose tablets, or soft drinks if the patient is conscious; and glucose 0.5 g/kg IV or glucagon 0.5–1 mg IV, intramuscularly, or subcutaneously if the patient is unconscious.

Complications

Diabetic Ketoacidosis

Diabetic ketoacidosis (DKA) is a complication of decompensated diabetes mellitus. The signs and symptoms of DKA are primarily the result of abnormalities in carbohydrate and fat metabolism. Episodes of DKA occur more commonly in patients with type 1 diabetes and are precipitated by infection or acute illness. High glucose levels exceed the threshold for renal tubular absorption, which creates a significant osmotic diuresis with marked hypovolemia. A tight metabolic coupling between hepatic gluconeogenesis and ketogenesis leads to overproduction of ketoacids by the liver. An increase in production of ketoacids (β-hydroxybutyrate, acetoacetate, acetone) creates an anion-gap metabolic acidosis (Table 23.4). Substantial deficits of water, potassium, and phosphorus exist, although laboratory values of these electrolytes may be normal or increased. Hyponatremia results from the effect of hyperglycemia and hyperosmolarity on water distribution. The deficit of potassium is usually substantial (3–5 mEq/kg), and the deficit of phosphorus can lead to diaphragmatic and skeletal muscle dysfunction and impaired myocardial contractility.

Treatment of DKA consists of administration of large amounts of normal saline, effective doses of insulin, and electrolyte supplementation. An IV loading dose of 0.1 unit/kg of regular insulin plus a low-dose insulin infusion of 0.1 unit/kg/h

is initiated. Insulin administration must be continued until a normal acid-base status is achieved. The insulin rate is reduced when hyperglycemia is controlled, blood pH is higher than 7.3, and bicarbonate level exceeds 18 mEq/L. Potassium and phosphate are replaced with KCl and K$_2$PO$_4$. Magnesium is replaced as needed. Sodium bicarbonate is administered if blood pH is less than 7.1. The infrequent but devastating development of cerebral edema can result from correction of hyperglycemia without simultaneous correction of serum sodium level.

Hyperglycemic Hyperosmolar Syndrome

Hyperglycemic hyperosmolar syndrome is characterized by severe hyperglycemia, hyperosmolarity, and dehydration. It usually occurs in the context of an acute illness in patients with type 2 diabetes who are older than 60 years. The syndrome evolves over days to weeks, with a persistent glycosuric diuresis. The patient experiences polyuria, polydipsia, hypovolemia, hypotension, tachycardia, and organ hypoperfusion. Hyperosmolarity (>340 mOsm/L) is responsible for mental obtundation or coma (Table 23.5). Patients may have some degree of metabolic acidosis but do not demonstrate ketoacidosis.

Treatment includes significant fluid resuscitation, insulin administration, and electrolyte supplementation. If plasma osmolarity is greater than 320 mOsm/L, large volumes of hypotonic saline (1000–1500 mL/h) should be administered until the osmolarity is less than 320 mOsm/L, at which time large volumes of isotonic saline (1000–1500 mL/h) can be given. Insulin therapy is initiated with an IV bolus of 15 units of regular insulin followed by a 0.1-unit/kg/h infusion. The insulin infusion is decreased to 2–3 units/h when the glucose level decreases to approximately 250–300 mg/dL. Electrolyte deficits are significant but usually less severe than in DKA.

Microvascular Complications

Microvascular dysfunction is unique to diabetes and characterized by nonocclusive microcirculatory disease and impaired autoregulation of blood flow and vascular tone. Chronic hyperglycemia is essential for development of these changes, and intensive glycemic control delays the onset and slows the progression of microvascular effects.

Nephropathy

Approximately 30%–40% of individuals with type 1 diabetes and 5%–10% of those with type 2 diabetes develop end-stage renal disease. The clinical course is characterized by hypertension, albuminuria, peripheral edema, and a progressive decrease in glomerular filtration rate (GFR). When the GFR decreases to less than 15–20 mL/min, the ability of the kidneys to excrete potassium and acids is impaired, and patients develop hyperkalemia and metabolic acidosis. Hypertension, hyperglycemia, hypercholesterolemia, and microalbuminuria accelerate the decrease in GFR. Treatment of hypertension can markedly slow the progression of renal dysfunction. ACE inhibitors are particularly beneficial in diabetic patients because they retard the progression of proteinuria and the decrease in GFR.

Peripheral Neuropathy

More than 50% of patients who have had diabetes for longer than 25 years develop a peripheral neuropathy. A distal symmetric diffuse sensorimotor polyneuropathy is the most common form. Sensory deficits usually overshadow motor abnormalities and appear in the toes or feet and progress proximally toward the chest in a "stocking-glove" distribution. Loss of large sensory and motor fibers produces loss of light touch and proprioception as well as muscle weakness. Loss of small fibers decreases the perception of pain and temperature and produces dysesthesia, paresthesia, and neuropathic pain. Foot ulcers develop from mechanical and traumatic injury as a result of loss of cutaneous sensitivity to pain and temperature and impaired perfusion. Significant morbidity results from recurrent infection, foot fractures (Charcot joint), and subsequent amputations. Treatment of peripheral neuropathy includes optimal glucose control as well as use of nonsteroidal antiinflammatory drugs, antidepressants, and anticonvulsants for pain control.

Retinopathy

Diabetic retinopathy results from a variety of microvascular changes. Visual impairment can range from minor changes in color vision to total blindness. Strict glycemic control and blood pressure control can reduce the risk of development and progression of retinopathy.

Autonomic Neuropathy

Diabetic autonomic neuropathy can affect any part of the autonomic nervous system. Symptomatic autonomic neuropathy is rare and present in fewer than 5% of diabetics. The pathogenesis is not completely understood but may involve metabolic, microvascular, and/or autonomic abnormalities. Cardiovascular signs of autonomic neuropathy include abnormalities in heart rate control as well as central and peripheral vascular dynamics. A heart rate that fails to respond to exercise is indicative of significant cardiac denervation and is likely to result in substantially reduced exercise tolerance. The heart may demonstrate systolic and diastolic dysfunction with a reduced ejection fraction. Dysrhythmias may be responsible for sudden death. The presence of cardiovascular autonomic neuropathy can be demonstrated by measuring orthostatic changes in heart rate and blood pressure and the hemodynamic response to exercise.

Diabetic autonomic neuropathy may also impair gastric secretion and gastric motility, eventually causing gastroparesis diabeticorum in approximately 25% of diabetic patients. Although it is often clinically silent, symptomatic patients will have nausea, vomiting, early satiety, bloating, and epigastric pain. Treatment of gastroparesis includes strict blood glucose control, consumption of multiple small meals, reduction of the fat content of meals, and use of prokinetic agents such as metoclopramide. Diarrhea and constipation are also common among diabetic patients and may be related to diabetic autonomic neuropathy.

Macrovascular Complications

Cardiovascular disease is a major cause of morbidity and the leading cause of mortality in diabetic individuals. Patients with poorly controlled diabetes demonstrate elevated triglyceride levels, low levels of high-density lipoprotein cholesterol, and an abnormally small, dense, more atherogenic low-density lipoprotein cholesterol. Measures to prevent coronary artery disease include maintaining lipid levels, glucose level, and blood pressure within normal limits. Aspirin and statin therapy should be considered for all diabetic patients.

Management of Anesthesia

Preoperative Evaluation

Preoperative evaluation should emphasize the cardiovascular, renal, neurologic, and musculoskeletal systems. The index of suspicion should be high for myocardial ischemia and infarction. Silent ischemia is possible if autonomic neuropathy is present, and stress testing should be considered in patients with multiple cardiac risk factors and poor or indeterminate exercise tolerance. For renal disease, control of hypertension is important. Meticulous attention to hydration status, avoidance of nephrotoxins, and preservation of renal blood flow are also essential. The presence of autonomic neuropathy predisposes the patient to perioperative dysrhythmias and intraoperative hypotension. In addition, loss of compensatory sympathetic responses interferes with detection and treatment of hemodynamic insults. Preoperative evaluation of the musculoskeletal system should look for limited joint mobility caused by nonenzymatic glycosylation of proteins and abnormal cross-linking of collagen. Gastroparesis may increase the risk of aspiration, regardless of nothing-by-mouth status.

Management of insulin in the preoperative period depends on the type of insulin the patient takes and the timing of dosing. If a patient takes subcutaneous insulin each night at bedtime, two-thirds of this dose (NPH and regular) should be administered the night before surgery, and one-half of the usual morning NPH dose should be given on the day of surgery. The daily morning dose of regular insulin should be held. If the patient uses an insulin pump, the overnight rate should be decreased by 30%. On the morning of surgery, the pump can be kept infusing at the basal rate or discontinued and replaced with a continuous insulin infusion at the same rate. Alternatively the patient can be given subcutaneous glargine and the pump discontinued 60–90 minutes after administration. If the patient uses glargine and lispro or aspart

TABLE 23.6	Inpatient Insulin Algorithm

Goal BG: _____ mg/dL
Standard drip: Regular insulin 100 units/100 mL 0.9% NaCl via infusion device
Initiation of infusion:
    Bolus dose: Regular insulin 0.1 unit/kg = _____ units
    Algorithm 1: Start here for most patients.
    Algorithm 2: Start here if patient has undergone CABG, solid organ transplant, or islet cell transplant; is receiving glucocorticoids or vasopressors; or is diabetic and receiving >80 units/day of insulin as an outpatient.

Algorithm 1		Algorithm 2		Algorithm 3		Algorithm 4	
BG	Units/h	BG	Units/h	BG	Units/h	BG	Units/h
<60 = Hypoglycemia (see below for treatment)							
<70	Off	<70	Off	<70	Off	<70	Off
70–109	0.2	70–109	0.5	70–109	1	70–109	1.5
110–119	0.5	110–119	1	110–119	2	110–119	3
120–149	1	120–149	1.5	120–149	3	120–149	5
150–179	1.5	150–179	2	150–179	4	150–179	7
180–209	2	180–209	3	180–209	5	180–209	9
210–239	2	210–239	4	210–239	6	210–239	12
240–269	3	240–269	5	240–269	8	240–269	16
270–299	3	270–299	6	270–299	10	270–299	20
300–329	4	300–329	7	300–329	12	300–329	24
330–359	4	330–359	8	330–359	14	>330	28
>360	6	>360	12	>360	16		

MOVING FROM ALGORITHM TO ALGORITHM

Moving up: Move to higher algorithm when current algorithm fails, defined as BG outside goal range for 2 h (see above goal) and failure of level to change by at least 60 mg/dL within 1 h.

Moving down: Move to lower algorithm when BG is <70 mg/dL for two checks OR BG decreases by >100 mg/dL in 1 h.

Tube feeds or TPN: Decrease infusion by 50% if nutrition (tube feeds or TPN) is discontinued or significantly reduced. Reinstitute hourly BG checks every 4 h.

Patient monitoring: Check capillary BG every hour until it is within goal range for 4 h, then decrease to every 2 h for 4 h, and if it remains at goal, may decrease to every 4 h.

TREATMENT OF HYPOGLYCEMIA (BG < 60 mg/dL)

Discontinue insulin drip
    and
Give D$_{50}$W IV
    Patient conscious: 25 mL (½ amp)
    Patient unconscious: 50 mL (1 amp)
    Recheck BG every 20 min and repeat 25 min of D$_{50}$W IV if <60 mg/dL. Restart drip once BG is >70 mg/dL for two checks. Restart drip with lower algorithm (see Moving Down).

INTRAVENOUS FLUIDS

Most patients will need 5–10 g of glucose per hour (D$_5$W or D$_5$ ½ NS at 100-200 mL/h or equivalent [TPN, enteral feeds]).

amp, Ampule; *BG,* blood glucose; *CABG,* coronary artery bypass graft; *D$_5$W,* 5% dextrose in water; *D$_5$ ½ NS,* 5% dextrose in half-normal saline; *D$_{50}$W,* 50% dextrose in water; *IV,* intravenously; *TPN,* total parenteral nutrition.

for daily glycemic control, he or she should take two-thirds of the glargine dose and the entire lispro or aspart dose the night before surgery and hold all morning dosing. Oral hypoglycemics should be discontinued 24–48 hours preoperatively. It is advised that sulfonylureas be avoided during the *entire* perioperative period because they block the myocardial potassium adenosine triphosphate (ATP) channels responsible for ischemia- and anesthetic-induced preconditioning.

Intraoperative Management

Aggressive glycemic control is important intraoperatively (Table 23.6). Ideally a continuous infusion of insulin should be initiated at least 2 hours before surgery. Intraoperative serum glucose levels should be maintained between 120 and 180 mg/dL. Levels above 200 mg/dL are likely to cause glycosuria and dehydration and to inhibit wound healing. Typically 1 unit of insulin lowers glucose approximately 25–30 mg/dL. The initial hourly rate for a continuous insulin infusion is determined by dividing the total daily insulin requirement by 24. A typical rate is 0.02 unit/kg/h, or 1.4 units/h in a 70-kg patient. An insulin infusion can be prepared by mixing 100 units of regular insulin in 100 mL of normal saline (1 unit/mL). Insulin infusion requirements are higher for patients undergoing coronary artery bypass graft surgery, patients receiving steroids, patients with severe infection, and patients receiving hyperalimentation or vasopressor infusions. An insulin infusion should be accompanied by an infusion of 5% dextrose in half-normal saline with 20 mEq KCl at 100–150 mL/h to provide enough carbohydrate (at least 150 g/day) to inhibit hepatic glucose production and protein catabolism. Serum glucose levels should be monitored at least every hour and even every 30 minutes in patients undergoing coronary artery bypass surgery or patients with high insulin requirements. Glucose determination is preferentially made using venous plasma or serum samples; arterial and capillary blood yields glucose values approximately 7% higher than those for venous blood, and whole-blood determinations are usually 15% lower than plasma or serum values. Urine glucose monitoring is not reliable.

Avoidance of hypoglycemia is especially critical, since recognition of hypoglycemia may be delayed in patients receiving anesthetics, sedatives, analgesics, β-blockers, or sympatholytics and in those with autonomic neuropathy. If hypoglycemia does occur, treatment consists of administration of 50 mL of 50% dextrose in water, which typically increases the glucose level 100 mg/dL or 2 mg/dL/mL.

Postoperative Care

Postoperative management of diabetic patients requires meticulous monitoring of insulin requirements. Hyperglycemia has been associated with poor outcomes in postoperative and critically ill patients. However, the optimal target for blood glucose level in the perioperative period has not yet been defined. In addition, this target may be different for patients with newly diagnosed hyperglycemia than for those with preexisting diabetes. The risks of hypoglycemia must also be considered. Currently the ADA recommends that glucose levels be maintained between 140 and 180 mg/dL in critically ill patients and that insulin treatment be initiated if serum glucose levels exceed 180 mg/dL.

INSULINOMA

Insulinomas are rare, benign, insulin-secreting pancreatic islet cell tumors. They usually occur as an isolated finding but may present as part of multiple endocrine neoplasia syndrome type I (MEN I; insulinoma, hyperparathyroidism, and a pituitary tumor). They occur in women twice as often as in men and usually in the fifth or sixth decade of life. The diagnosis is made by demonstrating Whipple's triad: (1) symptoms of hypoglycemia with fasting, (2) a glucose level below 50 mg/dL with symptoms, and (3) relief of symptoms with administration of glucose. An inappropriately high insulin level (>5–10 microunits/mL) during a 48- to 72-hour fast confirms the diagnosis.

Preoperatively, patients are often managed with diazoxide, an agent that directly inhibits insulin release from beta cells. Other medical therapies include verapamil, phenytoin, propranolol, glucocorticoids, and the somatostatin analogues octreotide and lanreotide. Surgical treatment is curative. Ninety percent of insulinomas are benign, and tumor

enucleation is the procedure of choice. Laparoscopic resection is used in selected cases.

Profound hypoglycemia can occur intraoperatively, particularly during manipulation of the tumor; however, marked hyperglycemia can follow removal of the tumor. In a few medical centers, an artificial pancreas that continuously analyzes the blood glucose concentration and automatically infuses insulin or glucose has been used for intraoperative management of these patients. In most cases, serial blood glucose measurements (every 15 minutes) are taken using a standard glucometer. Since evidence of hypoglycemia may be masked under anesthesia, it is probably wise to include glucose in intravenously administered fluids.

THYROID DISEASE

The thyroid gland weighs approximately 20 g and is composed of two lobes joined by an isthmus. The gland is closely affixed to the anterior and lateral aspects of the trachea, with the upper border of the isthmus located just below the cricoid cartilage. A pair of parathyroid glands is located on the posterior aspect of each lobe. The gland is innervated by the adrenergic and cholinergic nervous systems. The recurrent laryngeal nerve and external motor branch of the superior laryngeal nerve are in intimate proximity to the gland. Histologically the thyroid is composed of numerous follicles filled with proteinaceous colloid. The major constituent of colloid is thyroglobulin, an iodinated glycoprotein that serves as the substrate for thyroid hormone synthesis. The thyroid gland also contains parafollicular C cells that produce calcitonin.

Production of normal quantities of thyroid hormones depends on the availability of exogenous iodine. The diet is the primary source of iodine. Iodine is reduced to iodide in the GI tract, rapidly absorbed into the blood, then actively transported from the plasma into thyroid follicular cells (Fig. 23.10). Binding of iodine to thyroglobulin (i.e., organification) is catalyzed by an iodinase enzyme and yields inactive monoiodotyrosine and diiodotyrosine. Approximately 25% of the monoiodotyrosine and diiodotyrosine undergo coupling via thyroid peroxidase to form the active compounds triiodothyronine (T_3) and thyroxine (T_4). The remaining 75% never becomes hormones, and eventually the iodine is cleaved and recycled. T_3 and T_4 remain attached to thyroglobulin and are stored as colloid until they are released into the circulation. Since the thyroid contains a large store of hormones and has a low turnover rate, there is protection against depletion if synthesis is impaired or discontinued.

The T_4:T_3 ratio of secreted hormones is 10:1. Upon entering the blood, T_4 and T_3 bind reversibly to three major proteins: thyroxine-binding globulin (80% of binding), prealbumin (10%–15%), and albumin (5%–10%). Only the small amount of free fraction of hormone, however, is biologically active. Although only 10% of thyroid hormone secretion is T_3, T_3 is three to four times more active than T_4 per unit of weight and may be the only active thyroid hormone in peripheral tissues. Thyroid hormones stimulate virtually all metabolic processes.

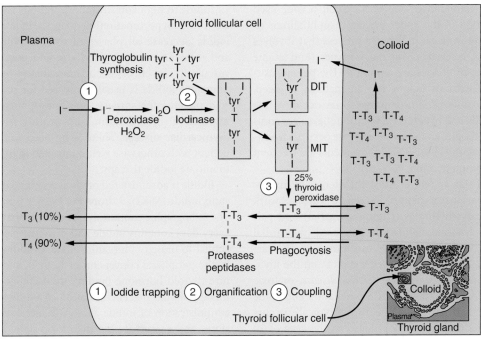

FIG. 23.10 Thyroid follicular cell. *DIT,* Diiodotyrosine; *MIT,* monoiodotyrosine; *T,* thyroglobulin; *T$_3$,* 3,5,3′-triiodothyronine (triiodothyronine); *T$_4$,* 3,5,3′,5′-tetraiodothyronine (thyroxine); *tyr,* tyrosine.

They influence growth and maturation of tissues, enhance tissue function, and stimulate protein synthesis and carbohydrate and lipid metabolism.

Thyroid hormone acts directly on cardiac myocytes and vascular smooth muscle cells. Thyroid hormone increases myocardial contractility directly, decreases systemic vascular resistance via direct vasodilation, and increases intravascular volume. Most recent studies emphasize the direct effects of T$_3$ on the heart and vascular smooth muscle as responsible for the exaggerated hemodynamic effects of hyperthyroidism.

Regulation of thyroid function is controlled by the hypothalamus, pituitary, and thyroid glands, which participate in a classic feedback control system. Thyrotropin-releasing hormone (TRH) is secreted from the hypothalamus, traverses the pituitary stalk, and promotes release of thyrotropin-stimulating hormone (TSH) from the anterior pituitary. TSH binds to specific receptors on the thyroid cell membrane and enhances all processes of synthesis and secretion of T$_4$ and T$_3$. A decrease in TSH causes a reduction in synthesis and secretion of T$_4$ and T$_3$, a decrease in follicular cell size, and a decrease in the gland's vascularity. An increase in TSH yields an increase in hormone production and release and an increase in gland cellularity and vascularity. TSH secretion is also influenced by plasma levels of T$_4$ and T$_3$ via a negative feedback loop. In addition to the feedback system, the thyroid gland has an autoregulatory mechanism that maintains a consistent level of hormone stores.

Diagnosis

The third generation of the TSH assay is now the single best test of thyroid hormone action at the cellular level. Small changes in thyroid function cause significant changes in TSH secretion. The normal level of TSH is 0.4–5.0 milliunits/L. A TSH level of 0.1–0.4 milliunits/L with normal levels of free T$_3$ (FT$_3$) and free T$_4$ (FT$_4$) is diagnostic of subclinical hyperthyroidism. A TSH level below 0.03 milliunits/L with elevated T$_3$ and T$_4$ is diagnostic of overt hyperthyroidism. A TSH level of 5.0–10 milliunits/L with normal levels of FT$_3$ and FT$_4$ is diagnostic of subclinical hypothyroidism. A TSH level higher than 20 milliunits/L (may be as high as 200 or even 400 milliunits/L) with reduced levels of T$_3$ and T$_4$ is diagnostic of overt hypothyroidism.

The TRH stimulation test assesses the functional state of the TSH-secreting mechanism in response to TRH and is used to test pituitary function. Thyroid scans using iodine 123 (^{123}I) or technetium 99m (^{99m}Tc) evaluate thyroid nodules as "warm" (normally functioning), "hot" (hyperfunctioning), or "cold" (hypofunctioning). Ultrasonography is 90%–95% accurate in determining whether a lesion is cystic, solid, or mixed.

Hyperthyroidism

Signs and Symptoms

Hyperthyroidism refers to hyperfunctioning of the thyroid gland, with excessive secretion of active thyroid hormones. The majority of cases of hyperthyroidism result from one of three pathologic processes: Graves disease, toxic multinodular goiter, or a toxic adenoma. Regardless of the cause, the signs and symptoms of hyperthyroidism are those of a hypermetabolic state. The patient is anxious, restless, and hyperkinetic and may be emotionally unstable. The skin is warm and moist, the face is flushed, the hair is fine, and the nails are soft and fragile. The patient may demonstrate increased sweating and complain of heat intolerance. The eyes exhibit a wide-eyed stare, with retraction of the upper eyelids (exophthalmos or proptosis) resulting from an infiltrative process that involves retrobulbar fat and the eyelids. Wasting, weakness, and fatigue of the proximal limb muscles are common. The patient usually complains of extreme fatigue but an inability to sleep. Increased bone turnover and osteoporosis may occur. A fine tremor of the hands and hyperactive tendon reflexes are common. Weight loss despite an increased appetite occurs secondary to increased calorigenesis. Bowel movements are frequent and diarrhea is not uncommon.

The cardiovascular system is most threatened by hypermetabolism of peripheral tissues, increased cardiac work with tachycardia, dysrhythmias (commonly atrial) and palpitations, a hyperdynamic circulation, increased myocardial contractility and cardiac output, and cardiomegaly. The cardiac responses are due to the direct effects of T_3 on the myocardium and peripheral vasculature. *Graves disease,* or toxic diffuse goiter, occurs in 0.4% of the US population and is the leading cause of hyperthyroidism. The disease typically occurs in females (female/male ratio is 7:1) between the ages of 20 and 40 years. Although the etiology is unknown, Graves disease appears to be a systemic autoimmune disease caused by thyroid-stimulating antibodies that bind to TSH receptors in the thyroid, activating adenylcyclase and stimulating thyroid growth, vascularity, and hypersecretion of T_4 and T_3. The thyroid is usually diffusely enlarged, becoming two to three times its normal size. An ophthalmopathy occurs in 30% of cases and may include upper lid retraction, a wide-eyed stare, muscle weakness, proptosis, and an increase in intraocular pressure. The diagnosis of Graves disease is confirmed by the presence of thyroid-stimulating antibodies in the context of a low TSH level and elevated T_4 and T_3 levels.

Toxic multinodular goiter usually arises from long-standing simple goiter and occurs mostly in patients older than age 50. It may present with extreme thyroid enlargement that can cause dysphagia, globus sensation, and possibly inspiratory stridor from tracheal compression. The latter is especially common when the mass extends into the thoracic inlet behind the sternum. In severe cases, superior vena cava obstruction syndrome may also be present. The diagnosis is confirmed by a thyroid scan demonstrating "hot" patchy foci throughout the gland or one or two "hot" nodules. Radioactive iodine uptake and serum T_4 and T_3 levels may only be slightly elevated. The goiter must be differentiated from a neoplasm, and a computed tomography (CT) scan and biopsy may be necessary.

Treatment

The first line of treatment for hyperthyroidism is an antithyroid drug, either methimazole or propylthiouracil (PTU). These agents interfere with the synthesis of thyroid hormones by inhibiting organification and coupling. PTU has the added advantage of inhibiting the peripheral conversion of T_4 to T_3. A euthyroid state can almost always be achieved in 6–8 weeks with either drug if a sufficient dosage is used.

Iodide in high concentrations inhibits release of hormones from the hyperfunctioning gland. High concentrations of iodide decrease all phases of thyroid synthesis and release and result in reduced gland size and possibly a decrease in vascularity. Its effects occur immediately but are short-lived. Therefore iodide is usually reserved for preparing hyperthyroid patients for surgery, managing patients with actual or impending thyroid storm, and treating patients with severe thyrocardiac disease. There is no need to delay surgery in a patient with otherwise well-controlled thyrotoxicosis in order to initiate iodide therapy.

Iodide is administered orally as a saturated solution of potassium iodide (SSKI), 3 drops PO every 8 hours for 10–14 days. The radiographic contrast dye ipodate or iopanoic acid (0.5–3.0 g every day) contains iodide and demonstrates beneficial effects similar to those of inorganic iodide. In addition, ipodate inhibits the peripheral conversion of T_4 to T_3 and may also antagonize thyroid hormone binding to receptors. Antithyroid drug therapy should precede initiation of iodide treatment, because administration of iodide alone will increase thyroid hormone stores and exacerbate the thyrotoxic state. Lithium carbonate 300 mg PO every 6 hours may be given in place of potassium iodide or ipodate to patients who are allergic to iodide.

β-Adrenergic antagonists do not affect the underlying thyroid abnormality but may relieve signs and symptoms of increased adrenergic activity such as anxiety, sweating, heat intolerance, tremors, and tachycardia. Propranolol offers the added features of impairing the peripheral conversion of T_4 to T_3.

Ablative therapy with radioactive iodine 131 (^{131}I) or surgery is recommended for patients with Graves disease for whom medical management has failed, as well as for patients with toxic multinodular goiter or a toxic adenoma. The remission rate is 80%–98%. A major disadvantage of therapy is that 40%–70% of treated patients become hypothyroid within 10 years.

Surgery (i.e., subtotal thyroidectomy or possibly total thyroidectomy) results in prompt control of disease and is associated with a lower incidence of hypothyroidism (10%–30%) than radioactive iodine therapy. Subtotal thyroidectomy corrects thyrotoxicosis in over 95% of patients.

Hyperthyroidism during pregnancy is treated with low dosages of antithyroid drugs. However, these drugs do cross the placenta and can cause fetal hypothyroidism. If the mother remains euthyroid while taking small dosages of an antithyroid drug, the occurrence of fetal hypothyroidism is rare. Radioactive iodine treatment is contraindicated during pregnancy, as is oral iodide therapy, because it can cause fetal goiter and hypothyroidism. Long-term use of propranolol during pregnancy is controversial, since intrauterine growth retardation has been attributed to its use. Thyroid storm occurring in pregnancy is managed in the same way as in nonpregnant patients.

Management of Anesthesia

In hyperthyroid patients undergoing surgery, euthyroidism should definitely be established preoperatively. In elective cases this may mean waiting a substantial time (6–8 weeks) for antithyroid drugs to become effective. In emergency cases the use of an IV β-blocker, ipodate, glucocorticoids, and PTU is usually necessary. No IV preparation of PTU is available, so the drug must be taken orally, via a nasogastric tube, or rectally. Glucocorticoids (dexamethasone 2 mg IV every 6 hours) should be administered to decrease hormone release and reduce the peripheral conversion of T_4 to T_3.

Evaluation of the upper airway for evidence of tracheal compression or deviation caused by a goiter is an important part of the preoperative evaluation. Examination of chest radiographs and CT scans is often helpful in this regard. Intraoperatively the need for invasive monitoring is determined on an individual basis and depends on the type of surgery to be performed and the medical condition of the patient. Controlled studies in hyperthyroid animals demonstrate no clinically significant increase in anesthetic requirements (i.e., minimum alveolar concentration). Establishment of adequate anesthetic depth is extremely important to avoid exaggerated sympathetic nervous system responses. Drugs that stimulate the sympathetic nervous system (i.e., ketamine, pancuronium, atropine, ephedrine, epinephrine) should be avoided. Eye protection (eyedrops, lubricant, eye pads) is critical, especially for patients with proptosis.

For maintenance of anesthesia, any of the potent inhalation agents may be used. A concern in hyperthyroid patients is organ toxicity secondary to an increase in drug metabolism. Nitrous oxide and opioids are safe and effective in hyperthyroid patients. Hyperthyroid patients may have co-existing muscle disease (e.g., myasthenia gravis) with reduced requirements for the nondepolarizing muscle relaxants; therefore careful titration is required. For treatment of intraoperative hypotension, a direct-acting vasopressor (phenylephrine) is preferred. Ephedrine, epinephrine, norepinephrine, and dopamine should be avoided or administered in extremely low doses to prevent exaggerated hemodynamic responses. Regional anesthesia can be safely performed and in fact may be a preferred technique. Epinephrine-containing local anesthetic solutions should be avoided.

Removal of the thyrotoxic gland does not mean immediate resolution of thyrotoxicosis. The half-life of T_4 is 7–8 days; therefore β-blocker therapy may need to be continued in the postoperative period.

Thyroid Storm

Thyroid storm is a life-threatening exacerbation of hyperthyroidism precipitated by trauma, infection, medical illness, or surgery. Thyroid storm and malignant hyperthermia can present with similar intraoperative and postoperative signs and symptoms (i.e., hyperpyrexia, tachycardia, hypermetabolism); differentiation between the two may be extremely difficult.

Thyroid storm most often occurs in the postoperative period in untreated or inadequately treated hyperthyroid patients after emergency surgery. Patients manifest extreme anxiety, fever, tachycardia, cardiovascular instability, and altered consciousness. Treatment includes rapid alleviation of thyrotoxicosis and general supportive care. Dehydration is

managed with IV administration of glucose-containing crystalloid solutions, and cooling measures (e.g., cooling blanket, ice packs, administration of cool humidified oxygen) are used to counter the fever. β-Blockers should be titrated to decrease heart rate to less than 90 beats per minute. Dexamethasone 2 mg every 6 hours or cortisol 100–200 mg every 8 hours can be used to decrease hormone release and conversion of T_4 to T_3. Antithyroid drugs (PTU 200–400 mg every 8 hours) may be administered through a nasogastric tube, orally, or rectally. If circulatory shock is present, IV administration of a direct vasopressor (phenylephrine) is indicated. A β-adrenergic blocker or digitalis is recommended for atrial fibrillation accompanied by a fast ventricular response. Serum thyroid hormone levels generally return to normal within 24–48 hours, and recovery occurs within 1 week. The mortality rate for thyroid storm remains surprisingly high at approximately 20%.

Hypothyroidism

Signs and Symptoms

Hypothyroidism, or *myxedema,* is a relatively common disease affecting 0.5%–0.8% of the adult population. Primary hypothyroidism results in decreased production of thyroid hormones despite adequate or increased levels of TSH and accounts for 95% of all cases of hypothyroidism. The most common cause in the United States is ablation of the gland by radioactive iodine or surgery. The second most common type of hypothyroidism is idiopathic and probably autoimmune in origin, with autoantibodies blocking TSH receptors in the thyroid. *Hashimoto thyroiditis* is an autoimmune disorder characterized by goitrous enlargement and hypothyroidism that usually affects middle-aged women.

In adults, hypothyroidism has a slow, insidious, progressive course. There is gradual slowing of mental and physical activity. In mild cases, patients tire easily and experience weight gain. In moderate to severe cases, patients develop fatigue, lethargy, apathy, and listlessness. Speech becomes slow and the intellect becomes dull. With time, patients experience cold intolerance, decreased sweating, constipation, menorrhagia, and slowing of motor function secondary to muscle stiffness and cramping. They gain weight despite a decrease in appetite. Physically they demonstrate dry thickened skin, coarse facial features, dry brittle hair, a large tongue, a deep hoarse voice, and periorbital and peripheral edema.

Physiologically, cardiac output is decreased secondary to reductions in stroke volume and heart rate. Baroreceptor function is also impaired. The electrocardiogram (ECG) in patients with overt hypothyroidism shows flattened or inverted T waves, low-amplitude P waves and QRS complexes, and sinus bradycardia; ventricular dysrhythmias may also be present. Peripheral vascular resistance is increased and blood volume is reduced, which results in pale, cool skin. Pericardial effusions are common. Hypothyroid patients usually have hypercholesterolemia and hypertriglyceridemia and may have coronary artery disease. Hyponatremia and impairment of free water excretion are also common, related to inappropriate secretion of antidiuretic hormone (ADH). Gastrointestinal function is slow, and an adynamic ileus may occur. Deep tendon reflexes demonstrate a prolonged relaxation phase.

Twenty percent of women older than 60 years have subclinical hypothyroidism. Subclinical disease is associated with an increased risk of coronary heart disease in patients with a TSH level above 10 milliunits/L. Even though changes are reversible with L-thyroxine therapy, use of thyroid replacement for subclinical disease remains controversial.

Secondary hypothyroidism is diagnosed by reduced levels of FT_4, T_4, and T_3, as well as a reduced TSH level. A TRH stimulation test can confirm pituitary abnormality as the cause. In primary hypothyroidism, basal levels of TSH are elevated, and the elevation is exaggerated after TRH administration. With pituitary dysfunction there is a blunted or absent response to TRH.

Euthyroid sick syndrome is the occurrence of abnormal results on thyroid function tests in critically ill patients with significant nonthyroidal illness. Characteristic findings include low levels of T_3 and T_4 and a normal TSH level. As illness increases in severity, T_3 and T_4 levels decrease further. The etiology of this response is not understood. Euthyroid sick syndrome may be a physiologic response to stress, and it can be induced by surgery. No treatment for thyroid function is necessary. Differentiating hypothyroidism from euthyroid sick syndrome can be extremely difficult. A serum TSH level is the best aid. Levels higher than 10 milliunits/L indicate hypothyroidism, whereas levels lower than 5.0 milliunits/L indicate euthyroidism.

Changes in thyroid function test results have also been documented following uncomplicated acute myocardial infarctions, congestive heart failure, and cardiopulmonary bypass. Significant depression of T_3 levels occurs, but administration of T_3 does not appear efficacious. In addition, the use of T_3 as an inotrope has not been shown to result in any substantial improvement in cardiac performance.

Treatment

L-Thyroxine (levothyroxine sodium) is usually administered for the treatment of hypothyroidism. The first evidence of a therapeutic response to thyroid hormone is sodium and water diuresis and a reduction in the TSH level. In patients with hypothyroid cardiomyopathy, a measurable improvement in myocardial function is often achieved with therapy.

Although angina is uncommon in hypothyroidism, it can appear or worsen during treatment of the hypothyroid state with thyroid hormone. Medical management of such patients is particularly difficult.

Management of Anesthesia

Hypothyroid patients may be at increased risk for a number of reasons when undergoing either general or regional anesthesia. Airway compromise secondary to a swollen oral cavity, edematous vocal cords, or goitrous enlargement may be present. Decreased gastric emptying increases the risk of regurgitation and aspiration. A hypodynamic cardiovascular system

characterized by decreased cardiac output, stroke volume, heart rate, baroreceptor reflexes, and intravascular volume may be compromised by surgical stress and cardiac-depressant anesthetic agents. Decreased ventilatory responsiveness to hypoxia and hypercarbia is enhanced by anesthetic agents. Hypothermia occurs quickly and is difficult to treat. Hematologic abnormalities such as anemia (25%–50% of patients) and dysfunction of platelets and coagulation factors (especially factor VIII), electrolyte imbalances (hyponatremia), and hypoglycemia are common and require close monitoring intraoperatively. Decreased neuromuscular excitability is exacerbated by anesthetic drugs.

These patients can be extremely sensitive to narcotics and sedatives and may even be lethargic secondary to their disease; therefore preoperative sedation should be undertaken with caution. Hypothyroid patients also appear to have an increased sensitivity to anesthetic drugs, although the effect of thyroid activity on the minimum alveolar concentration of volatile anesthetics is negligible. Increased sensitivity is probably secondary to reduced cardiac output, decreased blood volume, abnormal baroreceptor function, decreased hepatic metabolism, and decreased renal excretion of drugs. In patients with a hypodynamic cardiovascular system, invasive monitoring and/or transesophageal echocardiography may be needed to monitor intravascular volume and cardiac status.

General anesthetics should be administered through an endotracheal tube following either rapid-sequence induction or awake intubation if a difficult airway is present. Hypothyroid patients are very sensitive to the myocardial-depressant effects of the potent inhalational agents. Vasodilation in the presence of possible hypovolemia and impaired baroreceptor activity can produce significant hypotension. Pharmacologic support for intraoperative hypotension is best provided with ephedrine, dopamine, or epinephrine and *not* a pure α-adrenergic agonist (phenylephrine). Unresponsive hypotension may require supplemental steroid administration.

Controlled ventilation is recommended in all cases, since these patients tend to hypoventilate if allowed to breathe spontaneously. Dextrose in normal saline is the recommended IV fluid to avoid hypoglycemia and minimize hyponatremia secondary to impaired free water clearance.

If emergency surgery is necessary, the potential for severe intraoperative cardiovascular instability and myxedema coma in the postoperative period is high. Intravenous thyroid replacement therapy should be initiated as soon as possible. Although IV L-thyroxine takes 10–12 days to yield a peak basal metabolic rate, IV triiodothyronine is effective in 6 hours, with a peak basal metabolic rate seen in 36–72 hours. L-Thyroxine 300–500 μg IV or L-triiodothyronine 25–50 μg IV is an acceptable initial dose. Steroid coverage with hydrocortisone or dexamethasone is necessary, since decreased adrenal cortical function often accompanies hypothyroidism. Phosphodiesterase inhibitors such as milrinone may be effective in the treatment of reduced myocardial contractility, because their mechanism of action does not depend on β receptors, whose number and sensitivity may be reduced in hypothyroidism.

Myxedema Coma

Myxedema coma is a rare severe form of hypothyroidism characterized by delirium or unconsciousness, hypoventilation, hypothermia (80% of patients), bradycardia, hypotension, and a severe dilutional hyponatremia. It occurs most commonly in elderly women with a long history of hypothyroidism. Infection, trauma, cold, and central nervous system (CNS) depressants predispose hypothyroid patients to myxedema coma. Ironically most patients are not comatose. Hypothermia (as low as 27°C) is a cardinal feature and results from impaired thermoregulation caused by defective function of the hypothalamus (a target tissue of thyroid hormone). Myxedema coma is a medical emergency with a mortality rate higher than 50%. Intravenous L-thyroxine or L-triiodothyronine is the treatment of choice. Intravenous hydration with glucose-containing saline solutions, temperature regulation, correction of electrolyte imbalances, and stabilization of the cardiac and pulmonary systems are necessary. Mechanical ventilation is frequently required. Heart rate, blood pressure, and temperature usually improve within 24 hours, and a relative euthyroid state is achieved in 3–5 days. Hydrocortisone 100–300 mg/day IV is also prescribed to treat possible adrenal insufficiency.

Goiter and Thyroid Tumors

A goiter is a swelling of the thyroid gland that results from compensatory hypertrophy and hyperplasia of follicular epithelium secondary to a reduction in thyroid hormone output. The cause may be a deficient intake of iodine, ingestion of a dietary (e.g., cassava) or pharmacologic (e.g., phenylbutazone, lithium) goitrogen, or a defect in the hormonal biosynthetic pathway. The size of the goiter is determined by the level and duration of hormone insufficiency. In most cases a goiter is associated with a euthyroid state, with the increased mass and cellular activity eventually overcoming the impairment in hormone synthesis. However, hypothyroidism or hyperthyroidism occurs in some cases. Patients with simple nontoxic goiter are euthyroid. Nevertheless, simple nontoxic goiter is a forerunner of toxic multinodular goiter. In the United States, most cases of simple nontoxic goiter are of unknown cause and are treated with L-thyroxine. Surgery is indicated only if medical therapy is ineffective and the goiter is compromising the airway or is cosmetically unacceptable.

Anesthetic management of a patient undergoing surgical removal of a large goiter or thyroid mass that compromises the airway presents a major challenge. Examination of a CT scan of the neck will demonstrate anatomic abnormalities. Sedatives and narcotics should be avoided or used with great caution before and during endotracheal tube placement. Awake intubation with an armored (anode) tube using fiberoptic bronchoscopy is probably the safest method to assess the degree of obstruction and establish the airway. Surgical removal of the mass may reveal underlying tracheomalacia and a collapsible airway. Tracheal extubation should be performed with as much caution and concern as intubation.

If the mass extends into the substernal regional (i.e., anterior mediastinal mass), superior vena cava obstruction, major airway obstruction, and/or cardiac compression may occur. The latter two may become apparent only upon induction of general anesthesia. Airway obstruction appears to result from changes in lung and chest wall mechanics that occur with changes in patient position or with the onset of muscle paralysis. During spontaneous respiration, the larger airways are supported by negative intrathoracic pressure, and the effects of extrinsic compression may be apparent in only the most severe cases. With cessation of spontaneous respiration, compensatory mechanisms are removed and airway obstruction occurs. In addition, positive pressure ventilation may demonstrate total airway occlusion. A preoperative history of dyspnea in the upright or supine position is predictive of possible airway obstruction during general anesthesia. A CT scan must be examined to assess the extent of the tumor. Echocardiography with the patient in the upright and supine positions can indicate the degree of cardiac compression.

If practical, local anesthesia is recommended for patients requiring surgery. If general anesthesia is necessary, preoperative shrinkage of a thyroid tumor by radiation or chemotherapy is recommended unless the altered histologic appearance would prevent an accurate diagnosis, as when a biopsy specimen is required for diagnosis. Unfortunately, goiters are not sensitive to radiation therapy. In such patients an awake intubation with fiberoptic bronchoscopy using an anode tube is recommended. The patient is placed in semi-Fowler position, and volatile anesthetic with nitrous oxide and oxygen is administered using spontaneous ventilation. Muscle relaxants are avoided. It must be possible to change the patient's position.

Following tumor resection the airway should be examined by fiberoptic bronchoscopy to detect tracheomalacia and determine whether and when tracheal extubation is appropriate. A rigid bronchoscope should be available to reestablish the airway if collapse occurs. Cardiopulmonary bypass equipment should be on standby during the case.

Complications of Thyroid Surgery

Morbidity from thyroid surgery approaches 13%. Recurrent laryngeal nerve injury may be unilateral or bilateral and temporary or permanent. The injury may result from excess trauma to the nerve(s) (abductor and/or adductor fibers of the recurrent laryngeal nerve), inadvertent ligation, or transection. When paralysis of the abductor muscles to the vocal cord occurs, the involved cord assumes a median or paramedian position. If trauma is unilateral, the patient experiences hoarseness but no airway obstruction, and function usually returns in 3–6 months. Ligation or transection of the nerve results in permanent hoarseness. Bilateral involvement is more serious, since the patient usually experiences airway obstruction and problems with coughing and respiratory toilet. Depending on the degree of damage, a temporary or permanent tracheostomy is usually necessary. Injury to the adductor fibers of the recurrent laryngeal nerve(s) results in paralysis of the adductor muscle(s) and increases the risk of pulmonary aspiration. Injury to the motor branch of the superior laryngeal nerve, which innervates the inferior pharyngeal constrictor and cricothyroid muscles, can also occur during thyroid dissection. This injury results in weakening of the voice and inability to create high tones.

Hypoparathyroidism is also a complication of thyroid surgery. It usually results from damage to the blood supply of the parathyroid glands rather than inadvertent removal. One functioning parathyroid gland with an adequate blood supply is all that is necessary to avoid hypoparathyroidism. The signs and symptoms of hypocalcemia occur in the first 24–48 hours postoperatively. Anxiety, circumoral numbness, tingling of the fingertips, muscle cramping, and positive Chvostek and Trousseau signs are indicative of hypocalcemia. Stridor can occur and can proceed to laryngospasm. Immediate treatment with IV calcium gluconate (1 g, 10 mL of a 10% solution) or calcium chloride (1 g, 10 mL of a 10% solution) is necessary. A continuous infusion of calcium for several days is also recommended. For long-term management, oral calcium and vitamin D_3 are prescribed, or autotransplantation of parathyroid tissue may be performed.

Tracheal compression from an expanding hematoma may cause rapid respiratory compromise in the period immediately after thyroid surgery. Immediate hematoma evacuation is the first line of treatment. If time permits, the patient should be returned to the operating room. If necessary, the wound should be opened at the bedside, clots evacuated, and bleeding vessels secured to relieve airway obstruction. A thyroid tray including a tracheostomy set should always be available at the bedside during the postoperative period so that sutures or clips can be removed and the wound opened emergently.

PHEOCHROMOCYTOMA

Pheochromocytomas are catecholamine-secreting tumors that arise from chromaffin cells of the sympathoadrenal system. Although pheochromocytomas account for fewer than 0.1% of all cases of hypertension in adults, their detection is imperative, since they have lethal potential and are one of the few truly curable forms of hypertension. Uncontrolled catecholamine release can result in malignant hypertension, cerebrovascular accident, and myocardial infarction.

The precise cause of a pheochromocytoma is unknown. Pheochromocytomas are usually an isolated finding (90% of cases); 10% are inherited (familial) as an autosomal dominant trait. Familial pheochromocytomas usually occur as bilateral adrenal tumors or as extraadrenal tumors that appear in the same anatomic site over successive generations. Both sexes are equally affected, and the peak incidence is in the third to fifth decades of life. Familial pheochromocytomas can also be part of the MEN syndromes and can occur in association with several neuroectodermal dysplasias (e.g., von Hippel-Lindau syndrome). Patients with MEN IIA have a pheochromocytoma, medullary carcinoma of the thyroid, and hyperparathyroidism. Patients with MEN IIB have a pheochromocytoma,

medullary carcinoma of the thyroid, alimentary tract ganglioneuromatosis, thickened corneal nerves, and a marfanoid habitus. Almost 100% of patients with MEN II have or will develop bilateral benign adrenal medullary pheochromocytomas.

Eighty percent of pheochromocytomas are located in the adrenal medulla. The organ of Zuckerkandl near the aortic bifurcation is the most common extraadrenal site. Two percent of extraadrenal pheochromocytomas occur in the neck and thorax. Most extraadrenal pheochromocytomas follow a benign course. Malignant pheochromocytomas usually spread via venous and lymphatic channels, with a predilection for liver and bone. The 5-year survival rate for patients with malignancy is 44%. Following resection of benign tumors, 5%–10% of patients have a benign recurrence.

Most pheochromocytomas secrete norepinephrine, either alone or, more commonly, in combination with a smaller amount of epinephrine in a ratio of 85:15—the inverse of the secretion ratio in the normal adrenal gland. Approximately 15% of tumors secrete predominantly epinephrine.

Signs and Symptoms

The clinical presentation of pheochromocytoma is variable; attacks range from infrequent (i.e., once a month or fewer) to numerous (i.e., many times per day) and may last from less than a minute to several hours. They may occur spontaneously or be precipitated by physical injury, emotional stress, or medications. Hypertension, either continuous or paroxysmal, is the most frequent manifestation of pheochromocytoma. Headache, sweating, pallor, and palpitations are other classic signs and symptoms. Orthostatic hypotension is also a common finding and is considered to be secondary to hypovolemia and impaired vasoconstrictor reflex responses.

Hemodynamic signs depend on the predominant catecholamine secreted. With norepinephrine, α-adrenergic effects predominate and patients usually have systolic and diastolic hypertension and a reflex bradycardia. With epinephrine, β-adrenergic effects predominate and patients usually have systolic hypertension, diastolic hypotension, and tachycardia. Despite the 10-fold higher levels of circulating catecholamines, the hemodynamics are not greatly different in patients with pheochromocytomas and those with essential hypertension.

Cardiomyopathy is a complication of pheochromocytoma. In addition, high catecholamine levels result in coronary vasoconstriction through α-adrenergic pathways, which reduces coronary blood flow and potentially creates ischemia. Dilated and hypertrophic cardiomyopathies as well as left ventricular outflow tract obstruction have been demonstrated echocardiographically. ECG abnormalities may include elevation or depression of the ST segment, flattening or inversion of T waves, prolongation of the QT interval, high or peaked P waves, left axis deviation, and dysrhythmias. The cardiomyopathy appears reversible if catecholamine stimulation is removed early before fibrosis has occurred. Pheochromocytoma patients may also develop cardiac hypertrophy with congestive heart failure secondary to sustained hypertension.

Although pheochromocytoma patients rarely have primary diabetes, most have an elevated blood glucose level secondary to catecholamine stimulation of glycogenolysis and inhibition of insulin release.

Diagnosis

When a pheochromocytoma is clinically suspected, excess catecholamine secretion must be demonstrated. For patients with a low probability of having a pheochromocytoma, a 24-hour urine collection for measurement of metanephrines and catecholamines is a useful screening test. However, the most sensitive test for patients at high risk (familial pheochromocytoma or classic symptoms) is measurement of plasma free metanephrines. Catecholamines are metabolized to free metanephrines within tumor cells, and these metabolites are continuously released into the circulation. A plasma free normetanephrine level higher than 400 pg/mL and/or a metanephrine level higher than 220 pg/mL confirms the diagnosis of pheochromocytoma. A pheochromocytoma is excluded if the normetanephrine level is less than 112 pg/mL and the metanephrine level is less than 61 pg/mL.

Results are equivocal in 5%–10% of patients, and in these cases the clonidine suppression test may be used. In patients with a pheochromocytoma, increased plasma catecholamines result from tumor release that bypasses normal storage and release mechanisms. Clonidine acts to lower plasma catecholamine levels in patients without a pheochromocytoma but has no effect on catecholamine levels in patients with a pheochromocytoma.

In the past, provocative testing with histamine or tyramine was used to elicit excess catecholamine release from the tumor. However, owing to the relatively high incidence of morbidity, these tests have been abandoned. A glucagon stimulation test is now considered to be the safest and most specific provocative test. Glucagon acts directly on the tumor to induce release of catecholamines. A positive response to the test yields a plasma catecholamine increase of at least three times the baseline values or more than 2000 pg/mL within 1–3 minutes of glucagon administration. This test should be performed only in patients with a diastolic blood pressure below 100 mm Hg.

Tumor location can be predicted by the pattern of catecholamine production (Table 23.7). CT detects more than 95% of adrenal masses larger than 1 cm in diameter. Magnetic resonance imaging (MRI) offers advantages over CT, including better identification of small adrenal lesions, better differentiation of various types of adrenal lesions, no need for IV contrast, and lack of radiation exposure. Positron emission scanning and selective venous catheterization with sampling of catecholamines from the adrenal veins and other sites are additional useful tests.

Management of Anesthesia

Preoperative Management
Since most pheochromocytomas secrete predominantly norepinephrine, medical therapy has depended on α-blockade to

TABLE 23.7 Pattern of Catecholamine Production by Site of Pheochromocytoma

	Adrenal	Extraadrenal	Adrenal + Extraadrenal
Norepinephrine	61%	31%	8%
Epinephrine	100%	—	—
Norepinephrine + epinephrine	95%	—	5%

Adapted from Kaser H. Clinical and diagnostic findings in patients with chromaffin tumors: pheochromocytomas, pheochromoblastomas. *Recent Results Cancer Res.* 1990;118:97-105.

lower blood pressure, increase intravascular volume, prevent paroxysmal hypertensive episodes, allow resensitization of adrenergic receptors, and decrease myocardial dysfunction. Although a significantly reduced intravascular volume may accompany a pheochromocytoma, the majority of patients have a normal or only slightly decreased intravascular volume. α-Blockade appears to protect myocardial performance and tissue oxygenation from the adverse effects of catecholamines.

Phenoxybenzamine is the most frequently prescribed α-blocker for preoperative use. It is a noncompetitive α1-antagonist with some α2-blocking properties. Because it is a noncompetitive blocker, it is difficult for excess catecholamines to overcome the blockade. Its long duration of action permits oral dosing only twice daily. The goal of therapy is normotension, resolution of symptoms, elimination of ST-segment and T-wave changes on the ECG, and elimination of dysrhythmias. Overtreatment can result in severe orthostatic hypotension. The optimal duration of α-blockade therapy is undetermined and may range from 3 days to 2 weeks or longer. Because of the prolonged effect of phenoxybenzamine on α receptors, the recommendation has been to discontinue its use 24–48 hours before surgery to avoid vascular unresponsiveness immediately following removal of the tumor. Some anesthesiologists administer only one-half to two-thirds of the morning dose preceding surgery to address similar concerns. Some surgeons request its discontinuation 48 hours preoperatively so they can use hypertensive episodes intraoperatively as cues in localizing areas of metastasis. Prazosin and doxazosin, pure α1-competitive blockers, are alternatives to phenoxybenzamine. They are shorter acting, cause less tachycardia, and are easier to titrate to a desired end point than phenoxybenzamine.

If tachycardia (i.e., heart rates > 120 beats per minute) or other dysrhythmias result after α-blockade with phenoxybenzamine, a β-adrenergic blocker is prescribed. A nonselective β-blocker should *never* be administered before α-blockade, because blockade of vasodilatory β2-receptors results in unopposed α-agonism, leading to vasoconstriction and hypertensive crises. The degree of α- and β-blockade provided by labetalol (i.e., β effects exceed α effects) may *not* be appropriate for certain pheochromocytoma patients. In very rare circumstances, β-blockade may be initiated before α-blockade. A patient with a pheochromocytoma secreting solely epinephrine and with coronary artery disease may benefit greatly from the β1-selective antagonist esmolol.

α-Methylparatyrosine (metyrosine) inhibits the rate-limiting enzyme tyrosine hydroxylase of the catecholamine synthetic pathway and may decrease catecholamine production by 50%–80%. In combination with phenoxybenzamine, it has been shown to facilitate intraoperative hemodynamic management. It is especially useful for malignant and inoperable tumors. Side effects that include extrapyramidal reactions and crystalluria have limited its application.

Calcium channel blockers and ACE inhibitors may also be used to control hypertension. Calcium is a trigger for catecholamine release from the tumor, and excess calcium entry into myocardial cells contributes to a catecholamine-mediated cardiomyopathy. Nifedipine, diltiazem, and verapamil have all been used to control preoperative hypertension, as has captopril. An α_1-blocker plus a calcium channel blocker is an effective combination in treatment-resistant cases.

Intraoperative Management

Optimal preparation for pheochromocytoma resection involves preoperative administration of an α-adrenergic blocker with or without a β-blocker with or without α-methylparatyrosine, as well as correction of possible hypovolemia. Intraoperative goals include avoidance of drugs or maneuvers that may provoke catecholamine release or potentiate catecholamine actions, and maintenance of cardiovascular stability, preferably with short-acting drugs. Hypertension frequently occurs during pneumoperitoneum, as well as during tumor manipulation. On the other hand, significant hypotension may develop following ligation of the tumor's venous drainage. Intraoperative monitoring should include standard plus invasive monitoring methods. An arterial catheter enables monitoring of blood pressure on a beat-to-beat basis. A central venous pressure catheter is usually sufficient for patients without cardiac symptoms or other clinical evidence of cardiac involvement. A pulmonary artery catheter or transesophageal echocardiography may be necessary to manage the large fluid requirements, major volume shifts, and possible underlying myocardial dysfunction in patients with very active tumors. A large positive fluid balance is usually required to manage hypotension and keep intravascular volumes within a normal range.

Intraoperative ultrasonography can be used to localize small functional tumors and perform adrenal-sparing procedures or partial adrenalectomies. Adrenal-sparing procedures are particularly valuable when bilateral adrenal pheochromocytomas must be removed. Laparoscopy can be used for tumors smaller than 4–5 cm and is becoming the surgical approach of choice for many endocrine surgeons.

Factors that stimulate catecholamine release (e.g., fear, stress, pain, shivering, hypoxia, hypercarbia) must be minimized in the perioperative period. Although all anesthetic drugs have been used with some degree of success, certain drugs should theoretically be avoided to prevent possible adverse hemodynamic responses. Morphine and atracurium can cause histamine release, which may provoke release of catecholamines from the tumor. Atropine, pancuronium, and succinylcholine are examples of vagolytic or sympathomimetic drugs that may stimulate the sympathetic nervous system.

Virtually all patients exhibit increases in systolic arterial pressure in excess of 200 mm Hg for periods of time intraoperatively, irrespective of preoperative initiation of α-blockade. A number of antihypertensive drugs must be prepared and ready for immediate administration. Sodium nitroprusside (if available), a direct vasodilator, is the agent of choice because of its potency, immediate onset of action, and short duration of action. Phentolamine, a competitive α-adrenergic blocker and direct vasodilator, is effective, although tachyphylaxis and tachycardia are associated with its use. Nitroglycerin is effective, but large doses are often required and may cause tachycardia. Labetalol, with more β- than α-blocking properties, is preferred for predominantly epinephrine-secreting tumors. Magnesium sulfate inhibits release of catecholamines from the adrenal medulla and peripheral nerve terminals, reduces sensitivity of α receptors to catecholamines, is a direct vasodilator, and is an antidysrhythmic. However, like all antihypertensive medications, it is suboptimal in controlling hypertension during tumor manipulation. Mixtures of antihypertensive drugs such as nitroprusside (if available), esmolol, diltiazem, and phentolamine have been recommended to control refractory hypertension. Increasing the depth of anesthesia is also an option, although this approach may accentuate the hypotension accompanying tumor vein ligation.

Dysrhythmias are usually ventricular in origin and are managed with either lidocaine or β-blockers. Lidocaine is short acting and has minimal negative inotropic action. Although propranolol has been widely used, esmolol, a selective β_1-blocker, offers several advantages. Esmolol has a rapid onset and is short acting, which allows adequate control of heart rate; it may also provide protection against catecholamine-induced ischemia and development of postoperative hypoglycemia. Amiodarone, an antidysrhythmic agent that prolongs the duration of the action potential of atrial and ventricular muscle, has been used as an alternative to β-blockers to treat supraventricular tachycardia associated with hypercatecholaminemia.

Hypotension following tumor vein ligation is usually significant and occurs secondary to a combination of factors, including an immediate decrease in plasma catecholamine levels (half-lives of norepinephrine and epinephrine are ≈1–2 minutes), vasodilation from residual α-blockade with phenoxybenzamine, intraoperative fluid and blood loss, and increased anesthetic depth. Hypotension with systolic pressures in the range of 70–79 mm Hg is not infrequent. To prevent precipitous hypotension, volume expansion should be attained before tumor vein ligation. Lactated Ringer solution and physiologic saline are the recommended fluids for use before tumor removal. Vasopressors and inotropes should be viewed as a secondary treatment modality. Residual α-adrenergic blockade and downregulation of receptors make patients relatively less responsive to vasopressors. Intraoperative administration of blood salvage products has resulted in postresection hypertension secondary to the catecholamine content of the blood. A decrease in anesthetic depth will also aid in controlling hypotension. With a decrease in plasma catecholamine levels immediately following resection, insulin levels increase and hypoglycemia may occur. Therefore dextrose-containing solutions should be added after tumor removal. Glucocorticoid therapy should be administered if a bilateral adrenalectomy is performed or if hypoadrenalism is a possibility.

Postoperative Management

The majority of patients become normotensive following complete tumor resection. However, plasma catecholamine levels do not return to normal until 7–10 days after surgery because of a slow release of stored catecholamines from peripheral nerves. Fifty percent of patients are hypertensive for several days after surgery, and 25%–30% remain hypertensive indefinitely. In these patients, hypertension is sustained rather than paroxysmal, lower than before surgery, and not accompanied by the classic features of hypercatecholaminemia. The differential diagnosis of persistent hypertension includes a missed pheochromocytoma, surgical complications with subsequent renal ischemia, and underlying essential hypertension.

Hypotension is the most frequent cause of death in the period immediately after surgery. Large volumes of fluid are necessary, since the peripheral vasculature is poorly responsive to reduced levels of catecholamines. Vasopressors are a secondary consideration. Steroid supplementation may be necessary if hypoadrenalism is present. Dextrose-containing solutions should be included as part of the fluid therapy, and plasma glucose levels should be monitored for 24 hours.

ADRENAL GLAND DYSFUNCTION

Each adrenal gland consists of two components, the adrenal cortex and the adrenal medulla. The *adrenal cortex* is responsible for synthesis of three groups of hormones, classified as glucocorticoids, mineralocorticoids (aldosterone), and androgens. Corticotropin (ACTH) is secreted by the anterior pituitary gland in response to corticotropin-releasing hormone (CRH), which is synthesized in the hypothalamus and carried to the anterior pituitary in the portal blood. ACTH stimulates the adrenal cortex to produce cortisol. Maintenance of systemic blood pressure by cortisol reflects the importance of this hormone in facilitating conversion of norepinephrine to epinephrine in the adrenal medulla. Hyperglycemia in response to cortisol secretion reflects gluconeogenesis and inhibition of the peripheral use of glucose by cells. Retention of sodium and excretion of potassium are facilitated by cortisol. The antiinflammatory effects of cortisol and other glucocorticoids (cortisone, prednisone, methylprednisolone, dexamethasone, triamcinolone) are particularly apparent in the presence of high serum concentrations of these hormones. Aldosterone secretion is regulated by the renin-angiotensin system and serum concentrations of potassium.

The *adrenal medulla* is a specialized part of the sympathetic nervous system that is capable of synthesizing norepinephrine and epinephrine. The only important disease process associated with the adrenal medulla is pheochromocytoma. Adrenal medullary insufficiency is not known to occur.

Surgery is one of the most potent and best-studied activators of the hypothalamic-pituitary-adrenal (HPA) axis. The degree of activation of the axis depends on the magnitude and duration of surgery and the type and depth of anesthesia. Deep general anesthesia or regional anesthesia blunts but does not eliminate this response. Increases in ACTH begin with surgical incision and remain elevated during surgery, with the peak level occurring with pharmacologic reversal of muscle relaxants and extubation of the patient at the end of the procedure. Hormone levels remain elevated for several days postoperatively.

Hypercortisolism (Cushing Syndrome)

Cushing syndrome results from chronic exposure to excess glucocorticoids. The disorder may be ACTH dependent, ACTH independent, or iatrogenic. ACTH-dependent etiologies include pituitary corticotrope adenomas (known as *Cushing disease*) and ectopic secretion of ACTH from nonpituitary tumors (predominantly carcinoid tumors, especially lung). ACTH-independent etiologies include adrenocortical adenomas and carcinomas or adrenal hyperplasia. Medical use of glucocorticoids for immunosuppression or treatment of inflammatory disorders represents the iatrogenic cause. Medical use of glucocorticoids aside, the majority of patients with Cushing syndrome have an ACTH-producing corticotrope adenoma of the pituitary. Only 10% of patients with Cushing syndrome have a primary adrenal (autonomous release of cortisol) cause of their disease. Cushing syndrome generally occurs in the third or fourth decade of life. On clinical presentation, patients demonstrate an upregulation of gluconeogenesis, lipolysis, and protein catabolism. They also demonstrate signs of mineralocorticoid excess. Signs and symptoms include obesity (central adiposity), hyperglycemia (overt diabetes in <20%), diastolic hypertension, hirsutism, amenorrhea, osteoporosis, and emotional liability and depression, with unique/specific features of fragile skin, easy bruising, broad purple striae, and signs of proximal myopathy with thin extremities.

Diagnosis is made by first excluding exogenous glucocorticoid use and demonstrating an elevated 24-hour urinary free cortisol level. Patients also demonstrate a failure to suppress morning cortisol after overnight exposure to dexamethasone, and loss of diurnal cortisol secretion with high levels at midnight. A plasma ACTH level follows; if normal or elevated, the patient has ACTH-dependent Cushing syndrome. Further testing will include a pituitary MRI, chest CT, corticotropin-releasing hormone (CRH) test, and high-dose dexamethasone test. These patients demonstrate a decrease in cortisol and 17-hydroxycorticosteroid levels after high-dose dexamethasone because the pituitary tumor retains some negative feedback control, which adrenal tumors do not possess. A low ACTH level confirms the diagnosis of ACTH-independent Cushing syndrome, and a CT scan of the adrenal glands is performed.

Treatment for Cushing disease requires removal of the pituitary corticotrope tumor via a transsphenoidal hypophysectomy. Treatment for ACTH-independent disease requires removal of the adrenal tumor. Preoperative medical control of excess cortisol includes metyrapone (which inhibits cortisol synthesis), ketoconazole (which inhibits steroidogenesis), mitotane (which is an adrenolytic agent and reduces cortisol), and a low-dose IV infusion of etomidate. A hydrocortisone replacement regimen is initiated at the time of surgery and slowly tapered postoperatively.

There are no specific anesthetic techniques or medications recommended for these cases. Muscle relaxants should be used cautiously when significant skeletal muscle weakness is present. Perioperative management of hypertension, hyperglycemia, intravascular fluid volume (usually elevated), and electrolytes (hypokalemia is common) is extremely important. Preoperative diuresis with spironolactone is helpful. The patient's cardiac reserve dictates the use of intraoperative invasive monitoring. A pneumothorax is possible during adrenal surgery. Careful positioning is necessary for osteopenic patients. If bilateral adrenalectomy is performed, fludrocortisone will be necessary in the postoperative period (usually day 3–5) to provide mineralocorticoid activity. Delayed wound healing and increased susceptibility to infection can result from increased levels of glucocorticoids.

Primary Hyperaldosteronism (Conn Syndrome)

Primary hyperaldosteronism, or Conn syndrome, is the most common cause of mineralocorticoid (aldosterone) excess. Bilateral micronodular adrenal hyperplasia is a more common cause (60%) than unilateral adrenal adenoma (40%). Rarely, adrenocortical carcinoma is responsible. Hypokalemic hypertension is the common presentation. Clinical features include sodium retention, potassium depletion, hydrogen depletion with metabolic alkalosis, and cardiac remodeling. Muscle weakness and cramps occur secondary to hypokalemia. The diagnosis is made by demonstrating an elevated level of plasma aldosterone and low plasma renin (renin secretion is inhibited by the high aldosterone levels). A specific aldosterone-renin ratio (ARR) confirms the diagnosis. Localization studies include adrenal CT and MRI and adrenal vein sampling. A unilateral adrenal lesion is treated surgically. Bilateral adrenal hyperplasia is managed with spironolactone and eplerenone (competitive aldosterone antagonist) or amiloride. An adrenocortical carcinoma (ACC) is rare, highly malignant, requires staging, and carries a poor prognosis. With successful surgical removal, adjuvant treatment with mitotane is necessary.

Anesthetic management requires preoperative restoration of intravascular volume, electrolyte levels, renal function, and control of hypertension. Restricting sodium intake and administering spironolactone (an aldosterone antagonist) and potassium (significant total deficit) are necessary. A preoperative echocardiogram will determine the effects of long-standing hypertension. Excess preoperative diuresis may render the patient hypovolemic. No specific anesthetic technique or medications are recommended for these cases. An arterial line should be used, and other invasive monitors should be determined on a case-by-case basis. Patients with Conn syndrome have a high incidence of ischemic heart disease. Surgical excision of a solitary adrenal adenoma should not require exogenous cortisol administration, but bilateral manipulation of the adrenal glands to excise multiple functional tumors may require supplemental cortisol if transient hypocortisolism is a consideration.

Hypoaldosteronism

Hyperkalemia in the absence of renal insufficiency suggests the presence of hypoaldosteronism. Hyperchloremic metabolic acidosis is a predictable finding in the presence of hypoaldosteronism. Heart block secondary to hyperkalemia, orthostatic hypotension, and hyponatremia may also be present.

Isolated deficiency of aldosterone secretion may reflect congenital deficiency of aldosterone synthetase or hyporeninemia, resulting from defects in the juxtaglomerular apparatus, or treatment with ACE inhibitors, leading to loss of angiotensin stimulation. Hyporeninemic hypoaldosteronism typically occurs in patients older than age 45 with chronic renal disease and/or diabetes mellitus. Treatment of hypoaldosteronism includes liberal sodium intake and daily administration of fludrocortisone.

Adrenal Insufficiency

Signs and Symptoms

There are two types of adrenal insufficiency (AI): primary and secondary. In *primary* disease (Addison's disease) the adrenal glands are unable to elaborate sufficient quantities of glucocorticoid, mineralocorticoid, and androgen hormones. The most common cause of this rare endocrinopathy is bilateral adrenal destruction from autoimmune disease. More than 90% of the glands must be involved before signs of AI appear. The insidious onset of Addison's disease is characterized by fatigue, weakness, anorexia, nausea and vomiting, cutaneous and mucosal hyperpigmentation, hypovolemia, hyponatremia, and hyperkalemia. *Secondary* AI results from a failure in production of CRH or ACTH caused by hypothalamic-pituitary disease or suppression of the hypothalamic-pituitary axis. Unlike in Addison's disease, there is only a glucocorticoid deficiency in secondary disease. In the majority of cases the cause is iatrogenic, such as pituitary surgery, pituitary irradiation, or most commonly the use of synthetic glucocorticoids. These patients lack cutaneous hyperpigmentation and may demonstrate only mild electrolyte abnormalities.

Cortisol is one of the few hormones essential for life. It participates in carbohydrate and protein metabolism, fatty acid mobilization, electrolyte and water balance, and the antiinflammatory response. It facilitates catecholamine synthesis and action; modulates β-receptor synthesis, regulation, coupling, and responsiveness; and contributes to normal vascular permeability, tone, and cardiac contractility. Cortisol accounts for 95% of the adrenal gland's glucocorticoid activity, with corticosterone and cortisone contributing some activity.

TABLE 23.8	Glucocorticoid Preparations		
	Potency		
Steroid	Antiinflammatory (Glucocorticoid)	Na⁺ Retention (Mineralocorticoid)	Equivalent Dose (Oral or IV, mg)
SHORT ACTING			
Cortisol (hydrocortisone)	1	1	20
Cortisone	0.8	0.8	25
INTERMEDIATE ACTING			
Prednisone	4	0.8	5
Prednisolone	4	0.8	5
Methylprednisolone	5	0.5	4
Triamcinolone	5	0	4
LONG ACTING			
Dexamethasone	30–40	0	0.75

Adapted from Stoelting RK, Dierdorf SF. Endocrine disease. In: Stoelting RK, ed. *Anesthesia and Co-Existing Disease*. New York, NY: Churchill Livingstone; 1993:358.
IV, Intravenous.

Diagnosis

The classic definition of AI includes a baseline plasma cortisol concentration of less than 20 μg/dL and a cortisol level of less than 20 μg/dL after ACTH stimulation. The short 250-μg ACTH stimulation test is a reliable test of the integrity of the entire HPA axis. All steroids except dexamethasone must be discontinued for 24 hours before testing. A normal ACTH stimulation test result is a plasma cortisol level greater than 25 μg/dL. A positive test finding demonstrates a poor response to ACTH and indicates an impairment of the adrenal cortex. *Absolute AI* is characterized by a low baseline cortisol level and a positive result on the ACTH stimulation test. *Relative AI* is indicated when the baseline cortisol level is higher, but the result on the ACTH stimulation test is positive.

Treatment

The most common cause of AI is exogenous steroids (Table 23.8). Those who take steroids long term may exhibit signs and symptoms of AI during periods of stress, such as surgery or acute illness. For patients with a history of long-term steroid use, it may take 6–12 months from the time of discontinuation of the steroids for the adrenal glands to recover full function. Recovery from short courses of steroids may take several days. Preoperative glucocorticoid coverage should be provided for patients with a positive result on the ACTH stimulation test, Cushing syndrome, or AI, as well as for those at risk of HPA axis suppression or AI based on prior glucocorticoid therapy. Adrenal suppression is much more common than AI and is of concern because overt AI, although uncommon, may occur under the stressful conditions of surgery and anesthesia. Patients taking prednisone in dosages of less than 5 mg/day (morning dose) for any length of time, even years, do not demonstrate clinically significant HPA axis suppression and do not require perioperative supplementation, although they should receive their normal daily steroid dose. Any patient who received a glucocorticoid in dosages equivalent to more than 20 mg/day of

TABLE 23.9	Perioperative Steroid (Hydrocortisone) Supplementation
Superficial surgery (e.g., dental surgery, biopsy)	None
Minor surgery (e.g., inguinal hernia repair)	25 mg IV
Moderate surgery (e.g., cholecystectomy, colon resection)	50–75 mg IV, taper 1–2 days
Major surgery (e.g., cardiovascular surgery, Whipple procedure)	100–150 mg IV, taper 1–2 days
Intensive care unit (e.g., sepsis, shock)	50–100 mg q6–8h for 2 days to 1 week, followed by slow taper

IV, Intravenous.

prednisone for more than 3 weeks within the previous year is at risk of AI and should receive perioperative supplementation. Patients receiving dosages of steroids between these two extremes may have HPA axis suppression and should probably receive supplementation. Similarly, patients receiving more than 2 g/day of topical steroids or more than 0.8 mg/day of inhaled steroids on a long-term basis should probably receive supplementation.

Patients with known or suspected adrenal suppression or AI should receive their baseline steroid therapy plus supplementation in the perioperative period. Supplementation is individualized based on the surgery (Table 23.9). When more than 100 mg/day of hydrocortisone is administered, it may be wise to consider substituting methylprednisolone for hydrocortisone; given its lower mineralocorticoid activity, it is less likely to cause fluid retention, edema, and hypokalemia.

Management of Anesthesia

Acute AI should be considered in the differential diagnosis of hemodynamic instability, especially in patients unresponsive to the usual therapeutic interventions. Therapy includes treatment of the cause, repletion of circulating glucocorticoids, and replacement of water and sodium deficits. Glucocorticoid replacement may include IV hydrocortisone, methylprednisolone, or dexamethasone. A bolus of 100 mg of hydrocortisone followed by a continuous infusion at 10 mg/h is a recommended prescription. A 100-mg bolus of hydrocortisone every 6 hours is also an acceptable option. When the patient's condition stabilizes, the steroid dosage is reduced, with eventual conversion to an oral preparation. Volume deficits may be substantial (2–3 L), and 5% dextrose in normal saline is the replacement fluid of choice. Hemodynamic support with vasopressors may be necessary. Metabolic acidosis and hyperkalemia usually resolve with fluid and steroid administration. In primary disease, administration of the mineralocorticoid fludrocortisone is not necessary acutely because isotonic saline replaces sodium loss.

No specific anesthetic agent(s) and/or technique(s) are recommended in managing patients with or at risk of AI. However, etomidate transiently inhibits cortisol synthesis and should be avoided in this patient population. Patients with untreated AI undergoing emergency surgery should be managed aggressively with invasive monitoring, IV corticosteroids, and fluid and electrolyte resuscitation. Minimal doses of anesthetic agents and drugs are recommended, since myocardial depression and skeletal muscle weakness are frequently part of the clinical presentation.

PARATHYROID GLAND DYSFUNCTION

Four parathyroid glands are located on the posterior aspect of the thyroid gland. They produce and release parathormone (PTH), the primary regulator of extracellular fluid calcium concentration. PTH secretion is determined by the ionized fraction of calcium in blood. PTH increases calcium levels by interacting with bone (increases resorption), kidney (increases renal tubular absorption), and the GI tract (increases absorption via 1,25 dihydroxyvitamin D). Serum PTH levels are tightly regulated by a negative feedback loop. Low ionized calcium and vitamin D levels increase PTH synthesis and release, and vice versa. An immediate increase in blood calcium occurs secondary to PTH effects on bone resorption and, to a lesser extent, on renal absorption. Maintenance of steady-state calcium balance is provided by GI absorption. Continuous exposure to elevated PTH levels, usually from a parathyroid adenoma or hyperplasia, results in osteoclast-mediated bone resorption and hypercalcemia.

Hyperparathyroidism

Hyperparathyroidism is characterized by excess production of PTH. It is the most common cause of *hypercalcemia*, defined as total serum calcium above 10.4 mg/dL. Hyperparathyroidism may be primary, secondary, or ectopic. *Primary hyperparathyroidism* is most common and usually results from a parathyroid adenoma or parathyroid hyperplasia. Peak incidence is between the third and fifth decades of life. A solitary benign adenoma is responsible for 80% of primary

hyperparathyroidism cases. Hyperplasia, with all four glands hyperfunctioning, is present in 15% of cases; it is usually hereditary and may be associated with other endocrine abnormalities (MEN I and MEN IIA). Adenomas are mostly located in the inferior parathyroid glands. They are 0.5–5 grams in size (normal gland weighs 25 mg). Although over 50% of patients are asymptomatic, manifestations of hypercalcemia involve primarily the kidneys and skeletal system. Renal pathology includes calcium deposits in renal parenchyma or recurrent nephrolithiasis, and skeletal pathology. Signs and symptoms of hypercalcemia include CNS (confusion, depression), neuromuscular (weakness, fatigue), and GI (anorexia, nausea, vomiting, constipation, peptic ulcer disease) manifestations (Table 23.10). Symptoms are more common at calcium levels above 2.9–3 mmol/L (11.5–12 mg/dL).

Diagnostic tests include a third-generation PTH immunometric assay and a simultaneous calcium level. Patients with hyperparathyroidism have increased PTH and serum calcium. Localization studies can include a ^{99m}Tc sestamibi scan with single-photon emission CT scan. Surgical excision of the abnormal parathyroid tissue is the definitive treatment. Medical management can be safely followed in patients with mild asymptomatic disease by quarterly monitoring of blood pressure, serum calcium and creatinine, and bone density. For an adenoma, the one abnormal gland is removed and a second parathyroid gland is sought, biopsied, and confirmed to be histologically normal (without hyperplasia) to conclude the operation. An intraoperative PTH assay is measured before and at 5-minute intervals after adenoma removal to confirm a rapid fall to normal. For multiple-gland hyperplasia, all glands must be identified and either: (1) three are removed, with partial excision of the fourth (leaving a good blood supply),

TABLE 23.10	Signs and Symptoms of Hypercalcemia Due to Hyperparathyroidism
Organ System	Signs and Symptoms
Neuromuscular	Skeletal muscle weakness
Renal	Polyuria and polydipsia
	Decreased glomerular filtration rate
	Kidney stones
Hematopoietic	Anemia
Cardiac	Prolonged PR interval
	Shortened QT interval
	Systemic hypertension
Gastrointestinal	Vomiting
	Abdominal pain
	Peptic ulcer
	Pancreatitis
Skeletal	Skeletal demineralization
	Collapse of vertebral bodies
	Pathologic fractures
Nervous	Somnolence
	Decreased pain sensation
	Psychosis
Ocular	Calcifications (band keratopathy)
	Conjunctivitis

or (2) total parathyroidectomy is performed, with immediate transplantation of a removed, minced parathyroid gland into the forearm muscles. There is no preferred anesthetic technique and no special intraoperative monitoring. The effects of neuromuscular blocking agents are unpredictable secondary to hypercalcemia. Careful positioning is necessary to avoid bone injuries. Postoperative complications are similar to thyroid surgery (recurrent laryngeal nerve injury, hematoma, hypocalcemia). A decline in serum calcium occurs within 24 hours postoperatively. Acute hypocalcemia should occur only if severe bone deficits are present or injury to all normal parathyroid glands occurred during surgery. In such cases, parenteral calcium is necessary at 0.5–2 mg/kg/h for several days, with possible addition of a vitamin D analogue (calcitriol) and/or oral calcium. Hypophosphatemia and hypomagnesemia may also occur postoperatively and require phosphate and magnesium.

Parathyroid carcinoma is rare and usually not aggressive. Calcium values are frequently high (3.5–3.7 mmol/L [14–15 mg/dL]) and provide a preoperative clue for carcinoma, which requires removal of the entire gland with capsule intact.

The most common cause of hypercalcemia in hospitalized patients is malignancy (occurs in as many as 20% of cancer patients). Breast cancer accounts for 25%–50% of malignancy-related hypercalcemia. Unlike hypercalcemia from primary hyperparathyroidism, which is usually detected coincidentally on laboratory testing, the symptoms of malignancy bring the patient to medical attention, and hypercalcemia is then detected. In addition to a significant elevation in serum calcium, patients have a low PTH and an elevated PTH-related peptide (PTHrP) assay and require localization studies to include chest x-ray, CT of the chest and abdomen, and a bone scan. Less than 10% of cases of hypercalcemia are caused by disorders other than hyperparathyroidism and malignancy.

Medical treatment of hypercalcemia varies with its severity. Mild hypercalcemia (<3 mmol/L [12 mg/dL]) is managed with hydration. Moderate to severe hypercalcemia (3.2–3.7 mmol/L [13–15 mg/dL]) is aggressively treated with IV saline hydration and furosemide or ethacrynic acid to promote a Na/Ca diuresis. Serum calcium usually falls 1–3 mg/dL in 24 hours. Phosphate should be given to treat hypophosphatemia. Bisphosphonates (pamidronate, zolendronate), calcitonin, glucocorticoids, phosphates, mithramycin, plicamycin, and dialysis are also valuable. Bisphosphonates are powerful inhibitors of bone resorption, and calcitonin is a hypocalcemic hormone.

Hypoparathyroidism

Hypoparathyroidism results from absence or deficiency in PTH secretion or resistance of peripheral tissues to the effects of the hormone. The clinical features of hypoparathyroidism are those of hypocalcemia.

Normal total (bound and free) serum calcium concentration is 9.5–10.5 mg/dL. Normal ionized calcium is 4.75–5.7 mg/dL (1.19–1.33 mmol/L). Approximately 50% of serum calcium is bound to albumin, 40% is ionized, and 10% is bound to chelating agents (phosphate, citrate, sulfate). If the serum protein concentration decreases, so does the total serum calcium concentration. An increase in serum proteins yields an increase in serum calcium. Acidosis increases serum calcium, and alkalosis decreases serum calcium.

The most common cause of acquired hypoparathyroidism is iatrogenic (i.e., inadvertent removal of all parathyroid glands during thyroid or parathyroid surgery). Clinical signs of hypocalcemia include neuronal irritability, skeletal muscle spasms, tetany, and possibly seizures. Fatigue and mental status changes including depression are common symptoms. Acute hypocalcemia can present with stridor and apnea. Congestive heart failure, hypotension, and decreased responsiveness to β-agonists may occur. A prolonged QT interval is present on ECG. There are a number of other causes of hypoparathyroidism (Table 23.11). Treatment for hypoparathyroidism is electrolyte replacement. Calcium supplements and vitamin D analogues are the primary treatment of hypocalcemia. Hypomagnesemia is managed with oral or IV magnesium. Hyperphosphatemia is treated with phosphate-binding resins and possibly dialysis. Severe symptomatic hypocalcemia requires 10–20 mL of 10% calcium gluconate or 3–5 mL of 10% calcium chloride followed by a continuous infusion of calcium (1–2 mg/kg/h).

Hypoparathyroid patients may present to the operating room for an unrelated surgical condition. Patients with symptomatic hypocalcemia must be treated aggressively preoperatively. Calcium, phosphate, and magnesium levels should be measured preoperatively and postoperatively. Serum ionized calcium levels should maintained in the low-normal range intraoperatively. The QT interval may be used as an indirect guide of the serum calcium level. No specific anesthetic agents or techniques are recommended. Respiratory alkalosis must be avoided because it lowers ionized calcium levels.

TABLE 23.11	Causes of Hypoparathyroidism

DECREASED OR ABSENT PARATHYROID HORMONE
Accidental removal of parathyroid glands during thyroidectomy
Parathyroidectomy to treat hyperplasia
Idiopathic (DiGeorge syndrome)

RESISTANCE OF PERIPHERAL TISSUES TO EFFECTS OF PARATHYROID HORMONE
Congenital
  Pseudohypoparathyroidism
Acquired
  Hypomagnesemia
  Chronic renal failure
  Malabsorption
  Anticonvulsive therapy (phenytoin)
  Osteoblastic metastases
  Acute pancreatitis

TABLE 23.12	Hypothalamic and Related Pituitary Hormones		
Hypothalamic Hormone	Action	Pituitary Hormone or Organ Affected	Action
Corticotropin-releasing hormone	Stimulatory	Corticotropin	Stimulates secretion of cortisol and androgens
Thyrotropin-releasing hormone	Stimulatory	Thyrotropin	Stimulates secretion of thyroxine and triiodothyronine
Gonadotropin-releasing hormone	Stimulatory	Follicle-stimulating hormone, luteinizing hormone	Stimulate secretion of estradiol and progesterone,[a] stimulate ovulation,[a] stimulate secretion of testosterone,[b] stimulate spermatogenesis[b]
Growth hormone–releasing hormone	Stimulatory	Growth hormone	Stimulates production of insulinlike growth factor
Dopamine	Inhibitory	Prolactin	Stimulates lactation[a]
Somatostatin	Inhibitory	Pituitary, gastrointestinal tract, pancreas	Inhibits secretion of growth hormone and thyroid-stimulating hormone, suppresses release of gastrointestinal and pancreatic hormones
Vasopressin (antidiuretic hormone)	Stimulatory	Kidneys	Stimulates free water reabsorption
Oxytocin	Stimulatory	Uterus	Stimulates uterine contractions[a]
		Breasts	Stimulates milk ejection[a]

[a]Actions in females.
[b]Actions in males.
Adapted from Vance ML. Hypopituitarism. *N Engl J Med*. 1994;330:1651-1662.

PITUITARY GLAND DYSFUNCTION

The pituitary gland, located in the sella turcica at the base of the brain, consists of the anterior pituitary and posterior pituitary. The *anterior pituitary* secretes six hormones under the control of the hypothalamus (Table 23.12). The hypothalamus controls the function of the anterior pituitary by means of vascular connections (hormones travel via the hypophyseal portal veins to reach the anterior pituitary). The hypothalamic–anterior pituitary–target organ axis is composed of tightly coordinated systems in which hormonal signals from the hypothalamus stimulate or inhibit secretion of anterior pituitary hormones, which in turn act on target organs and modulate hypothalamic and anterior pituitary activity (closed-loop, negative feedback system). The *posterior pituitary* is composed of terminal neuron endings that originate in the hypothalamus. Vasopressin (ADH) and oxytocin are synthesized in the hypothalamus and are subsequently transported along the hypothalamic neuronal axons for storage in the posterior pituitary. The stimulus for the release of these hormones from the posterior pituitary arises from osmoreceptors in the hypothalamus that sense plasma osmolarity.

Overproduction of anterior pituitary hormones is most often associated with hypersecretion of ACTH (Cushing syndrome) by anterior pituitary adenomas. Hypersecretion of other tropic hormones rarely occurs. Underproduction of a single anterior pituitary hormone is less common than generalized pituitary hypofunction (panhypopituitarism). The anterior pituitary gland is the only endocrine gland in which a tumor, most often a chromophobe adenoma, causes destruction by compressing the gland against the bony confines of the sella turcica. Metastatic tumor, most often from the breast or lung, also occasionally produces pituitary hypofunction. Endocrine features of panhypopituitarism are highly variable and depend on the rate at which the deficiency develops

and the patient's age. Gonadotropin deficiency (amenorrhea, impotence) is typically the first manifestation of global pituitary dysfunction. Hypocortisolism occurs 4–14 days after hypophysectomy, whereas hypothyroidism is not likely to manifest before 4 weeks. CT and MRI are useful for radiographic assessment of the pituitary gland.

Acromegaly

Acromegaly is due to excessive secretion of growth hormone in adults, most often by an adenoma in the anterior pituitary gland. Failure of plasma growth hormone concentrations to decrease 1–2 hours after ingestion of 75–100 g of glucose is presumptive evidence of acromegaly, as are growth hormone concentrations higher than 3 ng/mL. A skull radiograph and CT are useful for detecting enlargement of the sella turcica, which is characteristic of anterior pituitary adenomas.

Signs and Symptoms

Manifestations of acromegaly reflect parasellar extension of the anterior pituitary adenoma and peripheral effects produced by the presence of excess growth hormone (Table 23.13). Headache and papilledema reflect increased intracranial pressure resulting from expansion of the anterior pituitary adenoma. Visual disturbances are due to compression of the optic chiasm by the expanding overgrowth of surrounding tissues.

Overgrowth of soft tissues of the upper airway (enlargement of the tongue and epiglottis) makes patients susceptible to upper airway obstruction. Hoarseness and abnormal movement of the vocal cords or paralysis of a recurrent laryngeal nerve may result from stretching caused by overgrowth of the surrounding cartilaginous structures. In addition, involvement of the cricoarytenoid joints can result in alterations in the patient's voice resulting from impaired movement of the vocal cords.

TABLE 23.13	Manifestations of Acromegaly

PARASELLAR TUMOR
Enlarged sella turcica
Headache
Visual field defects
Rhinorrhea

EXCESS GROWTH HORMONE
Skeletal overgrowth (prognathism)
Soft tissue overgrowth (lips, tongue, epiglottis, vocal cords)
Connective tissue overgrowth (recurrent laryngeal nerve paralysis)
Peripheral neuropathy (carpal tunnel syndrome)
Visceromegaly
Glucose intolerance
Osteoarthritis
Osteoporosis
Hyperhidrosis
Skeletal muscle weakness

Peripheral neuropathy is common and likely reflects trapping of nerves by skeletal, connective, and soft tissue overgrowth. Flow through the ulnar artery may be compromised in patients exhibiting symptoms of carpal tunnel syndrome. Even in the absence of such symptoms, approximately half of patients with acromegaly have inadequate collateral blood flow through the ulnar artery in one or both hands.

Glucose intolerance and, on occasion, diabetes mellitus requiring treatment with insulin reflect the effects of growth hormone on carbohydrate metabolism. The incidence of systemic hypertension, ischemic heart disease, osteoarthritis, and osteoporosis seems to be increased in these patients. Lung volumes are increased, and ventilation/perfusion mismatching may be present. The patient's skin becomes thick and oily, skeletal muscle weakness may be prominent, and complaints of fatigue are common.

Treatment

Transsphenoidal surgical excision of pituitary adenomas is the preferred initial therapy. When adenomas have extended beyond the sella turcica, surgery or radiation therapy is no longer feasible; medical treatment with suppressant drugs (bromocriptine) may be an option in these cases.

Management of Anesthesia

Management of anesthesia in patients with acromegaly is complicated by changes induced by excessive secretion of growth hormone. Particularly important are changes in the upper airway. Distorted facial anatomy may interfere with placement of an anesthesia face mask. Enlargement of the tongue and epiglottis predisposes to upper airway obstruction and interferes with visualization of the vocal cords by direct laryngoscopy. The distance between the lips and vocal cords is increased secondary to overgrowth of the mandible. The glottic opening may be narrowed because of enlargement of the vocal cords. This, in addition to subglottic narrowing, may necessitate use of a tracheal tube with a smaller internal diameter than would

be predicted based on the patient's age and size. Nasal turbinate enlargement may preclude the passage of nasopharyngeal or nasotracheal airways. A preoperative history of dyspnea on exertion or the presence of hoarseness or stridor suggests involvement of the larynx by acromegaly. In this instance, indirect laryngoscopy may be indicated to quantitate the extent of vocal cord dysfunction. When a catheter is placed in the radial artery, it is important to consider the possibility of inadequate collateral circulation at the wrist. Monitoring blood glucose concentrations is useful if diabetes mellitus or glucose intolerance accompanies acromegaly. Peripheral nerve stimulation is used to guide dosing of nondepolarizing muscle relaxants, particularly if skeletal muscle weakness is present. Skeletal changes associated with acromegaly may make use of regional anesthesia technically difficult or unreliable. There is no evidence that hemodynamic instability or alterations in pulmonary gas exchange accompany anesthesia in acromegalic patients.

Diabetes Insipidus

The posterior pituitary gland produces antidiuretic hormone (ADH). Secretion is regulated by the osmotic pressure of the intravascular volume. ADH increases permeability of cells lining the distal tubule and medullary collecting ducts of the kidney to promote water absorption.

Diabetes insipidus (DI) occurs from a decrease of synthesis and release of vasopressin (neurogenic DI) or from a resistance or insensitivity of renal tubules to vasopressin (nephrogenic DI). Secretion or action of vasopressin is decreased 80%–85% below normal. Neurogenic DI can be differentiated from nephrogenic DI based on response to desmopressin (DDAVP [1-deamino-8-D-arginine-vasopressin]). This vasopressin analogue concentrates urine in the presence of neurogenic DI but *not* nephrogenic DI. Neurogenic DI often occurs following damage or destruction to the pituitary gland by trauma, infiltrating lesions, or surgery. Patients present with polydipsia, hypernatremia, and high output of poorly concentrated urine despite increased serum osmolality. Clinically, patients demonstrate altered mental status/seizures, fatigue, weakness, and hemodynamic instability. Hypernatremia and hypovolemia can become severe enough to be life threatening. A 24-hour urine collection is required to make the diagnosis. The 24-hour urine volume must exceed 50 mL/kg of body weight, and the urine osmolality must be less than 300 mOsm/L to confirm DI. An increase in plasma osmolality (normal = 283–285 mOsm/L) also occurs. DI from pituitary surgery usually appears within 24 hours and may last a few days to 6 months. Desmopressin (DDAVP) is the treatment for neurogenic DI. During surgery an IV infusion of 100–200 m U/h is administered in combination with an isotonic crystalloid solution. Frequent monitoring of serum Na and plasma osmolality is required. DDAVP can also be administered IM or intranasally. Treatments for nephrogenic DI include chlorpropamide, clofibrate, and thiazide diuretics.

Anesthetic management includes continuous monitoring of urine output and hourly measurement of serum Na and plasma osmolality. The goal for plasma osmolality is less than 290 mOsm/L. Patients with complete DI and a total lack of ADH require a preoperative dose of desmopressin intranasally or an IV bolus of 100 mU (0.1 unit) of aqueous vasopressin followed by a continuous infusion of 100–200 mU/h (0.1–0.2 units/h). Isotonic fluids should be used for volume resuscitation. If plasma osmolality exceeds 290 mOsm/L, hypotonic fluid should be used for resuscitation and the vasopressin infusion should be increased above 200 mU/h. Since vasopressin causes vasoconstriction of arteriolar beds, close monitoring for myocardial ischemia is recommended.

Syndrome of Inappropriate Antidiuretic Hormone Secretion (SIADH)

Inappropriate (i.e., excessive) secretion of antidiuretic hormone yields hyponatremia (Na < 135 mEq/L) from the expansion of intravascular fluid volume secondary to hormone-induced resorption of water by renal tubules. Ectopic production of vasopressin by tumors is a common cause of SIADH. Small cell lung carcinoma (50% of these patients develop SIADH) and carcinoid tumors are the most common sources. Other types of lung cancer and tumors of the CNS, head and neck, GI tract, genitourinary tract, and ovary can also produce vasopressin. CNS trauma, infections, certain medications (chlorpropamide, clofibrate, thiazides, antineoplastic agents), hypothyroidism, and major surgery can also result in SIADH. Most patients are asymptomatic. Clinical signs and symptoms may include nausea, weakness, lethargy, confusion, depressed mental status, and seizures. Although hyponatremia usually develops slowly (over weeks to months), the rapidity of onset and degree of hyponatremia determine the severity of symptoms. The diagnosis is made by demonstrating hyponatremia (<130 mEq/L), reduced serum osmolality (<270 mOsm/L), normal or increased urine Na excretion (>20 mEq/L), and inappropriately normal or increased urine osmolality (hypertonic relative to plasma).

SIADH is a diagnosis of exclusion, and other causes of hyponatremia should be excluded first. SIADH is corrected gradually unless mental status is altered and/or the patient appears at risk for seizures. Treatment of the malignancy is primary. Free water restriction is required. Fluid intake is limited to 500–1000 mL/day. Demeclocycline inhibits the action of ADH on the renal distal tubule. Conivaptan, a vasopressin-2 receptor (V2R) antagonist, may be effective. Severe hyponatremia (Na < 115 mEq/L) may require 3% hypertonic saline or normal saline plus furosemide. The rate of sodium correction should be *slow* (0.5 mEq/L/h) until Na concentration is 125 mEq/L, then proceed *more slowly* to prevent central pontine myelinolysis and possibly permanent brain damage.

Anesthetic management of patients with SIADH involves careful administration and monitoring of fluids and electrolytes. If SIADH results from malignancy, anemia and malnutrition may be present. Perioperatively, these patients usually have low urine output and can demonstrate delayed awakening or awakening with mental confusion. Measurement of intravascular volume status with a central venous pressure catheter may be indicated. Cautious fluid resuscitation with normal saline is recommended. Frequent measures of urine osmolality, plasma osmolality, and serum Na are necessary perioperatively. It is not unusual to see patients in the neurosurgical intensive care unit with this syndrome.

KEY POINTS

- Diabetes mellitus results from inadequate supply of and/or inadequate tissue response to insulin, which leads to increased circulating glucose levels.
- The effects of chronic hyperglycemia are many and include hypertension, coronary artery disease, congestive heart failure, peripheral vascular disease, cerebrovascular accident, chronic renal failure, and autonomic neuropathy.
- Aggressive perioperative glucose control has been shown to limit infection risk, improve wound healing, and result in overall reductions in morbidity and mortality.
- The direct effects of T_3 on the heart and vascular smooth muscle are responsible for the exaggerated hemodynamic effects of hyperthyroidism.
- The third-generation TSH assay is the single best test of thyroid hormone action at the cellular level.
- Every effort should be made to render patients euthyroid before surgery. When caring for surgical patients with hyperthyroidism or hypothyroidism, the clinician must be prepared to manage thyroid storm or myxedema coma during the perioperative period.
- Since most pheochromocytomas secrete predominantly norepinephrine, preoperative α-blockade is necessary to lower blood pressure, increase intravascular volume, prevent paroxysmal hypertensive episodes, allow resensitization of adrenergic receptors, and decrease myocardial dysfunction.
- During surgical excision of a pheochromocytoma, the patient often exhibits an exaggerated hypertensive response to anesthetic induction, intubation, surgical excision, and particularly tumor manipulation. Conversely, hypotension may occur following ligation of the tumor's venous drainage.
- The physiologic response to surgical stress is an increase in CRH, ACTH, and cortisol secretion that begins at surgical incision and continues into the postoperative period.
- The most common cause of AI is administration of exogenous steroids.
- Patients who received glucocorticoids in dosages equivalent to more than 20 mg/day of prednisone for longer than 3 weeks within the previous year are considered to have adrenal suppression and are at increased risk of AI. Such patients require perioperative corticosteroid supplementation.
- Hydrocortisone 200–300 mg/day for a minimum of 5–7 days, followed by a tapering regimen over 5–7 days, results in overall improvement in patients with vasopressor-dependent septic shock.

- Primary hyperparathyroidism is the most common cause of hypercalcemia in the general population and usually results from a benign parathyroid adenoma. Hypercalcemia can be treated medically by saline infusion, furosemide, and/or bisphosphonates before surgery.
- Overproduction of anterior pituitary hormones is most commonly manifested as Cushing syndrome caused by ACTH hypersecretion by an adenoma in the anterior pituitary.
- SIADH is common in the postoperative period and usually responds to fluid restriction.

RESOURCES

Akhtar S, Barash PG, Inzucchi SE. Scientific principles and clinical implications of perioperative glucose regulation and control. *Anesth Analg.* 2010;110:478-497.

Axelrod L. Perioperative management of patients treated with glucocorticoids. *Endocrinol Metab Clin North Am.* 2003;32:367-383.

Bravo EL. Evolving concepts in the pathophysiology, diagnosis, and treatment of pheochromocytoma. *Endocr Rev.* 1994;15:356-368.

Burch HB, Wartofsky L. Life-threatening thyrotoxicosis: thyroid storm. *Endocrinol Metab Clin North Am.* 1993;22:263-277.

Cooper MS, Stewart PM. Corticosteroid insufficiency in acutely ill patients. *N Engl J Med.* 2003;348:727-734.

DeWitt DE, Hirsch IB. Outpatient insulin therapy in type 1 and type 2 diabetes mellitus. *JAMA.* 2003;289:2254-2264.

Inzucchi S. *The Diabetes Mellitus Manual: a Primary Care Companion to Ellenberg and Rifkin's Sixth Edition.* New York: McGraw-Hill; 2005.

Klein I, Ojamma K. Thyroid hormone and the cardiovascular system. *N Engl J Med.* 2001;344:501-509.

Mathur A, Gorden P, Libutti SK. Insulinoma. *Surg Clin North Am.* 2009;89:1105-1121.

Stathatos N, Wartofsky L. Perioperative management of patients with hypothyroidism. *Endocrinol Metab Clin North Am.* 2003;32:503-518.

Surks MI, Ortiz E, Daniels GH, et al. Subclinical thyroid disease: scientific review and guidelines for diagnosis and management. *JAMA.* 2004;291:228-238.

CHAPTER 24

Hematologic Disorders

ADRIANA D. OPREA

Disease states related to erythrocytes include anemia and polycythemia. *Anemia* is characterized by a decrease in the red cell mass, with the main adverse effect being a decrease in the oxygen-carrying capacity of blood. *Polycythemia (erythrocytosis)* represents an increase in hematocrit (Hct). Its consequences are primarily related to an expanded red cell mass and a resulting increase in blood viscosity.

PHYSIOLOGY OF ANEMIA

Anemia is a disease sign manifesting clinically as a reduced absolute number of circulating red blood cells (RBCs). Although a decrease in Hct is used most often as an indicator, *anemia* has been defined as a reduction in one or more of the major RBC indices: hemoglobin (Hb) concentration, Hct, and RBC count. In adults the World Health Organization defines

anemia as Hb concentration less than 12 g/dL for women and less than 13 g/dL for men. In pregnancy a decreased Hct reflects the increase in plasma volume in relationship to the RBC mass (*physiologic anemia*). However, Hb less than 11 g/dL in a pregnant patient is considered truly anemic. In *acute blood loss* the Hct may initially be unchanged. Decreases in Hct that exceed 1% every 24 hours can only be explained by acute blood loss or intravascular hemolysis.

The most important adverse effect of anemia is the reduction in arterial oxygen concentration and the potential for decreased tissue oxygen delivery. For example, a decrease in Hb concentration from 15 g/dL to 10 g/dL result in a 33% decrease in arterial oxygen content. The initial compensation for this decrease in oxygen content is an increase in cardiac output. This occurs via enhanced sympathetic nervous system activity and the decrease in blood viscosity that accompanies anemia. There is also a rightward shift of the oxyhemoglobin dissociation curve, which facilitates release of oxygen from Hb to tissues. This is followed by redistribution of blood flow to the myocardium, lungs, and brain. Muscle and skin blood flow decrease (which results in pallor), as does blood flow to the kidneys (which stimulates erythroid precursors in bone marrow to produce additional RBCs). Fatigue and low exercise tolerance indicate the inability of cardiac output to increase further to maintain tissue oxygenation. This is most notable in anemic patients who are physically active or in patients with coronary artery disease. Orthopnea and dyspnea on exertion, cardiomegaly, pulmonary congestion, ascites, and edema can occur as a consequence of high-output heart failure in chronic severe anemia.

There are many causes and forms of anemia. The most common causes of *chronic anemia* are iron deficiency, anemia of chronic disease, thalassemia, and ongoing blood loss.

The Transfusion Trigger

Preoperative transfusion for the sole purpose of facilitating elective surgery is rarely justified in an *asymptomatic* anemic patient. During the perioperative period, transfusion should be considered based on the lost circulating blood volume, Hb level, ongoing bleeding, and the risk of end-organ dysfunction due to inadequate oxygenation.

The most appropriate Hb level to serve as the trigger for perioperative blood transfusion is uncertain. The "10/30 rule" (transfuse if the Hb level is <10 g/dL or the Hct is <30%) was once a commonly cited reference point. However, there is *no* evidence that Hb values below this level mandate the need for perioperative RBC transfusion, but there *is* clear evidence that patients with Hb levels of 6 g/dL benefit from red cell transfusion. Patients with *compensated chronic anemia* with Hb values between 6 and 10 g/dL can tolerate these levels without evidence of end-organ ischemia.

The strongest evidence regarding perioperative transfusion comes from the Transfusion Requirements in Critical Care (TRICC) trial, which found no significant difference in 30-day mortality rates between a group managed using a "restrictive" transfusion strategy (transfusions were administered as necessary to keep Hb values between 7 and 8 g/dL) and a group treated using a "liberal" strategy (Hb was kept between 10 and 12 g/dL). The restrictive regime did *not* cause a significant increase in mortality, cardiac morbidity, or duration of hospitalization. Other studies also show no short- or long-term mortality benefit when a liberal transfusion strategy (transfusion when Hb was <10 g/dL) is used in patients with underlying coronary artery disease undergoing hip surgery (vs. a more restrictive strategy [i.e., transfusion when Hb < 8 g/dL]). However, the potential benefits of a restrictive transfusion plan may not be present in patients undergoing cardiac surgery. Recent data do not demonstrate a superior outcome with a restrictive transfusion strategy (when Hb < 7.5 g/dL) versus a liberal one (transfusion when Hb < 10 g/dL). Patients in the restrictive transfusion group

had a higher mortality rate but no increase in serious postoperative ischemic events.

RBC transfusions have been associated with direct transmission of infectious diseases such as hepatitis B, hepatitis C, and human immunodeficiency virus (HIV) infection. In critically ill and trauma patients, transfusions are independently associated with longer intensive care unit and hospital lengths of stay, higher mortality rates, an increased incidence of ventilator-associated pneumonia, and increased mortality. The immunomodulatory effects of RBC transfusion can lead to cancer recurrence, postoperative bacterial infection, transfusion-related acute lung injury, and hemolytic transfusion reactions.

An expected blood loss of 15% or less of total blood volume usually requires no blood replacement during surgery. A loss of up to 30% can be replaced exclusively with crystalloid solutions. A loss of more than 30%–40% generally requires RBC transfusion to restore oxygen-carrying capacity. The transfusion is given with crystalloid or colloid solutions to restore intravascular volume and maintain tissue perfusion. In cases of massive transfusion (>50% of blood volume replaced within 24 hours), RBC transfusion may need to be accompanied by administration of fresh frozen plasma and platelets at a ratio of 1:1:1.

Patients with active coronary artery disease (unstable angina or acute myocardial infarction) merit special consideration. The literature suggests that Hct of 28%–30% may be an appropriate transfusion trigger in patients with unstable coronary syndromes.

Management of Anesthesia: General Concepts for Anemia

If elective surgery is performed in the presence of chronic anemia, it is prudent to minimize the likelihood of significant changes that could further interfere with oxygen delivery to tissues. For example, drug-induced decreases in cardiac output or a leftward shift of the oxyhemoglobin dissociation curve due to respiratory alkalosis from iatrogenic hyperventilation could interfere with tissue oxygen delivery. Decreased body temperature also shifts the oxyhemoglobin dissociation curve to the left (i.e., there is less oxygen release to tissues). Decreased tissue oxygen requirements may accompany the myocardial depressant effects of anesthetic drugs and hypothermia. These offset the decrease in tissue oxygen delivery associated with anemia but to an unpredictable degree. Signs and symptoms of inadequate tissue oxygen delivery due to anemia may be difficult to appreciate during general anesthesia. Effects of anesthesia on the sympathetic nervous system and cardiovascular responses may blunt the usual increase in cardiac output associated with acute normovolemic anemia. Efforts to offset the impact of surgical blood loss by measures such as normovolemic hemodilution and intraoperative blood salvage can be considered in selected patients.

Volatile anesthetics may be *less soluble* in the plasma of anemic patients because of the decrease in concentration of lipid-rich RBCs. As a result, uptake of volatile anesthetics might be accelerated. However, the effect of this decreased solubility is likely offset by an increased cardiac output. Therefore it seems *unlikely* that clinically detectable differences in the rate of induction of inhalation anesthetics or vulnerability to an anesthetic overdose would be present in anemic patients compared to patients without anemia.

EVALUATION AND CLASSIFICATION OF ANEMIA

Anemia can be classified based on erythrokinetic mechanisms—that is, anemia due to ineffective erythropoiesis, anemia due to increased destruction of RBCs, and anemia due to blood loss. Anemia can also be classified based on morphologic characteristics—that is, microcytic, normocytic, or macrocytic based on mean corpuscular volume.

Initial evaluation of an anemic patient should include a complete blood cell count (CBC) with RBC count and standard indices, white blood cell (WBC) count, and platelet count. In addition, special indices such as RBC distribution width (RDW), which represents a measure of variation in red cell size (>14 is abnormal) and a reticulocyte count (>2% is abnormal) can indicate increased RBC destruction. Analysis of the peripheral blood smear is essential to evaluate RBC morphology.

Microcytic Anemias

Microcytic anemias are those with a mean corpuscular volume less than 80 fL. The most common causes of microcytic anemia are iron deficiency and the thalassemias. Sideroblastic anemia and (rarely) anemia of chronic disease can also present as microcytic anemias.

Iron Deficiency Anemia

Nutritional deficiency of iron as a cause of anemia is found only in infants and small children. In adults, *iron deficiency anemia (IDA) reflects depletion of iron stores caused by chronic blood loss.* Typically these losses are from the gastrointestinal (GI) tract or from the female genital tract (menstruation). Pregnant women are susceptible to development of IDA because of the increased RBC mass required during gestation and the needs of the fetus for iron.

Diagnosis

Patients experiencing chronic blood loss may not be able to absorb sufficient iron from the diet to form Hb as rapidly as RBCs are lost. As a result, RBCs are produced with too little Hb. Most cases of IDA in the United States are mild, with Hb concentrations of 9–12 g/dL. There is a concomitant decrease in serum ferritin concentration (<41 ng/mL), a low reticulocyte count, a decreased serum iron level, and a reduced transferrin saturation (<20%). The absence of stainable iron in a bone marrow aspirate is confirmatory evidence for IDA.

Treatment

Ideally IDA should be treated with ferrous iron salts administered orally and the iron stores replenished slowly. Oral iron should be considered if elective surgery can be postponed for 2–4 months to allow correction of the iron deficiency. Evidence of a favorable response to iron therapy is an increase in Hb concentration of approximately 2 g/dL in about 3 weeks and a return of Hb concentration to normal in about 6 weeks. Continued bleeding is indicated by reticulocytosis and failure of the Hb concentration to increase in response to iron therapy. Oral iron therapy should be continued for at least 1 year after the source of blood loss that caused the iron deficiency has been corrected.

If surgery is scheduled within just a few weeks, intravenous (IV) iron preparations can be used for correction of anemia. The efficacy of IV iron is superior to that of oral preparations. A total dose of 1000–1500 mg iron is usually adequate to replenish stores preoperatively and decrease the need for perioperative transfusion.

Thalassemia

Globin chains are assembled in the final globin molecule, which is a tetramer of two α-globin and two non–α-globin chains. In the adult, almost all Hb is made up of two α-globin and two β-globin chains (HbA), with minor components of HbF and HbA_2.

An inherited defect in globin chain synthesis known as *thalassemia* is one of the leading causes of microcytic anemia in children and adults. This disorder shows a strong geographic influence, with β-thalassemia predominating in Africa and the Mediterranean area, and α-thalassemia and HbE in Southeast Asia.

Thalassemia differs from IDA in several ways: presence of a family history of thalassemia, iron stores and ferritin are normal or increased, and RBC production is maintained or even disproportionately high. The diagnosis is confirmed by Hb electrophoresis, which determines the types of globin chains present.

Thalassemia Minor

Most individuals with thalassemia have *thalassemia minor* and are heterozygous for either an α-globin (α-thalassemia trait) or β-globin (β-thalassemia trait) gene mutation. Although the mutations may decrease synthesis of the affected globin chain by up to 50%, producing hypochromic and microcytic RBCs, the anemia is usually modest with relatively little accumulation of the unaffected globin. Therefore morbidity associated with chronic hemolysis and ineffective erythropoiesis is rarely encountered.

Thalassemia Intermedia

Patients with *thalassemia intermedia* show more severe anemia and prominent microcytosis and hypochromia. They have symptoms attributable to both anemia and hepatosplenomegaly, cardiomegaly, and skeletal changes secondary to bone marrow expansion. These individuals may have a mild form of homozygous β-thalassemia, a combined α- and β-thalassemia defect, or β-thalassemia with high levels of HbF.

Thalassemia Major

Patients with *thalassemia major* develop severe life-threatening anemia during the first few years of life. To survive childhood, they require repeated transfusion therapy to correct anemia and suppress the high level of ineffective erythropoiesis. The severity of this form of thalassemia is remarkably variable, even among patients with seemingly identical genetic mutations. In the most severe forms, patients exhibit three defects that markedly depress their oxygen-carrying capacity: (1) ineffective erythropoiesis, (2) hemolytic anemia, and (3) hypochromia with microcytosis. The deficit in oxygen-carrying capacity produces maximum erythropoietin release, and marrow erythroblasts respond by increasing their unbalanced globin synthesis. The accumulating unpaired globin chains aggregate and precipitate, forming inclusion bodies that cause membrane damage to the RBCs. Some of these defective red cells are destroyed within the marrow, which results in ineffective erythropoiesis. Some abnormal erythrocytes escape into the circulation, where their altered morphology causes accelerated clearance (hemolytic anemia) or, at best, reduced oxygen-carrying capacity resulting from the lower Hb content (hypochromia with microcytosis). Other features of severe thalassemia include those attributable to bone marrow hyperplasia, such as frontal bossing, maxillary overgrowth, overall stunted growth, osteoporosis, and extramedullary hematopoiesis (hepatomegaly). Hemolytic anemia may produce splenomegaly with dyspnea and orthopnea, which over time results in congestive heart failure and intellectual disability. Transfusion therapy will ameliorate many of these changes, but complications resulting from iron overload (e.g., cirrhosis, right-sided heart failure, endocrinopathy) frequently require zinc or chelation therapy. Some patients will demonstrate a reduced transfusion requirement after splenectomy. However, the risk of postsplenectomy sepsis in very young patients argues for deferring this surgery until after age 5 if possible. For patients receiving adequate transfusion and chelation therapy, splenectomy may not be indicated. Bone marrow transplantation was first performed for thalassemia major in 1982 and is a therapeutic option for young patients with an HLA-identical sibling.

Management of Anesthesia

The severity of thalassemia is the critical determinant of the amount of end-organ damage and anesthetic risk. In its mildest forms a chronic compensated anemia is a concern. With more severe forms the anemia is much more significant, as are the associated features of splenomegaly and hepatomegaly, skeletal malformations, congestive heart failure, intellectual disability, and complications of iron overload such as cirrhosis, right-sided heart failure, and endocrinopathies. Skeletal malformations can make tracheal intubation and regional anesthesia difficult.

Normocytic Anemias

Normocytic anemias have a mean corpuscular volume of 80–100 fL. Evaluation of normocytic anemia includes examination of the peripheral blood smear (for the presence of abnormally shaped RBCs), measuring the reticulocyte count (which will be low in cases of bone marrow suppression but high with a hemolytic anemia), and measuring other indices of hemolysis such as increased lactate dehydrogenase (LDH), haptoglobin, and indirect bilirubin levels. Creatinine levels will be elevated with the anemia of kidney disease. A search for a source of acute blood loss should also be undertaken.

The most common normocytic anemias are hemolytic anemias, anemia of chronic disease, anemia of kidney disease, aplastic anemia, and acute blood loss.

Hemolytic Anemias

Hemolytic anemia represents accelerated destruction (hemolysis) of erythrocytes, caused most often by hemoglobinopathies and immune disorders. In hemolytic anemias, either RBCs are removed from the circulation by the reticuloendothelial system *(extravascular hemolysis)* or the cells are lysed within the circulation *(intravascular hemolysis)*. Therefore RBC lifespan is shorter than the normal 120 days.

Hemolytic anemia is characterized by reticulocytosis, an increased mean corpuscular volume (reflecting the presence of immature erythrocytes), unconjugated hyperbilirubinemia, increased LDH levels, and decreased serum levels of haptoglobin. Confirmation of a hemolytic anemia should be followed by examination of a peripheral blood smear and a direct antiglobulin test (DAT) also known as the Coombs test to rule out an immunologic cause.

Disorders of Red Cell Structure

The mature RBC has the shape of a biconcave disk. It lacks a nucleus and mitochondria, and one-third of its mass is made up of a single protein, Hb. Intracellular energy requirements are supplied by glucose metabolism, which is targeted at maintaining Hb in a soluble reduced state, providing appropriate amounts of 2,3-diphosphoglycerate (2,3-DPG) and generating adenosine triphosphate (ATP) to support membrane function. Without a nucleus or protein metabolic pathway, the cell has a limited lifespan of about 120 days. However, the unique structure of the adult RBC provides maximum flexibility as the cell travels throughout the microvasculature.

Hereditary Spherocytosis. Abnormalities in membrane protein composition can result in lifelong hemolytic anemia. Hereditary spherocytosis is inherited in an autosomal dominant pattern. It is the most common inherited hemolytic anemia in Europe and the United States, with a frequency of 1 in 5000 individuals. The principal defect is a deficiency in membrane skeletal proteins, usually spectrin and ankyrin. Affected cells show abnormal osmotic fragility and a shortened circulation half-life. Hereditary spherocytosis can be clinically silent, and about one-third of patients have only a very mild hemolytic anemia and spherocytes rarely visible on peripheral blood smear. Some patients, however, have a more severe degree of hemolysis and anemia, but fewer than 5% of patients with spherocytosis develop life-threatening anemia. Patients with hereditary spherocytosis often have splenomegaly and experience easy fatigability that is out of proportion to the degree of anemia. These patients are at risk for episodes of hemolytic crisis, often precipitated by viral or bacterial infection. These crises worsen the chronic anemia and may be associated with jaundice. Infection with parvovirus B19 can produce a transient (10–14 days) but profound aplastic crisis. The risk of pigment gallstones is high in patients with hereditary spherocytosis and should be considered in patients complaining of biliary colic.

Management of Anesthesia. Anesthetic risk in these patients is dictated by the severity of the anemia and whether the hemolysis is stable or in a period of exacerbation due to concurrent infection.

Episodic anemia, often triggered by viral or bacterial infection and cholelithiasis, must be considered in the preoperative evaluation. Patients undergoing cardiac surgery with cardiopulmonary bypass merit special consideration. The use of cardiopulmonary bypass may lead to excessive hemolysis because spherocytes are more susceptible to mechanical and shear stress than normal erythrocytes. Mechanical heart valves should be avoided, but "short-term" use of cardiopulmonary bypass may be safe. In addition, patients with spherocytosis who have undergone splenectomy are at increased risk of arterial and venous thromboembolism.

Hereditary Elliptocytosis. Hereditary elliptocytosis is caused by an abnormality in one of the membrane proteins, spectrin or glycophorin, which makes the erythrocyte less pliable. Hereditary elliptocytosis is inherited as an autosomal dominant disorder and is prevalent in regions where malaria is endemic. In those areas the incidence may reach 3 in 100 people. Hereditary elliptocytosis is most often diagnosed as an incidental finding. The majority of RBCs demonstrate an elliptical or even rodlike appearance. Most patients with hereditary elliptocytosis are heterozygous and only rarely experience hemolysis. In contrast, those with homozygous or compound heterozygous defects may demonstrate greater degrees of hemolysis and more severe anemia.

Acanthocytosis. Acanthocytosis is another defect in membrane structure found in patients with a congenital lack of β-lipoprotein *(abetalipoproteinemia)* and infrequently in patients with cirrhosis or severe pancreatitis. It results from cholesterol or sphingomyelin accumulation on the outer membrane of the erythrocyte. This accretion gives the membrane a spiculated appearance and signals the splenic macrophages of the reticuloendothelial system to remove the red cell from the circulation, which produces hemolysis.

Paroxysmal Nocturnal Hemoglobinuria. Paroxysmal nocturnal hemoglobinuria (PNH) is a *stem cell disorder* that may arise in hematopoietic cells any time from the second to the eighth decade of life. Classically, patients pass dark-colored urine in the morning owing to the presence of hemosiderin. PNH causes complement-activated RBC hemolysis. This is caused by a mutation in the *PICA* gene located on the X chromosome, thus affecting both males and females equally. Besides hemolytic anemia, patients are at risk for other complications of Hb release such as smooth muscle dystonia, pulmonary hypertension, renal insufficiency, and

hypercoagulability. Hemolytic anemia can be either intravascular or extravascular because patients with PNH lack a surface-bound complement-regulating protein that normally protects RBCs and WBCs from complement-mediated lysis. Thromboses occur in approximately 40% of patients and can involve the hepatic and portal veins as well as other veins. The basis of the tendency to develop thromboses is unclear. About one-third of patients develop aplastic anemia.

Treatment of PNH. In the past, the life expectancy of patients with PNH was 8–10 years after diagnosis. In 2007 the US Food and Drug Administration (FDA) approved eculizumab for transfusion-dependent patients and for those with other disabling symptoms of the disease such as fatigue, smooth muscle dystonia, thrombosis, and significant renal insufficiency. Eculizumab is a monoclonal antibody against complement factor C5, which is essential for the complement system to develop membrane attack complexes. Patients with severe aplastic anemia and patients unresponsive to eculizumab are candidates for allogeneic bone marrow transplantation as a definitive treatment.

Management of Anesthesia. The nocturnal manifestation of hemolysis is thought to result from carbon dioxide retention and the subsequent respiratory acidosis. Therefore during anesthesia, predisposing factors such as hypoxemia, hypoperfusion, and hypercarbia that can lead to acidosis and complement activation must be avoided. If perioperative transfusion is deemed necessary, washed RBCs should be administered to decrease the risk of complement activation. Prophylaxis against venous thrombosis should be administered perioperatively.

Disorders of Red Cell Metabolism

Lacking a nucleus and having a limited life expectancy, the erythrocyte maintains only the very narrow spectrum of activities necessary to carry out its oxygen transport function. The stability of the RBC membrane and the solubility of intracellular Hb depend on four glucose-supported metabolic pathways. These four pathways are illustrated in Fig. 24.1. The most clinically relevant pathways are described in the following sections.

Embden-Meyerhof Pathway. The Embden-Meyerhof pathway (nonoxidative or anaerobic pathway) is responsible for generation of the ATP necessary for membrane function and the maintenance of cell shape and pliability. Defects in anaerobic glycolysis are associated with increased red cell rigidity and decreased survival, which produces a hemolytic anemia. Deficiencies of the glycolytic pathway are not associated with any typical morphologic red cell changes, nor do they lead to hemolytic crisis after exposure to oxidants. The severity of hemolysis is highly variable and largely unpredictable.

Phosphogluconate Pathway. The phosphogluconate pathway couples oxidative metabolism with nicotinamide adenine dinucleotide phosphate (NADP) and glutathione reduction. It counteracts environmental oxidants and prevents globin denaturation. When patients lack either glucose-6-phosphate dehydrogenase (G6PD) or glutathione reductase, denatured Hb precipitates on the inner surface of the RBC membrane.

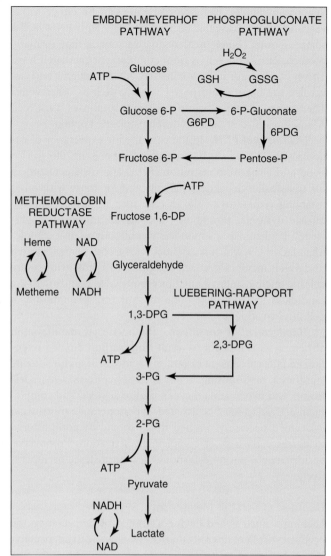

FIG. 24.1 Diagrammatic representation of the four pathways involved in the most common disorders affecting red blood cell metabolism. *ATP,* Adenosine triphosphate; *1,6-DP,* 1,6-diphosphate; *1,3-DPG,* 1,3-diphosphoglycerate; *2,3,-DPG,* 2,3-diphosphoglycerate; *G6PD,* glucose-6-phosphate dehydrogenase; *GSH,* glutathione reductase; *GSSG,* oxidized glutathione; *NAD,* nicotinamide adenine dinucleotide; *NADH,* reduced form of nicotinamide adenine dinucleotide; *6-P,* 6-phosphate; *6PDG,* 6-phosphogluconate dehydrogenase; *2-PG,* 2-phosphoglycerate; *3-PG,* 3-phosphoglycerate; *6-P-Gluconate,* 6-phosphogluconate; *Pentose-P,* pentose phosphate.

This is visible on the peripheral blood smear as Heinz bodies and results in membrane damage and hemolysis.

Glucose-6-Phosphate Dehydrogenase Deficiency. G6PD deficiency is an X-linked genetic disease and is the most common enzymatic disorder of RBCs, with more than 400 million people affected worldwide. G6PD activity is normally highest in young red cells and declines with the age of these cells. The half-life of erythrocytes in G6PD deficiency is approximately 60 days. Clinical manifestations depend on the amount of the enzyme present, with five classes described by the World Health Organization. Patients can have chronic hemolytic anemia (class I, <10% G6PD activity), intermittent hemolysis (class II, 10% G6PD activity), and hemolysis only with stressors (class III, 10%–60% G6PD activity). Classes IV and V have *increased* G6PD activity. There is no hemolysis in class IV or V.

Hemolysis is the result of the inability of a G6PD-deficient RBC to protect itself from oxidative damage. Events that can precipitate new or aggravate preexisting hemolysis include infection, certain metabolic conditions such as diabetic ketoacidosis, certain drugs, and ingestion of fava beans.

Anesthetic risk is largely a function of the severity and acuity of this anemia. The goal is to avoid the risk of hemolysis by not exposing the patient to oxidative drugs. In vitro studies show that codeine, benzodiazepines (except for diazepam), propofol, fentanyl, and ketamine are safe, but that it might be wise to avoid isoflurane, sevoflurane, metoclopramide, and penicillin, all of which depress G6PD activity in vitro. Methylene blue is a particular concern. If a patient with methemoglobinemia (with already compromised oxygen delivery) is also G6PD deficient, methylene blue administration may be life threatening. Drugs that can induce methemoglobinemia (e.g., lidocaine, prilocaine, silver nitrate) should be avoided. Many antibiotics and vitamin K should also be avoided. Hypothermia, acidosis, hyperglycemia, and infection can precipitate hemolysis in the G6PD-deficient patient, and these conditions need to be aggressively treated in the perioperative period.

Pyruvate Kinase Deficiency. Pyruvate kinase deficiency, an autosomal recessive disorder, is the most common erythrocyte enzyme defect causing *congenital hemolytic anemia.* Pyruvate kinase deficiency is found worldwide but shows a higher prevalence among people of Northern European extraction and individuals from some regions of China. Although less prevalent than G6PD deficiency, pyruvate kinase deficiency is much more likely to produce a chronic hemolytic anemia. The severity of the clinical presentation ranges from a mild fully compensated process without anemia to life-threatening, transfusion-requiring hemolytic anemia at birth. Severely affected individuals may have chronic jaundice, develop pigmented gallstones, and manifest splenomegaly. Splenectomy does not totally prevent hemolysis but does decrease the rate of RBC destruction and may even eliminate the need for transfusion.

Methemoglobin Reductase Pathway. The methemoglobin reductase pathway uses the pyridine nucleotide–reduced nicotinamide adenine dinucleotide (NADP) generated from anaerobic glycolysis to maintain heme iron in its ferrous state. An inherited mutation of the methemoglobin reductase enzyme results in an inability to counteract oxidation of Hb to methemoglobin. The ferric form of Hb does not transport oxygen. Patients with type I enzyme deficiency accumulate small amounts of methemoglobin in circulating red cells, whereas patients with type II disease have severe cyanosis and intellectual disability.

Luebering-Rapoport Pathway. The Luebering-Rapoport pathway is responsible for production of 2,3-DPG. A single enzyme—2,3 bisphosphoglycerate mutase—mediates both the synthesis of 2,3-DPG and the phosphatase activity that then converts 2,3-DPG to 3-phosphoglycerate, returning it to the glycolytic pathway. The balance of formation versus metabolism of 2,3-DPG is pH sensitive, with alkalosis favoring synthetic activity and acidosis favoring metabolic breakdown. The 2,3-DPG response is also influenced by the supply of phosphate. Severe phosphate depletion in patients with diabetic ketoacidosis or nutritional deficiency can result in reduced 2,3-DPG production.

Disorders of Hemoglobin

Inherited defects in Hb structure can interfere with its affinity for oxygen and the process of binding/unloading oxygen. Most defects are substitutions of a single amino acid in either the α- or β-globin chains. Some interfere with molecular movement, restricting the molecule to either a low- or high-affinity state, whereas others change the valency of heme iron from ferrous to ferric or reduce the solubility of the Hb molecule. HbS (the abnormal Hb in sickle cell disease) is an example of an Hb with a single amino acid substitution that results in reduced solubility, which causes precipitation of the abnormal Hb.

Sickle S Hemoglobin. Sickle cell disease is a disorder caused by the substitution of valine for glutamic acid in the β-globin subunit. In the deoxygenated state, HbS undergoes conformational changes that expose a hydrophobic region of the molecule. In states of severe deoxygenation the hydrophobic regions aggregate, and this results in distortion of the erythrocyte membrane, oxidative damage to the membrane, impaired deformability, and a shortened lifespan of only 10–20 days.

Sickle cell anemia, the homozygous form of HbS disease, presents early in life with severe hemolytic anemia and progresses to significant end-organ damage involving the bone marrow, spleen, kidneys, and central nervous system. Patients experience episodic painful crises (vasoocclusive crises) characterized by bone and joint pain that may or may not be associated with concurrent illness, stress, or dehydration. The severity and progression of the disease can vary remarkably. Organ damage can start early in childhood, with recurrent splenic infarction culminating in loss of splenic function in the first decade of life. The kidney can demonstrate painless hematuria and loss of concentrating ability as an early feature and then progress to chronic renal failure in the third or fourth decade of life. Pulmonary and neurologic complications are the major causes of morbidity and mortality. Lung damage results from chronic persistent inflammation. *Acute chest syndrome,* a pneumonia-like complication, is characterized by the presence of a new pulmonary infiltrate involving at least one entire lung segment *plus* at least one of the following: chest pain, fever, tachypnea, wheezing, or cough. Neurologic complications include stroke, usually as a result of arterial disease rather than sickling. Adolescents present with cerebral infarction, whereas adults typically develop hemorrhagic strokes.

Management of Anesthesia. Sickle cell trait does not cause an increase in perioperative morbidity or mortality. However, sickle cell disease is associated with a high incidence of perioperative complications. Risk factors include advanced age, frequent and severe recent episodes of sickling, evidence of end-organ damage (e.g., low baseline oxygen saturation, elevated

creatinine level, cardiac dysfunction, history of stroke), and concurrent infection. Risks intrinsic to the type of surgery are also important considerations, with minor procedures considered to be low risk, intraabdominal operations categorized as intermediate risk, and intracranial and intrathoracic procedures classified as high risk. Among orthopedic procedures, hip surgery and hip replacement in particular are associated with a high risk of complications, including excessive blood loss and sickling events.

The goals of preoperative management in patients with sickle cell disease have changed in recent years. Studies examining the effects of aggressive transfusion strategies aimed at increasing the *ratio of normal Hb to sickle Hb* appear to show *no benefit* compared with the more conservative goal of achieving an overall preoperative Hct of 30% (HbS combined with HbA or HbF). The aggressive strategy had necessitated significantly more transfusions, and complications from these transfusions have been significant.

Patients undergoing low-risk procedures now rarely require any preoperative transfusion, and patients undergoing moderate- to high-risk operations need only have preoperative anemia corrected to a target Hct (all Hb types) of 30%. However, some suggest that HbS levels below 30% are desirable for major noncardiac surgery, and HbS levels below 5% are desirable for cardiac surgery involving cardiopulmonary bypass, which is associated with several factors that can promote sickling and hemolysis. In such patients, exchange transfusion can be used perioperatively in conjunction with hydroxyurea (which increases levels of HbF) to achieve the desired low concentration of HbS.

Anesthetic technique *does not* appear to significantly affect the risk of complications stemming from sickle cell disease. Secondary goals like avoiding dehydration, acidosis, and hypothermia *do* help reduce the risk of perioperative sickling events. Use of occlusive orthopedic tourniquets is not contraindicated, but the incidence of perioperative complications is increased with their use. Postoperative pain requires aggressive, typically multimodal, pain management. Patients often have a degree of tolerance to opioids, and a subset of patients may even have opiate addiction, but these facts must not interfere with appropriate perioperative pain management.

Despite concerns that regional anesthesia might have detrimental effects in sickle cell patients, it is not contraindicated and may offer an advantage in pain control.

Acute chest syndrome may develop 2–3 days postoperatively and requires treatment of hypoxemia, pain, hypovolemia, anemia, likely infection, and possible venous thrombosis. Mild cases may respond to simple transfusion. Exchange transfusion may be needed in severely affected patients.

Sickle C Hemoglobin. The prevalence of HbC is about one-fourth that of HbS. HbC causes the erythrocyte to lose water via enhanced activity of the potassium chloride cotransport system. This results in cellular dehydration that in the homozygous state may produce a mild to moderate hemolytic anemia. *HbS trait or HbC trait in isolation cause no symptoms.* However, when they are present *together* (HbSC disease) they can produce sickling and complications similar to those of HbSS disease. It appears that the dehydration produced by HbC increases the concentration of HbS within the erythrocyte, exacerbating its insolubility and tendency to polymerize.

Management of Anesthesia. The anesthetic risks of HbSC disease have not been as well studied as those of HbSS disease. However, one investigation suggested that perioperative transfusion may reduce the incidence of sickling complications.

Sickle Hemoglobin–β-Thalassemia. Among African Americans, the frequency of the β-thalassemia gene is only one-tenth that of the gene for HbS. The clinical presentation of this compound heterozygous state is largely determined by whether it is associated with reduced amounts of HbA (sickle cell–β⁺-thalassemia) or no HbA whatsoever (sickle cell–β⁰-thalassemia). In the absence of any HbA, patients experience acute vasoocclusive crises, acute chest syndrome, and other sickling complications at rates approaching those of patients with HbSS.

Unstable Hemoglobins. Hbs are made unstable by structural changes that reduce their solubility or render them more susceptible to oxidation of amino acids within the globin chains. More than 100 unique unstable Hb variants have been documented, most associated with minimal clinical impact. The mutations typically impair the globin folding or hemoglobin binding that stabilizes the heme moiety within the hydrophobic globin pocket. Once freed from its cleft, the heme binds nonspecifically to other regions of the globin chains. This causes formation of precipitates called *Heinz bodies* that contains globin chains, chain fragments, and heme. Heinz bodies interact with the red cell membrane, reducing its deformability and favoring its removal by macrophages in the spleen. Unstable Hbs vary in their propensity to form Heinz bodies and also in the severity of any associated anemia. Hemolysis may be aggravated by the development of additional oxidative stresses, such as infection or ingestion of oxidizing drugs. Patients with recurring bouts of severe hemolysis or significant morbidity from the chronic anemia should be considered candidates for splenectomy, which is usually effective in reducing or even eliminating symptoms and signs.

Management of Anesthesia. Anesthetic management of patients with unstable Hbs is largely dictated by the degree of hemolysis. Transfusion during bouts of severe hemolysis and avoidance of oxidizing drugs are important. These patients may have severe anemia and Hb-induced renal injury.

Autoimmune Hemolytic Anemias

Autoimmune hemolytic anemias result from RBC cell lysis due to *warm agglutinins* (mostly immunoglobulin [Ig]G-mediated lysis at *body temperature*) or *cold agglutinins* (IgM-mediated lysis at lower temperatures). Antibodies against RBCs can be detected by a DAT (Coombs test). Warm autoimmune hemolytic anemia (WAHA) is associated with lupus (10% of lupus patients develop warm agglutinins), hematologic malignancies (non-Hodgkin lymphoma, chronic lymphocytic leukemia), viral infections (HIV) or drugs (penicillins, cephalosporins, quinine, quinidine, nonsteroidal antiinflammatory drugs [NSAIDs]). WAHA episodes are managed supportively and/or with corticosteroids.

Patients who are not responsive to steroids are candidates for splenectomy, rituximab, or other cytotoxic drugs.

Cold agglutinin disease manifests as hemolytic episodes that occur at lower temperatures. Pathologic cold agglutinins can be a result of certain infections (*Mycoplasma pneumoniae*, infectious mononucleosis) or of neoplastic/paraneoplastic processes. Avoidance of cold temperatures is the mainstay of therapy in such patients. Although the majority of patients do not require treatment, more severe cases may benefit from treatment with rituximab with or without fludarabine. *Glucocorticoids and splenectomy have no value in cold agglutinin disease.* Plasmapheresis should be considered in patients about to undergo surgery (especially surgery involving cardiopulmonary bypass), since plasmapheresis can remove up to 80% of these antibodies.

Anemia of Chronic Disease

Anemia of chronic disease (ACD) manifests as a normocytic, normochromic, hypoproliferative anemia due to decreased production of RBCs coupled with somewhat shortened RBC survival. ACD is thought to result from several mechanisms: trapping of iron in macrophages (resulting in a lower level of circulating iron available for hematopoiesis), a decrease in erythropoietin concentrations resulting in a decreased in bone marrow red cell production, and shorter RBC lifespan due to increased macrophage activity.

Patients with ACD present with low iron levels, normal to low transferrin levels, normal to high ferritin levels, but a *normal* transferrin saturation. This is in particular contrast to IDA, in which there is a *low* transferrin saturation. Markers of active inflammation may be present, such as an elevated sedimentation rate and C-reactive protein level. The CBC may support a diagnosis of infection with a high WBC count.

The diagnosis of ACD is supported by the clinical picture, with most patients already carrying a diagnosis of a chronic inflammatory or infectious disease or malignancy at the time the anemia is discovered.

Treatment

The ideal treatment for ACD is cure of the underlying disease, which unfortunately is not often possible. Preoperative treatment of patients with ACD may involve administration of iron with erythropoiesis-stimulating drugs such as darbepoetin and erythropoietin. Iron alone should *never* be given to patients with ACD due to malignancy and infection, since iron can worsen the underlying disease(s). Erythropoiesis-stimulating drugs should be avoided in patients with ACD due to cancer (especially during active treatment), but they are approved for treatment of significant anemia due to chemotherapy. The minimum effective dose should be administered to avoid thromboembolic complications. These drugs can also be used in patients with rheumatoid arthritis and HIV with low erythropoietin levels.

Anemia of Chronic Kidney Disease

The anemia of chronic kidney disease results from decreased erythropoietin production. Therefore these patients benefit from administration of erythropoiesis-stimulating drugs. The target Hb should be 10–12 g/dL, even with patients on hemodialysis, since these patients benefit with a reduction in their symptoms and a better quality of life. Concurrent iron deficiency should be investigated and treated to ensure optimal red cell production.

Aplastic Anemia

Congenital aplastic anemia (Fanconi anemia) is an autosomal recessive disorder that presents in the first 2 decades of life with severe pancytopenia that often progresses to acute leukemia. When the gene is fully expressed (as occurs in 1 per 100,000 live births), this disorder is associated with progressive bone marrow failure, a number of physical defects, chromosomal abnormalities, and a predisposition to cancer. Not all patients have the classic physical defects, so the diagnosis should be considered in all children and young adults with acute myelogenous leukemia.

Acquired aplastic anemia is due to bone marrow toxicity, typically from drugs. Anemia due to bone marrow damage is a predictable side effect of chemotherapy, and this anemia is usually mild unless high-dose multidrug chemotherapy that can cause pancytopenia is used. So long as the drugs do not irreversibly damage the bone marrow, recovery is usually complete. High-energy radiation can also produce anemia from bone marrow damage, the degree of which is predictable from the type of radiation, the dose, and the extent of bone marrow exposure. Long-term exposure to low levels of external radiation or ingested radioisotopes can produce aplastic anemia.

Several drugs have been associated with the development of severe, often irreversible, aplastic anemia. Table 24.1 lists many classes of these drugs. Some (e.g., chloramphenicol) can produce severe irreversible aplastic anemia after only a few doses, but most (e.g., phenylbutazone, propylthiouracil, tricyclic antidepressants) are associated with a more gradual onset of pancytopenia, which is reversible if the offending drug is withdrawn.

Immunosuppression of stem cell growth can also produce anemia, even aplastic anemia. This can be seen following viral

TABLE 24.1 Classes of Drugs Associated With Marrow Damage

Antibiotics (chloramphenicol, penicillin, cephalosporins, sulfonamides, amphotericin B, streptomycin)
Antidepressants (lithium, tricyclics)
Antiepileptics (phenytoin, carbamazepine, valproic acid, phenobarbital)
Antiinflammatory drugs (phenylbutazone, nonsteroidals, salicylates, gold salts)
Antidysrhythmics (lidocaine, quinidine, procainamide)
Antithyroidal drugs (propylthiouracil)
Diuretics (thiazides, pyrimethamine, furosemide)
Antihypertensives (captopril)
Antiuricemics (allopurinol, colchicine)
Antimalarials (quinacrine, chloroquine)
Hypoglycemics (tolbutamide)
Platelet inhibitors (ticlopidine)
Tranquilizers (prochlorperazine, meprobamate)

illnesses such as viral hepatitis, Epstein-Barr virus infection, HIV infection, and rubella. Parvovirus B19 infection can cause an acute reversible pure red cell aplasia in patients with congenital hemolytic anemia. Although most of these anemias are reversible, some infections can produce fatal aplastic anemia.

Management of Anesthesia

Patients may come for surgery with anemia and thrombocytopenia severe enough that transfusion is necessary preoperatively. The severity of the neutropenia will affect the need for and choice of antibiotic coverage. The use of granulocyte colony-stimulating factor preoperatively to increase neutrophil counts is controversial.

Macrocytic/Megaloblastic Anemias

Disruption of the erythroid precursor maturation sequence can result from deficiencies in vitamins such as folic acid and vitamin B_{12}, exposure to chemotherapeutic agents, or a preleukemic state. Since these are all defects in *nuclear maturation*, patients have *macrocytic anemia* and *megaloblastic* bone marrow morphology.

Folate and Vitamin B_{12} Deficiency Anemia

Folic acid and vitamin B_{12} deficiency are primary causes of macrocytic anemia in adults. Both vitamins are essential for normal DNA synthesis, and high-turnover tissues such as bone marrow are the first to be affected when these vitamins are in short supply. In deficiency states the marrow precursors appear much larger than normal and are unable to complete cell division. Therefore the marrow becomes megaloblastic, and macrocytic red cells are released into the circulation. The prevalence of deficiency of these vitamins varies considerably in different parts of the world. In developed countries, alcoholism is a frequent cause of folate deficiency, both because of the poor dietary habits of alcoholic individuals and because of alcohol's interference with folate metabolism. In developing countries where tropical and nontropical sprue are more widespread, malabsorption may increase the frequency of vitamin B_{12} deficiency.

Sustained exposure to nitrous oxide can produce an impairment of vitamin B_{12} activity. Nitrous oxide can oxidize the cobalt atom of the vitamin, which reduces its cofactor activity and causes impairment in both methionine synthesis and *S*-adenosylmethionine synthesis. This action requires *long* exposure to *high* concentrations of nitrous oxide and pertains only to situations in which scavenging systems are inadequate or there is recreational use of this gas.

The macrocytic anemia caused by folate or vitamin B_{12} deficiency may result in Hb levels below 8–10 g/dL, a mean red cell volume of 110–140 fL (normal, 90 fL), a normal reticulocyte count, and increased levels of LDH and bilirubin. In addition to causing megaloblastic anemia, vitamin B_{12} deficiency is associated with peripheral neuropathy due to degeneration of the lateral and posterior columns of the spinal cord. There are symmetrical paresthesias with loss of proprioceptive and vibratory sensations, especially in the lower extremities. Gait is unsteady, and deep tendon reflexes are diminished. Memory impairment and depression may be prominent. These neurologic deficits are progressive unless vitamin B_{12} is provided. Abuse of nitrous oxide may be associated with neurologic findings similar to those that accompany vitamin B_{12} deficiency and pernicious anemia.

Folate and/or vitamin B_{12} deficiency can be corrected by vitamin administration. In cases of intestinal malabsorption the parenteral route is preferred. Emergency correction of life-threatening anemia or preparation for urgent surgery requires red cell transfusion.

OTHER HEMOGLOBIN-RELATED DISORDERS

Hemoglobins With Increased Oxygen Affinity

Hb mutations that increase the oxygen-binding avidity of the heme moiety cause the oxyhemoglobin dissociation curve to shift to the left, which reduces the P_{50}, the partial pressure of oxygen at which Hb is 50% saturated with oxygen. Many types of mutations can *increase* oxygen affinity. *These Hbs bind oxygen more readily than normal and retain more oxygen at lower Po_2 levels.* Accordingly they deliver less oxygen to tissues at normal capillary Po_2, and blood returns to the lungs still partially saturated with oxygen. The net result is mild tissue hypoxia that triggers increased erythropoietin production, leading to polycythemia.

Management of Anesthesia

Tissue oxygen delivery at baseline may be barely adequate, so even a modest decrease in Hct is potentially dangerous. Patients with only mild erythrocytosis do not require intervention. Patients with high Hcts (>55%–60%), whose blood viscosity may further compromise oxygen delivery, will require hydration and possibly preoperative exchange transfusion.

Hemoglobins With Decreased Oxygen Affinity

Methemoglobinemia

Methemoglobin (HbM) is formed when the iron moiety in Hb is oxidized from the ferrous (Fe^{2+}) to the ferric (Fe^{3+}) state. Normal Hb, when bound to oxygen, partially transfers an electron from the iron to the oxygen, which moves the iron close to its ferric state, and the oxygen resembles a superoxide. Deoxygenation ordinarily returns the electron to the iron, but methemoglobin forms if the electron is not returned. The normal erythrocyte maintains methemoglobin levels at 1% or less by the methemoglobin reductase enzyme system. Methemoglobin moves the oxyhemoglobin dissociation curve markedly to the left and therefore delivers little oxygen to the tissues. Methemoglobin levels below 30% of total Hb content may cause no compromise in tissue oxygenation. However, levels between 30% and 50% do cause symptoms and signs of oxygen deprivation, and levels above 50% can result in coma and death.

Methemoglobinemia of clinical importance can arise from three mechanisms: globin chain mutations favoring the formation of methemoglobin, mutations impairing the efficacy of the methemoglobin reductase system, and toxic exposure to substances that oxidize normal Hb iron at a rate that exceeds the capacity of the normal reducing mechanisms.

HbM arises from mutations that stabilize heme iron in the ferric (Fe^{3+}) state, making it relatively resistant to reduction by the methemoglobin reductase system. The methemoglobin has a brownish blue color that does not change to red on exposure to oxygen, which gives patients a cyanotic appearance *(pseudocyanosis)* independent of their Pao_2. Patients with M-type Hb are usually asymptomatic, since their methemoglobin levels rarely exceed 30% of total Hb.

Mutations impairing the methemoglobin reductase system usually result in methemoglobinemia levels below 25%. Therefore these affected patients may also exhibit slate-gray pseudocyanosis despite normal Pao_2 levels. Exposure to chemical materials that directly oxidize Hb or produce reactive oxygen intermediates that oxidize Hb may produce an *acquired methemoglobinemia* in which life-threatening amounts of methemoglobin accumulate. Since infants have lower levels of methemoglobin reductase in their erythrocytes, they manifest greater susceptibility to oxidizing agents.

Management of Anesthesia

Management of anesthesia in patients with methemoglobinemia focuses on avoiding any tissue hypoxia. Pulse oximetry is unreliable in this setting because most pulse oximeters cannot detect methemoglobin. An intraarterial catheter should be inserted to be able to measure blood pressure, methemoglobin levels, and arterial blood gas concentrations. Any acidosis should be corrected, and the electrocardiogram must be closely monitored for signs of ischemia. Patients with HbM may be very sensitive to exposure to oxidizing agents. Therefore local anesthetics, nitrates, and nitric oxide should be avoided.

Methylene blue is the treatment for toxic methemoglobinemia. The dosage is 1–2 mg/kg infused over 3–5 minutes. A single treatment is usually effective but might need to be repeated after 30 minutes. Methylene blue acts through the methemoglobin reductase system and requires the activity of G6PD. Patients who are G6PD deficient and patients severely affected by methemoglobin may require exchange transfusion instead.

POLYCYTHEMIA

Sustained hypoxia usually results in a compensatory increase in RBC mass and Hct. Although this increases the oxygen-carrying capacity of the blood, it also increases blood viscosity. Tissue *oxygen delivery* is maximal at a Hct of 33%–36% (Hb concentration, 11–12 g/dL), assuming no changes occur in cardiac output or regional blood flow. With higher Hcts there is an increase in blood viscosity that will tend to slow blood flow and decrease oxygen delivery. This effect is relatively minor until the Hct exceeds 55%–60%, at which time blood flow to vital organs can be significantly reduced.

Physiology of Polycythemia

Polycythemia and *erythrocytosis* are terms that describe an abnormally high Hct. Even modest increases in the Hct can have a major impact on whole-blood viscosity. An increase in Hct can result from a reduction in plasma volume *(relative polycythemia)* without an actual increase in red cell mass. An acute decrease in plasma volume, as may be seen with preoperative fasting, can convert an asymptomatic polycythemia into one in which hyperviscosity threatens tissue perfusion. When the Hct rises to levels above 55%–60%, whole-blood viscosity increases *exponentially,* affecting blood flow especially in small blood vessels such as capillaries with low flow/ shear rates. The cerebral circulation is particularly vulnerable to reductions in blood flow resulting from increased viscosity (Figs. 24.2 and 24.3).

The signs and symptoms of a high Hct vary depending on the underlying disease process and the rate of development of the erythrocytosis. Patients with modest chronic polycythemia have few complaints until the Hct exceeds 55%–60%. Headaches and easy fatigability then occur. Hct levels above 60% can be life threatening because the increase in viscosity threatens vital organ perfusion. Patients with such high Hcts are also at significant risk of venous and arterial thromboses.

Polycythemia Vera

Primary polycythemia, also known as *polycythemia vera* (PV), is a stem cell disorder characterized by proliferation of a clone of hematopoietic precursors, nearly all of which arise from a mutation in the *JAK2* (Janus kinase 2) gene. This clonal expansion most commonly produces an excess of erythrocytes, but the number of platelets and leukocytes may also be increased. The criteria for a diagnosis of polycythemia vera include an elevated Hb level (>18.5 g/dL in men, >16.5 g/dL in women) and either the presence of the *JAK2* mutation or two of the following: hypercellularity of bone marrow, subnormal serum erythropoietin level, or endogenous erythroid colony formation. Polycythemia vera may appear at any age, but most patients develop the disease in their sixth or seventh decade. Patients can have a number of symptoms. Budd-Chiari syndrome (hepatic vein occlusion) is a common presentation, as is generalized pruritus and erythromelalgia. Coronary or cerebral thrombosis is also a common presenting sign. Pulmonary hypertension occurs with increased frequency in this population. Patients generally require regular phlebotomy and may also require treatment with myelosuppressive drugs such as hydroxyurea to control the Hct. Ruxolitinib, a JAK1/JAK2 inhibitor, is also now used to treat PV. Approximately 30% of patients with PV will die of thrombotic

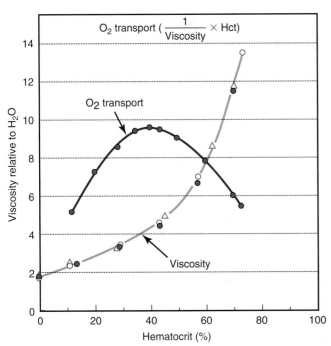

FIG. 24.2   Viscosity of heparinized normal human blood as a function of hematocrit (Hct). Viscosity is measured with an Ostwald viscosimeter at 37°C and expressed in relation to the viscosity of saline solution. Oxygen transport is computed from Hct and oxygen flow (1/viscosity) and is recorded in arbitrary units. (Data from Murray JF, Gold P, Johnson BL Jr, et al. Clinical manifestations and classification of erythrocyte disorders. In: Kaushansky K, Lichtman M, Beutler E, et al., eds. *Williams Hematology.* 8th ed. New York: McGraw-Hill Medical; 2010.)

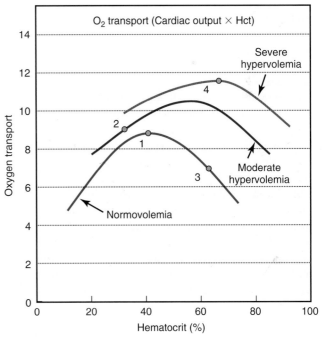

FIG. 24.3   Oxygen transport at various hematocrit (Hct) levels in normovolemia, moderate hypervolemia, and severe hypervolemia. Oxygen transport is estimated by multiplying Hct by cardiac output. (Adapted from Murray JF, Gold P, Johnson BL Jr, et al. Clinical manifestations and classification of erythrocyte disorders. In: Kaushansky K, Lichtman M, Beutler E, et al., eds. *Williams Hematology.* 8th ed. New York: McGraw-Hill Medical; 2010.)

complications and another 30% will succumb to cancer, most commonly myelofibrosis and acute leukemia.

Patients with PV who are undergoing surgery are at risk of perioperative thrombosis and (paradoxically) hemorrhage. This increased risk of thrombosis is due to the combination of baseline hypercoagulability augmented by the prothrombotic state of surgery. Hemorrhage is attributable to an acquired von Willebrand disease caused by abnormally low amounts of the ultralarge von Willebrand factor (vWF) multimers essential to normal platelet adhesion. The hyperviscosity associated with a high Hct favors a conformational change in vWF that renders it vulnerable to enzymatic cleavage. Therefore the most hemostatically effective large multimers become depleted, which then creates the risk of bleeding. Phlebotomy and absolute avoidance of dehydration lower the risk of both thrombosis and hemorrhage during the perioperative period.

Management of Anesthesia
Polycythemia vera patients are at risk for perioperative thromboses and hemorrhage. Reducing the Hct before surgery to 45% in men and 42% in women via phlebotomy and hydration may reduce the risk of thrombohemorrhagic complications. Thrombocytosis, if present, should be decreased to below 400,000 platelets/mm^3. Cytoreduction with hydroxyurea is recommended in patients older than 60 years or with a prior history of thrombosis. Hydroxyurea can often resolve the acquired vWF disease. Aspirin therapy should be withheld for 7 days before surgery. Desmopressin and vWF factor concentrates can be beneficial in improving levels of vWF and thus in reducing bleeding.

Secondary Polycythemia Due to Hypoxia

An increase in the RBC mass without evidence of a change in other hematopoietic cell lines is a normal physiologic response to hypoxia, regardless of cause. Individuals living at high altitudes develop a compensatory polycythemia that is physiologically appropriate and not associated with clinical abnormalities. At altitudes over 7000 feet, humans are at risk of both acute and chronic mountain sickness.

Significant cardiopulmonary disease can also result in enough tissue hypoxia to induce polycythemia. Congenital heart disease with a significant right-to-left shunt and cyanosis is a good example. Extremely low cardiac output, whether congenital or acquired, may stimulate release of erythropoietin and be associated with an increased Hct. Pulmonary disease can result in hypoxia-induced polycythemia. Extreme obesity with development of the obesity-hypoventilation syndrome (Pickwickian syndrome) is another classic example. Inherited defects of Hb, such as Hbs with a high-affinity for oxygen and defects in the amount or function 2,3-DPG, may cause polycythemia due to reduced tissue oxygen delivery and a leftward shift in the oxyhemoglobin dissociation curve. Defects or drugs producing significant methemoglobinemia can also lead to a compensatory polycythemia.

Secondary Polycythemia Due to Increased Erythropoietin Production

Renal disease and several erythropoietin-secreting tumors have been associated with secondary polycythemia. Hydronephrosis, polycystic kidney disease, renal cysts, and both benign and malignant renal tumors can result in increased erythropoietin production. Uterine myomas, hepatomas, and cerebellar hemangiomas have also been shown capable of secreting erythropoietin. After renal transplantation, patients can develop erythrocytosis that is unrelated to erythropoietin production. Angiotensin-converting enzyme inhibitors will reverse this particular form of polycythemia. Surreptitious use of erythropoietin by high-performance athletes may also produce polycythemia.

Management of Anesthesia in Secondary Polycythemia
Management of patients with secondary polycythemia depends on the specific cause of the polycythemia. Patients with mild hypoxic polycythemia require no specific treatment. Patients with a very high Hct may require phlebotomy to reduce the potential for perioperative thrombotic and hemorrhagic complications.

DISORDERS OF HEMOSTASIS

Normal Hemostasis

Any disruption of vascular endothelium is a potent stimulus to clot formation. As a localized process, clotting acts to seal the break in vascular continuity, limit blood loss, and begin the process of wound healing. Prevention of an exuberant response that would result in pathologic thrombosis relies on several counterbalancing mechanisms, including the anticoagulant properties of intact endothelial cells, circulating inhibitors of activated coagulation factors, and localized fibrinolytic enzymes. Most abnormalities in hemostasis involve a defect in one or more of the steps in the coagulation process, so it is important to understand the physiology of hemostasis.

Cascade Coagulation Model
The cascade model of coagulation was described during the 1960s and consists of an extrinsic and an intrinsic pathway (Fig. 24.4). The extrinsic system was represented by factor VIIa and tissue factor. By contrast, the intrinsic system was thought to be entirely intravascular. Both pathways could activate factor X which, when complexed with factor Va, could convert prothrombin to thrombin. The prothrombin time (PT) used to guide warfarin therapy reflects the extrinsic pathway, whereas the activated partial thromboplastin time (aPTT) used to guide heparin therapy reflects the intrinsic pathway. Although this model correlates well with clotting measurements, it does not accurately represent in vivo clotting.

New Coagulation Model
In vivo coagulation follows exposure of blood to a source of tissue factor, typically from subendothelial cells, following

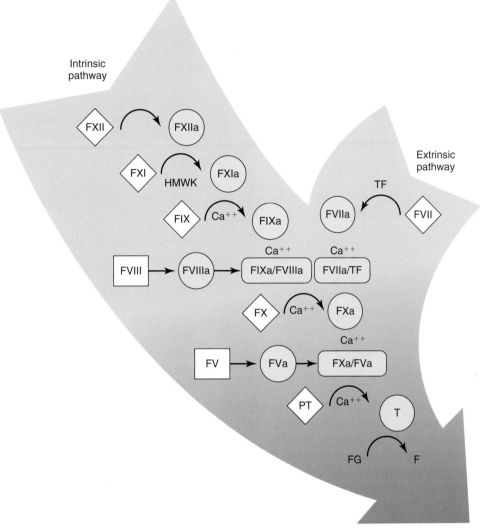

FIG. 24.4 Coagulation cascade. Glycoprotein components of the intrinsic pathway include factors XII, XI, IX, VIII, X, and V; prothrombin; and fibrinogen. Glycoprotein components of the extrinsic pathway, initiated by the action of tissue factor located on cell surfaces, include factors VII, X, and V; prothrombin; and fibrinogen. Cascade reactions culminate in conversion of fibrinogen to fibrin and formation of a fibrin clot. Certain reactions, including activation of factor X and prothrombin, take place on membrane surfaces. Diamonds indicate proenzymes; squares indicate pro-cofactors; circles indicate enzymes and cofactors; shaded rectangles indicate macromolecular complexes on membrane surfaces. *F,* Fibrin; *FG,* fibrinogen; *HMWK,* high-molecular-weight kininogen; *PT,* prothrombin; *T,* thrombin; *TF,* tissue factor. (From Furie B, Furie BC. Molecular basis of blood coagulation. In: Hoffman R, Benz EJ, Shattil SJ, et al., eds. *Hematology: Basic Principles and Practice.* 5th ed. Philadelphia: Churchill Livingstone; 2009: Fig. 118.1.)

damage to a blood vessel. The intrinsic, or contact, pathway of coagulation has no role in this earliest clotting event. Tissue factor–initiated coagulation has three phases: an *initiation phase, an amplification phase,* and a *propagation phase.*

The initiation phase begins as exposed tissue factor binds to factor VIIa (Fig. 24.5). This factor VIIa–tissue factor complex catalyzes the conversion of small amounts of factor X to Xa, which in turn generates similarly small amounts of thrombin. During the amplification phase, platelets, factor V, and factor XI are activated by the small amount of thrombin (Fig. 24.6). The propagation phase is initiated by the activation of factor X by factors VIII

and IX and calcium on the platelet surface (Fig. 24.7). During this phase, thrombin increases its own formation by activating platelets and factors V and VIII. This sets the stage for formation of the factor VIIIa-IXa complex. Formation of this complex allows factor Xa generation to switch from a reaction catalyzed by the factor VIIa–tissue factor complex to one produced by the intrinsic Xase pathway. This switch is of enormous kinetic advantage, since the intrinsic Xase complex is 50 times more efficient at factor Xa generation. The bleeding diathesis associated with hemophilia, with its intact initiation phase and absent propagation phase, is evidence of the hemostatic importance of the propagation phase.

Commonly used laboratory tests of soluble coagulation factors measure only the kinetics of the initiation phase. The PT and aPTT both have as end points the first appearance of fibrin gel. This occurs after completion of less than 5% of the total reaction. These tests are sensitive in detecting severe deficiencies in clotting factors such as hemophilia and in guiding warfarin or heparin therapy. However, they *do not* model the sequence of events necessary for actual hemostasis and do not necessarily predict the risk of intraoperative bleeding.

In the venous circulation the kinetic advantage of the coagulation cascade assembly on the platelet surface is readily apparent. However, relatively small numbers of platelets are needed to perform this function. To increase the risk of venous bleeding, the platelet count must decrease to very low levels (i.e., <10,000/mm^3). This contrasts sharply with the arterial circulation, in which the minimum platelet count needed to ensure hemostasis for surgery is at least five times higher.

Hemostatic Disorders Affecting Coagulation Factors of the Initiation Phase

Table 24.2 lists both inherited and acquired hemostatic disorders.

Factor VII Deficiency

Hereditary deficiency of factor VII is a rare autosomal recessive disease with highly variable penetrance and clinical severity. Only patients with a homozygous deficiency have factor VII levels low enough (<15%) to have symptomatic bleeding. These patients are easily recognized by their laboratory testing: they have a prolonged PT but normal partial thromboplastin time (PTT).

Management of Anesthesia

The treatment of a single-factor deficiency depends on the severity of the deficiency. For surgery, individual clotting factor levels of 20%–25% provide adequate hemostasis. Several products are available to treat factor VII deficiency. Patients with factor VII levels below 1% generally require treatment with a concentrated source of factor VII. For prophylaxis, factor VII concentrate (30–40 international units/kg) and recombinant factor VIIa (NovoSeven) are preferred to fresh frozen plasma. The concentrates consist of a low-volume infusion and have a low risk of infection. Actively bleeding patients can

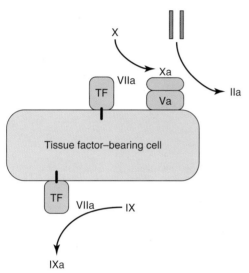

FIG. 24.5 Initiation phase of the blood coagulation cascade. *TF,* Tissue factor. (From Hoffmann M. Remodeling the blood coagulation cascade. *J Thromb Thrombolysis.* 2003;16:17-20, Fig. 2.)

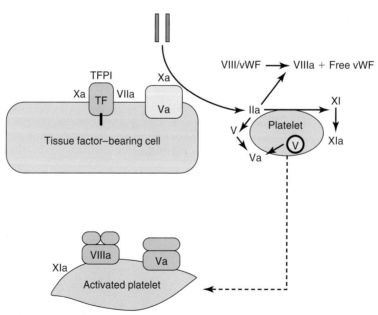

FIG. 24.6 Amplification phase of the blood coagulation cascade. *TF,* Tissue factor; *TFPI,* tissue factor pathway inhibitor; *vWF,* von Willebrand factor. (From Hoffmann M. Remodeling the blood coagulation cascade. *J Thromb Thrombolysis.* 2003;16:17-20, Fig. 3.)

be treated with factor VII concentrates, recombinant factor VIIa, or fresh frozen plasma.

Congenital Deficiencies in Factor X, Factor V, and Prothrombin (Factor II)

Congenital deficiencies in factor X, factor V, and prothrombin are inherited as autosomal recessive traits. Severe deficiencies are quite rare. However, patients with a severe deficiency in

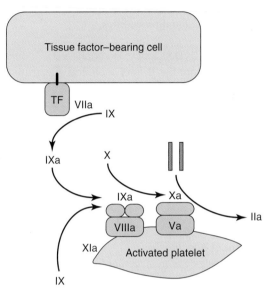

FIG. 24.7 Propagation phase of the blood coagulation cascade. *TF,* Tissue factor. (From Hoffmann M. Remodeling the blood coagulation cascade. *J Thromb Thrombolysis.* 2003;16:17-20, Fig. 4.)

TABLE 24.2	Categorization of Coagulation Disorders

HEREDITARY CAUSES
Hemophilia A
Hemophilia B
Von Willebrand disease
Afibrinogenemia
Factor V deficiency
Hereditary hemorrhagic telangiectasia
Protein C deficiency
Antithrombin III deficiency

ACQUIRED CAUSES
Disseminated intravascular coagulation
Perioperative anticoagulation
Intraoperative coagulopathies
Dilutional thrombocytopenia
Dilution of procoagulants
Massive blood transfusion
Certain types of surgery (cardiopulmonary bypass, brain surgery, orthopedic surgery, urologic surgery, obstetric delivery)
Drug-induced hemorrhage
Drug-induced platelet dysfunction
Idiopathic thrombocytopenic purpura
Thrombotic thrombocytopenic purpura
Catheter-induced thrombocytopenia
Vitamin K deficiency

any of these factors will demonstrate prolongation of both the PT and PTT.

Deficiencies in factor X, factor V, and prothrombin could be corrected with fresh frozen plasma. However, to obtain a significant increase in the level of any factor, a considerable volume of fresh frozen plasma must be infused. As a rule of thumb, 15–20 mL/kg of fresh frozen plasma is needed to obtain a 20% to 30% increase in the level of any clotting factor. This may present a significant cardiovascular challenge to some patients. The duration of effect of this replacement therapy depends on the turnover time of each factor, which then dictates how often another infusion of fresh frozen plasma will be needed. Factor V is stored in platelet granules, and in a bleeding patient, platelet transfusion is an alternate way to deliver missing factor V to the site of bleeding.

For factor X and prothrombin deficiency in patients about to undergo surgery with a significant risk of blood loss, several prothrombin complex concentrates are available. Some of these concentrates contain three clotting factors and some contain four. The advantage of these products is that factor levels of 50% or more can be achieved without the risk of volume overload. The disadvantages of prothrombin complex concentrates are significant, however, and include the risk of inducing widespread thrombosis, thromboembolism, and disseminated intravascular coagulation. Also it is important to recognize that the factor levels in the different products vary considerably.

Factor X deficiency can also be corrected with factor X concentrate.

Hemostatic Disorders Affecting Coagulation Factors of the Propagation Phase

Defects in the propagation phase of coagulation are associated with a significant bleeding tendency. Some of these propagation phase defects are detected by an isolated prolongation of the aPTT. The X-linked recessive disorders hemophilia A and B are the principal examples of this type of abnormality. A marked reduction in either factor VIII or factor IX is associated with spontaneous and/or excessive hemorrhage, commonly presenting as hemarthroses and muscle hematomas. A deficiency in factor XI also prolongs the aPTT but typically results in a less severe bleeding tendency.

Not all factor deficiencies causing prolongation of the aPTT are associated with bleeding. The initial activation stimulus for this laboratory test is surface contact activation of factor XII (Hageman factor) to produce XIIa. This reaction is facilitated by the presence of high-molecular-weight kininogen and the conversion of prekallikrein to the active protease kallikrein. Deficiency in any of these chemicals causes prolongation of the aPTT. However, these contact activation factors play *no role* in either the initiation phase or the propagation phase of clotting in vivo. Thus deficiencies of factor XII, high-molecular-weight kininogen, and prekallikrein are *not* associated with clinical bleeding. Patients with deficiencies of these particular factors require no special management.

Congenital Factor VIII Deficiency: Hemophilia A

The factor VIII gene is a very large gene on the X chromosome. Patients with very severe hemophilia generally have an inversion or deletion of major portions of the X chromosome genome or a missense mutation resulting in factor VIII activity below 1% of normal. Other mutations, including point mutations and minor deletions, generally result in milder disease with factor VIII levels above 1%. In some patients a functionally abnormal protein is produced that causes a discrepancy between results on the immunologic assay of factor VIII antigen and results on the coagulation test of factor VIII activity.

The clinical severity of hemophilia A is best correlated with the factor VIII activity level. Patients with severe hemophilia have factor VIII activity levels below 1% of normal and are usually diagnosed during childhood because of frequent spontaneous hemorrhage into joints, muscles, and vital organs. They require frequent treatment with factor VIII concentrates.

Factor VIII levels as low as 1%–5% of normal are enough to reduce the severity of hemophilia in everyday life, but such patients are at increased risk of hemorrhage with surgery or trauma. Patients with factor levels of 6%–30% have only mild disease that may go undiagnosed until adulthood. Nevertheless, they are at risk for excessive bleeding when undergoing a major surgical procedure. Female carriers of hemophilia A can also be at risk of excessive surgical bleeding. About 10% of female carriers have factor VIII activity below 30%.

Patients with severe hemophilia A have a significantly prolonged aPTT, whereas those with milder disease may an aPTT that is only a few seconds longer than normal. The PT is normal.

Management of Anesthesia

Whenever major surgery is necessary in a patient with hemophilia A, the factor VIII level must be brought close to normal (100%) prior to the procedure.

For patients with mild hemophilia A, an infusion of DDAVP may be sufficient. This should be administered 30–90 minutes prior to surgery. DDAVP increases the level of factor VIII threefold to fivefold, which may restore normal hemostasis. Preoperative use of DDAVP is only appropriate in patients who have had a trial demonstrating an adequate response to DDAVP infusion.

For patients with moderate to severe hemophilia A, correction of the coagulopathy requires an infusion of factor VIII concentrate preoperatively. There should also be preoperative assessment for the presence of factor VIII inhibitors, since up to 30% of patients with severe hemophilia A who have been exposed to factor VIII concentrate or recombinant factor VIII product will develop inhibitor antibodies that render administration of concentrate ineffective. The half-life of factor VIII is approximately 12 hours in adults, so repeated infusions every 8–12 hours will be needed to keep the factor VIII level above 50%. In children the half-life of factor VIII may be as short as 6 hours, which requires more frequent factor VIII infusions and laboratory assays to confirm efficacy. Peak and trough factor VIII levels should be measured to confirm the appropriate

amount of factor VIII to be infused and the dosing interval. Therapy must be continued for up to 2 weeks postoperatively to avoid bleeding that could disrupt wound healing. Even longer periods of therapy may be required in patients who undergo bone or joint surgery. In this situation, 4–6 weeks of replacement therapy may be needed.

Fresh frozen plasma and cryoprecipitate can also correct factor VIII levels. Fibrinolytic inhibitors such as ε-aminocaproic acid (EACA) and tranexamic acid, can be given as adjunctive therapy for bleeding from mucous membranes and are particularly useful for dental procedures.

Congenital Factor IX Deficiency: Hemophilia B

Patients with hemophilia B have a clinical spectrum of disease similar to that found in hemophilia A. Factor IX levels below 1% of normal are associated with severe bleeding, whereas more moderate disease is seen in patients with levels of 1%–5%. Patients with factor IX levels between 5% and 40% generally have very mild disease. Mild hemophilia (>5% factor IX activity) is often not detected until surgery is performed or the patient has a dental extraction. Similar to the laboratory findings in hemophilia A, patients with hemophilia B have a prolonged aPTT and a normal PT.

Management of Anesthesia

General guidelines for management of patients with hemophilia B do not differ significantly from those for management of hemophilia A patients. Recombinant or purified factor IX product or factor IX–prothrombin complex concentrate are used to treat mild bleeding episodes or are administered as prophylaxis for minor surgery. Caution is needed when using factor IX–prothrombin complex concentrates. These concentrates can contain activated clotting factors. When given in amounts sufficient to increase factor IX levels to above 50%, there is an increased risk of thromboembolic complications, especially in patients undergoing orthopedic procedures. *Therefore it is essential to use only purified factor IX or recombinant factor IX to treat patients undergoing major or orthopedic surgery and those with severe traumatic injuries or liver disease.*

Purified factor IX concentrates or recombinant factor IX is used for several days to treat bleeding in patients with hemophilia B. Because of absorption into collagen sites in the vasculature, factor IX is less available than factor VIII, so dosing is approximately double that for factor VIII concentrates. Factor IX has a half-life of 18–24 hours, so repeat infusion of half of the original dose every 12–24 hours is usually sufficient to keep the factor IX plasma level above 50%.

Acquired Factor VIII or IX Inhibitors

Patients with hemophilia A are at significant risk of developing circulating inhibitors to factor VIII. This occurs in 30%–40% of patients with severe hemophilia A. Patients with hemophilia B are less likely to develop inhibitors to factor IX, with only 3%–5% of patients with hemophilia B developing inhibitors. A severe hemophilia-like syndrome can occur in genetically normal individuals because of the appearance of an *acquired* autoantibody to either factor VIII or factor IX. Such patients are usually middle-aged or older, with no personal or family history of abnormal bleeding, who experience sudden onset of severe spontaneous hemorrhage.

A test known as a *mixing study* is required to detect the presence of an inhibitor. This study is performed by *mixing patient plasma and normal plasma* in a 1:1 ratio to determine whether this mix shortens the prolonged PTT. The mixing study in a patient with classic hemophilia A who has a deficiency of factor VIII activity but *no* circulating factor VIII inhibitor will usually show a shortening of the PTT to within 4 seconds of normal. In contrast the mixing test in a patient with a factor VIII inhibitor will not show any significant correction in the PTT.

Management of Anesthesia

Management of a hemophilia A patient with circulating factor VIII inhibitors will vary depending on whether the patient is a high or low responder. *Low responders* have low titers of inhibitors and do not show anamnestic responses to factor VIII concentrates. *High responders* have high titers of inhibitors and have dramatic anamnestic responses to therapy. Patients in the low-responder category can usually be managed with factor VIII concentrates. Larger initial and maintenance doses of factor VIII will be required, and frequent assays of factor VIII levels will be essential to guide therapy.

High responders *cannot* be treated with factor VIII concentrate. These patients represent a clinical challenge, and the use of *inhibitor bypassing drugs* is required. Such inhibitor bypassing drugs include activated prothrombin complex concentrates and recombinant factor VIIa (NovoSeven). NovoSeven (90–120 μg/kg preoperatively, then every 2 hours for the first 28 hours) and FEIBA (factor VIII inhibitor bypassing agent) in doses of 75–100 units/kg, then 70 units/kg every 6–8 hours for 3 days are FDA approved for use in patients with factor VIII antibodies.

Although the thrombin formed via factor VIIa is not as strong as that seen with factor VIII therapy, recombinant factor VIIa therapy is successful in controlling bleeding in more than 80% of patients with factor VIII inhibitors.

Hemophilia B patients with factor IX inhibitors can be managed in acute situations using recombinant VIIa or a prothrombin complex concentrate.

Patients *without* a history of hemophilia can develop an acquired autoantibody to factor VIII or IX and experience life-threatening hemorrhage. Often they exhibit very high inhibitor levels. Treatment with recombinant factor VIIa or an activated prothrombin concentrate *is required*. Administration of factor VIII or IX alone will *not* be effective.

Factor XI Deficiency

The only other coagulation factor defect causing an isolated prolongation of the PTT and a bleeding tendency is factor XI deficiency. It is inherited as an autosomal recessive trait. Factor XI deficiency is much rarer than either hemophilia A or B, but it affects up to 5% of Jews of Ashkenazi descent from Eastern Europe. Generally the bleeding tendency is mild and may be apparent only during a surgical procedure. Hematomas and hemarthroses are very unusual, even in patients with factor XI levels below 5%.

Management of Anesthesia

The treatment of factor XI deficiency depends on the severity of the deficiency and the bleeding history. Patients undergoing dental procedures can be treated exclusively with antifibrinolytic agents (tranexamic acid or ε-aminocaproic acid). Since factor XI concentrates are not available in the United States, infusion of fresh frozen plasma should be used to treat factor XI–deficient patients with active bleeding.

Congenital Abnormalities in Fibrinogen
Hypofibrinogenemia and Afibrinogenemia

Congenital abnormalities in fibrinogen production interfere with the final step in the generation of a fibrin clot. Disorders with decreased fibrinogen levels, either hypofibrinogenemia or afibrinogenemia, are relatively rare conditions inherited as autosomal recessive traits. Patients with *afibrinogenemia* have a severe bleeding diathesis with both spontaneous and posttraumatic bleeding. The bleeding can begin during the first few days of life, and this condition may initially be confused with hemophilia. *Hypofibrinogenemic* patients usually do not have spontaneous bleeding but may have bleeding with surgery. Severe bleeding can be anticipated in patients with plasma fibrinogen levels below 50–100 mg/dL.

Dysfibrinogenemia

Production of an abnormal fibrinogen is a more common defect than very low levels of fibrinogen. Fibrinogen is synthesized in the liver under the control of three genes on chromosome 4. More than 300 different mutations producing dysfunctional and/or reduced amounts of fibrinogen have been reported. Many of these mutations are inherited as autosomal dominant traits. The clinical presentation of *dysfibrinogenemia* is highly variable. Patients who have *both* a reduced amount of fibrinogen and a dysfunctional fibrinogen *(hypodysfibrinogenemia)* usually have excessive bleeding. Most dysfibrinogenemic patients have abnormal coagulation tests but do not have clinical bleeding. Overall, approximately 60% of dysfibrinogenemias are clinically silent. The remainder can present as either a bleeding diathesis or, paradoxically, a thrombotic tendency. A small number of dysfibrinogenemias have been associated with spontaneous abortion and poor wound healing.

Laboratory evaluation of fibrinogen involves measurement of both the concentration and function of fibrinogen. The most accurate quantitative measurement of total fibrinogen is provided by immunoassay or a protein precipitation technique. Screening tests for fibrinogen dysfunction include the thrombin time and clotting time using a venom enzyme such as reptilase.

Management of Anesthesia. Most patients with dysfibrinogenemia have no clinical disease. Those who are symptomatic and at risk of bleeding during or after surgery require treatment with cryoprecipitate or fresh frozen plasma. Cryoprecipitate is used in a dose of 1 unit/10 kg of body weight for procedures with a minor risk of bleeding and 1 unit/5 kg of body weight for procedures with a higher risk of bleeding. The goal is to achieve fibrinogen levels between 100 and 200 mg/dL, ensuring adequate hemostasis. Human fibrinogen concentrates are available in Europe for treatment of dysfibrinogenemia. However, in the United States, human fibrinogen concentrate (RiaSTAP) is approved for treating hypofibrinogenemia but not dysfibrinogenemia.

Factor XIII Deficiency

The stability of the fibrin clot is very important in hemostasis. Deficiency of factor XIII (fibrin-stabilizing factor) is a rare autosomal recessive disorder, with patients manifesting either A subunit or B subunit deficiency. Newborns may have persistent umbilical cord or circumcision-related bleeding. Others may demonstrate a severe bleeding diathesis characterized by recurrent soft tissue bleeding, poor wound healing, and a high incidence of intracranial hemorrhage. Blood clots form but are weak and therefore unable to maintain hemostasis. Fetal loss in women with factor XIII deficiency approaches 100% without replacement therapy.

Factor XIII deficiency should be considered in patients with a severe bleeding diathesis who have normal results on coagulation screening tests, including PT, PTT, fibrinogen level, platelet count, and platelet function assay. Clot dissolution in urea can be used as a screening test. Patients at risk of severe hemorrhage have factor XIII levels only 1% of normal. Those with factor XIII levels of 50% or more usually have no bleeding tendency.

Management of Anesthesia

Several factor XIII concentrates are available for use as prophylaxis or treatment of these patients. Recombinant A subunit factor XIII (Tretten) and factor XIII concentrated and purified from plasma (Corifact) are available in the United States. The long half-life of factor XIII (11–14 days) allows it to be used once a month. Patients who have no access to factor XIII concentrate can be treated with fresh frozen plasma or cryoprecipitate.

ARTERIAL COAGULATION

Disorders Affecting Platelet Number

The normal circulating platelet count is maintained within relatively narrow limits. Approximately one-third of platelets are sequestered in the spleen at any given time. Since a platelet has a lifespan of about 9–10 days, some 15,000–45,000 platelets/mm^3 must be produced each day to maintain a steady state.

General Concepts for Treating Thrombocytopenia

Regardless of the cause of thrombocytopenia, platelet transfusion is appropriate if the patient is experiencing a life-threatening hemorrhage, is bleeding into a closed space such as the cranium, or requires emergency surgery. Long-term management of the thrombocytopenia may require other therapeutic maneuvers to either improve platelet production or to decrease platelet destruction.

Platelet transfusion therapy must be tailored to the severity of the thrombocytopenia, the presence of bleeding complications, and the patient's underlying disease. For minor surgery a platelet count as low as 20,000–30,000/mm^3 may be adequate. For major surgery the platelet count should be increased to 50,000/mm^3. However, for neurosurgical, eye, and neuraxial procedures, platelets should be approximately 100,000/mm^3. Each unit of single-donor apheresis platelets or 6 units of random-donor platelets increases the platelet count in a normal-sized adult by about 50,000/mm^3. If there is alloimmunization or increased platelet consumption, measurement of platelet counts 1 hour after transfusion and at frequent intervals thereafter is important in planning further platelet transfusion needs.

One unit of single-donor apheresis platelets is equivalent to a random-donor pool of 4–8 units of platelets. For patients who become alloimmunized to random-donor platelets, blood banks can provide HLA-matched single-donor platelets. Random- and single-donor platelets do not need to be ABO compatible. However, sufficient RBCs are transfused in the platelet pool to increase the risk of sensitization in Rh-negative patients. Therefore such patients, particularly women of childbearing age, should receive platelets from Rh-negative donors or be treated with Rh$_O$(D) immune globulin (RhoGAM) after transfusion of Rh-positive product.

Patients with very low platelet counts (<15,000/mm^3) can experience significant bleeding from multiple sites including the nose, mucous membranes, GI tract, skin, and vessel puncture sites. One sign that strongly suggests thrombocytopenia is the appearance of a petechial rash involving the skin or mucous membranes. This condition is most pronounced in the lower extremities because of the increased hydrostatic pressure in the legs. The differential diagnosis of thrombocytopenia is best organized according to the physiology of (1) platelet production, (2) distribution in the circulation, and (3) platelet destruction.

Congenital Disorders Resulting in Platelet Production Defects

Platelet production disorders may be caused by megakaryocyte hypoplasia or aplasia in the bone marrow.

Congenital hypoplastic thrombocytopenia with absent radii (TAR syndrome) is inherited in an autosomal recessive manner. Thrombocytopenia develops in the third trimester or soon after birth. The thrombocytopenia is initially severe (<30,000 platelets/mm^3) but gradually improves, approaching the normal range by age 2. These patients often have bilateral radial anomalies, and abnormalities of other bones may also occur.

The hematologic manifestations of *Fanconi anemia* do not usually appear until about age 7. Bone marrow shows reduced cellularity and reduced numbers of megakaryocytes. Stem cell transplantation is curative in the majority of children once severe bone marrow failure has developed.

Patients with *May-Hegglin anomaly* typically have giant platelets in the circulation and Döhle bodies (basophilic inclusions) in WBCs. Platelet production is variably ineffective, with one-third of patients having significant thrombocytopenia.

Wiskott-Aldrich syndrome is an X-linked disorder that presents with a combination of eczema, immunodeficiency, and thrombocytopenia. Circulating platelets are smaller than normal, function poorly because of granule defects, and have a reduced survival. Ineffective thrombopoiesis is the principal abnormality.

Patients with *autosomal dominant thrombocytopenia* have an increased megakaryocyte mass but ineffective platelet production and release macrocytic platelets into the circulation. Many of these patients also have nerve deafness and nephritis (Alport syndrome).

Acquired Disorders Resulting in Platelet Production Defects

A failure in platelet production can result from bone marrow damage. All aspects of normal hematopoiesis can be depressed, even to the point of bone marrow aplasia (aplastic anemia). A reduction in the marrow megakaryocyte mass can be seen in response to radiation therapy or cancer chemotherapy, as a result of exposure to toxic chemicals (benzene, insecticides) or alcohol, and as a complication of viral hepatitis. Infiltration of bone marrow by a malignant process can also disrupt thrombopoiesis. Hematopoietic malignancies, including multiple myeloma, acute leukemia, lymphoma, and myeloproliferative disorders, frequently produce platelet production defects.

Ineffective thrombopoiesis is also seen in patients with vitamin B_{12} or folate deficiency (caused by alcoholism) and defective folate metabolism. Marrow megakaryocyte mass is increased, but effective platelet production is reduced. This failure of platelet production is rapidly reversed by appropriate vitamin therapy. Recovery of the platelet count to normal occurs within days of initiating vitamin therapy, which makes platelet transfusion unnecessary in all but the most acute situations.

Management of Anesthesia
Platelet transfusions are the mainstay in management of patients with platelet production disorders. Patients with ineffective thrombopoiesis due to an intrinsic abnormality of megakaryocytes are treated like those with a production disorder when there is need for urgent surgery.

Nonimmune Platelet Destruction Disorders

Platelet consumption as a part of intravascular coagulation can be seen in several clinical settings. If the entire coagulation pathway is activated, the process is referred to as *disseminated intravascular coagulation* (DIC). DIC can be fulminant, with severe thrombocytopenia and markedly abnormal coagulation factor assays accompanied by bleeding, or it can be low grade, with little or no thrombocytopenia and less tendency for bleeding. Platelet consumption can also occur as an isolated process, so-called platelet DIC. Viral infection, bacteremia, malignancy, high-dose chemotherapy, and vasculitis can result in sufficient endothelial cell damage to dramatically increase the rate of platelet clearance without full activation of the coagulation pathway. Basically this is an accentuation of the normal blood vessel repair process in which platelets adhere to exposed subendothelial surfaces and then aggregate with fibrinogen binding. With marked endothelial disruption, enough platelets can be consumed to result in thrombocytopenia. Blood vessel occlusion by platelet thrombi is unusual but can occur with severe vasculitis. Patients with acquired immunodeficiency syndrome (AIDS) can develop a consumptive thrombocytopenia with end-organ damage due to arterial thrombosis.

Thrombotic thrombocytopenic purpura, hemolytic uremic syndrome, and HELLP syndrome (see later discussion) are the most important examples of nonimmune platelet destruction. Although the underlying pathophysiology of each of these disorders is distinctly different, all of these entities can lead to thrombus formation and end-organ damage.

Thrombotic Thrombocytopenic Purpura
Thrombotic thrombocytopenic purpura (TTP) is characterized by formation of platelet-rich thrombi in the arterial and capillary microvasculature, leading to thrombocytopenia and microangiopathic hemolytic anemia. TTP is caused by a deficiency of ADAMTS 13 protease, whose usual function is to cut ultralarge vWF multimers into smaller pieces and prevent them from triggering formation of unnecessary blood clots. Its deficiency leads to accumulation of large vWF multimers and development of a microvasculopathy. Although this disease was classically described as a complex of five signs—fever, renal failure, thrombocytopenia, microangiopathic hemolytic anemia, and neurologic abnormalities—not all patients with TTP have all five signs. The presence of at least thrombocytopenia and microangiopathic hemolytic anemia suggest the diagnosis of TTP. The diagnosis is confirmed by measuring a reduced ADAMTS 13 activity level (<10% of normal). TTP can occur as a familial disease, sporadic illness without apparent cause (idiopathic), chronic relapsing condition, or as a complication of bone marrow transplantation or treatment with certain drugs such as quinine, ticlopidine, mitomycin C, interferon alfa, pentostatin, gemcitabine, tacrolimus, and cyclosporine. Preeclampsia with HELLP syndrome can evolve into TTP postpartum.

TTP is a medical emergency, and plasma exchange with fresh frozen plasma or administration of Octaplas (solvent- and detergent-treated pooled human plasma) should be initiated as soon as the diagnosis is suspected, without waiting for ADAMTS 13 levels. Glucocorticoids are also administered, and both the plasma exchange and steroid therapy should be continued until platelet counts return to normal. Rituximab may be useful in severe cases that are resistant to plasma exchange.

Hemolytic Uremic Syndrome

Hemolytic uremic syndrome (HUS) is a disorder similar to TTP that is typically seen in children who come for treatment of bloody diarrhea due to infection with a particular strain of *Escherichia coli* that produces a Shiga-like toxin. Acute renal failure dominates the presentation. Thrombocytopenia and anemia are less severe than with TTP, and neurologic signs are absent. Patients are treated with fluids and RBC and platelet transfusion as necessary. Most children recover spontaneously but may require hemodialysis for a period. The mortality rate is less than 5%. Adults infected with this strain of *E. coli* can have features of both HUS and TTP but usually with less renal involvement. Since the mortality rate in older children and adults is higher than it is in young children, they often need to be treated with plasma exchange and/or hemodialysis.

HELLP Syndrome

Thrombocytopenia is a frequent complication of pregnancy. Mild thrombocytopenia (platelet counts between 70,000 and 150,000/mm^3) is seen in about 6% of women nearing delivery, and this represents a physiologic change similar to the dilutional anemia of pregnancy. *Thrombocytopenia associated with hypertension* is observed in 1%–2% of pregnancies, and about half of these women with preeclampsia will develop a DIC-like condition with severe thrombocytopenia (platelet counts of 20,000–40,000/mm^3) at the time of delivery. This is referred to as *HELLP syndrome* when the combination of red cell hemolysis **(H),** elevated liver enzyme levels **(EL),** and low platelet count **(LP)** is present. Physiologically, HELLP syndrome resembles TTP. Control of the hypertension and delivery of the child are usually enough to bring this process to a halt. However, a few patients will go on to develop TTP following delivery. Postpartum TTP is a life-threatening illness with a poor prognosis. Treatment with both plasma exchange and IV immunoglobulin has yielded variable results.

Management of Anesthesia in Nonimmune Platelet Destruction Disorders

Proper management of patients with platelet destruction disorders depends on the diagnosis of the hematologic disorder. Individuals who have nonimmune destruction as a part of DIC may require supportive therapy with platelet and plasma transfusions, but the only truly effective therapy is treatment of the underlying cause of DIC. If the primary condition causing DIC can be corrected, the levels of coagulation factors and the platelet count will return to normal.

Patients with TTP or HUS should receive platelet transfusion only for life-threatening bleeding. There is potential for significant harm from platelet transfusion with these conditions. Platelet transfusion may cause further thrombosis and end-organ damage due to marked platelet activation and aggregation. Surgery should be delayed whenever possible until the underlying disorder is controlled.

HUS and HELLP syndrome present a different therapeutic challenge. HUS in children can usually be managed without plasmapheresis, although dialysis may be necessary if renal failure is severe. HELLP syndrome, like preeclampsia, typically resolves with delivery of the baby. However, a small number of women will develop a TTP-like syndrome postpartum.

Autoimmune Platelet Destruction Disorders

Thrombocytopenia is a common manifestation of autoimmune disease. The severity of this thrombocytopenia is highly variable. In some conditions the platelet count be as low as 1000–2000/mm^3. In other conditions the ability of megakaryocytes to increase platelet production can result in a compensated state, with platelet counts ranging from 20,000/mm^3 to near-normal levels.

The diagnosis of immune platelet destruction is usually made from the clinical presentation, the finding of an increased number of reticulated (RNA-containing) platelets in the peripheral blood smear, and demonstration of an increase in both the marrow megakaryocyte number and the number of chromosomes sets in these megakaryocytes (ploidy). Expansion of the megakaryocyte mass in the marrow is evidence that platelet production has increased markedly in an attempt to compensate for shortened platelet survival in the circulation.

Thrombocytopenic Purpura in Adults

The differential diagnosis of autoimmune thrombocytopenia in adults includes exposure to potentially toxic drugs, receipt of blood products, and viral infection.

Posttransfusion Purpura

Adults can develop posttransfusion purpura after exposure to a blood product, usually RBCs or platelets. Although multiparous women negative for platelet antigen A1 (PlA1) are at greatest risk, posttransfusion purpura has been reported in both men and women. Usually a potent alloantibody with PlA1 specificity is detected in the plasma.

Drug-Induced Autoimmune Thrombocytopenia

Several drugs can produce immune thrombocytopenia. Quinine and quinidine are the best known and studied. Clinically, patients show severe thrombocytopenia, with platelet counts below 20,000/mm^3. These drugs act as haptens to trigger antibody formation and then serve as obligate molecules for antibody binding to the platelet surface. Thrombocytopenia can also occur within hours of a *first* exposure to a drug because of preformed antibodies. This has been reported with varying frequency with abciximab (ReoPro) and other glycoprotein IIb/IIIa inhibitors. Other drugs, such as α-methyldopa, sulfonamides, and gold salts also stimulate autoantibody production.

Heparin-Induced Thrombocytopenia. The association of heparin with thrombocytopenia deserves special discussion. Heparin-induced thrombocytopenia (HIT) can take one of several forms. A modest decrease in the platelet count, HIT type 1 *(nonimmune HIT)* may be observed in most patients during the first day of therapy with full-dose unfractionated heparin. This condition is caused by passive heparin binding to platelets, which results in a modest shortening of the platelet lifespan. The effect is transient and clinically insignificant.

A second form of HIT, HIT type 2 *(immune-mediated HIT),* is much more important. In this type of HIT, antibodies form to the heparin–platelet factor 4 complex, and these antibodies are capable of binding to platelet receptors and inducing platelet activation and aggregation. Platelet activation results in further release of heparin–platelet factor 4 and the appearance of platelet microparticles in the circulation. These exacerbate this procoagulant state. In addition, heparin–platelet factor 4 complex binds to endothelial cells and stimulates thrombin production. This leads to both an increased clearance of platelets, with resultant thrombocytopenia, and venous and/or arterial thrombus formation, with the potential for severe end-organ damage and the potential for thromboses in unusual sites such as the adrenal gland, portal vein, and skin.

The incidence of HIT type 2 varies with the type and dose of heparin and the duration of heparin therapy. Between 10% and 15% of patients receiving *bovine* unfractionated heparin develop an antibody. Fewer than 6% of patients receiving *porcine* heparin develop antibodies. The risk of heparin-induced thrombosis is lower than the incidence of antibody formation. Fewer than 10% of those who *develop an antibody* to the heparin–platelet factor 4 complex will experience a thrombotic event. However, the risk varies considerably with the clinical situation and can exceed 40% in the period after orthopedic surgery. Some studies have suggested that the presence of the HIT antibody has a negative impact on clinical outcome even in the absence of overt thrombosis. HIT antibody–positive patients undergoing coronary artery bypass surgery or receiving heparin therapy for unstable angina have been reported to have a significantly higher incidence of adverse events, including stroke, myocardial infarction, prolonged hospitalization, and death.

Immune-mediated HIT occurs between days 5 and 10 of heparin use. There are two variants: an early-onset HIT that occurs in patients exposed to heparin within the previous 3 months and a delayed-onset HIT that appears after heparin is discontinued. The diagnosis of HIT is based on a scoring method called the *4Ts system* that considers the degree of **T**hrombocytopenia, the **T**iming of the platelet reduction, the presence of **T**hrombosis or other sequelae, and the presence of other causes of **T**hrombocytopenia (Table 24.3). A high index of suspicion should prompt performance of an anti–PF4–heparin enzyme immunoassay and a platelet function assay.

Patients who receive full-dose unfractionated heparin for longer than 5 days or who have previously received heparin should be routinely monitored with measurement of the platelet count every other day. A decrease in the platelet count of more than 50%, *even if the absolute platelet count remains within the normal range,* can signal the appearance of HIT type 2 antibodies. These significant decreases in platelet count mandate discontinuation of heparin therapy and substitution of a direct thrombin inhibitor for continued anticoagulation. If heparin is continued, even at low doses, or even if a low-molecular-weight heparin (LMWH) were to be substituted, there is still significant risk of a major thrombotic event. To prevent life-threatening thromboembolic events in patients with HIT type 2, all forms of heparin must be stopped immediately. Any delay can put a patient at increased risk of thrombosis. *Substitution of LMWH for unfractionated heparin is not an option* because there is significant antibody cross-reactivity. Patients with a suspected or confirmed episode of HIT should be started immediately on a direct thrombin inhibitor (argatroban, bivalirudin) or anti-Xa inhibitor (fondaparinux) even in the absence of a thrombotic event. *Oral* anticoagulants should *never* be started until there is continuous and successful thrombosis prophylaxis in place.

TABLE 24.3	4Ts Scoring System for Heparin-Induced Thrombocytopenia (HIT)		
Category	2 Points	1 Point	0 Points
Thrombocytopenia	Platelet count decreased >50% from baseline *and* platelet nadir ≥ 20,000/mm³	Platelet count decreased 30%–50% from baseline *or* platelet nadir 10,000–19,000/mm³	Platelet count decreased <30% from baseline *or* platelet nadir < 10,000/mm³
Timing of platelet decrease	Clear onset between days 5 and 10 of heparin exposure *or* platelet decrease in <1 day with heparin exposure within prior 30 days	Decrease in platelet counts consistent with onset between days 5 and 10 of heparin exposure, but timing is not clear because of missing platelet counts *or* onset after day 10 of heparin exposure *or* decrease in platelet counts in <1 day with prior heparin exposure between 30 and 100 days earlier	Platelet count decrease within 4 days of heparin exposure
Thrombosis or other sequelae	New thrombosis, skin necrosis, or acute systemic reaction after unfractionated heparin exposure	Progressive/recurrent thrombosis or unconfirmed but clinically suspected thrombosis	No thrombosis or previous heparin exposure
Other causes of **T**hrombocytopenia	None apparent	Possible other causes present	Probable other causes present

The 4Ts score is assigned by summing the values for each of the four categories. A score of 1, 2, or 3 is considered to indicate low probability of HIT; 4 or 5 indicates intermediate probability of HIT; and 6, 7, or 8 indicates high probability of HIT.
Data from Crowther MA, Cook DJ, Albert M, et al. The 4Ts scoring system for heparin-induced thrombocytopenia in medical-surgical intensive care unit patients. *J Crit Care.* 2010;25:287-293.

An acute form of HIT type 2 can occur when heparin therapy is restarted within 20 days of a previous exposure. If HIT antibodies are present, the patient in whom heparin therapy is restarted can exhibit an acute drug reaction with abrupt onset of severe dyspnea, rigors, diaphoresis, hypertension, and tachycardia. Such patients are at extreme risk of fatal thromboembolism if heparin administration is continued.

Management of Anesthesia. Platelet transfusions are appropriate if a patient with thrombocytopenia is experiencing life-threatening hemorrhage or is bleeding into a closed space. Platelet transfusion therapy must be tailored to the severity of the thrombocytopenia, the presence of bleeding complications, and the patient's underlying disease. Prophylactic platelet transfusion should be avoided in patients with HIT type 2, since transfused platelets can *increase* the risk of thrombosis. In patients with autoimmune thrombocytopenia due to drug ingestion, the most important management step is discontinuation of the offending drug. Corticosteroid therapy may speed recovery in patients with an idiopathic thrombocytopenic purpura–like presentation. The speed of recovery depends on both the clearance rate of the offending drug and the ability of marrow megakaryocytes to proliferate and increase platelet production. Even if the platelet count is very low, bleeding is unlikely and patients can be allowed to recover without platelet transfusion.

HIV-infected thrombocytopenic patients who require urgent surgery should be given platelet transfusions as appropriate. In preparation for elective surgery in patients who develop thrombocytopenia early in their HIV/AIDS disease course, consideration may be given to treatment with zidovudine for a period before surgery. About 60% of these patients will have a favorable response, and up to 50% will have long-lasting improvement in their platelet counts. The effect, however, is not immediate. It can take up to 2 months before the platelet count improves. If patients do not respond to zidovudine, splenectomy can be helpful in reducing significant thrombocytopenia in more than 85% of patients, especially if done early in the course of the thrombocytopenia. Corticosteroids, IV immunoglobulin, and IV Rh$_O$(D) immune globulin have also been used in patients with AIDS. Later in their disease progression, HIV-infected patients can develop a platelet production defect that responds only to platelet transfusion therapy.

Cardiac surgery represents a particular challenge for patients with HIT, since heparin is the ideal anticoagulant for use during cardiopulmonary bypass. Cardiac surgery should be delayed until the HIT episode resolves; if this is not possible, bivalirudin, a direct thrombin inhibitor, should be used for anticoagulation during cardiopulmonary bypass. In situations in which the HIT episode has resolved, antibodies have disappeared, and sufficient time has passed since the diagnosis (>100 days), heparin could be safely used just for the cardiopulmonary bypass period, since the likelihood of an anamnestic response is low.

Idiopathic Thrombocytopenic Purpura
Thrombocytopenia *unrelated* to drug exposure, infection, or autoimmune disease is generally classified as *autoimmune idiopathic thrombocytopenic purpura* (ITP). This diagnosis is made only by excluding all other causes of nonimmune and immune platelet destruction. Most adults with the disorder proceed to a chronic form of ITP in which a continued high level of marrow platelet production is required to maintain a chronically low to near-normal platelet count in the face of a shortened platelet lifespan. This condition is characterized by a high level of platelet destruction that is balanced by high marrow production of platelets that have *better-than-normal* function. Severe bleeding does not occur until the platelet count drops below 10,000/mm^3. Patients with chronic ITP have platelet counts of 20,000–100,000/mm^3.

Platelet survival in severely affected patients can be measured in hours rather than days, with destruction occurring mainly in the spleen. Transfused platelets also have a shortened lifespan. Some patients demonstrate only a modest shortening of platelet survival. Although most ITP patients receiving platelet transfusions rapidly destroy the infused platelets, up to 30% of patients do demonstrate near-normal posttransfusion platelet survival.

Management of Anesthesia. Severe ITP associated with bleeding in adults should be treated as a medical emergency, with administration of high-dose corticosteroids. If there is a need for emergency surgery or clinical evidence of intracranial hemorrhage, the patient should also be given IV immunoglobulin and platelet transfusions at least every 8–12 hours, *regardless of the effect on the platelet count.* Some patients who receive platelet transfusions will show a relatively normal posttransfusion platelet count and reasonable platelet survival. However, even when there is no posttransfusion improvement in the platelet count, sufficient numbers of the transfused platelets may survive and improve hemostasis.

Some adults do not respond to corticosteroids and develop chronic ITP. If ITP persists for longer than 3–4 months, it is extremely unlikely the patient will spontaneously recover. Splenectomy should be considered if the platelet count is less than 10,000–20,000/mm^3 because about half of patients will achieve a permanent remission after splenectomy. If splenectomy is being considered, it is important to immunize the patient with pneumococcal, meningococcal, and *Haemophilus influenzae* vaccines before surgery to reduce the risk of postsplenectomy sepsis.

Management of chronic ITP in pregnancy deserves special attention. Most pregnant women with chronic ITP can be managed with no medication, modest amounts of prednisone, or intermittent use of IV immunoglobulin. If the thrombocytopenia becomes more severe, a higher daily dose of corticosteroids together with weekly immunoglobulin infusion, especially during the last few weeks of pregnancy, may be needed to prevent maternal bleeding. Even though the mother has severe ITP, most children are born with normal platelet counts. Platelet counts in neonates normally decrease for about a week after delivery. Therefore in children at risk, platelet counts should be checked every 2–3 days until the platelet count begins to increase.

Qualitative Platelet Disorders

Abnormalities in platelet function are often noted for the first time as a complication of an acute illness or surgery. However, there may be several factors that could play a role in determining the severity of the bleeding tendency. Initial treatment should address as many potential contributing factors as possible and include discontinuation of drugs that inhibit platelet function, empirically replacing vWF or treating with desmopressin, and even transfusing platelets. Although this approach lacks precision, it is usually effective. Then after the acute event is over a precise diagnosis of the cause of the bleeding can be made.

Congenital Disorders Affecting Platelet Function
Von Willebrand Disease

Von Willebrand disease (vWD) is the most common inherited abnormality affecting platelet function. It is inherited as either an autosomal dominant or autosomal recessive trait. *Severe vWD with life-threatening bleeding is seen in fewer than 5 individuals per million in Western countries.*

Patients with vWD usually experience mucocutaneous bleeding (typically epistaxis), easy bruising, menorrhagia, and gingival and GI bleeding. The number of patients with mild to moderate reductions in vWF activity far exceeds the number of patients with overt clinical bleeding. Hence there will be a marked *overdiagnosis* of vWD if the measured vWF level is the sole criterion used for diagnosis. The diagnosis of "clinically important" vWD should be limited to those cases in which abnormal bleeding occurs. If vWD is considered to be a contributing factor in a bleeding patient, it should be treated empirically. Laboratory evaluation can be postponed until the patient is in stable condition and has not received blood products or drugs for several weeks.

The bleeding time, formerly considered a decent test of platelet function, has been shown to have poor reproducibility, sensitivity, and specificity. It has now been supplanted by the rapid platelet function assay (RPFA). Screening laboratory evaluation for vWD should include RPFA, platelet count, PT, and aPTT. Patients with mild vWD generally have near-normal test results. In those with more severe disease the RPFA is prolonged, but the platelet count is normal. Patients with a severe deficiency of vWF or defective binding of factor VIII to vWF have a prolonged PTT due to low levels of factor VIII in plasma. Specific assays of vWF levels and function are then necessary to confirm the diagnosis.

Full evaluation of these patients requires measurements of factor VIII coagulant activity, vWF antigen, vWF activity, and vWF multimer distribution. These studies are of diagnostic importance in the classification of vWD and in turn are essential in providing appropriate clinical management.

Type 1 Disease. Type 1 vWD (80% of cases) represents a *quantitative* defect in plasma vWF levels. Clinical severity is quite variable but generally correlates with the plasma levels of vWF and factor VIII. In patients/families with a history of repeated and severe bleeding episodes, vWF antigen and vWF activity are usually reduced to less than 15%–25% of normal.

These individuals with a history of severe disease should be treated for any bleeding episode and given prophylactic treatment for even minor surgical procedures.

Type 2 Disease. Type 2 vWD is characterized by a qualitative defect in plasma vWF. This can involve a reduction in the number of large vWF multimers or variable changes in vWF antigen and factor VIII binding. The absence of large multimers results in a significant decrease in vWF activity.

Type 3 Disease. Type 3 vWD is characterized by the virtual absence of circulating vWF antigen and very low levels of both vWF activity and factor VIII (3%–10% of normal). These patients experience severe bleeding with mucosal hemorrhage, hemarthroses, and muscle hematomas reminiscent of those seen in hemophilia A or B.

Management of Anesthesia. The type of vWD and its severity, as well as the nature, urgency, and location of the surgical procedure, factor into therapeutic management of a patient with vWD. Treatments for this disorder include desmopressin, a drug that increases plasma levels of endogenous vWF, and blood products that contain vWF in high concentrations.

Desmopressin (DDAVP) is a synthetic analogue of the antidiuretic hormone vasopressin; when given intravenously, it stimulates release of vWF from endothelial cells to produce an immediate increase in plasma vWF and factor VIII activity. This improves platelet function. It can be very effective in correcting the bleeding defect in vWD. Platelet function abnormalities resulting from aspirin, glycoprotein IIb/IIIa inhibitors, uremia, or liver disease can also be partially corrected by desmopressin-stimulated release of very large vWF multimers.

Success in treating vWD patients with desmopressin depends on the disease type. Patients with type 1 vWD show the best response. The value of treatment with desmopressin in patients with type 2 disease is less certain. Patients with type 3 vWD *do not* respond to desmopressin because these patients lack endothelial stores of vWF. Both vWF and factor VIII must be provided to treat bleeding in patients with type 3 vWD.

Desmopressin is available in both IV and intranasal preparations. It can be administered intravenously in a dose of 0.3 μg/kg. A highly concentrated nasal spray (Stimate) is also available and can be self-administered by women with type 1 vWD for management of menorrhagia. This nasal spray can also be effective in controlling bleeding associated with tooth extraction or minor surgery.

Desmopressin therapy is most effective in treating mild bleeding episodes or in preventing bleeding during minor surgery. Patients with baseline vWF and factor VIII levels above 10–20 IU/dL do best with this drug, demonstrating a threefold to fivefold increase in vWF levels. However, even if the response is suboptimal, bleeding may be partially contained and total blood loss and the need for transfusion can be reduced. A disadvantage of desmopressin is its relatively short-lived effect. Improvement in the RPFA and vWF levels is limited to 12–24 hours. The response can decrease with repeated doses because of development of tachyphylaxis. In situations where control of bleeding is critical (e.g., following major surgery), desmopressin administration by itself may be inadequate and vWF replacement may be necessary.

Replacement of vWF can be achieved with purified factor VIII concentrates containing the vWF–factor VIII complex. This is useful for patients with type 2 and 3 vWD and severe cases of type 1 vWD.

Three preparations are available in the United States to treat vWD that requires more than desmopressin therapy. They are Humate-P, Alphanate, and Wilate, and they all contain vWF/factor VIII replacement therapy prepared from pooled human plasma. They differ in their vWF/factor VIII ratios and the content of large vWF multimers. Humate-P is the only formulation approved for use in all three types of vWD and particularly for use prior to oral surgery in patients with type 3 vWD. Once bleeding is controlled, a single daily dose of concentrate is sufficient, since the half-life of the factor VIII–vWF complex in patients with vWD is about 24 hours.

Antifibrinolytics can be used as adjunctive therapy, and recombinant factor VII is useful in patients with vWD type 3 who have developed antibodies to vWF from treatment with concentrates.

Acquired Abnormalities of Platelet Function

Acquired platelet dysfunction is seen in association with hematopoietic disease, as part of a systemic illness, or as a result of drug therapy.

Myeloproliferative Disease

Patients with myeloproliferative disorders such as polycythemia vera, myeloid metaplasia, idiopathic myelofibrosis, essential thrombocythemia, and chronic myelogenous leukemia frequently exhibit abnormal platelet function. Some patients have very high platelet counts and can demonstrate either abnormal bleeding or a tendency for arterial or venous thrombosis. In patients with polycythemia vera, expansion of the total blood volume and an increase in blood viscosity may contribute to the thrombotic risk. The most consistent laboratory abnormalities in patients with myeloproliferative disorders and bleeding are defects in epinephrine-induced platelet aggregation and in dense granule and α-granule function. Bleeding from an acquired form of vWD (due to loss of higher-molecular-weight vWF multimers) may also be observed.

Dysproteinemia

Abnormal platelet function, including defects in adhesion, aggregation, and procoagulant activity, are observed in patients with dysproteinemia. Almost one-third of patients with Waldenström macroglobulinemia or IgA myeloma have a demonstrable defect in platelet function. Multiple myeloma patients are less often affected. The concentration of the monoclonal protein spike appears to correlate with the abnormality in platelet function.

Uremia

Uremic patients consistently show a defect in platelet function that correlates with the severity of the uremia and anemia. It appears that the uncleared metabolic product guanidinosuccinic acid acts as an inhibitor of platelet function by inducing endothelial cell nitric oxide release. Platelet adhesion, activation, and aggregation are abnormal, and thromboxane A_2 generation is decreased.

The abnormal bleeding in most patients with uremia is corrected by hemodialysis. Interestingly, measures of platelet function improve with either RBC transfusion or erythropoietin therapy. For acute bleeding episodes, desmopressin can transiently improve platelet function.

Liver Disease

The most likely cause of hemorrhage in severe liver disease is a discrete anatomic defect such as bleeding varices or a gastric or duodenal ulcer. However, if a cirrhotic patient has widespread bleeding, including ecchymoses and oozing from puncture sites, a coagulopathy should be considered. Such patients can have multiple defects in coagulation. Thrombocytopenia related to hypersplenism is common. Platelet dysfunction resulting from high levels of circulating fibrin degradation products can increase the bleeding tendency. In addition, reduced production of factor VII and/or low-grade chronic DIC with increased fibrinolysis can add to the coagulopathy.

Inhibition by Drugs

Several classes of drugs can affect platelet function (Table 24.4). Aspirin and other NSAIDs have a well-recognized impact on platelet function. Aspirin is a powerful inhibitor of platelet thromboxane A_2 synthesis because of its irreversible inhibition of cyclooxygenase function. NSAIDs such as indomethacin, ibuprofen, and sulfinpyrazone also inhibit platelet cyclooxygenase, but their effect is reversible and lasts only as long as the particular drug is in the circulation. Such drugs are

TABLE 24.4	Drugs That Inhibit Platelet Function

STRONG ASSOCIATION

Aspirin (and aspirin-containing medications)
Clopidogrel, ticlopidine
Abciximab
Nonsteroidal antiinflammatory drugs: naproxen, ibuprofen, indomethacin, phenylbutazone, piroxicam, ketorolac

MILD TO MODERATE ASSOCIATION

Antibiotics, usually only in high dosages
    Penicillins including carbenicillin, penicillin G, ampicillin, ticarcillin, nafcillin, mezlocillin
    Cephalosporins
    Nitrofurantoin
Volume expanders: dextran, hydroxyethyl starch
Heparin
Fibrinolytic agents: ε-aminocaproic acid

WEAK ASSOCIATION

Oncologic drugs: daunorubicin, mithramycin
Cardiovascular drugs: β-blockers, calcium channel blockers, nitroglycerin, nitroprusside, quinidine
Alcohol

weak inhibitors of platelet function and are not usually associated with significant clinical bleeding. However, they can contribute to bleeding when other aggravating factors such as treatment with anticoagulants, a GI disorder, or surgery are present. Certain foods, food additives, vitamins, and herbal products (e.g., vitamins C and E, omega-3 fatty acids, Chinese black tree fungus) can also reversibly inhibit platelet function through the cyclooxygenase pathway.

The impact of antibiotics on platelet function can be a major contributor to hemorrhage in critically ill patients. The penicillins, including carbenicillin, penicillin G, ticarcillin, ampicillin, nafcillin, and mezlocillin, can interfere with both platelet adhesion and platelet activation and aggregation. They bind to the platelet membrane and interfere with vWF binding and the response of platelets to agonists such as ADP and epinephrine. Significant clinical bleeding can occur if these antibiotics are administered in high dosages.

Volume expanders such as dextran can interfere with platelet aggregation and procoagulant activity when infused in large amounts. This can be a significant disadvantage in the trauma setting but can be very advantageous in the vascular surgery setting to prevent vascular thrombosis. Hydroxyethyl starch is less likely to interfere with platelet function but can cause a detectable defect if given in amounts in excess of 2 liters.

Management of Anesthesia in Patients With Qualitative Platelet Disorders

The therapeutic goal in treating qualitative platelet disorders is less exact than in disorders of thrombocytopenia. Because platelets are dysfunctional, the absolute platelet number does not predict bleeding risk. Treatment with desmopressin may improve a mild to moderate platelet defect, especially if the risk of bleeding is relatively minor. If the bleeding risk is more substantial, platelet transfusion may be required. Platelet function assays or the thromboelastogram may be used to measure the status of coagulation but may not guarantee adequacy of platelet function for the challenge of surgery. As a general rule, sufficient platelet transfusions to increase the percentage of *normally functioning platelets* to about 10%–20% of all platelets should be sufficient to provide adequate overall platelet function for surgery.

Platelets become quite dysfunctional in the setting of hypothermia (temperature < 35°C) and acidosis (pH < 7.3), and

platelets transfused into a patient with either or both of these conditions will rapidly become dysfunctional as well.

HYPERCOAGULABLE DISORDERS

Causes of hypercoagulability can be divided into two major classes: (1) congenital hypercoagulability caused by one or more genetic abnormalities, often referred to as *thrombophilia,* and (2) acquired or environmentally induced hypercoagulability.

Heritable Causes of Hypercoagulability

Hereditary conditions predisposing to venous thromboembolism (VTE) can be divided into conditions that *decrease* endogenous antithrombotic proteins or *increase* prothrombotic proteins (Table 24.5).

Thrombophilia Due to Decreased Antithrombotic Proteins
Hereditary Antithrombin Deficiency
Antithrombin (AT) III is the most important defense against clot formation in healthy blood vessels or at the perimeter of a site of active bleeding. AT III deficiency is inherited as an autosomal dominant trait. Homozygous AT deficiency is not compatible with life. Heterozygous patients have an AT III level between 40% and 70% of normal. Individuals who are heterozygous for AT III deficiency are about 20 times more likely than normal individuals to develop venous thromboembolism at some point in their lives. The thrombotic event usually occurs in association with some trigger that further increases hypercoagulability.

In addition to anticoagulation, anesthetic management for these patients should include maintaining the AT III level above 80% until 5 days after surgery. This is done by administering AT III concentrates. Thrombate III is made from human plasma, and ATryn is a recombinant form of AT III produced by genetically engineered goats that have been modified so they secrete AT III in their milk.

Hereditary Protein C and Protein S Deficiency
Hereditary deficiency of protein C and protein S adversely affects thrombin regulation by restricting the activity of thrombin already formed and interfering with the ability to

TABLE 24.5	Major Hereditary Disorders Linked to Hypercoagulability[a]		
Disorder	Prevalence in Healthy Controls (%)	Prevalence in Patients With First DVT (%)	Likelihood of DVT by Age 60 (%)
Antithrombin deficiency	0.2	1.1	62
Protein C deficiency	0.8	3	48
Protein S deficiency	0.13	1.1	33
Factor V Leiden	3.5	20	6
Prothrombin 20210A	2.3	18	<5

[a]All values pertain to the heterozygous state of the given condition.
DVT, deep vein thrombosis.

limit the amount of thrombin generated. The risk of VTE is about the same as with AT III deficiency.

Synthesis of both protein C and protein S is vitamin K dependent, so individuals who are protein C deficient are at particular risk of thrombosis *if warfarin therapy is initiated in the absence of protective anticoagulation with heparin.* Specifically, during the first days of warfarin treatment, before inhibition of the vitamin K–dependent clotting factors is sufficient to provide the intended anticoagulation, modest suppression of protein C synthesis may compound the already subnormal protein C levels and result in *greater hypercoagulability.* In addition to therapy to prevent or treat VTE, patients with protein C and S deficiency may require infusion of fresh frozen plasma and prothrombin complex concentrates to correct the levels of these proteins. In patients with protein C deficiency, purified plasma-derived protein C concentrate (Ceprotin) and activated protein C (Xigris) can be used.

Thrombophilia Due to Increased Prothrombotic Proteins
Factor V Leiden
Factor V Leiden differs from normal factor V because of a genetic mutation that makes it very resistant to inactivation. Therefore factor V Leiden stays active in the circulation longer than normal and promotes more thrombin generation.

Factor V Leiden carries a low to intermediate procoagulant risk. Patients who are heterozygous for factor V Leiden have a fivefold to sevenfold increased risk of VTE, whereas the risk in homozygous individuals is increased up to 80-fold. The prevalence of factor V Leiden varies considerably in different ethnic populations. It is present in 5% of people of Northern European descent but only rarely in those of African or Asian descent. Therefore depending on the ethnic makeup of the community, up to 1 in 20 patients coming for routine surgery could be expected to have some degree of increased risk of VTE attributable to factor V Leiden.

Prothrombin Gene Mutation
Another thrombophilia that operates via an increase in prothrombotic proteins is known as the *prothrombin gene mutation* (prothrombin 20210A), which causes levels of prothrombin to be much higher in affected individuals than in the general population. If this mutation is the only thrombophilic risk factor present, the VTE risk is relatively low. The importance of this thrombophilia is similar to that of factor V Leiden and lies in the frequency of the gene rather than its potency. Also as with factor V Leiden, ethnicity plays a significant role in the prevalence of this gene. It occurs in about 4% of individuals of European descent but rarely in persons of African or Asian descent.

Acquired Causes of Hypercoagulability

Myeloproliferative Disorders
Myeloproliferative disorders, especially polycythemia vera, essential thrombocytosis, and paroxysmal nocturnal hemoglobinuria, are associated with an increased incidence of thrombophlebitis, pulmonary embolism, and arterial occlusion. Patients with these conditions are also at risk of splenic, hepatic, portal vein, and mesenteric blood vessel thrombosis. The pathogenesis of these thromboses is unclear, but increased activation and aggregation of platelets may be important.

Malignancies
Patients with certain malignancies demonstrate a marked thrombotic tendency. Adenocarcinoma of the pancreas, colon, stomach, and ovaries are the tumors most often associated with thromboembolic events. Indeed, these malignancies often present with an episode of deep vein thrombosis or migratory superficial thrombophlebitis. Of all patients who develop primary thrombophlebitis, 25%–30% will have a recurrence, and 20% of these will turn out to have cancer. The pathogenesis of the thrombotic tendency appears to relate to the combination of release of one or more procoagulant factors by the tumor that can directly activate factor X, endothelial damage by tumor invasion, and blood stasis. Laboratory testing may show no abnormalities or some combination of thrombocytosis, elevation of the fibrinogen level, and low-grade DIC.

Pregnancy and Oral Contraceptive Use
Pregnancy and oral contraceptive use have been reported to increase the risk of thrombosis. The overall incidence of thrombosis is approximately 1 in 1500 pregnancies but is higher in women who have an inherited hypercoagulable state, a history of deep vein thrombosis or pulmonary embolism, or a family history of thromboembolic disease. The incidence is also higher in women who are obese, kept on bed rest for a prolonged period, or require cesarean section. The risk of pulmonary embolism is highest during the third trimester and immediately postpartum and is a significant cause of maternal death. AT III–deficient women are at greatest risk and should receive anticoagulant therapy throughout pregnancy. Factor V Leiden and the prothrombin mutation are associated with a much lower risk. Women with these inherited traits do not need to receive anticoagulant treatment.

The association of oral contraceptive use with thrombosis and thromboembolism appears to be multifactorial. Women who also smoke, have a history of migraine headaches, or have an inherited hypercoagulable defect are at a 30-fold increased risk of venous thrombosis, pulmonary embolism, and cerebrovascular thrombosis. There appears to be a weaker relationship between estrogen use at the time of menopause and the occurrence of thromboses.

Nephrotic Syndrome
Patients with nephrotic syndrome are at risk of thromboembolic disease, including renal vein thrombosis. The reason is unclear, but lower-than-normal levels of AT III or protein C due to renal loss of coagulation proteins, factor XII deficiency, platelet hyperactivity, abnormal fibrinolytic activity, and higher-than-normal levels of other coagulation factors may be implicated. Hyperlipidemia and hypoalbuminemia have also been proposed as possible contributing factors.

Antiphospholipid Antibodies

The presence of antiphospholipid antibodies does not necessarily correlate with thrombosis. Patients with hepatitis C, mononucleosis, syphilis, Lyme disease, multiple sclerosis, or HIV infection can have circulating antiphospholipid antibodies but do not have a propensity for thrombosis.

The term *antiphospholipid antibody syndrome* is used to describe patients who experience thromboses or pregnancy complications *and* have laboratory evidence of antiphospholipid antibodies in their blood. Antiphospholipid antibody syndrome can be primary (the sole manifestation of an autoimmune disease) or secondary (i.e., in association with systemic lupus erythematosus). The diagnosis requires the following clinical findings: thrombosis or pregnancy-related morbidity, and the presence of one of the antiphospholipid antibodies (anticardiolipin, anti–β_2-glycoprotein I, or the lupus anticoagulant).

The antibodies are clinically defined by the method of their detection. *Lupus anticoagulant antibodies* are detected by prolongation of the PTT and the dilute Russell viper venom time, whereas *anticardiolipin* and *anti–β_2-glycoprotein I antibodies* are measured directly by immunoassay. The risk of thrombosis appears to be greater with lupus anticoagulants and antibodies specifically directed at β_2-glycoprotein I.

The mechanism of the thrombotic action of these antibodies has yet to be defined. The antibodies might activate endothelial cells to increase the expression of vascular adhesion molecule 1 and E-selectin. This would increase the binding of WBCs and platelets to the endothelial surface and lead to thrombus formation.

Patients with lupus anticoagulants have an increased propensity for thrombosis, with 30%–60% of patients experiencing one or more thrombotic events during their lifetime. Isolated venous thrombosis or thromboembolism make up two-thirds of these events, and cerebral thrombosis accounts for the other third. Up to 20% of patients who have a VTE *not associated* with a disease, surgery, or trauma are found to have antiphospholipid antibodies. As with factor V Leiden and the prothrombin gene mutation, the presence of an antiphospholipid antibody must be considered as a likely cause of thromboembolic disease in younger individuals. Patients can also develop *catastrophic antiphospholipid syndrome* characterized by multiorgan failure resulting from widespread small vessel thrombosis, thrombocytopenia, acute respiratory distress syndrome, DIC, and occasionally an autoimmune hemolytic anemia. This clinical picture is indistinguishable from that of TTP. Bacterial infection is often the triggering event.

Optimal management of patients with antiphospholipid antibodies but *no history* of thrombotic events is unclear, but low-dose aspirin can be considered. The mainstay of therapy for patients *with a history* of thrombotic events consists of heparin, LMWH, and warfarin (contraindicated in pregnancy). Eculizumab (Soliris), a complement inhibitor, has been used to treat some cases of catastrophic antiphospholipid syndrome.

Management of Anesthesia in Venous Hypercoagulable Disorders

Patients with a history of thrombotic events should be managed based on the anticoagulant they are receiving and the risk of bleeding of the proposed surgery. If the patient is receiving antithrombotic treatment and there is a history of severe thrombophilia, a bridging regimen with parenteral antithrombotics may be considered preoperatively. In cases of mild thrombophilic disease, standard VTE prophylaxis should be sufficient.

Patients with heterozygous or homozygous mutations for inherited thrombophilia but no history of thrombotic events should not receive long-term anticoagulation. However, prophylactic anticoagulation should be used during the perioperative period. VTE prophylaxis can be achieved by using oral or parenteral anticoagulants, compression boots, and early ambulation. Very low-risk patients scheduled for general, abdominopelvic, or reconstructive/plastic procedures with no other risk factors for thrombosis have a very low risk of thrombosis (<0.5%) and can be managed with early ambulation. Minor low-risk procedures (thrombotic risk ≈ 1.5%) benefit from intermittent pneumatic compression or elastic stockings. Unless there are contraindications to anticoagulation, all other procedures with a high (>3%) and very high (>6%) thrombotic risk benefit from pharmacologic thromboprophylaxis. Regimens often include LMWH, subcutaneous heparin, or fondaparinux.

Patients undergoing orthopedic surgery merit special attention. In this patient population, thromboprophylaxis can be achieved with warfarin, oral direct thrombin inhibitors (dabigatran), or oral anti-Xa inhibitors (rivaroxaban, edoxaban, or apixaban). In patients undergoing major orthopedic surgeries or complex intraabdominal interventions for cancer, thromboprophylaxis should be continued for 1 month after the surgery.

Patients with cancer also represent a special category. For them, LMWH is the preferred antithrombotic for treatment of VTE in the acute setting but is also superior to warfarin in the ambulatory setting as long-term prophylaxis.

Since routine antithrombotic prophylaxis is used daily in the operating room, the advantages of regional anesthesia compared with general anesthesia are less clear in patients at high risk of VTE. Recent meta-analyses have found that regional and general anesthesia for hip surgery produce comparable results in most outcomes. Although there appears to be a slight reduction in VTE incidence with regional anesthesia and also a decreased need for transfusion, this does not translate into a significant difference in mortality. Regional anesthetics techniques can be safely performed in patients who are taking or who will be taking anticoagulants for thromboprophylaxis, without an increased risk of spinal/epidural hematoma so long as enough time has passed since the last dose of the anticoagulant for its effect to have dissipated. Similar precautions must be taken prior to catheter removal. Postoperative pharmacologic prophylaxis for VTE is very effective, so it may not be prudent to withhold these drugs just to use epidural analgesia for a longer period of time postoperatively.

Patients with an absolute contraindication to anticoagulant therapy or those with a major bleeding complication who have sustained a thrombotic event may benefit from placement of a vena cava filter to prevent recurrent pulmonary emboli. The filters are effective and reduce the incidence of pulmonary embolism to less than 4%.

Anesthetic Considerations in Patients Receiving Long-Term Anticoagulant Therapy

Perioperative management of patients receiving anticoagulant therapy requires special attention. The risk of perioperative thrombosis must be weighed against the risk of bleeding during and after surgery. Certain operations such as dental, dermatologic, and endoscopic procedures that can be done without disrupting mucosa can be accomplished without interruption of chronic anticoagulation therapy.

For most surgery, however, long-term oral anticoagulation needs to be temporarily discontinued. Patients at medium or high risk of thrombosis may receive bridging therapy with unfractionated heparin or LMWH. Many of the newer novel oral anticoagulants (NOACs) have much shorter half-lives than warfarin, so bridging may not be needed. Basic information about selected NOACs is presented in Table 24.6.

Resumption of anticoagulation postoperatively requires evaluation of the risk of recurrent thrombosis and consideration of the degree to which surgery itself increases hypercoagulability. These factors must be weighed against the bleeding risk associated with resumption of anticoagulation. Since there is a delay of approximately 24 hours after warfarin administration before the international normalized ratio (INR) begins to increase, warfarin therapy can generally be resumed soon after surgery except in patients at high risk of bleeding. Patients can also be managed with bridging therapy (subcutaneous heparin or LMWH), which can usually be started the day after surgery if surgical hemostasis has been achieved. Bridging can be stopped once the INR has been in the therapeutic range for 48 hours.

Acquired Hypercoagulability of the Arterial Vasculature

Heart Disease

Patients with acute anterior wall myocardial infarction who, because of a wall motion abnormality, are likely to form a mural thrombus should receive warfarin for 2–3 months after the infarction. After that time there is little risk of thromboembolism. Patients with atrial fibrillation, particularly atrial fibrillation associated with valvular disease, a dilated left atrium, and evidence of heart failure or a history of a prior embolus, generally require moderate-dose warfarin therapy indefinitely. The need for anticoagulation in patients with atrial fibrillation is determined using the CHADS$_2$ scoring system, which takes into account stroke risk factors such as congestive heart

TABLE 24.6 Mechanism of Action and Potential Antidotes for Commonly Used Anticoagulants

Generic Name	Brand Name	Mechanism	Route	Antidote
Unfractionated heparin		Antithrombin III–dependent inhibition of factor Xa	SQ or IV	Protamine
Low-molecular-weight heparins	Lovenox, Fragmin	Antithrombin III–dependent inhibition of factor Xa	SQ or IV	Protamine (partial reversal)
Warfarin	Coumadin	Depletion of vitamin K–dependent clotting factors	PO	Vitamin K; Fresh frozen plasma; Prothrombin complex concentrate (Kcentra)
Clopidogrel	Plavix	P2Y$_{12}$ ADP receptor platelet inhibitor	PO	Platelet transfusion
Prasugrel	Effient	P2Y$_{12}$ ADP receptor platelet inhibitor	PO	Platelet transfusion
Ticagrelor	Brilinta	P2Y$_{12}$ ADP receptor platelet inhibitor	PO	Platelet transfusion
Anagrelide	Agrylin	Inhibits platelet maturation cAMP PDE-III inhibitor	PO	Platelet transfusion
Fondaparinux	Arixtra	Factor Xa inhibitor	SQ	No reversal drug; Factor VIIa, antifibrinolytics
Rivaroxaban	Xarelto	Factor Xa inhibitor	PO	Andexanet alfa (in phase 3 trials)
Apixaban	Eliquis	Factor Xa inhibitor	PO	Andexanet alfa (in phase 3 trials)
Edoxaban	Savaysa	Factor Xa inhibitor	PO	Andexanet alfa (in phase 3 trials)
Dabigatran	Pradaxa	Direct thrombin inhibitor	PO	Idarucizumab (Praxbind)
Argatroban	Acova	Direct thrombin inhibitor	PO	No reversal drug; Factor VIIa
Bivalirudin	Angiomax	Direct thrombin inhibitor	IV	No reversal drug; Hemofiltration or hemodialysis, factor VIIa, fibrinogen, antifibrinolytics

ADP, Adenosine diphosphate; *cAMP,* cyclic adenosine monophosphate; *IV,* intravenous; *PDE,* phosphodiesterase; *PO,* oral; *SQ,* subcutaneous.

failure, hypertension, age 75 years or older, diabetes mellitus, and prior stroke (Table 24.7). Recently the safety of bridging in such patients has been challenged. It appears that patients who clearly benefit from bridging are those with $CHADS_2$ scores of 4–6 and those with a recent stroke.

Patients undergoing device placement (pacemaker or defibrillator) and those undergoing ablative procedures seem to have a higher risk of bleeding *with bridging* than with continuation of their usual anticoagulation medication. Therefore in these instances, oral anticoagulation should be continued perioperatively.

Perioperative and periprocedural management of patients receiving the newer oral anticoagulants have been incorporated into guidelines and protocols, and this information has been disseminated primarily by the American Society of Regional Anesthesia. *Regional Anesthesia in the Patient Receiving Antithrombotic or Thrombolytic Therapy: American Society of Regional Anesthesia and Pain Medicine Evidence-Based Guidelines (Third Edition)* was published in 2010. Work is underway on a fourth edition of these guidelines, and a prepublication executive summary was added to their website in 2015. Also in 2015, *Interventional Spine and Pain Procedures in Patients on Antiplatelet and Anticoagulation Medications:*

Guidelines From the American Society of Regional Anesthesia and Pain Medicine, the European Society of Regional Anesthesia and Pain Therapy, the American Academy of Pain Medicine, the International Neuromodulation Society, the North American Neuromodulation Society and the World Institute of Pain was published and is available on their website. Since recommendations on the subject of anticoagulation and anesthetic/pain management are constantly being reviewed, it is prudent to go to www.asra.com and review the latest information in deciding on a course of action for a particular patient.

In summary, hypercoagulability—a state of exaggerated activation of the coagulation system—plays a major role in the pathogenesis of VTE, a process that affects some 2 million Americans annually, with an estimated annual mortality of 150,000 from pulmonary embolism. New heritable causes of hypercoagulability are being identified, and some genetic predispositions to thrombosis can be identified in more than half of patients with deep vein thrombosis. The perioperative period represents a time of high risk for VTE (Table 24.8). Some kinds of surgery are associated with a more than 100-fold increase in the risk of thrombosis. Knowledge of the optimum operative management of these patients is evolving, but understanding the mechanisms of the hypercoagulable states and the mechanism of action of the many anticoagulants now available is a necessary part of the knowledge base for every anesthesiologist.

KEY POINTS

- The erythrocyte and its major protein constituent, Hb, are highly specialized so that oxygen delivery can be rapidly adjusted to meet local tissue needs. Disorders affecting the formation, structure, metabolism, and turnover of RBCs can impair their ability to perform this vital task in patients undergoing surgery.

TABLE 24.7	$CHADS_2$ Scoring System for Estimating Risk of Stroke in Nonrheumatic Atrial Fibrillation	
	Condition	Points
C	Congestive heart failure	1
H	Hypertension	1
A	Age ≥ 75 yr	1
D	Diabetes mellitus	1
S_2	Prior stroke or transient ischemic attack	2

TABLE 24.8	Suggested Risk Stratification for Perioperative Thromboembolic Events		
Risk Category	Mechanical Heart Valve	Atrial Fibrillation	VTE
High	Any mitral valve prosthesis Caged-ball or tilting-disc aortic valve prosthesis Recent (within 6 mo) stroke or TIA	$CHADS_2$ score of 5 or 6 Recent (within 3 mo) stroke or TIA Rheumatic heart disease	Recent (within 3 mo) VTE Severe thrombophilia, e.g., deficiency of protein C, protein S, or antithrombin III; presence of antiphospholipid antibodies; or multiple abnormalities
Moderate	Bileaflet aortic valve prosthesis and one of the following: atrial fibrillation, prior stroke or TIA, hypertension, diabetes, congestive heart failure, age > 75 yr	$CHADS_2$ score of 3 or 4	VTE within past 3–12 mo Mild to moderate thrombophilic condition Recurrent VTE Active cancer (treated within 6 mo or with palliative care)
Low	Bileaflet aortic valve prosthesis without atrial fibrillation and no other risk factors for stroke	$CHADS_2$ score of 0–2 No prior stroke or TIA	Single VTE occurring >12 mo earlier No other risk factors

CHADS_2, System for predicting stroke likelihood based on the risk factors of congestive heart failure, hypertension, age ≥ 75 yr, diabetes mellitus, and prior stroke (see Table 24.7); *TIA,* transient ischemic attack; *VTE,* venous thromboembolism.
Data from Douketis JD, Berger PB, Dunn AS, et al. The perioperative management of antithrombotic therapy: American College of Chest Physicians Evidence-Based Clinical Practice Guidelines (8th edition). *Chest.* 2008;133(6 Suppl):299S-339S.

- Preoperative management of patients with sickle cell disease no longer mandates exchange transfusion to decrease the ratio of sickle Hb to normal Hb. Instead, transfusions are required only as needed to achieve a preoperative Hct (total of all forms of Hb) of 30%.

- Recent advances in cell-based coagulation models have changed our fundamental understanding of in vivo clotting. This improved understanding allows a better appreciation of how specific defects in coagulation components affect the balance of hemostasis and what therapeutic interventions offer the best risk/benefit ratio.

- Sources of hypercoagulability can be divided into two major classes: a congenital predisposition that is usually lifelong and an acquired or environmental hypercoagulability such as may occur during the perioperative period. In patients experiencing a first-time venous thromboembolism, some congenital predisposition to hypercoagulability can be identified in up to 50% of cases. However, almost always, some acquired or environmental hypercoagulable condition seems to be necessary to trigger the thromboembolic event.

- Most disorders producing a state of *venous* hypercoagulability affect the production and disposition of thrombin, whereas hypercoagulability in the *arterial* circulation is affected by platelet and endothelial function and regulation in addition to abnormalities in thrombin generation and breakdown.

RESOURCES

American Society of Anesthesiologists Task Force on Perioperative Blood Management. Practice guidelines for perioperative blood management: an updated report by the American Society of Anesthesiologists Task Force on Perioperative Blood Management. *Anesthesiology*. 2015;122:241-275.

Auerbach M, Adamson J, Bircher A, et al. On the safety of intravenous iron, evidence trumps conjecture. *Haematologica*. 2015;100:e214-e215.

Avni T, Bieber A, Grossman A, et al. The safety of intravenous iron preparations: systematic review and meta-analysis. *Mayo Clin Proc*. 2015;90:12-23.

Carson JL, Terrin ML, Noveck H, et al. Liberal or restrictive transfusion in high-risk patients after hip surgery. *N Engl J Med*. 2011;365:2453-2462.

Chighizola CB, Raschi E, Borghi MO, et al. Update on the pathogenesis and treatment of the antiphospholipid syndrome. *Curr Opin Rheumatol*. 2015;27:476-482.

Crowther MA, Cook DJ, Albert M, et al. Canadian Critical Care Trials Group. The 4Ts scoring system for heparin-induced thrombocytopenia in medical-surgical intensive care unit patients. *J Crit Care*. 2010;25:287-293.

Douketis JD, Spyropoulos AC, Spencer, et al. The perioperative management of antithrombotic therapy: antithrombotic therapy and prevention of thrombosis. American College of Chest Physicians Evidence-Based Clinical Practice Guidelines (9th edition). *Chest*. 2012;141(2 Suppl):e326S-350S.

Elliott MA, Tefferi A. Thrombosis and haemorrhage in polycythaemia vera and essential thrombocythaemia. *Br J Haematol*. 2005;128:275-290.

Elyassi AR, Rowshan HH. Perioperative management of the glucose-6-phosphate dehydrogenase deficient patient: a review of the literature. *Anesth Prog*. 2009;56:86-91.

Firth PG, Head CA. Sickle cell disease and anesthesia. *Anesthesiology*. 2004;101:766-785.

Greinacher A. Heparin-Induced thrombocytopenia. *N Engl J Med*. 2015;373:252-261.

Gutt CN, Oniu T, Wolkener F, et al. Prophylaxis and treatment of deep vein thrombosis in general surgery. *Am J Surg*. 2004;189:14-22.

Hébert PC, Wells G, Blajchman MA, et al. A multicenter, randomized, controlled clinical trial of transfusion requirements in critical care. Transfusion Requirements in Critical Care Investigators, Canadian Critical Care Trials Group. *N Engl J Med*. 1999;340:409-417.

Hoffmann M. Remodeling the blood coagulation cascade. *J Thromb Thrombolysis*. 2003;16:17-20.

Horlocker TT, Wedel DJ, Rowlingson JC, et al. Regional anesthesia in the patient receiving antithrombotic or thrombolytic therapy: American Society of Regional Anesthesia and Pain Medicine Evidence-Based Guidelines (third edition). *Reg Anesth Pain Med*. 2010;35:64-101.

Khatri V, Holak EJ, Pagel PS. Perioperative implications of hereditary spherocytosis in coronary artery surgery. *J Cardiothorac Vasc Anesth*. 2010;24:636-638.

Levy JH, Key NS, Azran MS. Novel oral anticoagulants: implications in the perioperative setting. *Anesthesiology*. 2010;113:726-745.

Mensah PK, Gooding R. Surgery in patients with inherited bleeding disorders. *Anaesthesia*. 2015;70(Suppl 1):112-120, e39-40.

Murphy GJ, Pike K, Rogers CA, et al. Liberal or restrictive transfusion after cardiac surgery. *N Engl J Med*. 2015;372:997-1008.

Padhi S, Glen J, Pordes BA, et al. Management of anaemia in chronic kidney disease: summary of updated NICE guidance. *BMJ*. 2015;350: h2258.

Raut MS, Khanuja JS, Srivastava S. Perioperative considerations in a sickle cell patient undergoing cardiopulmonary bypass. *Indian J Anaesth*. 2014;58:319-322.

Shah A, Stanworth SJ, McKechnie S. Evidence and triggers for the transfusion of blood and blood products. *Anaesthesia*. 2015;70(Suppl 1):10-19, e3-5.

Schafer A, Levine M, Konkle B, Kearon C. Thrombotic disorders: diagnosis and treatment. *Hematology Am Soc Hematol Educ Program*. 2003:520-539.

Tefferi A. Annual clinical updates in hematological malignancies: polycythemia vera and essential thrombocythemia: 2011 Update on diagnosis, risk-stratification, and management. *Am J Hematol*. 2011;86:292-301.

Turpie AGG, Chin BSP, Lip GLH. Venous thromboembolism: pathophysiology, clinical features, and prevention. The ABCs of antithrombotic therapy. *BMJ*. 2002;325:887-890.

Weiss G. Pathogenesis and treatment of anaemia of chronic disease. *Blood Rev*. 2002;16:87-96.

Whitlock EL, Kim H, Auerbach AD. Harms associated with single unit perioperative transfusion: retrospective population-based analysis. *BMJ*. 2015;350: h3037.

Skin and Musculoskeletal Diseases

KATHERINE E. MARSCHALL

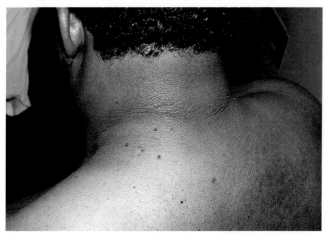

FIG. 25.1   The velvety hyperpigmentation of acanthosis nigricans in a neck crease in a patient with diabetes mellitus. (From Fitzpatrick JE, Morelli JG, eds. *Dermatology Secrets Plus.* 5th ed. Philadelphia: Elsevier; 2016. With permission.)

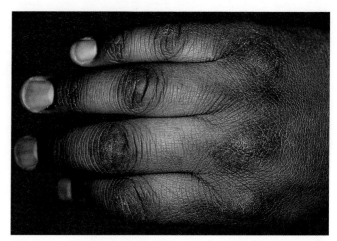

FIG. 25.2   Acanthosis nigricans over the knuckles in a patient with insulin resistance and obesity. (From Bolognia JL, Jorizzo JL, Schaffer JV, eds. *Dermatology.* 3rd ed. Philadelphia: Elsevier; 2012. With permission.)

SKIN DISEASES

Several dermatologic diseases have significance for the anesthesiologist. These include skin manifestations of systemic diseases where the skin lesions may not be themselves problematic but are markers of "internal" disease. Such rashes include acanthosis nigricans and atopic dermatitis. The dermal manifestations of scleroderma and dermatomyositis are, however, problematic. Vesicular/bullous or pustular skin lesions can be important because of issues with fluid balance from extensive weeping skin lesions and/or the risk of generalized infection. Stevens-Johnson syndrome and toxic epidermal necrolysis are typical examples. Finally, there are skin diseases which can be significantly worsened by various elements of anesthetic management. These include epidermolysis bullosa, pemphigus, mastocytosis, and various forms of urticaria.

Acanthosis Nigricans

Acanthosis nigricans produces a rash characterized by darkened, thickened "velvety" skin, usually in areas of skin creases such as the axillae, neck, and groin (Figs. 25.1 and 25.2). It is itself a benign skin condition, but it is typically a marker of insulin resistance, diabetes mellitus type II, polycystic ovarian syndrome, obesity, and gastric, colonic, or hepatic cancer. Thus hyperglycemia and the complications of obesity may influence anesthetic management.

Atopic Dermatitis

Atopic dermatitis is the cutaneous manifestation of the atopic state. It is characterized by dry, scaly, eczematous, pruritic patches on the face, neck, and flexor surfaces of the arms and legs. Pruritus is the primary symptom. Systemic antihistamines are effective in decreasing pruritus, and corticosteroids may be indicated for short-term treatment of

severe cases. Pulmonary manifestations of the atopic state (e.g., asthma, hay fever, otitis media, sinusitis) may influence anesthetic management.

Epidermolysis Bullosa

Epidermolysis bullosa is a group of *genetic diseases* of mucous membranes and skin, particularly the oropharynx and esophagus. Epidermolysis bullosa can be categorized as simplex, junctional, and dystrophic. In the *simplex type,* epidermal cells are fragile because of mutations of genes encoding for the keratin of basal epithelial cells. In the *junctional type* there are mutations in the genes for components of the dermal-epidermal junction. In the *dystrophic types* the genetic mutations appear to be in the genes encoding type VII collagen, the major component of anchoring fibrils for the basement membrane.

Signs and Symptoms

Epidermolysis bullosa is characterized by bulla formation (blistering) resulting from intercellular separation within the epidermis followed by fluid accumulation. Bulla formation is typically initiated when lateral shearing forces are applied to the skin. Pressure applied perpendicular to the skin is not as great a hazard. Bullae can form after even minimal trauma and can even develop spontaneously.

The *simplex form of epidermolysis bullosa* has a benign course, and development is normal. By contrast, patients with the *junctional form of epidermolysis bullosa* rarely survive beyond early childhood. Most die of sepsis, but metastatic squamous cell cancer is not uncommon. Features that distinguish junctional epidermolysis bullosa from other forms are generalized blistering beginning at birth, absence of scar formation, and generalized mucosal involvement (gastrointestinal (GI), genitourinary, respiratory tracts).

Manifestations of *epidermolysis bullosa dystrophica* include severe scarring with fusion of the digits (pseudosyndactyly), constriction of the oral aperture (microstomia), and esophageal stricture. The teeth are often dysplastic. Malnutrition, anemia, electrolyte derangements, and hypoalbuminemia are common, most likely reflecting chronic infection, debilitation, and renal dysfunction. Survival beyond the second decade is unusual.

Diseases associated with epidermolysis bullosa include porphyria cutanea tarda, amyloidosis, multiple myeloma, diabetes mellitus, and hypercoagulable states.

Treatment
Treatment of epidermolysis bullosa is symptomatic and supportive. Many of these patients are receiving corticosteroids. Infection of bullae with *Staphylococcus aureus* or β-hemolytic streptococci is common.

Management of Anesthesia
Supplemental corticosteroids may be indicated during the perioperative period if patients have been receiving long-term treatment with these drugs. However, the main anesthetic concerns in patients with epidermolysis bullosa center on the serious complications that can occur if proper precautions are not taken during any form of patient manipulation or instrumentation. Avoidance of trauma to the skin and mucous membranes is crucial. Bulla formation can be caused by trauma from tape, blood pressure cuffs, tourniquets, adhesive electrodes, and rubbing of the skin with alcohol wipes. Blood pressure cuffs should be padded with a loose cotton dressing. Electrodes should have the adhesive portion removed. Petroleum jelly gauze can help hold the electrodes in place. Anything that touches a patient should be well padded. Intravenous (IV) and intraarterial catheters should be sutured or held in place with gauze wraps rather than tape. A nonadhesive pulse oximetry sensor should be used. A soft foam, sheepskin, or gel pad should be placed under the patient. All creases should be removed from the linen.

Trauma from the anesthetic face mask can be minimized by gentle application against the face. Lubrication of the face and mask with cortisol ointment or another lubricant can be helpful. Upper airway instrumentation should be minimized because the squamous epithelium lining the oropharynx and esophagus is very susceptible to trauma. Frictional trauma to the oropharynx, such as that produced by an oral airway, can result in formation of large intraoral bullae and/or extensive hemorrhage from denuded mucosa. Nasal airways are equally hazardous. Esophageal stethoscopes should be avoided. Hemorrhage from ruptured oral bullae has been treated successfully by application of epinephrine-soaked gauze directly to the bullae.

Interestingly, endotracheal intubation has *not* been associated with laryngeal or tracheal complications in patients with epidermolysis bullosa dystrophica. Indeed, laryngeal involvement is rare in this form of the disease, and tracheal bullae have not been reported. This finding is consistent with the greater resistance of columnar epithelium (laryngotracheal lining) to disruption compared with fragile squamous epithelium (lining of oropharynx). Generous lubrication of the laryngoscope blade with cortisol ointment and/or petroleum jelly and selection of a smaller-than-usual endotracheal tube are recommended. Chronic scarring of the oral cavity can result in a narrow oral aperture and immobility of the tongue, which may make tracheal intubation difficult. After intubation the tube must be carefully immobilized with soft cloth bandages to prevent movement in the oropharynx, and the tube must be positioned so that it does not exert lateral forces at the corners of the mouth. Tape is not used to hold the endotracheal tube in place. Oropharyngeal suctioning can lead to life-threatening bulla formation. The risk of pulmonary aspiration may be increased in the presence of esophageal stricture.

Porphyria cutanea tarda has been reported to occur with increased frequency in patients with epidermolysis bullosa, but this type of porphyria does not precipitate attacks of acute porphyria. Any anesthetic drugs may be used.

Propofol and ketamine are useful for avoiding airway manipulation when the operative procedure does not require controlled ventilation or skeletal muscle relaxation. Despite the presence of dystrophic skeletal muscle, there is no evidence these patients are at increased risk of a hyperkalemic response when treated with succinylcholine. There are no known contraindications to the use of volatile anesthetics in these patients. As alternatives to general anesthesia, regional anesthetic techniques (spinal, epidural, brachial plexus block) have been recommended.

Pemphigus

Pemphigus refers to a group of chronic *autoimmune* blistering (vesiculobullous) diseases that may involve extensive areas of the skin and mucous membranes. The cause is the presence of autoantibodies to desmogleins, which are adherence molecules in the skin. *Paraneoplastic pemphigus* is an autoimmune blistering mucocutaneous disease that can be seen with non-Hodgkin's lymphoma, chronic lymphocytic leukemia, thymoma, spindle cell tumors, and Waldenström macroglobulinemia. As with epidermolysis bullosa, there may be an absence of intercellular bridges that normally prevent the separation of epidermal cells. Therefore frictional trauma can result in bulla formation. *Pemphigus vulgaris* is the most common form of pemphigus and also the most significant because of its high incidence of oropharyngeal lesions.

Pemphigus closely resembles the oral manifestations of epidermolysis bullosa dystrophica. Involvement of the oropharynx is present in approximately 50% of patients with pemphigus (Fig. 25.3). Extensive oropharyngeal involvement makes eating painful, and patients may decrease oral intake to the point that malnutrition develops. Denuding of skin and bulla formation can result in significant fluid and protein losses. The risk of secondary infection is substantial.

Treatment
Treatment of pemphigus with corticosteroids has decreased the mortality associated with this disease from 70% to 5%. Biologic and immunosuppressive therapy with mycophenolate

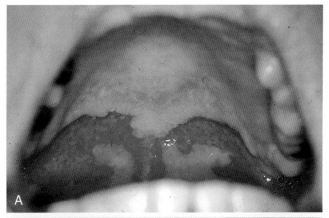

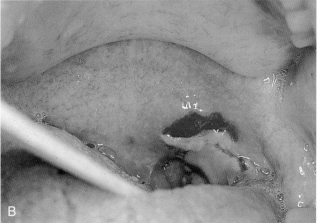

FIG. 25.3   A and B, Two images of pemphigus with lesions of the palate. Essentially all patients with pemphigus develop painful oral mucosal erosions, with the most common sites being the buccal and palatine mucosa. These lesions are flaccid, thin-walled, easily ruptured blisters. (From Bolognia JL, Jorizzo JL, Schaffer JV, eds. *Dermatology.* 3rd ed. Philadelphia: Elsevier; 2012. With permission.)

mofetil, azathioprine, methotrexate, and cyclophosphamide has also been used successfully for early treatment of pemphigus. Resistant disease may respond well to rituximab, IV immunoglobulin, or plasmapheresis.

Management of Anesthesia

Management of anesthesia in patients with pemphigus and epidermolysis bullosa is similar. Preoperative evaluation must consider current drug therapy. "Stress-dose" supplementation with corticosteroids may be necessary. Electrolyte derangements due to chronic fluid losses through bullous skin lesions may be present. Dehydration and hypokalemia are not uncommon.

Airway management may be difficult because of bullae in the oropharynx. Airway manipulation, including direct laryngoscopy and endotracheal intubation, can result in acute bulla formation, upper airway obstruction, and bleeding. Regional anesthesia, although controversial, has been used successfully in these patients. Skin infection at the site selected for regional anesthesia is possible. Infiltration with a local anesthetic solution is usually avoided because of the risk of skin sloughing

and bulla formation at the injection site. Propofol and ketamine are useful for general anesthesia in selected patients.

Mastocytosis

Mastocytosis is a rare disorder of mast cell proliferation that can occur in a cutaneous or systemic form. *Urticaria pigmentosa,* the lesion of the cutaneous form, is usually benign and asymptomatic. Children are most often affected. In nearly half of affected children, the small red-brown macules that are present on the trunk and extremities disappear by adulthood. In the systemic form of mastocytosis, mast cells may proliferate in all organs but not in the central nervous system (CNS). Degranulation of mast cells with release of histamine, leukotrienes, prostaglandins, proteases (tryptases, hydrolases), and proteoglycans (heparin and chondroitin sulfate) may occur spontaneously or be triggered by nonimmune factors, including temperature changes, exercise, psychological stimuli, alcohol, spicy foods, and drugs known to release histamine. There are several forms of systemic mastocytosis, ranging in character from indolent to aggressive. Some forms may progress to myelodysplastic or myeloproliferative disorders or even to mast cell leukemia. These may be characterized by diffuse mast cell proliferation in parenchymal organs, especially bone marrow and liver. Bone marrow aspiration and biopsy are required to categorize systemic forms of mastocytosis.

Signs and Symptoms

Classic signs and symptoms of mastocytosis reflect degranulation of mast cells, with responses characterized by pruritus, urticaria, flushing, nausea and vomiting, abdominal cramping, and diarrhea. These changes may be accompanied by hypotension and tachycardia. Hypotension may be so severe as to be life threatening. Although symptoms are usually attributed to histamine release from mast cells, histamine H_1- and H_2-receptor antagonists are not always protective, suggesting that some vasoactive substances other than histamine are also involved. The incidence of bronchospasm is low. Bleeding is unusual in these patients, even though mast cells contain heparin. In addition to antihistamine receptor antagonists, patients may also be taking oral cromolyn sodium, which inhibits mast cell degranulation and leukotriene receptor–binding inhibitors to help relieve itching, abdominal pain, and diarrhea.

Management of Anesthesia

Management of anesthesia is influenced by the possibility of intraoperative mast cell degranulation. Preoperative discussion with the patient, surgeon, and an allergist may be very helpful for perioperative planning. Although the intraoperative period is usually uneventful, there are reports of life-threatening anaphylactoid reactions with even minor surgical procedures, which emphasizes the need to have resuscitation drugs such as epinephrine immediately available. Preoperative administration of H_1- and H_2-receptor antagonists should be considered to decrease the clinical response to histamine release. Oral cromolyn sodium may also be used preoperatively.

TABLE 25.1	Features of Common Types of Chronic Urticaria			
Type of Urticaria	Age Range (yr)	Clinical Features	Angioedema	Diagnostic Test
Chronic idiopathic urticaria	20–50	Pink or pale edematous papules or wheals, wheals often annular; pruritus	Yes	
Symptomatic dermatographism	20–50	Linear wheals with a surrounding bright red flare at sites of stimulation; pruritus	No	Light stroking of skin causes wheal
PHYSICAL URTICARIAS				
Cold	10–40	Pale or red swelling at sites of contact with cold surfaces or fluids; pruritus	Yes	Application of ice pack causes wheal within 5 minutes of removing ice (cold stimulation test)
Pressure	20–50	Swelling at sites of pressure (soles, palms, waist) lasting ≥2–24 hours; pain, pruritus	No	Application of pressure perpendicular to skin produces persistent red swelling after a latent period of 1–4 hours
Solar	20–50	Pale or red swelling at site of exposure to ultraviolet or visible light; pruritus	Yes	Radiation by solar simulator for 30–120 seconds causes wheals in 30 minutes
Cholinergic	10–50	Monomorphic pale or pink wheals on trunk, neck, and limbs; pruritus	Yes	Exercise or hot shower elicits wheals

Adapted from Greaves MW. Chronic urticaria. *N Engl J Med.* 1995;332:1767-1772.

Some recommend preoperative skin testing of anesthesia-related drugs to help define which anesthetics would provoke mast cell degranulation. Fentanyl, propofol, and vecuronium have been administered to these patients without causing mast cell degranulation, as have succinylcholine and meperidine. However, drugs known to stimulate histamine release (e.g., morphine, some muscle relaxants) are best avoided. Volatile anesthetics appear to be acceptable in these patients. Monitoring serum tryptase concentration during the perioperative period may be useful for detecting the occurrence of mast cell degranulation. An elevated serum or plasma tryptase level may be noted for up to 3 hours after either nonimmunologic mast cell degranulation or classic anaphylaxis (the tryptase concentration cannot distinguish between these two entities).

Episodes of profound hypotension have been observed with administration of radiocontrast media to patients with mastocytosis. Therefore it is prudent to pretreat these patients with H_1- and H_2-histamine receptor antagonists and a glucocorticoid before procedures involving contrast dye.

Urticaria

Urticaria may be characterized as *acute urticaria, chronic urticaria,* or *physical urticaria.* Acute urticaria (hives) affects 10%–20% of the US population at one time or another. In most people the cause cannot be determined and the lesions resolve spontaneously or after administration of antihistamines. Only a minority of patients have lesions for a long period of time. With physical urticaria, physically stimulating the skin causes formation of local wheals, itching, and in some cases angioedema. *Cold urticaria* accounts for 3%–5% of all physical urticarias (Table 25.1). Urticarial vasculitis may be a presenting symptom of systemic lupus erythematosus (SLE) and Sjögren syndrome.

Chronic Urticaria

Chronic urticaria is characterized by circumscribed wheals and localized areas of edema produced by extravasation of fluid through blood vessel walls. It is often idiopathic in origin. The wheals are smooth, pink to red, and surrounded by a bright red flare. They are usually intensely pruritic, can be found anywhere on hairless or hairy skin, and last less than 24 hours. Wheals lasting longer than 24 hours raise the possibility of other diagnoses, including urticarial vasculitis. Chronic urticaria affects approximately twice as many women as men and often follows a remitting and relapsing course, with symptoms typically increasing at night. Mast cells and basophils regulate urticarial reactions. When they are stimulated by certain nonimmunologic events or by immunologic factors (drugs, inhaled allergens), storage granules in these cells release histamine and other vasoactive substances such as bradykinin. These substances result in localized vasodilation and transudation of fluid characteristic of urticarial lesions.

Except in patients with chronic urticaria for whom avoidable causes can be identified, treatment is symptomatic. A tepid shower temporarily alleviates pruritus. Antihistamines (H_1-receptor antagonists) are the principal treatment for mild cases of recurring chronic urticaria. Terfenadine has a low potential for sedation and is a common treatment for mild cases of chronic urticaria. If antihistamines do not control chronic urticaria, a course of systemic corticosteroids may be considered. The period of treatment is usually limited to 21 days; prolonged use of corticosteroids is invariably associated with a decrease in efficacy and an increase in side effects. Omalizumab (Xolair) has been developed to treat very symptomatic chronic idiopathic urticaria. It is an anti–immunoglobulin E (anti-IgE) antibody and binds to IgE and lowers free IgE levels. This results in downregulation of IgE receptors on mast cells and basophils. Omalizumab is given by monthly subcutaneous injection. A 2% topical spray of ephedrine is useful for treating oropharyngeal edema. Swelling involving the tongue may require urgent treatment with epinephrine.

All patients with chronic urticaria should be advised to avoid angiotensin-converting enzyme (ACE) inhibitors, aspirin, and other nonsteroidal antiinflammatory drugs (NSAIDs).

Cold Urticaria

Cold urticaria exists in a familial and an acquired form and is characterized by development of urticaria and angioedema following exposure to cold. The most common triggering factors are cold air currents, rain, aquatic activities, snow, consumption of cold foods and beverages, and contact with cold objects. Severe cold urticaria may be life-threatening, with laryngeal edema, bronchospasm, and hypotension. The diagnosis is based on skin stimulation at a temperature of 0°–4°C for 1–5 minutes (cold stimulation test). Immunologic mechanisms may be associated with the development of cold urticaria. IgE concentrations may be increased. Cutaneous mast cells rather than intravascular basophils seem to be the target cells for degranulation.

The primary objective of treatment of cold urticaria is to prevent systemic reactions caused by known triggers. Antihistamines may decrease the incidence of urticarial events and prolong the time a cold stimulus is tolerated before a reaction occurs. Doxepin, a tricyclic antidepressant with antihistaminic properties, can be used topically with very good results in cold urticaria.

Management of Anesthesia

Management of anesthesia includes avoidance of drugs likely to evoke histamine release. Drugs requiring cold storage should be avoided or warmed before injection. Other prophylactic measures include warming IV fluids and increasing the ambient temperature of the operating room. Preoperative administration of H_1- and H_2-receptor antagonists and corticosteroids has been recommended, especially when intraoperative hypothermia is unavoidable, as may be the case during cardiac surgery. Patients with cold urticaria undergoing cardiac surgery have been managed in three ways: off-pump coronary artery bypass grafting in patients with suitable coronary anatomy, use of cardiopulmonary bypass under normothermic conditions with isothermic cardioplegia, and cardiopulmonary bypass with systemic hypothermia and cold cardioplegia. If the patient is exposed to cold, clinical manifestations of cold urticaria are typically manifested *during rewarming rather than during cooling.*

Erythema Multiforme

Erythema multiforme is a recurrent disease of the skin and mucous membranes characterized by lesions ranging from edematous macules and papules to vesicular or bullous lesions that may ulcerate. (Vesicles are ≤0.5 cm in size, and bullae are >0.5 cm in size). Attacks are associated with viral infection

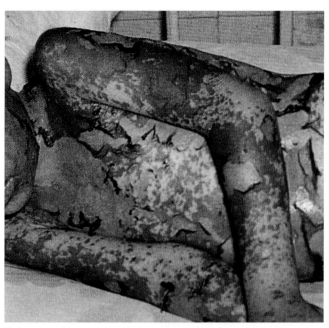

FIG. 25.4   Large areas of desquamation in Stevens-Johnson syndrome. (From Baren JM, Rothrock SG, Brennan J, Brown L. *Pediatric Emergency Medicine.* Philadelphia: Saunders; 2008. With permission.)

(especially infection with herpes simplex), infection with hemolytic streptococci, cancer, collagen vascular disease, and drug-induced hypersensitivity.

Stevens-Johnson syndrome (SJS) and *toxic epidermal necrolysis* (TEN) are severe manifestations of erythema multiforme associated with multisystem dysfunction. High fever, tachycardia, and tachypnea may occur. There may be skin sloughing (Figs. 25.4 and 25.5). SJS is typically associated with skin involvement of less than 10%, SJS/TEN overlap syndrome has 10%–30% skin involvement, and TEN involves over 30% of the skin surface. Mortality correlates with the amount of skin involved and is less than 5% for SJS and up to 50% for TEN.

Drugs associated with the onset of these syndromes include antibiotics, analgesics, and certain over-the-counter medications. Corticosteroids are used in the management of severe cases.

Management of Anesthesia

The hazards of administering anesthesia to patients with SJS or any degree of TEN may be similar to those encountered in anesthetizing patients with epidermolysis bullosa or pemphigus. For example, involvement of the upper respiratory tract can make management of the airway and tracheal intubation difficult. Patients with moderate to severe disease should be treated in a burn unit.

Scleroderma

Scleroderma (also known as *systemic sclerosis*) is characterized by three interrelated processes: (1) inflammation and autoimmunity, (2) vascular injury with eventual vascular

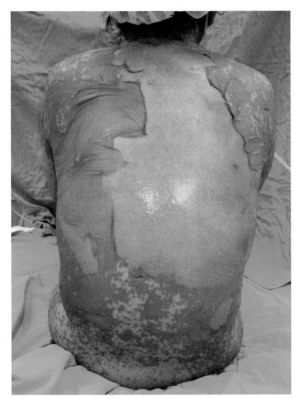

FIG. 25.5 Back lesion in a woman presenting with toxic epidermal necrolysis involving 48% of total body surface area. (From Huang SH, Yang PS, Wu SH, et al. Aquacel Ag with Vaseline gauze in the treatment of toxic epidermal necrolysis [TEN]. *Burns.* 2010;36:121-126. Copyright Elsevier and ISBI with permission.)

obliteration, and (3) fibrosis and accumulation of excess matrix in many organs and tissues. Its etiology is unclear but may include triggers such as exposure to toxins, drugs, and perhaps some microbial pathogens. Microvascular changes produce tissue fibrosis and organ sclerosis. Injury to vascular endothelial cells results in widespread capillary loss and vascular obliteration and leakage of serum proteins into the interstitial space. These vascular structures *do not* regenerate. These proteins produce tissue edema, lymphatic obstruction, and ultimately fibrosis. In some patients the disease evolves into *CREST syndrome* (*c*alcinosis, *R*aynaud phenomenon, *e*sophageal hypomotility, *s*clerodactyly, *t*elangiectasia). The prognosis is poor and related to the extent of visceral involvement. No drugs or treatments have proved safe and effective in altering the underlying disease process.

The typical age at onset is 20–40 years, and women are most often affected. Pregnancy accelerates the progression of scleroderma in about half of patients. The incidence of spontaneous abortion, premature labor, and perinatal mortality is high.

Signs and Symptoms

Manifestations of scleroderma occur in the skin and musculoskeletal system, nervous system, cardiovascular system, lungs, kidneys, and GI tract.

Skin exhibits mild thickening and diffuse nonpitting edema. As scleroderma progresses the skin becomes taut, which results in limited mobility and flexion contractures, especially of the fingers. Skeletal muscles may develop myopathy manifested as weakness, particularly of proximal skeletal muscle groups. The plasma creatine kinase concentration is typically increased. Mild inflammatory arthritis can occur, but most limitation to joint movement is due to the thickened, taut skin. Avascular necrosis of the femoral head may occur.

Peripheral or cranial nerve neuropathy has been attributed to nerve compression by thickened connective tissue surrounding the nerve sheath. Facial pain suggestive of trigeminal neuralgia may occur as a result of this thickening. Keratoconjunctivitis sicca (dry eyes) exists in some patients and may predispose to corneal abrasions.

Changes in the myocardium reflect sclerosis of small coronary arteries and the conduction system, replacement of cardiac muscle with fibrous tissue, and the indirect effects of systemic and pulmonary hypertension. These changes result in cardiac dysrhythmias, cardiac conduction abnormalities, and congestive heart failure. Intimal fibrosis of pulmonary arteries is associated with a high incidence of pulmonary hypertension, which may progress to cor pulmonale. Pulmonary hypertension is often present, even in asymptomatic patients. Pericarditis and pericardial effusion with or without cardiac tamponade are not infrequent. Changes in the peripheral portion of the vascular tree are common and typically involve intermittent vasospasm in the small arteries of the digits. Raynaud phenomenon occurs in most cases and may be the initial manifestation of scleroderma. Oral or nasal telangiectasias may be present.

The effects of scleroderma on the lungs are a major cause of morbidity and mortality. Diffuse interstitial pulmonary fibrosis may occur independent of the vascular changes that lead to pulmonary hypertension. Arterial hypoxemia resulting from a decreased diffusion capacity is not unusual in these patients even at rest. Although dermal sclerosis does not decrease chest wall compliance, pulmonary compliance is diminished by fibrosis.

Renal artery stenosis is a result of arteriolar intimal proliferation, leading to decreased renal blood flow and systemic hypertension. Development of malignant hypertension and irreversible renal failure used to be the most common cause of death in patients with scleroderma. Now, however, the 10%–15% of people who develop a scleroderma renal crisis can be treated effectively with ACE inhibitors. These drugs will control the hypertension and improve the impaired renal function that accompanies the hypertension. Corticosteroids can precipitate a renal crisis in patients with scleroderma.

Involvement of the GI tract by scleroderma may manifest as dryness of the oral mucosa (xerostomia). Progressive fibrosis of the GI tract causes hypomotility of the lower esophagus and small intestine. Dysphagia is a common complaint. Lower esophageal sphincter tone is decreased, and reflux of gastric fluid into the esophagus is common. Small intestine bacterial overgrowth resulting from intestinal hypomotility can produce a malabsorption syndrome. Coagulation disorders reflecting malabsorption of vitamin K may be present. Broad-spectrum antibiotics are effective in treating this type of malabsorption syndrome. Intestinal hypomotility can also manifest as intestinal pseudo-obstruction. Somatostatin analogues such as octreotide may improve refractory hypomotility of the small intestine. Prokinetic drugs such as metoclopramide are not effective.

With the exception of the use of ACE inhibitors to treat scleroderma renal crisis, no other drug therapy has been shown to alter the course of this disease. Treatment consists of monitoring disease activity, alleviating symptoms, and managing complications (e.g., administering drugs to treat systemic and/or pulmonary hypertension).

Management of Anesthesia

Preoperative evaluation of patients with scleroderma must focus attention on the organ systems likely to be involved by this disease. Decreased mandibular motion and narrowing of the oral aperture resulting from taut skin must be appreciated before induction of anesthesia. Fiberoptic laryngoscopy may be necessary to facilitate endotracheal intubation through a small oral aperture. Oral or nasal telangiectasias may bleed profusely if traumatized during tracheal intubation. IV access may be impeded by dermal thickening. Intraarterial catheterization for blood pressure monitoring introduces the same concerns as in patients with Raynaud phenomenon. Cardiac evaluation may provide evidence of pulmonary hypertension. Because of chronic systemic hypertension and vasomotor instability, patients with scleroderma may have a contracted intravascular volume. This may produce hypotension during induction of anesthesia when anesthetic drugs with vasodilating properties exert their effects. Hypotonia of the lower esophageal sphincter puts patients at risk of regurgitation and pulmonary aspiration. Efforts to increase gastric fluid pH with antacids, H_2-receptor antagonists, or proton pump inhibitors prior to induction of anesthesia are needed.

Intraoperatively, decreased pulmonary compliance may require higher airway pressures to ensure adequate ventilation. Supplemental oxygen is indicated in view of the impaired diffusion capacity and vulnerability to the development of arterial hypoxemia. Events known to increase pulmonary vascular resistance (e.g., respiratory acidosis, arterial hypoxemia) must be prevented. These patients may be particularly sensitive to the respiratory depressant effects of opioids, and a period of postoperative ventilatory support may be required in patients with significant pulmonary disease.

The degree of renal dysfunction must be considered when selecting anesthetic drugs dependent on renal elimination. Regional anesthesia may be technically difficult because of the skin and joint changes that accompany scleroderma. Attractive features of regional anesthesia include peripheral vasodilation and postoperative analgesia. Measures to minimize peripheral vasoconstriction include maintenance of the operating room temperature above 21°C and administration of warmed IV fluids. The eyes should be protected to prevent corneal abrasions.

DISORDERS OF ELASTIN AND COLLAGEN

Pseudoxanthoma Elasticum

Pseudoxanthoma elasticum is a rare hereditary disorder of elastic tissue that is most notable because it is associated with premature arteriosclerosis. Elastic fibers degenerate and calcify over time. The most striking feature of this condition, and often the basis for the diagnosis, is the appearance of *angioid streaks* in the retina. Substantial loss of visual acuity may result from these ocular changes. Additional visual impairment may occur when vascular changes predispose to vitreous hemorrhage. Skin changes consisting of a leathery, cobblestone-like appearance of the skin in the axilla, neck creases, and groin are among the earliest clinical features. Interestingly, some tissues rich in elastic fibers (e.g., lungs, aorta, palms, soles) are *not* affected by this disease process.

GI hemorrhage is a frequent occurrence, occurring in about 10% of patients with this disorder. Degenerative changes in the arteries supplying the GI tract are thought to prevent vasoconstriction of these blood vessels in response to mucosal injury. The incidence of hypertension and ischemic heart disease is increased in these patients. Endocardial calcification can involve the conduction system and predispose to cardiac dysrhythmias and sudden death. Involvement of cardiac valves is frequent. Progressive occlusion of peripheral arteries, including the radial and ulnar arteries, may lead to loss of pulses.

Management of Anesthesia

Management of anesthesia in patients with pseudoxanthoma elasticum is based on an appreciation of the abnormalities associated with this disease. Cardiovascular derangements are probably the most important considerations. The increased incidence of ischemic heart disease must be considered when establishing limits for acceptable changes in blood pressure and heart rate, as well as whether or not invasive hemodynamic monitoring is needed. Electrocardiographic (ECG) monitoring is particularly important in view of the potential for cardiac dysrhythmias. Trauma to the mucosa of the upper GI tract, as may be produced by a gastric tube or esophageal stethoscope, should be minimized. There are no specific recommendations regarding the choice of anesthetic drugs or techniques.

Ehlers-Danlos Syndrome

Ehlers-Danlos syndrome consists of a group of inherited connective tissue disorders caused by abnormal production of procollagen and collagen. It is estimated that 1 in 5000 people is affected by this syndrome. The only form of Ehlers-Danlos syndrome associated with an increased risk of death is the vascular type. This form may be complicated by rupture of large blood vessels, the bowel, and the uterus.

Signs and Symptoms

All forms of Ehlers-Danlos syndrome cause signs and symptoms of joint hypermobility, skin fragility or hyperelasticity, bruising and scarring, musculoskeletal discomfort, and susceptibility to osteoarthritis. The GI tract, uterus, and vasculature are normally particularly well endowed with type III collagen, which accounts for complications such as spontaneous rupture of the bowel, uterus, or major arteries. These ruptured arteries are notoriously difficult to repair because of the marked fragility of the arterial wall. Uterine or large-artery rupture during pregnancy, premature labor, and excessive bleeding at the time of delivery are common obstetric problems. Dilatation of the trachea is often present, and the incidence of pneumothorax is increased. Mitral regurgitation and cardiac conduction abnormalities are occasionally seen. Patients may exhibit extensive ecchymoses with even minimal trauma, although a specific coagulation defect has not been identified.

Management of Anesthesia

Management of anesthesia in patients with Ehlers-Danlos syndrome must consider the cardiovascular manifestations of this disease and the propensity of these patients to bleed excessively. Avoidance of intramuscular injections or instrumentation of the nose or esophagus is important in view of the bleeding tendency. Trauma during direct laryngoscopy must be minimized. The decision regarding placement of an arterial or central venous catheter must consider the fact that hematoma formation may be extensive, so these forms of monitoring are often avoided. Extravasation of IV fluids resulting from a displaced venous cannula may go unnoticed because of the extreme laxity of the skin. Maintenance of low airway pressure during assisted or controlled mechanical ventilation seems prudent in view of the increased incidence of pneumothorax. There are no specific recommendations for the selection of drugs to provide anesthesia. Regional anesthesia is not recommended because of the tendency of these patients to bleed and form extensive hematomas. Surgical complications may include hemorrhage and postoperative wound dehiscence.

Marfan Syndrome

Marfan syndrome, a connective tissue disorder due to defects in the large glycoprotein fibrillin-1, is inherited as an autosomal dominant trait. The incidence is 4–6 per 100,000 live births. Characteristically these patients have long tubular bones, giving them a tall stature and an "Abe Lincoln" appearance. Additional skeletal abnormalities include a high-arched palate, pectus excavatum or carinatum, kyphoscoliosis, and hyperextensibility of the joints. Early development of emphysema is characteristic and may further accentuate the impact of lung disease related to kyphoscoliosis. There is a high incidence of spontaneous pneumothorax. Ocular changes such as lens dislocation, myopia, and retinal detachment occur in more than half of patients with Marfan syndrome.

Cardiovascular System

Cardiovascular abnormalities are responsible for nearly all premature deaths in patients with Marfan syndrome. Defective connective tissue in the aorta and heart valves can lead to aortic dilation, dissection, or rupture and to prolapse of cardiac valves, especially the mitral valve. Mitral regurgitation resulting from mitral valve prolapse is a common abnormality. The risk of bacterial endocarditis is increased in the presence of this valvular heart disease. Cardiac conduction abnormalities, especially bundle branch block, are common. Prophylactic β-blocker therapy is recommended for patients with a dilated thoracic aorta. This therapy should begin at a young age and continue throughout life to slow the rate of aortic dilation and the risk of aortic dissection. Surgical replacement of the aortic valve and ascending aorta is indicated in Marfan syndrome when the diameter of the ascending aorta exceeds 4.5 cm and substantial aortic regurgitation is present. Pregnancy poses a unique risk of rupture or dissection of the aorta in women with Marfan syndrome.

Management of Anesthesia

Preoperative evaluation of patients with Marfan syndrome should focus on cardiopulmonary abnormalities. In most patients, skeletal abnormalities have little impact on the airway. However, a high-arched palate may be associated with crowded teeth. Care should be exercised to avoid temporomandibular joint dislocation, to which these patients are susceptible. In view of the risk of aortic dissection, it is prudent to *avoid* any sustained increase in systemic blood pressure, as can occur during direct laryngoscopy or in response to painful surgical stimulation. Invasive monitoring including transesophageal echocardiography may be a consideration in selected patients. A high index of suspicion must be maintained for development of a pneumothorax.

INFLAMMATORY MYOPATHIES

Polymyositis and Dermatomyositis

Polymyositis and dermatomyositis are multisystem diseases manifesting as inflammatory myopathies. Dermatomyositis has characteristic skin changes in addition to muscle weakness. These cutaneous changes include discoloration of the upper eyelids (a blue-purple periorbital heliotrope), periorbital edema, a scaly erythematous malar rash, and symmetrical erythematous to violaceous raised papules overlying the metacarpal and interphalangeal joints (Gottron papules). Abnormal immune responses may be responsible for the slowly progressive skeletal muscle damage of dermatomyositis and polymyositis. Up to 30% of patients with dermatomyositis will develop cancer (typically breast, colon, and lung cancer), so many consider dermatomyositis a *paraneoplastic syndrome.*

Signs and Symptoms

Muscle weakness involves proximal skeletal muscle groups, especially the flexors of the neck, shoulders, and hips. Patients may have difficulty climbing stairs. Dysphagia, pulmonary aspiration, and pneumonia can result from paresis of pharyngeal and respiratory muscles. Diaphragmatic and intercostal muscle weakness may contribute to ventilatory insufficiency. Increased serum creatine kinase concentrations parallel the extent and rapidity of skeletal muscle destruction. These diseases *do not* affect the neuromuscular junction.

Heart block secondary to myocardial fibrosis or atrophy of the conduction system, left ventricular dysfunction, and myocarditis can occur. Polymyositis can also be associated with SLE, scleroderma, and rheumatoid arthritis.

Diagnosis

The diagnosis of polymyositis or dermatomyositis is considered when proximal skeletal muscle weakness, an increased serum creatine kinase concentration, and the characteristic skin rash are present (dermatomyositis) or absent (polymyositis). Electromyography may demonstrate the triad of spontaneous fibrillation potentials, decreased amplitude of voluntary contraction potentials, and repetitive potentials on needle insertion. Skeletal muscle biopsy findings confirm the clinical diagnosis. The symptoms of dermatomyositis may overlap those of scleroderma and mixed connective tissue disorder.

Treatment

Corticosteroids are the usual treatment for dermatomyositis and polymyositis. Immunosuppressive therapy with methotrexate, azathioprine, cyclophosphamide, mycophenolate, or cyclosporine may be effective when the response to corticosteroids is inadequate. Cyclophosphamide and tacrolimus may be particularly helpful if there is co-existing interstitial lung disease. IV immunoglobulin may be useful in refractory cases. Biologic agents that have been approved to treat other immune diseases may be considered as experimental treatments if there has been an inadequate response to steroids, immunoglobulins, and traditional immunosuppressive therapy.

Management of Anesthesia

Management of anesthesia must consider the vulnerability of patients with polymyositis to pulmonary aspiration. In view of the skeletal muscle weakness, there has been concern that these patients could display abnormal responses to muscle relaxants. However, *responses to nondepolarizing muscle relaxants and succinylcholine are normal in patients with polymyositis.*

MUSCULAR DYSTROPHY

Muscular dystrophy is a group of hereditary diseases characterized by *painless degeneration* of muscle fibers, usually due to a breakdown of the dystrophin-glycoprotein complex, which is a series of proteins that bind myofibrils to the matrix and stabilize the sarcolemma during contraction and relaxation (Table 25.2). Loss of this protein complex leads to myonecrosis and fibrosis. There is progressive symmetrical skeletal muscle weakness and wasting but no evidence of skeletal muscle denervation. Sensation and reflexes are

TABLE 25.2	Muscular Dystrophies

Duchenne muscular dystrophy
Becker muscular dystrophy
Limb-girdle muscular dystrophy
Facioscapulohumeral muscular dystrophy
Emery-Dreifuss muscular dystrophy
Myotonic muscular dystrophy

intact. Increased permeability of skeletal muscle membranes precedes clinical evidence of muscular dystrophy. In order of decreasing frequency, muscular dystrophy can be categorized as *pseudohypertrophic* (Duchenne muscular dystrophy), *limb-girdle, facioscapulohumeral* (Landouzy-Dejerine dystrophy), or *oculopharyngeal.*

Pseudohypertrophic Muscular Dystrophy (Duchenne Muscular Dystrophy)

Pseudohypertrophic muscular dystrophy is the most common and most severe form of childhood progressive muscular dystrophy and is caused by a mutation in the dystrophin gene located on the X chromosome. This disease becomes apparent in 2- to 5-year-old boys. Initial symptoms include a waddling gait, frequent falling, and difficulty climbing stairs, and these reflect involvement of the proximal skeletal muscle groups of the pelvic girdle. Affected muscles become larger as a result of fatty infiltration, and this accounts for the designation of this disorder as *pseudohypertrophic.* There is progressive deterioration in skeletal muscle strength, and typically these boys are confined to a wheelchair by age 8–10. Kyphoscoliosis can develop. Skeletal muscle atrophy can predispose to long bone fractures. Intellectual disability is often present. Serum creatine kinase concentrations are 20–100 times normal even early in the disease, reflecting increased permeability of skeletal muscle membranes and skeletal muscle necrosis. Approximately 70% of the female carriers of this disease also exhibit increased serum creatine kinase concentrations. Skeletal muscle biopsy specimens early in the course of the disease may demonstrate necrosis and phagocytosis of muscle fibers. Death usually occurs at 20–25 years of age as a result of congestive heart failure and/or pneumonia.

Degeneration of cardiac muscle invariably accompanies this muscular dystrophy. Characteristically the ECG reveals tall R waves in V_1, deep Q waves in the limb leads, a short PR interval, and sinus tachycardia. Mitral regurgitation may occur as a result of papillary muscle dysfunction or decreased myocardial contractility.

Chronic weakness of the respiratory muscles and a weakened cough result in loss of pulmonary reserve and accumulation of secretions. These abnormalities predispose to recurrent pneumonia. However, respiratory insufficiency often remains covert because overall activity is so limited. As the disease progresses, kyphoscoliosis contributes to further lung disease. Sleep apnea may occur and contribute to development of pulmonary hypertension. Approximately 30% of deaths in individuals with pseudohypertrophic muscular dystrophy are due to respiratory causes.

Management of Anesthesia

Children with pseudohypertrophic muscular dystrophy may require anesthesia for muscle biopsy or correction of orthopedic deformities. Preparation for anesthesia must take into consideration the implications of increased skeletal muscle membrane permeability and decreased cardiopulmonary reserve. Hypomotility of the GI tract may delay gastric emptying and, in the presence of weak laryngeal reflexes, can increase the risk of pulmonary aspiration. *Use of succinylcholine is contraindicated because of the risk of rhabdomyolysis, hyperkalemia, and/or cardiac arrest.* Cardiac arrest may be due to hyperkalemia or to ventricular fibrillation. Indeed, ventricular fibrillation during induction of anesthesia that included succinylcholine administration has been observed in patients later discovered to have this form of muscular dystrophy. *The response to nondepolarizing muscle relaxants is normal.*

Rhabdomyolysis, with or without cardiac arrest, has been observed in association with administration of volatile anesthetics to these patients, even in the absence of succinylcholine administration. *Dantrolene should be available because there is an increased incidence of malignant hyperthermia in these patients.* Malignant hyperthermia has been observed after even brief periods of halothane administration, although most cases have been triggered by succinylcholine or prolonged inhalation of halothane. Regional anesthesia avoids the unique risks of general anesthesia in these patients. During the postoperative period, neuraxial analgesia may facilitate chest physiotherapy.

Monitoring is directed at early detection of malignant hyperthermia and cardiac depression. Postoperative pulmonary dysfunction should be anticipated and attempts made to facilitate clearance of secretions. Delayed pulmonary insufficiency may occur up to 36 hours postoperatively even though skeletal muscle strength has apparently returned to its preoperative level.

Becker Muscular Dystrophy

Becker muscular dystrophy is a milder form of Duchenne muscular dystrophy. It is typically diagnosed in boys older than age 5, in teenagers, and even in adults. It too has the symmetrical proximal muscle weakness and prominent calf pseudohypertrophy seen in Duchenne dystrophy but to a lesser degree. Some patients may have a normal lifespan, but others develop heart or respiratory failure and die younger.

Limb-Girdle Muscular Dystrophy

Limb-girdle muscular dystrophy is a slowly progressive but relatively benign disease. Onset occurs from the second to the fifth decade. Shoulder girdle or hip girdle muscles may be the only skeletal muscles involved.

Facioscapulohumeral Muscular Dystrophy

Facioscapulohumeral muscular dystrophy is the third most common muscular dystrophy after Duchenne and myotonic muscular dystrophy, with an incidence of about 1:15,000. It is characterized by a slowly progressive wasting of facial, pectoral, and shoulder girdle muscles that begins during adolescence. Eventually the lower limbs are also involved. Early symptoms include difficulty raising the arms above the head and difficulty smiling or whistling. There is no involvement of cardiac muscle, and serum creatine kinase concentration is usually normal. Progression of this muscular dystrophy is slow, and a normal lifespan is likely in many patients.

Oculopharyngeal Dystrophy

Oculopharyngeal dystrophy is a rare variant of muscular dystrophy characterized by progressive dysphagia and ptosis. It typically occurs in people aged 40–60 years. These patients are at risk of aspiration during the perioperative period. Their sensitivity to muscle relaxants may be increased.

Emery-Dreifuss Muscular Dystrophy

Emery-Dreifuss muscular dystrophy is an X-linked recessive disorder characterized by development of *skeletal muscle contractures* that precede the onset of *skeletal muscle weakness.* These contractures are typically in a scapuloperoneal distribution. Respiratory function is usually maintained. Cardiac involvement may be life-threatening and present as congestive heart failure, thromboembolism, or as a cardiac conduction disorder such as bradycardia. Female carriers of this disorder may experience weakness and cardiac disease.

Myotonic Dystrophy

The term *myotonic dystrophy* designates a group of hereditary degenerative diseases of skeletal muscle characterized by persistent contracture (myotonia) after voluntary contraction of a muscle or following electrical stimulation. Clinically a patient may be unable to relax the fingers after a firm handshake or other grip, relax a muscle after it is tapped with a reflex hammer, or open the eyelids after one forcibly closes them. These disorders are the second most common inherited muscle diseases. Peripheral nerves and the neuromuscular junction are *not* affected. Electromyographic findings are diagnostic and characterized by prolonged discharges of repetitive muscle action potentials. This inability of skeletal muscle to relax after voluntary contraction or stimulation results from abnormal calcium metabolism. Intracellular adenosine triphosphatase (ATPase) fails to return calcium to the sarcoplasmic reticulum, so unsequestered calcium remains available to produce sustained skeletal muscle contraction. Interestingly, *general anesthesia, regional anesthesia, and neuromuscular blockade are not able to prevent or relieve this skeletal muscle contraction.* Infiltration of contracted skeletal muscles with local anesthetic may induce relaxation. Quinine (300–600 mg IV) has also been reported to be effective in some cases. Increasing the ambient temperature of the operating room decreases the severity of myotonia and the incidence of postoperative shivering, which can precipitate skeletal muscle contraction.

Most patients with myotonia survive to adulthood with little impairment, and it is common for them to conceal their symptoms, so they may come for surgery without the underlying myotonia being appreciated.

Myotonia Dystrophica

Myotonia dystrophica (myotonic dystrophy type 1) is the most common and most serious form of myotonic dystrophy affecting adults. It is inherited as an autosomal dominant trait, with the onset of symptoms during the second or third decade. Unlike other myotonic syndromes, myotonia dystrophica is a multisystem disease, although skeletal muscles are affected most. Death from pneumonia or heart failure often occurs by the sixth decade of life. This reflects progressive involvement of skeletal, cardiac, and smooth muscle. Cardiac conduction system defects are common and could lead to sudden death. Perioperative morbidity and mortality rates are high and principally due to cardiopulmonary complications.

Treatment is symptomatic and may include use of mexiletine, which can improve muscle relaxation. Quinine and procainamide also have antimyotonic properties but can worsen cardiac conduction abnormalities. These three drugs depress sodium influx into skeletal muscle cells and delay the return of membrane excitability.

Signs and Symptoms

Type 1 myotonic dystrophy usually manifests as facial weakness (expressionless facies), wasting and weakness of sternocleidomastoid muscles, ptosis, dysarthria, dysphagia, and inability to relax the hand grip (myotonia). Other characteristic features include the triad of intellectual disability, frontal baldness, and cataracts. Endocrine gland involvement may be indicated by gonadal atrophy, diabetes mellitus, hypothyroidism, and adrenal insufficiency. Delayed gastric emptying and intestinal pseudo-obstruction may be present. Central sleep apnea may occur and account for the frequent presence of hypersomnolence. There is an increased incidence of cholelithiasis, especially in men. Exacerbation of symptoms during pregnancy is common, and uterine atony and retained placenta often complicate vaginal delivery.

Cardiac dysrhythmias and conduction abnormalities presumably reflect myocardial involvement by the myotonic process. First-degree atrioventricular heart block is common and is often present before the clinical onset of the disease. Up to 20% of patients have asymptomatic mitral valve prolapse. Reports of sudden death may reflect development of complete heart block. Pharyngeal and thoracic muscle weakness makes these patients vulnerable to pulmonary aspiration.

Management of Anesthesia

Preoperative evaluation and management of anesthesia in patients with myotonia dystrophica must consider the likelihood of cardiomyopathy, respiratory muscle weakness, and the potential for abnormal responses to anesthetic drugs. Even asymptomatic patients have some degree of cardiomyopathy, so the myocardial depression produced by volatile anesthetics

TABLE 25.3	Inherited Myopathies

Nemaline rod myopathy
Myotonia congenita
Paramyotonia congenita
Periodic paralysis
Central core disease
Multicore myopathy
Centronuclear myopathy

may be exaggerated. Cardiac dysrhythmias may need treatment. Anesthesia and surgery could aggravate cardiac conduction problems by increasing vagal tone.

Succinylcholine should not be administered, because prolonged skeletal muscle contraction can result. However, the response to *nondepolarizing* neuromuscular blocking drugs is *normal.* Theoretically, reversal of neuromuscular blockade could precipitate skeletal muscle contraction, but adverse responses do not predictably occur with neostigmine use. Careful titration of short-acting nondepolarizing muscle relaxants may obviate the need for reversal of neuromuscular blockade.

Patients with myotonia dystrophica are sensitive to the respiratory depressant effects of barbiturates, opioids, benzodiazepines, and propofol. This is most likely due to drug-induced central respiratory depression acting in tandem with weak and/or atrophic respiratory muscles. In addition, hypersomnolence and central sleep apnea contribute to increased sensitivity to respiratory depressant drugs.

Myotonic contraction during surgical manipulation and/or use of electrocautery may interfere with surgical access. Drugs such as phenytoin and procainamide, which stabilize skeletal muscle membranes, may be helpful in this situation. High concentrations of volatile anesthetics can also abolish myotonic contractions but at the expense of myocardial depression. Maintenance of normothermia and avoidance of shivering are very important, since cold may induce myotonia.

INHERITED MYOPATHIES

Congenital myopathies are primarily muscle disorders. They are characterized by structural abnormalities of muscle fibers and accumulation of abnormal proteins in the sarcoplasm (Table 25.3). In contrast to congenital muscular dystrophies, these disorders *do not* show muscle necrosis or fibrosis on muscle biopsy. Some of these muscle disorders involve abnormal chloride, sodium, and calcium channel genes.

Nemaline Rod Myopathy

Nemaline rod myopathy is an autosomal dominant disease characterized by slowly progressive or nonprogressive symmetrical weakness of skeletal and smooth muscle. In particular there is weakness and hypotonia in the muscles of the face, neck, and arms and often the respiratory muscles as well. The diagnosis is confirmed by skeletal muscle biopsy. Histologic

TABLE 25.4	Clinical Features of Familial Periodic Paralysis		
Type	Serum Potassium Concentration During Symptoms (mEq/L)	Precipitating Factors	Other Features
Hypokalemic	<3.0	High-carbohydrate meal, strenuous exercise, glucose infusion, stress, menstruation, pregnancy, anesthesia, hypothermia	Cardiac dysrhythmias, electrocardiographic signs of hypokalemia
Hyperkalemic	>5.5	Exercise, potassium infusion, metabolic acidosis, hypothermia	Skeletal muscle weakness may be localized to tongue and eyelids

examination demonstrates the presence of rods between normal myofibrils. These rods are composed of muscle proteins. Some forms of nemaline rod myopathy are associated with an abnormal ryanodine receptor 1 (RYR1).

Affected individuals experience delayed motor development, generalized skeletal muscle weakness, a decrease in muscle mass, hypotonia, and loss of deep tendon reflexes. There are typical dysmorphic features and an abnormal gait, but intelligence is usually normal. Affected infants may present with hypotonia, dysphagia, respiratory distress, and cyanosis. Micrognathia and dental malocclusion are common. Other skeletal deformities include kyphoscoliosis and pectus excavatum. Restrictive lung disease may result from the myopathy and/or scoliosis. Cardiac failure resulting from dilated cardiomyopathy has been described.

Management of Anesthesia
Tracheal intubation may be difficult because of anatomic abnormalities such as micrognathia and a high-arched palate. Awake fiberoptic intubation may be prudent. The respiratory depressant effects of drugs may be exaggerated secondary to respiratory muscle weakness and chest wall abnormalities. Ventilation/perfusion mismatching is increased, and the ventilatory response to carbon dioxide may be blunted. Bulbar palsy associated with regurgitation and aspiration may further complicate anesthetic management.

The response to succinylcholine and nondepolarizing neuromuscular blockers is unpredictable. There is no conclusive evidence that administration of succinylcholine evokes excessive potassium release. Indeed, resistance to succinylcholine has been described in some patients. Myocardial depression may accompany administration of volatile anesthetics if the disease process involves the myocardium. Plans for regional anesthesia must consider the possible respiratory compromise that could accompany a high motor block. In addition, the exaggerated lumbar lordosis and/or kyphoscoliosis may make neuraxial anesthesia technically difficult.

Myotonia Congenita

Myotonia congenita is transmitted as an autosomal dominant trait and becomes manifest at birth or during early childhood. Skeletal muscle involvement is widespread, but other organ systems are not usually involved. Muscle hypertrophy and myotonia are present. The disease does not progress, nor

does it result in a decreased life expectancy. Patients with myotonia congenita respond to phenytoin, mexiletine, or quinine therapy. *The response to succinylcholine administration is abnormal.*

Paramyotonia Congenita

Paramyotonia congenita is a rare autosomal dominant disorder characterized by generalized myotonia that is recognized during early childhood. It is due to sodium channel dysfunction. Generalized muscle hypertrophy may occur. In contrast to other myotonias, the skeletal muscle stiffness in paramyotonia congenita is often *exacerbated* by exercise, whereas in other myotonias, sustained exercise *improves* myotonia *(warm-up phenomenon)*. Cold markedly aggravates the myotonia, and flaccid paralysis may be present after the muscles are warmed. Some patients develop muscle paralysis independent of myotonia. This could be related to serum potassium concentration and may be the reason why many researchers consider paramyotonia congenita to be a form of hyperkalemic periodic paralysis. The electromyogram may be normal when recorded at room temperature, but typical myotonic discharges become evident as muscles are cooled.

Periodic Paralysis

Periodic paralysis is a spectrum of diseases characterized by intermittent acute attacks of skeletal muscle weakness or paralysis (sparing only a few muscles such as the muscles of respiration) and associated with hypokalemia or hyperkalemia (Table 25.4). The hyperkalemic form is much rarer than the hypokalemic form. Attacks generally last for a few hours but may persist for days. Muscle strength is normal between attacks.

Etiology
The causes of familial periodic paralysis are inherited mutations in one or more voltage-dependent calcium channel genes or in some inward rectifier potassium channels. It is recognized that the mechanism of this disease is not related to any abnormality at the neuromuscular junction but rather to loss of muscle membrane excitability. Skeletal muscle weakness provoked by a glucose-insulin infusion confirms the presence of *hypokalemic* familial periodic paralysis, and skeletal muscle weakness after oral administration of

potassium confirms the presence of *hyperkalemic* familial periodic paralysis. Acetazolamide is recommended for treatment of *both forms* of familial periodic paralysis. Acetazolamide produces a nonanion gap acidosis that protects against hypokalemia and promotes renal potassium excretion, which protects against hyperkalemia as well.

Management of Anesthesia

A principal goal of anesthetic management is avoidance of any events that can precipitate skeletal muscle weakness. Hypothermia must be avoided in patients with periodic paralysis, regardless of the nature of the potassium sensitivity. In patients undergoing cardiac surgery, it may be necessary to maintain normothermia during cardiopulmonary bypass. Nondepolarizing muscle relaxants can be safely administered.

Hypokalemic Periodic Paralysis

Preoperative considerations include maintenance of carbohydrate balance, correction of electrolyte abnormalities, and avoidance of events known to trigger hypokalemic attacks (psychological stress, cold, carbohydrate loads). High-carbohydrate meals can trigger hypokalemic episodes and should be avoided during the 24 hours preceding surgery. Glucose-containing solutions and drugs known to cause intracellular shifts of potassium (e.g., β-adrenergic agonists) must also be avoided. Mannitol can be administered in lieu of a potassium-wasting diuretic should the operative procedure require diuresis. Frequent perioperative monitoring of serum potassium concentration is useful, and aggressive intervention to increase the serum potassium concentration (infusion of potassium chloride at a rate of up to 40 mEq/h) may occasionally be needed. Hypokalemia may precede the onset of muscle weakness by several hours, so timely potassium supplementation may help avoid muscle weakness. Short-acting neuromuscular blockers are preferable if skeletal muscle relaxation is required for the surgery. Regional anesthesia has also been safely used.

Hyperkalemic Periodic Paralysis

Management of anesthesia in patients with hyperkalemic periodic paralysis includes preoperative potassium depletion with diuretics, prevention of carbohydrate depletion by administration of glucose-containing solutions, and avoidance of potassium-containing solutions and potassium-releasing drugs such as succinylcholine. Frequent monitoring of serum potassium concentration is indicated, as is ready availability of calcium for IV administration should signs of hyperkalemia appear on the ECG.

Central Core Disease

Central core disease is named for the muscle biopsy findings of damaged areas—cores—within muscle cells. The cores represent disorganized myofibrils and missing mitochondria. There is a defect in sodium channels and a mutation in *RYR1* genes. *The risk of malignant hyperthermia is very high.*

Multicore Myopathy

Multicore myopathy is a histologic diagnosis. On muscle biopsy there are multifocal well-circumscribed areas with a reduction in oxidative staining and low ATPase. There is also a paucity of mitochondria. These "minicores" do not extend the entire length of the muscle fiber as they do in central core disease. There may be mutations in the selenoprotein-N gene and/or the skeletal muscle *RYR1* gene. This myopathy represents a heterogeneous group of diseases characterized by proximal skeletal muscle weakness, a decrease in muscle mass, and musculoskeletal abnormalities such as scoliosis and high-arched palate. There is typically respiratory impairment. Recurrent pulmonary infection is common and may be related to the severity of the associated kyphoscoliosis. Cardiomyopathy may accompany this myopathy. Unlike in other myopathies, serum creatine kinase concentration is usually normal and intelligence is normal.

Management of Anesthesia

Preoperative assessment of respiratory function is necessary in all patients, especially those with kyphoscoliosis and recurrent lung infection. Difficulty swallowing and an inability to clear secretions may reflect pharyngeal and laryngeal muscle involvement. Postoperative aspiration may be associated with impaired upper airway reflexes and the lingering effects of drugs administered during anesthesia. *It is important to recognize the relationship between multicore myopathy and malignant hyperthermia.* Dantrolene, a ryanodine receptor antagonist, must be immediately available.

Centronuclear Myopathy

Centronuclear myopathy is a rare congenital myopathy characterized by progressive muscle weakness of extraocular, facial, neck, and limb muscles. The defect is a mutation in a gene important for muscle cell growth and differentiation. There are severe neonatal forms of this disease, as well as slowly progressive forms that can begin anytime from birth to adulthood. Development of scoliosis with restrictive lung disease is an important manifestation of disease severity. Serum creatine kinase concentration is usually normal. The association of ptosis and strabismus with this myopathy increases the likelihood that affected children will undergo surgery.

Management of Anesthesia

Management of anesthesia is influenced by the degree of skeletal muscle weakness, the presence of restrictive lung disease, and gastroesophageal reflux. Muscle relaxants are avoided and a nontriggering general anesthetic technique used.

MITOCHONDRIAL MYOPATHIES

Mitochondrial myopathies are a heterogeneous group of disorders of skeletal muscle energy metabolism. Mitochondria produce the energy required by skeletal muscle cells through

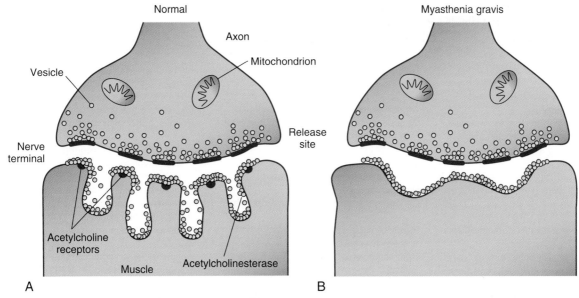

FIG. 25.6   Normal (A) and myasthenic (B) neuromuscular junctions. Compared with normal neuro-muscular junctions, myasthenic neuromuscular junctions have fewer acetylcholine receptors, simplified synaptic folds, and widened synaptic spaces. (From Drachman DB. Myasthenia gravis. *N Engl J Med.* 1994;330:1797-1810. Copyright 1994 Massachusetts Medical Society. All rights reserved.)

the oxidation-reduction reactions of the electron transfer chain and oxidative phosphorylation, thereby generating ATP. Defects in this process result in abnormal fatigability with sustained exercise, skeletal muscle pain, and progressive weakness. The hallmark lesions are large subsarcolemmal accumulations of abnormal mitochondria that appear as red-staining granules (ragged-red fibers) on histologic analysis. Disorders of mitochondrial metabolism may also involve other organ systems with high energy demands, such as the brain, heart, liver, and kidneys.

Kearns-Sayre Syndrome

Kearns-Sayre syndrome is a rare mitochondrial myopathy accompanied by progressive external ophthalmoplegia, retinitis pigmentosa, heart block, hearing loss, short stature, peripheral neuropathy, and impaired ventilatory drive. Dilated cardiomyopathy and congestive heart failure may be present.

Management of Anesthesia
Management of general anesthesia in these patients must consider the risk of drug-induced myocardial depression, development of cardiac conduction defects, and hypoventilation during the early postoperative period.

OTHER MYOPATHIES

Alcoholic Myopathy

Acute and chronic forms of proximal skeletal muscle weakness occur frequently in alcoholic patients. Differentiation of alcoholic myopathy from alcoholic neuropathy is based on

the presence of proximal rather than distal skeletal muscle involvement, an increased serum creatine kinase concentration, myoglobinuria in acute cases, and rapid recovery after cessation of alcohol consumption.

Floppy Infant Syndrome

Floppy infant syndrome is a term used to describe weak, hypotonic skeletal muscles in infants. A diminished cough reflex and difficulty swallowing predispose to aspiration, and recurrent pneumonia is common. Progressive weakness and atrophy of skeletal muscles leads to contractures and kyphoscoliosis.

Management of Anesthesia
Anesthesia may be associated with increased sensitivity to nondepolarizing muscle relaxants and hyperkalemia with cardiac arrest after administration of succinylcholine. These infants are also susceptible to malignant hyperthermia. Ketamine can be useful for anesthesia because it does not cause significant respiratory depression.

DISEASES OF THE NEUROMUSCULAR JUNCTION

Myasthenia Gravis

Myasthenia gravis is the most common disease affecting the neuromuscular junction. It is a chronic autoimmune disorder caused by a decrease in functional acetylcholine receptors at the neuromuscular junction resulting from their destruction or inactivation by circulating antibodies (Fig. 25.6). As many as 80% of functional acetylcholine receptors can be

TABLE 25.5	Differential Diagnosis of Myasthenia Gravis	
Condition	Symptoms and Characteristics	Comments
Congenital myasthenic syndromes	Rare, early onset, not autoimmune	Electrophysiologic and immunocytochemical tests required for diagnosis
Drug-induced myasthenia gravis		
Penicillamine	Triggers autoimmune myasthenia gravis	Recovery within weeks of discontinuing drug
Nondepolarizing muscle relaxants, aminoglycosides, procainamide	Weakness in normal persons; exacerbation of myasthenia	Recovery after drug discontinuation
Eaton-Lambert syndrome	Small cell lung cancer, fatigue	Incremental response on repetitive nerve stimulation, antibodies to calcium channels
Hyperthyroidism	Exacerbation of myasthenia gravis	Thyroid function abnormal
Graves disease	Diplopia, exophthalmos	Thyroid-stimulating immunoglobulin present
Botulism	Generalized weakness, ophthalmoplegia	Incremental response on repetitive nerve stimulation, mydriasis
Progressive external ophthalmoplegia	Ptosis, diplopia, generalized weakness in some cases	Mitochondrial abnormalities
Intracranial mass compressing cranial nerves	Ophthalmoplegia, cranial nerve weakness	Abnormalities on computed tomography or magnetic resonance imaging

Adapted from Drachman DB. Myasthenia gravis. *N Engl J Med*. 1994;330:1797-1810. Copyright 1994 Massachusetts Medical Society. All rights reserved.

lost. This accounts for the weakness and easy fatigability of these patients and their marked sensitivity to nondepolarizing muscle relaxants. Indeed, the hallmarks of this disease are weakness and rapid exhaustion of voluntary muscles with repetitive use, followed by partial recovery with rest. Skeletal muscles innervated by cranial nerves (ocular, pharyngeal, and laryngeal muscles) are especially vulnerable, as indicated by the appearance of ptosis, diplopia, and dysphagia, which are often the initial symptoms of the disease. Myasthenia gravis is not a rare disease. It has a prevalence of 1 in 7500. Women aged 20–30 years are most often affected; men with myasthenia gravis are often older than 60 when the disease presents. Acetylcholine receptor-binding antibodies are present in more than 85% of patients with myasthenia gravis. The origin of these antibodies is unknown, but a relationship to the thymus gland is suggested by the association of myasthenia gravis with thymus gland abnormalities. For example, thymic hyperplasia is present in two-thirds of patients with myasthenia gravis, and 10%–15% of these patients have thymomas.

About 10% of patients with myasthenia gravis will not have acetylcholine receptor antibodies but rather antibodies to muscle-specific kinase (MuSK), a tyrosine kinase specifically present at the neuromuscular junction and crucial in the formation and maintenance of the postsynaptic membrane. MuSK antibodies cause loss of acetylcholine receptors and a change in the structure of postsynaptic folds. Patients with MuSK antibodies do not have associated thymic disease.

Other conditions that cause weakness of the cranial and somatic musculature must be considered in the differential diagnosis of myasthenia gravis (Table 25.5).

Classification

Myasthenia gravis is classified based on the skeletal muscles involved and the severity of symptoms. Type I is limited to involvement of the extraocular muscles. Approximately 10% of patients show signs and symptoms confined to the extraocular muscles and are considered to have ocular myasthenia gravis. Patients in whom the disease has been confined to the ocular muscles for longer than 2 years are unlikely to experience any progression in their disease. Type IIa is a slowly progressive, mild form of skeletal muscle weakness that spares the muscles of respiration. The response to anticholinesterase drugs and corticosteroids is good in these patients. Type IIb is a more rapidly progressive and more severe form of skeletal muscle weakness. The response to drug therapy is not as good, and the muscles of respiration may be involved. Type III is characterized by acute onset and rapid deterioration of skeletal muscle strength within 6 months. It is associated with a high mortality rate. Type IV is a severe form of skeletal muscle weakness that results from progression of type I or type II myasthenia.

Signs and Symptoms

The clinical course of myasthenia gravis is marked by periods of exacerbation and remission. Muscle strength may be normal in well-rested patients, but weakness occurs promptly with exercise. Ptosis and diplopia resulting from extraocular muscle weakness are the most common initial complaints. Weakness of pharyngeal and laryngeal muscles can result in dysphagia, dysarthria, and difficulty handling saliva. Patients with myasthenia gravis are at high risk of pulmonary aspiration. Arm, leg, or trunk weakness can occur in any combination and is usually asymmetrical. Muscle atrophy does not occur. Myocarditis can result in atrial fibrillation, heart block or cardiomyopathy. Other autoimmune diseases may occur in association with myasthenia gravis. For example, hyperthyroidism is present in approximately 10% of patients with myasthenia gravis. Rheumatoid arthritis, SLE, and pernicious anemia occur more commonly in patients with myasthenia than in those without myasthenia. Approximately 15% of neonates born to mothers with myasthenia gravis demonstrate transient (2–4 weeks) skeletal muscle weakness. Infection, electrolyte abnormalities, pregnancy, emotional stress, and surgery may precipitate or exacerbate muscle weakness. Antibiotics, especially aminoglycosides, can aggravate muscle weakness. Isolated respiratory failure may occasionally be the presenting manifestation of myasthenia gravis.

Treatment

Treatment modalities for myasthenia gravis include anticholinesterase drugs to enhance neuromuscular transmission, thymectomy, immunosuppression, and short-term immunotherapy, including plasmapheresis and administration of immunoglobulin.

Anticholinesterase drugs are the first line of treatment for myasthenia gravis. These drugs are effective because they inhibit the enzyme responsible for hydrolysis of acetylcholine and thus increase the amount of neurotransmitter available at the neuromuscular junction. Pyridostigmine is the most widely used anticholinesterase drug for this purpose. Its onset of effect occurs in 30 minutes, and peak effect is achieved in approximately 2 hours. Oral pyridostigmine lasts longer (3–6 hours) and produces fewer side effects than neostigmine. Pyridostigmine dosing is tailored to response, but the maximal dosage of pyridostigmine rarely exceeds 120 mg every 3 hours. Higher dosages may actually induce more muscle weakness (*cholinergic crisis*). The presence of significant muscarinic side effects (salivation, miosis, bradycardia) plus accentuated muscle weakness after administration of edrophonium (1–2 mg IV) confirms the diagnosis of a cholinergic crisis. Although anticholinesterase drugs benefit most patients, the improvements may be incomplete and wane after weeks or months of treatment.

Thymectomy is intended to induce remission or at least allow the doses of immunosuppressive medications to be reduced. Patients with generalized myasthenia gravis are candidates for thymectomy. Preoperative preparation should include optimizing strength and respiratory function. Immunosuppressive drugs should be avoided if possible because they can increase the risk of perioperative infection. If the vital capacity is less than 2 L, plasmapheresis can be performed before surgery to improve the likelihood of adequate spontaneous respiration during the perioperative period. A surgical approach via median sternotomy optimizes visualization and removal of all thymic tissue. Mediastinoscopy through a cervical incision has been advocated as an alternative because it is associated with a smaller incision and less postoperative pain. The use of neuraxial analgesia minimizes postoperative pain and thus improves postoperative ventilation. The need for anticholinesterase medication may be decreased for a few days

postoperatively, but the full benefit of thymectomy is often delayed for months. The mechanism by which thymectomy produces improvement is uncertain, although acetylcholine receptor antibody levels usually decrease after thymectomy.

Immunosuppressive therapy (corticosteroids, azathioprine, cyclosporine, mycophenolate) is indicated when skeletal muscle weakness is not adequately controlled by anticholinesterase drugs. Corticosteroids are most commonly used and are the most consistently effective immunosuppressive drugs for the treatment of myasthenia gravis.

Plasmapheresis removes antibodies from the circulation and produces short-term clinical improvement in patients with myasthenia gravis who are experiencing *myasthenic crises* or are being prepared for thymectomy. The beneficial effects of plasmapheresis are transient, and repeated treatment introduces the risk of infection, hypotension, and pulmonary embolism. The indications for administration of *immunoglobulin* are the same as for plasmapheresis. The effect is temporary, and this treatment has no effect on circulating concentrations of acetylcholine receptor antibodies.

Management of Anesthesia

Patients with myasthenia gravis often require ventilatory support after surgery. Therefore it is important to advise these patients during the preoperative interview that they may be intubated and ventilated when they awaken. Factors that may correlate with the need for mechanical ventilation during the postoperative period following *transsternal thymectomy* include (1) disease duration longer than 6 years, (2) presence of chronic obstructive pulmonary disease unrelated to myasthenia gravis, (3) a daily dose of pyridostigmine of more than 750 mg, and (4) vital capacity less than 2.9 L. These factors are less predictive of the need for ventilatory support following *transcervical thymectomy,* which indicates that this less invasive surgical approach produces less respiratory depression.

The acetylcholine receptor–binding antibodies of myasthenia gravis decrease the number of functional acetylcholine receptors, and this results in an increased sensitivity to nondepolarizing muscle relaxants. The balance between active and nonfunctional acetylcholine receptors modulates the sensitivity to nondepolarizing muscle relaxants. The initial muscle relaxant dose should be titrated according to response at the neuromuscular junction as monitored using a peripheral nerve stimulator. Monitoring these responses at the orbicularis oculi muscle may *overestimate* the degree of neuromuscular blockade but may help to avoid unrecognized persistent neuromuscular blockade in these patients.

It is possible that drugs used to treat myasthenia gravis can influence the response to muscle relaxants independent of the disease process. For example, anticholinesterase drugs inhibit not only true cholinesterase but also impair plasma pseudocholinesterase activity, which introduces the possibility of a prolonged response to succinylcholine. They could also antagonize the effects of nondepolarizing muscle relaxants. However, neither of these effects is seen clinically. Corticosteroid therapy does not alter the dose requirement for

TABLE 25.6 | Comparison of Myasthenic Syndrome and Myasthenia Gravis

Characteristic	Myasthenic Syndrome	Myasthenia Gravis
Manifestations	Proximal limb weakness (legs more than arms), exercise improves strength, muscle pain common, reflexes absent or decreased	Extraocular, bulbar, and facial muscle weakness; exercise causes fatigue; muscle pain uncommon; reflexes normal
Gender	Affects males more often than females	Affects females more often than males
Co-existing pathologic conditions	Small cell lung cancer	Thymoma
Response to muscle relaxants	Sensitive to succinylcholine and nondepolarizing muscle relaxants	Resistant to succinylcholine, sensitive to nondepolarizing muscle relaxants
	Poor response to anticholinesterases	Good response to anticholinesterases

succinylcholine but has been reported to produce resistance to the neuromuscular blocking effects of steroidal muscle relaxants such as vecuronium.

Measurement of neuromuscular function in patients with myasthenia gravis treated with pyridostigmine demonstrates *resistance* to the effects of succinylcholine. The ED_{95} dose is approximately 2.6 times higher than normal. Because the dose of succinylcholine often administered to patients without myasthenia gravis (1–1.5 mg/kg) represents 3–5 times the ED_{95}, it is likely that adequate intubating conditions can be achieved in patients with myasthenia gravis using these typical doses of succinylcholine. The mechanism for the resistance to succinylcholine is unknown, but the decreased number of acetylcholine receptors at the postsynaptic junction may play a role.

However, in contrast to the resistance to succinylcholine, *patients with myasthenia gravis exhibit marked sensitivity to nondepolarizing muscle relaxants*. Even small doses of nondepolarizing muscle relaxant, such as those intended to block succinylcholine-induced fasciculations, can produce profound skeletal muscle weakness in some patients. In patients with mild to moderate myasthenia gravis, the potency of atracurium and vecuronium is increased at least twofold compared with the response in patients without the disease. Despite the increase in potency, the duration of action of intermediate-acting muscle relaxants is short enough that adequate skeletal muscle paralysis can be achieved intraoperatively and yet be predictably reversed at the conclusion of surgery.

Induction of anesthesia with a short-acting IV anesthetic is acceptable for patients with myasthenia gravis. However, the respiratory depressant effects of these drugs may be accentuated. Tracheal intubation can often be accomplished without neuromuscular blockers because of intrinsic muscle weakness and the relaxant effect of volatile anesthetics on skeletal muscle.

Maintenance of anesthesia is often provided with a volatile anesthetic with or without nitrous oxide. Use of volatile anesthetics can decrease the required dose of muscle relaxant or even eliminate the need for them altogether. Should administration of a nondepolarizing neuromuscular blocker be necessary, the initial dose should be decreased by one-half to two-thirds and the response monitored using a peripheral nerve stimulator. The relatively short duration of action of intermediate-acting muscle relaxants is a desirable

characteristic in this patient group. The respiratory effects of opioids, which can linger into the postoperative period, detract from their use for maintenance of anesthesia.

At the conclusion of surgery, it is important to postpone extubation until clear evidence of good respiratory function is present. Skeletal muscle strength often seems adequate during the early postoperative period but may deteriorate a few hours later. The need for mechanical ventilation during the postoperative period should be anticipated in those patients meeting the criteria known to correlate with inadequate ventilation after surgery.

Myasthenic Syndrome

Myasthenic syndrome (Eaton-Lambert syndrome) is a disorder of neuromuscular transmission that resembles myasthenia gravis (Table 25.6). This syndrome of skeletal muscle weakness, originally described as a paraneoplastic syndrome in patients with small cell carcinoma of the lung, has subsequently been described in some patients without cancer. Myasthenic syndrome is an *acquired autoimmune disease* characterized by the presence of IgG antibodies to voltage-sensitive calcium channels that causes a deficiency of these channels at the motor nerve terminal. This deficiency restricts calcium entry when the terminal is depolarized. Anticholinesterase drugs effective in the treatment of myasthenia gravis *do not* produce an improvement in patients with myasthenic syndrome. The drug 3,4-diaminopyridine (3,4 DAP), which increases acetylcholine release at the neuromuscular junction, *does* improve muscle strength but has not yet been approved by the US Food and Drug Administration (FDA) for use in this country. IV immunoglobulin, plasmapheresis, immunosuppressive therapy, and treatment of the underlying cancer can all cause improvement in this condition.

Management of Anesthesia

Patients with myasthenic syndrome are sensitive to the effects of both depolarizing and nondepolarizing muscle relaxants. Antagonism of neuromuscular blockade with anticholinesterase drugs may be inadequate. The potential presence of myasthenic syndrome and the need to decrease doses of muscle relaxants should be considered in patients undergoing bronchoscopy, mediastinoscopy, or thoracoscopy for suspected lung cancer.

SKELETAL DISEASES

Osteoarthritis

Osteoarthritis is by far the most common joint disease in the United States, one of the leading chronic diseases of the elderly and a major cause of disability. Osteoarthritis is a degenerative process that affects articular cartilage. This process is different from rheumatoid arthritis because there is minimal inflammatory reaction in the joints. The pathogenesis is likely related to joint trauma from biomechanical stresses, joint injury, or abnormal joint loading resulting from neuropathy, ligamentous injury, muscle atrophy, or obesity. Pain is usually present on motion and is relieved by rest. Stiffness tends to disappear rapidly with joint motion, in contrast to the morning stiffness associated with rheumatoid arthritis, which can last for several hours.

One or several joints can be affected by osteoarthritis. The knees and hips are common sites of involvement. Bony enlargements referred to as *Heberden nodes* are seen at the distal interphalangeal joints of the fingers. There may be degenerative disease of the vertebral bodies and intervertebral disks, which can be complicated by protrusion of the nucleus pulposus and compression of nerve roots. Degenerative changes are most significant in the middle to lower cervical spine and the lumbar area. Radiographic findings include narrowing of the intervertebral disk spaces and osteophyte formation.

Although often overlooked, physical therapy and exercise programs can provide benefits for patients with osteoarthritis. Maintaining muscle function is important for both cartilage integrity and pain reduction. Pain can also be relieved by application of heat, use of simple analgesics such as acetaminophen, and treatment with antiinflammatory drugs. Symptomatic improvement with application of heat may be due to an increase in pain threshold in warm tissues compared with that in cold tissues. Transcutaneous nerve stimulation and acupuncture can be effective in some patients. Systemic corticosteroids have no place in the treatment of osteoarthritis. Joint replacement surgery may be recommended when pain caused by osteoarthritis is persistent and disabling or significant limitation of joint function is present.

Kyphoscoliosis

Kyphoscoliosis is a spinal deformity characterized by anterior flexion *(kyphosis)* and lateral curvature *(scoliosis)* of the vertebral column. Idiopathic kyphoscoliosis, which accounts for 80% of cases, commonly begins during late childhood and may progress in severity during periods of rapid skeletal growth. The incidence of idiopathic kyphoscoliosis is approximately 4 per 1000 population. There may be a familial predisposition to this disease, and females are affected four times more often than males. Diseases of the neuromuscular system (e.g., poliomyelitis, cerebral palsy, muscular dystrophy) may also be associated with kyphoscoliosis.

Signs and Symptoms

Spinal curvature of more than 40 degrees is considered severe and is likely to be associated with physiologic derangements in cardiac and pulmonary function. Restrictive lung disease and pulmonary hypertension progressing to cor pulmonale are the principal causes of death in patients with kyphoscoliosis. As the scoliosis curvature worsens, more lung tissue is compressed, which results in a decrease in vital capacity and dyspnea on exertion. The work of breathing is increased because of the abnormal mechanical properties of the distorted thorax and the increased airway resistance that results from small lung volumes. The alveolar-arterial oxygen difference is increased. Pulmonary hypertension is the result of increased pulmonary vascular resistance due to compression of lung vasculature and the response to arterial hypoxemia. The $Paco_2$ is usually maintained at normal levels, but an insult such as bacterial or viral upper respiratory tract infection can result in hypercapnia and acute respiratory failure. A poor cough contributes to frequent pulmonary infection.

Management of Anesthesia

Preoperatively it is important to assess the severity of the physiologic derangements produced by this skeletal deformity. Pulmonary function test results reflect the magnitude of restrictive lung disease. Arterial blood gas values are helpful for detecting unrecognized hypoxemia or acidosis that could be contributing to pulmonary hypertension. These patients may have preoperative pulmonary infection resulting from chronic aspiration. Certainly any reversible component of pulmonary dysfunction such as infection or bronchospasm should be corrected before elective surgery.

Although no specific drug or drug combination can be recommended as optimal for patients with kyphoscoliosis, it should be remembered that nitrous oxide may increase pulmonary vascular resistance. This could be particularly problematic in patients with pulmonary hypertension. Monitoring central venous pressure may provide data suggesting an increase in pulmonary vascular resistance.

When a patient is undergoing surgery to correct the spinal curvature, special anesthetic considerations include the potential for blood loss and the risk of surgically induced spinal cord damage. Controlled hypotension as a way of decreasing blood loss should be used with caution because of the risk of ischemic optic neuropathy and spinal cord ischemia. Prolonged surgery and a high transfusion threshold could increase the risk of ischemia. At the time the spinal curvature is straightened or distracted, excessive traction on the spinal cord can result in spinal cord ischemia, which can produce paralysis. There are several maneuvers designed to detect spinal cord ischemia. One is the *wake-up test,* which entails determining that no significant neuromuscular blockade is present by discontinuing the anesthetic until the patient is sufficiently awake to move both legs on command and thus confirm that spinal cord motor pathways are intact. Anesthesia is then reestablished and the operation completed. Another method to confirm an intact spinal cord is to monitor somatosensory and/or

TABLE 25.7 Comparison of Rheumatoid Arthritis and Ankylosing Spondylitis

Characteristic	Rheumatoid Arthritis	Ankylosing Spondylitis
Family history	Rare	Common
Gender	Female (30–50 yr)	Male (20–30 yr)
Joint involvement	Symmetrical polyarthropathy	Asymmetrical oligoarthropathy
Sacroiliac involvement	No	Yes
Vertebral involvement	Only cervical	Total *(ascending from lumbosacral region)*
Cardiac changes	Pericardial effusion, aortic regurgitation, cardiac conduction abnormalities, cardiac valve fibrosis, coronary artery arteritis	Cardiomegaly, aortic regurgitation, cardiac conduction abnormalities
Pulmonary changes	Pulmonary fibrosis, pleural effusion	Pulmonary fibrosis
Eyes	Keratoconjunctivitis sicca	Conjunctivitis, uveitis
Rheumatoid factor	Positive	Negative
HLA-B27	Negative	Positive

motor evoked potentials. The advantage of this monitoring is that patients need not be awakened intraoperatively. However, many anesthetic drugs, especially volatile anesthetics and nitrous oxide, interfere with the monitoring of evoked potentials, and neuromuscular blockers cannot be used if motor evoked potentials are being monitored. Therefore total IV anesthesia with an opioid and propofol or the combination of an opioid, propofol, and low-dose (0.33 MAC) volatile anesthetic is usually chosen to provide general anesthesia. These techniques make it easier to interpret changes in amplitude and latency resulting from spinal cord ischemia. A wake-up test may still be necessary if abnormalities persist. Measurement of evoked potentials is used much more frequently than a wake-up test. At the conclusion of surgery a principal concern is restoration of adequate ventilation. Postoperative mechanical ventilation may be necessary in some patients with severe kyphoscoliosis.

Back Pain

Low back pain is the most common musculoskeletal complaint requiring medical attention. Risk factors for low back pain include male gender, frequent lifting of heavy objects, and smoking. In many patients the cause of the back pain cannot be determined with certainty, and it is usually attributed to muscular or ligamentous strain, facet joint arthritis, or disk pressure on the annulus fibrosus, vertebral end plate, or nerve roots.

Acute Low Back Pain

Back pain improves within 30 days in 90% of patients. Continuing ordinary activities within the limits permitted by the pain can lead to more rapid recovery than bed rest or back-mobilizing exercises. NSAIDs are often effective for analgesia for acute back pain. Pain arising from inflammation initiated by mechanical or chemical insult to a nerve root may be responsive to epidural administration of corticosteroids, but few patients experience symptomatic relief from epidural corticosteroids if the radicular pain has been present for longer than 6 months or if laminectomy has been performed. A herniated disk should be considered in any patient with a

radiculopathy. They will describe pain radiating down a leg, and often their symptoms can be reproduced by a straight leg–raising test. Most lumbar disk herniations producing sciatica occur at the L4-5 and L5-S1 levels. Magnetic resonance imaging (MRI) can confirm a herniated disk, but findings should be interpreted with caution because many asymptomatic people also have disk abnormalities. Surgical intervention is indicated in patients with persistent radiculopathy or neurologic deficits. Patients who have persistent back pain after 30 days of conservative treatment (NSAIDs) should be evaluated for systemic illness.

Lumbar Spinal Stenosis

Lumbar spinal stenosis is a narrowing of the spinal canal or its lateral recesses. It typically results from hypertrophic degenerative changes in spinal structures (extensive degenerative disk disease and/or osteophyte formation) and occurs most often in elderly patients with chronic back pain and sciatica. Symptoms include pain, numbness, and weakness in the buttocks that can extend down one or both legs. Symptoms often worsen with standing or walking and improve in the flexed or supine position. The diagnosis of lumbar spinal stenosis is confirmed by MRI or myelography. Conservative measures may be helpful in some patients, but surgical decompression and fusion are needed for those with progressive functional deterioration.

Rheumatoid Arthritis

Rheumatoid arthritis (RA), the most common chronic inflammatory arthritis, affects approximately 1% of adults. The incidence is two to three times higher in women than in men. The etiology of RA is unknown, but it is suspected to be a complex interaction between genetic and environmental factors and the immune system. The disease is characterized by symmetrical polyarthropathy and significant systemic involvement (Table 25.7). Involvement of the proximal interphalangeal and metacarpophalangeal joints of the hands and feet helps distinguish RA from osteoarthritis, which typically affects weight-bearing joints and distal interphalangeal joints. The disease course is

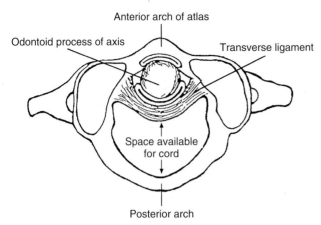

FIG. 25.7 The atlantoaxial articulation seen from above. With atlantoaxial subluxation the odontoid process is no longer positioned close to the anterior arch of the atlas and can move posteriorly to compress the spinal cord. It can also move vertically through the foramen magnum. (From Atlee JL, ed. *Complications in Anesthesia.* 2nd ed. Philadelphia: Saunders; 2007. With permission.)

characterized by exacerbations and remissions. Rheumatoid nodules are typically present at pressure points, particularly under the elbows. *Rheumatoid factor* is an immunoglobulin antibody that is present in the serum of in roughly 90% of patients with RA but *not* present in osteoarthritis. However, the presence of rheumatoid factor is not specific to RA. It is also present in patients with viral hepatitis, SLE, bacterial endocarditis, sarcoidosis, and Sjögren syndrome.

Signs and Symptoms

The onset of RA in adults may be acute, involving single or multiple joints, or insidious with symptoms such as fatigue, anorexia, and weakness preceding overt arthritis. In some patients the onset of RA coincides with trauma, a surgical procedure, childbirth, or exposure to extremes of temperature.

Morning stiffness is a hallmark of RA. Several joints—often the hands, wrists, knees, and feet—are affected in a symmetrical distribution. Fusiform swelling is typical when there is involvement of the proximal interphalangeal joints. These joints are swollen and painful and remain stiff for several hours after the start of daily activity. Synovitis of the temporomandibular joint can produce marked limitation of mandibular motion. When the disease is progressive and unremitting, nearly every joint is affected except for the thoracic and lumbosacral spine.

Cervical spine involvement is frequent and can result in pain and neurologic complications. The most significant abnormality of the cervical spine is atlantoaxial subluxation and consequent separation of the atlanto-odontoid articulation (Fig. 25.7). Normally, with the neck flexed the separation of the anterior margin of the odontoid process from the posterior margin of the anterior arch of the atlas is less than 3 mm. When this separation is severe, the odontoid process can protrude into the foramen magnum and exert pressure on the spinal cord or impair blood flow through the vertebral arteries. Since the odontoid process is often eroded, effects on the

spinal cord may be minimized. Subluxation of other cervical vertebrae can also occur. MRI has confirmed the frequency of cervical spine involvement in RA.

Cricoarytenoid arthritis is common in patients with generalized RA. With acute cricoarytenoid arthritis, hoarseness, pain on swallowing, dyspnea, and stridor may accompany tenderness over the larynx. Redness and swelling of the arytenoids can be seen on direct laryngoscopy. With chronic cricoarytenoid arthritis, patients may be asymptomatic or manifest variable degrees of hoarseness, dyspnea, and upper airway obstruction. Cricoarytenoid arthritis may make endotracheal intubation difficult. Osteoporosis is ubiquitous in patients with RA.

Many of the systemic manifestations of RA are a result of small and medium-sized artery vasculitis due to deposition of immune complexes. Systemic involvement is usually most obvious in patients with severe arthritis.

In the cardiovascular system, RA may manifest as pericarditis, myocarditis, coronary artery arteritis, accelerated coronary atherosclerosis, cardiac valve fibrosis, and formation of rheumatoid nodules in the cardiac conduction system. Aortitis with dilatation of the aortic root may result in aortic regurgitation. Pericardial thickening or effusion is present in about one-third of patients.

Vasculitis in small synovial blood vessels is an early finding in patients with RA, but more widespread vascular inflammation may occur, especially in older men. Patients may demonstrate a neuropathy *(mononeuritis multiplex),* skin ulcerations, and purpura. The neuropathy is presumably due to deposition of immune complexes in the vasa nervorum. Manifestations of visceral ischemia, including bowel perforation, myocardial infarction, and cerebral infarction, are possible.

The most common pulmonary manifestation is pleural effusion. Many of these effusions are small and asymptomatic. Rheumatoid nodules can develop in the pulmonary parenchyma and on pleural surfaces and may mimic tuberculosis or cancer on chest radiographs. Progressive pulmonary fibrosis associated with cough, dyspnea, and diffuse honeycomb changes on chest radiographs is rare. Costochondral involvement may affect chest wall motion and produce restrictive lung changes, with a decrease in vital capacity and lung volumes. This may result in ventilation/perfusion mismatching and decreased arterial oxygenation.

Neuromuscular involvement can be seen, with loss of strength in skeletal muscles adjacent to joints with active synovitis. Peripheral neuropathies resulting from nerve compression, carpal tunnel syndrome, and tarsal tunnel syndrome are common.

The most common hematologic abnormality in patients with RA is *anemia of chronic disease,* the severity of which usually parallels the severity of the RA. *Felty syndrome* consists of RA with splenomegaly and leukopenia. *Keratoconjunctivitis sicca* (dry eyes) occurs in approximately 10% of patients with RA. The cause is lack of tear formation due to impaired lacrimal gland function. A similar pathologic process may involve the salivary glands, resulting in *xerostomia* (dry mouth). These are both manifestations of Sjögren syndrome.

Mild abnormalities of liver function are common in patients with RA. Renal dysfunction may be due to amyloidosis, vasculitis, or drug therapy.

Treatment

Treatment of RA includes measures to relieve pain, preserve joint function and strength, prevent deformities, and attenuate systemic complications. These objectives may be met by a combination of drugs, physical therapy, occupational therapy, and orthopedic surgery. Drug therapy is used to provide analgesia, control inflammation, and produce immunosuppression.

NSAIDs are important for symptomatic relief of RA but have little role in changing the underlying disease process. They should not be used without the concomitant use of *disease-modifying antirheumatic drugs* (DMARDs). NSAIDs decrease swelling in affected joints and relieve stiffness, but associated GI irritation and inhibition of platelet cyclooxygenase 1 (COX-1) may necessitate discontinuation of these drugs. Selective COX-2 inhibitors are as effective as COX-1 inhibitors in producing analgesia and reducing inflammation, and they may evoke fewer GI side effects and do not interfere with platelet function. It appears, however, that some COX-2 inhibitors increase the risk of coronary artery disease and stroke. Both COX-1 and COX-2 drugs can adversely affect renal blood flow and glomerular filtration rate.

Corticosteroids are potent antiinflammatory drugs that decrease joint swelling, pain, and morning stiffness in patients with RA. However, the dosages of systemic corticosteroids necessary to maintain desirable effects are often associated with significant long-term side effects, including osteoporosis, osteonecrosis, increased susceptibility to infection, myopathy, hyperglycemia, and poor wound healing. Intraarticular corticosteroids produce beneficial effects lasting about 3 months, but repeated injections may result in cartilage destruction and osteonecrosis. Corticosteroids are indicated as bridge therapy (i.e., therapy to decrease inflammation rapidly) while DMARDs are starting to work in controlling the disease process. Prednisone dosages greater than 10 mg/day are rarely indicated for joint disease, but higher dosages may be needed to treat other manifestations of RA, especially vasculitis.

DMARDs are a group of drugs that have the potential to modify or change the course of RA. They can slow or halt progression of the disease. Included in this group are methotrexate, sulfasalazine, leflunomide, antimalarials, D-penicillamine, azathioprine, and minocycline. These drugs generally take 2–6 months to achieve their effects. Patients who show no response to one drug may respond to another. *Methotrexate* is the preferred DMARD in the treatment of RA. It is given in a once-a-week dosing regimen. Methotrexate is primarily antiinflammatory. Monitoring of hematologic parameters and liver function test results is necessary in individuals being treated with methotrexate because of the risk of bone marrow suppression and cirrhosis. Daily folic acid therapy can decrease methotrexate toxicity.

It appears that cytokines, especially tumor necrosis factor (TNF)-α and interleukin (IL)-1, play a central role in the pathogenesis of RA. Interference with the function of TNF-α either by drug-induced receptor blockade or by monoclonal antibodies is effective in treating RA. Drugs such as infliximab and etanercept, TNF-α inhibitors, are quite effective in treating RA and act more rapidly than other DMARDs. Long-term toxicities such as infection (tuberculosis) and demyelinating syndromes are a concern. Anakinra, an IL-1 receptor antagonist, is effective against the signs and symptoms of RA, but its onset of action is slower and its overall effect is less than that of the TNF-α inhibitors.

Gold, the traditional DMARD, is extremely effective therapy for some patients with RA, but it is not commonly used because of its toxicities.

Indications for surgery in patients with RA include intractable pain, impairment of joint function, and the need for joint stabilization. Eroded cartilage, ruptured ligaments, and progressive bone destruction can lead to impairments that are only amenable to surgical treatment. Arthroscopic surgery can be used to remove cartilaginous fragments and to perform partial synovectomy. When joints are destroyed by the disease process, total replacement of large and small joints can be considered.

Management of Anesthesia

The multiorgan involvement and side effects of drugs used to treat RA must be appreciated when planning anesthetic management. Preoperatively, patients should be evaluated for airway involvement by this disease process. Compromise of the airway may occur at the cervical spine, temporomandibular joint, and cricoarytenoid joint. Flexion deformity of the cervical spine may make it difficult if not impossible to straighten the neck. Atlantoaxial subluxation may be present. Radiographic evidence (during neck extension) that the distance from the anterior arch of the atlas to the odontoid process exceeds 3 mm confirms the presence of atlantoaxial subluxation. This abnormality is important because the displaced odontoid process can compress the cervical spinal cord or medulla or occlude the vertebral arteries. *When atlantoaxial subluxation is present, care must be taken to minimize movement of the head and neck during direct laryngoscopy to avoid further displacement of the odontoid process and damage to the brainstem or spinal cord.* It is helpful to evaluate preoperatively whether there is interference with vertebral artery blood flow during flexion, extension, or rotation of the head and cervical spine. This can be accomplished by having the awake patient demonstrate head movement or positioning that can be tolerated without discomfort or symptoms.

Limitation of temporomandibular joint movement must be recognized before induction of anesthesia. The combination of limited mobility of these joints plus cervical spine stiffness may make visualizing the glottic opening by direct laryngoscopy difficult or impossible. Endotracheal intubation by fiberoptic laryngoscopy or by use of a videolaryngoscope may be indicated if preoperative evaluation suggests that direct visualization of the glottic opening will be difficult. Involvement of the cricoarytenoid joints by arthritic changes is suggested by the preoperative presence of hoarseness or stridor or by the observation of erythema or edema of the vocal cords during direct laryngoscopy. Diminished movement of these joints can result in narrowing of the glottic opening and interference with passage of the endotracheal tube or an increased risk of cricoarytenoid joint dislocation.

Preoperative pulmonary function studies and assessment of arterial blood gas values may be indicated if severe rheumatoid lung disease is suspected. Postoperative ventilatory support might be needed in the subset of patients with such disease. The effect of aspirin or NSAIDs on platelet function must be considered. Corticosteroid supplementation may be indicated in patients being treated long term with these drugs. Postextubation laryngeal obstruction may occur in patients with cricoarytenoid arthritis.

Systemic Lupus Erythematosus

SLE is a multisystem chronic inflammatory disease characterized by antinuclear antibody production. Interestingly these antinuclear antibodies have not been documented to be directly involved in the pathogenesis of this disease. SLE typically occurs in young women and may affect as many as 1 in 1000 women. Stresses such as infection, pregnancy, or surgery may exacerbate SLE. The onset of SLE can also be drug-induced, with procainamide, hydralazine, isoniazid, D-penicillamine, and α-methyldopa being the most frequently associated drugs. Susceptibility to the development of SLE with exposure to hydralazine or procainamide is related to acetylator phenotype. The disease is more likely to develop in those who metabolize these drugs slowly (slow acetylators). The clinical presentation of drug-induced SLE is similar to that of the naturally occurring form of the disease, but the progression is usually slower and the symptoms are usually milder and consist of arthralgias, a maculopapular rash, fever, anemia, and leukopenia. The natural history of SLE is highly variable. The presence of nephritis and hypertension heralds a worse prognosis. Pregnancy in patients with SLE, especially those with nephritis or hypertension, is associated with a substantial risk of disease exacerbation and/or a poor fetal outcome.

Diagnosis

Detection of antinuclear antibodies is a sensitive screening test for SLE. These antibodies occur in over 95% of SLE patients. The diagnosis is very likely if patients have three of five typical manifestations: antinuclear antibodies, characteristic rash, thrombocytopenia, serositis, and nephritis. However, presentation may not always be so clear, and features such as arthralgias, vague CNS symptoms, rash, Raynaud phenomenon, and/or a weakly positive antinuclear antibody test may make the diagnosis more difficult.

Signs and Symptoms

Clinical manifestations of SLE can be categorized as *articular* or *systemic*. Polyarthritis and dermatitis are the most common signs and symptoms. Many of the clinical manifestations of SLE are the result of tissue damage from a vasculopathy mediated by immune complexes. Others, such as thrombocytopenia and antiphospholipid syndrome, are a direct result of antibodies to cell surface molecules or serum components.

Symmetrical arthritis involving the hands, wrists, elbows, knees, and ankles is common and occurs in 90% of patients. This arthritis is characteristically episodic and migratory, with pain that is out of proportion to the apparent degree of synovitis present. Lupus arthritis does not involve the spine. Another form of skeletal involvement is avascular necrosis, which most often involves the head or condyle of the femur.

Systemic manifestations of SLE can appear in the CNS, heart, lungs, kidneys, liver, neuromuscular system, and skin. Neurologic complications can affect any part of the CNS. Cognitive dysfunction occurs in approximately one-third of individuals. Psychological changes ranging from depression and anxiety to psychosomatic complaints to signs of organic psychosis with deterioration in intellectual capacity are seen in more than half of patients. Most serious CNS manifestations appear to be the result of vasculitis. Fluid and electrolyte disturbances, fever, hypertension, uremia, infection, and drug-induced effects may contribute to CNS dysfunction. Atypical migraine headaches are common and may be accompanied by cortical visual disturbances.

Pericarditis resulting in chest pain, a friction rub, ECG changes, and pericardial effusion is the most common cardiac manifestation of SLE. Myocarditis may result in abnormalities of cardiac conduction. Congestive heart failure can develop with extensive cardiac involvement. Valvular abnormalities can be identified by echocardiography. These include verrucous endocarditis (Libman-Sacks endocarditis) that can involve the aortic and/or mitral valves.

Pulmonary involvement can manifest as lupus pneumonia characterized by diffuse pulmonary infiltrates, pleural effusion, dry cough, dyspnea, and arterial hypoxemia. Pulmonary function testing typically shows restrictive lung disease. Recurrent atelectasis can result in *shrinking* or *vanishing lung syndrome*. This may be a result of diaphragmatic weakness or elevation caused by phrenic neuropathy. Pulmonary angiitis with lung hemorrhage may complicate severe SLE. Pulmonary hypertension is present in some patients.

The most common renal abnormality is glomerulonephritis with proteinuria, which can result in hypoalbuminemia. Hematuria is a frequent finding. The glomerular filtration rate can decrease dramatically and result in oliguric renal failure.

Liver function test findings are abnormal in approximately 30% of patients. Severe liver disease is most likely due to infection or to undiagnosed autoimmune hepatitis or primary biliary cirrhosis.

Neuromuscular manifestations include myopathy with proximal skeletal muscle weakness and increased serum creatine kinase concentration. Tendinitis is common and can result in tendon rupture.

Hematologic abnormalities may be present. Thromboembolism associated with antiphospholipid antibodies can be an important cause of CNS dysfunction. Leukopenia, granulocyte dysfunction, decreased complement levels, and functional asplenia have been implicated in an increased risk of infection. Thrombocytopenia and hemolytic anemia are seen in some patients. The presence of circulating anticoagulants is reflected in a prolonged aPTT. Patients with circulating anticoagulants often manifest a false-positive test result for syphilis.

Some patients with lupus have cutaneous manifestations. The classic butterfly-shaped malar rash occurs in approximately half of patients. This rash can be transient and is often exacerbated by sunlight. Discoid lesions on the face, scalp, and upper trunk develop in approximately 25% of patients with SLE but may occur in the absence of any other features of SLE. Alopecia is common.

Treatment

Treatment is determined by individual disease manifestations. Arthritis and serositis can often be controlled with aspirin or NSAIDs. Antimalarial drugs such as hydroxychloroquine and quinacrine are also effective in treating the dermatologic and arthritic manifestations of SLE. Patients should use sunscreens and avoid intense sun exposure. Thrombocytopenia and hemolytic anemia usually respond to corticosteroid therapy. Danazol, vincristine, cyclophosphamide or splenectomy can be used if thrombocytopenia does not respond to glucocorticoid administration. In view of the increased susceptibility to infection, the risk/benefit ratio of splenectomy must be carefully considered.

Corticosteroids are the principal treatment for severe manifestations of SLE. Corticosteroids effectively suppress glomerulonephritis and cardiovascular abnormalities. However, corticosteroid therapy can be a major cause of morbidity in patients with SLE. Death during the course of SLE may be due to coronary atherosclerosis. The development and progression of coronary atherosclerosis is accelerated by treatment with corticosteroids. Immunosuppressive treatment with alternative drugs such as methotrexate, cyclophosphamide, azathioprine, or mycophenolate mofetil may be preferable to prolonged treatment with high-dose corticosteroids.

Management of Anesthesia

Management of anesthesia is influenced by the magnitude of organ system dysfunction and the drugs used to treat SLE. Laryngeal involvement, including mucosal ulceration, cricoarytenoid arthritis, and recurrent laryngeal nerve palsy, may be present in up to one-third of patients.

Spondyloarthropathies

Spondyloarthropathies are a group of nonrheumatic arthropathies that include ankylosing spondylitis, reactive arthritis (Reiter syndrome), juvenile chronic polyarthropathy, psoriatic arthritis, and enteropathic arthritis. These diseases are characterized by involvement of the spine, especially the sacroiliac joints; asymmetrical peripheral arthritis and synovitis; and absence of rheumatoid nodules or detectable circulating rheumatoid factor (see Table 25.7). There is a shared predilection for new bone formation at sites of chronic inflammation, and joint ankylosis often results. There is also a predilection for ocular inflammation. Causes of these seronegative spondyloarthropathies are unknown, but there is a strong association with HLA-B27.

Ankylosing Spondylitis

Ankylosing spondylitis is a chronic, usually progressive, inflammatory disease involving the articulations of the spine and adjacent soft tissues. It is the most common inflammatory disease of the axial skeleton. Spinal disease begins in the sacroiliac joints and moves cranially. The degree of spinal disease can range from just sacroiliac involvement to complete ankylosis of the spine. Hip involvement occurs in approximately one-third of patients. Back pain characterized as morning stiffness that improves with activity and exercise (rather than rest) plus radiographic evidence of sacroiliitis is highly suggestive of this diagnosis. The disease occurs predominantly in men and often begins in young adulthood. The strong familial incidence is supported by the finding that 90% of patients with ankylosing spondylitis are HLA-B27 positive compared with only 6% of the general population. Ankylosing spondylitis is often erroneously diagnosed as back pain caused by lumbar disk degeneration. Examination of the spine may demonstrate skeletal muscle spasm, loss of lordosis, and decreased mobility of the vertebral column.

Systemic involvement can manifest as weight loss, fatigue, and low-grade fever. Conjunctivitis and uveitis occur in about 40% of patients. The uveitis is usually unilateral and presents as visual impairment, photophobia, and eye pain. Distinctive pulmonary abnormalities associated with ankylosing spondylitis include apical cavitary lesions and pleural thickening that mimic tuberculosis. Cardiovascular involvement (e.g., aortic regurgitation, bundle branch block) is observed in 40% of patients. Arthritic involvement of the thoracic spine and costovertebral articulations can result in a decrease in chest wall compliance and a consequent decrease in vital capacity.

Treatment

Treatment of ankylosing spondylitis consists of exercises designed to maintain joint mobility and posture plus antiinflammatory drugs. NSAIDs are commonly used. Infliximab and etanercept may cause profound improvement in this disease, but patients often experience relapse when treatment is discontinued. For uveitis, topical corticosteroid eye drops are an integral part of management.

Management of Anesthesia

Management of anesthesia in patients with ankylosing spondylitis is influenced by the magnitude of spinal involvement. The spinal column can be stiff and deformed and prevent appropriate cervical spine motion for endotracheal intubation. Fiberoptic or videolaryngoscope assistance may be needed for endotracheal intubation. Restrictive lung disease from costochondral rigidity and flexion deformity of the thoracic spine must be appreciated. Sudden or excessive increases in systemic vascular resistance are poorly tolerated if significant aortic regurgitation is present. Management of aortic regurgitation includes keeping the heart rate at 90 beats per minute or higher and the systemic vascular resistance lower than normal. Neurologic monitoring is a consideration for patients undergoing corrective spinal surgery. Epidural or spinal anesthesia is an acceptable alternative to general anesthesia for perineal or lower limb surgery, but regional anesthesia may be technically difficult owing to limited joint mobility and closed interspinous spaces. Ossification of the ligamentum flavum is uncommon, however. A paramedian approach for spinal or epidural anesthesia may be easier than a midline approach.

Reactive Arthritis

Reactive arthritis is an aseptic arthritis that occurs after an extraarticular infection, especially infection with *Chlamydia, Salmonella,* and *Shigella* species. When reactive arthritis is accompanied by extraarticular features such as urethritis, uveitis or conjunctivitis, and skin lesions, the term *Reiter syndrome* is often used. Predisposing factors include genetic makeup (HLA-B27 positivity). Most of the signs of Reiter syndrome persist for only a few days, but arthritis progresses to sacroiliitis and spondylitis in approximately 20% of patients. Cricoarytenoid arthritis can also occur. Hyperkeratotic skin lesions cannot be distinguished from those of psoriasis, and the two diseases frequently overlap. Management consists of antibiotic treatment for the initial infection and NSAIDs or sulfasalazine for symptomatic relief of the arthritis.

Chronic Juvenile Polyarthropathy

The pathologic process in chronic juvenile polyarthropathy is similar to that in adult RA. Growth abnormalities may occur if arthritis appears before puberty. Hepatic dysfunction may be present, but cardiac involvement is unusual. An acute form of polyarthritis that presents as fever, rash, lymphadenopathy, and splenomegaly in young children who test negative for rheumatoid factor and HLA-B27 is designated *Still's disease.* Aspirin is commonly used to treat this disorder. Corticosteroids can effectively control the disease, but their use is limited because of concerns about drug-induced growth retardation in these young patients.

Enteropathic Arthritis

Approximately 10%–20% of patients with Crohn's disease and 2%–7% of patients with ulcerative colitis will have an inflammatory polyarthritis, most often involving the large joints of the lower extremities. In general, this arthritis activity parallels the activity of the GI inflammation, and measures that control the gut disease usually control this joint disease as well. This arthritis is *not* linked to the presence of HLA-B27.

Inflammatory bowel disease can also be associated with sacroiliitis and spondylitis, which follow a pattern in which the joint inflammation waxes and wanes *independently* of the GI inflammation. HLA-B27 is found in 50% of these patients. This arthritis is usually chronic and may become ankylosing spondylitis. Treatment is as described for ankylosing spondylitis.

Paget's Disease

Paget's disease of bone is characterized by excessive *osteoblastic* and *osteoclastic* activity that results in abnormally thick but weak bones. The cause is unknown but may involve an excess of parathyroid hormone or a deficiency of calcitonin. A familial tendency is present, with white men older than age 40 affected most often. Bone pain is the most common symptom. Complications of Paget's disease involve bones (fractures and neoplastic degeneration), joints (arthritis), and the nervous system (nerve compression, paraplegia). Hypercalcemia and renal calculi may also occur. The most characteristic radiographic feature of Paget's disease is localized bone enlargement. Lytic and sclerotic bone changes may involve the skull. If the skull is affected, it may be grossly enlarged, and irreversible hearing loss may occur. A radionuclide bone scan is the most reliable test to identify lesions caused by Paget's disease. Serum alkaline phosphatase concentration (reflecting *bone formation*) and urinary hydroxyproline excretion (reflecting *bone resorption*) are usually increased.

Treatment of Paget's disease is designed to alleviate bone pain and to minimize or prevent progression of the disease. Bisphosphonates, particularly nitrogen-containing bisphosphonates (aminobisphosphonates, which are more potent), can induce marked and prolonged inhibition of bone resorption by decreasing osteoclastic activity. Often disease activity remains low for many months, sometimes years, after treatment with bisphosphonates is discontinued. Radiographically confirmed repair of osteolytic lesions may occur in response to treatment with bisphosphonates. Analgesics, antiinflammatory drugs, and drugs to treat neuropathic pain may also be needed, especially if there is nerve compression or concomitant osteoarthritis.

Conservative treatment of fractures in patients with Paget's disease is associated with a high risk of delayed union. Patients with Paget's disease who have severe arthritis of the hips or knees often benefit from joint replacement. Rarely, osteotomy must be performed to correct bowing deformities of long bones. Patients with evidence of peripheral nerve compression, radiculopathy, or spinal cord compression require decompressive surgery.

Dwarfism

Dwarfism can occur in two forms: *proportionate dwarfism,* in which the limbs, trunk, and head size are in the same relative proportions as those of a normal adult, and *disproportionate dwarfism,* in which the limbs, trunk, and head size are not in the usual proportions of those in a normal adult.

Proportionate dwarfism is typically due to medical illnesses at birth or in early childhood that limit overall growth and development. Disproportionate dwarfism is due to disorders that limit bone development.

TABLE 25.8	Characteristics of Achondroplastic Dwarfism That May Influence Management of Anesthesia

Difficulty exposing the glottic opening
Foramen magnum stenosis
Odontoid hypoplasia with cervical instability
Kyphoscoliosis
Restrictive lung disease
Obstructive sleep apnea
Central sleep apnea
Pulmonary hypertension
Cor pulmonale
Hydrocephalus

Achondroplasia

Achondroplasia is the most common cause of disproportionate dwarfism. It occurs predominantly in females, with an incidence of 1.5 per 10,000 births. Transmission is by an autosomal dominant gene, although an estimated 80% of cases represent spontaneous mutations. The basic defect is a decrease in the rate of endochondral ossification that, when coupled with normal periosteal bone formation, produces short tubular bones. The anticipated height of achondroplastic males is 132 cm (52 inches) and that of females is 122 cm (48 inches). Kyphoscoliosis and genu varum are common. Premature fusion of the bones at the base of the skull can result in a shortened skull base and a stenotic foramen magnum. In addition, there may be functional fusion of the atlanto-occipital joint with odontoid hypoplasia, atlantoaxial instability, bulging disks, and severe cervical kyphosis. These changes may result in hydrocephalus or damage to the cervical spinal cord. Central sleep apnea in individuals with achondroplasia may be a result of brainstem compression due to foramen magnum stenosis. Pulmonary hypertension leading to cor pulmonale is the most common cardiovascular disturbance that develops in individuals with dwarfism. Mental and skeletal muscle development are normal, as is life expectancy for those who survive the first year of life.

Management of Anesthesia

Management of anesthesia in patients with achondroplastic dwarfism is influenced by potential airway difficulties, cervical spine instability, and the potential for spinal cord trauma with neck extension (Table 25.8).

Patients with achondroplasia may undergo a number of specific operations, including suboccipital craniectomy for foramen magnum stenosis, laminectomy for spinal stenosis or nerve root compression, and ventriculoperitoneal shunt placement. A history of obstructive sleep apnea may predispose to development of upper airway obstruction after sedation or induction of anesthesia. Abnormal bone growth can result in several potential anesthetic problems. Facial features, including a large protruding forehead, short maxilla, large mandible, flat nose, and large tongue, may result in difficulty obtaining a good mask fit and in maintaining a patent upper airway. Despite these anatomic characteristics, clinical experience has not confirmed difficulty with upper airway patency or endotracheal intubation in most patients.

In achondroplastic patients with cervical kyphosis, tracheal intubation may be difficult because of inability to align the axes of the airway. Hyperextension of the neck during direct laryngoscopy should be avoided because of the likely presence of foramen magnum stenosis. Fiberoptically guided tracheal intubation may be considered in selected patients. Weight rather than age is the best guide for selecting the proper size of endotracheal tube.

Excess skin and subcutaneous tissue may make peripheral venous access technically difficult. Patients with achondroplastic dwarfism undergoing suboccipital craniectomy, especially in the sitting position, are at risk of venous air embolism. Insertion of a right atrial catheter is desirable should an air embolism occur, but placing such a catheter may be technically difficult because of the short neck and the difficulty of identifying landmarks, which may be obscured by excess soft tissue. Evoked potential monitoring is useful during surgery that may be associated with brainstem or spinal cord injury. Achondroplastic patients respond normally to anesthetic drugs and neuromuscular blockers. Anesthetic techniques that permit rapid awakening may be desirable for prompt evaluation of neurologic function.

Delivery by cesarean section is necessary in women with achondroplasia, because a small, contracted maternal pelvis combined with an infant of near-normal birth weight leads to cephalopelvic disproportion. Regional anesthesia might be considered, but technical difficulties may occur secondary to kyphoscoliosis and a narrow epidural space and spinal canal. The small epidural space may make it difficult to introduce an epidural catheter. Osteophytes, prolapsed intervertebral disks, or deformed vertebral bodies can also contribute to difficulties with neuraxial blockade. There are no data confirming appropriate doses of local anesthetics for epidural or spinal anesthesia in these patients. Epidural anesthesia may be preferable to spinal anesthesia because it permits titration of the local anesthetic drug to achieve the desired level of sensory blockade.

Russell-Silver Syndrome

Russell-Silver syndrome is a form of dwarfism characterized by intrauterine growth retardation with subsequent severe postnatal growth impairment, dysmorphic facial features (including mandibular and facial hypoplasia), limb asymmetry, congenital heart defects, and a constellation of endocrine abnormalities including hypoglycemia, adrenocortical insufficiency, and hypogonadism. Developmental and hormonal abnormalities tend to normalize with age, and individuals with this syndrome can achieve adult heights near 150 cm (≈60 inches). Rapid depletion of limited hepatic glycogen stores, especially in small-for-gestational-age neonates, may predispose to hypoglycemia. The risk of hypoglycemia diminishes as the child grows and usually disappears after about age 4.

Management of Anesthesia

Preoperative evaluation should consider the serum glucose concentration, especially in neonates at risk of hypoglycemia. IV infusions containing glucose may be indicated preoperatively. Facial manifestations of this syndrome (similar to those in Goldenhar and Treacher-Collins syndromes) may make direct laryngoscopy and exposure of the glottic opening difficult. An endotracheal tube smaller than the predicted size may be needed. Obtaining a good mask fit may also be difficult because of facial asymmetry. Administration of some drugs (e.g., muscle relaxants) based on body weight rather than body surface area may result in relative underdosing. Infants with Russell-Silver syndrome may be especially prone to intraoperative hypothermia because of their large surface-to-volume ratio. Unexplained tachycardia, diaphoresis, or somnolence after emergence from anesthesia may indicate hypoglycemia.

Tumoral Calcinosis

Tumoral calcinosis is a rare genetic disorder that presents as metastatic calcifications adjacent to large joints. Joint motion is unaffected, but the masses may enlarge and interfere with skeletal muscle function. Treatment consists of complete excision of the masses. The principal anesthetic consideration is the rare involvement of the hyoid bone, hypothyroid ligament, or cervical intervertebral joints by this disease process, which leads to difficulty exposing the glottic opening during direct laryngoscopy.

Disorders of the Shoulder

Rotator cuff tear is the most common pathologic entity involving the shoulders. The prevalence of partial- or full-thickness rotator cuff tears is 5%–40% as determined at postmortem examinations of adults older than 40 years. The incidence of rotator cuff tears increases with age. As many as half of individuals older than 55 have arthrographically detectable rotator cuff tears. Other pathologic shoulder conditions are less common. Adhesive capsulitis (frozen shoulder) occurs in approximately 2% of the adult population and in 11% of the adult diabetic population. The incidence of calcific tendinitis ranges from 3%–7%. Shoulder pain ranks just behind back and neck pain as a cause of disability in workers.

Corticosteroid injection into the subacromial space may provide symptomatic relief in patients with impingement syndromes with or without rotator cuff tears, adhesive capsulitis, or supraspinatus tendinitis. Arthroscopic release or manipulation under anesthesia may be used in an attempt to restore shoulder motion. Total shoulder replacement (replacement of humeral and glenoid articular surfaces) reduces shoulder pain in most patients.

Management of Anesthesia

Brachial plexus anesthesia via the interscalene approach with continuous infusion of local anesthetic can provide anesthesia for shoulder surgery as well as postoperative analgesia.

Ipsilateral hemidiaphragmatic paralysis virtually always occurs with an interscalene block, because the phrenic nerve lies close to the area into which the local anesthetic is injected for this block. For this reason, interscalene block may be problematic and is best avoided in patients with severe chronic obstructive pulmonary disease or with neuromuscular diseases associated with weakness of the respiratory muscles. Wound infiltration or lavage with solutions containing a long-acting local anesthetic such as bupivacaine or ropivacaine can also provide postoperative analgesia following major shoulder surgery.

Tracheomegaly

Tracheomegaly is characterized by marked dilatation of the trachea and bronchi resulting from a congenital defect in elastin and smooth muscle fibers in the tracheobronchial tree or to the destruction of these elements by radiotherapy. The diagnosis is confirmed by measuring a tracheal diameter of more than 30 mm on a chest radiograph. Symptoms include a chronic productive cough and frequent pulmonary infection, perhaps related to chronic aspiration. The tracheal and bronchial walls are abnormally flaccid and may collapse during vigorous coughing. Aspiration during general anesthesia is possible, especially if maximal inflation of the endotracheal tube cuff does not produce a seal.

Prader-Willi Syndrome

Prader-Willi syndrome manifests at birth as hypotonia, which may be associated with a weak cough, swallowing difficulties, and upper airway obstruction. Nasogastric feeding may be necessary during infancy. The syndrome progresses during childhood and is characterized by hyperphagia leading to obesity, plus endocrine abnormalities including hypogonadism and diabetes mellitus. Pickwickian syndrome may develop in some patients. There is little growth in height, so patients remain short. Intellectual disabilities are often severe. There is a deletion in chromosome 15 in this syndrome, and an autosomal recessive mode of inheritance has been proposed.

Micrognathia, a high-arched palate, strabismus, a straight ulnar border, and congenital dislocation of the hip may be present. Dental caries are common and may be related to chronic regurgitation of gastric contents. Seizures are associated with this syndrome, but cardiac dysfunction *does not* accompany Prader-Willi syndrome.

Management of Anesthesia

The principal anesthetic concerns in these patients center on hypotonia and altered metabolism of carbohydrates and fat. Weak skeletal musculature is associated with a poor cough and an increased incidence of pneumonia. Intraoperative monitoring of blood glucose concentration is necessary, and exogenous glucose administration may be needed because these patients use circulating glucose to manufacture fat rather than to meet basal energy needs. When calculating drug doses, one should consider the decreased skeletal muscle mass and increased fat content in these patients. Muscle relaxant requirements may be decreased in the presence of hypotonia. Succinylcholine has been administered without incident to these patients.

Disturbances in thermoregulation, often characterized by intraoperative hyperthermia and metabolic acidosis, have been observed, but a relationship to malignant hyperthermia has not been established. There is an increased incidence of perioperative aspiration pneumonia.

Prune-Belly Syndrome

Prune-belly syndrome is characterized by congenital agenesis of the lower central abdominal musculature and the presence of urinary tract anomalies, including gross ureteral dilatation, hypotonic bladder, prostatic hypoplasia, and bilateral undescended testes. The full syndrome appears only in males, but up to 3% of patients with an incomplete syndrome are female. Recurrent respiratory tract infections are seen and reflect an impaired ability to cough effectively. It is unlikely that muscle relaxants will be necessary during the management of anesthesia in these patients.

Meige Syndrome

Meige syndrome is an idiopathic dystonic disorder that manifests as blepharospasm and oromandibular dystonia. It most often affects middle-aged to elderly women. Facial muscle spasms are characterized by symmetrical dystonic contractions of the facial muscles. Dystonia is aggravated by stress and disappears during sleep. The pathophysiology of this disease is unknown but may be related to dopamine hyperactivity or dysfunction of the basal ganglia. Drug therapy (antidopaminergics, anticholinergics, acetylcholine agonists, γ-aminobutyric acid agonists) may have some effect, and facial nerve block has been reported to provide sustained relief.

Spasmodic Dysphonia

Spasmodic dysphonia is a laryngeal disorder characterized by adductor or abductor dystonic spasms of the vocal cords. This syndrome typically manifests as abnormal phonation but on rare occasions is associated with respiratory distress. Stress can exacerbate it, and associated neurologic symptoms (tremors, weakness, dystonia of other skeletal muscle groups) are present in most patients. Botulinum toxin, which blocks neuromuscular transmission, may be effective for treating the spasms of torticollis, blepharospasm, and spasmodic dysphonia.

Management of Anesthesia

Preoperative fiberoptic or direct laryngoscopy may be necessary to define anatomic abnormalities and estimate airway dimensions. The presence of laryngeal stenosis may necessitate use of smaller-than-usual endotracheal tubes. The risk of pulmonary aspiration may be increased by vocal cord dysfunction caused by therapeutic interventions such as botulinum toxin injection or recurrent laryngeal nerve interruption.

Continued monitoring during the postoperative period is important because these patients may experience respiratory difficulties.

Chondrodysplasia Calcificans

Chondrodysplasia calcificans is a rare congenital syndrome caused by dysfunctional peroxisomes. It manifests as erratic cartilage calcification resulting in bone and skin lesions, cataracts, and cardiac malformations. In surviving children, abnormal growth leads to dwarfism, kyphoscoliosis, and subluxation of the hips. There is no available treatment. Orthopedic procedures are often necessary to offset functional limitations of the disease and to stabilize spine and limb malformations. Tracheal cartilage may be involved by the disease process; this results in tracheal stenosis that may complicate perioperative airway management.

Erythromelalgia

Erythromelalgia literally means "red, painful extremities." Erythema, intense burning pain, and increased temperature of the involved extremities are hallmarks of the disease. The feet, especially the soles, are most often involved, and males are affected twice as often as females. The pain is triggered by exposure to heat or exercise and is relieved with cooling. Primary erythromelalgia occurs more frequently than secondary erythromelalgia, which is associated with myeloproliferative disorders such as polycythemia vera. Intravascular platelet aggregation may be prominent. Aspirin is the most effective treatment for secondary erythromelalgia resulting from myeloproliferative diseases. Patients may seek relief by exposing the affected extremity to a cooler environment, such as immersing the extremity in cold water. Neuraxial opioids and local anesthetics may provide some symptom relief.

Farber Lipogranulomatosis

Farber lipogranulomatosis is an inherited disorder caused by a deficiency of ceramidase that results in accumulation of ceramide in tissues (pleura, pericardium, synovial lining of joints, liver, spleen, lymph nodes). Progressive arthropathy, psychomotor retardation, and nutritional failure are present, and most affected individuals die by age 2 as a result of airway and respiratory problems. Acute renal and hepatic failure may reflect accumulation of ceramide in these organs. Difficulty in airway management is a common problem because of lipogranuloma formation in the pharynx or larynx. Tracheal intubation is best avoided in patients with upper airway involvement, because laryngeal edema or bleeding from laryngeal granulomas is possible.

Klippel-Feil Syndrome

Klippel-Feil syndrome is characterized by a short neck resulting from fusion of two or more cervical vertebrae. Movement of the neck is limited. Associated skeletal abnormalities include spinal stenosis and kyphoscoliosis. Mandibular malformations and micrognathia may be present. There is an increased incidence of cardiac and genitourinary anomalies. Cervical spine instability and the risk of neurologic damage during direct laryngoscopy are important considerations that affect management of anesthesia. Preoperative lateral neck radiographs help in evaluating cervical spine stability.

Osteogenesis Imperfecta

Osteogenesis imperfecta is a rare, autosomal dominant, inherited disease of connective tissue that affects bones, sclera, and the inner ear. Bones are very brittle because of a defect in type I collagen production. The incidence of osteogenesis imperfecta is higher in females. There are several types of osteogenesis imperfecta, with some types being mild and others so severe that death occurs within the first year of life. The less severe form typically manifests during childhood or early adolescence with blue sclerae, fractures after minor trauma, kyphoscoliosis, development of bow legs, and gradual onset of otosclerosis and deafness. Impaired platelet function may produce a mild bleeding tendency. Hyperthermia with hyperhidrosis can occur in patients with osteogenesis imperfecta. An increased serum thyroxine concentration associated with an increase in oxygen consumption occurs in at least 50% of patients with this disease. Treatment consists of bisphosphonates to strengthen bones. This treatment also reduces both bone pain and the number of fractures.

Management of Anesthesia

Management of anesthesia is influenced by the co-existing orthopedic deformities and the potential for additional fractures during the perioperative period. Patients with osteogenesis imperfecta often have a decreased range of motion of the cervical spine resulting from remodeling of bone. Tracheal intubation must be accomplished with as little manipulation and trauma as possible because cervical and mandibular fractures may easily occur. Awake fiberoptic intubation or videolaryngoscopy may be prudent if orthopedic deformities suggest that it will be difficult to visualize the glottic opening with direct laryngoscopy. Dentition is often defective, and teeth are vulnerable to damage during direct laryngoscopy. Succinylcholine-induced fasciculations may produce fractures. Kyphoscoliosis and pectus excavatum decrease vital capacity and chest wall compliance and can result in arterial hypoxemia caused by ventilation/perfusion mismatching. Use of automated blood pressure cuffs may be hazardous, since inflation can result in fractures. Regional anesthesia is acceptable in selected patients; it avoids the need for endotracheal intubation, but it may be technically difficult because of kyphoscoliosis. The coagulation status should be evaluated before a regional anesthetic technique is selected, because osteogenesis imperfecta may be associated with *platelet function abnormalities* despite a normal platelet count. These may be due to impairment in

platelet-endothelial cell adhesion. Desmopressin may be effective in normalizing this platelet dysfunction. These patients may have mild hyperthermia intraoperatively, but it is not a forerunner of malignant hyperthermia.

Fibrodysplasia Ossificans

Fibrodysplasia ossificans is a rare inherited autosomal dominant disease that usually presents before age 6. Muscle and connective tissue (including tendons and ligaments) are gradually replaced by bone. Thus there is bone formation outside of the skeleton. Body parts become rigid. Ectopic bone formation typically affects the muscles of the elbows, hips, and knees, leading to serious limitations of joint movement. Cervical spine involvement is common. There may be varying degrees of cervical fusion, and atlantoaxial subluxation is possible. Temporomandibular joint involvement is also common and can result in malnutrition from inability to open the mouth to eat. Muscles of the face, larynx, eyes, anterior abdominal wall, diaphragm, and heart usually escape involvement.

During the early stages of the disease, fever may occur at the same time that localized lumps appear in affected skeletal muscles. Alkaline phosphatase activity is increased during active phases of the disease. A restrictive breathing pattern can result from limitation of rib movement, but progression to respiratory failure is rare. Pneumonia, however, is a common complication. Abnormalities on ECG include ST-segment changes and right bundle branch block. Deafness may occur, but intellectual disability is unlikely. There is no effective therapy.

Deformities of the Sternum

Pectus carinatum (outward protuberance of the sternum) and pectus excavatum (inward concavity of the sternum) produce cosmetic problems, but functional impairment is unusual. Considerable narrowing of the distance between the posterior sternum and the anterior border of the vertebral bodies can be tolerated with little effect on cardiopulmonary function. Rarely is pectus excavatum associated with increased cardiac filling pressures or dysrhythmias. Obstructive sleep apnea may be more common in young children with pectus excavatum, perhaps because of greater inward movement of the sternum and the pliable costochondral apparatus.

Macroglossia

Macroglossia is an infrequent but potentially lethal postoperative complication that is most often associated with posterior fossa craniotomy performed in the sitting position. Possible causes of macroglossia include arterial compression, venous compression resulting from excessive neck flexion or a head-down position, and mechanical compression of the tongue by the teeth, an oral airway, or an endotracheal tube. Macroglossia may also have a neurogenic origin. When the onset of macroglossia is immediate, it is easily recognized, and airway obstruction does not occur because tracheal extubation is delayed. In some patients, however, obstruction to venous outflow from the tongue leads to development of regional ischemia from compression of the lingual arteries. This is followed by a reperfusion injury that does not occur until the outflow obstruction is relieved. As a result the development of macroglossia may be delayed for 30 minutes or longer. There is then the risk of complete airway obstruction occurring at an unexpected time during the postoperative period.

KEY POINTS

- Epidermolysis bullosa and pemphigus are characterized by bulla formation (blistering) that can involve extensive areas of skin and mucous membranes. Even minor frictional trauma can result in bulla formation. Airway management may be difficult because of bullae in the oropharynx. Airway manipulation, including direct laryngoscopy and endotracheal intubation, can result in acute bulla formation, upper airway obstruction, and bleeding.

- Patients with scleroderma can present several problems in anesthetic management. Decreased mandibular motion and narrowing of the oral aperture caused by taut skin may make endotracheal intubation difficult. Oral or nasal telangiectasias may bleed profusely if traumatized. Intravenous access may be impeded by dermal thickening. Systemic or pulmonary hypertension may be present. Hypotonia of the lower esophageal sphincter puts patients at risk of regurgitation and aspiration.

- Muscular dystrophy is characterized by progressive symmetrical skeletal muscle weakness and wasting but no evidence of skeletal muscle denervation. Sensation and reflexes are intact. Increased permeability of skeletal muscle membranes precedes clinical evidence of muscular dystrophy. *Patients with muscular dystrophy are susceptible to malignant hyperthermia.*

- The term *myotonic dystrophy* designates hereditary degenerative diseases of skeletal muscle characterized by persistent contracture (myotonia) after voluntary contraction of a muscle or electrical stimulation of the muscle. Peripheral nerves and the neuromuscular junction are not affected. This inability of skeletal muscle to relax after voluntary contraction or stimulation results from abnormal calcium metabolism.

- The clinical course of myasthenia gravis is marked by periods of exacerbation and remission. Muscle strength may be normal in well-rested patients, but weakness occurs promptly with exercise. Ptosis and diplopia resulting from extraocular muscle weakness are the most common initial signs. Weakness of pharyngeal and laryngeal muscles results in dysphagia, dysarthria, and difficulty handling saliva. Patients with myasthenia gravis are at high risk of pulmonary aspiration.

- The acetylcholine receptor–binding antibodies of myasthenia gravis decrease the number of functional acetylcholine receptors, and this results in an increased *sensitivity* to nondepolarizing muscle relaxants. However, patients with myasthenia gravis demonstrate *resistance* to the effects of succinylcholine.

- Myasthenic syndrome (Eaton-Lambert syndrome) is a disorder of neuromuscular transmission that resembles myasthenia gravis. Myasthenic syndrome is an acquired autoimmune disease characterized by the presence of IgG antibodies to voltage-sensitive calcium channels that causes a deficiency of these channels at the motor nerve terminal. Anticholinesterase drugs effective in the treatment of myasthenia gravis *do not* produce an improvement in patients with myasthenic syndrome.

- Cervical spine involvement is frequent in patients with rheumatoid arthritis and may result in pain and neurologic complications. The most significant abnormality of the cervical spine is atlantoaxial subluxation and consequent separation of the atlanto-odontoid articulation. When this separation is severe, the odontoid process may protrude into the foramen magnum and exert pressure on the spinal cord or impair blood flow through the vertebral arteries.

- Involvement of the cricoarytenoid joints by rheumatoid arthritis is suggested by the presence of hoarseness or stridor or by the observation of erythema or edema of the vocal cords during direct laryngoscopy. Diminished movement of these joints can result in narrowing of the glottic opening and interference with passage of the endotracheal tube or an increased risk of cricoarytenoid joint dislocation.

- The spondyloarthropathies are a group of nonrheumatic arthropathies characterized by involvement of the spine, especially the sacroiliac joints; asymmetrical peripheral arthritis; synovitis; and absence of rheumatic nodules or detectable circulating rheumatoid factor. These diseases have a shared predilection for new bone formation at sites of chronic inflammation, and joint ankylosis often results. Ocular inflammation is frequently present.

- Osteoarthritis is by far the most common joint disease, one of the leading chronic diseases of the elderly and a major cause of disability. Osteoarthritis is a degenerative process that affects articular cartilage. Both the cervical and lumbar spine may be involved. This process is different from rheumatoid arthritis in that there is minimal inflammatory reaction in osteoarthritic joints. The pathogenesis is likely related to joint trauma from biomechanical stresses, joint injury, or abnormal joint loading resulting from neuropathy, ligamentous injury, muscle atrophy, or obesity. Pain is usually present on motion but relieved by rest.

- Kyphoscoliosis is a spinal deformity characterized by anterior flexion (kyphosis) and lateral curvature (scoliosis) of the vertebral column. Spinal curvature of more than 40 degrees is considered severe and is likely to be associated with physiologic derangements in cardiac and pulmonary function. Restrictive lung disease and pulmonary hypertension progressing to cor pulmonale are the principal causes of death in patients with kyphoscoliosis. During corrective surgery for scoliosis or kyphosis, spinal cord monitoring now utilizes measurement of evoked potentials (sensory and motor) much more frequently than the wake-up test.

RESOURCES

Ben-Menachem E. Systemic lupus erythematosus: a review for anesthesiologists. *Anesth Analg.* 2010;111:665-676.

Berkowitz ID, Raja SN, Bender KS, et al. Dwarfs: pathophysiology and anesthetic considerations. *Anesthesiology.* 1990;73:739-759.

Berman BM, Langevin HM, Witt CM, et al. Acupuncture for chronic low back pain. *N Engl J Med.* 2010;363:454-461.

Dalakas MC, Hohlfeld R. Polymyositis and dermatomyositis. *Lancet.* 2003;362:971-982.

Davis PJ, Brandon BW. The association of malignant hyperthermia and unusual diseases: when you're hot you're hot, or may not. *Anesth Analg.* 2009;109:1001-1003.

Dillon FX. Anesthesia issues in the perioperative management of myasthenia gravis. *Semin Neurol.* 2004;24:83-94.

Ferschl M, Moxley R, Day JW, Gropper M. Practical suggestions for the anesthetic management of a myotonic dystrophy patient. Myotonic Dystrophy Foundation website. www.myotonic.org.

Hirsch NP. The neuromuscular junction in health and disease. *Br J Anaesth.* 2007;99:132-138.

Kuczkowski KM. Labor analgesia for the parturient with an uncommon disorder: a common dilemma in the delivery suite. *Obstet Gynecol Surv.* 2003;58:800-803.

Muscular dystrophy association website. www.mda.org.

Nandi R, Howard R. Anesthesia and epidermolysis bullosa. *Dermatol Clin.* 2010;28:319-324.

O'Neill GN. Acquired disorders of the neuromuscular junction. *Int Anesthesiol Clin.* 2006;44:107-121.

Whyte MP. Paget's disease of bone. *N Engl J Med.* 2006;355:593-600.

Infectious Diseases

ANTONIO HERNANDEZ CONTE

Great advances have been made in modern medicine in the treatment of cardiovascular disease and certain kinds of cancer, but infectious diseases remain a major obstacle to good health worldwide. The advent of antibiotics to treat some bacterial diseases was a major advance, as was the development of vaccines against a number of infectious diseases. But for every step forward, a substantial obstacle has appeared. For example, microorganisms have developed resistance to some antibiotic drugs, and they continue to mutate in ways that make their eradication ever more difficult. Development of vaccines to treat some of the most common and potentially deadly infectious diseases in the world have been stymied by the ability of some infectious agents to mutate much more quickly than lab personnel can change their vaccine formulations. Malaria and human immunodeficiency virus (HIV) disease are examples of this. In addition, about one new infectious disease organism has been discovered annually over the past 50 years. Some have been discovered in regions far removed from our country, but easy travel has brought the opportunity for nearly anyone anywhere to become infected with what were formerly thought to be "exotic" diseases.

Healthcare facilities, long thought to be havens for the very ill, are now also reservoirs of several infectious diseases due to resistant microorganisms or to infection by microorganisms that can only manifest disease when other more virulent organisms have been reduced in number or eradicated. Thus the presence of infectious agents as a comorbid condition in patients coming for surgery remains a significant issue for the perioperative physician. Additionally, the development of hospital-acquired infections remains a significant cause of morbidity and mortality in the perioperative period. Patients may have co-existing infectious diseases that impact perioperative care when they come for surgery; these infections may be manifest or occult. Preexisting infectious diseases may be the reason for the surgery or may alter the risks associated with the surgery. In addition, every patient undergoing surgery is at risk of acquiring an infectious disease during the perioperative period. Patients undergoing surgery are vulnerable to infection both at the surgical site and where natural defenses are breached, such as the respiratory tract, urinary tract, bloodstream, and sites of invasive monitoring. These infectious diseases can be passed on to other patients and to health professionals in the perioperative period, and healthcare workers themselves may serve as active agents in transmitting infectious diseases to patients.

INFECTION PREVENTION OVERVIEW

Antibiotic Resistance

Prior to the development of microscopic biology, humans had little understanding of infection and were subject to many devastating pandemics, such as the Black Death of the 14th century. Since the discovery of penicillin in 1928, bacteria have undergone thousands of mutations, resembling a darwinian "survival-of-the-fittest" evolutionary response to antibiotic exposure that has perpetuated the need for ever-new antibiotics. Most classes of antibiotics were discovered in the 1940s and 1950s, and these drugs are directed at a few specific aspects of bacterial physiology: biosynthesis of the cell wall, DNA, and proteins. During the past 40 years, only two new chemical classes of antibiotics have been developed.

One reason for the widespread drug resistance among bacterial pathogens is the limited choice of antibiotics that manipulate only a narrow range of bacterial functions. Another is overprescription and inappropriate use of current antibiotics.

Infectious diseases that were presumably eradicated (e.g., tuberculosis [TB]) are demonstrating a resurgence. Some reemerging pathogens, such as multidrug-resistant (MDR) TB and extensively drug-resistant (XDR) TB, have resistance to previously successful antimicrobial therapies. MDR organisms cause an increasing number of bacterial infections in hospitals, and bacteria are emerging with resistance to *all* available antibiotics. Much of the attention is presently focused on *resistant gram-positive organisms,* such as methicillin-resistant *Staphylococcus aureus* (MRSA). However, there is virtually no development of antibiotics active against *resistant gram-negative pathogens.* New antibiotic development has dramatically slowed owing to regulatory disincentives, market failures, and lack of profitability compared to other pharmacologic pursuits.

Surgical Site Infections

Surgical site infections (SSIs) have been the focus of much attention during the past 30 years, and the major emphasis has been on completely preventing the occurrence of surgery-related infections and their associated morbidity and mortality. In 2002 the Centers for Medicare and Medicaid Services (CMS), in collaboration with the Centers for Disease Control and Prevention (CDC), implemented the national Surgical Infection Prevention Project (SIPP). The key measures being monitored by this project are: (1) the proportion of patients who receive parenterally administered antibiotics within 1 hour prior to incision (within 2 hours for vancomycin and fluoroquinolones), (2) the proportion of patients who receive prophylactic antimicrobial therapy consistent with published guidelines, and (3) the proportion of patients whose prophylactic antibiotic is discontinued within 24 hours after surgery.

Despite the implementation of numerous sets of drug and policy guidelines, SSIs continue to occur at a rate of 2%–5% for extraabdominal surgery and up to 20% for intraabdominal surgery, and affect approximately 500,000 patients annually. SSIs are among the most common causes of nosocomial infection, accounting for 14%–16% of all nosocomial infections in hospitalized patients. SSIs are a major source of morbidity and mortality, rendering patients 60% more likely to spend time in the intensive care unit (ICU), five times more likely to require hospital readmission, and twice as likely to die. A recent resurgence in SSIs may be attributable to bacterial resistance, increased implantation of prosthetic and foreign materials, or the poor immune status of many patients undergoing surgery. Universal adoption of simple measures, including frequent handwashing and appropriate administration of prophylactic antibiotics, has been emphasized as a method of decreasing the incidence of SSIs.

SSIs are divided into *superficial infections* (involving skin and subcutaneous tissues), *deep infections* (involving fascial and muscle layers), and *infections of organs or tissue spaces* (any area opened or manipulated during surgery) (Fig. 26.1). *S. aureus,* including MRSA, is the predominant cause of SSIs. The increased proportion of SSIs caused by resistant pathogens and *Candida* species may reflect the increasing numbers of severely ill and immunocompromised surgical patients and the impact of widespread use of broad-spectrum antimicrobial drugs.

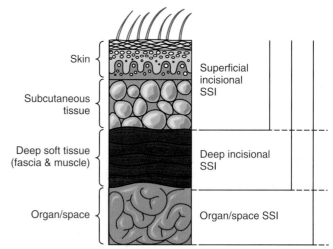

FIG. 26.1 Cross-section of abdominal wall, showing the CDC classification of surgical site infection (SSI). (Adapted from Horan TC, Gaynes RP, Martone WJ, et al. CDC definitions of nosocomial surgical site infections, 1992: a modification of CDC definitions of surgical wound infections. *Infect Control Hosp Epidemiol.* 1992;13:606-608.)

Risk Factors for Surgical Site Infections

The risk of developing an SSI is affected by patient-related, microbe-related, and wound-related factors. Patient-related factors include chronic illness, extremes of age, baseline immunocompetence or inherent or acquired immunocompromise, diabetes mellitus, and corticosteroid therapy. These factors are associated with an *increased risk* of developing an SSI.

Microbial factors include pathogen enzyme production, possession of a polysaccharide capsule, and the ability to bind to fibronectin in blood clots. These are some of the mechanisms by which microorganisms exploit weakened host defenses and initiate infection. *Biofilm formation* is particularly important in the development of prosthetic material infections (i.e., prosthetic joint infection). Coagulase-negative staphylococci produce a glycocalyx and an associated component called *slime* that physically shield bacteria from phagocytes or inhibit antimicrobial agents from binding with or penetrating into the bacteria.

Devitalized tissue, dead space, and hematomas are wound-related features associated with the development of SSIs. Historically, wounds have been described as *clean, contaminated,* and *dirty* according to the expected number of bacteria entering the surgical site. The presence of a foreign body (i.e., sutures or mesh) reduces the number of organisms required to induce an SSI. Interestingly the implantation of major devices such as prosthetic joints and cardiac devices is not associated with a higher risk of SSIs. Risk factors for SSI are summarized in Table 26.1.

Signs and Symptoms

SSIs typically present within 30 days of surgery with localized inflammation at the surgical site and evidence of poor wound healing. Systemic features of infection, such as fever and malaise, may occur soon thereafter.

Diagnosis

There may be nonspecific evidence of infection, such as an elevated white blood cell count, poor blood glucose control, and elevated levels of inflammatory markers such as C-reactive protein. However, surgery is a great confounder because surgery itself causes inflammation and thus renders surrogate markers of infection less reliable. Purulence at the wound site is highly suggestive of infection. The gold standard in documenting a wound infection is growth of organisms in an aseptically obtained culture specimen. Approximately one-third of organisms cultured are staphylococci (*S. aureus* and *Staphylococcus epidermidis*); *Enterococcus* species make up more than 10%, and Enterobacteriaceae make up the bulk of the remaining culprits. Table 26.2 lists the criteria for diagnosing an SSI.

Management of Anesthesia
Preoperative

Active infections should be treated aggressively before surgery, and when possible, surgery should be postponed until infection has resolved. If a localized area of infection is present at the intended surgical site, surgery should be postponed until the localized infection is treated and/or resolves spontaneously. If a patient has clinical evidence of infection, such as fever, chills, or malaise, efforts should be made to identify the source of the infectious process. Several studies have shown that smoking may increase not only the incidence of respiratory tract infection but also the incidence of wound infections. Preoperative cessation of smoking for 4–8 weeks before orthopedic surgery decreases the incidence of wound-related complications. Significant preoperative alcohol consumption may result in generalized immunocompromise. One month of preoperative alcohol abstinence reduces postoperative morbidity in alcohol users.

Diabetes mellitus is an independent risk factor for infection, and optimization of preoperative diabetes treatment may decrease perioperative infection. Malnutrition, whether manifesting as cachexia or obesity, is associated with an increased perioperative infection rate. Appropriate diet and/or weight loss may be beneficial before major surgery.

S. aureus is the organism most commonly implicated in SSIs, and many individuals are carriers of *S. aureus* in the anterior nares. This carrier state has been identified as a risk factor for *S. aureus* wound infections. Topical mupirocin applied to the anterior nares has been successful in eliminating the carrier state of *S. aureus* and decreasing the risk of infection. However, there is concern that this practice may promote development of mupirocin-resistant *S. aureus*. Active surveillance programs to eliminate nasal colonization in hospital surgical personnel have controlled outbreaks of *S. aureus* SSIs.

Hair clipping at the planned surgical site is acceptable, but shaving increases the risk of SSI, probably because microcuts serve as entry portals for microorganisms. Preoperative skin cleansing with chlorhexidine has been shown to reduce the incidence of SSIs.

Intraoperative

Prophylactic Antibiotics. It was recognized many years ago that prophylactic administration of antimicrobial agents prevents postoperative wound infections. This is particularly

TABLE 26.1	Risk Factors for Surgical Site Infection	
Patient-Related Factors	Microbial Factors	Wound-Related Factors
Extremes of age	Enzyme production	Devitalized tissue
Poor nutritional status	Polysaccharide capsule	Dead space
ASA physical status score > 2	Ability to bind to fibronectin	Hematoma
Diabetes mellitus	Biofilm and slime formation	Contaminated surgery
Smoking		Presence of foreign material
Obesity		
Co-existing infections		
Colonization		
Immunocompromise		
Longer preoperative hospital stay		

ASA, American Society of Anesthesiologists.

TABLE 26.2 Criteria for Diagnosis of Surgical Site Infection (SSI)

Type of SSI	Time Course	Criteria (At Least One Must Be Present)
Superficial incisional SSI	Within 30 days of surgery	Superficial pus drainage Organisms cultured from superficial tissue or fluid Signs and symptoms (pain, redness, swelling, heat)
Deep incisional SSI	Within 30 days of surgery or within 1 yr if prosthetic implant present	Deep pus drainage Dehiscence or wound opened by surgeon (for temperature >38°C, pain, tenderness) Abscess (e.g., radiographically diagnosed)
Organ/space SSI	Within 30 days of surgery or within 1 yr if prosthetic implant present	Pus from a drain in the organ/space Organisms cultured from aseptically obtained specimen of fluid or tissue in the organ/space Abscess involving the organ/space

true when the inoculum of bacteria is high, such as in colon, rectal, or vaginal surgery, or when the procedure involves insertion of an artificial implant such as a hip prosthesis or heart valve. The organisms implicated in SSIs are usually those carried by the patient in the nose or on the skin. Unless the patient has been in the hospital for some time before surgery, these are usually community organisms that have not developed multiple drug resistance. Timing of antibiotic prophylaxis (within 1 hour of surgical incision) is important, since these organisms are introduced into the bloodstream at the time of incision. For most procedures, a single dose of antibiotic is adequate. Prolonged surgery (>4 hours) may necessitate a second dose. Prophylaxis should be discontinued within 24 hours of the procedure. For cardiac surgery, the Joint Commission has recommended that the duration of prophylaxis be increased to 48 hours. A first-generation cephalosporin, such as cefazolin, is effective for many types of surgery. In general the spectrum of bacteria against which cephalosporins are effective, their low incidence of side effects, and the tolerability of these drugs have made them an ideal choice for prophylaxis. For high-risk patients and procedures, selection of another appropriate antibiotic plays a critical role in decreasing the incidence of SSIs.

When the small bowel is entered, coverage for gram-negative organisms is important, and for procedures involving the large bowel and the female genital tract, the addition of coverage against anaerobic organisms is appropriate. Infections associated with *clean* surgery are caused by staphylococcal species, whereas infections associated with *contaminated* surgery are polymicrobial and involve the flora of the viscus entered. Guidelines for antimicrobial prophylaxis for those considered at risk of infective endocarditis are published by the American Heart Association. Additional considerations are listed in Table 26.3.

Physical and Physiologic Preventive Measures. Several simple physical measures have been studied to determine their effects on the incidence of postoperative infection. Much of the work has focused on the oxygen tension at the wound site. Destruction of organisms by oxidation, or *oxidative killing,* is the most important defense against surgical pathogens and depends on the partial pressure of oxygen in contami-

TABLE 26.3 Surgical Infection Prevention Guidelines

1. Give prophylactic antibiotics within 1 hour of surgical incision.
2. Stop prophylactic antibiotics at 24 hours (or 48 hours for cardiac surgery).
3. Increase dose of antibiotics for larger patients.
4. Repeat dose when surgery exceeds 4 hours.
5. Administer antibiotic(s) appropriate for local resistance patterns.
6. Follow American Heart Association guidelines for patients at risk of infective endocarditis.
7. Adhere to procedure-specific antibiotic recommendations.

nated tissue. In patients with normal peripheral perfusion, the subcutaneous oxygen tension is linearly related to the arterial oxygen tension. An inverse correlation has been demonstrated between subcutaneous tissue oxygen tension and the rate of wound infections. Tissue hypoxia appears to increase the vulnerability to infection.

Hypothermia has been shown to increase the incidence of SSI. In a study in which patients were randomly assigned to hypothermia and normothermia groups, SSI was found in 19% of patients in the hypothermia group but in only 6% of those in the normothermia group. Radiant heating to 38°C increases subcutaneous oxygen tension. This may be one of the mechanisms for the decreased infection risk associated with increased body temperature.

Oxygen. An easy method of improving oxygen tension is to increase the concentration of inspired oxygen. Studies of patients undergoing colorectal resection have demonstrated that perioperative administration of 80% oxygen decreases the incidence of SSI in this patient group. It is unknown whether perioperative administration of 80% oxygen decreases the incidence of SSI in other surgical settings. Universal adoption of this treatment protocol remains controversial, since a prolonged period of high inspired oxygen tension might cause pulmonary damage.

Analgesia. Superior treatment of surgical pain is associated with increased postoperative subcutaneous oxygen partial pressures at wound sites. Adequate analgesia may therefore be associated with a decreased incidence of SSI.

Carbon Dioxide. *Hypocapnia* occurs frequently during anesthesia and can be deleterious for many reasons, particularly because of the vasoconstriction it causes. Such vasoconstriction could impair perfusion of vital organs. *Hypercapnia* causes vasodilation and increases skin perfusion. Intriguing research has shown that mild intraoperative hypercapnia increases the oxygen tension in subcutaneous tissue and the colon.

Glucose. The results of studies to date suggest that in the perioperative period, the ideal blood glucose goal should be in the normal range with minimal variability. A high blood glucose concentration is thought to inhibit leukocyte function and provide a favorable environment for bacterial growth. Interestingly the therapy for hyperglycemia may itself have beneficial effects. Administration of glucose, insulin, and potassium stimulates lymphocytes to proliferate and attack pathogens. Glucose, insulin, and potassium may play an important role in restoring immunocompetence to patients with immunocompromise.

Wound-Probing Protocols. Current studies suggest that infection of contaminated wounds can be decreased by following wound-probing protocols. Wound probing is a bedside technique that combines the benefits of primary and secondary wound closure. Use of this technique has been shown to decrease length of stay and SSIs, but the exact mechanism of its effect is not clearly understood.

BLOODBORNE INFECTIONS

Bloodstream Infections

Bloodstream infections (BSIs) are among the top three nosocomial infections in incidence. Anesthesiologists may play an important role in the prevention and often the treatment of BSIs. Central venous catheters are the major cause of nosocomial bacteremia and fungemia. Catheter-related bloodstream infections are common, costly, and potentially lethal. These infections are monitored by the National Nosocomial Infections Surveillance (NNIS) System of the CDC. A total of 80,000 cases of central venous catheter–associated BSI are estimated to occur annually in the United States. Mortality risk related to these is estimated to be 12%–25% for each bloodstream infection.

Signs and Symptoms
Patients typically have nonspecific signs of infection with no obvious source. There is no cloudy urine, purulent sputum, pus drainage, or wound inflammation. There is only an indwelling catheter. Inflammation at the catheter insertion site is suggestive of infection. A sudden change in a patient's condition, such as mental status changes, hemodynamic instability, altered tolerance for nutrition, and generalized malaise, can indicate a BSI.

Diagnosis
Catheter-associated BSIs are defined as bacteremia or fungemia in a patient with an intravascular catheter with at least one blood culture positive for a recognized pathogen not related

TABLE 26.4	Common Pathogens Associated With Bloodstream Infections

Gram-positive bacteria (59%)
  Coagulase-negative staphylococci
  Staphylococcus aureus
  Enterococci
  Streptococcus pneumoniae
Gram-negative bacteria (31%)
  Escherichia coli
  Enterobacter species
  Klebsiella pneumoniae
  Acinetobacter baumanii
Fungi (10%)
  Candida species

From Orsini J, Mainardi C, Muzylo E, et al. Microbiological profile of organisms causing bloodstream infection in critically ill patients. *J Clin Med Res*. 2012;4:371-377.

to another infection in that patient, clinical manifestations of infection, and no other apparent source for the BSI except the catheter. BSIs are considered to be associated with a central line if the line was in use during the 48-hour period before the development of the BSI. If the time interval between the onset of infection and device use is longer than 48 hours, other sources of infection must be considered. The diagnosis is more compelling if after catheter removal the same organisms that grew in the blood culture grow from the catheter tip. Table 26.4 lists pathogens commonly associated with BSI.

Treatment
The best "treatment" of central venous catheter–related BSIs is prevention. However, if infection is suspected, the source of the infection should be removed as soon as possible, and broad-spectrum antimicrobial therapy should be initiated. Once culture results are available, antibiotic therapy can be targeted to the specific organism. Because of antibiotic resistance patterns, it is difficult to strike a compromise between providing appropriate initial empirical coverage and not exhausting the last-line antimicrobial agents with the first salvo of antibiotic therapy. Treatment of patients with BSIs is similar to treatment of patients with sepsis.

Management of Anesthesia
Preoperative
Many central venous catheters are placed by anesthesiologists who may not be informed about BSIs that develop days later. Preventing BSIs related to central venous catheter use can be minimized by implementing a series of evidence-based steps shown to reduce catheter-related infection. A recent interventional study targeted *five evidence-based procedures* recommended by the CDC and identified as having the greatest effect in reducing the rate of catheter-related BSIs and the fewest barriers to implementation. The five interventions are (1) handwashing with soap and water or an alcohol cleanser by the operator before catheter insertion or maintenance, (2) using full-barrier precautions (hat, mask, sterile gown, sterile area covering) during central venous catheter insertion, (3) cleaning the skin with chlorhexidine, (4) avoiding the femoral site

and peripheral arms if possible, and (5) conducting routine daily inspection of catheters and removing them as soon as deemed unnecessary. In this study, use of these evidence-based interventions resulted in a large and sustained reduction (up to 66%) in rates of catheter-related BSIs that was maintained throughout the 18-month study period. The subclavian and internal jugular venous routes carry less risk of infection than the femoral route, but the decision regarding anatomic location also has to consider the higher risk of pneumothorax with a subclavian catheter. During insertion, catheter contamination rates can be further reduced by rinsing gloved hands in a solution of chlorhexidine in alcohol before handling the catheter. Sterility must be maintained with frequent hand decontamination and cleaning of catheter ports with alcohol before accessing them. The same high standards of sterility should be applied with regional anesthetic catheters. Central venous catheters may be coated or impregnated with antimicrobial or antiseptic agents. These catheters have been associated with a lower incidence of BSIs. Concerns about widespread adoption of drug-impregnated catheters are based on increased costs and promotion of antimicrobial resistance. However, use of such catheters may be indicated for the most vulnerable patients, such as those with severe immunocompromise.

Intraoperative

Transfusion of red blood cells and blood components increases the incidence of postoperative infection via two mechanisms: direct transmission of organisms from the blood product and immunosuppression. Even autologous blood transfusion results in natural killer cell inhibition and is intrinsically immunosuppressive. The mechanism of immunosuppression may be related to infusion of donor leukocytes or their byproducts. Blood transfusion–associated immunosuppression may be decreased by leukodepletion.

Transfusion of cellular blood components has been implicated in transmission of viral, bacterial, and protozoal diseases. Over the past 20 years, reductions in the risk of viral infection from blood components have been achieved. Minipool nucleic acid amplification testing detects HIV and hepatitis B and C virus during the time before antibodies develop. This sensitive and specific test has decreased the risk of HIV-1 and hepatitis C virus transmission to 1 in 2 million blood transfusions.

Because of the success in detecting viral infection, bacterial contamination of blood products has emerged as the greatest residual source of transfusion-transmitted disease. Each year, approximately 9 million units of platelet concentrates are transfused in the United States. An estimated 1 in 1000–3000 platelet units is contaminated with bacteria. Platelets, to maintain viability and function, must be stored at room temperature, which creates an excellent growth environment for bacteria. The prevalence of episodes of transfusion-associated bacterial sepsis is approximately 1 in 50,000 for platelet units and 1 in 500,000 for red blood cell units. Implementation of bacterial detection methods will improve the safety and extend the shelf life of platelets. The best way to avoid infectious complications related to transfusion is simply to avoid or minimize the use of transfusions.

Postoperative

Several postoperative management strategies can decrease the incidence of catheter-related BSI: (1) removal of central lines and pulmonary artery catheters as soon as possible, and (2) avoidance of unnecessary parenteral nutrition and dextrose-containing fluid, since these may be associated with an increased risk of BSI. Food and glucose can usually be withheld for a short period or delivered into the gut rather than into a vein.

Sepsis

Sepsis is an umbrella term encompassing those conditions in which there are pathogenic microorganisms in the body. Sepsis may be life threatening because of complications precipitated by an organism, its toxins, and the body's own defensive inflammatory response. (A similar response may occur in the absence of infection, and this is sometimes called *systemic inflammatory response syndrome* [SIRS].) Sepsis is a spectrum of disorders on a continuum, with localized inflammation at one end and a severe generalized inflammatory response with multiorgan failure at the other (Fig. 26.2). *Severe sepsis* is defined as acute organ dysfunction secondary to infection,

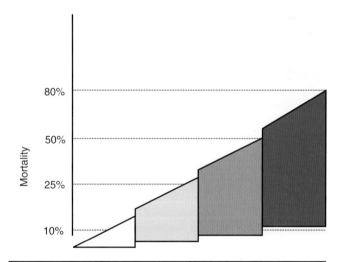

	Infection	Sepsis	Severe sepsis	Septic shock
Definition	Pathogens detected in blood or tissue	Infection plus systemic inflammatory response syndrome (SIRS)	Sepsis plus organ dysfunction: Lactic acidosis Oliguria Confusion Hepatic dysfunction	Severe sepsis plus hypotension (systolic BP < 90 mm Hg despite adequate fluid resuscitation)
Estimated mortality	0%-10%	10%-25%	25%-50%	50%-80%

FIG. 26.2 Continuum of sepsis, with definitions and approximate mortality rates. *BP,* Blood pressure. (Adapted from Bone RC. Toward an epidemiology and natural history of systemic inflammatory response syndrome. *JAMA.* 1992;268:3452-3455.)

and *septic shock* is severe sepsis with hypotension not reversed by fluid administration.

Surgery and anesthesia should be postponed until sepsis is at least partially treated. However, sometimes the underlying cause of sepsis requires urgent surgical intervention. Such surgery may be termed *source control surgery*. Examples of septic sources are abscesses, infective endocarditis, bowel perforation or infarction, infected prosthetic device (e.g., intravenous [IV] catheter, intrauterine device, or pacemaker), endometritis, and necrotizing fasciitis.

Bacterial components such as endotoxin, through their action on neutrophils and macrophages, can induce a wide range of proinflammatory factors and counterregulatory host responses that turn off production of proinflammatory cytokines. As a result the proinflammatory reaction (SIRS) can become exaggerated by associated activation of the complement system and coagulation cascade, widespread arterial vasodilation, and altered capillary permeability. This may result in multiorgan dysfunction and death.

Signs and Symptoms

Signs and symptoms of sepsis are often nonspecific, and presentation varies according to the initial source of infection. SIRS is an important component of sepsis (Table 26.5).

Sepsis may result in multiorgan failure. Features of infection include fever, altered mental status, and encephalopathy. Hyperglycemia may be present. *Septic shock* refers to hemodynamic instability that may accompany sepsis and the perfusion abnormalities that may include (but are not limited to) lactic acidosis, oliguria, or a change in mental status. Classically, hypotension, bounding pulses, and a wide pulse pressure are present. These are characteristic signs of high-output cardiac failure and distributive shock, both of which may occur with sepsis. Patients who are receiving inotropic drugs or vasopressor support may not be hypotensive.

Diagnosis

A diagnosis of sepsis is surmised from history, signs, and symptoms. Confirmation is based on isolation of a specific causative pathogen. It is important to identify the culprit microbe to ensure that antimicrobial therapy is appropriate and targeted. Specimens for culture should be sent from all sources where organism growth is suspected. Blood, urine, and sputum specimens are a minimum. Tissue sampling from specific sources such as heart valves, bone marrow, and cerebrospinal fluid can also be important.

Treatment

Initial treatment of sepsis involves broad antimicrobial coverage coupled with supportive care of failing organs. The speed and appropriateness of therapy administered in the initial hours of sepsis can dramatically influence outcome. The replication of virulent bacteria can be so rapid that every minute may be crucial. As soon as specific microbiological information is available, therapy should be tailored to the specific organism and its sensitivities. Choice of an antibiotic must also take into account the ability of the drug to penetrate various tissues, including bone, cerebrospinal fluid, lung tissue, and abscess cavities.

In addition to targeted antimicrobial therapy, supportive treatment relating to organ system dysfunction is essential. Early goal-directed optimization that targets oxygen delivery and cardiac output may improve outcome in sepsis.

Prognosis

Prognosis in sepsis depends on the virulence of the infecting pathogen(s), stage at which appropriate treatment is initiated, inflammatory response of the patient, immune status of the patient, and extent of organ system dysfunction. It is impossible to predict the outcome for any individual patient.

Management of Anesthesia
Preoperative

The most important considerations for a patient with sepsis requiring surgery are whether the surgery may be postponed pending treatment of sepsis and whether the patient's condition may be improved before surgery. A treatment algorithm for septic patients (Fig. 26.3) suggests goal-directed optimization of the patient's condition. Resuscitation should be targeted to achieve mean arterial pressure above 65 mm Hg, central venous pressure of 8–12 mm Hg, adequate urine output, a pH without a metabolic (lactic) acidosis, and a mixed venous oxygen saturation above 70%.

Intraoperative

Intraoperative management of patients with sepsis is challenging. Patients with sepsis may have limited physiologic reserve that renders them vulnerable to hypotension and hypoxemia with induction of anesthesia. Invasive monitoring, such as intraarterial blood pressure and central venous pressure monitoring, is usually indicated. Establishment of sufficient IV access to allow for volume resuscitation as well as transfusion of blood and blood components is essential. Antimicrobial prophylaxis appropriate for surgery is indicated. Ideally this would be combined with the treatment regimen for the pathogen thought to be responsible for the sepsis. Prophylactic antibiotics should be administered within 30 minutes of skin incision.

Postoperative

Patients with sepsis invariably require ICU admission after surgery. In the ICU the priorities include support of failing

TABLE 26.5	Systemic Inflammatory Response Syndrome (SIRS)

Diagnosis of SIRS requires fulfillment of two or more of the following criteria in a variety of clinical scenarios, *not necessarily involving infection:*
White blood cell count > 12,000/mm³ or < 4000/mm³ or more than 10% band forms
Heart rate > 90 beats/min
Temperature > 38°C or < 36°C
Respiratory rate > 20 breaths/min or $Paco_2$ < 32 mm Hg

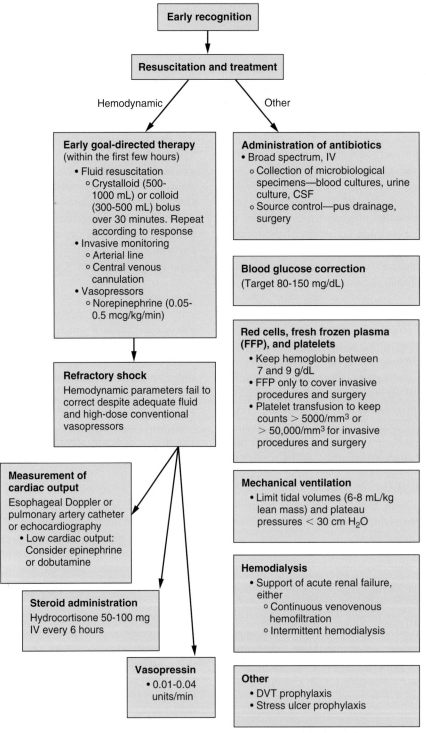

FIG. 26.3   Management of sepsis. *APACHE,* Acute Physiology and Chronic Health Evaluation II (score); *CSF,* cerebrospinal fluid; *DVT,* deep vein thrombosis; *IV,* intravenous(ly).

organ systems, targeted antimicrobial therapy, and minimizing the likelihood of new infections, such as a fungal infection, infection with *Clostridium difficile,* or the emergence of a resistant organism. Another important postoperative priority is continuation of antimicrobial therapy for only as long as it is indicated. Broad guidelines for treatment of patients with sepsis in the ICU have been published by the Society of Critical Care Medicine in the Surviving Sepsis Campaign Guidelines for Management of Severe Sepsis and Septic Shock.

GASTROINTESTINAL INFECTIONS

Clostridium Difficile Infection

C. difficile is an anaerobic, gram-positive, spore-forming bacterium that is the major identifiable cause of *antibiotic-associated* diarrhea and pseudomembranous colitis. It is clear today that most antibiotics can alter bowel flora, facilitating the growth of *C. difficile.* With the frequent use of broad-spectrum antibiotics, the incidence of *C. difficile* diarrhea has risen dramatically.

C. difficile infection is the most common cause of diarrhea in healthcare settings, resulting in increased hospital stays and higher morbidity and mortality among patients. The prevalence of asymptomatic colonization in the hospital, especially in older people, is over 20%. It is transmitted by spores that are resistant to heat, acid, and antibiotics. *C. difficile* is extremely hardy, can survive in the environment for prolonged periods of time, and is resistant to common disinfectants, which leads to transmission from contaminated surfaces and airborne spores. In approximately one-third of those colonized, *C. difficile* produces toxins that cause diarrhea. The two principal toxins are toxin A and toxin B. Toxin B is approximately 1000 times more cytotoxic than toxin A. Toxin A activates macrophages and mast cells. Activation of these cells causes production of inflammatory mediators, which leads to loss of intestinal barrier function and neutrophilic colitis. Toxin A is also an enterotoxin in that it loosens the tight junctions between the epithelial cells that line the colon, which helps toxin B enter these colonic cells.

A number of risk factors for *C. difficile*–associated diarrhea have been identified: advanced age (>65 years), severe underlying disease, gastrointestinal surgery, presence of a nasogastric tube, use of antiulcer medications such as proton pump inhibitors, admission to an ICU, long duration of hospital stay, long duration of antibiotic administration (risk doubles after 3 days), use of multiple antibiotics, immunosuppressive therapy or general immunocompromise, recent surgery, and sharing of a hospital room with a *C. difficile*–infected patient. Some antibiotics are frequently associated with *C. difficile* infection (Table 26.6).

Signs and Symptoms

The most frequent symptoms of *C. difficile* infection are diarrhea and abdominal pain. Patients may be febrile with

TABLE 26.6	Antibiotic Therapy Most Commonly Associated With *C. Difficile* Infection[a]
Clindamycin	
Fluoroquinolones	
Cephalosporins, carbapenems, monobactams	
Macrolides	
Sulfonamides	
Penicillins	
Tetracyclines	

[a]Listed in order of highest to lowest risk.

abdominal tenderness and distention. With perforation, patients may have an acute abdomen.

Diagnosis

The gold standard for diagnosis *C. difficile* infection is detection of *C. difficile* toxins A and B in stool. The detection of *C. difficile* antibody does not indicate current infection.

Treatment

Therapy for patients with *C. difficile*–associated diarrhea consists of fluid and electrolyte replacement, withdrawal of current antibiotic therapy if possible, and institution of targeted antibiotic treatment to eradicate *C. difficile.* Antibiotic treatment should be given orally if possible. The first-line regimen is oral metronidazole 500 mg three times daily. An alternative is oral vancomycin 125 mg four times daily. Vancomycin has a theoretical advantage over metronidazole, since it is poorly absorbed and may therefore be present in higher concentrations at the site of infection. The major downside to vancomycin is that it may promote the growth of vancomycin-resistant enterococci. In 2011 fidaxomicin was approved by the US Food and Drug Administration (FDA) for treatment of *C. difficile* infection. It appears to be equivalent in effect to vancomycin in curing infection and is superior to vancomycin in reducing the risk of recurrent *C. difficile* infection. It is, however, even more expensive than vancomycin therapy. Fecal microbial transplantation is another treatment for *C. difficile* infection. Transplantation of feces from a healthy tested donor administered in a solution via a nasoduodenal tube and the cessation of all antibiotics are successful in treating over 90% of recurrent *C. difficile* infections.

Additional therapies might include probiotics to restore normal bowel flora, but their usefulness has yet to be defined.

Prognosis

C. difficile infection accounts for considerable increases in length of hospital stays and more than $1.1 billion in healthcare costs each year in the United States. The condition is a common cause of significant morbidity and even death in elderly, debilitated, and immunocompromised patients.

Management of Anesthesia
Preoperative

It is generally the sickest patients with *C. difficile* colitis, including those whose infection does not improve with conventional therapy, who come for surgery such as subtotal colectomy and ileostomy. If the patient is hemodynamically unstable, major surgery should be deferred and an ileostomy, cecostomy, or colostomy performed as a temporizing intervention. Surgery is associated with high mortality. Resuscitation and preoperative treatment of metabolic derangements may be needed. Patients with *C. difficile* infection should be scheduled for surgery at the end of the surgical day so the operating room can undergo additional cleaning to minimize the risk of transmission to subsequent patients.

Intraoperative

Patients with fulminant *C. difficile* colitis are very ill, and hemodynamic instability is likely during anesthesia. Invasive monitoring, including an intraarterial catheter and central venous catheter, may guide fluid administration and the use of inotropes and vasopressors. Dehydration, acid base abnormalities, and electrolyte imbalances may be present because of the diarrhea. Opiates decrease intestinal motility, which may exacerbate toxin-mediated disease.

Postoperative

One of the most important considerations perioperatively is prevention of the spread of *C. difficile*. The spores are hardy and not destroyed by alcohol, so use of alcohol-based solutions for hand cleansing is *not* effective in removing *C. difficile* spores. Strict contact and isolation precautions, routine use of gloves and gowns, and *vigorous handwashing with soap and water* will remove spores and help prevent spread of this disease. Stethoscopes and neckties are potential repositories for spores.

CUTANEOUS INFECTIONS

Necrotizing Soft Tissue Infection

Necrotizing soft tissue infection is a nonspecific term that may encompass such diagnoses as gas gangrene, Fournier's gangrene, severe cellulitis, and "flesh-eating" infections. One of the most important aspects of these infections is that the severity of the infection may be underappreciated at the time of presentation. The responsible organisms are highly virulent, the clinical course is fulminant, and mortality is high (up to 75%). *Fournier's gangrene* was eponymously named for the French physician Jean Alfred Fournier, who described scrotal gangrene in five young men. He noted a sudden onset of symptoms, rapid progression to gangrene, and absence of a definite cause. Necrotizing soft tissue infections are surgical emergencies and represent a subclass of severe sepsis.

Signs and Symptoms

At presentation, patients may have general features of infection including malaise, fever, sweating, and altered mental status. Pain is invariable and may be out of proportion to the physical signs. Specific features may include scrotal swelling and erythema, vaginal discharge, tissue inflammation, pus, or subcutaneous air (crepitus). The cutaneous signs are often surprisingly mild and do not reflect the extent of tissue necrosis, because necrotizing skin infections begin in *deep* tissue planes. Hypotension is an ominous sign and may presage progression to septic shock. Resolution of pain may also be ominous, since this may occur with progression to gangrene.

Diagnosis

History is important in suggesting a diagnosis. Older patients and patients with a history of alcohol use, malnutrition, obesity, trauma, cancer, burns, vascular disease, and diabetes are more susceptible, as are patients taking immunosuppressant medication or those infected with HIV. There may be a high white blood cell count, thrombocytopenia, coagulopathy, electrolyte abnormalities, acidosis, hyperglycemia, elevated levels of markers of inflammation such as C-reactive protein, and radiographic evidence of extensive necrotic inflammation/necrosis with subcutaneous air. Ultrasonography, computed tomography (CT), or magnetic resonance imaging (MRI) may be used to delineate the extent of tissue necrosis. Blood, urine, and tissue samples should be sent to the laboratory for culture. Organisms most frequently grown from necrotic tissue include *Streptococcus pyogenes, S. aureus, S. epidermidis, Bacteroides* species, *Clostridium perfringens,* and gram-negative organisms, especially *Escherichia coli.* Polymicrobial infection is common.

Treatment

The definitive treatment is extensive débridement of necrotic tissue coupled with antimicrobial therapy, which typically includes coverage of gram-positive, gram-negative, and anaerobic organisms. Empirical broad-spectrum antibiotic coverage is provided initially, and treatment can subsequently be targeted to the specific organism(s) based on culture results.

Prognosis

Necrotizing soft tissue infection has a high mortality. If patients survive the initial insult, they remain vulnerable to secondary infection. They may require repeated anesthesia for débridements, skin grafts, and reconstructive surgery.

Management of Anesthesia
Preoperative

The anesthesiologist should treat patients with necrotizing soft tissue infection as having severe sepsis and should resuscitate preoperatively with goal-directed therapy, including administration of IV fluids and optimization of global oxygen delivery, with success reflected by resolution of lactic acidosis or an increase in mixed venous oxygen saturation. However, surgical débridement should *not* be postponed; any delay is associated with increased mortality.

Intraoperative

Concern has been raised about the use of etomidate for induction of anesthesia in patients with septic shock, since they may already have adrenal insufficiency, which theoretically may be worsened by even a single dose of etomidate. Major fluid shifts, blood loss, and release of cytokines occur intraoperatively.

Good IV access is essential, and invasive intraarterial and central venous monitoring may provide valuable information. Blood should be cross-matched and readily available. Patients are at risk of developing both hypovolemic and septic shock.

Postoperative
Like patients with sepsis, patients with necrotizing soft tissue infection are at risk of multiple organ failure. Postoperative admission to an ICU is prudent. Antibiotic therapy and fluid resuscitation should be continued in the postoperative period.

Tetanus

Tetanus is caused by the gram-negative bacillus *Clostridium tetani* and occurs when a wound or entry site becomes contaminated with bacterial spores. Production of the neurotoxin *tetanospasmin* is responsible for the clinical manifestations of tetanus. With the exception of botulinum toxin, tetanospasmin is the most powerful microbe-produced poison known. Tetanospasmin, when absorbed into wounds, spreads centrally along motor nerves to the spinal cord or enters the systemic circulation to reach the central nervous system (CNS). The toxin migrates into synapses, where it binds to presynaptic nerve terminals and inhibits or stops the release of certain inhibitory neurotransmitters such as glycine and γ-aminobutyric acid (GABA). Because the motor nerve has no inhibitory signals from other nerves, the chemical signal to the motor nerve of the muscle intensifies, causing the muscle to tighten up in a continuous contraction or spasm.

Tetanospasmin affects the nervous system in several areas. In the spinal cord, tetanospasmin suppresses inhibitory internuncial neurons, which results in generalized skeletal muscle contractions (spasms), and in the brain there is fixation of toxin by gangliosides. The fourth ventricle is believed to have selective permeability for tetanospasmin, which results in early manifestations of trismus and neck rigidity. Sympathetic nervous system hyperactivity may manifest as the disease progresses.

Signs and Symptoms
Trismus is the presenting symptom of tetanus in most patients. The greater strength of the masseter muscles compared with the opposing digastric and mylohyoid muscles results in *lockjaw*, and these patients may initially seek dental attention. Rigidity of the facial muscles results in the characteristic appearance described as *risus sardonicus*. Spasm of laryngeal muscles can occur at any time. Intractable pharyngeal spasms following tracheal extubation have been described in patients with unrecognized tetanus. Dysphagia may be due to spasm of the pharyngeal muscles. Spasm of the intercostal muscles and diaphragm interfere with adequate ventilation. The rigidity of abdominal and lumbar muscles accounts for the opisthotonic posture. Skeletal muscle spasms are tonic and clonic in nature and are excruciatingly painful. The increased skeletal muscle work is associated with dramatic increases in oxygen consumption, and peripheral vasoconstriction can contribute to hyperthermia.

External stimulation (e.g., sudden exposure to bright light, unexpected noise, tracheal suctioning) can precipitate generalized skeletal muscle spasms, leading to inadequate ventilation and death. Hypotension has been attributed to myocarditis. Isolated and unexplained tachycardia may be an early manifestation of hyperactivity of the sympathetic nervous system, but more often this hyperactivity is manifested as systemic hypertension. Sympathetic nervous system responses to external stimuli are exaggerated, as demonstrated by tachydysrhythmias and labile blood pressure. In addition, excessive sympathetic nervous system activity is associated with intense peripheral vasoconstriction and diaphoresis.

Treatment
Treatment of patients with tetanus is directed toward controlling the skeletal muscle spasms, preventing sympathetic hyperactivity, supporting ventilation, neutralizing circulating toxin, and surgically débriding the affected area to eliminate the source of the toxin. Diazepam or lorazepam are preferred for controlling skeletal muscle spasms. Administration of nondepolarizing muscle relaxants and mechanical ventilation may be necessary. Indeed, early protection of the upper airway is important, since laryngospasm may accompany generalized skeletal muscle spasms. Overactivity of the sympathetic nervous system can be managed with IV administration of β-blockers. The circulating exotoxin may be neutralized by intrathecal or intramuscular administration of human antitetanus immunoglobulin. This neutralization does not alter the symptoms already present but does prevent additional exotoxin from reaching the CNS. Penicillin or metronidazole can destroy the toxin-producing vegetative forms of *C. tetani*.

Management of Anesthesia
General anesthesia including tracheal intubation is a useful approach for surgical débridement. Surgical débridement is delayed until several hours after the patient has received antitoxin, because tetanospasmin is mobilized into the systemic circulation during surgical resection. Invasive monitoring is indicated and should include continuous recording of systemic blood pressure and measurement of central venous pressure. Volatile anesthetics are useful for maintenance of anesthesia if excessive sympathetic nervous system activity is present. Drugs such as lidocaine, esmolol, metoprolol, magnesium, nicardipine, and nitroprusside should be readily available during the perioperative period.

RESPIRATORY INFECTIONS

Pneumonia

Community-Acquired Pneumonia
Combined with influenza, community-acquired pneumonia is one of the 10 leading causes of death in the United States. *Streptococcus pneumoniae* is by far the most frequent cause of bacterial pneumonia in adults. *S. pneumoniae* causes *typical* pneumonia. Influenza virus, *Mycoplasma pneumoniae,*

chlamydia, legionella, adenovirus, and other microorganisms may cause *atypical* pneumonia. These latter pneumonias are considered atypical because the organisms are not common pneumonia-producing bacteria, do not respond to common antibiotics, and can cause uncommon symptoms.

Aspiration Pneumonia

Patients with *depressed consciousness* may experience aspiration that in the presence of underlying diseases that impair host defense mechanisms may manifest as aspiration pneumonia. Alcohol- and drug-induced alterations of consciousness, head trauma, seizures, other neurologic disorders, and administration of sedatives are most often responsible for the development of aspiration pneumonia. Patients with *abnormalities of swallowing or esophageal motility* resulting from placement of nasogastric tubes, esophageal cancer, bowel obstruction, or repeated vomiting are also prone to aspiration. Poor oral hygiene and periodontal disease predispose to development of pneumonia after aspiration because of the increased bacterial flora in the aspirate. Induction and recovery from anesthesia may place patients at increased risk of aspiration.

Clinical manifestations of pulmonary aspiration depend on the nature and volume of aspirated material. Aspiration of large volumes of acidic gastric fluid produces fulminant pneumonia and arterial hypoxemia. Aspiration of particulate material may result in airway obstruction, and smaller particles may produce atelectasis. Infiltrates are most common in those areas of the lungs that were in a dependent position at the time of aspiration. Penicillin-sensitive anaerobes are the most likely cause of aspiration pneumonia. Hospitalization or antibiotic therapy alters the usual oropharyngeal flora, so aspiration pneumonia in hospitalized patients often involves pathogens that are uncommon in community-acquired pneumonia.

Postoperative Pneumonia

Postoperative pneumonia occurs in approximately 20% of patients undergoing major thoracic, esophageal, or upper abdominal surgery but is rare after other procedures in previously fit patients. Chronic lung disease increases the incidence of postoperative pneumonia threefold. Other risk factors include obesity, age older than 70 years, and operations lasting longer than 2 hours.

Lung Abscess

Lung abscess may develop after bacterial pneumonia. Alcohol abuse and poor dental hygiene are important risk factors. Septic pulmonary embolization, which is most often seen in IV drug abusers, may also result in formation of a lung abscess. The finding of an air-fluid level on the chest radiograph signifies rupture of the abscess into the bronchial tree. Foul-smelling sputum is characteristic. Antibiotics are the mainstay of treatment of a lung abscess. Surgery is indicated only when complications such as empyema occur. Thoracentesis is necessary to establish the diagnosis of empyema, and treatment requires chest tube drainage and antibiotics. Surgical drainage may be necessary to treat chronic empyema.

Diagnosis

An initial chill followed by abrupt onset of fever, chest pain, dyspnea, fatigue, rigors, cough, and copious sputum production often characterize bacterial pneumonia. Nonproductive cough is a feature of atypical pneumonia. A detailed history may suggest possible causative organisms. Hotels and whirlpools are associated with outbreaks of legionnaires disease. Fungal pneumonia may occur with cave exploration and diving. *Chlamydia psittaci* pneumonia may follow contact with birds, and Q fever may follow contact with sheep. Alcoholism increases the risk of aspiration. Patients who are immunocompromised, such as those with acquired immunodeficiency syndrome (AIDS), are at risk of fungal pneumonia, such as *Pneumocystis* pneumonia.

Chest radiography may be extremely helpful in diagnosing pneumonia. Diffuse infiltrates are suggestive of an atypical pneumonia, whereas a lobar opacification is suggestive of a typical pneumonia. Atypical pneumonia occurs more frequently in young adults. Radiography is useful for detecting pleural effusions and multilobar involvement. Leukocytosis is typical, and arterial hypoxemia may occur in severe cases of bacterial pneumonia. Arterial hypoxemia reflects intrapulmonary shunting resulting from perfusion of alveoli filled with inflammatory exudates.

Microscopic examination of sputum plus cultures and sensitivity testing may be helpful in suggesting the cause of the pneumonia and in guiding antibiotic treatment. Unfortunately, sputum specimens are frequently inadequate, and organisms do not always grow from sputum. Interpretation of sputum culture results may be challenging. If there is suspicion of TB, sputum specimens should be sent for testing for acid-fast bacilli. Antigen detection in urine is a good test for *Legionella,* whereas blood antibody titers are helpful in diagnosing *Mycoplasma* pneumonia. Sputum polymerase chain reaction (PCR) testing is useful for diagnosing *Chlamydia* infection. Blood cultures usually yield negative results but are important to rule out bacteremia. HIV infection is an important risk factor for pneumonia and should be ruled out when pneumonia is suspected.

Treatment

For severe pneumonia, empirical therapy is typically a combination of antibiotic drugs. However, local patterns of antibiotic resistance should always be considered before initiating therapy.

Therapy is advised for 10 days for pneumonia caused by *S. pneumoniae* and for 14 days for that caused by *M. pneumoniae* or *Chlamydia pneumoniae.* When symptoms resolve, therapy can be switched from the IV to the oral route. Inappropriate prescription of antibiotics for *nonbacterial* respiratory tract infections is common and promotes antibiotic resistance. It has recently been demonstrated that even brief administration of a macrolide antibiotic such as azithromycin to healthy subjects promotes resistance of oral streptococcal flora that lasts for months. Resistance of *S. pneumoniae* to antibiotics is becoming a problem. In 2013 30% of pneumococcal bacteria

TABLE 26.7 Elements of Pneumonia Severity Index

Age in years
Gender
Nursing home resident
Neoplastic disease history
Liver disease
Congestive heart failure
Cerebrovascular disease
Renal disease
Altered mental status
Respiratory rate > 29 breaths/min
Systolic blood pressure < 90 mm Hg
Temperature < 35°C or > 39.9°C
Pulse > 124 beats/min
pH < 7.35
Blood urea nitrogen > 29 mg/dL
Sodium < 130 mmol/L
Glucose > 249 mg/dL
Hematocrit < 30%
Pa_{O_2} < 60 mm Hg
Pleural effusion on radiograph

were resistant to one or more antibiotics. Expanded use of pneumococcal vaccines may slow or reverse this emerging drug resistance.

Prognosis

The Pneumonia Severity Index (Table 26.7) is a useful tool for aiding clinical judgment, guiding appropriate management, and suggesting prognosis. Old age and co-existing organ dysfunction have a negative impact. **Physical examination findings** associated with worse outcome are:

T temperature ≤ 35°C or ≥ 40°C

R respiratory rate ≥ 30 breaths/min

A altered mental status

S systolic blood pressure < 90 mm Hg

H heart rate ≥ 125 beats/min

Laboratory findings and other test results indicative of a poorer prognosis are:

H hypoxia (Po_2 < 60 mm Hg or saturation < 90% on room air)

E effusion

A anemia (hematocrit < 30%)

R renal: blood urea nitrogen > 29 mg/dL

G glucose > 250 mg/dL

A acidosis (pH < 7.35)

S sodium < 130 mmol/L

Management of Anesthesia

Anesthesia and surgery should ideally be deferred if acute pneumonia is present. Patients with acute pneumonia are often dehydrated and may have renal insufficiency. Fluid management can be challenging, since overhydration may worsen gas exchange and morbidity. If general anesthesia is used, a protective ventilation strategy is appropriate, with tidal volumes of 6–8 mL/kg ideal body mass and mean airway pressures of less than 30 cm H_2O. The anesthesiologist can perform pulmonary hygiene, including actively removing secretions during

the period of intubation, even with bronchoscopy if needed. Endotracheal intubation offers the opportunity to obtain distal sputum specimens for Gram stain and culture.

Ventilator-Associated Pneumonia

Ventilator-associated pneumonia (VAP) is the most common nosocomial infection in the ICU and makes up one-third of all nosocomial infections. *VAP is defined as pneumonia developing more than 48 hours after mechanical ventilation has been initiated via endotracheal tube or tracheostomy.* Between 10% and 20% of patients who have endotracheal tubes and undergo mechanical ventilation for longer than 48 hours acquire VAP, with mortality rates ranging from 5%–50%. VAP increases a patient's hospital stay by approximately 7–9 days and can increase hospital costs by an average of $40,000 per patient.

Several simple interventions may decrease the occurrence of VAP: ensuring meticulous hand hygiene for all caregivers, providing oral care, limiting patient sedation, positioning patients semi-upright, performing repeated aspiration of subglottic secretions, limiting intubation time if feasible, and considering the appropriateness of *noninvasive ventilatory support.*

Diagnosis

VAP is difficult to differentiate from other common causes of respiratory failure such as acute respiratory distress syndrome (ARDS) and pulmonary edema. VAP is usually suspected when a patient develops a new or progressive infiltrate on chest radiograph, together with leukocytosis and purulent tracheobronchial secretions. An endotracheal tube or a tracheostomy tube provides a foreign surface that rapidly becomes colonized with upper airway flora. However, the mere presence of potentially pathogenic organisms in tracheal secretions is not diagnostic of VAP. A standardized diagnostic algorithm for VAP was developed in 2004, employing clinical and microbiological data into a Clinical Pulmonary Infection Score (CPIS) to promote diagnostic consistency among clinicians and investigators. However, the sensitivity and specificity of the CPIS are lower than is desirable. As a result the CPIS has been modified in various ways to both simplify data collection and improve its utility. One such modification is shown in Table 26.8. However, the accurate diagnosis of VAP remains elusive.

Treatment and Prognosis

Treatment of VAP includes supportive care for respiratory failure plus antibiotics against the organism most likely to be implicated. The most common pathogens are *Pseudomonas aeruginosa* and *S. aureus.* Prognosis is improved if treatment is initiated early. Therefore despite the high rate of false-positive diagnoses, broad-spectrum antibiotic therapy should be initiated to cover resistant organisms such as MRSA and *P. aeruginosa.* Treatment should be narrowed to target specific organisms once results of culture and sensitivity testing are available and should be stopped at 48 hours if culture results are negative. Fig. 26.4 presents an algorithm to guide treatment.

TABLE 26.8	A Modified Clinical Pulmonary Infection Score	
Parameter	Options	Score
Temperature (°C)	≥36.5 and ≤ 38.4	0
	≥38.5 and ≤ 38.9	1
	≥39 or ≤ 36	2
Blood leuko-cytes (per mm³)	≥4000 and ≤ 11,000	0
	<4000 or >11000	1
	+ Band forms ≥ 50%	Add 1
Tracheal secre-tions	No secretions	0
	Abundant secretions	1
	Abundant and purulent secretions	2
Oxygenation: Pao₂/Fio₂ (mm Hg)	>240 or ARDS	0
	≤240 and no ARDS	2
Pulmonary radio-graph	No infiltrate	0
	Diffuse (or patchy) infiltrate	1
	Localized infiltrate	2
Culture of tra-cheal aspirate	Negative	0
	Positive	2

ARDS, Acute respiratory distress syndrome; *Pao₂/Fio₂;* ratio of arterial oxygen pressure to fraction of inspired oxygen.

Management of Anesthesia

Patients with VAP frequently require anesthesia for tracheostomy. Major surgery should be deferred until the pneumonia has resolved and respiratory function has improved. Tracheostomy is not an emergency procedure, and it may be ill advised to proceed when the patient has minimal pulmonary reserve. One of the major goals for the anesthesiologist in this situation is to ensure that patients with VAP do not experience a setback following anesthesia and tracheostomy. Because patients with respiratory failure may be positive end-expiratory pressure (PEEP) dependent, a PEEP valve should be used to decrease the likelihood of "de-recruitment" of alveoli during transport to the operating room. In the operating room, protective mechanical ventilation should be used. Ideally the same ventilator settings, mode of ventilation, and PEEP that were used in the ICU should be continued.

Severe Acute Respiratory Syndrome and Influenza

Influenza pandemics have been described throughout history and typically occur several times each century. The influenza pandemic of 1918 was one of the major plagues to have affected humankind. It is estimated that this "Spanish flu" infected as many as 500 million people worldwide and led to the deaths of as many as 50–100 million people in just 25 weeks. The Spanish flu was caused by an H1N1 strain of influenza virus that continues to cause human influenza pandemics. The 1957 and 1968 pandemics did not approach the catastrophic level of the 1918 pandemic.

H1N1 influenza (so named for the specific types of capsular peptides—*hemagglutinin* and *neuraminidase*—found on

the virus) continues to impact society to this day, and CDC estimates for the 2009 pandemic of influenza A (H1N1) in the United States from April 2009 to January 2010 was 57 million cases, 257,000 hospitalizations, and 11,700 deaths. In seasonal influenza the greatest mortality is among the very young and the very old. In contrast the 1918 and 2009 epidemics affected children and younger adults.

Influenza A virus and the virus causing *severe acute respiratory syndrome* (SARS) are examples of respiratory viruses that may be associated with rampant courses, high virulence, and high mortality. From 2002–2003, SARS occurred without any warning and was a grim reminder of our vulnerability to new infectious diseases. SARS affected populations in Asia, the Pacific Rim, and Canada. The causative agent for SARS was thought to be an RNA coronavirus that was passed along through direct contact and droplet spread. This virus is viable ex vivo for 24–48 hours. Twenty percent of the victims of the 2003 SARS coronavirus outbreak were healthcare workers. There were over 8000 documented cases of SARS coronavirus infection and approximately 700 deaths in 29 countries.

A new strain of avian influenza or "bird flu," the H5N1 strain, which is a subtype of influenza A, is now threatening humankind. Influenza is an RNA orthomyxovirus; like other RNA viruses, it mutates at an alarming rate. The World Health Organization (WHO) has reported that 478 human cases of avian influenza occurred between 2003 and 2010, with 286 deaths. Many cases were in young children. Currently, H5N1 influenza A is passed from bird to human. This virus has not developed a high affinity for human respiratory tract receptors. Therefore human-to-human transmission is not sustained, and cases have occurred only in small clusters.

Signs and Symptoms

Symptoms include nonspecific complaints of viral infection such as cough, sore throat, headache, diarrhea, arthralgias, and muscle pain. In more severe cases, patients may show respiratory distress, confusion, and hemoptysis. Signs may include fever, tachycardia, sweating, conjunctivitis, rash, tachypnea, use of accessory respiratory muscles, cyanosis, and pulmonary features of pneumonia, pleural effusion, or pneumothorax. A chest radiograph may show patchy infiltrates, areas of opacification, pneumothoraces, and/or evidence of pleural effusion. Both H5N1 influenza A virus and SARS coronavirus infection may cause acute lung injury and ARDS. Viruses that exhibit a propensity to bind to receptors in the lower respiratory tract may cause hemorrhagic bronchitis and pneumonia with diffuse alveolar damage and destruction. Complications include sepsis and multiple organ failure.

Diagnosis

In the context of an outbreak, history, symptoms, and presentation are usually sufficient to suggest the diagnosis. A definitive diagnosis is made by detection of the virus in

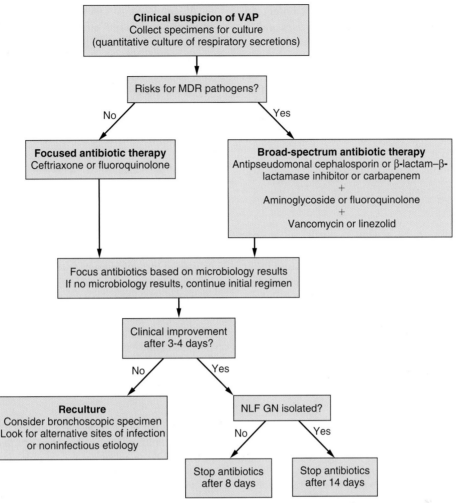

FIG. 26.4 Management of ventilator-associated pneumonia (VAP). *GN,* Gram-negative (organism); *NLF,* non–lactose fermenting; *MDR,* multidrug-resistant. (Adapted from Porzecanski I, Bowton DL. Diagnosis and treatment of ventilator-associated pneumonia. *Chest.* 2006;130:597-604.)

sputum. The problem with serologic testing is that it may take 2–3 weeks for seroconversion (development of antibodies) after infection. PCR tests can detect genetic material from these viruses in various body fluids and tissues and are useful for diagnosing both SARS coronavirus infection and H5N1 influenza A.

Treatment
Vaccine development is a key component in preventing widespread viral infection and reducing morbidity and mortality associated with viral infection. Thus far there is no vaccine for either the SARS coronavirus or the H5N1 influenza A virus. For H5N1 influenza, neuraminidase inhibitors have been developed, including zanamivir and oseltamivir. These drugs may decrease the severity of infection, but sufficient quantities of these drugs are not likely to be available in the event of a major outbreak. Other pharmacologic treatments for influenza include amantadine and rimantadine. Antiviral drugs are of modest benefit and help only if administered within the first 48 hours of symptoms. There is no proven drug therapy that attenuates the course of SARS.

The mainstay of treatment for influenza and SARS is supportive care.

Prognosis
Prognosis depends on the virulence of the infecting virus as well as the susceptibility of the infected person. Influenza and SARS may trigger a marked inflammatory response and a cytokine storm. A clinical picture indistinguishable from severe bacterial sepsis may result. Superinfection with bacteria has been described and considerably worsens the outcome.

Management of Anesthesia
Preoperative
The anesthesiologist should assess the patient with an appreciation of the potentially deadly nature of the infection. Both patient and family should be counseled about the high risks associated with SARS coronavirus infection. Since primary transmission is via direct and indirect respiratory droplet spread, these viruses are highly contagious. Strict patient isolation should be enforced, and precautions

to protect healthcare workers must be taken. Contact precautions are also necessary because the viruses can be spread via fomites such as clothing, contaminated surfaces, and exposed skin.

Ideally, infected patients should be cared for in rooms with negative pressure to decrease aerosolized spread and contagion. Barrier precautions include use of full-body disposable oversuits, double gloves, goggles, and powered air-purifying respirators with high-efficiency particulate air filters. If these are not available, N95 masks (which block 95% of particles) should be used rather than regular surgical masks.

Intraoperative

Aerosolized particles may be generated during all invasive airway procedures, ventilation with noninvasive and positive pressure ventilator support modes, suctioning, sputum induction, high-flow oxygen delivery, aerosolized or nebulized medication delivery, and interventions that stimulate coughing. If mechanical ventilation is required, protective ventilation is indicated. Tidal volumes should be limited to 6–8 mL/kg lean body mass, and mean airway pressure should be less than 30 cm H_2O. Sudden cardiorespiratory compromise could indicate an expanding pneumothorax. Drainage of pleural effusions may improve ventilation and gas exchange.

Postoperative

Precautions to prevent spread of infection should be ongoing. The same treatment principles as for ARDS and sepsis should apply.

Tuberculosis

Mycobacterium tuberculosis is the obligate aerobe responsible for TB. This organism survives and thrives in tissues with high oxygen concentrations, which is consistent with the increased presentation of TB in the apices of the lungs.

In the past, many cases of TB in the United States were due to reactivation of infection, especially in elderly individuals. However, from 1985–1992, the United States was confronted with an unprecedented resurgence in TB. This resurgence was accompanied by a rise in *MDR TB,* defined as TB caused by *M. tuberculosis* strains resistant to the most effective first-line drugs—isoniazid and rifampin. In addition, virtually untreatable strains of the TB organism are emerging worldwide. *XDR strains* of *M. tuberculosis* are resistant to second-line therapeutic agents including fluoroquinolones and at least one of three injectables used to treat TB—amikacin, kanamycin, and capreomycin. Mortality rates for patients with XDR TB are similar to those for TB patients in the preantibiotic era. Unfortunately, drug-resistant TB is a manmade problem resulting from poor adherence of infected patients to their medical regimens or improper treatment regimen designs. Worldwide, approximately 2 billion persons are infected with *M. tuberculosis*. In 2015 the WHO estimated that 480,000 new cases of MDR TB occurred worldwide.

At present most cases of TB in the United States occur in minority racial and ethnic groups, foreign-born individuals from areas where TB is endemic (Asia, Africa), IV drug abusers, and patients who are HIV seropositive or have AIDS. Any patient with TB should be tested for HIV, since there is a high association between the two infections. However, even in patients who are HIV negative, MDR TB has a 26% mortality rate. The epidemiologic increase in the incidence of TB coincided with the initial AIDS epidemic in the early 1980s.

Almost all *M. tuberculosis* infections result from inhalation of aerosolized droplets. It has been estimated that up to 600,000 droplet nuclei are expelled with each cough and that the expelled organisms remain viable for several days. Although a single infectious unit is capable of causing infection in susceptible individuals, prolonged exposure in closed environments is optimal for transmission of infection. An estimated 90% of patients infected with *M. tuberculosis* never become symptomatic and are identified only by conversion of the tuberculin skin test or by results on an interferon release assay. Often patients who acquire the infection early in life do not become symptomatic until much later. Patients who are HIV seropositive or immunocompromised with AIDS are at much higher risk of becoming symptomatic, especially after initiation of highly active antiretroviral therapy (HAART).

Diagnosis

The diagnosis of TB is based on the presence of clinical symptoms, the epidemiologic likelihood of infection, and the results of diagnostic tests. Symptoms of pulmonary TB often include persistent nonproductive cough, anorexia, weight loss, chest pain, hemoptysis, and night sweats. The most common test for TB is the tuberculin skin test (Mantoux test). The skin reaction is read in 48–72 hours, and a positive reaction is generally defined as induration of more than 10 mm. For patients with severe immunocompromise, including but not limited to AIDS, a reaction of 5 mm or more is considered positive. Because the skin test is nonspecific, its utility is limited. The tuberculin skin test result may be positive if the individual has received a bacille Calmette-Guérin (BCG) vaccine or has been exposed to TB or other mycobacteria, even if no viable mycobacteria are present at the time of the test. The CDC and WHO have now accepted two interferon release assays as equivalent to—and possibly even better than—the tuberculin skin test in sensitivity and specificity. These are the QuantiFERON TB Gold In-Tube test and the T-SPOT.*TB* test. Both are blood tests that measure release of interferon (IFN)-γ from sensitized lymphocytes that are incubated with two peptides from the TB bacillus. Results of these tests are not affected by prior BCG immunization, nor do the tests cross-react with common environmental mycobacteria or *Mycobacterium avium-intracellulare.*

Chest radiographs are important for the diagnosis of TB. Apical or subapical infiltrates are highly suggestive of TB. Bilateral upper lobe infiltration with cavitation is also common. Patients with AIDS may demonstrate a less classic picture on chest radiography, which may be further confounded by the presence of *Pneumocystis* pneumonia. Tuberculous vertebral osteomyelitis (Pott's disease) is a common manifestation of extrapulmonary TB.

Sputum smears and cultures are used to diagnose TB. Smears are examined for the presence of acid-fast bacilli. This test is based on the ability of mycobacteria to take up and retain neutral red stains after an acid wash. It is estimated that 50%–80% of individuals with active TB have positive sputum smear results. Although the absence of acid-fast bacilli does not rule out TB, a sputum culture positive for *M. tuberculosis* provides a definitive diagnosis.

Healthcare workers are at increased risk for occupational acquisition of TB; TB is twice as prevalent in physicians as in the general population. Nosocomial outbreaks of TB have occurred, especially among patients with AIDS. Anesthesiologists are at increased risk of nosocomial TB by virtue of events surrounding the induction and maintenance of anesthesia that may induce coughing (tracheal intubation, tracheal suctioning, mechanical ventilation). Bronchoscopy is a particularly high-risk procedure for anesthesiologists and has been associated with conversion of the tuberculin skin test. As a first step in preventing occupational acquisition of TB, anesthesia personnel should participate in annual tuberculin screening so that those who develop a positive skin test result may be offered chemotherapy. The decision to initiate TB chemotherapy is not trivial, since treatment may cause significant toxicity. A baseline chest radiograph is indicated at the time of the first positive tuberculin skin test result.

Treatment

Antituberculous chemotherapy has decreased mortality from TB by more than 90%. With adequate treatment, more than 90% of patients who have susceptible strains of *M. tuberculosis* have bacteriologically negative sputum smears within 3 months.

Some argue that for the protection of the community, people who have positive results on a skin test should receive chemotherapy with isoniazid. However, isoniazid is a potentially toxic drug; its toxicity is manifested in the peripheral nervous system and liver. Neurotoxicity may be prevented by daily administration of pyridoxine. Hepatotoxicity is most likely to be related to metabolism of isoniazid by hepatic acetylation. Depending on genetically determined traits, patients may be characterized as slow or rapid acetylators. Hepatitis appears to be more common in rapid acetylators, consistent with their greater production of hydrazine, a potentially hepatotoxic metabolite of isoniazid. Persistent elevations of serum transaminase concentrations mandate that isoniazid be discontinued, but mild transient increases do not.

Other first-line drugs used to treat TB include rifampicin, pyrazinamide, streptomycin, and ethambutol. Adverse effects of rifampicin include thrombocytopenia, leukopenia, anemia, and renal failure. Hepatitis associated with increases in serum transaminase concentrations occurs in approximately 10% of patients being treated with rifampicin. *To be curative, treatment for pulmonary TB should continue for 6 months.*

Extrapulmonary TB usually requires a longer course of antituberculous therapy.

Management of Anesthesia

Preoperative assessment of patients considered to be at risk of having TB includes taking a detailed history with questions concerning the presence of a persistent cough and tuberculin test status. Patients with HIV or AIDS should undergo a thorough review of systems to elicit a possible history of TB.

Elective surgical procedures should be postponed until patients are no longer considered infectious. Patients are considered noninfectious if they have received antituberculous chemotherapy, are improving clinically, and have had three consecutive negative findings on sputum smears. If surgery cannot be delayed, it is important to limit the number of involved personnel, and high-risk procedures (bronchoscopy, tracheal intubation, and suctioning) should be performed in a negative-pressure environment whenever possible. Patients should be transported to the operating room wearing a tight-fitting N95 face mask to prevent casual exposure of others to airborne bacilli. Staff should also wear N95 masks.

A high-efficiency particulate air filter should be placed in the anesthesia delivery circuit between the Y connector and the mask, laryngeal mask airway, or tracheal tube. Bacterial filters should be placed on the exhalation limb of the anesthesia delivery circuit to decrease the discharge of tubercle bacilli into the ambient air. Anesthesia equipment should be sterilized with standard methods, using a disinfectant that destroys tubercle bacilli. Use of a dedicated anesthesia machine and ventilator is recommended. Postoperative care should, if possible, take place in a negative-pressure isolation room.

INFECTIOUS DISEASES IN SOLID ORGAN TRANSPLANT RECIPIENTS

Each year, over 16,000 patients in the United States receive solid organ transplants, and this number is expected to continue rising. Patients who have received solid organ transplants (liver, kidney, heart, lung) present unique perioperative challenges to the anesthesiologist. Because of advances in surgical technique, immunosuppressive therapy, and medical management, this patient population has a 1-year survival rate of 80%–90%, so these patients are coming for additional surgical procedures not necessarily related to their organ transplant.

To prevent allograft rejection, solid organ transplant recipients commonly receive a combination of immunosuppressive drugs. The mechanisms of action of immunosuppressants include blunting of general antibody responses, depression of cell-mediated immunity, down-modulation of lymphocyte and macrophage function, inhibition of cell proliferation, blocking of T-cell activation, and depletion of T-cells. Regardless of the effect, immunosuppression is variable and depends on dosage, duration of therapy, and time since transplantation. Immunosuppression is most intense in the first few months after transplantation and becomes progressively less intense as immunosuppressive therapy is gradually withdrawn over time.

Immunosuppression in transplant recipients can also be affected by metabolic abnormalities, damage to mucocutaneous barriers, foreign bodies that interrupt these barriers (e.g., surgical incisions, chest tubes, biliary drains, endotracheal tubes, urinary catheters), and the possible presence of immunomodulating viruses such as cytomegalovirus and HIV. Therefore the resultant state of immunosuppression in the posttransplantation patient is a dynamic condition that impacts the development of infectious diseases and/or cancer.

Infectious Disease Occurrence

The best approach to infection control in the solid organ transplant recipient is prevention. If prevention is not possible, immediate diagnosis and treatment are essential. Challenges in managing infectious diseases in organ transplant recipients are many and include:

1. The spectrum of infective organisms is diverse and unusual.
2. The inflammatory response is blunted because of immunosuppressive therapy, so clinical and radiologic findings may be limited.
3. Antimicrobial coverage is complex and typically empirically based.

There are three major time periods during which specific infectious disease processes occur in the posttransplantation patient: the first month, the second through sixth months, and beyond the sixth month. In addition, these periods may be influenced by surgical factors, the net level of immunosuppression present, and environmental exposures. Defining the time period after transplantation will assist the clinician in determining likely infectious processes.

During the first month after transplantation, active infections can be harbored within the allograft and are typically bacterial or fungal. In addition, anatomic defects related to surgery (e.g., devitalized tissue, undrained fluid collections at high risk for microbial seeding) must be addressed if they foster infection. The only common viral infection during the first month after transplantation is reactivated herpes simplex virus infection in individuals positive for this virus before transplantation.

The period from the second through the sixth month after transplantation may be marked by unusual infections. These may be either community-acquired or opportunistic infections. Opportunistic pathogens possess very little virulence in healthy hosts but can cause serious infections in patients with immunocompromise. Trimethoprim-sulfamethoxazole is commonly given as prophylaxis for *Pneumocystis* pneumonia during the first 6 months after transplantation in all solid organ graft recipients and for longer periods in heart and lung transplant recipients.

In addition, high-dose immunosuppression may lead to *reactivation disease syndromes* caused by organisms present in the recipient before transplantation. TB has become especially common and occurs in 1% of the posttransplant population.

From 6 months after transplantation onward, most transplant recipients do fairly well from an infectious disease standpoint and usually only sustain infections paralleling those seen in the community at large. However, another group of patients may have chronic or progressive viral infections with hepatitis B virus, hepatitis C virus, cytomegalovirus, or Epstein-Barr virus. The most commonly occurring viral infection is varicella-zoster virus infection manifesting as herpes zoster.

Patients with chronic or recurrent rejection are generally taking high dosages of immunosuppressants and are predisposed to acquiring the opportunistic infections typically seen in posttransplantation patients during the second to sixth months. In addition, posttransplantation patients with HIV and/or AIDS must be more closely followed for evidence of infections, both common and opportunistic. HIV HAART regimens must be maintained and can complicate immunosuppressive drug dosing.

Management of Anesthesia

Preoperative

Patients who have received solid organ transplants comprise a wide clinical spectrum, and it is difficult to make any generalizations about this patient population. Overall the preoperative assessment should focus on determining the degree of immunosuppression and allograft function, examining for the presence of any infection, and evaluating any co-existing medical diseases. Laboratory evaluation should include a complete blood cell count (CBC), full metabolic panel, liver function tests, viral panels with viral loads as indicated, chest radiograph, and electrocardiogram (ECG). If patients are currently receiving immunosuppressants, blood levels of immunosuppressive agents should also be obtained when possible. Findings elicited on history taking, review of systems, and physical examination may serve as indicators for additional laboratory testing or further specialist evaluations. Evidence of active rejection is a contraindication to elective surgery. However, one may be faced with managing anesthesia in a posttransplantation patient with active rejection who requires explantation of the transplanted organ. This is considered an emergent procedure.

All medications and antimicrobial drugs taken by the patient should be noted, and these drugs should be continued during the perioperative period. If the posttransplantation patient manifests *any* active infection, surgery should be delayed or cancelled until additional consultation is obtained.

Intraoperative

All anesthetic techniques—general anesthesia, regional anesthesia, and sedation—have been used successfully in posttransplantation patients. Selection of anesthetic technique should be based on the type of surgery to be performed, the patient's associated comorbid conditions, the presence of contraindications for specific anesthetic techniques, and the potential for interactions between immunosuppressive and anesthetic drugs.

Use of regional anesthesia in immunosuppressed patients remains controversial, since studies have demonstrated that infections may occur secondary to neuraxial blockade. However, few studies have evaluated the frequency of epidural abscess or meningitis in the immunocompromised population. Information on the incidence of infection during peripheral nerve blockade and pain procedures in immunocompromised posttransplantation patients is scant. With regard to general anesthesia, nasal intubation should be avoided because it may introduce nasal bacterial flora into the systemic circulation. Overall, general anesthesia is considered to create more generalized immunosuppressant effects than regional anesthesia, although levels of specific and nonspecific biological markers indicating immune suppression are not consistently depressed. Cyclosporine may delay the metabolism of neuromuscular blockers, specifically pancuronium and vecuronium. Invasive monitoring may be warranted, but strict use of aseptic technique during insertion of catheters is critical in this patient population.

Postoperative

Because of the high potential for further immunosuppression secondary to anesthesia and surgery, the posttransplantation patient must be observed for any clinical deterioration in graft function or any indication of an infectious process. All antibiotic regimens must be strictly followed and monitored closely. Because of the blunted inflammatory response in immunosuppressed patients, signs and symptoms of active infection are often difficult to detect.

HIV INFECTION AND AIDS

The disease syndrome now known as *AIDS* was first described in 1981 and initially termed *gay-related immune disorder* because it was identified in a group of homosexual men in Los Angeles, California. The etiologic mechanism was initially unknown. However, severe immune dysfunction was present and was manifested clinically by the occurrence of unusual malignancies and opportunistic infections in previously healthy individuals. The disease was later reclassified as *acquired immunodeficiency syndrome* (AIDS). In 1984 the cause of AIDS was elucidated and found to be a retrovirus that was named *human immunodeficiency virus (HIV) type 1* and *type 2*.

Thirty years later, HIV infection and the associated AIDS pandemic continue to pose a major threat to global health. It is estimated that more than 50 million people worldwide ($\approx$0.6% of the world's population) are infected with HIV, and AIDS is thought to have caused more than 26 million deaths worldwide. There are approximately 1.2 million people in the United States living with HIV infection and/or AIDS, and 1 in 8 is unaware of their infection. HIV disease continues to spread. The most rapid increases are being observed in southern and central Africa and in Southeast Asia. Throughout the world, the predominant mode of HIV transmission is by heterosexual sex, with women representing a large proportion of the new infections. Other sources of infection globally include IV drug use, vertical transmission from pregnant mother to child, and blood transfusion. However,

TABLE 26.9	Routes of Transmission of HIV Infection in United States
Transmission Category	New Cases of HIV (%)
Men who have sex with men (MSM)	63
Heterosexual sex (twice as many women as men get infected)	25
Injection drug use	8
MSM with injection drug use	3
Other	<1

Data from Centers for Disease Control and Prevention 2010 Statistics.

in the United States the largest population of persons infected with HIV is men who have sex with men (Table 26.9). HIV antiretroviral therapy has decreased the rate of disease progression, but there is no cure available. Research continues into development of a vaccine to prevent the acquisition of HIV infection.

Treatment modalities known as *highly active antiretroviral therapy* (HAART) have been effective in halting HIV replication and thereby delaying the transition from HIV infection to AIDS or delaying the progression of AIDS itself. An increasing number of patients coming for surgery are HIV seropositive or may have had a diagnosis of AIDS in the past. Therefore anesthesiologists should be familiar with this infectious disease and syndrome and its impact on anesthetic management. An understanding of the pathogenesis of HIV, the multiple organ system involvement of HIV and AIDS, the possible drug interactions occurring with HIV therapy, side effects related to HAART, and associated opportunistic infections will serve to better guide preoperative assessment and anesthetic planning.

Signs and Symptoms

Acute seroconversion illness occurs approximately 2–3 weeks after inoculation with the HIV virus. The acute viral phase is typically marked by a flulike illness associated with fever, fatigue, headache, night sweats, pharyngitis, myalgias, and arthralgias. Therefore signs and symptoms during the period after the initial infection may mimic those of any common flulike illness. Within 1–2 weeks after inoculation with HIV, the virus initiates rapid replication. After several months there is a gradual decrease in the viremia. As the immune system responds, viral replication decelerates and a balance develops between host immune defenses and viral replication. The resulting viral level can be described as a steady-state rate of viral production equal to the rate of viral destruction and suppression. Generalized lymphadenopathy is a hallmark of HIV infection and may persist until HAART is initiated. An HIV-positive individual is *not* considered to have AIDS unless one of the AIDS-defining diagnoses is present.

As noted earlier, HIV belongs to the family of retroviruses. It is characteristically cytopathic (cell damaging), with a long latency period and a chronic course of infection. When the first cases of AIDS appeared, its pathogenesis was frustratingly elusive because the disease does not appear immediately after infection with HIV. It has been shown that the steady-state viral level is a reliable predictor of the rate of progression from HIV positivity to the development of AIDS. In general, higher basal viral levels correspond to more rapid disease progression. Weight loss and failure to thrive are among the first manifestations patients display as HIV infection progresses from the chronic latent phase to the development of AIDS.

Diagnosis

With the advent of HAART, the prognosis of those infected with HIV has dramatically improved. Therefore it is important that the stigma attached to HIV infection be removed so that high-risk individuals feel comfortable undergoing testing. The standard test to diagnose HIV infection is an enzyme-linked immunosorbent assay (ELISA), the results of which become positive when antibodies to HIV are present. This is typically 4–8 weeks after infection. This test is not a measure of viral load but simply indicates the presence of antibodies to HIV. During the initial period of infection, there is significant viremia and patients are highly infectious, but antibodies may *not* be present. Therefore a false-negative test result may occur. If a positive diagnosis is made, infection is confirmed with a Western blot test or by direct measurement of HIV viral load in the blood. HIV viral load is measured via PCR RNA analysis. If a patient is tested within a very short period after the initial infection, the ELISA test result may be negative or inconclusive. Nucleic acid testing of HIV RNA is the most specific and sensitive test for HIV.

Since HIV is lymphotropic and has a particular affinity for $CD4^+$ cells, measurement of these cells is useful in assessing the degree of HIV progression. $CD4^+$ cell levels are measured as cells per cubic millimeter (cells/mm^3). Ninety-eight percent of helper T lymphocytes ($CD4^+$ T cells) are located in lymph nodes, which are the major site of viral replication and T-cell destruction. During the acute infectious period, $CD4^+$ cell counts decline dramatically then rise again. Over the course of 8–12 years, there is a gradual involution of lymph nodes, with a concomitant slow decrease in $CD4^+$ T-cell counts that is accompanied by an increase in viral load as the inexorable onset of AIDS occurs (Fig. 26.5).

After the diagnosis of HIV infection is confirmed, a patient will undergo further testing to determine viral genotype and phenotype. In addition, HIV sensitivity and resistance to existing HAART agents as well as coreceptor usage will be determined. These testing modalities have been extremely effective in minimizing resistance when HAART is initiated, because selection of HAART agents is tailored to each individual patient. For the purposes of disease surveillance and disease severity estimation and management, patients who are HIV positive are classified as having AIDS *only* when at least *one* of the AIDS-defining diagnoses is present (Table 26.10).

HIV Infection Clinical Continuum

Patients who are HIV positive are typically asymptomatic and will not demonstrate any external evidence of clinical immunosuppression. However, HIV infection is a disease that encompasses a continuum of clinical signs from acute infection to clinical latency, then to clinical progression, and eventually to development of AIDS with associated opportunistic infections and ultimately death. However, the clinical continuum from HIV infection to AIDS can be interrupted, delayed, or altered by the institution of HAART. Opportunistic infections are caused by pathogens with no intrinsic virulence and require a compromised or defective immune system to proliferate. Because subclinical and clinical multiple organ system involvement is a hallmark of HIV infection, the anesthesiologist should be adept at eliciting a history and reviewing systems to detect any of the myriad co-existing diseases that can be present, as well as performing a thorough physical examination to detect pertinent pathologic conditions.

Cardiac Manifestations

Cardiac involvement in the course of HIV infection is common but often subclinical. Up to 50% of HIV-positive patients have abnormal echocardiographic findings at some point during their disease. HIV is an extremely trophic virus with a high affinity for the myocardium, and evidence has demonstrated the presence of HIV in myocardial cells. Left ventricular dilatation and cardiac dysfunction may result. In addition, pulmonary hypertension is present in about 1% of patients with HIV infection or AIDS. Cardiac disease may be exacerbated by HAART, especially when protease inhibitors are used. Protease inhibitors may cause premature atherosclerosis and diastolic dysfunction leading to heart failure. Myocardial infarction has been reported even in young patients with HIV infection. Approximately 25% of patients with HIV infection have a pericardial effusion. Myocarditis, which is more common in advanced disease, may be caused by toxoplasmosis, disseminated cryptococcosis, coxsackievirus B infection, cytomegalovirus infection, lymphoma, aspergillosis, and HIV infection itself. In addition, HIV is trophic for vascular structures and has been implicated in the development of multifocal abdominal aortic aneurysms in adults and children, as well as aortic arch aneurysms and aortic dissection in adults.

Central and Peripheral Nervous System Manifestations

Neurologic disease, ranging from AIDS dementia to infectious and neoplastic involvement, may be common, especially as AIDS progresses. HIV enters the CNS early in the course of infection, and the CNS is considered a reservoir for HIV. Three diagnoses comprise the majority of predominantly focal cerebral diseases complicating AIDS: cerebral toxoplasmosis, primary CNS lymphoma, and progressive multifocal leukoencephalopathy. *Cryptococcus neoformans*, HIV, and the TB bacillus can cause meningitis. Aggressive generalized cerebrovascular disease may occur as a complication of HAART. Increased intracranial pressure may develop with active HIV infection, resulting from the presence of intracranial masses or opportunistic infections. Peripheral neuropathy is the most frequent neurologic complication in HIV-positive patients. Approximately 35%

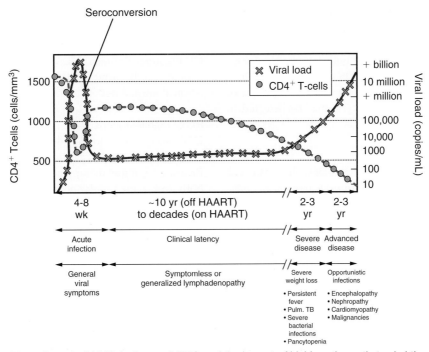

FIG. 26.5 Course of HIV infection and AIDS and the impact of highly active antiretroviral therapy (HAART). *Pulm. TB,* Pulmonary tuberculosis.

TABLE 26.10	AIDS-Defining Diagnoses in HIV-Seropositive Patients

Bacterial infection, multiple or recurrent
Burkitt lymphoma
Candidiasis of the bronchi, trachea, lungs, or esophagus
CD4+ T-lymphocyte cell count < 200 cells/mm3
Cervical cancer, invasive
Coccidiomycosis, disseminated or extrapulmonary
Cryptococcosis, extrapulmonary
Cryptosporidiosis, chronic intestinal (>1 mo)
Cytomegalovirus retinitis or cytomegalovirus infection (with loss of vision)
Herpes simplex with chronic ulcers (>1 mo), bronchitis, pneumonitis, or esophagitis
HIV-related encephalopathy
Histoplasmosis, disseminated or extrapulmonary
Isosporiasis, chronic (>1 mo)
Kaposi sarcoma
Immunoblastic lymphoma
Lymphoma of the brain, primary
Mycobacterium avium-intracellulare complex or *Mycobacterium kansasii* infection, disseminated or extrapulmonary
Mycobacterium tuberculosis infection, any site
Mycobacterium infection, any other species, pulmonary or extrapulmonary
Pneumocystis jiroveci pneumonia (PCP)
Pneumonia, recurrent
Progressive multifocal leukoencephalopathy (PML)
Recurrent *Salmonella* septicemia
Toxoplasmosis of the brain
Wasting syndrome due to HIV

AIDS, Acquired immunodeficiency syndrome; *HIV,* human immunodeficiency virus.

of patients with AIDS show clinical evidence of polyneuropathy or myopathy. Autonomic nervous system dysfunction may also appear with or without the presence of CNS involvement.

Pulmonary Manifestations
Pulmonary manifestations in HIV-positive patients are typically caused by opportunistic infections. Complications include respiratory failure, pneumothorax, and chronic pulmonary disease. Cavitary lung disease can be due to pyogenic bacterial lung abscess, pulmonary TB, fungal infection, or *Nocardia* infection. Kaposi sarcoma and lymphoma can also affect the lungs. Adenopathy can lead to tracheobronchial obstruction or compression of the great vessels. Endobronchial Kaposi sarcoma may cause massive hemoptysis. HIV directly affects the lungs and may cause a destructive pulmonary syndrome similar to emphysema.

Pneumocystis jiroveci pneumonia (PCP) does not usually occur until the CD4+ count falls below 200 cells/mm3 and fortunately has become less common with the use of HAART. With PCP, an AIDS-defining illness, the chest radiograph can be normal but typically shows bilateral ground-glass opacities. Pneumothoraces may be evident, or there may be several pneumatoceles. High-resolution CT scans reveal a ground-glass appearance even when chest radiograph findings appear normal. Pulmonary function tests show reduced lung volumes with decreased compliance and diminished diffusing capacity. Measurements of oxygen saturation during exercise may be more helpful than pulmonary function tests. If PCP is suspected, fiberoptic bronchoscopy and bronchoalveolar lavage should be performed. The advantage of an early diagnosis compensates for the high frequency of negative examination findings.

Disseminated TB is a potential cause of severe respiratory failure, and respiratory secretions should be examined routinely for acid-fast bacilli in HIV/AIDS patients with pulmonary infiltrates. Bacterial pneumonia may also be the cause of severe acute respiratory failure. Bacteria may be detected in sputum or bronchial washings.

Endocrine Manifestations

Adrenal insufficiency should be considered, since this may occur with advanced HIV infection. Random measurement of cortisol levels and tests of adrenal stimulation may reveal absolute or relative adrenal insufficiency. This is the most serious endocrine complication in HIV-positive patients. In HIV-positive patients taking protease inhibitor therapy, glucose intolerance, disorders of lipid metabolism, and fat redistribution are common.

Hematologic Manifestations

The hematopoietic system is widely affected by HIV infection, and the most common early finding of HIV infection is anemia. Lymphocytosis, with an increase mainly in $CD8^+$ T lymphocytes, may appear within 2 weeks of initial HIV infection. Bone marrow involvement can occur secondary to HIV infection itself and/or to opportunistic infection. This can produce leukopenia, lymphopenia, and thrombocytopenia. In addition, bone marrow suppression may develop after initiation of zidovudine therapy. Thrombocytopenia typically worsens as $CD4^+$ counts diminish to less than 250 cells/mm^3. HIV-positive patients may be prone to either hypercoagulable states or coagulation abnormalities.

Renal Manifestations

HIV-positive patients may develop renal disease secondary to HIV infection, viral hepatitis, associated drug use, or HAART. Protease inhibitor therapy has been specifically implicated in both toxic acute tubular necrosis and nephrolithiasis. In addition, nephrotic syndrome may occur as a result of HIV-associated nephropathy. HIV-associated nephropathy is especially common in African American men and commonly leads to end-stage renal disease.

Treatment

HAART targets the various steps in the HIV replication cycle (Fig. 26.6). Six major classes of antiretroviral drugs are currently in use, and another two groups of drugs are undergoing clinical investigation.

There is continued interest in developing treatment regimens that have a higher safety profile, lower rates of adverse

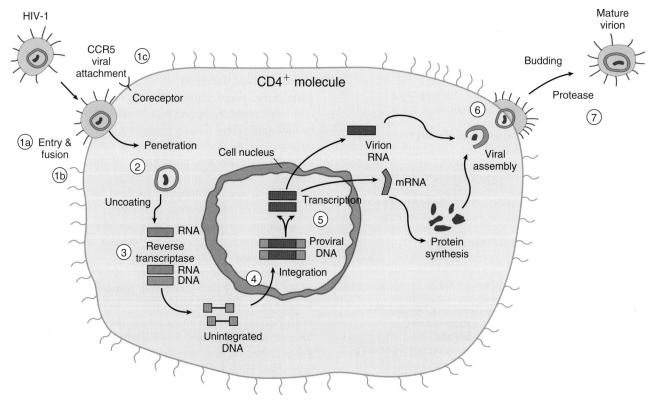

FIG. 26.6 Life cycle of HIV and targets of action of antiretroviral therapy (indicated by circled numbers). *1a,* Fusion inhibitors; *1b,* entry inhibitors; *1c,* chemokine receptor 5 (CCR5) antagonists/blockers; *2,* no antivirals available for "uncoating"; *3,* nucleoside and nonnucleoside reverse transcriptase inhibitors; *4,* integrase strand transfer inhibitors; *5,* no antivirals available for RNA transcription; *6,* maturation inhibitors; *7,* protease inhibitors; *mRNA,* messenger RNA.

effects, and easier dosing regimens. Antiretroviral drugs used to treat HIV infection are *always* employed in combinations of *at least three drugs*. Patients who have developed resistance to commonly used HAART regimens or have advanced AIDS may require four drugs and possibly additional booster medications designed to increase drug bioavailability.

The decision to initiate HAART is based on several factors, and once begun, treatment entails a lifelong commitment. Nonadherence to the medical regimen for any reason is one of the main causes of the development of viral resistance and treatment failure. Initiation of HAART is not necessarily a benign process, and implementation of HAART may result in a host of drug-related complications. Some patients who are in the early phase of HIV infection may decide, in conjunction with their physicians, *not* to immediately implement therapy and choose simply to be monitored.

Patients begin HAART immediately when there is evidence that CD4+ cell counts are diminishing rapidly, counts have already fallen below 200 cells/mm^3, or a patient with newly diagnosed HIV infection already meets AIDS-defining criteria. Recommendations advocate that HAART be instituted when CD4+ cell counts approach 500 cells/mm^3 or as soon after the initial HIV diagnosis that the patient can realistically begin HAART. Early institution of HAART is linked to greater long-term survival and lower morbidity.

A typical antiretroviral regimen consists of at least three drugs, and drug selection is based on viral sensitivity, resistance patterns, coreceptor subtypes, and virulence subtypes. In some circumstances, combinations of four or more drugs are used, such as when drug resistance patterns are evident with a patient undergoing a rapid clinical decline. The aim of therapy in treatment-naïve patients is to achieve an undetectable viral load in 24 weeks and to improve and extend the length and quality of life. Numerous side effects and drug interactions complicate such regimens and decrease adherence. Patients may develop a myriad of adverse drug reactions, and some are potentially fatal (Table 26.11).

Patients who begin HAART may also develop a reaction known as *immune reconstitution inflammatory syndrome* (IRIS). IRIS occurs as a result of restoration of basic immune competence with HAART and the gradual improvement and strengthening of the immune system. IRIS leads to a paradoxical deterioration of general clinical symptoms in the context of improving CD4+ counts and a reduced viral load. IRIS is marked by the appearance and/or exacerbation of previously silent clinical diseases such as hepatitis A, B, and C; PCP; TB; and any other dormant opportunistic infection.

Concurrent use of zidovudine and corticosteroids may result in severe myopathy and respiratory muscle dysfunction. In addition, reports have documented several cases of respiratory failure related to HAART initiation. Of particular importance to anesthesiologists is that patients receiving HAART are subject to long-term metabolic complications,

Class	Common Drug-HAART Interactions	Anesthetic-Specific Drug-HAART Interactions
TABLE 26.11 Highly Active Antiretroviral Therapy (HAART) Drug Interactions		
Nucleoside reverse transcriptase inhibitors (NRTIs)	Interactions with: *Anticonvulsant:* phenytoin *Antifungals:* ketoconazole, dapsone *Alcohol* *H$_2$ blocker:* cimetidine	HAART potentially changes drug clearance and effects of: *Opiate:* methadone
Nonnucleoside reverse transcriptase inhibitors (NNRTIs)	Interactions with: *Anticoagulant:* warfarin *Anticonvulsants:* carbamazepine, phenytoin, phenobarbital *Anti-TB drug:* rifampin *Herbal:* St. John's wort	HAART prolongs half-life and/or effects of: *Sedatives:* diazepam, midazolam, triazolam *Opiates:* fentanyl, meperidine, methadone
Protease inhibitors (PIs)	Interactions with: *Anticoagulant:* warfarin *Anticonvulsants:* carbamazepine, phenytoin, phenobarbital *Antidepressant:* sertraline *Calcium channel blockers* *Anti-TB drug:* rifampin *Herbal:* St. John's wort *Immunosuppressant:* cyclosporine	HAART prolongs half-life and/or effects of: *Antidysrhythmics:* amiodarone, digoxin, quinidine *Sedatives:* diazepam, midazolam, triazolam *Opiates:* fentanyl, meperidine, methadone *Local anesthetic:* lidocaine
Integrase strand transfer inhibitors (INSTIs)	Interactions with: *Proton pump inhibitor:* omeprazole *Anti-TB drug:* rifampin	None
Entry inhibitors	Interactions with: *Anticonvulsant:* carbamazepine *Anti-TB drug:* rifampin *Oral contraceptives* *Proton pump inhibitor:* omeprazole *Herbal:* St. John's wort	HAART potentially changes drug clearance and effects of: *Sedative:* midazolam

TB, Tuberculosis.

including lipid abnormalities and glucose intolerance, which may result in development of diabetes, coronary artery disease, and cerebrovascular disease. HAART has also been implicated in fat redistribution to the neck, back of the neck, and abdomen. This phenomenon may make airway management more difficult or increase intraabdominal pressure.

Protease inhibitors, particularly ritonavir and saquinavir, act as inhibitors of cytochrome P450. In contrast, drugs such as nevirapine are inducers of hepatic microsomal enzymes. These variable effects on liver enzyme mechanics further complicate the dosing of HAART drugs and other drugs that undergo hepatic metabolism, including anesthetic and analgesic drugs. Therefore caution must be used when administering pharmacologic agents that may be metabolized via these pathways, because drug duration and anticipated effect may be highly variable.

Prognosis

Before 1995 the prospects for successful treatment of HIV infection were dismal, and a diagnosis of HIV infection was inevitably followed by death. Several independent factors dramatically changed the situation: (1) improved understanding of the pathogenesis of HIV infection, (2) availability of surrogate markers of immune function and plasma viral burden to determine whether HAART is effective (specifically $CD4^+$ cell counts and HIV viral load quantification), (3) use of $CD4^+$ cell counts and viral load determinations by researchers to determine minimal effective concentrations of HAART and thereby improve its risk/benefit profile, (4) development of viral genotype/phenotype profiling, coreceptor subtyping, and sensitivity and resistance pattern analysis, which has enabled optimal selection of specific HAART regimens, (5) continued development of new and more powerful drugs, and (6) completion of several large clinical end-point trials that have conclusively demonstrated that antiretroviral combinations significantly delay the progression of HIV disease and improve long-term survival.

Management of Anesthesia

Preoperative

Patients with HIV infection and/or AIDS are usually managed by an internist, primary care provider, or infectious disease specialist. Although a medical evaluation by one of these physicians immediately before surgery is not mandatory, it may be helpful to obtain a consultation if the patient is unable to delineate pertinent medical history and management specifically related to HIV infection and/or AIDS. Additional information from primary care and infectious disease specialists may be especially pertinent in patients who present with advanced AIDS.

Not all patients with HIV/AIDS are receiving HAART, and it is important to understand what current treatment strategies are being used for a specific patient. Some patients may be waiting for further deterioration in clinical and immune status before initiating HAART, whereas a subset of patients may be on physician-approved "drug holidays," and other patients may simply be unable to tolerate the adverse effects of HAART. HAART treatment strategies in the 21st century typically include initiation of antiviral therapy immediately after diagnosis and confirmation of genotype/phenotype.

Whether or not a patient is receiving HAART and has an undetectable viral load, patients with HIV/AIDS should *always* be considered a potential source of disease transmission. In patients who are not receiving HAART, initiating HAART to minimize viral load and improve overall clinical condition in the period immediately before surgery is not indicated. Studies have indicated that HAART has no protective effect in reducing perioperative risk, and initiation of HAART within 6 months of surgery actually *increases* overall morbidity and mortality in patients with HIV infection. The occurrence of IRIS after HAART is begun may paradoxically worsen the patient's overall condition and further delay surgery.

Since HIV infection, AIDS, and HAART can all potentially impact multiple organ systems, it is advisable to order a CBC, basic metabolic panel including renal function studies, liver function tests, and coagulation studies. A chest radiograph and ECG are also useful preoperatively regardless of age or evidence of cardiopulmonary disease. If a patient with HIV infection or AIDS has any signs or symptoms of cardiac dysfunction, echocardiography or stress testing may also be indicated, with additional consultation by a cardiologist as indicated.

There is little specific information concerning the overall risk of anesthesia and surgery in the HIV-positive patient. The American Society of Anesthesiologists (ASA) physical status assessment and the inherent surgical risk probably provide a measure of global risk assessment. An ASA status of 2 is typically assigned to HIV-positive patients *without* any clinical evidence of immunocompromise or acute deterioration; these patients *may or may not be receiving HAART*. Patients with AIDS may be classified as having an ASA status of either 3 or 4 depending on the severity of co-existing disease processes either related or unrelated to HIV infection. In addition, patients with advanced AIDS may be receiving HAART but for all practical purposes may be minimally responsive to it; $CD4^+$ cell counts may be low and viral load may range from undetectable to low, moderate, or high. This information, when combined with the stage of the HIV infection, degree of clinical immunosuppression, and presence and severity of opportunistic infections or neoplasms, may offer the best predictor of global perioperative risk in the HIV-positive patient.

The utility of obtaining a $CD4^+$ cell count and viral load determination before surgery has not been demonstrated. Studies have shown that there is no significant difference in perioperative outcomes in HIV-positive or AIDS patients whose $CD4^+$ cell counts are higher than 50 cells/mm^3 compared with outcomes in patient populations without HIV/AIDS matched for the same surgery, comorbid conditions, and ASA status. Viral load level is not a predictor of perioperative outcome unless viral load exceeds 30,000 copies/mL. Owing to the overall improved effectiveness of HAART, CD4$^+$ cell counts and viral load are usually monitored every 6 months. HAART does not offer any real protective effects or decrease the overall morbidity and mortality associated with surgery and anesthesia. However, patients with HIV infection and AIDS do demonstrate a higher overall mortality 1 year after surgery than similar cohorts without HIV/AIDS. This has been attributed to HIV infection and/or AIDS itself and not to the surgical procedure performed or the anesthetic used.

In general if a patient is HIV positive and has never met AIDS-defining criteria, one can presume the patient's CD4$^+$ cell count is higher than 200 cells/mm^3. However, patients with AIDS-defining diagnoses or a history of AIDS (with or without HAART) may have widely varying CD4$^+$ cell counts. Not all HIV-positive patients receiving HAART have undetectable viral loads, so viral load quantification does not assist the anesthesiologist in any meaningful way during the perioperative period. In addition, even if viral load is undetectable, universal precautions must still be employed because the absence of a measurable viral load does not imply that HIV cannot be transmitted. HIV persistence is a known phenomenon, and HIV can remain dormant in lymph nodes and CNS reservoirs.

Since patients with HIV infection or AIDS can manifest a wide array of co-existing diseases, every patient should undergo a thorough history, review of systems, and physical examination focused particularly on subclinical or clinical manifestations of cardiac, pulmonary, neurologic, renal, and hepatic disorders related to HIV or AIDS. With regard to selection of anesthetic method, any anesthetic technique is acceptable unless there is a specific contraindication to regional anesthesia. Consideration should be given to addressing potential HAART-drug interactions when selecting anesthetic drugs and analgesics in the perioperative period.

Overall, HIV infection and AIDS do not increase the risk of postsurgical complications, including death, up to 30 days postoperatively. Thus surgical intervention should not be restricted because of HIV status and concern for subsequent complications. During anesthesia, however, tachycardia is more frequently seen in HIV-positive patients; postoperatively, fever, anemia, and tachycardia are more frequent.

Intraoperative

Selection of a particular anesthetic technique should take into account both HIV/AIDS-related comorbidities and any other clinical issues. Overall, no specific anesthetic technique has been shown to be superior or inferior in patients with HIV infection or AIDS. Specifically in patients with AIDS, focal neurologic lesions may increase intracranial pressure, which precludes neuraxial anesthesia. Spinal cord involvement, peripheral neuropathy, and myopathy may occur with cytomegalovirus or HIV infection itself. Therefore succinylcholine could conceivably be hazardous in this setting. HIV infection may be associated with autonomic neuropathy, and this can produce hemodynamic instability during anesthesia or in the ICU. Invasive hemodynamic monitoring may be helpful in

patients with severe autonomic dysfunction. Steroid supplementation may decrease hemodynamic instability and should be considered in cases of unexplained persistent hypotension.

Several studies indicate that general anesthesia and opiates may have a negative effect on immune function. Although this immunosuppressive effect may be of little clinical importance in healthy individuals, the implications for the HIV-infected patient are uncertain. Immunosuppression resulting from general anesthetics occurs within 15 minutes of induction and may persist for as long as 3–11 days. The psychological stress of undergoing anesthesia and surgery may also lead to some degree of generalized immunosuppression. However, no studies have been undertaken to determine specific effects in HIV-positive patients. Aside from CD4$^+$ cell count and viral load, there are no specific markers of immune status in this patient population.

The prevalence of HIV infection and AIDS is increasing in women of childbearing age, and there has been much study of this patient population. Although research has demonstrated the effectiveness of zidovudine in parturient women, monotherapy has limited long-term benefit because HIV resistance develops rapidly. Therefore during pregnancy, combination therapy is preferable, and acceptable multidrug regimens are available. Data suggest that cesarean section decreases the incidence of vertical transmission of HIV from mother to child. A combination of antiretroviral therapy and elective cesarean section reduces the rate of vertical transmission to 2%. However, cesarean section is a major surgical intervention with many potential complications. Many practitioners in the past did not recommend elective cesarean section for HIV-infected women who were adherent to antiretroviral treatment regimens and had undetectable HIV viral loads. However, studies demonstrate that cesarean section can proceed safely. Unfortunately, HIV-positive women with low CD4$^+$ counts whose infants would likely benefit most from caesarean delivery are also the women who are most likely to experience perioperative complications.

HIV-positive parturient women who are given regional anesthesia have not had neurologic or infectious complications related to the anesthetic or obstetric course. In the immediate postpartum period, immune function has remained essentially unchanged, as has the severity of the preexisting HIV disease. There have been concerns that access to the epidural space and lumbar puncture in HIV-positive patients might allow entry of the virus into the CNS. However, the natural history of HIV infection includes CNS involvement early in its clinical course. The safety of epidural blood patches for treatment of postdural puncture headache has been reported in HIV-positive patients. Fear of disseminating HIV from the bloodstream into the CNS is not warranted.

Postoperative

A limited number of retrospective studies have evaluated the long-term consequences of undergoing anesthesia and surgery in HIV-positive and AIDS patients, but many of the studies conducted in the pre-HAART era yielded conflicting results. Current studies are examining surgical and anesthetic-related morbidity and mortality in HIV-positive patients who had been receiving HAART. Therefore it is important to understand the impact HAART has had on overall well-being in the HIV-positive population.

It appears that patients with HIV infection and AIDS do not experience any statistically significant increases in perioperative complications compared with similar cohorts who are not HIV positive. No statistically significant differences have been noted with regard to wound healing, SSI rates, wound dehiscence, number of complications, length of hospital stay, number of follow-up visits to the surgeon, or need for further operative procedures to treat surgical complications. However, 1-year mortality is higher overall in patients who are HIV positive and/or have AIDS. This is felt to be due to HIV infection itself. Patients with CD4+ cell counts of less than 50 cells/mm^3 and patients with viral loads of more than 30,000 copies/mL fare the worst in terms of postoperative mortality. Patients with HIV infection may have a higher incidence of postoperative pneumonia than non–HIV-positive patients. Proper diagnosis and treatment typically lead to resolution of the pulmonary infection without sequelae.

Acute Physiology and Chronic Health Evaluation II (APACHE II) scoring *significantly underestimates* mortality risk in HIV-positive patients admitted to the ICU with a total lymphocyte count below 200 cells/mm^3. This is particularly true of patients admitted with pneumonia or sepsis. There is a diverse range of indications for critical care in patients with HIV infection. Historically, respiratory failure caused by PCP was the most common reason for ICU admission and accounted for a third of ICU admissions in HIV-positive patients. The need for mechanical ventilation for PCP and other pulmonary disorders is associated with a mortality rate over 50%. In contrast, admission to the ICU and mechanical ventilation for nonpulmonary disorders is associated with a mortality rate below 25%. In patients with septic shock, however, HIV infection is an independent predictor of poor outcome. In the era of HAART, fewer patients with HIV infection are admitted to the ICU with AIDS-defining illnesses. Many patients are now admitted to the ICU with unrelated critical illnesses and are found coincidentally to be infected with HIV.

EBOLA VIRUS DISEASE

Incidence

Ebola virus disease (EVD), also called *Ebola hemorrhagic fever* or simply *Ebola,* is a disease of humans and other primates caused by Ebola viruses. The disease was first identified in 1976 in two simultaneous outbreaks, one in Nzara and the other in Yambuku, a village near the Ebola River from which the disease takes its name. EVD outbreaks occur intermittently in tropical regions of sub-Saharan Africa. Between 1976 and 2013 the WHO reported a total of 24 outbreaks involving 1716 cases. The largest outbreak ever reported was the epidemic that began in 2014 in West Africa. As of January 17, 2016, this outbreak had resulted in 28,638 reported cases and 11,316 deaths.

Some healthcare experts astutely predicted that Ebola fever would appear in patients outside the original epidemic zone because of the importation of healthcare workers from Europe and the United States for treatment and control maneuvers. Although the incidence and presence in the United States is quite rare, identification and containment of patients with Ebola virus is absolutely essential to infection control.

EVD in humans is caused by four of five viruses of the genus *Ebolavirus.* The four are Bundibugyo virus, Sudan virus, Taï Forest virus, and one simply called *Ebola virus* (formerly Zaire Ebola virus). Ebola, species *Zaire ebolavirus,* is the most dangerous of the known EVD-causing viruses and is responsible for the largest number of outbreaks. The fifth virus, Reston virus, is not thought to cause disease in humans but has caused disease in other primates.

Early diagnosis is difficult, since signs and symptoms of fever and flulike illness are nonspecific and similar to early findings in malaria and typhoid fever (Table 26.12). Diagnosis of Ebola infection can be made via antigen-capture ELISA, immunoglobulin M (IgM) ELISA, PCR testing, and/or virus isolation.

Infection Control

Because of the small group of patients (who were healthcare workers infected with Ebola virus) that were medically evacuated to the United States for treatment during the 2014 Ebola outbreak, the majority of healthcare institutions in the United States had to reevaluate their infectious disease identification measures, as well as their prevention strategies, to deal with persons potentially exposed to Ebola virus during travel. Healthcare institutions initiated a three-point screening process aimed at identifying patients possibly infected with Ebola virus. Patients being admitted to a hospital or healthcare facility are currently asked (1) if they have traveled in the last 21 days to an area associated with EVD, (2) if they have been directly exposed to a person (or the human remains of any person) with known or suspected Ebola virus infection, and (3) if they have had recent clinical symptoms of high fever, nausea, and/or vomiting. If patients respond "yes" to any of the listed questions, appropriate steps are

TABLE 26.12	Symptoms of Ebola Virus Disease Infection

Fever
Severe headache
Muscle pain
Weakness
Fatigue
Diarrhea
Vomiting
Abdominal (stomach) pain
Unexplained hemorrhage (bleeding or bruising)

taken to perform further testing to determine whether exposure to Ebola virus is likely. Any suspected cases are immediately reported to the epidemiology department of the institution.

To minimize the risk of EVD, existing standard precautions should be strengthened and carefully applied when providing care to any patient, regardless of the presenting signs and symptoms. Hand hygiene is the most important measure. Gloves should be worn for any contact with blood or bodily fluids. Medical masks and goggles or face shields should be used if there is any potential for splashes of blood or bodily fluids to the face, and cleaning of contaminated surfaces is paramount. These same precautions should also be taken for contact with corpses.

During EVD outbreaks, every healthcare facility should have a dedicated and well-equipped triage area at the entrance to evaluate any patients presenting with high fever who are seeking care in the facility. This area should be staffed with professionals (i.e., doctor or nurse) trained in basic infection control principles and specific precautions for EVD, and on the use of a standard algorithm to identify EVD cases. Staff in the triage area should wear a scrub suit, a gown, examination gloves, and a face shield. The area should be large enough to keep the potentially infected EVD patient at a 1-meter distance from staff and should be equipped with an easily accessible hand hygiene facility (alcohol-based disinfectant dispensers; sink with running water, liquid soap, and single-use towels), thermometer, bin with lid and infectious waste plastic bags, and a sharps container (if rapid diagnostic testing is meant to be performed there). Triage staff should follow a "no-touch" process while interviewing patients.

Suspected or confirmed cases must be placed in single isolation rooms with an adjoining dedicated toilet or latrine, showers, sink (equipped with running water, soap, and single-use towels), alcohol-based handrub dispensers, stocks of personal protective equipment (PPE), stocks of medicines, adequate ventilation, closed doors, and restricted access. If single isolation rooms are unavailable, EVD patients should be put together in confined areas while rigorously *keeping suspected and confirmed patients separated.*

It is important to ensure that clinical and nonclinical personnel are assigned exclusively to EVD patient care areas, and *do not* move freely between the EVD isolation areas and other clinical areas during the outbreak. All nonessential staff must be kept from EVD patient care areas. If a patient with EVD were to require surgery, a specifically designated operating room should be used and maintained for this patient population, with *only* designated staff accompanying the patient to the operating room. After the procedure, additional cleaning measures should include "terminal" cleaning of all devices and surfaces, including the anesthesia machine, with bleach/chlorine. Personal protection equipment should be worn according to current WHO guidelines for Ebola outbreaks. All waste material, linens, and nondisposable materials should be decontaminated according to WHO guidelines. Fortunately, to date there are no reported cases of patients infected with the Ebola virus who have undergone surgery in the United States.

Treatment

Symptoms of Ebola and complications are treated as they appear. The following basic interventions, when used early, can significantly improve the chances of survival: (1) providing IV fluids and creating electrolyte balance, (2) maintaining satisfactory oxygen saturation and blood pressure, and (3) treating other infections if they occur. Experimental vaccines and treatments for Ebola are under development, but they have not yet been fully tested for safety or effectiveness. Recovery from Ebola depends on strong supportive care and an adequate immune response by the patient. Those who recover from Ebola infection develop antibodies that last for at least 10 years, possibly longer. It is not known whether people who recover are immune for life or if they can become infected with a different species of Ebola. Some patients who have recovered from Ebola infection have developed long-term complications such as joint and vision problems.

KEY POINTS

- The 21st century is likely to be marked by a proliferation of infectious viral illnesses.
- There are few new antibiotics under development to combat resistant gram-negative organisms.
- Multidisciplinary protocols focusing on preoperative, intraoperative, and postoperative prevention of SSI do decrease the likelihood of patients developing such infections.
- Frequent hand decontamination with either alcohol or soap and water may be the single most effective intervention in decreasing nosocomial infection.
- Administration of antibiotics at the right time, in the right dosage, and for an appropriate duration of time effectively treats infection and retards development of antibiotic drug resistance.
- The growing epidemic of virulent *C. difficile*–associated diarrhea among hospitalized patients may be associated with widespread use of broad-spectrum antibiotics.
- To minimize widespread resistance of organisms to all antimicrobial agents, therapy *must* be narrowed as soon as organisms are identified and susceptibility testing is completed.
- Specimens for culture should be obtained from all likely sources if sepsis is suspected.
- With necrotizing soft tissue infections, superficial cutaneous signs typically do not reflect the extent of tissue necrosis.
- Between 10% and 20% of patients requiring endotracheal intubation and mechanical ventilation for longer than 48 hours develop ventilator-associated pneumonia, which is associated with significant mortality.
- Respiratory viruses may have high virulence, a fulminant infectious course, and high mortality.

- Allogeneic red blood cell transfusion creates generalized immunosuppression and can reactivate latent viruses.
- The development of extremely drug-resistant (XDR) TB, caused by *M. tuberculosis* strains that are not only resistant to antibiotic therapy but also more virulent and more frequently lethal, has become a large public health problem.
- Posttransplantation patients are especially susceptible to infectious diseases, and strict adherence to immunosuppression regimens, antimicrobial prophylaxis, and surgical infection prophylaxis is critical in preventing new infections.
- HIV infection is a modern pandemic and has acute, latent, and end-stage phases. HAART has transformed HIV into a manageable chronic disease; however, significant HAART-induced and/or HIV-related morbidity continues to exist.
- Healthcare workers must recognize that they are potential agents of infection transmission.

RESOURCES

Bartzler DW, Dellinger EP, Olsen KM, et al. Clinical practice guidelines for antimicrobial prophylaxis in surgery. *Am J Health Syst Pharm.* 2013;70:195-283.

Bartzler DW, Hunt DR. The Surgical Infection Prevention and Surgical Care Improvement projects: national initiatives to improve outcomes for patients having surgery. *Clin Infect Dis.* 2006;43:322-330.

Chalmers JD, Taylor JK, Singanayagam A, et al. Epidemiology, antibiotic therapy, and clinical outcomes in health care–associated pneumonia: a UK cohort study. *Clin Infect Dis.* 2011;53:107-113.

Dellinger EP. Prophylactic antibiotics: administration and timing before operation are more important than administration after operation. *Clin Infect Dis.* 2007;44:928-930.

Dellinger RP, Levy MM, Rhodes A, et al. Surviving Sepsis Campaign: international guidelines for management of sever sepsis and shock: 2012. *Intensive Care Med.* 2013;39:165-228.

Horberg MA, Hurley LB, Klein DB, et al. Surgical outcomes in human immunodeficiency virus–infected patients in the era of highly active antiretroviral therapy. *Arch Surg.* 2006;141:1238-1245.

Leffler DA, Lamont JT. *Clostridium difficile* infection. *N Engl J Med.* 2015;372:1539-1548.

Mauermann WJ, Nemergut EC. The anesthesiologist's role in the prevention of surgical site infections. *Anesthesiology.* 2006;105:413-421.

Musher DM, Thorner AR. Community-acquired pneumonia. *N Engl J Med.* 2014;371:1619-1628.

O'Grady NP, Alexander M, Burns LA, et al. Guidelines for the prevention of intravascular catheter-related infections. *Clin Infect Dis.* 2011;52:e162-e193.

Plan to combat extensively drug-resistant tuberculosis: recommendations of the Federal Tuberculosis Task Force. *MMWR Recomm Report.* 2009;58(RR-3):1-43.

Interim infection prevention and control guidance for care of patients with suspected or confirmed filovirus haemorrhagic fever in health care settings with a focus on Ebola. World Health Organization; December 2014. WHO reference number WHO/HIS/SDS/2014.4 Rev.1.

World Wide Web Links

Facts about antibiotic resistance:
http://www.idsociety.org/AR_Facts/.

Information about surgical site infection:
http://www.hopkinsmedicine.org/heic/infection_surveillance/ssi.html.

Perioperative management of HIV-infected patients. NY State Department of Health AIDS Institute's Clinical Guidelines Development Program. January 2012. http://www.hivguidelines.org.

Diseases Related to Immune System Dysfunction

NATALIE F. HOLT

The human immune system has evolved from both invertebrate and vertebrate organisms. It has become a highly sophisticated system that can not only recognize an enormous number of pathogens but also develop memory so that a rapid-recall response can be used on reexposure to some antigens. It does all of this with minimal impact on normal or "self" tissue.

The human immune system is traditionally viewed as consisting of two pathways: *innate immunity* and *adaptive immunity* (also known as *acquired immunity*). Each comprises a series of unique components, all of which function to protect the host against invading microorganisms. The innate immune response that has evolved from invertebrate precursors is rapid and nonspecific—that is, it recognizes pathogen-associated molecular patterns (targets common to many pathogens) and requires no prior exposure to elicit an immune response. Innate immunity is passed on to each generation, apparently to protect the *species.* Its noncellular elements include physical barriers (epithelial and mucous membrane surfaces), complement factors, acute-phase proteins, and proteins of the contact activation pathway. Cellular elements include neutrophils, macrophages, monocytes, and a subset of lymphocytes called *natural killer (NK) cells* (Fig. 27.1).

The adaptive immune response is a more mature system present only in vertebrates. Each individual must develop their own adaptive immunity. This system seems designed to protect a particular *member* of the species. Adaptive immunity has a more delayed onset of activation but is capable of developing memory and very specific antigenic responses. It consists of a humoral component mediated by B lymphocytes that produce antibodies and a cellular component composed of T lymphocytes. T cells are divided into two main subsets—cytotoxic (T_C) cells and helper-modulatory (T_H) cells—and are distinguished by their different combinations of surface antigens. T_C cells express a predominance of CD8 antigen, whereas T_H cells express a predominance of CD4 antigen. Precursor helper T lymphocytes differentiate into four distinct cell lines: T_H1, T_H2, T_H17, and regulatory T (T_{reg}) cells. T_H1 cells produce interferon and promote cell-mediated immune responses. T_H2 cells produce specific interleukins, including interleukin (IL)-4 and IL-10, which favor a humoral immune response and suppress cell-mediated immunity. T_H17 cells are proinflammatory and appear to play a role in chronic inflammatory conditions, including some cell-mediated autoimmune diseases. In contrast, T_{reg} cells promote tolerance and minimize autoimmune and allergic or inflammatory responses. As a general rule, cytotoxic and helper T-cell responses are most important in mounting an effective response to trauma,

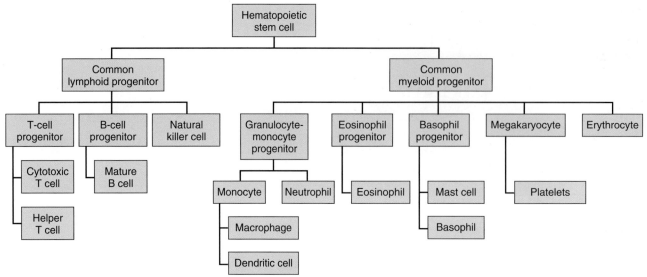

FIG. 27.1 Hematopoietic stem cell differentiation. A pluripotent hematopoietic stem cell gives rise to all blood cell types via two main lineages: lymphoid and myeloid. A common myeloid progenitor differentiates into the granule-containing cells of the immune system (monocytes, macrophages, neutrophils, eosinophils, basophils) as well as megakaryocytes and erythrocytes. A common lymphoid progenitor differentiates into the non–granule-containing cells of the immune system (T cells, B cells, and natural killer cells).

infection, and tumorigenesis. IL-4, IL-10, and T_H2 cells tend to promote the humoral immune system and help protect against immune-mediated tissue injury; however, they may also activate immunoglobulin (Ig)E and contribute to hypersensitivity reactions (Table 27.1).

Immune dysfunction can be divided into three categories: (1) an inadequate immune response, (2) an excessive immune response, and (3) a misdirection of the immune response.

INADEQUATE INNATE IMMUNITY

Neutropenia

Neutropenia is defined as a neutrophil granulocyte count of less than 1500/mm³. Normal neutrophil counts vary somewhat by age and ethnicity. For example, newborns tend to have higher granulocyte counts in the first few days of life, and African Americans tend to have lower average granulocyte counts in general compared with whites. It is not until the granulocyte count decreases to less than 500/mm³ that a patient is at significantly increased risk of pyogenic infections. Common infecting organisms include *Staphylococcus aureus*, *Pseudomonas aeruginosa*, *Escherichia coli*, and *Klebsiella* species, which frequently produce infections of the skin, mouth, pharynx, and lung. Broad-spectrum parenteral antibiotics are indicated in the management of these patients.

Neutropenia in Pediatric Patients
Several neutropenic syndromes can be observed in newborns and children. Neonatal sepsis is the most common cause of severe

TABLE 27.1	T-Lymphocyte Differentiation	
Subset	Main Functions	Cytokines
HELPER T CELLS		
T_H1	Macrophage activation	IFN-γ
	Cellular cytotoxicity	IL-2
	Protection against intracellular	IL-10
	microorganisms	TNF-β
T_H2	IgE production	IL-4
	Eosinophil proliferation	IL-5
	Protection against parasitic	IL-6
	infection	IL-9
		IL-10
		IL-13
T_H17	Protection against extracellular	IL-17
	bacteria and fungi	IL-21
	Aberrant regulation leads to	IL-22
	chronic inflammation, allergy,	
	autoimmune diseases	
T_{reg}	Maintenance of tolerance	IL-19
	Downregulation of immune	TGF-β
	response	IL-35
CYTOTOXIC T CELLS	Induction of apoptosis in infected or tumor cells	IFN-γ
	Inhibition of microbial replication	TNF-β

Ig, Immunoglobulin; *IL,* interleukin; *IFN,* interferon; *TNF,* tumor necrosis factor; *TGF,* transforming growth factor; T_{reg}, regulatory T cell.

neutropenia within the first few days of life. A transient neutropenia may be seen in children born to mothers with autoimmune diseases and may also occur as a result of maternal hypertension or drug ingestion. Persistent neutropenia can occur as a result of defects in neutrophil production, maturation, or survival.

The autosomal dominant disorder *cyclic neutropenia* is a particularly well-studied cause of childhood neutropenia. It is characterized by recurrent episodes of neutropenia that are not always associated with infection but occur in regular cycles every 3–4 weeks. Each episode is characterized by 1 week of reduced granulocyte production followed by a period of reactive mastocytosis and then spontaneous recovery of normal granulocyte production. The granulocytopenia can be severe enough to result in recurrent severe bacterial infection that requires antibiotic therapy. As the child grows up, chronic persistent granulocytopenia may result. The postulated mechanism of this disorder is a defect in a feedback mechanism that normally stimulates precursor cells to respond to growth factors such as granulocyte colony-stimulating factor (G-CSF).

Kostmann syndrome is an autosomal recessive disorder of neutrophil maturation. Patients with Kostmann syndrome appear to have a normal population of early progenitor cells that somehow become suppressed, which inhibits normal maturation. If the disorder is left untreated, mortality in the first year of life approaches 70%. Treatment with G-CSF is effective in 90% of patients. Bone marrow transplantation may be required in patients who show no response to G-CSF.

Neutropenia in Adults

Acquired defects in the production of neutrophils in adults are very common. Typical causes include cancer chemotherapy and treatment of human immunodeficiency virus (HIV) infection with zidovudine. Neutropenia usually reflects the impact of a drug on proliferation of stem cells and early myelocytic progenitors. In most cases the marrow recovers once the drug is withdrawn. Many drugs have been associated with neutropenia. Among the most prominent of these are injectable gold salts, chloramphenicol, antithyroid medications (carbimazole and propylthiouracil), analgesics (indomethacin, acetaminophen, and phenacetin), tricyclic antidepressants, and phenothiazines. However, virtually any drug can, on occasion, produce severe life-threatening neutropenia. Therefore when neutropenia occurs in the course of medical treatment, the possibility that it is drug induced must be considered.

Autoimmune-related neutropenia can be observed as an isolated disorder or in the context of another known autoimmune condition. Antineutrophil antibodies are sometimes present. The two most common associated conditions are systemic lupus erythematosus (SLE), in which the neutropenia can occur alone or be accompanied by thrombocytopenia, and rheumatoid arthritis (RA). Conditions associated with splenomegaly often lead to granulocytopenia resulting from white cell sequestration in the spleen. *Felty syndrome* is the triad of RA, splenomegaly, and neutropenia. Other causes of splenomegaly and neutropenia include lymphoma, myeloproliferative disease, and severe liver disease with portal hypertension. In these latter situations it is often difficult to decide whether the granulocytopenia is caused simply by splenic sequestration or whether it also has an autoimmune component. In some patients, splenectomy has been reported to significantly improve neutrophil counts.

Acute life-threatening granulocytopenia can occur as a result of certain infections. A decreasing white cell count in a patient with sepsis is a bad prognostic sign. It reflects a rate of granulocyte use that exceeds the marrow's ability to produce new cells. Alcoholic patients are especially susceptible to infection-induced granulocytopenia. Both folic acid deficiency and direct toxic effects of ethanol on marrow precursor cells compromise the host's ability to produce new neutrophils in response to infection. HIV infection is a common cause of T-cell dysfunction. In these patients, loss of the T_H subset and overexpression of the T_{reg} subset is associated with abnormalities of neutrophil production and function.

Chronic benign neutropenia is a condition characterized by markedly reduced neutrophil counts, often as low as 200–500/mm^3. Although the clinical course is variable, most patients have a benign course.

Abnormalities of Phagocytosis

Chronic granulomatous disease is a genetic disorder in which granulocytes lack the ability to generate reactive oxygen species. The granulocytes can migrate to a site of infection and ingest organisms but are unable to kill them. *S. aureus* and certain gram-negative bacteria such as *Serratia marcescens* and *Burkholderia cepacia* that are normally killed by phagocytosis and lysosomal digestion are responsible for most infections in patients with this disorder. The condition is usually diagnosed during childhood or early adult life when patients have recurrent microabscesses and chronic granulomatous inflammation. Persistent inflammation and granuloma formation can lead to multiorgan dysfunction, including intestinal obstruction, glomerulonephritis, and chorioretinitis. Aggressive treatment of infectious complications, prophylaxis with antibiotics and antifungal agents, and use of recombinant interferon gamma has significantly improved survival in patients with this disease.

The primary substrate for the enzymatic generation of reactive oxygen species is the reduced form of nicotinamide adenine dinucleotide phosphate (NADPH). Patients with *neutrophil glucose-6-phosphate dehydrogenase (G6PD) deficiency* are unable to generate large amounts of NADPH, which limits their ability to produce the oxidase needed to kill ingested microorganisms. Like patients with chronic granulomatous disease, neutrophil G6PD-deficient patients are at lifelong risk of infection with catalase-positive microorganisms.

Leukocyte adhesion deficiency is a relatively rare deficiency of a subunit of the integrin family of leukocyte adhesion molecules. This subunit is critical for cellular adhesion and chemotaxis. Although clinical severity varies, patients with leukocyte adhesion deficiency experience a higher risk of recurrent bacterial infections. Persistent granulocytosis is often present; however, the absence of pus is the most characteristic feature of this disease.

Chédiak-Higashi syndrome is a rare multisystem disease characterized by partial oculocutaneous albinism, frequent bacterial infections, a mild bleeding diathesis, progressive neuropathy, and cranial nerve defects. The neutrophils of these patients contain characteristic giant granules. Patients exhibit multiple defects of immune function, including impairment in neutrophil chemotaxis, phagocytosis, NK cell activity, and T-cell cytotoxicity. Many white blood cells are destroyed before leaving the bone marrow. In most patients an accelerated lymphoproliferative syndrome leads to death. However, bone marrow transplantation can reverse immunologic dysfunction in some patients.

Neutrophil-specific granule deficiency syndrome is another rare congenital disorder characterized by neutrophils that exhibit impaired chemotaxis and bactericidal activity. Patients are prone to recurrent bacterial and fungal infections with abscess formation. Skin and pulmonary infections appear to predominate, and most of these respond well to aggressive antibiotic therapy. Affected patients frequently survive into their adult years.

Management of Patients With Neutropenia or Abnormalities of Phagocytosis

Patients with neutropenia or a qualitative disorder of granulocyte function often benefit significantly from treatment with G-CSF. Recombinant G-CSF therapy reduces the duration of absolute neutropenia in patients receiving ablative chemotherapy and autologous bone marrow transplantation. It also shortens the length of antibiotic therapy and reduces the risk of life-threatening bacteremia and fungal infections. G-CSF therapy has been approved for reversal of the neutropenia associated with HIV infection and prevention of worsening neutropenia in patients receiving HIV therapy. Neutropenic patients undergoing elective surgery may benefit from a course of G-CSF preoperatively to reduce the risk of perioperative infection.

Deficiencies in Components of the Complement System

Complement refers to a family of serum proteins that are critical to the host response to infection. Complement activation may occur by *pathogen-dependent (classical or lectin)* or *pathogen-independent (alternative)* pathways (Fig. 27.2). Complement proteins assist in clearing microorganisms by coating infectious agents with proteins that facilitate phagocytosis. Complement proteins also promote the inflammatory response. Certain complement components are unique to a particular pathway, but all pathways lead to formation of C3 and the membrane attack complex. Deficiencies in virtually all of the soluble complement components have been described. Defects in early components of the classical pathway of complement activation (C1q, C1r, C2, and C4) predispose to autoimmune inflammatory disorders resembling SLE. Deficiencies in the common pathway component C3 are usually fatal in

utero. Deficiencies in the terminal complement components C5 through C8 are associated with recurrent infection and rheumatic diseases. Patients with deficiencies in C9 and components of the alternative pathway (factor D and properdin) are predisposed to neisserial infection. Factor H deficiency is associated with familial relapsing hemolytic uremic syndrome. The liver is the primary organ of complement protein synthesis. Therefore patients with advanced liver disease are often at increased risk of infection, especially pneumonia and sepsis caused by *Streptococcus pneumoniae, S. aureus,* and *E. coli.* Prompt recognition and treatment of infection and careful maintenance of routine immunizations are key in the treatment of these patients.

Tight regulation of complement activation prevents misdirected activation of the inflammatory and immune response. The main inhibitor compound is C1 esterase inhibitor. Deficiency of C1 esterase inhibitor is responsible for *hereditary angioedema,* an autosomal dominant condition marked by episodes of subcutaneous and submucosal edema caused primarily by excessive concentrations of bradykinin, which increases vascular permeability.

Hyposplenism

Splenectomy is the most common cause of splenic dysfunction, although various clinical conditions may lead to impaired splenic functioning. Perhaps the most common of these is sickle cell anemia, which causes autoinfarction of the spleen as a result of vasoocclusive disease. *S. pneumoniae* is the most common cause of bacterial sepsis in postsplenectomy patients. Splenic dysfunction also increases the risk of infection with *Neisseria meningitidis, E. coli, Haemophilus influenzae,* and malaria. As recommended for patients with complement deficiencies, management of hyposplenic patients relies on prevention, mainly through immunization against *S. pneumoniae, H. influenzae* type b, and *N. meningitidis* in particular. These immunizations should be given prior to splenectomy.

EXCESSIVE INNATE IMMUNITY

Neutrophilia

The earliest response to an infection is migration of granulocytes out of the circulation and into the site of bacterial invasion. The rapidity and magnitude of the increase in the number of circulating granulocytes in response to infection is remarkable. Within hours of the onset of a severe infection, the granulocyte count increases twofold to fourfold. This increase represents a change in the marginated and circulating pools of granulocytes as well as delivery of new granulocytes from bone marrow. *Neutrophilia* is defined as an absolute neutrophil count higher than 7000/mm^3.

An increase in the granulocyte count does not produce specific symptoms or signs unless the count exceeds 100,000/mm^3. Such marked leukocytosis can produce leukostasis, resulting in splenic infarction and reduction in the oxygen-diffusing

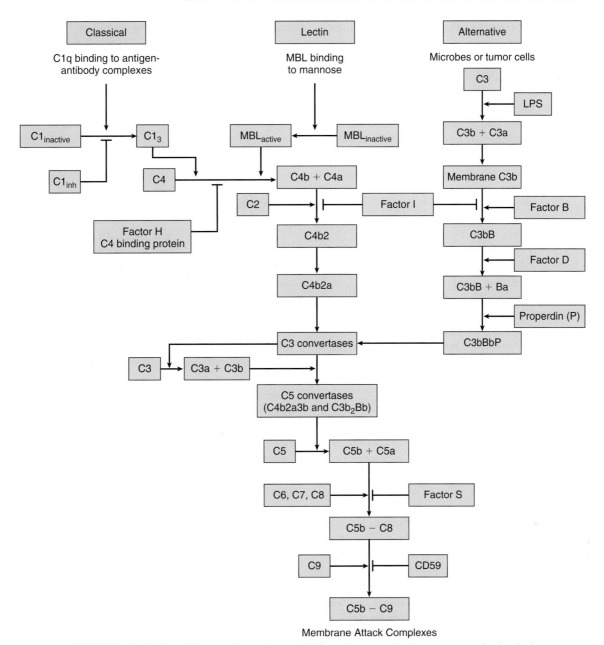

FIG. 27.2 Activation of the complement cascade. Complement activation can occur via classical and lectin pathways or by alternative pathways. In the classical pathway, binding of an antigen-antibody complex to C1q is the triggering event. In the lectin pathway, mannose residues on bacteria bind to mannose binding lectin (MBL), setting off complement activation. The alternative pathway can be activated by microbes or tumor cells. All pathways lead to formation of C3, which is important in immune complex modification, opsonization, and lymphocyte activation. The terminal common pathway that flows from all three activation pathways leads to production of the membrane attack complex C5b-9, which lyses cells. $C1_{inh}$, C1 inhibitor; *LPS*, lipopolysaccharide.

capacity of the lungs. Granulocytes can also accumulate in the skin to produce nontender purplish nodules called *chloromas.* Unlike immature blasts, mature granulocytes do not invade brain tissue, so neurologic complications do not result from reactive granulocytosis.

The clinical features associated with moderate granulocytosis vary depending on the primary disease underlying the condition. Deep-seated infections and peritonitis are associated

with granulocyte counts of 10,000–30,000/mm³ or more. Reactive monocytosis is seen in patients with tuberculosis, subacute bacterial endocarditis, or severe granulocytopenia. Parasitic infestations are typically associated with an elevated eosinophil count, whereas basophilia is seen in patients with chronic myeloid leukemia. As a general rule, sustained granulocyte counts of 50,000/mm³ or higher indicate a malignant disease process such as a myeloproliferative disorder. The appearance of very immature myelocytic cells in the circulation and accompanying changes in other cell lines (increased or decreased platelets or red blood cells) are also signs of hematologic malignancy.

Granulocytosis is an expected side effect of glucocorticoid therapy, because glucocorticoids interfere with the egress of granulocytes from the circulation into tissues. Patients receiving prednisone 60–100 mg/day often have white blood cell counts of 15,000–20,000/mm³. Other causes of granulocytosis include physiologic stress, exposure to certain drugs, and cigarette smoking.

Monocytosis

Monocytosis occurs in conjunction with inflammatory disorders such as SLE, RA, and sarcoidosis and in the context of certain infections, including tuberculosis, syphilis, and subacute bacterial endocarditis. Monocytosis can also be seen in patients with primary neutropenic disorders or hematologic malignancies. Although monocytes are important components of the immune system, the association between the circulating monocyte count and the propensity for infection is not as clear as in the case of neutrophils.

Asthma

Asthma is characterized by an exaggerated bronchoconstrictor response to certain stimuli (see Chapter 2, "Obstructive Respiratory Diseases"). Triggers for bronchospasm unrelated to the immune system produce *intrinsic* asthma. Placement of an endotracheal tube may trigger this type of asthma; other common triggers are cold, exercise, stress, and inhaled irritants. Mediators of intrinsic asthma are components of the innate immune system. By contrast, triggers that activate the immune system and release IgE produce *extrinsic* asthma and are part of adaptive immunity. Inhaled allergens such as pollen and pet dander are common causes of extrinsic asthma. Symptoms of extrinsic or allergic asthma are highly variable and can include cough, dyspnea, and wheezing. Treatment consists of administration of β-agonists, anticholinergics, corticosteroids, and leukotriene inhibitors.

MISDIRECTED INNATE IMMUNITY

Angioedema

Angioedema may be hereditary or acquired and is characterized by episodic subcutaneous and submucosal edema formation, often involving the face, extremities, and gastrointestinal tract. There are two types of angioedema. One is caused by release of mast cell mediators and is associated with urticaria, bronchospasm, flushing, and even hypotension. The other results from bradykinin release and does not cause allergic symptoms. The most common hereditary form of angioedema results from an autosomal dominant deficiency or dysfunction of *C1 esterase inhibitor*. This serine protease inhibitor (serpin) regulates complement, contact activation,

and fibrinolytic pathways. The absence of C1 esterase inhibitor also leads to the release of vasoactive mediators that increase vascular permeability and produce edema via bradykinin. Patients deficient in this regulatory enzyme experience repeated bouts of facial and/or laryngeal edema lasting 24–72 hours. These episodes usually begin in the second decade of life and may be triggered by menses, trauma, infection, stress, or estrogen-containing oral contraceptives. Dental surgery can be an important trigger of laryngeal attacks. Abdominal attacks usually present with excruciating pain, nausea, vomiting, and/or diarrhea.

C1 esterase inhibitor deficiency can be acquired by patients with lymphoproliferative disorders. These patients have antibodies to C1 inhibitor, and this gives rise to a syndrome that closely mimics hereditary angioedema. Angiotensin-converting enzyme (ACE) inhibitors used for the treatment of hypertension and heart failure can also precipitate angioedema. This drug-induced angioedema is thought to result from increased availability of bradykinin made possible by the ACE inhibitor–mediated blockade of bradykinin catabolism. Interestingly, angioedema provoked by ACE inhibitors may develop unexpectedly after prolonged drug use.

Androgens such as danazol and stanozolol have been the mainstay of prophylactic therapy, both long term and preoperatively, in patients with angioedema. Antifibrinolytic therapy (e.g., ε-aminocaproic acid, tranexamic acid, or aprotinin) has also been used. Anabolic steroids (androgens) are believed to increase hepatic synthesis of C1 esterase inhibitor, whereas antifibrinolytics are thought to act by inhibiting plasmin activation. There are several medications now available to treat an acute attack of angioedema: C1 inhibitor concentrate (plasma-derived or recombinant); icatibant, a synthetic bradykinin receptor antagonist; ecallantide, a recombinant plasma kallikrein inhibitor that blocks the conversion of kininogen to bradykinin; or fresh frozen plasma (2–4 units) to replace the deficient enzyme. It is important to note that androgens, catecholamines, antihistamines, and antifibrinolytics are *not* useful in the treatment of acute episodes of angioedema. Should upper airway obstruction develop during an acute attack, tracheal intubation until the edema subsides may be lifesaving. When laryngoscopy is undertaken, it is important to have personnel and equipment available to perform tracheostomy if needed, but tracheostomy itself may be extremely difficult or impossible in the face of severe airway edema.

Management of Anesthesia

Patients experiencing recurrent angioedema, whether hereditary or acquired, require prophylaxis before a stimulating procedure such as dental surgery or any surgery requiring endotracheal intubation. It is prudent to ensure ready availability of C1 inhibitor concentrates for intravenous (IV) infusion should an acute attack occur. Incidental trauma to the oropharynx, such as that produced by suctioning, should be minimized. Regional anesthetic techniques and intramuscular injections are well tolerated by these patients.

INADEQUATE ADAPTIVE IMMUNITY

Defects of Antibody Production

X-linked agammaglobulinemia is an inherited defect in maturation of B cells. Mature B cells are missing or reduced in the circulation, and lymphoid tissues have no plasma cells. Therefore functional antibody is not produced. Affected boys have recurrent pyogenic infections during the latter half of their first year of life as maternal antibodies wane. Treatment with IV immunoglobulin every 3–4 months to maintain plasma IgG levels near 500 mg/dL allows the majority of these children to survive into adulthood.

Selective IgA deficiency occurs in 1 in every 600–800 adults. In this condition, plasma IgA concentrations are less than 5 mg/dL, but concentrations of other immunoglobulins are normal. Recurrent sinus and pulmonary infections are common, although many patients are asymptomatic. When transfused with blood products containing IgA, a subset of patients with selective IgA deficiency may experience anaphylaxis due to antibody directed against IgA. Therefore these patients should receive blood or blood components obtained from IgA-deficient donors.

Waldenström macroglobulinemia is due to proliferation of a malignant plasma cell clone that secretes IgM, which results in marked increases in plasma viscosity. Bone marrow is infiltrated with malignant lymphocytes, as are the liver, spleen, and lungs. Anemia and an increased incidence of spontaneous hemorrhage are common findings in these patients. In contrast to multiple myeloma, Waldenström macroglobulinemia rarely involves the skeletal system. As a result, renal dysfunction resulting from hypercalcemia is uncommon. *Hyperviscosity syndrome* is a serious complication of this condition; it produces neurologic complaints such as blurring or loss of vision, headache, vertigo, nystagmus, dizziness, tinnitus, sudden deafness, diplopia, and ataxia. Treatment consists of urgent plasmapheresis to remove the abnormal proteins and reduce plasma viscosity. Chemoimmunotherapy may be instituted to decrease proliferation of the cells responsible for production of abnormal immunoglobulins.

Cold autoimmune diseases are characterized by the presence of abnormal circulating proteins (usually IgM or IgA antibodies) that agglutinate in response to a decrease in body temperature. These disorders include *cryoglobulinemia* and *cold hemagglutinin disease*. Plasma hyperviscosity is prominent, and microvascular thrombosis may cause acute end-organ damage during a period of hypothermia. Symptoms normally do not occur until body temperature falls below 33°C. Management of anesthesia in these patients includes strict maintenance of normothermia. Patients scheduled for surgery requiring cardiopulmonary bypass present significant challenges. Use of systemic hypothermia may be contraindicated, and cold cardioplegia solutions may precipitate intracoronary hemagglutination with consequent thrombosis, ischemia, or infarction. Alternatives to cold cardioplegia include fibrillatory arrest for brief time periods. Plasmapheresis may

also be helpful in reducing plasma concentrations of these immunoglobulins.

Amyloidosis encompasses several disorders characterized by accumulation of insoluble fibrillar proteins (amyloid) in various tissues including the heart, vascular smooth muscle, kidneys, adrenal glands, gastrointestinal tract, peripheral nerves, and skin. *Primary amyloidosis* is a plasma cell disorder marked by accumulation of immunoglobulin light chains. *Secondary amyloidosis* is observed in association with several other conditions, including multiple myeloma, RA, and a prolonged antigenic challenge such as that produced by chronic infection.

Macroglossia is a classic feature of patients with amyloidosis, occurring in about 20% of these patients. The enlarged stiff tongue may impair swallowing and speaking. Involvement of salivary glands and adjacent tissue may cause upper airway obstruction that mimics angioedema. Cardiac involvement is fairly common and may cause intraventricular conduction delays including heart block. Sudden death is not uncommon. Cardiac dysfunction classically involves right-sided heart failure, with relative sparing of left-sided heart function until late in the disease. Accumulation of amyloid in the kidneys may produce nephrotic syndrome. Deposition in joint spaces may lead to limited range of motion as well as peripheral nerve entrapments such as carpal tunnel syndrome. Amyloidosis of the gastrointestinal tract may lead to malabsorption, ileus, and impaired gastric emptying. Hepatomegaly is common, although hepatic dysfunction is rare. The diagnosis of amyloidosis is based on clinical suspicion confirmed by tissue biopsy. Since amyloid deposits are frequently found in the rectum, rectal biopsy is a common initial diagnostic procedure.

Treatment of amyloidosis is generally directed toward symptomatic improvement rather than a cure. Airway management may be challenging owing to an enlarged tongue. Perioperative management of these patients requires careful preoperative evaluation for signs of end-organ dysfunction such as renal insufficiency and heart failure or conduction defects. Gastric motility drugs may be useful in some patients. Of note, amyloid deposits have the potential to trap factor X or evoke fibrinolysis, which predisposes these patients to hemorrhagic complications.

Defects of T Lymphocytes

DiGeorge syndrome (thymic hypoplasia) is the result of a gene deletion. Features include absent or diminished thymus development, hypoplasia of the thyroid and parathyroid glands, cardiac malformations, and facial dysmorphisms. The degree of immunocompromise correlates with the amount of thymic tissue present. Complete absence of the thymus produces a severe combined immunodeficiency syndrome with the risk of bacterial, fungal, and parasitic infections. Complete DiGeorge syndrome is treated by thymus transplantation or infusion of mature T cells. Partial DiGeorge syndrome requires no therapy.

Combined Immune System Defects

Severe combined immunodeficiency syndromes are caused by a number of genetic mutations that affect T, B, or NK cell functions. The most common form of severe combined immunodeficiency syndrome is the *X-linked form,* which has a prevalence of approximately 1 in 58,000 live births and accounts for approximately half of severe combined immunodeficiency syndrome cases in the United States. The disease is caused by a mutation in a gene that encodes for a protein subunit shared by several of the interleukin receptors. Absence of these receptors results in defective interleukin signaling, which in turn blocks normal differentiation of NK, B, and T cells. The only treatment that substantially prolongs life expectancy is bone marrow or stem cell transplantation from an HLA-compatible donor.

Adenosine deaminase deficiency is another form of severe combined immunodeficiency syndrome, accounting for approximately 15% of cases. The adenosine deaminase enzyme is most abundant in lymphocytes, and deficiency allows toxic levels of purine intermediates to accumulate, which leads to T-cell death. There is profound lymphopenia together with skeletal abnormalities of the ribs and hips. Hematopoietic stem cell transplantation from an HLA-matched donor is the preferred treatment. When such a match is not an option, gene therapy or enzyme replacement with bovine adenosine deaminase enzyme is of benefit in prolonging life.

Ataxia-telangiectasia is a syndrome consisting of cerebellar ataxia, oculocutaneous telangiectasias, chronic sinopulmonary disease, and immunodeficiency. The genetic basis of this disorder is a mutation in the gene encoding ATM protein, which is important in surveillance and repair of double-strand DNA breaks. In this syndrome, DNA damage that occurs during cell division is missed, and defective cells are released into the circulation. One consequence of this defect is production of dysfunctional lymphocytes. These patients also have a very high risk of malignancy, especially leukemia and lymphoma, and in women, breast cancer. Patients with ataxia-telangiectasia are extremely susceptible to radiation-induced injury, so treatments such as bone marrow transplantation (which requires total body irradiation) are not possible. Supportive

therapy includes IV administration of immunoglobulin. Chronic lung disease is a major source of morbidity and mortality, and routine pulmonary function testing is part of ongoing management.

EXCESSIVE ADAPTIVE IMMUNITY

Allergic Reactions

Immune-mediated allergic reactions—which are in essence "overreactions" of the immune system—are classified according to their mechanism (Table 27.2). *Type I* allergic reactions are IgE mediated and involve mast cells and basophils. The majority of cases of anaphylaxis are IgE-mediated events. *Type II* reactions mediate cytotoxicity via IgG, IgM, and complement. Type II reactions usually manifest as hemolytic anemia, thrombocytopenia, or neutropenia, since these are the cell types most often affected. Clinical presentation and severity vary widely, and presentation may be delayed for several days. *Type III* reactions produce tissue damage via immune complex formation and deposition and often lead to glomerulonephritis, urticaria, vasculitis, and arthralgias. *Type IV* reactions are marked by T lymphocyte–mediated delayed hypersensitivity and are typically drug reactions.

Cutaneous symptoms are the most common physical manifestation of drug allergy. Clinical severity ranges from simple contact dermatitis to Stevens-Johnson syndrome and toxic epidermal necrolysis, two types of severe exfoliative dermatitis that can be life threatening. *Drug-induced hypersensitivity syndrome* (DIHS), also called *drug rash with eosinophilia and systemic symptoms* (DRESS), is another severe form of type IV delayed drug hypersensitivity, marked by eosinophilia, rash, fever, and multiple organ failure. This condition does not usually manifest until 2–6 weeks after drug exposure and appears to be associated with herpes reactivation. Patients with viral infections such as Epstein-Barr virus or cytomegalovirus infection experience an increased incidence of some type IV drug reactions.

Not all drug allergies are mediated by the immune system. *Nonimmune anaphylaxis* (formerly called *anaphylactoid*

| TABLE 27.2 | Classification of Immune-Mediated Allergic Reactions |

Reaction Type	Mediators	Timing	Examples
Type I Allergy	IgE	Immediate	Anaphylaxis Urticaria
Type II Cytotoxic, antibody dependent	IgG IgM Complement	May be delayed	Autoimmune hemolytic anemia Immune thrombocytopenia Incompatible blood reaction
Type III Immune complex disease	Immune complex formation and deposition	Delayed	Glomerulonephritis Serum sickness Vasculitis
Type IV T-lymphocyte–mediated delayed hypersensitivity	T lymphocytes	Delayed	Dermatitis Chronic transplant rejection Tuberculin test

reaction) occurs when mediator release from mast cells and basophils results from direct interaction with the offending drug rather than activation of the immune system.

Anaphylaxis

Anaphylaxis is a life-threatening condition marked by cardiovascular collapse, interstitial edema, and bronchospasm. Anaphylaxis may occur by immune-mediated or non–immune-mediated mechanisms. The most common type of immune-mediated anaphylaxis results when previous exposure to antigens in drugs or foods evokes production of antigen-specific IgE antibodies. Subsequent exposure to the same or a chemically similar antigen results in antigen-antibody interactions that initiate marked degranulation of mast cells and basophils. Approximately 60% of anaphylactic reactions are mediated by IgE antibodies. Less commonly, IgG or IgM antibody reactions are to blame. Non–immune-mediated anaphylaxis results from direct release of histamine and other mediators from mast cells and basophils. Initial manifestations of anaphylaxis usually occur within 5–10 minutes of exposure to the antigen. Vasoactive mediators released by degranulation of mast cells and basophils are responsible for the clinical indicators of anaphylaxis (Table 27.3). Urticaria and pruritus are common. Primary vascular collapse occurs in approximately 25% of cases of fatal anaphylaxis. Laryngeal edema, bronchospasm, and arterial hypoxemia may accompany anaphylaxis. Extravasation of up to 50% of the intravascular fluid volume into the extracellular space reflects the extent of microvascular permeability that can accompany anaphylaxis. Indeed, hypovolemia is the most likely cause of hypotension in these patients, although leukotriene-mediated negative inotropism may also be a factor.

The estimated incidence of all immune- and non–immune-mediated episodes of anaphylaxis during anesthesia is between 1 in 3500 and 1 in 20,000 anesthetic cases. The wide variability reflects the difficulty in determining the denominator (total number of anesthetic cases) as well as inconsistencies in event reporting. Estimated mortality from perioperative anaphylaxis ranges from 3%–9%. Risk factors include asthma, atopy, multiple past surgeries or procedures (especially for incidents involving latex), and the presence of certain systemic conditions such as hereditary angioedema or systemic mastocytosis.

Diagnosis

The diagnosis of anaphylaxis is suggested by the often dramatic nature of the clinical manifestations in close temporal relationship to exposure to a particular antigen. Cardiovascular, respiratory, and cutaneous manifestations are most common. Typical signs include tachycardia, bronchospasm, and laryngeal edema. Recognition of an allergic reaction that occurs during anesthesia may be compromised by the patient's inability to communicate early symptoms such as pruritus, and surgical drapes may obscure recognition of cutaneous signs. Consequently, cardiovascular collapse may be the first detectable signal of this event in the operating room.

Immunologic and biochemical evidence of anaphylaxis is provided by an increased plasma tryptase concentration within 1–2 hours of the suspected event. *Tryptase,* a neutral protease stored in mast cells, is liberated into the systemic circulation during immune-mediated but not during non–immune-mediated reactions. Its presence verifies that mast cell activation and mediator release have occurred and thus serves to distinguish immunologic from chemical reactions. Plasma histamine concentration returns to baseline within 30–60 minutes of an anaphylactic reaction, so plasma histamine concentration must be measured immediately after treatment of anaphylaxis to capture the change in plasma histamine concentration.

In cases of IgE-mediated anaphylaxis, identification of the offending agent can be established by a positive response to a skin prick or intradermal test (wheal-and-flare response), which confirms the presence of specific IgE antibodies. Skin testing should not be performed within 6 weeks of an anaphylactic reaction, because mast cell and basophil mediator depletion may lead to a false-negative result. Because of the risk of inducing a systemic reaction, testing must be done with a dilute preservative-free solution of suspected antigen and performed only by trained personnel with appropriate resuscitation equipment available. In vitro immunoassays for allergen-specific IgE are commercially available for some drugs. This type of testing is most commonly used in the evaluation of potential reactions to neuromuscular blockers, latex, penicillin, and other β-lactam antibiotics. Skin testing remains the more sensitive and preferred method of testing in the majority of cases.

Treatment

The immediate goals of treatment of anaphylaxis are reversal of hypotension and hypoxemia, replacement of intravascular volume, and inhibition of further cellular degranulation and release of vasoactive mediators (Table 27.4). Several liters of crystalloid and/or colloid solution must be infused to restore intravascular fluid volume and blood pressure. Epinephrine

TABLE 27.3	Vasoactive Mediators Released During Anaphylaxis
Mediator	Physiologic Effect
Histamine	Increased capillary permeability Peripheral vasodilation Bronchoconstriction Urticaria
Leukotrienes	Increased capillary permeability Bronchoconstriction Negative inotropy Coronary artery vasoconstriction
Prostaglandins	Bronchoconstriction
Eosinophil chemotactic factor	Attraction of eosinophils
Neutrophil chemotactic factor	Attraction of neutrophils
Platelet-activating factor	Platelet aggregation Release of vasoactive amines

TABLE 27.4	Management of Anaphylactic Reactions During Anesthesia

PRIMARY TREATMENT

General Measures
Inform the surgeon.
Request immediate assistance.
Stop administration of all drugs, colloids, blood products.
Maintain airway with 100% oxygen.
Elevate the legs if practical.

Epinephrine Administration
Titrate dose according to symptom severity and clinical response.
Adults: 10–100 µg by IV bolus, repeat every 1–2 min as needed
IV infusion starting at 0.05–1 µg/kg/min
Children: 1–10 µg/kg by IV bolus, repeat every 1–2 min as needed

Fluid Therapy
Crystalloid: normal saline 10–25 mL/kg over 20 min, more as needed
Colloid: 10 mL/kg over 20 min, more as needed

Anaphylaxis Resistant to Epinephrine
Glucagon: 1–5 mg IV bolus followed by 1–2.5 mg/h IV infusion
Norepinephrine: 0.05-0.1 µg/kg/min IV infusion
Vasopressin: 2–10 unit IV bolus followed by 0.01–0.1 unit/min IV infusion

SECONDARY TREATMENT

Bronchodilator
β_2-Agonist for symptomatic treatment of bronchospasm

Antihistamines
Histamine-1 antagonist: diphenhydramine 0.5–1 mg/kg IV
Histamine-2 antagonist: ranitidine 50 mg IV

Corticosteroids
Adults: hydrocortisone 250 mg IV or methylprednisolone 80 mg IV
Children: hydrocortisone 50–100 mg IV or methylprednisolone 2 mg/kg IV

AFTERCARE
Patient may experience relapse; admit for observation.
Obtain blood samples for diagnostic testing.
Arrange allergy testing at 6–8 weeks postoperatively.

Adapted from Mertes PM, Tajima K, Regnier-Kimmoun MA, et al. Perioperative anaphylaxis. *Med Clin North Am.* 2010;94:780.

is indicated in doses of 10–100 µg IV. Early intervention with epinephrine is critical for reversing the life-threatening events characteristic of anaphylaxis. Epinephrine, by increasing intracellular concentrations of cyclic adenosine monophosphate, restores membrane permeability and decreases the release of vasoactive mediators. The β-agonist effects of epinephrine relax bronchial smooth muscle and reverse bronchospasm. The dose of epinephrine can be doubled and repeated every 1–2 minutes until a satisfactory blood pressure response has been obtained. If anaphylaxis is not life threatening, intramuscular rather than IV epinephrine may be used in a dose of 0.3–0.5 mg. Injection into thigh muscle is preferred to injection into upper arm muscle because

absorption is more rapid. In cases where cardiovascular collapse is unresponsive to epinephrine, alternative vasopressors such as vasopressin, glucagon, or norepinephrine should be considered.

Antihistamines such as diphenhydramine compete with membrane receptor sites normally occupied by histamine and may decrease some manifestations of anaphylaxis, including pruritus and bronchospasm. However, administration of an antihistamine is not effective in treating anaphylaxis once vasoactive mediators have been released. β₂-Agonists such as albuterol delivered by metered-dose inhaler or nebulizer are useful for treatment of bronchospasm associated with anaphylaxis.

Corticosteroids are often administered intravenously to patients experiencing anaphylaxis. These drugs have no known effect on degranulation of mast cells or antigen-antibody interactions. In addition, they take several hours to take effect and therefore have no role in managing acute symptoms. There is no evidence from randomized trials that corticosteroids are useful in the treatment of anaphylaxis. The favorable impact sometimes observed with corticosteroid therapy may reflect enhancement of the β-agonist effects of other drugs or inhibition of the release of arachidonic acid responsible for production of leukotrienes and prostaglandins. Corticosteroids may, however, be uniquely helpful in patients experiencing life-threatening allergic reactions resulting from activation of the complement system.

Drug Allergy

Epidemiology

The incidence of allergic and anaphylactic drug reactions during anesthesia appears to be increasing, probably because of the frequent administration of several drugs to each patient and cross-sensitivity among drugs. It is not possible to reliably predict which patients are likely to experience anaphylaxis after administration of drugs that are usually innocuous. However, patients with a history of allergy (extrinsic asthma, allergy to tropical fruits or drugs) have an increased incidence of anaphylaxis, possibly related to a genetic predisposition to form increased amounts of IgE antibodies. A history of allergy to specific drugs elicited during the preoperative evaluation is helpful, but previous uneventful exposure to a drug does *not* eliminate the possibility of anaphylaxis on subsequent exposure. In addition, anaphylaxis can occur on first exposure to a drug because of cross-reactivity with other environmental agents.

Allergic drug reactions must be distinguished from drug intolerance, idiosyncratic reactions, and drug toxicity. The occurrence of undesirable pharmacologic effects at a low dose of drug reflects intolerance, whereas idiosyncratic reactions are undesirable responses to a drug independent of the dose administered. Evidence of histamine release along veins into which drugs are injected indicates localized and nonimmunologic release of histamine insufficient to evoke systemic symptoms. Patients manifesting such a localized response should *not* be categorized as allergic to a drug.

TABLE 27.5	Drugs Associated With Perioperative Anaphylaxis

COMMON

Muscle relaxants
Antibiotics (β-lactam drugs, sulfonamides, vancomycin, quinolones)
Latex

LESS COMMON

Hypnotics (barbiturates, propofol)
Opioids
Local anesthetics (esters more than amides)
Synthetic colloids (dextran, hydroxyethyl starch)
Blood and blood products
Protamine
Chlorhexidine
Vital dyes (isosulfan blue)
Nonsteroidal antiinflammatory drugs (COX-1 drugs)
Aspirin
Heparin
Insulin
Radiocontrast media
Povidone
Bacitracin
Streptokinase, urokinase
Hyaluronidase

Allergic Drug Reactions During the Perioperative Period

Allergic drug reactions to nearly all drugs administered during anesthesia have been reported (Table 27.5). Most drug-induced allergic reactions manifest within 5–10 minutes of exposure. An important exception is the allergic response to latex, which is typically delayed for 30 minutes or more.

Muscle Relaxants

Muscle relaxants are one of the most common causes of drug-induced allergic reactions during the perioperative period, with rocuronium and succinylcholine the most frequent offenders. Cross-sensitivity among muscle relaxants emphasizes the structural similarities of many drugs in this class. Approximately half of patients who experience an allergic reaction to one muscle relaxant are also allergic to other muscle relaxants. IgE antibodies develop to quaternary or tertiary ammonium ions. Many over-the-counter drugs and cosmetics contain these ammonium ions and are capable of sensitizing an individual. Consequently, anaphylaxis may develop on the first exposure to a muscle relaxant in a patient sensitized by one of these products. Neostigmine and morphine contain ammonium ions that are also capable of cross-reacting with antibodies to muscle relaxants. Antibodies that develop against muscle relaxants remain present for decades, so a patient with a history of anaphylaxis to *any* muscle relaxant should be *skin tested preoperatively* for all drugs likely to be used in future anesthetic management. Ideally an alternative drug to which the patient has been found to be nonallergic should be used. Avoidance is preferred if an alternative means of providing anesthesia is available. Desensitization is theoretically possible but is not practical, given that it would require prolonged exposure to a paralytic agent.

Nonimmune reactions to muscle relaxants include direct mast cell degranulation that causes release of histamine and other mediators. Benzylisoquinolinium compounds such as D-tubocurarine, metocurine, atracurium, and mivacurium are more likely to cause direct mast cell degranulation than aminosteroid compounds like pancuronium, vecuronium, and rocuronium. Skin testing is not useful in the investigation of non–immune-mediated allergic reactions. Reactions that are not IgE mediated may be reduced in frequency or intensity by pretreatment with antihistamines and glucocorticoids.

Antibiotics

Antibiotics are also a leading cause of anaphylaxis in the perioperative period. Penicillin allergy is most common, and in the general population, penicillin accounts for most fatal anaphylactic drug reactions. Approximately 10% of patients report a penicillin allergy; however, it has been estimated that up to 90% of these patients are in fact able to tolerate penicillin. This is due in part to an initial misattribution of clinical signs to a penicillin reaction rather than to the underlying medical illness being treated with the penicillin. In addition, IgE antibodies to penicillin wane over time, so many patients diagnosed as penicillin allergic in childhood are able to tolerate penicillin as adults. Elective skin testing should be considered for any patient with a convincing history of IgE-mediated penicillin allergy to avoid unnecessary use of more expensive and broader-spectrum antibiotics. The negative predictive value of penicillin skin testing is high—that is, a *negative skin test* result for penicillin reliably indicates that the patient is *not* allergic to penicillin. Patients with a positive skin test result are candidates for drug desensitization. This is accomplished by administration of escalating challenge doses of an allergen or drug to an allergic patient so the patient eventually becomes desensitized to that allergen or drug.

Penicillins contain two allergenic components also present in other antibiotics: the β-lactam ring (also found in cephalosporins, carbapenems, and monobactams) and the R-group side chain. The R-group side chain of the aminopenicillins amoxicillin and ampicillin is identical to that of some of the cephalosporins. In the United States, most penicillin-allergic patients are sensitive to the β-lactam ring, whereas in Europe, most patients react to the R-group side chain. As a result of these shared components, there is potential for patients allergic to penicillin to also be allergic to other antibiotics. However, the incidence of life-threatening allergic reactions following administration of cephalosporins is low (0.05%). Historically the incidence of allergic reaction to cephalosporins in patients with a history of penicillin allergy was reported to be in the range of 7%. More recent research suggests a much lower rate of cross-reactivity (2%). Patients with selective allergies to amoxicillin or ampicillin should not be given cephalosporins with identical R-group side chains (Table 27.6). Despite the common β-lactam ring, the incidence of carbapenem allergy

TABLE 27.6	Antibiotics to Avoid in Patients With Amoxicillin or Ampicillin Allergy
Amoxicillin Allergy	**Ampicillin Allergy**
Avoid:	*Avoid:*
Cefadroxil	Cefaclor
Cefprozil	Cephalexin
Cefatrizine	Cephradine
	Cephaloglycin

Adapted from Solensky R. Penicillin-allergic patients: use of cephalosporins, carbapenems, and monobactams. Available at www.uptodate.com.

in patients with penicillin allergy is less than 1%, and there is no cross-reactivity between penicillin and the only clinically available monobactam, aztreonam.

Allergy to sulfonamide antibiotics is the second most commonly reported antibiotic allergy after allergy to penicillins and cephalosporins. Reactions manifest most often as delayed cutaneous rashes, and sulfonamides are the most common cause of Stevens-Johnson syndrome. In HIV-positive patients, the incidence of rash due to sulfonamides is approximately 10 times higher than that in HIV-negative patients. Because trimethoprim-sulfamethoxazole is the drug of choice for treatment and prophylaxis of *Pneumocystis jiroveci* pneumonia in HIV-positive patients, drug desensitization is advised.

Most purported cases of vancomycin allergy are non–IgE-mediated reactions involving direct histamine release from mast cells and basophils and are directly related to the rate of drug infusion. In most cases these patients are able to tolerate repeat administration using slower infusion rates and antihistamine premedication. However, in rare cases, IgE-mediated allergy has been reported on repeat exposure to this drug.

Latex

Latex is a saplike substance produced by the commercial rubber tree *Hevea brasiliensis*. Several different *Hevea* proteins may cause an IgE-mediated antibody response that can lead to cardiovascular collapse during anesthesia and surgery. A feature that distinguishes latex-induced allergic reactions from other drug-induced allergic reactions is its delayed onset, typically longer than 30 minutes after exposure. This may reflect the time needed for the responsible antigen to be eluted from rubber gloves and absorbed across mucous membranes into the systemic circulation in amounts sufficient to cause an allergic reaction. Contact with latex at mucosal surfaces is the most significant route of latex exposure. However, inhalation of latex antigens is an alternative route. Cornstarch powder in gloves is not immunogenic but can act as an airborne vehicle for latex antigens.

Sensitized patients develop IgE antibodies directed specifically against latex antigens. Skin testing can confirm latex hypersensitivity, but anaphylaxis has occurred during skin testing, so this test must be performed with great caution. A radioallergosorbent test and an enzyme-linked immunosorbent assay are available for in vitro detection of latex-specific IgE antibodies. These tests are virtually equal in sensitivity and specificity and avoid the risk of anaphylaxis associated with skin testing.

Questions about itching, conjunctivitis, rhinitis, rash, or wheezing after inflating balloons or wearing latex gloves or after undergoing dental or gynecologic examinations performed using latex gloves may be helpful in identifying sensitized patients. Operating room personnel and patients with spina bifida have an increased incidence of latex allergy that is thought to reflect frequent exposure to latex devices such as bladder catheters and protective outerwear. Latex sensitivity most often manifests as contact dermatitis or bronchospasm resulting from inhalation of latex allergens.

Prevalence of latex allergy peaked in the 1990s and has declined since then. Factors responsible for the increase during that period probably included widespread adoption of universal precautions in the 1990s. Hence latex gloves were worn much more often than previously. In addition, the tapping of younger rubber trees and use of stimulant chemicals to increase latex production probably increased the amount of allergenic protein in the raw material and ultimately in the finished goods of production, which also contributed to the increase in allergic responses. Reduction in the frequency of latex allergy over the past several years is probably a result of the transition to latex-free products and avoidance of powdered latex gloves.

Patients at high risk of latex sensitivity (those with spina bifida, multiple previous operations, or history of fruit allergy, as well as healthcare workers) should be questioned for symptoms related to exposure to natural rubber during their daily routines or previous surgical procedures. Intraoperative management of these patients includes maintenance of a latex-free environment, including the use of nonlatex gloves (styrene, neoprene) by all personnel in contact with the patient. In addition, medications should not be drawn up through latex caps or injected through latex ports on IV delivery tubing.

Hypnotics

Approximately 5% of perioperative anaphylactic events are caused by hypnotic induction agents, more commonly by barbiturates than by nonbarbiturates. Most reported cases of barbiturate allergy have occurred in patients with a history of previous uneventful exposure to a barbiturate. Cross-reactivity among barbiturates is possible, but there is no evidence of cross-reactivity between barbiturate and nonbarbiturate agents. Propofol has been implicated in allergic reactions both on first and repeated exposure. It was formerly advised that propofol be used with caution in patients with a history of egg, soy, or peanut allergy, owing to the presence of lecithin and soybean oil as emulsifying agents in the propofol formulation. However, there is no evidence that patients with these food sensitivities are at increased risk of experiencing an allergic response to propofol. Allergic reactions to midazolam, etomidate, and ketamine are extremely rare.

Opioids

Anaphylaxis after administration of opioids is very rare, which perhaps reflects the similarity of these drugs to naturally occurring endorphins. Certain opioids (e.g., morphine, codeine, meperidine) may directly evoke release of histamine from mast cells and basophils that mimics an allergic response. These reactions are usually limited to cutaneous manifestations such as pruritus and urticaria, consistent with the fact that opioid receptors have been found on dermal mast cells but not on mast cells from any other organs. Fentanyl is unique among narcotics in that it lacks the ability to stimulate mast cell degranulation; this makes it a good option for patients with cutaneous reactions to other narcotics.

Local Anesthetics

True allergy to local anesthetics is rare, despite the common labeling of patients as allergic to drugs in this class. It is estimated that only about 1% of purported allergic reactions to local anesthetics are in fact truly allergic; the remainder represent adverse but known responses to inadvertent intravascular injection (hypotension and seizure) or systemic absorption of epinephrine added to local anesthetic (hypertension and tachycardia). Careful history and review of past medical records are most useful in discerning the true mechanism responsible for the event. Urticaria, laryngeal edema, and bronchoconstriction suggest a true allergic response.

Ester-type local anesthetics more commonly cause allergic reactions than amide-type anesthetics. Ester-type local anesthetics are metabolized to compounds related to para-aminobenzoic acid, which is a highly antigenic compound. Preservatives used in local anesthetic solutions such as methylparaben, propylparaben, and metabisulfite also produce allergic reactions. As a result, anaphylaxis may actually be due to stimulation of antibody production to the preservative rather than to the local anesthetic itself.

It is not uncommon to be presented with the question of the safety of administering a local anesthetic to a patient with a purported history of allergy to this class of drugs. It is generally agreed that cross-sensitivity does not exist between ester-type and amide-type compounds. It is advisable to use only preservative-free local anesthetic solutions, since preservatives may evoke allergic reactions. It is reasonable to recommend intradermal testing with preservative-free local anesthetic in the occasional patient with a convincing history of local anesthetic allergy in whom failure to document a safe local anesthetic drug would prevent use of local or regional anesthesia when clinically indicated.

Volatile Anesthetics

Clinical features of halothane-induced hepatitis suggest a drug-induced allergic reaction. These include eosinophilia, fever, rash, and previous exposure to halothane. The plasma of patients with a clinical diagnosis of halothane hepatitis may contain antibodies that react with halothane-induced liver antigens (neoantigens). These neoantigens are formed by covalent interaction of reactive oxidative trifluoroacetyl halide metabolites with hepatic microsomal proteins. Acetylation of liver proteins changes these metabolites so they are no longer recognized as "self" but rather are regarded as "nonself." As a result, antibodies are formed against these now foreign proteins. It is postulated that subsequent antigen-antibody interactions are responsible for the liver injury associated with halothane hepatitis. Similar oxidative halide metabolites are produced after exposure to enflurane, isoflurane, and desflurane, which suggests the possibility of cross-sensitivity to volatile anesthetics in susceptible patients. Based on the degree of metabolism of these volatile anesthetics, it is predictable that the likelihood of anesthetic-induced allergic hepatitis would be greatest for halothane, intermediate for enflurane, minimal for isoflurane, and remote for desflurane. Unlike the other volatile agents, sevoflurane does not produce these oxidative halide metabolites.

Aspirin and Other NSAIDs

Pseudoallergic reactions after administration of aspirin and other nonsteroidal antiinflammatory drugs (NSAIDs) are well documented. Patients with a history of asthma, hyperplastic sinusitis, and nasal polyps are at increased risk of experiencing these reactions. Common symptoms include rhinorrhea and bronchospasm; airway compromise and severe angioedema may also occur. For the most part these reactions are attributable to inhibition of the cyclooxygenase-1 (COX-1) enzyme that promotes synthesis of leukotrienes and subsequent release of mediators from basophils and mast cells. This is substantiated by the fact that reactions are far less severe when selective COX-2 inhibitor NSAIDs are employed.

Radiocontrast Media

Contrast media injected intravenously for radiographic studies evokes allergic reactions in approximately 3% of patients. The risk of an allergic reaction is increased in patients with a history of asthma or allergies to other drugs or foods. However, the pathogenesis of allergy to contrast material is unrelated to that of "seafood" allergy, which is attributed to high concentrations of iodine. Most reactions to contrast material appear to be non–immune mediated. Therefore in patients with a history of contrast agent allergy, pretreatment with corticosteroids and histamine antagonists is usually effective. A common regimen is oral prednisone 50 mg administered at 13 hours, 7 hours, and 1 hour before exposure, and diphenhydramine 50 mg administered 1 hour before contrast agent administration. Allergic reactions are most common with ionic contrast agents; use of nonionic agents substantially reduces the incidence of allergic reactions.

Although rare, severe progressive nephrogenic systemic fibrosis has been reported in patients exposed to gadolinium-based contrast agents. An immunologic reaction to gadolinium chelates appears to be involved in this disease, which results in fibrosis of the skin and internal organs. Delayed gadolinium excretion resulting from preexisting renal failure is the predisposing factor.

Dyes

Isosulfan blue and other dyes used in sentinel lymph node mapping have an estimated incidence of anaphylaxis of approximately 1%. It is hypothesized that the dye binds to endogenous protein to form a compound that elicits an IgE response. The structural similarity of the dye to compounds found in cosmetics, soaps, and other commonly used household products may lead to prior sensitization.

Chlorhexidine

Chlorhexidine is a commonly used hospital disinfectant. It has been associated with a variety of allergic reactions, including contact dermatitis, urticaria, and anaphylaxis. The incidence of reactions to chlorhexidine is thought to be underreported. Because chlorhexidine is found in household products, patients are capable of developing IgE sensitization.

Protamine

Protamine is capable of causing direct histamine release from mast cells and activating the complement pathway to produce thromboxane, which causes bronchoconstriction, pulmonary artery hypertension, and systemic hypotension. This is a predictable response and is directly related to the rate of injection. It is *not* an allergic reaction.

Immune-mediated anaphylactic reactions to protamine are rare. The presence of serum antiprotamine IgE and IgG antibodies can be demonstrated in these patients. Diabetic patients treated with protamine-containing insulin preparations such as neutral protamine Hagedorn (NPH) are pre-exposed to protamine and may develop antibodies against it. Although protamine is derived from salmon sperm or testis, there is no evidence that patients with fish allergies have an increased risk of experiencing an allergic reaction to protamine. After vasectomy, men develop circulating antibodies to spermatozoa; however, no clinically significant allergic reactions to protamine have been reported in men with vasectomies. Patients known to be allergic to protamine present a therapeutic challenge when neutralization of heparin is required, because no effective alternative to protamine is commonly available. In the rare instances when patients with protamine allergy require anticoagulation, use of a direct thrombin inhibitor such as bivalirudin instead of heparin can be considered. This obviates the use of protamine. Heparinase, a heparin-neutralizing enzyme from the gram-negative bacterium *Flavobacterium heparinum,* has also been used as a substitute for protamine.

Blood and Blood Products

Minor urticarial allergic reactions to properly cross-matched blood products may occur in 1%–3% of patients. The cause is unknown but may involve soluble antigens in the donor unit to which the recipient has been previously sensitized. Diphenhydramine is an effective treatment. *Febrile nonhemolytic reactions* are the result of cytokines in stored blood. The incidence of these reactions is reduced with the use of leukocyte-reduced blood products. Premedication with antihistamines and antipyretics is also effective. *Hemolytic transfusion reactions* occur in 1 in 10,000–50,000 blood component transfusions. These reactions appear to be mediated by immunoglobulins, particularly IgM and IgG. Acute hemolytic reactions are usually due to ABO incompatibility, whereas delayed reactions are often due to Kidd or Rh antibodies. Acute hemolytic reactions may lead to renal failure and disseminated intravascular coagulation (DIC). Hydration should be vigorous to maintain urine output, and dialysis is occasionally required; heparinization is also sometimes considered to prevent complications of DIC. Delayed hemolytic reactions usually require no treatment. *Anaphylactic reactions* are rare, occurring in approximately 1 in 20,000–50,000 transfusions. These may result from antibodies against IgA, HLA, or complement proteins. In addition to cessation of transfusion, anaphylaxis due to blood transfusion is treated with aggressive supportive care, including fluids, epinephrine, and other vasopressors as needed.

The leading cause of transfusion-related morbidity and mortality is *transfusion-related acute lung injury* (TRALI). Diagnostic criteria for TRALI include hypoxia and bilateral pulmonary edema that occur within 6 hours of transfusion and in the absence of intravascular fluid overload or heart failure. The pathogenesis of TRALI appears to be activation of neutrophils on the pulmonary vascular endothelium as a result of donor leukocyte antibodies, particularly anti-HLA and antineutrophil antibodies (Fig. 27.3). These antibodies are contained in the plasma component of transfused blood products. Therefore TRALI is most commonly seen after transfusion of plasma-rich components such as fresh frozen plasma and platelets. The reported incidence of TRALI varies significantly, since diagnostic criteria have only recently been agreed upon. The rate of TRALI in critically ill patients may approach 5%–8%. Treatment is supportive; neither steroid therapy nor diuresis is beneficial.

Synthetic Volume Expanders

The estimated incidence of allergic reactions to plasma volume expanders is 3%–4%. All synthetic colloids have been implicated, but reactions are more common with dextrans and gelatins than with albumin and hydroxyethyl starch. Both immune- and non–immune-mediated mechanisms have been implicated, with manifestations ranging from rash and modest hypotension to bronchospasm and shock.

Other Drugs

Several other drugs have been implicated in cases of perioperative drug allergy. These include heparin and insulin. This underscores the importance of including drug allergy as part of the differential diagnosis of *any* case of cardiovascular collapse that occurs during the perioperative period.

Eosinophilia

Clinically significant eosinophilia is defined as a sustained absolute eosinophil count over 1500/mm^3. Moderate eosinophilia is commonly seen in a wide spectrum of disorders, including

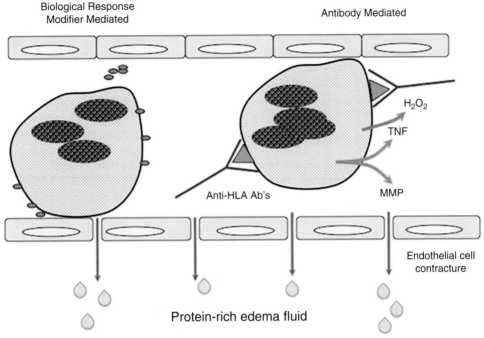

FIG. 27.3   Pathophysiology of TRALI. The pathogenesis of TRALI appears to be activation of neutrophils on the pulmonary vascular endothelium as a result of donor leukocyte antibodies, particularly anti-HLA and antineutrophil antibodies. This results in leakage of protein-rich fluid, which causes pulmonary edema and amplification of the inflammatory cascade. *Ab's,* Antibodies; *MMP,* matrix metalloproteinase; *TNF,* tumor necrosis factor. (From Gilliss BM, Looney MR, Gropper MA. Reducing noninfectious risks of blood transfusion. *Anesthesiology.* 2011;115:635-649, Fig. 2.)

parasitic infestations, systemic allergic disorders, collagen vascular diseases, various forms of dermatitis, drug reactions, and tumors. Hodgkin lymphoma and both B- and T-cell non-Hodgkin lymphomas can present with eosinophilia. Even when there is no obvious sign of an underlying lymphoma, up to 25% of patients with apparent idiopathic eosinophilia have an expanded clone of aberrant T cells that produce high levels of IL-5.

Hypereosinophilia is associated with tissue damage secondary to release of basic protein by the eosinophil. Irreversible endomyocardial fibrosis producing a restrictive cardiomyopathy is common in patients who maintain eosinophil counts higher than 5000/mm³. In patients with eosinophilic leukemia or idiopathic hypereosinophilic (Löffler) syndrome, eosinophil counts can reach 20,000–100,000/mm³. Widespread organ dysfunction and rapidly progressive heart disease are associated with these conditions. These patients need aggressive treatment with both corticosteroids and hydroxyurea. Interferon alfa is sometimes used as a substitute for hydroxyurea. The mechanism of action of these drugs in this situation is not fully understood. Leukapheresis can be used to acutely lower eosinophil counts.

MISDIRECTED ADAPTIVE IMMUNITY

Autoimmune Disorders

The challenge of adaptive immunity is the need for immune cells to be capable of responding efficiently to a wide variety of foreign antigens yet still be able to recognize and tolerate

"self" antigens. There is growing evidence that major immunologic stimuli such as certain infections can activate *self-reactive lymphocytes.* In general these primed self-reactive lymphocytes tend to undergo apoptotic elimination once the immunologic challenge has been controlled. Indeed, transient autoimmunity appears to be a relatively common byproduct of major immune system activation. The specific defects that cause autoimmunity to persist and develop into a chronic self-destructive immune disorder are not well understood. Genetic predisposition may play a role.

Anesthetic implications of autoimmune disorders can be divided into three categories. The first includes the anesthetic considerations involving certain vulnerable organs specific to the particular immune disorder. Examples include cervical instability with RA, renal injury with SLE, and liver failure with chronic autoimmune hepatitis. The second is related to the consequences of therapy used to treat the autoimmune disorder. The potential for addisonian crisis in patients treated long term with corticosteroids is well recognized. Newer therapies for autoimmune disorders inhibit specific facets of the immune response, which places patients who take these medications at increased risk of perioperative infection. The third category, especially in patients with long-standing autoimmune disorders, concerns the risk of accelerated atherosclerosis and associated cardiovascular complications such as heart disease and stroke. Some studies suggest that the risk of cardiovascular morbidity and mortality is increased by as much as 50-fold in the presence of an autoimmune disease. Some of this added risk may be due to the drugs used to treat the autoimmune disease itself. For example, long-term steroid therapy is associated with hypertension and diabetes mellitus, both of which are powerful risk factors for development of cardiovascular disease. Therefore patients with long-standing autoimmune conditions warrant thorough cardiovascular evaluation and consideration of the increased risk of perioperative cardiovascular complications.

ANESTHESIA AND IMMUNOCOMPETENCE

Many perioperative factors affect immunocompetence and therefore may alter the incidence of perioperative infection or the body's response to cancer.

Transfusion-Related Immunomodulation

In recent years it has come to be appreciated that transfusion of allogeneic blood products has a measurable impact on immune function. Such *transfusion-related immunomodulatory (TRIM) effects* include increased susceptibility to infection and promotion of tumor growth. Conversely a TRIM effect is likely to explain improved renal allograft survival in transplant patients. Specific TRIM effects include decreased NK cell and phagocytic function, impaired antigen presentation, and suppression of lymphocyte production. The mechanism underlying TRIM effects remains unclear but may involve donor leukocytes present in transfused blood products and soluble HLA class I peptides. Partial HLA compatibility between donor leukocytes and the recipient induces a state of microchimerism that prompts release of IL-4, IL-10, and other inflammatory mediators that impair cell-mediated immunity and cytotoxicity. An extreme manifestation of microchimerism is the development of transfusion-associated graft-versus-host disease, a rare but often fatal condition in which immunocompetent donor (graft) cells attack the recipient's cells, which leads to pancytopenia and liver failure. Application of leukoreduction techniques to stored blood appears to mitigate some but not all TRIM effects. The presence in stored blood of other soluble mediators such as histamine and other proinflammatory cytokines not removed by leukoreduction may account for the incomplete effect of leukoreduction in maintaining immune function.

Neuroendocrine Stress Response

By far the most important influence on immune function in the perioperative period is the neuroendocrine stress response initiated by activation of the autonomic nervous system and the hypothalamic-pituitary axis. Surgical stress induces release of catecholamines, corticotropin, and cortisol. Monocytes, macrophages, and T cells possess β_2-adrenergic and glucocorticoid receptors. Activation of these receptors results in net inhibition of T_H1 cytokine production and promotion of T_H2 antiinflammatory cytokine release. Monocyte and macrophage activation lead to release of cytokines such as IL-1, IL-6, and tumor necrosis factor (TNF)-α, which further stimulate

the hypothalamic-pituitary axis. The benefit of this immunosuppression is to minimize the inflammatory response caused by surgical trauma, but the downside is increased vulnerability to infection and tumor proliferation.

Numerous other perioperative factors weaken the immune system. Acute pain suppresses NK cell activity, probably as a result of activation of the hypothalamic-pituitary axis and autonomic nervous system. Hypothermia exacerbates the neuroendocrine stress response and induces thermoregulatory vasoconstriction. Tissue hypoxia impairs oxidative killing by neutrophils and prolongs wound healing. Hypothermia has also been shown to suppress NK cell activity and lymphocyte function. Elevated plasma cortisol and catecholamine concentrations during surgery result in hyperglycemia, which can provide a medium for bacterial growth. Hyperglycemia itself also has deleterious effects on the immune system. Hyperglycemia induces changes in the vascular endothelium that impede lymphocyte migration. It also reduces immune cell proliferation by interfering with critical enzymatic functions, and it impairs neutrophil phagocytosis.

Effects of Anesthetics on Immune Response

It is well established that immunocompetence is essential for a host to resist cancer. For example, recipients of solid organ transplants who have a history of cancer experience a higher rate of cancer recurrence following initiation of immunosuppressive therapy. Surgical excision remains the treatment of choice for most locally contained solid organ cancers, but there is concern that exposure to surgery and anesthesia may actually promote tumor progression.

Several mechanisms are likely at play. Surgical disruption of the tumor may release tumor cells into the circulation, providing the seeds for micrometastases. The presence of a primary tumor may itself inhibit angiogenesis; therefore tumor removal may paradoxically favor survival of minimal residual disease. Release of growth factors and suppression of antiangiogenic factors may also contribute. In addition, tissue injury depresses cell-mediated immunity, including the function of cytotoxic T cells and NK cells. Allogeneic red blood cell transfusion in the perioperative period may also play a role in increasing the risk of tumor recurrence. Laboratory investigation of TRIM has demonstrated a reduction in T_H and NK cell counts and decreased levels of the T_H1 cytokines IL-2 and interferon.

Considerable in vitro and in vivo evidence from animal studies suggests that anesthetics and analgesics also have an impact on the immune response (Table 27.7). The magnitude of this effect is probably considerably less than that of the surgical stress itself, but an additive effect may be important. Ketamine, thiopental, and all the volatile anesthetics appear to reduce NK cell activity and/or number. Volatile anesthetics also impair neutrophil function by inhibiting the respiratory oxidative burst mechanism and reducing lymphocyte proliferation. Nitrous oxide impairs DNA and nucleotide synthesis and has been observed to depress hematopoietic

TABLE 27.7	Effects of Anesthetic Drugs on Immune System Function
Drug	Effect on Immune System
Thiopental	Reduces NK cell activity and number in animal models
Propofol	Reduces NK cell number in animal models
Volatile agents	Inhibit stimulation of NK cell cytotoxicity in animal models
	Reduce NK cell number in humans
Nitrous oxide	Associated with acceleration in development of lung and liver metastases in animal models
	Inhibits hematopoietic cell formation
Local anesthetic drugs	Inhibit tumor cell proliferation
Morphine	Inhibits cellular and NK cell immunity in animal models
Fentanyl	Inhibits NK cell activity in humans
Tramadol	Stimulates NK cell activity in animal and human models
Cyclooxygenase-2 inhibitors	Display antiangiogenic and antitumor effects in animal models

NK, Natural killer.
Data from Snyder GL, Greenberg S. Effect of anaesthetic technique and other perioperative factors on cancer recurrence. *Br J Anaesth*. 2010;105:109.

and mononuclear cell synthesis and depress neutrophil chemotaxis. The impact of propofol on immune function is less clear, but propofol bears a chemical resemblance to the antioxidant α-tocopherol and may possess antiinflammatory and antioxidative properties that tend to inhibit neutrophil, monocyte, and macrophage activity. Recent interest has focused on propofol ester conjugates in the treatment of breast cancer; they have been shown in some studies to inhibit cellular adhesion and migration of breast cancer cells and have also shown direct cytotoxicity toward some cancer cells.

The immunosuppressive effects of opiates have been known for decades. Opioid receptors in the hypothalamic-pituitary axis promote release of corticotropin and cortisol. Sympathetic nervous system activation and catecholamine release further suppress NK cell, lymphocyte, neutrophil, and macrophage functions. Immune cells also possess a specific subset of μ receptors, the activation of which leads to increased intracellular calcium gradients and activation of nitric oxide synthase. High nitric oxide concentrations appear to mediate many of the antiinflammatory effects of naturally occurring opioids. Morphine also impairs antibody formation and synthesis of proinflammatory cytokines. As expected, many of the immunomodulatory effects of opioids can be blocked by administration of the μ-receptor antagonist naloxone. There is some evidence to suggest that synthetic opioids such as fentanyl and remifentanil have less impact on immune function, possibly related to their differential activation of specific opioid receptors.

Nonopioid analgesics seem to have less effect on immune function than opiates. In fact, some evidence suggests that tramadol, which has noradrenergic and serotoninergic activity in addition to μ-receptor affinity, may promote NK cell activity. NSAIDs that inhibit the COX enzyme have been shown

in an animal model to possess antitumor and antiangiogenic properties. COX-2 inhibitors such as etodolac and celecoxib may attenuate the deleterious effects of opioid-induced tumor growth.

Some retrospective studies have shown that use of regional anesthesia instead of IV morphine for postoperative pain control is associated with measurable reductions in cancer recurrence. Several mechanisms may account for this observation. Regional anesthesia attenuates the neuroendocrine surgical stress response by blocking afferent transmission to the hypothalamic-pituitary axis. In addition, patients who receive regional anesthesia or regional analgesia have reduced requirements for drugs with known immunosuppressive effects, such as general anesthetics and opioids. Local anesthetic drugs may also possess intrinsic antitumor properties. Both lidocaine and ropivacaine have been shown to exert antiproliferative effects on tumor cells. Not all research has supported a benefit of regional anesthesia over general anesthesia in terms of cancer prognosis. The impact may differ depending on tumor type. Therefore despite these promising findings, more research is needed before definitive conclusions can be drawn about the optimal anesthetic choice in cancer patients.

KEY POINTS

- The immune system is divided into *innate* and *adaptive* or *acquired* pathways.
- The innate immune pathway mounts the initial response to any infection, recognizes targets common to many pathogens, and has no specific memory. Its cellular components are neutrophils, macrophages, monocytes, and natural killer cells, and its main noncellular elements are the complement proteins.
- The adaptive immune pathway has a more delayed onset of action and may take days to activate when challenged by an unfamiliar antigen. However, adaptive immunity is capable of developing memory and is more rapidly induced by antigen when memory is present. Adaptive immunity consists of a humoral component mediated by B lymphocytes that produce antibodies and a cellular component dominated by T lymphocytes.
- Angioedema may be hereditary or acquired and is characterized by episodic edema resulting from increased vascular permeability. The condition commonly involves swelling of the face and oropharyngeal mucous membranes and may lead to airway compromise. The most common hereditary form results from an autosomal dominant deficiency of C1 esterase inhibitor, which results in a buildup of the vasoactive compound bradykinin. Treatment of acute episodes involves administration of C1 inhibitor concentrate (plasma-derived or recombinant); icatibant, a synthetic bradykinin B_2-receptor antagonist; ecallantide, a recombinant plasma kallikrein inhibitor; or fresh frozen plasma (2–4 units) to replace the deficient enzyme. Androgens, catecholamines, antihistamines, and antifibrinolytics are *not* useful in the treatment of acute episodes of angioedema.

- Anaphylaxis is a life-threatening condition caused by massive release of vasoactive mediators via degranulation of mast cells and basophils through either immune- or non–immune-mediated mechanisms. Treatment requires reversal of hypotension through replacement of intravascular fluid volume and inhibition of further release of vasoactive mediators. Early intervention with epinephrine is critical. Epinephrine increases intracellular cyclic adenosine monophosphate and thereby reduces vasoactive mediator release. It also relaxes bronchial smooth muscle and relieves bronchospasm.
- Muscle relaxants, antibiotics, and latex are the leading causes of drug-induced allergic reactions in the perioperative period. Reaction may occur on first exposure (presumably caused by sensitization from other environmental chemicals) or after previous uneventful exposure.
- In 90% of cases, patients who report a penicillin allergy are able to tolerate penicillin. Although cross-reactivity between penicillin and other antibiotics exists, only about 2% of patients with a penicillin reaction will have an allergic response to a cephalosporin, and less than 1% will react adversely to a carbapenem.
- Almost all allergic reactions occur within 5–10 minutes of exposure to an antigen. An important exception to this rule is the allergic response to latex, which often occurs at least 30 minutes after exposure. Preoperative referral for skin testing is appropriate for patients with a strong clinical history of previous latex allergic reaction. Latex sensitivity is an occupational hazard for healthcare workers. Other groups with a higher-than-average risk of latex allergy are patients with a history of spina bifida, multiple prior surgeries, or fruit allergy.
- Autoimmune disorders result in immune-mediated end-organ dysfunction because of inappropriate activation of antibody against self-antigens. Each disorder is accompanied by a distinct set of multisystem features. Patients with autoimmune disorders also have an increased risk of cardiovascular disease. Therefore careful preoperative evaluation is imperative to prevent excess perioperative morbidity and mortality. Many of these patients are treated with exogenous glucocorticoids and may require "stress-dose" steroids prior to major surgery to prevent addisonian crisis.
- Many factors related to surgery and anesthesia impair immune function, which may precipitate infection and cancer progression in susceptible patients. The principal factor appears to be the neuroendocrine response to surgical stress, which includes release of catecholamines and glucocorticoids that impair both innate and adaptive immune responses. Anesthetic agents, including volatile anesthetics and opioids, also impair immune function. Regional and neuraxial anesthesia with local anesthetics *may* help preserve immune system function.

RESOURCES

Bonilla FA, Oettgen HC. Adaptive immunity. *J Allergy Clin Immunol.* 2010;125:S33-S40.

Bork K. An evidence based therapeutic approach to hereditary and acquired angioedema. *Curr Opin Allergy Clin Immunol.* 2014;14:354-362.

Cakmakkaya OS, Kolodzie K, Apfel CC, Pace NL. Anaesthetic techniques for risk of malignant tumour recurrence. *Cochrane Database Syst Rev.* 2014;11: CD008877.

Chaplin DD. Overview of the immune response. *J Allergy Clin Immunol.* 2010;125:S3-S23.

Gurrieri C, Weingarten TN, Martin DP, et al. Allergic reactions during anesthesia at a large United States referral center. *Anesth Analg.* 2011;113:1202-1212.

Gilliss BM, Looney MR, Gropper MA. Reducing noninfectious risks of blood transfusion. *Anesthesiology.* 2011;115:635-649.

Grumach AS, Kirschfink M. Are complement deficiencies really rare? Overview on prevalence, clinical importance and modern diagnostic approach. *Mol Immunol.* 2014;61:110-117.

Hart S, Cserti-Gazdewich CM, McCluskey SA. Red cell transfusion and the immune system. *Anaesthesia.* 2015;70(Suppl 1):38-45. e13-6.

Kannan JA, Berstein JA. Perioperative anaphylaxis. *Immunol Allergy Clin N Am.* 2014;35:321-334.

Lekstrom-Himes JA, Gallin JI. Immunodeficiency diseases caused by defects in phagocytes. *N Engl J Med.* 2000;343:1703-1714.

Mertes PM, Tajima K, Regnier-Kimmoun MA, et al. Perioperative anaphylaxis. *Med Clin North Am.* 2010;94:761-789.

Vamvakas E, Blajchman MA. Transfusion-related immunomodulation: an update. *Blood Rev.* 2007;21:327-348.

Walport MJ. Complement. *N Engl J Med.* 2001;344:1058-1066. 1140-1151.

Cancer

NATALIE F. HOLT

Cancer is a major cause of morbidity and mortality in the United States and causes more deaths than heart disease in persons younger than age 80 (Table 28.1). Approximately 40% of men and women will be diagnosed with cancer at some point in their lifetime. The lifetime risk of dying from cancer is one in four for men and one in five for women. About 90% of patients with cancer require surgery for reasons both related and unrelated to the cancer diagnosis. In addition, approximately 65% of patients diagnosed with cancer survive for at least 5 years, which means that a growing number of patients are coming to surgery after cancer treatment. Most of these individuals with a history of cancer are age 65 years or older.

The anesthetic implications of cancer stem not only from the cancer itself but also from the therapies employed for its treatment. In addition, because of the older age of the majority of patients with active cancer or a history of cancer, comorbid conditions in these patients can affect their perioperative course.

MECHANISM

Cancer results from an accumulation of genetic mutations that causes dysregulation of cellular proliferation. Genes are involved in carcinogenesis by virtue of inherited traits that predispose to cancer (e.g., altered metabolism of potentially carcinogenic compounds), mutation of a normal gene into an *oncogene* that promotes the conversion of normal cells into cancer cells, or inactivation of a tumor suppressor gene that allows a tumor to undergo malignant transformation. A critical gene related to cancer in humans is the tumor suppressor *p53*. This gene is not only essential for cell viability but critical for monitoring damage to DNA. Inactivation of *p53* is an early step in the development of many types of cancer. Stimulation of oncogene formation by carcinogens (tobacco, alcohol, sunlight) is estimated to be responsible for 80% of cancers in the United States. Tobacco accounts for more cases of cancer than all other known carcinogens combined.

The fundamental event that causes cells to become malignant is an alteration in their DNA structure. These mutations occur in cells of target tissues, and these cells then become the ancestors of the entire future tumor cell population. Evolution to more undifferentiated cells reflects high mutation rates and contributes to the development of tumors that are resistant to therapy.

Cancer cells must evade the host's immune surveillance system, which is designed to seek out and destroy tumor cells. Most mutant cancer cells stimulate the host's immune system to form antibodies. This protective role of the immune system is apparent in those with acquired immunodeficiency syndrome (AIDS) and recipients of organ transplants who are maintained on long-term immunosuppressive drugs. These groups have a higher incidence of cancer.

DIAGNOSIS

Most cancers produce solid tumors. Cancer often becomes clinically evident when tumor bulk compromises vital organ function. The initial diagnosis is frequently made by aspiration cytology or biopsy. Monoclonal antibodies that recognize antigens for specific cancers may aid in the diagnosis of cancer. A commonly used staging system for solid tumors is the TNM system based on tumor size (T), lymph node involvement (N), and distant metastases (M). This system groups cancers into stages ranging from I (best prognosis) to IV (poorest prognosis).

Tumor invasiveness is related to the release of various tumor mediators that modify the surrounding microenvironment in such a way as to permit cancer cells to spread along the lines of least resistance. Lymphatics lack a basement membrane, so local spread of cancer is influenced by the anatomy of the regional lymphatics. For example, regional lymph node involvement occurs late in squamous cell cancer of the vocal cords, because these structures have few lymphatics, whereas regional lymph node involvement is an early manifestation of supraglottic cancer, because this region is rich in lymphatics. Imaging techniques including computed tomography (CT), magnetic resonance imaging (MRI), and positron emission tomography (PET) are used to more clearly delineate tumor presence and spread.

TREATMENT

Most cancers are treated by a multimodal approach involving surgery, radiation therapy, and/or chemotherapies that vary by tumor type and stage. The development of more effective cancer treatments has dramatically improved survival from

TABLE 28.1	Leading Causes of Death[a] in United States in 2013		
Age (Years)	Accidents	Cancer	Heart Disease
1–4	X		
5–9	X		
10–14	X		
15–19	X		
20–24	X		
25–29	X		
30–34	X		
35–39	X		
40–44	X		
45–49		X	
50–54		X	
55–59		X	
60–64		X	
65–69		X	
70–74		X	
75–79		X	
≥80			X

[a]All races and both sexes.
Information from the Centers for Disease Control and Prevention, National Center for Health Statistics, Division of Vital Statistics, 2013.

cancer. Indeed, the number of deaths due to cancer is gradually decreasing. However, use of these powerful therapies is associated with toxicities and adverse effects that have the potential to affect nearly every organ system. Some of these effects are transient; others produce permanent sequelae. All of them have important potential consequences in the perioperative care of cancer patients.

Traditional Chemotherapy

Traditional chemotherapy involves the use of cytotoxic drugs that target rapidly dividing cells and interfere with replication. They are divided into classes based on mechanism of action: alkylating agents, antimetabolites, antibiotics, microtubule assembly inhibitors, hormonal agents, and various miscellaneous or mixed-mechanism drugs. *Alkylating agents* form reactive molecules that cause DNA cross-linking problems such as abnormal base pairing and strand breaks that interfere primarily with DNA but also with RNA and protein synthesis and replication. *Antimetabolites* are structural analogues of folic acid, purines, or pyrimidines that block enzymes necessary for nucleic acid and protein synthesis. *Antitumor antibiotics* form complexes with DNA or RNA that inhibit their subsequent synthesis. *Microtubule assembly inhibitors* include the vinca alkaloids and taxanes, both of which act on the mitotic process by interfering with microtubule assembly or disassembly. The growth of certain tumor types, notably breast and prostate, is responsive to *hormonal agents.* Hormones are not cytotoxic, so they often stimulate tumor regression but do not cause cell death. Several other drugs have been shown to have anticancer properties. Topoisomerase inhibitors act by inhibiting the topoisomerase II and I enzymes. This results in single strand and double strand DNA breaks that lead to apoptosis.

Targeted Chemotherapy

Targeted chemotherapy uses a set of chemotherapeutic drugs directed against specific processes involved in tumor cell proliferation and migration. The first targeted therapy was developed for estrogen receptors present in certain types of breast cancers. Binding of estrogen to estrogen receptors is an important step in the growth of these tumor cells, and estrogen receptor blockade turned out to be an effective way to reduce tumor spread.

Other targeted therapies have been developed against a number of cell processes, including secretion of growth factors that facilitate gene expression, angiogenesis (creation of new blood vessels), cell migration, and tumor growth. Growth factors such as endothelial growth factor (EGF), vascular endothelial growth factor (VEGF), and matrix metalloproteinases are involved in growth and differentiation of normal cells, but they are usually overexpressed or mutated on cancer cells. Binding of growth factors to receptors on the cell membrane induces a cascade of signal transduction events that often involve activation of the enzyme tyrosine kinase. Absence of these signals may lead to apoptosis. Drugs have now been developed that block these growth factors, their receptors, or their associated tyrosine kinases. Included among the targeted therapies are monoclonal antibodies that act on extracellular receptors such as EGF and VEGF, as well as small molecules that penetrate cell membranes and block intracellular signaling pathways. Cancer cells have the ability to mutate and develop resistance to targeted therapies, so targeted therapies are often used in conjunction with traditional chemotherapy.

Radiation Therapy

Radiation induces cell death by causing damage to DNA. The sensitivity of a cell to radiation injury is influenced by its phase in the cell cycle and its ability to repair DNA damage. For the treatment of cancer, radiation timing and delivery are adjusted to maximize therapeutic benefit and minimize damage to surrounding tissue. Radiation can be administered through external beam technology or through radioactive pellets implanted into a target organ (e.g., radioactive "seeds" for treatment of prostate cancer). *Stereotactic radiosurgery* (CyberKnife, Gamma Knife) uses advances in three-dimensional (3D) imaging and *conformal radiotherapy* (which allows radiation energy to be matched to tumor shape) to deliver high-dose radiation at a precise location. Contrary to the names Gamma Knife and CyberKnife, this procedure involves no incision and is not painful. However, it does require complete stillness and may involve use of a rigid head or body frame to localize the radiation beam. This technique is most commonly associated with treatment of brain and spine tumors but is also used for management of tumors of the prostate, liver, lung, and other sites. With newer technologies, whole brain radiation is now being applied to treat multiple brain lesions arising from advanced metastatic disease from distant organs (e.g., breast, lung, colon), offering a treatment option for patients who would have otherwise been considered terminal.

Ablation Therapy

Ablative cancer treatments involve localized destruction of cancer cells. The most popular of these techniques is *radiofrequency ablation* (RFA), which uses thermal energy to cause coagulative tissue destruction. First described in the 1990s for treating primary liver tumors and metastases, this technology has now been extended to treatment of localized lung, kidney, adrenal gland, and bone tumors. During the procedure a needle is inserted into the tumor, then a generator is used to deliver radiofrequency energy that coagulates the cells. *Microwave ablation* is an alternative technology that also uses heat to destroy cells. Relative to RFA, microwave ablation is beneficial for tumors larger than 4 cm and those that are close to major blood vessels. *Laser interstitial thermal therapy* (LITT) is another form of ablative cancer therapy that uses the energy of lasers to produce tissue coagulation. Advances in MRI and laser probe design have widened the applications for LITT, particularly in the treatment of inoperable brain tumors. Nd-YAG and diode lasers are most commonly used.

Cryotherapy uses cold instead of heat to cause tumor cell lysis. The most common approach is to use image guidance—often ultrasound—and an argon gas–driven unit to apply direct cooling (−160°C) to the tumor. Cryotherapy has been used to treat pancreas, liver, prostate, and renal tumors.

Electroporation is an evolving nonthermal therapy that uses an electric field to disrupt the phospholipid layer of tumor cells. There are two types of electroporation: *reversible* and *irreversible*. Reversible electroporation is used in conjunction with the delivery of chemotherapy, which can more easily enter the tumor cells owing to cell membrane disruption caused by electroporation. Subsequent cell death occurs as a result of the chemotherapeutic agent. Irreversible electroporation causes permanent cell membrane disruption and cell lysis without the aid of chemotherapy.

Adverse Effects of Cancer Treatment

Bone marrow suppression, cardiovascular and pulmonary toxicity, and central and peripheral nervous system damage are among the most serious adverse effects of cancer treatment. However, dysfunction of nearly every organ system has been described. The following sections present a system-specific review of toxicities related to cancer treatment. Tables 28.2 and 28.3 summarize the adverse effects of selected chemotherapies and radiation treatment.

Cardiovascular System

Anthracyclines like doxorubicin (Adriamycin), daunorubicin, epirubicin, and idarubicin are the chemotherapeutic drugs most often associated with cardiotoxicity. These drugs are commonly used to treat cancers such as leukemias and lymphomas. Anthracyclines impair myocyte function by forming free radicals that interfere with mitochondrial activation and cause lipid peroxidation. Cardiotoxicity may be acute or chronic. Acute toxicity begins early in treatment (with development of dysrhythmias, QT prolongation, and cardiomyopathy) and then reverses with discontinuation of therapy. Chronic toxicity (left ventricular dysfunction and cardiomyopathy) can occur in an early-onset form that usually appears within 1 year of treatment and a late-onset form that can emerge several years or decades after completion of therapy. Risk factors for cardiotoxicity include a large cumulative dose of drug (for doxorubicin, >300 mg/m^2), a history of high-dose

---

TABLE 28.2	Toxicities of Commonly Used Chemotherapeutic Agents
Chemotherapeutic Agent	**Adverse Effects**
Arsenic	Leukocytosis, pleural effusion, QT interval prolongation
Asparaginase (Elspar)	Coagulopathy, hemorrhagic pancreatitis, hepatic dysfunction, thromboembolism
Bevacizumab (Avastin)	Bleeding, congestive heart failure, gastrointestinal perforation, hypertension, impaired wound healing, thromboembolism
Bleomycin	Pulmonary hypertension, pulmonary fibrosis
Busulfan	Pulmonary fibrosis, alveolar hemorrhage, myelosuppression, venoocclusive disease, endocardial fibrosis
Carmustine (BiCNU)	Myelosuppression, pulmonary fibrosis
Chlorambucil (Leukeran)	Myelosuppression, chronic interstitial pneumonitis, SIADH
Cisplatin	Dysrhythmias, magnesium wasting, mucositis, ototoxicity, peripheral neuropathy, SIADH, renal tubular necrosis, thromboembolism
Cyclophosphamide (Cytoxan)	Encephalopathy/delirium, hemorrhagic cystitis, myelosuppression, pericarditis, pericardial effusion, SIADH, pulmonary fibrosis
Doxorubicin (Adriamycin)	Cardiomyopathy, myelosuppression
Erlotinib (Tarceva)	Deep vein thrombosis, interstitial lung disease
Etoposide	Myelosuppression, interstitial pneumonitis, vasospastic angina
Fluorouracil	Acute cerebellar ataxia, ischemic and nonischemic ECG changes, chest pain, gastritis, myelosuppression
Ifosfamide (Ifex)	Dysrhythmias, left ventricular dysfunction, hemorrhagic cystitis, renal insufficiency, SIADH
Methotrexate	Encephalopathy, hepatic dysfunction, mucositis, platelet dysfunction, hypersensitivity pneumonitis, renal failure, myelosuppression
Mitomycin	Myelosuppression, diffuse alveolar damage, interstitial pneumonitis, pulmonary venoocclusive disease
Mitoxantrone (Novantrone)	Left ventricular dysfunction, dysrhythmias, myelosuppression
Paclitaxel (Taxol)	Ataxia, autonomic dysfunction, myelosuppression, peripheral neuropathy, arthralgias, bradycardia
Sorafenib (Nexavar)	Left ventricular dysfunction, hypertension, impaired wound healing, thromboembolism
Sunitinib (Sutent)	Adrenal insufficiency, left ventricular dysfunction, hypertension, thromboembolism
Tamoxifen	Thromboembolism
Thalidomide	Bradycardia, neurotoxicity, thromboembolism
Trastuzumab (Herceptin)	Left ventricular dysfunction, dysrhythmias, hypertension, interstitial pneumonitis
Tretinoin	Myelosuppression, retinoic acid syndrome
Vinblastine	Hypertension, myocardial ischemia, myelosuppression, bronchospasm, SIADH
Vincristine	Autonomic dysfunction, myocardial ischemia peripheral neuropathy, bronchospasm, SIADH

bolus administration, and a history of concomitant radiation therapy or use of other cardiotoxic drugs. The cardiotoxicity of doxorubicin may be decreased by the use of free radical scavengers such as dexrazoxane or liposomal preparations.

Mitoxantrone, which is structurally similar to the anthracyclines, has also been associated with cardiomyopathy, as have other drugs including cyclophosphamide, clofarabine, and certain of the tyrosine kinase inhibitors, including imatinib and sorafenib. Baseline echocardiography is recommended for all patients before anthracycline treatment. Periodic echocardiography is advised in patients receiving high-dose therapy and those with underlying cardiac impairment or significant risk factors for heart disease.

Pericarditis, angina, coronary artery vasospasm, ischemia-related electrocardiographic (ECG) changes, and conduction defects are other cardiac complications related to cancer chemotherapy. Fluorouracil and capecitabine cause the highest incidence of chemotherapy-related ischemia. Estimates vary widely from 1%–68% for fluorouracil and from 3%–9% for capecitabine. Paclitaxel and thalidomide can cause severe bradycardia requiring pacemaker implantation. Arsenic, lapatinib, and nilotinib frequently cause QT prolongation.

Hypertension has emerged as a relatively common adverse effect of treatment with newer targeted chemotherapeutic drugs such as bevacizumab, trastuzumab, sorafenib, and sunitinib and occurs in as many as 35%–45% of patients. Vascular thromboembolic complications, including both symptomatic and asymptomatic pulmonary embolism, have also been associated with use of the VEGF inhibitors, as has left ventricular dysfunction, which is usually reversible upon drug discontinuation. The pathophysiology of the cardiovascular damage associated with these drugs is probably directly related to inhibition of EGF and VEGF. Although important to tumor cell proliferation, these growth factors also play a role in normal myocyte growth, repair, and adaptation to pressure loads.

Patients who receive radiation to the mediastinum are at risk for developing myocardial fibrosis, pericarditis, valvular fibrosis, conduction abnormalities, and accelerated development of coronary artery disease. Incidence is related to cumulative radiation exposure as well as concomitant administration of cardiotoxic chemotherapeutic agents.

Respiratory System

Pulmonary toxicity is a well-recognized complication of bleomycin therapy. Other agents associated with pulmonary damage include busulfan, cyclophosphamide, methotrexate, lomustine, carmustine, mitomycin, and the vinca alkaloids. The mechanism of injury differs for each drug. In the case of bleomycin, free radical formation seems to be a factor. Several of the targeted chemotherapies, including EGF receptor blockers and human epidermal growth factor receptor-2 (HER2) inhibitors, have been associated with pulmonary fibrosis or pneumonitis. Type II pneumocytes possess EGF receptors that play a role in alveolar repair, which may explain this type of alveolar cell damage.

Pneumonitis or bronchiolitis obliterans with organizing pneumonia occurs in 3%–20% of patients treated with bleomycin, depending on dose. Pulmonary fibrosis can develop decades after treatment. Risk factors include preexisting lung disease, smoking, and radiation exposure. Baseline and serial pulmonary function testing and chest radiography are often performed. Of note, evidence suggests that intraoperative exposure to high concentrations of oxygen may exacerbate preexisting bleomycin-induced lung injury and contribute to postoperative ventilatory failure. Perioperative corticosteroid administration may be of benefit in treating bleomycin-induced pneumonitis.

Interstitial pneumonitis and pulmonary fibrosis are complications of radiation to the thorax or total body irradiation. Symptoms typically begin within the first 2–3 months of treatment and generally regress within 12 months of treatment completion. However, subclinical abnormalities revealed by pulmonary function testing may occur in up to 50% of patients exposed to radiation for treatment of childhood cancers. *Radiation recall pneumonitis* is a recognized clinical syndrome in which patients with prior radiation exposure manifest symptomatic pneumonitis after exposure to a second pulmonary toxin.

Renal System

Many chemotherapeutic drugs can be nephrotoxic; among the most commonly cited are cisplatin, high-dose methotrexate, and ifosfamide. Renal insufficiency and hypomagnesemia are the typical presenting signs of cisplatin-related nephrotoxicity. Ifosfamide usually causes proximal tubule dysfunction marked by proteinuria and glucosuria. Leucovorin, a folic acid precursor, can be helpful in treating methotrexate-related renal failure. Renal insufficiency usually resolves with cessation of treatment and supportive therapy.

TABLE 28.3	Common Adverse Effects of Radiation Therapy	
System	Acute	Chronic
Skin	Erythema, rash, hair loss	Fibrosis, sclerosis, telangiectasias
Gastrointestinal	Malnutrition, mucositis, nausea, vomiting	Adhesions, fistulas, strictures
Cardiac		Conduction defects, pericardial effusion, pericardial fibrosis, pericarditis
Respiratory		Airway fibrosis, pulmonary fibrosis, pneumonitis, tracheal stenosis
Renal	Glomerulonephritis	Glomerulosclerosis
Hepatic	Sinusoidal obstruction syndrome	
Endocrine		Hypothyroidism, panhypopituitarism
Hematologic	Bone marrow suppression	Coagulation necrosis

Prehydration and avoidance of other nephrotoxins limit the risk of renal toxicity.

Cyclophosphamide is often associated with the syndrome of inappropriate antidiuretic hormone secretion (SIADH) via a direct effect on renal tubules, but this condition is usually benign. The most serious adverse effect of cyclophosphamide is hemorrhagic cystitis, which can cause hematuria severe enough to produce obstructive uropathy.

Induction chemotherapy or high-dose radiation therapy can induce tumor cell lysis that causes release of large amounts of uric acid, phosphate, and potassium. Hyperuricemia can cause uric acid crystals to precipitate in renal tubules, which leads to acute renal failure. Calcium phosphate deposition may exacerbate the condition. Radiation exposure can cause glomerulonephritis or glomerulosclerosis with permanent injury marked by chronic renal insufficiency and systemic hypertension.

Hepatic System

Antimetabolites such as methotrexate, as well as asparaginase, arabinoside, plicamycin, and streptozocin, have been associated with acute liver dysfunction. However, chronic liver disease is uncommon. Radiation-induced liver injury is also typically dose dependent and reversible.

The most severe form of liver dysfunction in cancer patients is *sinusoidal obstruction syndrome*. This usually occurs in patients receiving total body irradiation in preparation for hematopoietic stem cell transplantation; however, several chemotherapeutic agents have also been associated with this syndrome, including busulfan, cyclophosphamide, vincristine, and dactinomycin. Mortality ranges from 20%–50%.

Airway and Oral Cavity

Mucositis is a painful inflammation and ulceration of the mucous membranes of the digestive tract. Oral lesions begin as mucosal whitening followed by development of erythema and tissue friability. Oral mucositis is a relatively common adverse effect of high-dose chemotherapy and radiation to the head and neck. Mucositis can also occur in the context of hematopoietic stem cell transplantation. Chemotherapeutic drugs associated with mucositis include the anthracyclines, taxanes, and platinum-based compounds, as well as antimetabolites such as methotrexate and fluorouracil. Mucositis associated with chemotherapy often begins during the first week of treatment and typically resolves after treatment is terminated. Mucositis associated with radiation therapy usually has a more delayed onset. Patients with mucositis are at risk of infection from spread of oral bacteria. Narcotics are frequently required to achieve adequate analgesia. In its most severe form, pseudomembrane formation, edema, and bleeding may cause airway compromise or risk of aspiration.

Radiation to the head and neck can result in permanent tissue fibrosis that may limit mouth opening and neck and tongue mobility. Airway fibrosis and tracheal stenosis may result in difficulty in ventilation and intubation that is not recognized on physical examination.

Gastrointestinal System

Almost all chemotherapy and radiation therapy produces gastrointestinal (GI) adverse effects. Nausea, vomiting, diarrhea, and enteritis are common. Diarrhea is frequent with fluorouracil, melphalan, anthracyclines, and the topoisomerase inhibitors. In the short term, these symptoms can produce dehydration, electrolyte abnormalities, and malnutrition, but these effects are usually transient. Radiation, however, may produce permanent sequelae such as adhesions and stenotic lesions anywhere along the GI tract. *Hemorrhagic pancreatitis* is a unique complication associated with asparaginase.

Endocrine System

Hyperglycemia is a common adverse effect of glucocorticoid therapy, as is suppression of the hypothalamic-pituitary-adrenal axis, which may become evident during stress or surgery. Adrenal suppression is reversible, but it may take up to a year for adrenal function to return to normal. SIADH can be seen with cyclophosphamide, ifosfamide, cisplatin, and melphalan, although symptomatic hyponatremia is uncommon.

Total body irradiation in the context of hematopoietic stem cell transplantation and radiation therapy for head and neck cancers can cause panhypopituitarism and/or hypothyroidism, which typically becomes symptomatic during the first few *years* following treatment. Patients with a history of radiation exposure to the neck are also at increased risk of thyroid cancer.

Hematologic System

Myelosuppression is the most frequent adverse effect associated with chemotherapy. In most cases this effect is transient, and blood cell counts return to normal within a week following therapy.

Bleeding is relatively common in patients on chemotherapy and may be the result of thrombocytopenia and/or platelet dysfunction. Depletion of vitamin K–dependent coagulation factors contributes to this problem. Bleeding has also been associated with the angiogenesis inhibitor bevacizumab as well as several of the tyrosine kinase inhibitors, particularly when used in conjunction with other drugs. For this reason it has been recommended that bevacizumab therapy be withheld before major surgery.

Tumors release procoagulants such as tissue factor that create a hypercoagulable state. Some chemotherapeutic drugs can exacerbate this condition. Thalidomide and the related drug lenalidomide pose an especially high risk of venous thromboembolism, particularly when used in combination with glucocorticoids and doxorubicin. Other drugs associated with an increased risk of thromboembolism include cisplatin and tamoxifen. For high-risk patients, such as those who undergo major abdominal, pelvic, or orthopedic surgeries and are likely to be sedentary, both the American College of Chest Physicians and the American Society of Clinical Oncology advise that venous thromboembolism prophylaxis be continued for 4 weeks postoperatively.

Radiation-induced coagulation disorders occur as a delayed effect and involve coagulation necrosis of vascular endothelium. Postradiation bleeding in the rectum, vagina, bladder, lung, and brain has been reported.

Nervous System

Chemotherapy can cause a number of neurotoxic adverse effects, including peripheral neuropathy and encephalopathy. Virtually all patients treated with vincristine develop paresthesias in their hands and feet. Autonomic neuropathy may accompany the paresthesias. These changes are usually reversible. The platinum agents (cisplatin, carboplatin, oxaliplatin) cause dose-dependent large-fiber neuropathy by damaging dorsal root ganglia. Loss of proprioception may be sufficiently severe to interfere with ambulation. Consideration of regional anesthesia in patients being treated with these drugs must take into account the fact that subclinical neurotoxicity is present in a large percentage of patients and may extend several months beyond discontinuation of treatment. Paclitaxel causes dose-dependent ataxia that may be accompanied by paresthesias in the hands and feet and proximal skeletal muscle weakness. Corticosteroids (prednisone or its equivalent at 40–60 mg/day) may cause a myopathy characterized by weakness of the neck flexors and proximal weakness of the extremities. The first sign of corticosteroid-induced neuromuscular toxicity is difficulty rising from the sitting position. Respiratory muscles may also be affected. Corticosteroid-induced myopathy usually resolves when the drug is discontinued.

Cancer chemotherapeutic drugs can also cause encephalopathy, delirium, and/or cerebellar ataxia. Examples include high-dose cyclophosphamide and methotrexate. Prolonged administration of methotrexate, especially in conjunction with radiation therapy, can lead to progressive irreversible dementia. Small doses of brain irradiation alone have been shown to cause neurocognitive changes; however, large doses (>50 Gy) are needed to cause frank tissue destruction.

Tumor Lysis Syndrome

Tumor lysis syndrome is caused by sudden destruction of tumor cells by chemotherapy or radiation, leading to the release of large amounts of uric acid, potassium, and phosphate. This syndrome occurs most often after induction treatment for hematologic neoplasms such as acute lymphoblastic leukemia. Acute renal failure can develop because of uric acid crystal formation and/or calcium phosphate deposition in the kidney. Hyperkalemia and cardiac dysrhythmias are more likely in the presence of renal dysfunction. Hyperphosphatemia can lead to secondary hypocalcemia, which increases the risk of cardiac dysrhythmias from hypokalemia and can cause neuromuscular symptoms such as tetany.

CANCER IMMUNOLOGY

Diagnosis

The use of monoclonal antibodies to detect proteins encoded by oncogenes or other types of tumor-associated antigens (TAs) is a common method for identifying cancer. TAs such as α-fetoprotein (AFP), prostate-specific antigen (PSA), and carcinoembryonic antigen (CEA) are present on cancer cells and normal cells, but concentrations are higher on tumor cells. Monoclonal antibodies to various TAs can be labeled with radioisotopes and injected to monitor the spread of cancer. Because TAs are present on normal tissues, measurement of these antigens may be less useful for the diagnosis of cancer than for monitoring disease activity.

Immunomodulators

Tumor cells are antigenically different from normal cells, and evidence now confirms that the body is able to mount an immune response against tumor-associated antigens in a process similar to that which causes allograft rejection. However, because TAs also exist on normal cells, they are only weakly antigenic. Adjuvants are compounds that potentiate the immune response. Examples include bacille Calmette-Guérin (BCG) and naturally occurring interferons such as interleukin (IL)-2, interferon (IFN)-α, and granulocyte-macrophage colony-stimulating factor (GM-CSF). These agents are used to augment the host's intrinsic anticancer capabilities.

Cancer Vaccines

Appreciation of the role of tumor-associated antigens in eliciting an immune response is now driving the development of cancer vaccines. Two types of cancer vaccines exist: preventive and therapeutic. The *preventive vaccines* target infectious agents known to contribute to cancer development. Two preventive vaccines are currently marketed, one against human papillomavirus (HPV) types 6, 11, 16, 18 and another against hepatitis B virus (HBV). HPV types 16 and 18 are responsible for approximately 70% of cervical cancers and are also a causal factor in some cancers of the vagina, vulva, anus, penis, and oropharynx. Chronic HBV infection is a major risk factor for development of hepatocellular carcinoma. HBV vaccination is now recommended in childhood as part of a strategy to reduce not only the risk of HBV infection but also the incidence of hepatocellular cancer.

The premise behind *therapeutic cancer vaccines* is that injection of tumor antigen can be used to stimulate an immune system response against tumor cells. In 2010 the US Food and Drug Administration (FDA) approved the first therapeutic cancer vaccine, sipuleucel-T (Provenge) for the treatment of some cases of metastatic prostate cancer. Sipuleucel-T is an autologous vaccine produced by isolating antigen-presenting cells from the patient's own immune system, then culturing them with a protein consisting of prostatic acid phosphatase (an antigen found on most prostate cancer cells) linked to GM-CSF. Treatment elicits an immune response that has shown efficacy in reducing tumor progression. Vaccines are in development for a number of other cancers. Some of these are made from weakened or killed cancer cells that contain TAs, others from immune cells that have been modified to express TAs. Still others are being made synthetically. A novel type of cancer vaccine uses "naked" DNA or RNA that codes for TAs. Injection of the vaccine either directly or via a virus carrier induces massive TA production, which in turn promotes a robust immune response that is intended to halt tumor progression.

PARANEOPLASTIC SYNDROMES

Paraneoplastic syndromes are pathophysiologic disturbances that affect an estimated 8% of patients with cancer. Sometimes symptoms of a paraneoplastic syndrome manifest before the cancer diagnosis and may actually result in cancer detection. Certain of these conditions (superior vena cava obstruction, increased intracranial pressure) may manifest as life-threatening medical emergencies.

Fever and Cachexia

Fever may occur with any type of cancer but is particularly likely with metastases to the liver. Fever may accompany rapidly proliferating tumors such as leukemias and lymphomas. Fever may reflect tumor necrosis, inflammation, release of toxic products by cancer cells, or production of endogenous pyrogens.

Cancer cachexia is a frequent occurrence in cancer patients. In addition to the psychological effects of cancer on appetite, cancer cells compete with normal tissues for nutrients and may eventually cause nutritive death of normal cells. Tumor factors such as proteolysis-inducing factor and host response factors such as tumor necrosis factor (TNF)-α, IFN-γ, and IL-6 also contribute to muscle atrophy and lipolysis. Hyperalimentation is indicated for nutritional support when malnutrition is severe, especially if surgery is planned.

Neurologic Abnormalities

Paraneoplastic neurologic syndromes are the result of antibody-mediated damage to the nervous system. Antibodies produced by the host in response to tumor-associated antigens cross-react with elements of the nervous system, which leads to neurologic dysfunction. The vast majority of paraneoplastic neurologic syndromes (80%) manifest *before* the diagnosis of cancer. They can affect both the central and peripheral nervous systems. They are relatively rare—occurring in about 1% of cancer patients—but are seen disproportionately in those with small cell lung cancer (SCLC), lymphoma, and myeloma. Examples are limbic encephalitis, paraneoplastic cerebellar degeneration, Lambert-Eaton myasthenia syndrome, and myasthenia gravis. Lambert-Eaton syndrome is caused by antibodies to voltage-gated calcium channel receptors and is commonly associated with SCLC. Myasthenia gravis is caused by antibodies to the acetylcholine receptor and is often present in patients with thymoma. Potentiation of neuromuscular blocking agents may be observed in these myasthenic disorders.

These paraneoplastic neurologic syndromes often present a diagnostic challenge because symptoms are nonspecific and the underlying cancer diagnosis is usually unknown. Antibodies to tumor-associated material (called *onconeural antibodies*) are present in the serum of some but not all patients. Immunosuppression is the mainstay of treatment of these syndromes. Corticosteroids and immunoglobulin therapies are frequently employed. Plasmapheresis may also be required to reduce the antibody burden. Once the condition is diagnosed, screening for an underlying malignancy is indicated.

Endocrine Abnormalities

Paraneoplastic endocrine syndromes arise from hormone or peptide production within tumor cells (Table 28.4). Most occur after the diagnosis of cancer has been established. Treatment of the underlying tumor is the preferred management.

SIADH

SIADH affects approximately 1%–2% of cancer patients, with most cases related to SCLC. Headache and nausea are early symptoms that may progress to confusion, ataxia, lethargy, and seizures. Symptoms depend on the degree of hyponatremia

TABLE 28.4	Ectopic Hormone Production	
Hormone	Associated Cancer	Manifestations
Adrenocorticotropic hormone	Carcinoid, lung (small cell), thymoma, thyroid (medullary)	Cushing syndrome
Antidiuretic hormone	Duodenal, lung (small cell), lymphoma, pancreatic, prostate	Water intoxication
Erythropoietin	Hemangioblastoma, hepatic, renal cell, uterine myofibroma	Polycythemia
Human chorionic gonadotropin	Adrenal, breast, lung (large cell), ovarian, testicular	Gynecomastia, galactorrhea, precocious puberty
Insulinlike substances	Retroperitoneal tumors	Hypoglycemia
Parathyroid hormone	Lung (small cell, squamous cell), ovary, pancreas, renal	Hyperparathyroidism, hypercalcemia, hypertension, renal dysfunction, left ventricular dysfunction
Thyrotropin	Choriocarcinoma, testicular (embryonal)	Hyperthyroidism, thrombocytopenia
Thyrocalcitonin	Thyroid (medullary)	Hypocalcemia, hypotension, muscle weakness

and the rapidity with which it develops. SIADH resolves with treatment of the underlying tumor. Vasopressin receptor antagonists (tolvaptan and conivaptan) and demeclocycline (a tetracycline drug that produces a reversible form of nephrogenic diabetes insipidus) are the pharmacologic therapies available if symptoms are severe.

Hypercalcemia

Cancer is the most common cause of hypercalcemia in hospitalized patients and is considered a poor prognostic indicator. There are several different mechanisms for the hypercalcemia seen in cancer patients. The most common is secretion of a parathyroid hormone–like protein by tumor cells that binds to parathyroid hormone receptors in the bone and kidney. This occurs commonly with squamous cell cancers of the kidneys, lungs, pancreas, and ovaries. Hypercalcemia can also be caused by local osteolytic activity associated with bone metastases, especially from breast cancer, multiple myeloma, and some lymphomas. Occasionally tumors secrete vitamin D.

The rapid onset of hypercalcemia that occurs in patients with cancer may present as lethargy or coma. Polyuria accompanies hypercalcemia and may lead to dehydration. Treatment includes hydration with normal saline. Intravenous (IV) bisphosphonates or calcitonin may also be indicated.

Cushing Syndrome

Cushing syndrome is most commonly associated with neuroendocrine tumors of the lung, such as SCLC and carcinoid. It is caused by tumor secretion of either adrenocorticotropic hormone (ACTH) or corticotropin-releasing factor (CRF). Clinical symptoms include hypertension, weight gain, central obesity, and edema. The diagnosis can be confirmed by measuring serum concentrations of ACTH or CRF and by performing a dexamethasone suppression test, which involves administration of dexamethasone followed by measurement of urinary cortisol levels. Normally, administration of dexamethasone causes a marked reduction in urinary cortisol concentration. In patients with paraneoplastic Cushing syndrome, however, there is no reduction in urinary cortisol level after dexamethasone administration. Treatment includes agents that block steroid production (e.g., ketoconazole, mitotane). Antihypertensives and diuretics may also be needed for symptom management.

Hypoglycemia

Intermittent hypoglycemic episodes can occur with insulin-producing islet cell tumors in the pancreas or with non–islet cell tumors outside the pancreas that secrete insulinlike growth factor (IGF)-2. Patients with islet cell tumors demonstrate a *high* serum insulin level. In contrast, those with non–islet cell tumors that secrete insulinlike substances demonstrate a *low* serum insulin level and an elevated level of IGF-2.

Renal Abnormalities

Paraneoplastic glomerulopathies occur in a variety of different forms, including membranous glomerulonephritis, nephrotic syndrome, and amyloidosis. Many involve renal deposition of immunoglobulins or immune complexes containing tumor antigens with host antibodies. Amyloidosis is marked by deposition of a unique protein called *amyloid* and is most often associated with renal cell carcinoma. Glomerulopathies are relatively common in lymphoma and leukemia.

Dermatologic and Rheumatologic Abnormalities

Paraneoplastic dermatologic and rheumatologic conditions can occur without overt evidence of malignancy, but their appearance should initiate screening for an underlying cancer. *Acanthosis nigricans* is a skin pigmentation disorder recognized by dark patches of skin with a thick velvety texture usually occurring in the axilla or neck. This skin disorder is most commonly related to insulin resistance or other non–cancer-related conditions. However, when found on the palms (tripe palm), it is almost always associated with cancer, most often of GI origin. Dermatomyositis is an inflammatory condition that causes proximal muscle weakness as well as characteristic skin changes, including a rash on the eyelids and hands. It can be seen with ovarian, breast, lung, prostate, and colorectal cancers. Hypertrophic osteoarthropathy—commonly known as *clubbing*—involves subperiosteal bone deposition that causes a characteristic remodeling of the phalangeal shafts. It is classically associated with intrathoracic tumors or metastases to the lungs.

Hematologic Abnormalities

Paraneoplastic hematologic syndromes are rarely symptomatic, though they are usually present with advanced cancer. Paraneoplastic eosinophilia is related to production of specific interleukins that promote eosinophilic differentiation and is most often seen in leukemia and lymphoma. Eosinophilia can sometimes cause wheezing or occasionally end-organ damage resulting from eosinophilic infiltration. Granulocytosis usually occurs with solid tumors, particularly large cell lung cancer. Pure red cell aplasia is commonly associated with thymoma but also occurs with leukemia and lymphoma. Underlying malignancy is the diagnosis in about a third of patients with thrombocytosis (platelet count > 400,000/mm^3). It appears to be caused by tumor-released cytokines such as IL-6.

LOCAL EFFECTS OF CANCER AND METASTASES

Superior Vena Cava Syndrome/Superior Mediastinal Syndrome

Obstruction of the superior vena cava is caused by spread of cancer into the mediastinum or directly into the caval wall and is most often associated with lung cancer. Veins above the level of the heart, particularly the jugular veins and veins in the arms, become engorged. Edema of the face and upper extremities is usually prominent. Increased intracranial pressure manifests as nausea, seizures, and decreased levels of consciousness and is most likely due to an increase in cerebral venous pressure. Compression of the great vessels may cause syncope.

Superior mediastinal syndrome is the combination of superior vena cava syndrome and tracheal compression. Hoarseness, dyspnea, and airway obstruction may be present because of tracheal compression. Treatment consists of prompt radiation therapy or chemotherapy for symptomatic relief. Bronchoscopy and/or mediastinoscopy to obtain a tissue diagnosis can be very hazardous, especially in the presence of co-existing airway obstruction and increased pressure in the mediastinal veins.

Spinal Cord Compression

Spinal cord compression results from the presence of metastatic lesions in the epidural space, most often breast, lung, or prostate cancer or lymphoma. Symptoms include pain, skeletal muscle weakness, sensory loss, and autonomic dysfunction. CT and MRI can visualize the limits of compression. Radiation therapy is a useful treatment when neurologic deficits are only partial or in development. Corticosteroids are often administered to minimize the inflammation and edema that can result from radiation directed at tumors in the epidural space. Once total paralysis has developed, the results of surgical laminectomy or radiation treatment to decompress the spinal cord are poor.

Increased Intracranial Pressure

Metastatic brain tumors, most often from lung and breast cancer, present initially as mental deterioration, focal neurologic deficits, or seizures. Treatment of an acute increase in intracranial pressure caused by a metastatic lesion includes corticosteroids, diuretics, and mannitol. Radiation therapy is the usual palliative treatment, but surgery can be considered for patients with only a single metastatic lesion. Intrathecal administration of chemotherapeutic drugs is usually necessary when the tumor involves the meninges.

CANCER PAIN

Cancer patients may experience acute pain associated with pathologic fractures, tumor invasion, surgery, radiation treatment, and chemotherapy. Pain is frequently related to metastatic spread of the cancer, especially to bone. Nerve compression or infiltration may also cause pain. Patients with cancer who experience frequent and significant pain often exhibit signs of depression and anxiety.

Pathophysiology

Cancer pain resulting from organic causes may be subdivided into nociceptive and neuropathic pain. *Nociceptive pain* includes somatic and visceral pain and refers to pain caused by the peripheral stimulation of nociceptors in somatic or visceral structures. *Somatic pain* is related to tumor involvement of somatic structures such as bones or skeletal muscles and is often described as aching, stabbing, or throbbing. *Visceral pain* is related to lesions in a hollow or solid viscus and is described as diffuse, gnawing, or crampy if a hollow viscus is involved and as aching or sharp if a solid viscus is involved. Nociceptive pain is typically responsive to both nonopioid and opioid medication. *Neuropathic pain* involves peripheral or central afferent neural pathways and is commonly described as burning or lancinating pain. Patients experiencing neuropathic pain often respond poorly to opioids.

Trauma associated with surgery for removal of cancerous tissue may also be a cause of chronic pain. Scars and injury of soft tissue and of sensory afferents that innervate the surgical area may contribute to the development of chronic pain.

Drug Therapy

Drug therapy is the cornerstone of cancer pain management because of its efficacy, rapid onset of action, and relatively low cost. Mild to moderate cancer pain is initially treated with nonsteroidal antiinflammatory drugs (NSAIDs) and acetaminophen. NSAIDs are especially effective for managing bone pain, which is the most common type of cancer pain. The next step in management of cancer pain is the addition of codeine or one of its analogues. When cancer pain is severe, more potent opioids are employed. Morphine is commonly selected and can be administered orally. When the oral route of administration is inadequate, alternative routes (IV, subcutaneous, epidural, intrathecal, transmucosal, transdermal) are considered. Fentanyl is available in transdermal and transmucosal delivery systems. Tolerance to opioids does occur and may necessitate dosage adjustment. Fear of addiction is a major reason why opioids are underutilized, but addiction is rare in cancer patients when these drugs are correctly managed.

Tricyclic antidepressant drugs are indicated for patients with depressive symptoms. These drugs may also exhibit analgesic properties by potentiating the effects of opioids. Anticonvulsants are useful for the management of chronic neuropathic pain. Corticosteroids can decrease pain perception, have a sparing effect on opioid requirements, improve mood, increase appetite, and lead to weight gain. Multimodal analgesia with local anesthetics and adjunctive agents such as gabapentin and ketamine may be effective in preventing both acute and chronic pain and reducing analgesic use after surgery.

Neuraxial Analgesia

Neuraxial analgesia is an effective way to control pain in cancer patients undergoing surgery and may play a role in providing preemptive analgesia. Neuraxial analgesia with local anesthetics provides immediate pain relief in patients whose pain cannot be alleviated with oral or IV analgesics and is frequently employed for treatment of cancer pain. Neuraxial analgesia is not used in patients with local infection, bacteremia, and systemic infection because of the increased risk of epidural abscess. However, in the setting of intractable cancer pain, there may be a role for epidural analgesia despite the risk of meningeal infection. Morphine may be administered intrathecally or epidurally for management of acute and chronic cancer pain. Spinal opioids may be delivered for weeks to months via a long-term, subcutaneously tunneled, exteriorized catheter or an implanted drug delivery system. The implantable systems can be intrathecal or epidural and typically feature a drug reservoir and the capability for external programming. Patients are typically considered for neuraxial opioid administration when systemic opioid administration has failed because of the occurrence of intolerable side effects or inadequate analgesia. Neuraxial administration of opioids is usually successful, but some patients may require addition of a dilute concentration of local anesthetic to the infusate to achieve adequate pain control.

Neurolytic Procedures

Neurolytic procedures intended to destroy sensory components of nerves cannot be used without also destroying motor and autonomic nervous system fibers. Important considerations in determining the suitability of a destructive nerve block for control of cancer pain are the location and quality of the pain, effectiveness of less destructive treatment modalities, inherent risks associated with the block, availability of experienced anesthesiologists to perform the procedures, and the patient's anticipated life expectancy. In general, constant pain is more amenable to destructive nerve block than is intermittent pain. Neurolytic celiac plexus block with alcohol or phenol has been used to treat pain originating from abdominal viscera, especially in the context of pancreatic cancer. The block is associated with significant side effects, but analgesia usually lasts 6 months or longer.

Neuroablative or neurostimulatory procedures for managing cancer pain are reserved for patients whose pain is unresponsive to other less invasive procedures. Cordotomy involves interruption of the spinothalamic tract in the spinal cord and is considered for treatment of unilateral pain involving the lower extremity, thorax, or upper extremity. Dorsal rhizotomy involves interruption of sensory nerve roots and is used when pain is localized to specific dermatomal levels. Dorsal column stimulators or deep brain stimulators may be used in selected patients.

MANAGEMENT OF ANESTHESIA

Preoperative evaluation of patients with cancer includes consideration of the pathophysiologic effects of the disease and recognition of the potential adverse effects of cancer treatments (Table 28.5). In addition, the patient's underlying medical comorbidities must not be overlooked. Correction of nutrient deficiencies, electrolyte abnormalities, anemia, and coagulopathies may be needed preoperatively. In most cases, laboratory evaluation should include complete blood cell count (CBC), coagulation profile, serum electrolyte concentrations, and transaminase levels. Chest radiography, echocardiography, pulmonary function evaluation, and other specialized testing should be used if clinical suspicion warrants. There are no specific rules regarding preoperative management of chemotherapeutic drugs. However, most of them have the potential to impair wound healing, especially the growth factor and angiogenesis inhibitors. It has been suggested that surgery be delayed for 4–8 weeks after treatment with bevacizumab because of an increased risk of bleeding and postoperative wound complications.

Potential pulmonary or cardiac toxicity is a consideration in patients being treated with chemotherapeutic drugs known to be associated with these complications. The myocardial depressant effects of anesthesia can unmask cardiac dysfunction related to cardiotoxic chemotherapeutic drugs such as doxorubicin. Therefore when major surgery is planned, preoperative echocardiography may be indicated. Since several chemotherapeutic agents can cause ECG abnormalities such as QT prolongation, a baseline ECG should be reviewed.

A preoperative history of drug-induced pulmonary fibrosis (dyspnea, nonproductive cough) or congestive heart failure will influence subsequent management of anesthesia. In patients treated with bleomycin, it may be helpful to perform arterial blood gas monitoring in addition to oximetry and to carefully titrate intravascular fluid replacement, since these patients are at risk of developing interstitial pulmonary edema, presumably because of impaired lymphatic drainage in the lung. Bleomycin-associated pulmonary injury may be exacerbated by high oxygen concentrations; therefore it is prudent to adjust the delivered oxygen concentration to the minimum that provides adequate oxygen saturation. Nitrous oxide may augment the toxicity of methotrexate, so it is best avoided.

The presence of hepatic or renal dysfunction should influence the choice and dose of anesthetic drugs and muscle relaxants. Although it is not consistently observed, the possibility of a prolonged response to succinylcholine is a consideration in patients being treated with alkylating chemotherapeutic drugs like cyclophosphamide that cause drug-induced pseudocholinesterase deficiency. The presence of paraneoplastic syndromes (e.g., myasthenia gravis, Eaton-Lambert syndrome) may also affect the patient's response to muscle relaxants.

Attention to aseptic technique is important because immunosuppression occurs with most chemotherapeutic agents and is exacerbated by malnutrition. Immunosuppression produced by anesthesia, surgical stress, or blood transfusion during the perioperative period could have deleterious effects on the patient's subsequent response to his or her cancer. Adrenal suppression may be present in patients who are being treated with steroids. Those who have been receiving more than 20 mg of prednisone (or its equivalent) per day for longer than 3 weeks are considered most at risk. Recovery of the hypothalamic-pituitary-adrenal axis

TABLE 28.5	Preanesthetic Evaluation of Cancer Patients		
System	Risk Factors	Investigations	Anesthetic Considerations
Cardiovascular	Doxorubicin exposure Mediastinal radiation Anterior mediastinal mass	Chest radiograph Chest CT scan Echocardiogram	Left ventricular dysfunction Dysrhythmias Engorgement of great vessels
Pulmonary	Bleomycin, busulfan, chlorambucil exposure Radiation to thorax	Arterial blood gas analysis Chest radiograph Chest CT scan Flow-volume loops Pulmonary function tests	Obstructive/restrictive disease Avoid high concentrations of oxygen with history of bleomycin exposure.
Renal and hepatic	Induction chemotherapy or radiation therapy Tumor lysis syndrome	Renal and liver function tests Coagulation profile Uric acid level	Acute renal failure with tumor lysis syndrome Adjust drug dosages based on end-organ damage.
Hematologic	Metastatic disease Exposure to most chemotherapeutic drugs and radiation	CBC Coagulation profile	Infection risk Bleeding risk Thromboembolism prophylaxis
Neurologic	Cisplatin, vincristine, fluorouracil exposure Metastatic disease Paraneoplastic syndromes (myasthenia gravis, Eaton-Lambert syndrome)	Physical examination and documentation of preexisting sensorimotor defects	Elevated intracranial pressure, papilledema, spinal cord compression due to metastases Phrenic nerve palsy in presence of metastases or superior vena cava syndrome Exercise caution with peripheral nerve blocks, neuraxial anesthesia
Gastrointestinal	Exposure to all chemotherapeutic drugs and radiation Advanced cancer	Physical examination Serum electrolyte and prealbumin levels	Hypovolemia Electrolyte abnormalities Metabolic acidosis/alkalosis Mucositis/oral ulcerations that may predispose to bleeding with airway instrumentation Increased aspiration risk in presence of nausea/vomiting Increased infection risk, poor wound healing
Endocrine	Steroid exposure Paraneoplastic syndromes—SIADH, hypercalcemia	Preoperative medication history Serum electrolyte levels	Risk of electrolyte abnormalities (hyponatremia, hypercalcemia, hypocalcemia) Consider stress-dose steroids with adrenal insufficiency.
Airway	Airway	Physical examination Chest radiograph Chest CT scan Flow-volume loops	Difficult airway precautions Tracheal compression Airway collapse with cessation of spontaneous ventilation

CBC, Complete blood cell count; *CT,* computed tomography; *SIADH,* syndrome of inappropriate antidiuretic hormone secretion.
Adapted from Latham GJ, Greenberg RS. Anesthetic considerations for the pediatric oncology patient—part 3: pain, cognitive dysfunction, and preoperative evaluation. *Paediatr Anaesth.* 2010;20:486, Fig. 2.

may take up to a year. A typical steroid replacement regimen is hydrocortisone 100 mg IV administered at induction of anesthesia, followed by 100 mg IV every 8 hours for the first 24 hours after surgery.

Intubation in the presence of oral mucositis may cause bleeding. Patients with cancers of the head, neck, and anterior mediastinum may exhibit airway compromise. Patients with a history of radiation exposure may have airway abnormalities that are difficult to detect on physical examination.

Recent evidence suggests that anesthetics and analgesics have immunomodulatory properties (see Chapter 27, "Diseases Related to Immune System Dysfunction"). IV opioids tend to blunt natural killer (NK) cell activity, producing an immunosuppressive effect that supports proliferation of tumor cells. Use of neuraxial anesthesia may preserve the host's intrinsic anticancer defenses better than general anesthesia. However, coagulopathies may prevent use of these techniques in some cancer patients. Peripheral nerve blocks may be used, but baseline

peripheral neuropathies related to chemotherapeutic drugs such as vincristine and cisplatin should be well documented.

Postoperative care must include adequate attention to pain management. Many cancer patients have been treated for pain related to their underlying diagnosis. Therefore narcotic dosing must be adjusted to account for possible drug tolerance. Prophylaxis against infection and thromboembolism must also be considered.

COMMON CANCERS ENCOUNTERED IN CLINICAL PRACTICE

The most common cancers in adults encountered by anesthesiologists in the surgical setting are lung, breast, colon, and prostate cancers. Lung cancer is the second most common malignancy in men, surpassed only by prostate cancer; in women the incidence of lung cancer is increasing and is now exceeded only by breast cancer.

Lung Cancer

Lung cancer is the leading cause of cancer death among men and women. It is largely a preventable disease, since about 90% of lung cancer deaths are related to cigarette smoking. Five-year survival varies significantly based on cell type and stage of the disease. For those with non–small cell lung cancer (NSCLC), 50% of patients with only local disease may survive 5 years, but only 2% of those with distant metastases evident at the time of diagnosis will be alive 5 years later. For patients with SCLC, the disease is usually disseminated at presentation and survival rates are much lower—only about 10%–13% for patients with limited disease and 1%–2% for patients with extensive disease.

Etiology

The strong association between cigarette smoking and lung cancer is well established. Smoking marijuana produces a greater carbon monoxide and tar burden than smoking a similar quantity of tobacco, and thus its use may pose an additional risk factor for lung cancer in cigarette smokers. The mutagens and carcinogens present in cigarette smoke may cause chromosomal damage and over time may cause malignancy. Other carcinogens that cause lung cancer are ionizing radiation (byproduct of coal and iron mining), asbestos (increases the incidence of lung cancer in nonsmokers and acts as a cocarcinogen with tobacco smoke), and naturally occurring radon gas. Adjuvant radiation therapy for breast cancer following mastectomy is also associated with an increased risk of lung cancer.

There is a familial risk of lung cancer that is related to genetic and ecogenetic factors and to exposure to passive smoking. Inhalation of secondhand smoke increases the risk of lung cancer and contributes to development of childhood respiratory infections and asthma. Cigarette smokers who develop emphysema are at increased risk of developing lung cancer. AIDS may be associated with an increased incidence of lung cancer. Following cessation of cigarette smoking, the risk and incidence of lung cancer decreases to that of nonsmokers after approximately 10–15 years.

Signs and Symptoms

Patients with lung cancer have features related to the extent of the disease, including local and regional manifestations, signs and symptoms of metastatic disease, and various paraneoplastic syndromes related indirectly to the cancer. Cough, hemoptysis, wheezing, stridor, dyspnea, or pneumonitis from airway obstruction may be presenting clinical signs. Mediastinal metastases may cause hoarseness (recurrent laryngeal nerve compression), superior vena cava syndrome, cardiac dysrhythmias, or congestive heart failure from pericardial effusion and tamponade. Pleural effusion results in increasing dyspnea and often chest pain. Generalized weakness, fatigue, anorexia, and weight loss are common.

Histologic Subtypes

Clinical manifestations of lung cancer vary with the histologic subtype. NSCLC, which includes squamous cell carcinoma, adenocarcinoma, and large cell carcinoma, accounts for about 85% of all new cases of lung cancer.

Squamous cell cancers arise in major bronchi or their primary divisions (central origin) and are usually detected by cytologic analysis of sputum. These tumors tend to grow slowly and may reach a large size before they are finally detected. Hemoptysis, bronchial obstruction with associated atelectasis, dyspnea, and fever from pneumonia are common presenting signs. Cavitation may be evident on chest radiography.

Adenocarcinomas most often originate in the lung periphery. These tumors commonly present as subpleural nodules and have a tendency to invade the pleura and induce pleural effusions that contain malignant cells. Lung adenocarcinomas may be difficult to differentiate morphologically from malignant mesothelioma or adenocarcinoma that has metastasized from other sites such as breast, GI tract, or pancreas.

Large cell carcinomas are usually peripheral in origin and present as large bulky tumors. Like adenocarcinomas, these tumors metastasize early and preferentially to the central nervous system (CNS).

Small cell carcinomas are usually of central bronchial origin and have a high frequency of early lymphatic invasion, especially to lymph nodes in the mediastinum, and metastases to liver, bone, CNS, adrenal glands, and pancreas. Prominent mediastinal lymphadenopathy may lead to the erroneous diagnosis of malignant lymphoma. Superior vena cava syndrome may result from mediastinal compression. Small cell tumors have a marked propensity to produce polypeptides and ectopic hormones that result in metabolic abnormalities. The tumors are not usually detected in these patients until the disease process is widespread.

Diagnosis

Cytologic analysis of sputum is often sufficient for the diagnosis of lung cancer, especially when the cancer arises in proximal endobronchial locations where shedding of cells is likely to occur. Peripheral lesions as small as 3 mm can be detected by high-resolution CT. Lung cancer screening with low-dose computed tomography (LDCT) has been recommended for patients who are at highest risk for lung cancer—adults aged 55–80 years who have at least a 30-pack-year smoking history and who currently smoke or have quit smoking within the past 15 years.

Flexible fiberoptic bronchoscopy in combination with biopsy, brushings, or washings is a standard procedure for initial evaluation of lung cancer. Peripheral lung lesions can be diagnosed by percutaneous fine-needle aspiration guided by fluoroscopy, ultrasonography, or CT. Video-assisted thoracoscopic surgery is useful for diagnosing peripheral lung lesions and pleura-based tumors. CT and PET scanning are sensitive for detecting pulmonary metastases. Brain MRI and head CT are useful for detecting brain metastases even in patients without neurologic symptoms or signs. Mediastinoscopy and video-assisted thoracoscopy provide the opportunity to biopsy lymph nodes and stage the tumor.

Treatment

Treatments for lung cancer include surgery, radiation therapy, and chemotherapy. The preferred treatment depends on cell type, stage, and the patient's underlying health.

Pulmonary function testing is used to evaluate the patient's candidacy for lung resection. Forced expiratory volume in 1 second (FEV_1) and diffusing capacity for carbon monoxide (D_{LCO}) are considered among the most useful predictors of postoperative complications. If FEV_1 is more than 2 L and D_{LCO} is more than 80%, patients are at low risk of postoperative respiratory complications. When patients are not clearly in a low-risk category, predicted postoperative pulmonary function can be evaluated. Predicted postoperative pulmonary function takes into consideration preoperative lung function, the amount of lung tissue that will be resected, and the relative contribution of that tissue to overall lung function. Ideally its calculation is based on preoperative pulmonary function test results as well as some quantitative measure of differential lung function, such as ventilation/perfusion scanning. Predicted postoperative FEV_1 can also be estimated using a formula that takes into account the number of lung segments expected to be removed: predicted postoperative FEV_1 = preoperative FEV_1 × (number of segments remaining postoperatively/total number of lung segments). In general, if predicted postoperative FEV_1 is less than 0.8 L, patients are considered poor candidates for pneumonectomy. Cardiopulmonary exercise testing with measurement of maximum oxygen consumption is another test that can be used to evaluate high-risk patients.

Surgery has little effect on survival when the disease has spread to mediastinal lymph nodes or when metastases are present. Even among those considered to have surgically curable disease, recurrent or metastatic disease develops in half of patients within 5 years. For these reasons, many patients with NSCLC are candidates for chemotherapy alone or in combination with surgery or radiation therapy. Video-assisted thoracoscopy is the preferred surgical approach, especially for wedge resection and lobectomy. Standard thoracotomy is needed for more complex procedures or pneumonectomy. In most patients, radiation therapy is effective in palliating symptoms from tumor invasion.

Radiation therapy is the preferred treatment for small cell carcinoma, because it is particularly radiosensitive and the cancer is not detected in most patients until disease is extensive. Chemotherapy is used as an adjunct.

Management of Anesthesia
Management of anesthesia in patients with lung cancer includes preoperative consideration of tumor-induced effects such as malnutrition, pneumonia, pain, and ectopic hormone production leading to electrolyte imbalances like hyponatremia or hypercalcemia.

Hemorrhage and pneumothorax are the most frequently encountered complications of mediastinoscopy. The mediastinoscope can also exert pressure on the right innominate artery, causing loss of the radial pulse and an erroneous diagnosis of cardiac arrest. Likewise, unrecognized compression of the right innominate artery, of which the right carotid artery is a branch, may manifest as a postoperative neurologic deficit. Bradycardia during mediastinoscopy may be due to stretching of the vagus nerve or tracheal compression by the mediastinoscope. Lung resection requires the ability to perform differential lung ventilation, such as with a double-lumen tube or bronchial blocker.

Colorectal Cancer

Colon cancer is the third most common cause of cancer deaths in the United States. Almost all colorectal cancers are adenocarcinomas, and the disease generally occurs in adults older than 50 years.

Etiology
Most colorectal cancers arise from premalignant adenomatous polyps. Although adenomatous polyps are common (present in >30% of patients aged >50 years), fewer than 1% become malignant. Large polyps, especially those larger than 1.5 cm in diameter, are more likely to contain invasive cancer. It is thought that adenomatous polyps require 5–10 years of growth before they develop into a cancer. The evolution of normal colonic mucosa to a benign adenomatous polyp that contains cancer and then to life-threatening invasive cancer is associated with a series of genetic events that involve mutational activation of a protooncogene and the loss of several genes that normally suppress tumorigenesis.

Most colorectal cancers appear to be related to diet. There is a direct correlation between colorectal cancer incidence and the amount of calories, animal fat, and meat protein consumed. Family history of colorectal cancer, inflammatory bowel disease, and a 35 or more pack-year history of smoking are also risk factors.

Diagnosis
The rationale for colorectal cancer screening is that early detection and removal of localized superficial tumors and precancerous lesions in asymptomatic individuals increases the cure rate. Screening programs (digital rectal examination, examination of the stool for occult blood, colonoscopy) appear to be particularly useful for persons who have first-degree relatives with a history of the disease, especially if these relatives developed colorectal cancer before age 55.

Signs and Symptoms
The presenting signs and symptoms of colorectal cancer reflect the anatomic location of the cancer. Because stool is relatively liquid as it passes into the right colon through the ileocecal valve, tumors in the cecum and ascending colon can become large and markedly narrow the bowel lumen without causing obstructive symptoms. Ascending colon cancers frequently ulcerate, which leads to chronic blood loss in the stool. These patients experience symptoms related to anemia, including fatigue and, in some patients, angina pectoris.

Stool becomes more concentrated as it passes into the transverse colon. Transverse colon cancers cause abdominal cramping, occasional bowel obstruction, and even perforation. Abdominal radiographs reveal characteristic abnormalities in the colonic gas pattern, reflecting narrowing of the lumen ("napkin-ring lesion"). Colon cancers developing in the rectosigmoid portion of the large intestine result in tenesmus and thinner stools. Anemia is unusual despite the passage of bright red blood from the rectum (often attributable to hemorrhoids).

Colorectal cancers initially spread to regional lymph nodes and then through the portal venous circulation to the liver, which represents the most common visceral site of metastases. Colorectal cancers rarely spread to lung, bone, or brain in the absence of liver metastases. A preoperative increase in the serum concentration of carcinoembryonic antigen (CEA) suggests that the tumor will recur following surgical resection. CEA is a glycoprotein that is also increased in the presence of other cancers (stomach, pancreas, breast, lung) and certain nonmalignant conditions (alcoholic liver disease, inflammatory bowel disease, cigarette smoking, pancreatitis).

Treatment

The prognosis for patients with adenocarcinoma of the colorectum depends on the depth of tumor penetration into the bowel wall and the presence or absence of regional lymph node involvement and distant metastases (liver, lung, bone). Radical surgical resection, which includes the blood vessels and lymph nodes draining the involved bowel, offers the best potential for cure. Surgical management of cancers that arise in the distal rectum may necessitate a permanent colostomy (abdominoperineal resection). Because most recurrences occur within 3–4 years, the cure rate for colorectal cancer is often estimated by 5-year survival rates.

Radiation therapy is considered for patients with rectal tumors, since the risk of recurrence following surgery is significant. Postoperative radiation therapy causes transient diarrhea and cystitis, but permanent damage to the intestine and bladder is uncommon.

Management of Anesthesia

Management of anesthesia for surgical resection of colorectal cancers may be influenced by anemia and the effects of metastatic lesions in liver, lung, bone, or brain. Chronic large bowel obstruction probably does not increase the risk of aspiration during induction of anesthesia, although abdominal distention could interfere with adequate ventilation and oxygenation. It has been suggested that blood transfusion during surgical resection of colorectal cancers is associated with a decrease in the length of patient survival. This could reflect immunosuppression produced by transfused blood. For this reason, careful review of the risks and benefits of blood transfusion in these patients is prudent.

Prostate Cancer

The reported number of cases of prostate cancer has increased dramatically in recent years, which presumably reflects the widespread use of prostate-specific antigen (PSA) testing. The incidence of prostate cancer is highest in African Americans and lowest in Asians. The presence of the hereditary prostate cancer gene mutation (HPC1) greatly increases the risk of developing prostate cancer. The possibility that vasectomy may be associated with an increased risk of prostate cancer has not been substantiated. Prostate cancer is almost always an adenocarcinoma.

Diagnosis

The use of PSA-based screening has changed the way prostate cancer is diagnosed. An increased serum PSA concentration may indicate the presence of prostate cancer in asymptomatic men and prompt a digital rectal examination. Detection of a discrete nodule or diffuse induration on digital rectal examination raises suspicion of prostate cancer, especially in the presence of impotence or symptoms of urinary obstruction (frequency, nocturia, hesitancy, urgency). However, the rectal examination can evaluate only the posterior and lateral aspects of the prostate. If the rectal examination indicates the possible presence of cancer, transrectal ultrasonography and biopsy are needed regardless of the PSA concentration. There is a much greater likelihood of detecting cancer if the PSA level is higher than 10 ng/mL, regardless of the findings on rectal examination. Infrequently, patients have symptoms of metastatic disease, such as bone pain and weight loss, at presentation.

Treatment

There are several options available for treating prostate cancer. Important factors to consider are the: (1) Gleason score, (2) anatomic extent of disease (tumor size, nodes), (3) serum PSA, and (4) age as well as general health of the patient. Active surveillance with serial monitoring of PSA is an option for low-risk prostate cancer (serum PSA < 10 ng/mL, and Gleason score ≤ 6). Radical prostatectomy is a definitive treatment option for patients with localized disease. The majority of surgeries are performed using a minimally invasive (laparoscopic or robotic) approach. For patients with lymph node involvement, lymph node dissection is performed in connection with prostatectomy. A nerve-sparing approach allows for preservation of erectile function. Some degree of urinary incontinence is a common postoperative complication.

An alternative to radical prostatectomy is radiation therapy. Radiation therapy can be delivered either by an external beam or by implantation of radioactive seeds. Radiation therapy produces impotence less often than surgery, but debilitating cystitis or proctitis may develop. The decision to select surgery or radiation therapy is based on the adverse effects of each treatment and the patient's overall health.

Hormone therapy is indicated for management of metastatic prostate cancer, because these tumors are under the trophic influence of androgens. Androgen deprivation therapy (ADT) dramatically reduces testosterone levels and causes tumor regression. Androgen deprivation can be accomplished by surgical castration (bilateral orchiectomy), use of analogues of gonadotropin-releasing hormone (GNRH) that inhibit release of pituitary gonadotropins (e.g., leuprolide, goserlin), use of antiandrogens that block the action of androgens at target tissues (e.g., flutamide, bicalutamide), and/or a combination of drugs from both classes. For patients with high-volume disease, docetaxel is added to ADT.

Patients who experience a rising PSA or new metastases while being treated with ADT are said to have *castration-resistant disease*. At this point, several treatment options are available. These include use of alternative endocrine-modulating drugs such as abiraterone or enzalutamide, usually in combination with prednisone. Systemic chemotherapies used to treat advanced prostate cancer include the taxanes and mitoxantrone, which is generally reserved for patients who do not tolerate taxane treatment. In the terminal phases of the disease, administration of high doses of prednisone for short periods may produce subjective improvement in pain from bony metastases. Radium-223 is a bone-seeking particle that deposits radiation over a short distance and has been shown to increase survival and relieve symptoms in patients with advanced prostate cancer.

Breast Cancer

Women in the United States have a 12% lifetime risk of developing breast cancer. The risk of death from breast cancer is approximately 3%. Most women in whom breast cancer is diagnosed do not die of the disease.

Risk Factors
The principal risk factors for development of breast cancer are increasing age (75% of cases occur in patients > age 50 years) and family history (a first-degree relative diagnosed with breast cancer before age 50 increases the risk threefold to fourfold). Reproductive risk factors that increase the risk of breast cancer include early menarche, late menopause, late first pregnancy, and nulliparity, all of which are presumed to prolong exposure of the breasts to estrogen. Two breast cancer susceptibility genes (*BRCA1* and *BRCA2*) are mutations that are inherited as autosomal dominant traits.

Screening
Current recommended screening strategies for breast cancer include clinical breast examination by a professional and screening mammography. Interestingly it has been found that breast self-examination does not pick up more breast cancers but rather detects more benign breast disease. Annual screening mammography is generally recommended for all women beginning between the ages of 40 and 50 years. A small percentage of breast cancers are not detected by mammography, so alternative screening methods such as ultrasonography and/or MRI may be of value in selected patients.

Prognosis
Axillary lymph node invasion and tumor size are the two most important determinants of outcome in patients with early breast cancer. Other established prognostic factors include the estrogen, progesterone, and HER2 expression of the primary tumor and its histologic grade. The absence of estrogen and progesterone receptor expression is associated with a worse prognosis, whereas HER2 overexpression is a marker of unfavorable prognosis. Most tumors that express receptors are responsive to endocrine therapy.

Treatment
Although radical mastectomy (removal of the involved breast, axillary contents, and underlying chest wall musculature) was the principal treatment for invasive breast cancer in the past, it is seldom used in current practice. Breast conservation therapy, including lumpectomy with radiation therapy, simple mastectomy, and modified radical mastectomy provide similar survival rates. Because the likelihood of distant micrometastases is highly correlated with the number of lymph nodes invaded by tumor, axillary lymph node dissection provides prognostic information. Sentinel lymph node mapping involves injection of a radioactive tracer or isosulfan blue dye into the area around the primary breast tumor. The injected substance tracks rapidly to the dominant axillary lymph node (sentinel node). If the sentinel node is tumor free, the remaining lymph nodes are also likely to be tumor free, and further axillary surgery can be avoided. The morbidity associated with breast cancer surgery is now largely related to adverse effects of lymph node dissection, such as lymphedema and restricted arm motion. Obesity, weight gain, and infection in the arm are additional risk factors for development of lymphedema. To minimize the risk of lymphedema, it is reasonable to protect the arm from venipuncture, compression, infection, and exposure to heat. Use of isosulfan blue dye is associated with anaphylaxis in approximately 1% of cases. Treatment with corticosteroid, diphenhydramine, and famotidine before injection may reduce the severity of the reaction but not its incidence.

Radiation treatment is an important component of breast conservation therapy, since lumpectomy alone is associated with a high incidence of recurrence. Radiation therapy after a mastectomy is reserved for women with extensive local disease, such as skin and chest wall invasion and extensive lymph node involvement.

Systemic Treatment
Many women with early-stage breast cancer already have distant micrometastases at the time of diagnosis. Adjuvant systemic therapy is recommended to prevent or delay disease recurrence. The choice of drugs is driven by whether the tumor is positive or negative for the estrogen receptor, progesterone receptor, and HER2. In patients with hormone receptor–positive breast cancer, adjuvant endocrine therapy is recommended. *Tamoxifen* is a mixed estrogen agonist-antagonist often referred to as a *selective estrogen receptor modulator*. It acts as an estrogen antagonist on tumor cells but has agonist properties on some other targets. Five years of tamoxifen therapy in patients with estrogen receptor–positive tumors is associated with a significant reduction in the risk of recurrent breast cancer. This drug does *not* alter outcome in patients with minimal or no estrogen receptor expression on their tumors. Tamoxifen can cause body temperature disturbances (hot flashes), vaginal discharge, and an increased risk

of developing endometrial cancer. Megestrol (progestin) may be administered to decrease the severity of hot flashes associated with tamoxifen treatment. Tamoxifen lowers serum cholesterol and low-density lipoprotein concentrations, but the importance of these effects in reducing the risk of ischemic heart disease is unclear. Tamoxifen preserves bone density in postmenopausal women by its proestrogenic effects and may decrease the incidence of osteoporosis-related fractures of the hip, spine, and radius. There is an increased risk of thromboembolic events, including deep vein thrombosis, pulmonary embolism, and stroke with tamoxifen therapy. Another very useful drug in treating patients with estrogen receptor–positive breast cancer is exemestane, which is an irreversible aromatase inhibitor. In postmenopausal women, most estrogen is produced by conversion of androgens into estrogens peripherally. Exemestane prevents this conversion of androgens into estrogens.

Chemotherapy. Adjuvant chemotherapy is useful in patients with tumors larger than 0.5 cm, pathologically involved lymph nodes, and those with high tumor grade. For patients with HER2-negative tumors, commonly used treatments include doxorubicin and cyclophosphamide followed by paclitaxel in 2-week cycles. For those with HER2-positive lesions, trastuzumab, lapatinib, or pertuzumab (all monoclonal antibodies directed against HER2) are added to the regimen.

Chemotherapy for breast cancer has adverse effects such as nausea and vomiting, hair loss, and bone marrow suppression that typically resolve following treatment. The most serious late sequelae of chemotherapy are leukemia and doxorubicin-induced cardiac impairment. Patients with symptoms of cardiac disease or congestive heart failure should be evaluated with an ECG and echocardiography. Cardiac toxicity is also a side effect of the monoclonal antibodies, especially when used in conjunction with doxorubicin. Myelodysplastic syndromes or acute myeloid leukemia can occur after chemotherapy, but the incidence is low (0.2%–1%). High-dose radiation therapy may be associated with brachial plexopathy or nerve damage, pneumonitis, and/or pulmonary fibrosis.

Supportive Treatment

Palliation of symptoms and prevention of complications are primary goals when treating advanced breast cancer. The most common site of breast cancer metastasis is bone. Regular administration of bisphosphonates in addition to hormone therapy or chemotherapy can decrease bone pain and lower the incidence of bone complications by inhibiting osteoclastic activity. Adequate pain control is usually achieved with sustained-release oral and/or transdermal opioid preparations.

Management of Anesthesia

Preoperative evaluation includes a review of potential adverse effects related to chemotherapy. Placement of IV catheters in the arm at risk of lymphedema is *avoided* because of the potential to exacerbate lymphedema and the susceptibility to infection. It is also necessary to protect that arm from compression (as from a blood pressure cuff) and heat exposure.

The presence of bone pain and pathologic fractures is noted when considering regional anesthesia and when positioning the patient during surgery. Selection of anesthetic drugs, techniques, and special monitoring is influenced more by the planned surgical procedure than by the presence of breast cancer. Of note, if isosulfan blue dye is injected during the surgical procedure, it is likely that pulse oximetry will demonstrate a transient spurious decrease in the measured oxygen saturation, usually a 3% decrease.

LESS COMMON CANCERS ENCOUNTERED IN CLINICAL PRACTICE

Less commonly encountered cancers include cardiac tumors, head and neck cancers, and cancers involving the endocrine glands, liver, gallbladder, genitourinary tract, and reproductive organs. Lymphomas and leukemias are examples of cancers that involve the lymph glands and blood-forming elements.

Cardiac Tumors

Cardiac tumors may be primary or secondary, benign or malignant. Metastatic cardiac involvement—usually from adjacent lung cancer—occurs 20–40 times more often than primary malignant cardiac tumors. Cardiac myxomas account for 40%–50% of benign cardiac tumors in adults. About three-quarters of cardiac myxomas occur in the left atrium, and the remaining 25% occur in the right atrium. Myxomas often demonstrate considerable movement within the cardiac chamber during the cardiac cycle.

Signs and symptoms of cardiac myxomas reflect interference with filling and emptying of the involved cardiac chamber. Left atrial myxoma may mimic mitral valve disease with development of pulmonary edema. Right atrial myxoma often mimics tricuspid disease and can be associated with impaired venous return and evidence of right-sided heart failure. Emboli occur in about a third of patients with cardiac myxomas. These emboli are composed of myxomatous material or thrombi that have formed on the tumor. Because most myxomas are located in the left atrium, systemic embolism is particularly frequent and often involves the retinal and cerebral arteries. Cardiac myxomas may occur as part of a syndrome complex (Carney complex) that includes cutaneous myxomas, myxoid fibroadenomas of the breast, pituitary adenomas with acromegaly, and adrenocortical hyperplasia with Cushing syndrome. Echocardiography can determine the location, size, shape, attachment, and mobility of cardiac myxomas.

Surgical resection of cardiac myxomas is usually curative. After the diagnosis has been established, prompt surgery is indicated because of the possibility of embolic complications and sudden death. In most cases, cardiac myxomas can be removed easily because they are pedunculated. Intraoperative fragmentation of the tumor must be avoided. All chambers of the heart are examined to rule out the existence of multifocal disease. Mechanical damage to a heart valve or adhesion of the tumor to valve leaflets may necessitate valvuloplasty or valve replacement.

Anesthetic considerations in patients with cardiac myxomas include the possibility of low cardiac output and arterial hypoxemia resulting from obstruction at the mitral or tricuspid valve. Symptoms of obstruction may be exacerbated by changes in body position. The presence of a right atrial myxoma prohibits placement of right atrial or pulmonary artery catheters. Supraventricular dysrhythmias may follow surgical removal of atrial myxomas. In some patients, permanent cardiac pacing may be required because of atrioventricular conduction abnormalities.

Head and Neck Cancers

Head and neck cancers account for approximately 3% of all cancers in the United States, with a predominance in men older than 50 years. Most patients have a history of excessive alcohol and/or tobacco use including the use of chewing tobacco. Human papillomavirus (HPV) is now found in about 50% of younger patients with oropharyngeal cancer. The most common sites of metastases are lung, liver, and bone. Hypercalcemia may be associated with bony metastases, and altered liver function test results presumably reflect alcohol-induced liver disease. Preoperative nutritional therapy may be indicated before surgical resection. The goal of chemotherapy, if selected, is to decrease the bulk of the primary tumor or known metastases and thereby enhance the efficacy of subsequent surgery or radiation treatment. A secondary goal is eradication of occult micrometastases.

Anesthetic considerations in patients with head and neck cancers include the possibility of distorted airway anatomy that may not be appreciated on external airway examination. Available diagnostic images and the report of nasal fiberoptic examination should be reviewed preoperatively. Preparation must be made for the possibility of difficult ventilation and/or intubation.

Thyroid Cancer

Papillary and follicular thyroid carcinomas are among the most curable of all cancers. Thyroid cancers are more frequent in women. External radiation to the neck during childhood increases the risk of papillary thyroid cancer, as does a family history of the disease. Medullary thyroid cancers may be associated with pheochromocytomas in an autosomal dominant disorder known as *multiple endocrine neoplasia type II*. This type of thyroid cancer typically produces large amounts of calcitonin, which provides a sensitive measure of the presence of the disease as well as the success of treatment.

Subtotal and total thyroidectomy result in lower recurrence rates than more limited partial thyroidectomy. Even with total thyroidectomy, some thyroid tissue remains, as detected by postoperative scanning with radioactive iodine. Risks of total thyroidectomy include recurrent laryngeal nerve injury (2%) and permanent hypoparathyroidism (2%). Patients with papillary thyroid cancers require dissection of paratracheal and tracheoesophageal lymph nodes. The growth of papillary and follicular tumor cells is controlled by thyrotropin, and inhibition of thyrotropin secretion with thyroxine improves long-term survival. External beam radiation can be used for palliative treatment of obstructive and bony metastases.

Esophageal Cancer

Esophageal cancer has two histologic subtypes: squamous cell and adenocarcinoma. Excessive alcohol consumption and long-term cigarette smoking are independent risk factors for the development of squamous cell carcinoma of the esophagus. The risk of adenocarcinoma is highest in people with Barrett esophagus, a complication of gastroesophageal reflux disease. Dysphagia and weight loss are the initial symptoms of esophageal cancer in most patients. The dysphagia may be associated with malnutrition. Difficulty swallowing may result in regurgitation and increase the risk of aspiration. The disease has usually metastasized by the time clinical symptoms are present. The lack of a serosal layer around the esophagus and the presence of an extensive lymphatic system are responsible for the rapid spread of tumor to adjacent lymph nodes. However, in patients with Barrett esophagus who undergo routine endoscopic surveillance, the disease can be diagnosed at a very early stage.

When cancer is localized to the esophagus, 5-year survival may be as high as 40%. However, if regional lymph nodes are involved, 5-year survival drops to 20%. Esophagectomy is often performed for carcinoma of the esophagus and is associated with significant morbidity and mortality. Chemotherapy and radiation therapy may be instituted before surgical resection is attempted. Adenocarcinomas are radioinsensitive and generally associated with a slightly better prognosis, but chemotherapy and surgery may improve survival. In end-stage disease, palliation may include surgical placement of a feeding tube, bougienage, or endoscopic stent placement.

The likelihood of underlying alcohol-induced liver disease, chronic obstructive pulmonary disease from cigarette smoking, and cross-tolerance of anesthetic drugs in patients who abuse alcohol are considerations during anesthetic management of patients with esophageal cancer. Extensive weight loss often parallels a decrease in intravascular fluid volume and manifests as hypotension during induction and maintenance of anesthesia.

Gastric Cancer

The incidence of gastric cancer has decreased dramatically since 1930, when it was the leading cause of cancer-related death among men in the United States. It is still a leading cause of cancer deaths in less developed countries. Achlorhydria (loss of gastric acidity), pernicious anemia, chronic gastritis, and *Helicobacter* infection contribute to the development of gastric cancer. The presenting features of gastric cancer (indigestion, epigastric distress, anorexia) are indistinguishable from those of benign peptic ulcer disease. Approximately 90% of gastric cancers are adenocarcinomas, and approximately half of them occur in the distal portion of the stomach. Gastric cancer is usually far advanced when signs and symptoms such as weight loss, palpable epigastric mass, jaundice, and ascites appear.

Complete surgical eradication of gastric tumors with resection of adjacent lymph nodes is the only treatment that is curative. Resection of the primary lesion also offers the best palliation. Adjuvant chemoradiotherapy is used in some cases to minimize the risk of recurrence.

Liver Cancer

Liver cancer occurs most often in men with liver disease caused by hepatitis B or C virus, alcohol consumption, or hemochromatosis. Initial manifestations are typically abdominal pain, palpable abdominal mass, and constitutional symptoms such as anorexia and weight loss. There may be compression of the inferior vena cava and/or portal vein, lower extremity edema, ascites, and jaundice. Laboratory findings reflect the abnormalities associated with underlying chronic liver disease. Liver function test results are likely to be abnormal. CT and MRI can determine the anatomic location of the tumor, although angiography may be more useful for distinguishing hepatocellular cancer (hypervascular) from hepatic metastases (hypovascular) and for determining whether a tumor is resectable. Partial hepatectomy is the treatment of choice for patients with adequate liver reserve and single tumors. However, many patients with liver cancer are not candidates for surgical resection because of extensive cirrhosis, impaired liver function, and the presence of extrahepatic disease. RFA is a technique in which heat from an electric current is used to evaporate discreet tumor lesions and may be considered as an alternative to surgical resection in patients who are poor candidates for resections. Transarterial chemoembolization (TACE) involves injection of chemotherapy directly into the hepatic artery and is sometimes used in combination with RFA. For advanced hepatocellular carcinoma, therapeutic options include radioembolization or stereotactic radiation therapy as well as systemic chemotherapy.

Pancreatic Cancer

Pancreatic cancer, despite its low incidence, is the fourth most common cause of cancer-related death in men and women in the United States. There is no evidence linking this cancer to caffeine ingestion, cholelithiasis, or diabetes mellitus, but cigarette smoking, obesity, and chronic pancreatitis show a positive correlation. Approximately 95% of pancreatic cancers are ductal adenocarcinomas, with most occurring in the head of the pancreas. Abdominal pain, anorexia, and weight loss are the usual initial symptoms. Pain suggests retroperitoneal invasion and infiltration of splanchnic nerves. Jaundice reflects biliary obstruction in patients with tumor in the head of the pancreas. Diabetes mellitus is rare in patients who develop pancreatic cancer.

Pancreatic cancer may appear as a localized mass or as diffuse enlargement of the gland. Biopsy is needed to confirm the diagnosis. Complete surgical resection is the only effective treatment. Patients most likely to have resectable lesions are those with tumors in the head of the pancreas that cause painless jaundice. Extrapancreatic spread eliminates the possibility of surgical cure. The two most commonly employed surgical resection techniques are total pancreatectomy and pancreaticoduodenectomy (Whipple procedure). Total pancreatectomy is technically easier but has the disadvantage of producing diabetes mellitus and malabsorption. Even when surgical resection can be performed, 5-year survival of patients with node-negative disease is only about 25% and only about 10% for those with node-positive disease. Median survival for patients with unresectable tumors is 5 months. Palliative procedures include radiation therapy, chemotherapy, and surgical diversion of the biliary system to relieve obstruction. Celiac plexus block with alcohol or phenol is the most effective intervention for treating the pain associated with pancreatic cancer. A complication of celiac plexus block is hypotension resulting from sympathetic denervation in these often hypovolemic patients. CT guidance of a celiac plexus block may be used to confirm proper needle placement before any neurolytic solution is injected into the celiac plexus.

Renal Cell Cancer

Renal cell cancer most often manifests as hematuria, mild anemia, and flank pain. Risk factors include a family history of renal cancer and cigarette smoking. Renal ultrasonography can help identify renal cysts, and CT and MRI are useful for determining the presence and extent of disease. Laboratory testing may reveal eosinophilia and renal function abnormalities. Paraneoplastic syndromes, especially hypercalcemia caused by ectopic parathyroid hormone secretion and erythrocytosis resulting from ectopic erythropoietin production, are not uncommon. The only curative treatment for renal cell carcinoma confined to the kidneys is radical nephrectomy with regional lymphadenectomy. Radical nephrectomy is not helpful in patients with distant metastases, but molecular targeted chemotherapy may have some benefit. The most effective drugs are those that block the VEGF pathway or mammalian target of rapamycin (mTOR) inhibitors.

Bladder Cancer

Bladder cancer occurs more often in men and is associated with cigarette smoking and long-term exposure to chemicals used in the dye (aniline), leather, and rubber industries. The most common presenting feature is hematuria.

Treatment of noninvasive bladder cancer includes endoscopic resection and intravesical chemotherapy, often with BCG. Carcinoma in situ of the bladder often behaves aggressively and may require cystectomy to help prevent muscle invasion and metastatic spread. In men, radical cystectomy includes removal of the bladder, prostate, and proximal urethra. In women, hysterectomy, oophorectomy, and partial vaginectomy are required. Urinary diversion is either by ileal conduit or creation of a neobladder from segments of small bowel. Traditional treatments for metastatic disease include radiation therapy and chemotherapy.

Testicular Cancer

Although testicular cancer is rare, it is the most common cancer in young men and represents a tumor that can be cured even when distant metastases are present. Orchiopexy before age 2 is recommended for cryptorchidism to decrease the risk of testicular cancer. Testicular cancer usually presents as a painless testicular mass. When the diagnosis is suspected, an inguinal orchiectomy is performed and the diagnosis is histologically confirmed. A transscrotal biopsy is not performed because disruption of the scrotum may predispose to local recurrence and/or metastatic spread to inguinal lymphatics. Germ cell cancers, which account for 95% of testicular cancers, can be subdivided into seminomas and nonseminomas. Seminomas metastasize through regional lymphatics to the retroperitoneum and mediastinum, and nonseminomas spread hematogenously to viscera, especially the lungs.

Following surgery, patients may be treated with active surveillance, adjuvant chemotherapy, or radiation therapy. The choice of treatment is dependent on the degree of lymph node involvement.

Cervical and Uterine Cancer

Cancer of the uterine cervix is the most common gynecologic cancer in females aged 15–34 years. Infection with HPV types 16 and 18 are responsible for approximately 70% of cervical cancers. Vaccination against these viruses is expected to reduce the incidence of cervical cancers in future generations. Carcinoma in situ and cervical dysphasia detected by Papanicolaou test is treated with loop electrosurgical excision procedure (LEEP) or cone biopsy, whereas more extensive local disease or disease that has metastasized is treated with some combination of surgery, radiation therapy, and chemotherapy.

Cancer involving the uterine endometrium occurs most frequently in women aged 50–70 years and may be associated with estrogen replacement therapy at menopause, more than 5 years of tamoxifen treatment for breast cancer, obesity, hypertension, and diabetes mellitus. Endometrial cancer is often diagnosed at an early stage because more than 90% of patients have postmenopausal or irregular bleeding. Initial evaluation of these patients often includes fractional dilation and curettage. In the absence of metastatic disease, a total abdominal hysterectomy and bilateral salpingo-oophorectomy with or without radiation to the pelvic and periaortic lymph nodes is usually the treatment of choice. Hormone therapy with progesterone may be useful for metastatic disease. Metastatic endometrial cancer responds poorly to traditional chemotherapy.

Ovarian Cancer

Ovarian cancer is the most deadly of the gynecologic malignancies. It is most likely to develop in women who experience early menopause or have a family history of ovarian cancer. Early ovarian cancer is usually asymptomatic, so advanced disease is often present by the time the cancer is discovered. Widespread intraabdominal metastases to lymph nodes, omentum, and peritoneum are frequently present. Surgery is the treatment of choice for both early-stage and advanced ovarian cancer. Aggressive tumor debulking, even if all cancer cannot be removed, improves the length and quality of survival. Intraperitoneal chemotherapy is indicated postoperatively in most women and is usually well tolerated.

Skin Cancer

Skin cancer is a very common cancer in the United States. Skin cancers are either melanomas or nonmelanomas. Nonmelanomas include basal cell carcinomas and squamous cell carcinomas. Basal cell carcinoma is the most common type of skin cancer. Most of these cancers grow superficially and rarely metastasize, so local treatment (excision, topical chemotherapy, cryotherapy) is usually curative. Squamous cell carcinoma is the second most common type of skin cancer. Organ transplant patients are up to 250 times more likely than the general public to develop squamous cell carcinoma of the skin.

Melanoma accounts for only about 2% of all skin cancers but the majority of skin cancer deaths. The incidence of cutaneous melanoma is increasing. Sunlight (ultraviolet light) is an important environmental factor in the pathogenesis of melanoma. Initial treatment of a suspected lesion is wide and deep excisional biopsy, often with sentinel node mapping. Melanoma can metastasize to virtually any organ. Treatment of metastatic melanoma focuses on palliation and can include resection of a solitary metastasis, simple or combination chemotherapy, and/or immunotherapy.

Bone Cancer

Bone cancers include multiple myeloma, osteosarcoma, Ewing sarcoma, and chondrosarcoma.

Multiple Myeloma

Multiple myeloma (plasma cell myeloma) is a malignant neoplasm characterized by poorly controlled growth of a single clone of plasma cells that produce a monoclonal immunoglobulin. Multiple myeloma accounts for approximately 10% of hematologic cancers and 1% of all cancers in the United States. The disease is more common in elderly patients (median age at time of diagnosis is 69 years), and it occurs twice as often in African Americans as in Caucasians. The cause of multiple myeloma is unknown. Its extent, complications, sensitivity to drugs, and clinical course vary greatly.

The most frequent manifestations of multiple myeloma are bone pain (often from vertebral collapse), anemia, thrombocytopenia, neutropenia, hypercalcemia, renal failure, and recurrent bacterial infection. Most of these reflect bone marrow invasion by tumor cells. Extramedullary plasmacytomas can produce compression of the spinal cord; this occurs in approximately 10% of patients. Other extramedullary sites of tumor invasion include liver, spleen, ribs, and skull. Inactivation of plasma procoagulants by myeloma proteins may interfere with coagulation. These proteins coat platelets and interfere with platelet function. The presence of hypercalcemia from excessive bone destruction should be suspected in patients with myeloma who develop nausea, fatigue, confusion, or polyuria. Renal insufficiency occurs in up to 50% of patients with multiple myeloma resulting from either deposition of an abnormal protein (Bence Jones protein) in renal tubules or development of acute renal failure. Amyloidosis or immunoglobulin deposition can cause nephrotic syndrome or contribute to renal failure. The combination of hypogammaglobulinemia, granulocytopenia, and depressed cell-mediated immunity increases the risk of infection. Development of fever in patients with multiple myeloma is an indication for antibiotic therapy. In an estimated 20% of patients, multiple myeloma is diagnosed by chance in the absence of symptoms when screening laboratory studies reveal increased serum protein concentrations.

Treatment of overt symptomatic multiple myeloma most often includes autologous stem cell transplantation and chemotherapy. The majority of patients with multiple myeloma who survive initial treatment experience a relapse. Overall 5-year survival is approximately 47%. Palliative radiation therapy is used for patients who have disabling pain and a well-defined focal process that has not responded to chemotherapy. Chemotherapy reverses mild renal failure in many patients with multiple myeloma, but temporary hemodialysis may be necessary until chemotherapy becomes effective. Erythropoietin therapy may be indicated to treat anemia. Hypercalcemia requires treatment with volume expansion and saline diuresis. Bed rest is avoided because inactivity leads to further mobilization of calcium from bone and increased risk of deep vein thrombosis.

Signs of spinal cord compression resulting from an extramedullary plasmacytoma require early confirmation and prompt radiation therapy. Urgent decompressive laminectomy to avoid permanent paralysis may be needed if radiation treatment is not effective. The presence of compression fractures requires caution when positioning patients during anesthesia and surgery. Fluid therapy depends on the degree of renal insufficiency and/or hypercalcemia. Pathologic fractures of the ribs may impair ventilation and predispose to the development of pneumonia.

Osteosarcoma

Osteosarcoma accounts for 1% of tumors in the United States and has a bimodal age distribution, with peaks in incidence in adolescents and adults older than age 65. Characteristic lesions typically involve the distal femur and proximal tibia. A genetic predisposition is suggested by the association of this tumor with retinoblastoma. MRI is used to assess the extent of the primary lesion and the existence of metastatic disease, especially in the lungs. Serum alkaline phosphatase concentrations are likely to be increased, and the levels correlate with

prognosis. Treatment consists of combination chemotherapy followed by surgical excision or amputation. Successful chemotherapy may permit limb salvage procedures in selected patients. Pulmonary resection may be indicated in patients with solitary metastatic lesions. Nonmetastatic disease is associated with an 85%–90% survival rate.

Ewing Sarcoma

Ewing sarcoma usually occurs in children and young adults and most often involves the pelvis, femur, or tibia. Ewing sarcoma is highly malignant, and metastatic disease is often present at the time of diagnosis. Treatment consists of surgery, local radiation therapy, and combination chemotherapy.

Chondrosarcoma

Chondrosarcoma is a tumor notable for its production of cartilage and most commonly affects the axial skeleton. This tumor often grows slowly, and low-grade lesions rarely metastasize. The preferred treatment is radical surgical excision; radiation therapy is used when surgery is not feasible (e.g., skull base lesions) or after incomplete resections. Chemotherapy is rarely used.

LYMPHOMAS AND LEUKEMIAS

Hodgkin Lymphoma

Hodgkin lymphoma (HL) accounts for about 10% of all lymphomas, with peak incidences in young adults (15–34 years) and adults older than 80 years. HL seems to have infective (Epstein-Barr virus), genetic, and environmental associations. Another factor that appears to predispose to the development of Hodgkin lymphoma is impaired immunity, as seen in patients after organ transplantation or in patients infected with human immunodeficiency virus. The most useful diagnostic test in patients with suspected lymphoma is lymph node biopsy.

HL is a lymph node–based malignancy, and presentation consists of lymphadenopathy in predictable locations including the neck and anterior mediastinum. Characteristic systemic symptoms include pruritus, night sweats, and unexplained weight loss. Moderately severe anemia is often present. Peripheral neuropathy and spinal cord compression may occur as a direct result of tumor growth. Bone marrow and CNS involvement is unusual, unlike other lymphomas.

Staging of the disease is accomplished by CT and PET scanning of the chest, abdomen, and pelvis; biopsy of available nodes; and bone marrow biopsy. Precise definition of the extent of nodal and extranodal disease is necessary to select the proper treatment strategy. Most patients are treated with combination chemotherapy plus radiation therapy. Cure can be achieved, with 20-year survival rates approaching 90%.

Non-Hodgkin Lymphoma

Non-Hodgkin lymphomas are divided into subtypes based on cell type and immunophenotypic and genetic features. They can be of B-cell, T-cell, or NK-cell origin. Adenopathy and pancytopenia are commonly present at diagnosis. Treatment and prognosis vary widely depending on subtype. Chemotherapy is the first-line treatment for most non-Hodgkin lymphomas. Hematopoietic stem cell transplantation can be used in refractory cases.

Leukemia

Leukemia is the uncontrolled production of leukocytes owing to cancerous mutation of lymphogenous or myelogenous cells. Lymphocytic leukemias begin in lymph nodes, and myeloid leukemias begin in bone marrow with spread to extramedullary organs. The principal difference between normal hematopoietic stem cells and leukemia cells is the ability of the latter to continue to divide. The result is an expanding mass of cells that infiltrates bone marrow and renders patients functionally aplastic. Anemia may be profound. Eventually, bone marrow failure leads to fatal infection or hemorrhage caused by thrombocytopenia. Leukemia cells may also infiltrate the liver, spleen, lymph nodes, and meninges, producing signs of dysfunction at these sites. Extensive use of nutrients by rapidly proliferating cancerous cells depletes amino acid stores, which leads to patient fatigue and metabolic starvation of normal tissues.

Acute Lymphoblastic Leukemia

Acute lymphoblastic leukemia (ALL) is the most common leukemia in children but also occurs in adults. The most common presenting symptoms are fatigue related to anemia, easy bruising related to thrombocytopenia, and bone pain. Lymphadenopathy is a common finding. Affected patients are highly susceptible to life-threatening opportunistic infections, including infections caused by *Pneumocystis jiroveci* and cytomegalovirus. Five-year survival for children with ALL is better than 85%; for adults, 5-year survival is between 20% and 40%.

Chronic Lymphocytic Leukemia

Chronic lymphocytic leukemia (CLL) is the most common leukemia in adults. The median age at diagnosis is 71 years, and it is more common in men than in women. This form of leukemia rarely occurs in children. The diagnosis of CLL is confirmed by the presence of lymphocytosis and lymphocytic infiltrates in bone marrow. Signs and symptoms are highly variable, with the extent of bone marrow infiltration often determining the clinical course. Autoimmune hemolytic anemia and hypersplenism that results in pancytopenia may be prominent. Lymph node enlargement may obstruct the ureters. Corticosteroids may be useful in treating the hemolytic anemia, but splenectomy may occasionally be necessary. Single or combination chemotherapy is the usual treatment, with radiation therapy reserved for treatment of localized nodal masses or an enlarged spleen. Median survival for patients diagnosed with CLL is 8–10 years.

Acute Myeloid Leukemia

Acute myeloid leukemia (AML), also known as *acute myelocytic* or *acute myelogenous leukemia,* is characterized by an increase in the number of myeloid cells in bone marrow and arrest of their maturation, which frequently results in hematopoietic insufficiency (granulocytopenia, thrombocytopenia, anemia). It is a disease of adults, with a median age at diagnosis of 67 years. Clinical signs and symptoms of AML are diverse and nonspecific, but they are usually attributable to leukemic infiltration of bone marrow. Approximately one-third of patients with AML have significant or life-threatening infection when initially seen. Other patients present with complaints of fatigue, bleeding gums or nosebleeds, pallor, and/or headache. Dyspnea on exertion due to severe anemia is common. Leukemic infiltration of various organs (hepatomegaly, splenomegaly, lymphadenopathy), bones, gingiva, and the CNS can produce a variety of signs. Hyperleukocytosis (>100,000 cells/mm³) can result in signs of leukostasis with ocular and cerebrovascular dysfunction or bleeding. Metabolic abnormalities may include hyperuricemia and hypocalcemia.

Chemotherapy is administered to induce remission. Five-year survival varies from 15%–70% depending on tumor cell cytogenics and age at diagnosis. Bone marrow transplantation may be a consideration in patients who do not have an initial remission or who experience relapse after chemotherapy.

Acute promyelocytic leukemia (APL) is a distinct subset of AML that represents about 5%–20% of cases and is characterized by the presence of promyelocytes in bone marrow and blood. Patients with APL require immediate medical attention, since disseminated intravascular coagulation and bleeding can be deadly if treatment is not instituted promptly. The treatment of choice is usually all-*trans* retinoic acid (tretinoin). *Retinoic acid syndrome* is a unique, potentially lethal complication of induction therapy in patients with APL. Respiratory distress, pulmonary infiltrates, fever, and hypotension are common presenting symptoms. The etiology is unclear, but it may be related to release of cytokines from myeloid cells, which causes capillary leak syndrome. High-dose corticosteroid administration is the most commonly employed treatment for retinoic acid syndrome. With standard therapy, 70%–90% of patients with APL experience long-term remission.

Chronic Myeloid Leukemia

Chronic myeloid leukemia (CML), also known as *chronic myelogenous, myelocytic,* or *granulomatous leukemia,* manifests as myeloid leukocytosis with splenomegaly. The average age at diagnosis is approximately 64 years. In most cases there is a prolonged dormant phase in which patients are asymptomatic. The disease then progresses through an accelerated phase followed by a blast crisis. This latter condition resembles acute leukemia and signals a poor prognosis. High leukocyte counts may predispose to vascular occlusion. Hyperuricemia is common and is treated with allopurinol. Cytoreduction therapy with hydroxyurea, chemotherapy, leukapheresis, and splenectomy may be necessary. CML is treated with chemotherapeutic agents such as imatinib, which are targeted to the BCR-ABL tyrosine kinase inhibitor, a product of the Philadelphia chromosome, a unique marker of CML. Tyrosine kinase inhibitors such as imatinib are successful in the majority of patients. Hematopoietic stem cell transplantation or other combined chemotherapies are alternatives if primary treatment is unsuccessful.

HEMATOPOIETIC STEM CELL TRANSPLANTATION

Hematopoietic stem cell transplantation offers an opportunity for cure for several otherwise fatal diseases. Hematopoietic stem cells can be obtained from peripheral blood or bone marrow. Autologous bone marrow transplantation entails collection of the patient's own bone marrow for subsequent reinfusion, whereas allogeneic transplantation uses bone marrow or peripheral blood elements from an immunocompatible donor. Regardless of the type of bone marrow transplantation, recipients must undergo a preprocedural regimen designed to achieve functional bone marrow ablation. This is produced by a combination of total body irradiation and chemotherapy.

Bone marrow is usually harvested by repeated aspirations from the posterior iliac crest. For allogeneic bone marrow transplantation with major AB incompatibility between donor and recipient, it is necessary to remove mature erythrocytes from the graft to avoid a hemolytic transfusion reaction. Removal of T cells from the allograft can decrease the risk of graft-versus-host disease (GVHD). Processing of the harvested bone marrow may take 2–12 hours. The condensed volume of bone marrow (≈200 mL) is then infused into the recipient through a central venous catheter. From the systemic circulation, the bone marrow cells pass into the recipient's bone marrow, which provides the microenvironment necessary for maturation and differentiation of the cells. The time necessary for bone marrow engraftment is usually 10–28 days, during which time protective isolation of the patient is required.

Anesthesia for Bone Marrow Transplantation

General or regional anesthesia is used during aspiration of bone marrow from the iliac crests. Use of nitrous oxide might be avoided in the donor because of potential bone marrow depression associated with this drug. However, there is no evidence that nitrous oxide administered during bone marrow harvesting adversely affects marrow engraftment and subsequent function. Substantial fluid losses may accompany this procedure. Blood replacement may be necessary, either by autologous blood transfusion or by reinfusion of separated erythrocytes obtained during the harvest. Perioperative complications are rare, although discomfort at bone puncture sites is predictable.

Complications of Bone Marrow Transplantation

In addition to prolonged myelosuppression, bone marrow transplantation is associated with several specific complications.

Graft-Versus-Host Disease

GVHD is a life-threatening complication of bone marrow transplantation, manifesting as organ system dysfunction that most often involves the skin, liver, and GI tract (Table 28.6). Severe rash, jaundice, and diarrhea are usually seen. This response occurs when immunologically competent T lymphocytes from the donor graft target proteins on the recipient's cells. These proteins are usually human leukocyte antigens (HLAs) that are encoded by the major histocompatibility complex. Even when the patient and host are matched for HLAs, minor histocompatibility antigens can provoke GVHD.

GVHD can be divided into two somewhat distinct clinical entities: acute disease, which usually occurs during the first 30–60 days after bone marrow transplantation, and chronic disease, which develops at least 100 days after transplantation. The incidence of acute GVHD is directly associated with the degree of incompatibility between HLA proteins. It ranges from 35%–45% in fully matched sibling donors to 60%–80% in patients with a single HLA mismatch. Patients undergoing allogeneic bone marrow transplantation receive prophylaxis to prevent acute GVHD. These treatments are mainly directed at minimizing the host's immune response. Examples of agents used are tacrolimus and cyclosporine, which inhibit calcineurin, an enzyme important for T-cell activation. When it occurs, acute GVHD is usually treated with high-dose steroids. *Extracorporeal photopheresis* is an emerging treatment for acute GVHD that involves removal of a patient's white blood cells and their exposure to ultraviolet light, followed by reinfusion into the patient. This process induces cellular apoptosis, which in turn prompts an acute antiinflammatory response that appears to reduce the risk of graft rejection.

Chronic GVHD shares features typical of autoimmune diseases. Symptoms include sclerosis of the skin, xerostomia, fasciitis, myositis, transaminitis, pericarditis, nephritis, and restrictive lung disease. The pathophysiology of chronic GVHD is poorly understood, so treatments are limited. Prophylaxis against acute GVHD appears to reduce the risk of chronic GVHD. Extracorporeal photopheresis has shown benefit in some studies. Steroids remain the mainstay of treatment.

Graft Rejection

Graft rejection occurs when immunologically competent cells of host origin destroy the cells of donor origin. This is rarely seen with transplants from well-matched related donors but can occur with transplants from other donors.

TABLE 28.6 Manifestations of Acute Graft-Versus-Host Disease

Desquamation, erythroderma, maculopapular rash
Interstitial pneumonitis
Gastritis, diarrhea, abdominal cramping
Mucosal ulceration and mucositis
Hepatitis with coagulopathy
Glomerulonephritis, nephrotic syndrome
Immunodeficiency and pancytopenia

Pulmonary Complications

Pulmonary complications following hematopoietic stem cell transplantation include infection, adult respiratory distress syndrome, chemotherapy-induced lung damage, and interstitial pneumonitis. When interstitial pneumonitis occurs 60 days or longer after bone marrow transplantation, it is most likely due to cytomegalovirus or fungal infection.

Sinusoidal Obstruction Syndrome

Sinusoidal obstruction syndrome may occur following allogeneic and autologous hematopoietic stem cell transplantation and appears to be related to high-dose radiation exposure. Primary symptoms include jaundice, tender hepatomegaly, ascites, and weight gain. The syndrome can manifest within days or as late as a year after hematopoietic stem cell transplantation. Progressive hepatic and multiorgan failure can develop, and the mortality rate approaches 50%.

ANESTHESIA FOR UNIQUE CANCER PROCEDURES

New modalities of cancer treatment are being used with increasing frequency, either alone or in combination with surgery, each of which has unique considerations with respect to anesthesia.

Proton Radiotherapy

Proton radiotherapy is used to treat posterior fossa tumors as well as some prostate, bladder, and liver cancers. Protons travel in a straight line and deliver their maximal energy at the end of their path. As a result they are particularly useful for treating tumors in deep tissue. Patients must undergo a series of 10–30 treatments that can last up to 90 minutes. It is important that patients be immobilized in specially made cradles so that the proton beam is directly at the tumor site rather than the surrounding healthy site. As a result, anesthesia is required, especially for children. The standard technique is total IV sedation with propofol and supplemental oxygen via nasal cannula or face mask.

Hyperthermic Intraperitoneal Chemotherapy

Hyperthermic intraperitoneal chemotherapy (HIPEC) is a technique used to treat peritoneal surface malignancies as well as mesothelioma and desmoplastic small round-cell tumors, which typically occur as abdominal or pelvic masses. This technique combines regional administration of cytotoxic drugs with the direct toxic effects of hyperthermia. Chemotherapies commonly used for this purpose include oxaliplatin, cisplatin, mitomycin C, and doxorubicin. The goal is to maximize tumor exposure to high-dose chemotherapy while protecting surrounding tissue. First the tumor is debulked through extensive surgical resection, which often includes omentectomy. Then chemotherapeutic agents heated to 40°–43°C are delivered through an inflow cannula, typically a Tenckhoff catheter placed in the upper abdomen. The drug solution is drained via a pelvic outflow cannula and recirculated through a perfusion circuit driven by a roller pump heat exchanger. The process continues for 60–120 minutes. Prior to initiation of treatment the patient is cooled with forced air warmers, cooling mattresses, and ice packs to approximately 34°–35°C to minimize the risks of hyperthermia. During treatment it is typical to see an increase in central venous pressure, heart rate, and oxygen consumption, as well as a decrease in systemic vascular resistance and mean arterial pressure. There is also an increase in intraabdominal pressure as the chemotherapy solution is infused into the peritoneal cavity. In order to maintain adequate abdominal perfusion pressure, it is useful to maximize the administration of paralytic agents and increase mean arterial pressure either by increasing intravascular volume or systemic vascular resistance. The chemotherapeutic agents are administered in a carrier solution of isotonic saline or a dextrose-containing solution. Systemic absorption of these solutions may cause electrolyte changes including hyponatremia and hyperglycemia. It is important to keep patients well hydrated during the procedure, since between 1% and 5% of patients develop acute kidney injury as a result of treatment. Thoracic epidurals are commonly employed to facilitate intraoperative and postoperative pain management.

Isolated Limb Perfusion

Isolated limb perfusion (ILP) is a limb-salvage technique used to treat melanoma that has invaded the lymph nodes by delivery of concentrated chemotherapeutic agents to the affected limb through a cardiopulmonary bypass circuit. Melphalan is the most commonly used drug for this purpose. For upper extremity ILP the axillary vessels are cannulated, and for lower extremity ILP the external iliac vessels are used. The patient is heparinized so that the activated clotting time remains above 400 seconds for the duration of the procedure. Once the vessels are cannulated, the limb is also heated to 38°–40°C with sterile warming blankets. Complications of therapy include acidosis from ischemia of the isolated limb and leakage of chemotherapy in the systemic circulation.

Photodynamic Therapy

Photodynamic therapy is a technique most often used for palliation of head and neck cancers and locally advanced cholangiocarcinomas. Porfimer sodium, a photosensitizing agent, is administered intravenously and accumulates in malignant cells. After exposure to a particular laser, a photochemical reaction results in tumor necrosis. The treatment causes generalized photosensitivity; therefore the surgical suite and recovery area should be minimally illuminated. In addition, repeated exposure to the light of a standard laryngoscope blade or fiberscope poses the risk of airway burn. Patients and staff should wear wavelength-specific safety goggles to protect against ocular damage during laser therapy. The treatment can be very painful; a multimodal approach that uses NSAIDs along with local anesthetics and IV opiates is most appropriate. Postprocedure tissue necrosis and edema may result in airway compromise.

Robotic Surgery

Robotic surgery is a technique in which tools mounted on a robotic arm driven by a surgeon are used to perform complex surgeries through small incisions. The technique is being used with increasing frequency to treat gynecologic and urologic cancers, among other conditions. Positioning is an important consideration for the procedure. Robot docking requires that the patient be in a steep Trendelenburg and lithotomy position for most abdominal procedures. Careful attention must be given to padding pressure points to limit the risk of nerve injuries. The introduction of pneumoperitoneum results in a 30%–50% decrease in pulmonary compliance and functional residual capacity, which leads to increased peak airway pressures and hypercapnia. There is also an increase in systemic vascular resistance, mean arterial pressure, and central venous pressure. These changes may result in myocardial ischemia or respiratory acidosis in patients with significant cardiac or pulmonary disease. Pneumoperitoneum and Trendelenburg position also increase intracranial pressure and venous congestion in the upper extremities and head, introducing the risk of laryngeal edema. Postoperative visual loss has also been reported during robotic cases of long duration, presumably as a result of ischemia to the optic nerve.

KEY POINTS

- Stimulation of oncogene formation by carcinogens (tobacco, alcohol, sunlight) is estimated to be responsible for 80% of cancers in the United States. Tobacco accounts for more cases of cancer than all other known carcinogens combined. The fundamental event that causes cells to become malignant is an alteration in the structure of their DNA. The responsible mutations occur in cells of target tissues, with these cells then becoming the ancestors of the entire future tumor cell population.
- A commonly used staging system for solid tumors is the TNM system based on tumor size (T), lymph node involvement (N), and distant metastasis (M). This system further groups cancers into stages ranging from I (best prognosis) to IV (poorest prognosis).
- Drugs administered for cancer chemotherapy may produce significant adverse effects including cardiomyopathy, pulmonary fibrosis, and peripheral neuropathy. These adverse effects may have important implications for management of anesthesia during surgical procedures for cancer treatment, as well as during operations unrelated to the cancer.
- Many patients with cancer exhibit paraneoplastic syndromes, some of which are related to ectopic hormone production and others of which are caused by the host's immune response to the tumor cells. Examples include SIADH, Cushing syndrome, and Eaton-Lambert syndrome.
- Mass effects of tumors or metastases can cause life-threatening oncologic crises. Superior vena cava syndrome results from spread of cancer into the mediastinum or caval wall that causes engorgement of the jugular and upper extremity veins and diminished venous return to the heart. Increased intracranial pressure as a result of increased cerebral venous pressure can lead to nausea, seizures, and/or diminished consciousness. Superior mediastinal syndrome exists when tracheal compression accompanies superior vena cava syndrome. Other examples of mass-effect conditions are spinal cord compression and increased intracranial pressure resulting from metastases to the CNS.
- Cancer is the most common cause of hypercalcemia in hospitalized patients. It reflects local osteolytic activity from bone metastases (especially in breast cancer) or ectopic parathyroid hormonal activity associated with tumors that arise from the kidneys, lungs, pancreas, or ovaries. The rapid onset of hypercalcemia that occurs in patients with cancer may manifest as lethargy or coma. Polyuria and dehydration may accompany hypercalcemia.
- Induction chemotherapy or high-dose radiation therapy can destroy large numbers of tumor cells and result in tumor lysis syndrome, a major feature of which is acute hyperuricemic nephropathy resulting from precipitation of uric acid crystals and calcium phosphate in the renal tubules.
- Hematopoietic stem cell transplantation is a potentially lifesaving treatment for many types of cancer, but it has serious potential complications. Graft-versus-host disease occurs when immunologically competent T lymphocytes from a donor graft target proteins on the recipient's cells and incite a profound immune response. GVHD manifests as organ system dysfunction, most often involving the skin, liver, and GI tract. Sinusoidal obstruction syndrome is marked by sudden onset of jaundice, tender hepatomegaly, ascites, and weight gain. The syndrome can manifest within days or as late as a year after hematopoietic stem cell transplantation. Progressive hepatic and multiorgan failure can develop, and mortality is high.
- Cancer patients may experience acute pain associated with surgery, chemotherapy, radiation therapy, pathologic fractures, and tumor invasion. A frequent source of pain is metastatic spread of the cancer, especially to bone. Nerve compression or infiltration may also be a cause of pain. Patients with cancer who experience frequent and significant pain often exhibit signs of depression and anxiety.
- Drug therapy is the cornerstone of cancer pain management because of its efficacy, rapid onset of action, and relatively low cost. Mild to moderate cancer pain is initially treated with acetaminophen and/or NSAIDs. NSAIDs are particularly effective for managing bone pain. The next step in management is addition of codeine or one of its analogues. When cancer pain is severe, more potent opioids are employed.
- Spinal opioids may be delivered for weeks to months via a long-term, subcutaneously tunneled, exteriorized catheter or an implanted drug delivery system. Implantable systems can be intrathecal or epidural. Patients are typically considered

for neuraxial opioid administration when systemic opioid administration has failed as a result of intolerable adverse effects or inadequate analgesia. Neuraxial administration of opioids is usually successful, but some patients require addition of a dilute concentration of local anesthetic to the neuraxial infusion to achieve adequate pain control.

- Important aspects of determining the suitability of a destructive nerve block are the location and quality of the pain, effectiveness of less destructive treatment modalities, life expectancy, inherent risks associated with the block, and availability of experienced anesthesiologists to perform the procedure. In general, constant pain is more amenable to destructive nerve block than intermittent pain.
- Recently developed cancer treatments use a multimodal approach often involving surgery combined with targeted radiation or chemotherapy. These strategies call for unique anesthetic techniques and knowledge of the adverse effects associated with these treatments.

RESOURCES

Arunkumar R, Rebello E, Owusu-Agyemang P. Anaesthetic techniques for unique cancer surgery procedures. *Best Pract Res Clin Anaesthesiol.* 2013;27:513-526.

Auret K, Schug S. Pain management for the cancer patient—current practice and future developments. *Best Pract Res Clin Anaesthesiol.* 2013;27:545-561.

Holtan SG, Pasquini M, Weisdorf DJ. Acute graft-versus-host disease: a bench-to-bedside update. *Blood.* 2014;124:363-373.

Huitink JM, Teoh WH. Current cancer therapies—a guide for perioperative physicians. *Best Pract Res Clin Anaesthesiol.* 2013;27:481-492.

Kurosawa S. Anesthesia in patients with cancer disorders. *Curr Opin Anesthesiol.* 2012;25:376-384.

Latham GJ. Anesthesia for the child with cancer. *Anesthesiol Clin.* 2014;32:185-213.

Libert N, Tourtier J-P, Védrine L, et al. Inhibitors of angiogenesis: new hopes for oncologists, new challenges for anesthesiologists. *Anesthesiology.* 2010;113:704-712.

Raspe C, Piso P, Wiesenack W, et al. Anesthetic management in patients undergoing hyperthermic chemotherapy. *Curr Opin Anesthesiol.* 2012;25:347-355.

Sahai SK. Perioperative assessment of the cancer patient. *Best Pract Res Clin Anaesthesiol.* 2013;27:465-480.

Socie G, Ritz J. Current issues in chronic graft-versus-host disease. *Blood.* 2014;124:374-384.

Tarin D. Update on clinical and mechanistic aspects of paraneoplastic syndromes. *Can Metastasis Rev.* 2013;32:707-721.

Vahid B, Marik PE. Pulmonary complications of novel antineoplastic agents for solid tumors. *Chest.* 2008;133:528-538.

Yeh ET, Bickford CL. Cardiovascular complications of cancer therapy: incidence, pathogenesis, diagnosis, and management. *J Am Coll Cardiol.* 2009;53:2231-2247.

CHAPTER 29

Psychiatric Disease, Substance Abuse, and Drug Overdose

KATHERINE E. MARSCHALL, ROBERTA L. HINES

The prevalence of mental disorders and substance use disorders in the United States is about 30%, so these conditions are often present in patients undergoing anesthesia and surgery. Effects of and potential drug interactions with psychotropic medications are important perioperative considerations, as are potential behavioral issues. In addition, substance abuse and suicide represent significant occupational hazards for anesthesiologists.

MOOD DISORDERS

Mood is defined as a temporary state of mind or temper or feeling. Thus moods are transient. *Mood disorders* are characterized by disturbances in the regulation of mood, behavior, and affect that are longer-lasting or even lifelong. They are typically divided into three classes: (1) depressive disorders, (2) bipolar disorders, and (3) depression associated with medical illness or substance abuse.

Depression

Depression is a common psychiatric disorder, affecting 6%–7% of the population (Fig. 29.1). It is distinguished from normal sadness and grief by the severity and duration of the mood disturbance. There is a familial pattern to major depression, and females are affected more often than males. A significant number of patients with *major* depression attempt suicide, and about 15% are successful. Pathophysiologic causes of major depression are unknown, although abnormalities of amine neurotransmitter pathways are the most likely etiologic factors.

Diagnosis

The diagnosis of major depression is based on the persistent presence of at least five of the symptoms noted in Table 29.1 for a period of at least 2 weeks. There is a profound loss of pleasure in previously enjoyable activities *(anhedonia)*. Organic causes of irritability or mood changes and a normal reaction to a major loss (e.g., death of a loved one, loss of a job) must be excluded. *Depressive symptoms* often are present in patients with cardiac disease, cancer, neurologic diseases, diabetes mellitus, hypothyroidism, and human immunodeficiency virus (HIV) infection. This depression can be a "situational" depression caused by the patient's reaction to the health condition with which they are now confronted, which may compromise both the quality and quantity of their life. It could also be directly related to the medical illness itself or be a side effect of medications used to treat the medical illness.

All patients with depression should be evaluated for the potential to commit suicide. Suicide is the 10th leading cause of death among Americans, with about 45,000 deaths per year due to this cause. Interestingly, physicians have moderately higher to much higher suicide rates than the general population. Most individuals who commit suicide have been under the care of

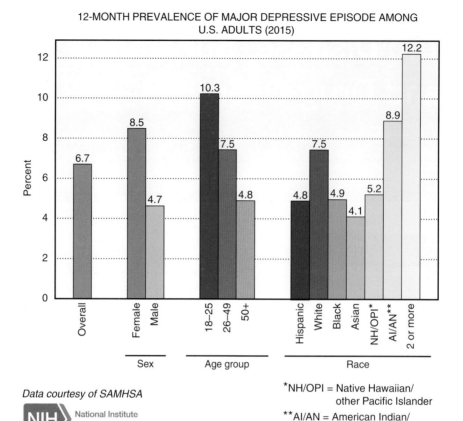

FIG. 29.1   Twelve-month prevalence of depressive episodes among US adults (2015). (Data courtesy of Substance Abuse and Mental Health Services Administration from the National Institute of Mental Health website. http://www.nimh.nih.gov/health/statistics/prevalence/.)

TABLE 29.1	Characteristics of Severe Depression

Depressed mood
Markedly diminished interest or pleasure in almost all activities
Fluctuations in body weight and appetite
Insomnia or hypersomnia
Restlessness
Fatigue
Feelings of worthlessness or guilt
Decreased ability to concentrate
Suicidal ideation

a physician (not necessarily a psychiatrist) *within the month before their death,* which emphasizes the need for physicians in *all* specialties to recognize patients at risk. Hopelessness is the most important aspect of depression associated with suicide.

Treatment

Depression can be treated with antidepressant medications, psychotherapy, electroconvulsive therapy (ECT), and other nonpharmacologic measures. An estimated 70%–80% of patients respond to pharmacologic therapy, and most who do not respond to antidepressants do respond favorably to ECT or one of the alternative measures. ECT is typically reserved

for patients with depression resistant to antidepressant drugs or those with medical contraindications to treatment with these drugs. Patients with depression plus psychotic symptoms (delusions, hallucinations, catatonia) require both antidepressant and antipsychotic drugs.

Approximately 50 years ago, neurochemical hypotheses regarding depression postulated that decreased availability of norepinephrine and serotonin at specific synapses in the brain is associated with depression and, conversely, that an increased concentration of these neurotransmitters is associated with mania. Subsequent studies have generally supported this hypothesis that norepinephrine and serotonin metabolism are important in mood states, although the exact mechanisms remain to be elucidated. Almost all drugs with antidepressant properties affect the availability of catecholamines and/or serotonin in the central nervous system (CNS) (Table 29.2). These include selective serotonin reuptake inhibitors (SSRIs), selective serotonin-norepinephrine reuptake inhibitors (SNRIs), norepinephrine-dopamine reuptake inhibitors (NDRIs), "atypical" antidepressants, monoamine oxidase inhibitors (MAOIs), and tricyclic antidepressants.

SSRIs block reuptake of serotonin at presynaptic membranes but have relatively little effect on adrenergic, cholinergic, histaminergic, or other neurochemical systems. As a result, they are associated with few side effects.

TABLE 29.2	Commonly Used Antidepressant Medications Listed by Class	
Drug Class	**Generic Name**	**Trade Name**
SSRIs	Fluoxetine	Prozac
	Paroxetine	Paxil
	Sertraline	Zoloft
	Citalopram	Celexa
	Escitalopram	Lexapro
SNRIs	Duloxetine	Cymbalta
	Venlafaxine	Effexor
	Desvenlafaxine	Pristiq
NDRI	Bupropion	Wellbutrin
MAOIs	Phenelzine	Nardil
	Tranylcypromine	Parnate
	Selegiline	Emsam
Atypical	Trazodone	Desyrel
	Vortioxetine	Trintellix
	Mirtazapine	Remeron

MAOIs, Monoamine oxidase inhibitors; *NDRI,* norepinephrine-dopamine reuptake inhibitor; *SNRIs,* serotonin-norepinephrine reuptake inhibitors; *SSRIs,* selective serotonin reuptake inhibitors.

Venlafaxine, desvenlafaxine, and duloxetine (SNRIs) are methylamine antidepressants that selectively inhibit reuptake of norepinephrine and serotonin without affecting other neurochemical systems. Bupropion inhibits of reuptake of serotonin and dopamine. Other atypical antidepressants have a diverse range of activity ranging from antagonism of specific serotonin receptors, dopamine receptor blockade, presynaptic α_2-blockade resulting in increases in norepinephrine and serotonin release, and histamine receptor blockade

MAOIs are inhibitors of either or both the A and B forms of brain MAO and change the concentration of neurotransmitters by preventing breakdown of catecholamines and serotonin. They are not considered first-line drugs in the treatment of depression because of their adverse effect profile, which includes the risk of hypertensive crises from consumption of tyramine-containing foods and the risk of serotonin syndrome if they are used concomitantly with SSRIs.

Before the availability of SSRIs, tricyclic antidepressants were the most commonly prescribed drugs for treatment of depression. They were thought to affect depression by inhibiting synaptic reuptake of norepinephrine and serotonin. However, they also affect other neurochemical systems, including histaminergic and cholinergic systems. They are now rarely used as first-line therapy for depression but are used more commonly as adjuvant therapy for patients with chronic pain syndromes. Their principal advantage is the existence of well-defined correlations between dosage, plasma concentration, and therapeutic response for nortriptyline, imipramine, and desipramine. Adverse effects include sedation, anticholinergic effects, and cardiovascular abnormalities, including orthostatic hypotension and cardiac dysrhythmias.

There has been a resurgence in the use of amphetamine and its congeners in treating depression. Typically these drugs are used in small dosages in combination with SSRIs. The effects on mood can be remarkable. However, because of their status as class II controlled substances, they are not widely used.

Selective Serotonin Reuptake Inhibitors

Serotonin is produced by hydroxylation and decarboxylation of L-tryptophan in presynaptic neurons, then stored in vesicles that are released and bound to postsynaptic receptors when needed for neurotransmission. A reuptake mechanism allows for return of serotonin to the presynaptic vesicles. Metabolism is by MAO type A. *Serotonin-specific reuptake inhibitors,* as their name implies, inhibit reuptake of serotonin from the neuronal synapse without having significant effects on reuptake of norepinephrine and/or dopamine.

SSRIs comprise the most widely prescribed class of antidepressants and are the drugs of choice to treat mild to moderate depression. These drugs are also effective for treating panic disorders, posttraumatic stress disorder, bulimia, dysthymia, obsessive-compulsive disorder, and irritable bowel syndrome. Common side effects include insomnia, agitation, headache, nausea, diarrhea, dry mouth, and sexual dysfunction. Appetite suppression is associated with fluoxetine therapy, though this effect is usually transient. Abrupt cessation of SSRI use, especially use of paroxetine and fluvoxamine, which have short half-lives and no active metabolites, can result in a *discontinuation syndrome* that can mimic serious illness and can be distressing and uncomfortable. Discontinuation symptoms typically begin 1–3 days after abrupt cessation of SSRI use and may include dizziness, irritability, mood swings, headache, nausea and vomiting, dystonia, tremor, lethargy, myalgias, and fatigue. Symptoms are relieved within 24 hours of restarting SSRI therapy.

Among SSRIs, fluoxetine is a potent inhibitor of certain hepatic cytochrome P450 enzymes. As a result this drug may increase plasma concentrations of drugs that depend on hepatic metabolism for clearance. For example, addition of fluoxetine to treatment with tricyclic antidepressant drugs may result in twofold to fivefold increases in plasma concentrations of tricyclic drugs. Some cardiac antidysrhythmic drugs and some β-adrenergic antagonists are also metabolized by this enzyme system, and fluoxetine inhibition of enzyme activity may result in potentiation of their effects.

Serotonin Syndrome. Serotonin syndrome is a potentially life-threatening adverse drug reaction that may occur with therapeutic drug use, overdose, or interactions between serotoninergic drugs. A large number of drugs have been associated with serotonin syndrome. These include SSRIs, atypical and cyclic antidepressants, MAOIs, opiates, cough medicine, antibiotics, antiemetic drugs, antimigraine drugs, drugs of abuse (especially "Ecstasy"), and herbal products (Table 29.3).

Typical symptoms of serotonin syndrome include agitation, delirium, autonomic hyperactivity, hyperreflexia, clonus, and hyperthermia (Fig. 29.2). Additional syndromes to consider in the differential diagnosis of serotonin syndrome are listed in Table 29.4. Treatment includes supportive measures and control of autonomic instability, excess muscle activity, and hyperthermia. Cyproheptadine, a 5-hydroxytryptamine (serotonin)

TABLE 29.3	Drugs Known to Be Associated With Serotonin Syndrome

Selective serotonin reuptake inhibitors
Selective serotonin-norepinephrine reuptake inhibitors
Bupropion
Atypical antidepressants
Monoamine oxidase inhibitors
Tricyclic antidepressants
Drugs of abuse: ecstasy, lysergic acid diethylamide (LSD), amphetamines
Antiemetic drugs: ondansetron, granisetron, metoclopramide, droperidol
Analgesics: meperidine, fentanyl, tramadol,
Lithium
"Muscle relaxant": cyclobenzaprine
Antimigraine drugs: triptans
Anticonvulsant drugs: valproate
Antibiotics: linezolid, ritonavir
Cough medicine: dextromethorphan
Dietary supplements: nutmeg, ginseng, St. John's wort

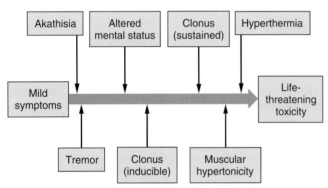

FIG. 29.2 Spectrum of clinical findings in serotonin syndrome. Manifestations range from mild to life threatening. Vertical arrows suggest the approximate point at which clinical findings initially appear in the spectrum of the disease. (Adapted from Boyer EW, Shannon M. The serotonin syndrome. *N Engl J Med.* 2005;352:1112-1120. Copyright 2005 Massachusetts Medical Society. All rights reserved.)

type 2A (5-HT$_{2A}$) antagonist, can be used to compete for and bind to serotonin receptors. It is available only for oral use.

Monoamine Oxidase Inhibitors

Patients whose depression does not respond to other antidepressant drugs may benefit from treatment with MAOIs. MAOIs inhibit norepinephrine and serotonin and tyramine breakdown, so there is more norepinephrine and serotonin available for release. Selegiline is a subtype A MAOI that is *reversible* and specifically catabolizes serotonin, norepinephrine, and tyramine, the substances most directly linked to MAOI antidepressant activity. It is used in a *transdermal* preparation that limits enterohepatic MAO inhibition and may help eliminate the need for dietary tyramine restriction.

The principal clinical problems associated with use of MAOIs, especially the nonselective irreversible forms, include the need for dietary restrictions, the potential for drug interactions, and adverse side effects. Probably the most dreaded occurrence is very significant systemic hypertension if patients ingest foods containing tyramine (cheeses, wines) or receive sympathomimetic drugs. Both tyramine and sympathomimetic drugs are potent stimuli for norepinephrine release. Interestingly, however, orthostatic hypotension is the most common adverse effect observed in patients being treated with MAOIs (Table 29.5). The mechanism for this hypotension is unknown, but it may involve accumulation of false neurotransmitters such as octopamine that are less potent than norepinephrine. This mechanism may also explain the *antihypertensive effects* observed with long-term use of MAOIs.

Adverse interactions between MAOIs and serotoninergic drugs have been observed. In the anesthetic environment the interaction between MAOIs and the opioid meperidine has been the most notable.

Management of Anesthesia. Anesthesia can be safely conducted in patients being treated with MAOIs despite earlier recommendations that these drugs be discontinued 14 days before elective surgery to permit time for regeneration of new enzyme. Proceeding with anesthesia and surgery in patients being treated with MAOIs influences selection and doses of

TABLE 29.4	Drug-Induced Hyperthermic Syndromes			
Syndrome	Time to Onset	Causative Drugs	Outstanding Features	Treatment
Malignant hyperthermia	Within minutes	Succinylcholine, inhalation anesthetics	Muscle rigidity, severe hypercarbia	Dantrolene, supportive care
Neuroleptic malignant syndrome	24–72 h	Dopamine antagonist antipsychotic drugs	Muscle rigidity, stupor or coma, bradykinesia	Bromocriptine or dantrolene, supportive care
Serotonin syndrome	Up to 12 h	Serotoninergic drugs	Clonus, hyperreflexia, agitation; possible muscle rigidity	Cyproheptadine, supportive care
Sympathomimetic syndrome	Up to 30 min	Cocaine, amphetamines	Agitation, hallucinations, myocardial ischemia, dysrhythmias, no rigidity	Vasodilators, α- and β-blockers, supportive care
Anticholinergic poisoning	Up to 12 h	Atropine, belladonna	Toxidrome of hot, red, dry skin; dilated pupils; delirium; no rigidity	Physostigmine, supportive care
Cyclic antidepressant overdose	Up to 6 h	Cyclic antidepressants	Hypotension, stupor or coma, polymorphic ventricular tachycardia, no rigidity	Serum alkalinization, magnesium

drugs to be administered. Benzodiazepines are acceptable for pharmacologic treatment of preoperative anxiety. Induction of anesthesia can be safely accomplished with most intravenous (IV) induction agents, but it should be kept in mind that CNS effects and depression of ventilation may be exaggerated. Ketamine, a sympathetic stimulant, should be avoided. Serum cholinesterase activity may decrease in patients treated with phenelzine, so the dose of succinylcholine may need to be reduced. A volatile anesthetic with or without nitrous oxide is acceptable for maintenance of anesthesia. Anesthetic requirements may be increased because of increased concentrations of norepinephrine in the CNS. Fentanyl has been administered intraoperatively to patients being treated with MAOIs without apparent adverse effects. The choice of nondepolarizing muscle relaxants is not influenced by treatment with MAOIs. Spinal or epidural anesthesia is acceptable, although the potential of these anesthetic techniques to produce hypotension and the consequent need for vasopressors may argue in favor of general anesthesia. Addition of epinephrine to local anesthetic solutions should probably be avoided.

During anesthesia and surgery, it is important to avoid stimulating the sympathetic nervous system as, for example, by light anesthesia, topical application of cocaine spray, or injection of indirect-acting vasopressors to decrease the incidence of systemic hypertension. If hypotension occurs and vasopressors are needed, use of a direct-acting drug such as phenylephrine is recommended. The dose should probably be decreased to minimize the likelihood of an exaggerated hypertensive response.

Postoperative Care. Provision of analgesia during the postoperative period is influenced by the potential adverse interactions between opioids, especially meperidine and MAOIs, which can result in serotonin syndrome. If opioids are needed for postoperative pain management, morphine is a preferred drug. Alternatives to opioid analgesics such as nonopioid analgesics, nonsteroidal antiinflammatory drugs (NSAIDs), and peripheral nerve blocks should be considered. Neuraxial opioids provide effective analgesia, but experience is too limited to permit recommendations regarding use of this approach in patients being treated with MAOIs.

Nonpharmacologic Treatments of Depression

For patients who do not respond well to antidepressant drug therapy, there are several forms of treatment for severe depression that do not include antidepressant medications but rather

rely on various forms of brain "stimulation." At the present time these alternatives include transcranial magnetic stimulation and ECT. Magnetic seizure therapy is in investigational trials.

Repetitive transcranial magnetic stimulation (rTMS) uses a magnet instead of electric current to activate the brain. An electromagnetic coil is placed against the forehead near the region of the brain thought to be involved in regulation of mood (Fig. 29.3). Then short electromagnetic impulses are administered through the coil. These cause small electric currents that stimulate cells in the targeted region. The impulses can apparently not travel farther than about 2 inches from the point of origin, so the treatment is localized to the area of interest, which is typically the left or right prefrontal cortex. The impulses have about the same strength as those in use during an MRI exam. A major advantage of this treatment is that anesthesia is not needed. Most complications consist of headaches and scalp discomfort. In 2008 the US Food and Drug Administration (FDA) approved rTMS for treatment of depression in patients who have failed treatment with at least one antidepressant medication.

Magnetic seizure therapy (MST) uses elements of both rTMS and ECT. It uses a magnetic pulse instead of electricity to stimulate a target area in the brain, but it uses a higher frequency of electromagnetic stimulation, with the aim of inducing a seizure. Because of this, an anesthetic is required in a manner similar to that needed for ECT. There is some evidence that MST may reduce the incidence and severity of cognitive side effects compared to traditional ECT.

Despite many decades of use of *ECT,* the exact mechanism for its therapeutic effect remains unknown. Alterations in neurophysiologic, neuroendocrine, and neurochemical systems are thought to be involved but have not been clearly elucidated. What is evident is that electrically induced seizures

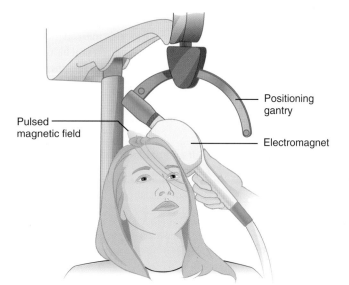

FIG. 29.3 Repetitive transcranial magnetic stimulation (rTMS). This modality uses a magnet instead of an electric current to activate the brain. Typically the magnetic field is centered over either prefrontal cortex.

TABLE 29.5	Adverse Effects of Monoamine Oxidase Inhibitors

Sedation
Blurred vision
Orthostatic hypotension
Tyramine-induced hypertensive crisis
Excessive effects of sympathomimetic drugs
Potential for serotonin syndrome

of at least 25 seconds' duration are necessary for a therapeutic effect. ECT is indicated for treatment of severe depression in patients who show no response to drug therapy, cannot tolerate the adverse effects of psychotropic drug therapy, or are suicidal. The electric current may be administered to both hemispheres or only to the nondominant hemisphere (which may reduce memory impairment). The electrical stimulus produces a grand mal seizure consisting of a brief tonic phase followed by a more prolonged clonic phase. The electroencephalogram shows changes similar to those present during spontaneous grand mal seizures. Typically patients undergo 6–12 induction treatments during hospitalization and then may continue weekly, biweekly, or monthly maintenance therapy. More than two-thirds of patients receiving ECT show significant improvement in their depressive symptoms.

In addition to the seizure and its neuropsychiatric effects, ECT produces significant cardiovascular and CNS effects (Table 29.6). The typical cardiovascular response to the ECT stimulus consists of 10–15 seconds of parasympathetic stimulation producing bradycardia with a reduction in blood pressure, followed by sympathetic nervous system activation resulting in tachycardia and hypertension lasting several minutes. These changes may be undesirable in patients with ischemic heart disease. Indeed, the most common causes of death associated with ECT are myocardial infarction and cardiac dysrhythmias, although overall mortality rates are extremely low, approximately 1 in 5000 treatments. Transient myocardial ischemia, however, is not an uncommon event. Other cardiovascular changes in response to ECT include decreased venous return caused by the increased intrathoracic pressure that accompanies the seizure and/or positive pressure ventilation and ventricular premature beats that presumably reflect excess sympathetic nervous system activity. Patients with acute coronary syndromes, decompensated congestive heart failure, significant dysrhythmias, and severe valvular heart disease require cardiologic consultation prior to initiation of ECT.

Cerebrovascular responses to ECT include marked increases in cerebral blood flow (up to sevenfold) and cerebral blood flow velocity (more than double) compared with pretreatment values. Cerebral oxygen consumption increases as well. The rapid increase in systemic blood pressure may transiently overwhelm

---

TABLE 29.6   Adverse Effects of Electroconvulsive Therapy

Parasympathetic nervous system stimulation
   Bradycardia
   Hypotension
Sympathetic nervous system stimulation
   Tachycardia
   Hypertension
Dysrhythmias
Increased cerebral blood flow
Increased intracranial pressure
Increased intraocular pressure
Increased intragastric pressure

---

cerebral autoregulation and result in a dramatic increase in intracranial pressure. Thus the use of ECT is *prohibited* in patients with known space-occupying lesions or head injury. The cerebral hemodynamic changes are also associated with increased wall stress on cerebral aneurysms, and intracranial aneurysm disease is another contraindication to ECT.

Increased intraocular pressure is an inevitable side effect of electrically induced seizures. Increased intragastric pressure also occurs during seizure activity. Transient apnea, postictal confusion or agitation, nausea and vomiting, and headache may follow the seizure. The most common long-term effect of ECT is memory impairment.

Management of Anesthesia. Anesthesia for ECT must be brief, provide the ability to monitor and limit the physiologic effects of the seizure, and minimize any interference with seizure activity or duration. Patients must fast before the procedure. IV administration of glycopyrrolate 1–2 minutes before induction of anesthesia and delivery of the electric current may be useful in decreasing excessive salivation and bradycardia. The magnitude of treatment-induced hypertension can be ameliorated with use of nitroglycerin intravenously, sublingually, or transdermally. Likewise, esmolol 1 mg/kg IV administered just before induction of anesthesia can attenuate the tachycardia and hypertension associated with ECT, and it does so better than labetalol. Many other drugs, including calcium channel blockers, ganglionic blockers, α_2-agonists and antagonists, and direct-acting vasodilators, have been used to treat the sympathetic overactivity during ECT, but they do not appear to offer any specific advantages over esmolol or nitroglycerin therapy.

Methohexital (0.5–1 mg/kg IV) is the traditional drug used for induction of anesthesia for ECT. It has a rapid onset, short duration of action, minimal anticonvulsant effects, and recovery is rapid. Because of shortages of barbiturates in the United States, other induction drugs are now commonly used for ECT. Propofol is an alternative to methohexital and is associated with a lower blood pressure and heart rate response to ECT. Recovery time is similar after administration of methohexital and propofol, but the anticonvulsant effect of propofol can be manifested as a shortened seizure duration. Ketamine and etomidate improve the quality and duration of the electrically induced seizure, but ketamine is associated with a prolonged reorientation time after the procedure, and etomidate is associated with more hypertension after the seizure and the possibility of spontaneous seizures before the electrical stimulus is delivered.

IV injection of succinylcholine promptly after induction is intended to attenuate the potentially dangerous skeletal muscle contractions and bone fractures that can result from seizure activity. Doses of 0.3–0.5 mg/kg IV are sufficient to attenuate skeletal muscle contractions and still permit visual confirmation of seizure activity. The most reliable method to confirm electrically induced seizure activity is the electroencephalogram. Alternatively, tonic and clonic movements in an extremity that has been isolated from the circulation by applying a tourniquet before administration of succinylcholine are evidence that a seizure has occurred. Succinylcholine-induced myalgias are remarkably uncommon, occurring in only about 2% of patients undergoing ECT. There is no evidence that succinylcholine-induced release of potassium is increased by ECT. Ventilatory support and oxygen supplementation are continued as necessary until there is complete recovery to pretreatment cardiopulmonary status. Because repeated administration of anesthetics is necessary, it is possible to establish the exact doses of the anesthetic induction drug and succinylcholine that produce the most predictable and desirable effects in each patient.

Occasionally ECT is necessary in a patient with a permanent cardiac pacemaker or cardioverter-defibrillator. Fortunately most of these devices are shielded and not adversely affected by the electric currents necessary to produce seizures, but it is prudent to have a magnet available to ensure the pacemaker can be converted to an asynchronous mode should malfunction occur in response to the delivered electric current or to myopotentials from the succinylcholine or the seizure. Monitoring the electrocardiogram (ECG) and the plethysmographic waveform of the pulse oximeter, and palpation of peripheral arterial pulses will document uninterrupted function of a cardiac pacemaker. Implantable cardioverter-defibrillators should be turned off before ECT and reactivated when the treatment is finished.

Safe and successful use of ECT has been described in patients following cardiac transplantation. In such patients, lack of vagal innervation to the heart eliminates the risk of bradydysrhythmias. However, the sympathetic responses still occur.

Bipolar Disorder

Bipolar disorder, previously called *manic-depressive disorder,* is characterized by marked mood swings from depressive episodes to manic or hypomanic episodes, with normal behavior often seen between these episodes. Between 8% and 10% of patients with bipolar disorder commit suicide. The manic phase of bipolar disorder is manifested clinically by sustained periods of expansive euphoric mood in which the patient expresses grandiose ideas and plans. The mood disturbance may be sufficiently severe to cause impairment in occupational functioning, social activities, and relationships, so there is risk of harm to self and others. Irritability and hyperactivity are also present; in severe cases, psychotic delusions and hallucinations may appear that are indistinguishable from those of schizophrenia (Table 29.7).

TABLE 29.7	Manifestations of Mania

Expansive euphoric mood
Inflated self-esteem
Decreased need for sleep
Flight of ideas
Greater talkativeness than usual
Distractibility
Psychomotor agitation

Genetic patterns in bipolar disorders suggest autosomal dominance with variable penetrance. Presumably there are abnormalities in neuroendocrine pathways that result in aberrant regulation of one or more amine neurotransmitter systems. Thus the pathophysiology of bipolar disorder—to the extent it is known—is similar to that of major depressive illness. Note that evaluation of mania must exclude the effects of substance abuse drugs, medications, and concomitant medical conditions.

Treatment

Mania necessitates prompt treatment, usually in a hospital setting to protect patients from potential harmful actions. Lithium remains a mainstay of treatment, but antiepileptic drugs such as carbamazepine and valproate are often used. Olanzapine is another treatment option. When manic symptoms are severe, lithium may be administered in combination with an antipsychotic drug until the acute symptoms abate.

Lithium

Lithium is an alkali metal, a monovalent cation, and is minimally protein bound. It does not undergo biotransformation and is excreted by the kidneys. Lithium is efficiently absorbed after oral administration. Its therapeutic serum concentration for acute mania and for prophylaxis is approximately 0.8–1.2 mEq/L. Because of this narrow therapeutic window, the serum lithium concentration must be monitored to prevent toxicity. The therapeutic effects of lithium are most likely related to actions on second-messenger systems based on phosphatidylinositol turnover. Lithium also affects transmembrane ion pumps and has inhibitory effects on adenylate cyclase.

Common adverse effects of lithium therapy include cognitive dysfunction, weight gain, and tremor. Lithium inhibits release of thyroid hormone and results in hypothyroidism in about 5% of patients. Long-term administration of lithium may also result in polyuria due to a form of vasopressin-resistant diabetes insipidus. Cardiac problems may include sinus bradycardia, sinus node dysfunction, atrioventricular block, T-wave changes, and ventricular irritability. Leukocytosis in the range of 10,000–14,000 cells/mm^3 is common.

Toxicity occurs when the serum lithium concentration exceeds 2 mEq/L, with signs of skeletal muscle weakness, ataxia, sedation, and widening of the QRS complex. Atrioventricular heart block, hypotension, and seizures may accompany severe lithium toxicity. Hemodialysis may be necessary in this medical emergency.

Lithium is excreted entirely by the kidneys. Reabsorption of lithium occurs in the proximal tubule in exchange for sodium, so diuretic use can affect the serum lithium concentration. Thiazide diuretics trigger an increase in lithium reabsorption in the proximal tubule, whereas loop diuretics do not promote lithium reabsorption. Administration of sodium-containing solutions or osmotic diuretics enhances renal excretion of lithium and results in lower lithium levels. Concomitant administration of NSAIDs and/or angiotensin-converting enzyme (ACE) inhibitors increases the risk of lithium toxicity.

Management of Anesthesia. Evidence of lithium toxicity is an important consideration during the preoperative evaluation. The most recent serum lithium concentration should be reviewed, and inclusion of a lithium level in measurements of the patient's serum electrolyte concentrations during the perioperative period is very useful. To prevent significant renal reabsorption of lithium, it is reasonable to administer sodium-containing IV solutions during the perioperative period. Stimulation of urine output with thiazide diuretics must be avoided. The ECG should be monitored for evidence of lithium-induced conduction defects or dysrhythmias. The association of sedation with lithium therapy suggests that anesthetic requirements may be decreased in these patients. Monitoring the effects of neuromuscular blockade is indicated because the duration of action of both depolarizing and nondepolarizing muscle relaxants may be prolonged in the presence of lithium.

SCHIZOPHRENIA

Schizophrenia (Greek for "split mind") is the major *psychotic* mental disorder. It is characterized by abnormal reality testing or thought processes. The essential features of the illness include two broad categories of symptoms. *Positive symptoms* are those that reflect distortion or exaggeration of normal behavior and include delusions and hallucinations. *Negative symptoms* represent a loss or diminution in normal function and include flattened affect, apathy, social or occupational dysfunction (including withdrawal), and changes in appearance and hygiene. Subtypes of schizophrenia include paranoid type, disorganized type, catatonic type, and undifferentiated type. In some patients the disorder is persistent, whereas in others there are exacerbations and remissions.

Treatment

The dopamine hypothesis concerning the etiology of schizophrenia suggests the disorder is a result of neurotransmitter dysfunction, specifically dysfunction of the neurotransmitter dopamine. This hypothesis is based on the discovery that agents that diminish dopaminergic activity also reduce the acute signs and symptoms of psychosis, especially agitation, anxiety, and hallucinations. Drugs that affect dopaminergic function by blocking dopamine receptors, especially D_2 and D_4 receptors, have demonstrated the ability to improve a variety of psychotic symptoms, especially positive symptoms. Conventional antipsychotic drugs have broad-spectrum dopamine receptor–blocking properties affecting all dopamine receptor subtypes. As a result these drugs have significant adverse motor effects. These troubling side effects include tardive dyskinesia (choreoathetoid movements), akathisia (restlessness), acute dystonia (contraction of skeletal muscles of the neck, mouth, and tongue), and parkinsonism. Some of these effects diminish over time, but some persist even after drug discontinuation. Concurrent administration of anticholinergic medication may lessen some of these motor abnormalities. Acute dystonia resolves with administration of diphenhydramine 25 to 50 mg IV.

Newer antipsychotic drugs, also called *atypical antipsychotic drugs,* have variable effects on dopamine receptor subtypes and serotonin receptors, especially the 5-HT$_{2A}$ receptor. These newer drugs appear to be quite effective in relieving the negative symptoms of schizophrenia and have fewer extrapyramidal side effects than traditional drugs.

Management of Anesthesia

For the anesthesiologist, important effects of antipsychotic medications include β-adrenergic blockade causing postural hypotension, prolongation of the QT interval (potentially producing ventricular dysrhythmias), seizures, elevations in hepatic enzyme levels, abnormal temperature regulation, and sedation. Drug-induced sedation may decrease anesthetic requirements.

Neuroleptic Malignant Syndrome

Neuroleptic malignant syndrome is a rare, potentially fatal complication of antipsychotic drug therapy that probably reflects dopamine depletion in the CNS. This syndrome can occur anytime during the course of antipsychotic treatment but often is manifest during the first few weeks of therapy or after an increase in drug dosage. Clinical manifestations usually develop over 24–72 hours and include hyperpyrexia, severe skeletal muscle rigidity, rhabdomyolysis, autonomic hyperactivity (tachycardia, hypertension, cardiac dysrhythmias), altered consciousness, and acidosis. Skeletal muscle spasm may be so severe that mechanical ventilation becomes necessary. Renal failure may occur as a result of myoglobinuria and dehydration.

Treatment of neuroleptic malignant syndrome requires immediate cessation of antipsychotic drug therapy and supportive therapy (mechanical ventilation, hydration, cooling). Bromocriptine (5 mg orally every 6 hours) or dantrolene (up to 10 mg/kg daily as a continuous infusion) may decrease skeletal muscle rigidity. Mortality rates approach 20% in untreated patients, with death resulting from cardiac dysrhythmias, congestive heart failure, hypoventilation, or renal failure. Patients who have had this syndrome are likely to experience a recurrence when treatment with antipsychotic drugs is resumed, so a switch is usually made to a less potent antidopaminergic drug or to an atypical antipsychotic medication.

Because there are similarities between neuroleptic malignant syndrome and malignant hyperthermia, the possibility that patients with a history of neuroleptic malignant syndrome are vulnerable to developing malignant hyperthermia is an important issue to consider. At the present time there is *no evidence* of a pathophysiologic link between the two syndromes, and there is no familial pattern or evidence of inheritance in neuroleptic malignant syndrome. However, until any association between neuroleptic malignant syndrome and malignant hyperthermia is clearly disproved, careful metabolic monitoring during general anesthesia is recommended. Note that succinylcholine has been used without problems for ECT in patients with a history of neuroleptic malignant syndrome.

ANXIETY DISORDERS

Anxiety disorders are the most prevalent form of psychiatric illness in the general community. *Anxiety* is defined as a subjective sense of unease, dread, or foreboding. It can be a primary psychiatric illness, a reaction to or result of a medical illness, or a medication side effect. Anxiety is associated with distressing symptoms such as nervousness, insomnia, hypochondriasis, and somatic complaints. It is useful clinically to consider anxiety disorders as occurring in two different patterns: (1) generalized anxiety disorder and (2) episodic, often situation-dependent, anxiety. The γ-aminobutyric acid (GABA) neurotransmitter system has been implicated in the pathogenesis of anxiety disorders.

Anxiety resulting from identifiable stressors is usually self-limited and rarely requires pharmacologic treatment. Performance anxiety (stage fright) is a type of situational anxiety that is often treated with β-blockers, which do not produce sedation or allay anxiety but do eliminate the motor and autonomic manifestations of anxiety. The presence of unrealistic or excessive worry and apprehension may be cause for drug therapy. Buspirone, a partial 5-HT$_{2A}$ receptor antagonist, is a nonbenzodiazepine anxiolytic drug that is not sedating and does not produce tolerance or drug dependence. However, its slower onset of action (several weeks until full effect is reached) and the need for thrice-daily dosing have limited its use. Short-term and often dramatic relief is afforded by almost any benzodiazepine, which is not surprising since these drugs bind to GABA receptors. Other drugs with GABAergic properties such as gabapentin, pregabalin, and divalproex may also be effective in treating anxiety disorders. Supplemental cognitive-behavioral therapy, relaxation techniques, hypnosis, and psychotherapy are also very useful in treating anxiety disorders.

Panic disorders are qualitatively different from generalized anxiety. The patient typically experiences recurrent and *unprovoked* episodes of intense fear and apprehension associated with physical symptoms and signs such as dyspnea, tachycardia, diaphoresis, paresthesias, nausea, chest pain, and fear of impending doom or dying. Such episodes can be confused with, or indeed caused by, certain medical conditions such as angina pectoris, epilepsy, pheochromocytoma, thyrotoxicosis, hypoglycemia and cardiac dysrhythmias. Several classes of medications are effective in reducing panic attacks, including SSRIs, benzodiazepines, cyclic antidepressants and MAOIs. These drugs have comparable efficacy. Psychotherapy and education increase the effectiveness of drug treatment.

EATING DISORDERS

Eating disorders are traditionally classified as anorexia nervosa, bulimia nervosa, and binge-eating disorder (Table 29.8). Bulimia nervosa and binge-eating disorder are more common than anorexia nervosa. All these disorders are characterized by serious disturbances in eating (fasting or binging) and excessive concerns about body weight. Eating disorders typically

TABLE 29.8	Diagnostic Criteria for Eating Disorders

ANOREXIA NERVOSA
Body mass index < 17.5 kg/m^2
Fear of weight gain
Inaccurate perception of body shape and weight
Amenorrhea

BULIMIA NERVOSA
Recurrent binge eating (twice weekly for 3 mo)
Recurrent purging, excessive exercise, or fasting
Excessive concern about body weight or shape

BINGE-EATING DISORDER
Recurrent binge eating (2 days/wk for 6 mo)
Eating rapidly
Eating until uncomfortably full
Eating when not hungry
Eating alone
Guilt feelings after a binge
No purging or excessive exercise

Adapted from Becker AE, Grinspoon SK, Klibanski A, et al. Eating disorders. *N Engl J Med*. 1999;340:1092-1098.

occur in adolescent girls or young women, although 5%–15% of cases of anorexia nervosa and bulimia and 40% of binge-eating disorders occur in boys and young men.

Anorexia Nervosa

Anorexia nervosa is a relatively rare disorder, with an incidence of 5–10 cases per 100,000 and a mortality rate of 5%–10%. Approximately half of deaths result from medical complications associated with malnutrition, and the remainder are due to suicide. The disease is characterized by a dramatic decrease in food intake and excessive physical activity in the obsessive pursuit of thinness. Bulimic symptoms may be part of the syndrome. Weight loss often exceeds 25% of normal body weight, but patients perceive that they are still obese despite this dramatic weight loss.

Signs and Symptoms

Marked unexplained weight loss in adolescent girls is suggestive of anorexia nervosa. Among the more serious medical complications seen in these patients are those that affect the cardiovascular system. Such changes include a decrease in cardiac muscle mass and depressed myocardial contractility. Cardiomyopathy due to starvation or to abuse of ipecac (used to induce vomiting) may be present. Sudden death has been attributed to ventricular dysrhythmias, presumably reflecting the effects of starvation or associated hypokalemia. ECG findings may include low QRS amplitude, nonspecific ST-T wave changes, sinus bradycardia, U waves, and a prolonged QT interval (another possible association with sudden death). Hyponatremia, hypochloremia, and hypokalemia can be present along with metabolic alkalosis from vomiting and laxative and diuretic abuse. Amenorrhea is often seen in patients with anorexia.

Physical examination reveals emaciation, dry skin that may be covered with fine body hair, and cold, cyanotic extremities. Decreased body temperature, orthostatic hypotension, bradycardia, and cardiac dysrhythmias may reflect alterations in autonomic nervous system activity. Bone density is decreased as a result of poor nutrition and low estrogen concentrations, and long bones or vertebrae may fracture as a result of osteoporosis. Gastric emptying may be slowed, which leads to complaints of gastric distress after eating. In addition, starvation may impair cognitive function. Occasionally patients develop a fatty liver and abnormal liver function tests. Renal complications may reflect long-term dehydration resulting in damage to the renal tubules. Parturient women are at increased risk of delivering low-birth-weight infants. Anorexic patients are often anemic, neutropenic, and thrombocytopenic.

Treatment

Treatment of patients with anorexia nervosa is complicated by the patient's denial of the condition. Pharmacologic treatment has not been predictably successful, but SSRIs that are effective in treating obsessive-compulsive disorder, particularly fluoxetine, may have some value. Most therapy involves medical management of the malnutrition-related symptoms and signs, dietary counseling, and family and/or individual psychotherapy.

Management of Anesthesia

There is a paucity of information relating to management of anesthesia in patients with this eating disorder. Preoperative evaluation is based on the known pathophysiologic effects of starvation. Electrolyte abnormalities, hypovolemia, and delayed gastric emptying are important preanesthetic considerations. There is a risk of perioperative cardiac dysrhythmias. Experience is too limited to permit recommendations regarding specific anesthetic drugs, muscle relaxants, and anesthetic techniques.

Bulimia Nervosa

Bulimia nervosa is characterized by episodes of binge eating, purging, and dietary restriction. Binges are most often triggered by a negative emotional experience. Purging usually consists of self-induced vomiting that may be facilitated by laxatives and/or diuretics. In most patients this disorder is chronic, with relapses and remissions. Depression, anxiety disorders, and substance abuse commonly accompany bulimia nervosa.

Signs and Symptoms

Findings on physical examination suggestive of bulimia nervosa include dry skin, evidence of dehydration, and bilateral painless hypertrophy of the salivary glands. Resting bradycardia is often present. The most common laboratory finding is an increased serum amylase concentration, presumably of salivary gland origin. Metabolic alkalosis due to purging is frequently seen. Dental complications are common, especially enamel loss from repeated vomiting and exposure of the lingual surface of the teeth to gastric acid.

Treatment

The most effective treatment of bulimia nervosa is cognitive-behavioral therapy. Pharmacotherapy may be helpful in selected patients. Potassium supplementation may be necessary in the presence of hypokalemia caused by recurrent self-induced vomiting.

Binge-Eating Disorder

Binge-eating disorder resembles bulimia nervosa, but in contrast to patients with bulimia, those with binge-eating disorder do not purge, and periods of dietary restriction are shorter. The diagnosis of binge-eating disorder should be suspected in morbidly obese patients, particularly obese patients with continued weight gain or marked weight cycling. The disease is chronic and accompanied by weight gain. Like anorexia nervosa and bulimia nervosa, this disorder is frequently accompanied by depression, anxiety, and personality disorders. The principal medical effects of binge-eating disorder are severe clinical obesity and its associated complications: hypertension, diabetes mellitus, hypercholesterolemia, and degenerative joint disease. Antidepressant medications may be useful for treatment of binge-eating disorders.

SUBSTANCE ABUSE

Substance abuse may be defined as drug use by self-administration that deviates from accepted medical or social use and, if sustained, can lead to physical and psychological dependence. Interestingly the incidence of substance abuse and drug-related deaths is high among physicians, especially during the first 5 years after medical school graduation. *Dependence* is diagnosed when patients manifest at least three of nine characteristic symptoms/signs, and these have persisted for at least 1 month or have occurred repeatedly (Tables 29.9 and 29.10). *Physical dependence* develops when the presence of a drug in the body is *necessary* for normal physiologic function and prevention of withdrawal symptoms. Typically the *withdrawal syndrome* consists of a rebound phenomenon in the physiologic systems modified by the drug. *Tolerance* is a state in which tissues become accustomed to the presence of a drug, so increased dosages of that drug become necessary to produce effects similar to those experienced initially with smaller dosages. Substance abusers can manifest *cross-tolerance* to drugs, which makes it difficult to predict analgesic or anesthetic requirements. Most often, *long-term* substance abuse results in increased analgesic and anesthetic requirements, whereas additive or even synergistic effects may occur in the presence of *acute* substance abuse. It is important to recognize the signs of drug withdrawal during the perioperative period. Certainly a detoxification program should *not* be attempted during the perioperative period.

TABLE 29.9	Characteristic Symptoms of Psychoactive Drug Dependence

Use of drug in higher dosages or for longer periods than intended
Unsuccessful attempts to reduce use of the drug
Increased time spent obtaining the drug
Frequent intoxication or withdrawal symptoms
Restricted social or work activities because of drug use
Continued drug use despite social or physical problems related to drug use
Evidence of tolerance to effects of the drug
Characteristic withdrawal symptoms
Drug use to avoid withdrawal symptoms

TABLE 29.10	Common Signs of Drug Abuse
Opioid drugs	Drowsiness, constricted pupils, sweating, poor appetite/weight loss, twitching/seizures, coma, needle marks
Marijuana	Loss of focus, weight loss or gain, bloodshot eyes, lethargy
Depressant drugs	Slurred speech, difficulty concentrating, constricted pupils
Stimulant drugs	Hyperactivity, dilated pupils, euphoria, anxiety, dry mouth

Diagnosis

Substance abuse is often first suspected or recognized during medical management of other conditions such as hepatitis, acquired immunodeficiency syndrome, or pregnancy. Patients often have a concomitant personality disorder and may display antisocial traits. Sociopathic characteristics (school dropout, criminal record, abuse of multiple drugs) seem to predispose to, rather than result from, drug addiction. Approximately 50% of patients admitted to hospitals with factitious disorders are drug abusers, as are some patients with chronic pain. *Psychiatric consultation is recommended in all cases of substance abuse.*

Drug overdose is the leading cause of unconsciousness in patients brought to emergency departments. Often more than one class of drug as well as some alcohol has been ingested. Since many conditions other than drug overdose may result in unconsciousness, laboratory testing is important (electrolyte levels, blood glucose concentration, arterial blood gas analysis, renal and liver function tests) in confirming the diagnosis. The depth of CNS depression can be estimated based on the response to painful stimulation, activity of the gag reflex, presence or absence of hypotension, respiratory rate, and size and responsiveness of the pupils.

Treatment

Regardless of the drug(s) ingested, the manifestations may be similar. Assessment and treatment proceed simultaneously. The first step is to secure the airway and support ventilation and circulation. Absence of a gag reflex is confirmatory evidence that protective laryngeal reflexes are dangerously depressed. In this situation a cuffed endotracheal tube should be placed to protect the lungs from aspiration. Body temperature is monitored, since hypothermia frequently accompanies unconsciousness as a result of drug overdose. Decisions to attempt removal of ingested substances (gastric lavage, forced diuresis, hemodialysis) depend on the drug ingested, time since ingestion, and degree of CNS depression. Gastric lavage may be beneficial if less than 4 hours have elapsed since ingestion. Gastric lavage or pharmacologic stimulation of emesis is not recommended when the ingested substances are hydrocarbons or corrosive materials or when protective laryngeal reflexes are not intact. After gastric lavage or emesis, activated charcoal can be administered to adsorb any drug remaining in the gastrointestinal tract. Hemodialysis may be considered when potentially fatal doses of drugs have been ingested, when there is progressive deterioration of cardiovascular function, or when normal routes of metabolism and excretion are impaired. Treatment with hemodialysis is of little value when the ingested drugs are highly protein bound or avidly stored in tissues because of high lipid solubility.

Drugs of Abuse

Alcohol

Alcoholism is defined as a chronic disease whose development and manifestations are influenced by genetic, psychosocial, and environmental factors. Alcoholism affects at least 10 million Americans and is responsible for 200,000 deaths annually. Up to one-third of adult patients have medical problems related to alcohol (Table 29.11). The diagnosis of alcoholism requires a high index of suspicion combined with nonspecific but suggestive symptoms such as gastritis, tremor, a history of falling, or unexplained episodes of amnesia. The possibility of alcoholism is often overlooked in the elderly.

Male gender and a family history of alcohol abuse are the two major risk factors for alcoholism. Adoption studies indicate that male children of alcoholic parents are more likely to become alcoholic, even when raised by nonalcoholic adoptive parents. Other forms of psychiatric disease such as depression and sociopathy are *not* increased in children of alcoholic parents.

Although alcohol appears to produce widespread nonspecific effects on cell membranes, there is evidence that many of its neurologic effects are mediated by actions at receptors for the inhibitory neurotransmitter γ-aminobutyric acid. When GABA binds to receptors it causes chloride channels in the receptors to open, which hyperpolarizes the neurons and makes the occurrence of depolarization less likely. Alcohol appears to increase GABA-mediated chloride ion conductance. A shared site of action for alcohol, benzodiazepines, and barbiturates is consistent with the ability of these different classes of drugs to produce cross-tolerance and cross-dependence.

TABLE 29.11   Medical Problems Related to Alcoholism

CENTRAL NERVOUS SYSTEM EFFECTS
Psychiatric disorders (depression, antisocial behavior)
Nutritional disorders (Wernicke-Korsakoff syndrome)
Withdrawal syndrome
Cerebellar degeneration
Cerebral atrophy

CARDIOVASCULAR EFFECTS
Cardiomyopathy
Cardiac dysrhythmias
Hypertension

GASTROINTESTINAL AND HEPATOBILIARY EFFECTS
Esophagitis
Gastritis
Pancreatitis
Hepatic cirrhosis
Portal hypertension

SKIN AND MUSCULOSKELETAL EFFECTS
Spider angiomata
Myopathy
Osteoporosis

ENDOCRINE AND METABOLIC EFFECTS
Decreased serum testosterone concentrations (impotence)
Decreased gluconeogenesis (hypoglycemia)
Ketoacidosis
Hypoalbuminemia
Hypomagnesemia

HEMATOLOGIC EFFECTS
Thrombocytopenia
Leukopenia
Anemia

Treatment

Treatment of alcoholism mandates total abstinence from alcohol. Disulfiram may be administered as an adjunctive drug along with psychiatric counseling. The unpleasantness of the symptoms that accompany alcohol ingestion in the presence of disulfiram (flushing, vertigo, diaphoresis, nausea, vomiting) is intended to serve as a deterrent to the urge to drink. These symptoms reflect the accumulation of acetaldehyde from oxidation of alcohol, which cannot be further oxidized because of disulfiram-induced inhibition of aldehyde dehydrogenase activity. Unfortunately, adherence to long-term disulfiram therapy is poor, and this drug has not been documented to have advantages over placebo for achieving total alcohol abstinence. Medical contraindications to disulfiram use include pregnancy, cardiac dysfunction, hepatic dysfunction, renal dysfunction and peripheral neuropathy. Emergency treatment of an alcohol-disulfiram interaction includes IV infusion of crystalloids and transient maintenance of systemic blood pressure with vasopressors if needed.

Management of anesthesia in patients being treated with disulfiram should consider the potential presence of disulfiram-induced sedation and hepatotoxicity. Decreased anesthetic drug requirements could reflect additive effects from co-existing sedation or the ability of disulfiram to inhibit metabolism of drugs other than alcohol. For example, disulfiram may potentiate the effects of benzodiazepines. Acute unexplained hypotension during general anesthesia could reflect inadequate stores of norepinephrine as a result of disulfiram-induced inhibition of dopamine β-hydroxylase. This hypotension might respond to ephedrine, but direct-acting sympathomimetics such as phenylephrine produce a more predictable response in the presence of norepinephrine depletion. Use of regional anesthesia may be influenced by the presence of disulfiram-induced or alcohol-induced polyneuropathy. Alcohol-containing solutions, such as those used for skin cleansing, should probably be avoided in disulfiram-treated patients.

Overdose

The intoxicating effects of alcohol parallel its blood concentration. In patients who are not alcoholics, blood alcohol levels of 25 mg/dL are associated with impaired cognition and coordination. At blood alcohol concentrations higher than 100 mg/dL, signs of vestibular and cerebellar dysfunction (nystagmus, dysarthria, ataxia) are likely. Autonomic nervous system dysfunction may result in hypotension, hypothermia, stupor, and coma. *Intoxication* with alcohol is often defined as a blood alcohol concentration of more than 80–100 mg/dL, and levels above 500 mg/dL are usually fatal as a result of respiratory depression. However, long-term tolerance from prolonged excessive alcohol ingestion may allow alcoholic patients to remain sober despite potentially fatal blood alcohol concentrations. The critical aspect of treating life-threatening alcohol overdose is maintenance of ventilation. Hypoglycemia may be profound if excessive alcohol consumption has been associated with food deprivation. It must be appreciated that other CNS-depressant drugs are often ingested simultaneously with alcohol.

Withdrawal Syndrome

Physiologic dependence on alcohol produces a withdrawal syndrome when the drug is discontinued or there is a significant decrease in intake.

The earliest and most common *alcohol withdrawal syndrome* is characterized by generalized tremors that may be accompanied by perceptual disturbances (nightmares, hallucinations), autonomic nervous system hyperactivity (tachycardia, hypertension, dysrhythmias), nausea, vomiting, insomnia, and mild confusion with agitation. These symptoms usually begin within 6–8 hours after a substantial decrease in blood alcohol concentration and are typically most pronounced at 24–36 hours. These withdrawal symptoms can be suppressed by resumption of alcohol ingestion or by administration of benzodiazepines, β-blockers, or α₂-agonists. In clinical situations, diazepam is often administered to produce sedation. A β-blocker is added if tachycardia is present. The ability of sympatholytic drugs to attenuate these symptoms suggests a role for autonomic nervous system hyperactivity in the etiology of the alcohol withdrawal syndrome.

Approximately 5% of patients experiencing alcohol withdrawal syndrome exhibit *delirium tremens,* a life-threatening medical emergency. Delirium tremens occurs 2–4 days after cessation of alcohol ingestion and manifests as hallucinations, combativeness, hyperthermia, tachycardia, hypertension or hypotension, and grand mal seizures. Treatment of delirium tremens must be aggressive, with administration of a benzodiazepine every 5 minutes until the patient becomes sedated but remains awake. Administration of β-blockers such as propranolol and esmolol is useful to suppress manifestations of sympathetic hyperactivity. The goal of β-blocker therapy is to decrease the heart rate to less than 100 beats per minute. Protection of the airway with a cuffed endotracheal tube may be necessary in some patients. Correction of fluid, electrolyte (magnesium, potassium), and metabolic (thiamine) derangements is also important. Lidocaine is effective if dysrhythmias occur despite correction of electrolyte abnormalities. Physical restraints may be necessary to decrease the risk of self-injury or injury to others. Even with aggressive treatment, mortality from delirium tremens is approximately 10%, resulting from hypotension, dysrhythmias or seizures.

Wernicke-Korsakoff syndrome reflects a loss of neurons in the cerebellum *(Wernicke encephalopathy)* and a loss of memory *(Korsakoff psychosis)* resulting from lack of thiamine (vitamin B_1), which is required for the intermediary metabolism of carbohydrates. This syndrome is not an alcohol withdrawal syndrome, but its occurrence establishes that a patient is, or has been, physically dependent on alcohol. In addition to ataxia and memory loss, many patients exhibit global confusion, drowsiness, nystagmus, and orthostatic hypotension. An associated peripheral polyneuropathy is almost always present.

Treatment of Wernicke-Korsakoff syndrome consists of IV administration of thiamine followed by normal dietary intake when possible. Because carbohydrate loads may precipitate this syndrome in thiamine-depleted patients, it is useful to administer thiamine before initiation of glucose infusions in malnourished or alcoholic patients.

Alcohol crosses the placenta and may result in decreased infant birth weight. High blood alcohol concentrations (>150 mg/dL) may lead to *fetal alcohol syndrome,* characterized by craniofacial dysmorphology, growth retardation, and intellectual disability. The incidence of cardiac malformations, including patent ductus arteriosus and septal defects, is increased in the children of alcoholic mothers.

Cocaine

Cocaine use for nonmedical purposes is a public health problem with important economic and social consequences. Myths associated with cocaine abuse state that the drug is sexually stimulating, nonaddictive, and physiologically benign. In fact, cocaine is *highly* addictive. Casual use is not possible once addiction occurs, and life-threatening adverse effects can accompany cocaine use. Cocaine produces sympathetic stimulation by blocking presynaptic uptake of norepinephrine and dopamine and thereby increases postsynaptic concentrations of these neurotransmitters. Because of this effect, dopamine is present in high concentrations in synapses, which produces the characteristic "cocaine high."

Acute cocaine administration has been known to cause coronary vasospasm, myocardial ischemia, myocardial infarction, and ventricular dysrhythmias, including ventricular fibrillation. Associated systemic hypertension and tachycardia further increase myocardial oxygen requirements at a time when coronary oxygen delivery is decreased by the effects of cocaine on coronary blood flow. Cocaine use can cause myocardial ischemia and hypotension that lasts as long as 6 weeks after discontinuation of cocaine use. Excessive sensitivity of the coronary vasculature to catecholamines after long-term exposure to cocaine may be due in part to cocaine-induced depletion of dopamine stores. Lung damage and pulmonary edema have been observed in patients who smoke cocaine. Cocaine-abusing parturient women are at higher risk of spontaneous abortion, abruptio placenta, and fetal malformations. Cocaine causes a dose-dependent decrease in uterine blood flow. It may also produce hyperpyrexia, which can contribute to seizures. There is a temporal relationship between recreational use of cocaine and cerebrovascular accidents. Long-term cocaine abuse is associated with nasal septal atrophy, agitated behavior, paranoid thinking, and heightened reflexes. Symptoms associated with cocaine withdrawal include fatigue, depression, and increased appetite. Death due to cocaine use has occurred with all routes of administration (intranasal, oral, IV, inhalational) and is usually due to apnea, seizures, or cardiac dysrhythmias. Persons with decreased plasma cholinesterase activity (elderly individuals, parturient women, those with severe liver disease) may be at risk of sudden death when using cocaine, because this enzyme is essential for metabolizing cocaine.

Cocaine overdose evokes overwhelming sympathetic stimulation. Uncontrolled hypertension may result in pulmonary and cerebral edema, and the effects of increased circulating catecholamines may include coronary artery vasoconstriction and platelet aggregation that can lead to myocardial infarction.

Treatment

Treatment of cocaine overdose includes administration of nitroglycerin to manage myocardial ischemia. Although esmolol has been recommended for treating the tachycardia caused by cocaine overdose, there is evidence that β-blockade can actually *accentuate* cocaine-induced coronary artery vasospasm. α-Adrenergic blockade is quite effective in the treatment of coronary vasoconstriction caused by cocaine, with no notable adverse effects. Administration of IV benzodiazepines is effective in controlling seizures associated with cocaine toxicity. Active cooling may be necessary if hyperthermia is significant.

Management of Anesthesia

Management of anesthesia in patients acutely intoxicated with cocaine must consider the vulnerability of these patients to myocardial ischemia and dysrhythmias. Any event or drug likely to increase already enhanced sympathetic activity must be avoided. It seems prudent to have nitroglycerin readily available to treat signs of myocardial ischemia associated with tachycardia or hypertension. Increased anesthetic requirements may be present in *acutely* intoxicated patients, which presumably reflects increased concentrations of catecholamines in the CNS. Thrombocytopenia associated with cocaine abuse may influence selection of regional anesthesia. Unexpected agitation during the postoperative period may also reflect the effects of cocaine ingestion.

In the absence of acute intoxication, long-term abuse of cocaine has not been shown to be associated with adverse anesthetic interactions, although the possibility of cardiac dysrhythmias remains a constant concern. Cocaine's rapid metabolism probably decreases the likelihood that an acutely intoxicated patient will come to the operating room.

Opioids

Contrary to common speculation, opioid dependence rarely develops from use of these drugs to treat acute postoperative pain. However, it is possible to become addicted to opioids in less than 14 days if the drug is administered daily in ever-increasing dosages. Opioids are abused orally, subcutaneously, or intravenously for their euphoric and analgesic effects. Numerous medical problems are encountered in patients addicted to opioids, especially those who take the drugs intravenously (Table 29.12). Evidence of these medical problems in patients addicted to opioids must be sought during the preoperative evaluation. Tolerance may develop to some of the effects of opioids (analgesia, sedation, emesis, euphoria, hypoventilation) but not to others (miosis, constipation). Fortunately, as tolerance increases, so does the lethal dose of the opioid. In general there is a high degree of cross-tolerance among drugs with morphine-like actions, although tolerance wanes rapidly when opioids are withdrawn.

Overdose

The most obvious manifestation of overdose of an opioid (usually heroin) is a slow respiratory rate with an increased tidal volume. Pupils are typically miotic, although mydriasis

TABLE 29.12	Medical Problems Associated With Chronic Opioid Abuse

Hepatitis
Cellulitis
Superficial skin abscesses
Septic thrombophlebitis
Endocarditis
Systemic septic emboli
Acquired immunodeficiency syndrome
Aspiration pneumonitis
Malnutrition
Tetanus
Transverse myelitis

may occur if hypoventilation results in severe hypoxemia. CNS manifestations range from dysphoria to unconsciousness. Seizures are unlikely. Pulmonary edema occurs in a large proportion of patients with heroin overdose. The cause of this pulmonary edema is poorly understood, but hypoxemia, hypotension, neurogenic mechanisms, drug-related pulmonary endothelial damage, or the effects of other materials (contaminants) injected with the heroin may be responsible. Gastric atony is a predictable accompaniment of acute opioid overdose. Fatal opioid overdose is most often an outcome of fluctuations in the purity of street products or the combination of opioids with other CNS depressants. Naloxone is the specific opioid antagonist administered to maintain an acceptable respiratory rate. Currently it is customary for first responders—police, fire personnel, emergency medical technicians, and others—to carry naloxone nasal spray so it can be administered *immediately* to anyone suspected of a narcotic drug overdose.

Withdrawal Syndrome

Although withdrawal from opioids is rarely life threatening, it is unpleasant and may complicate management during the perioperative period. In this regard it is useful to consider the time to onset, peak intensity, and duration of withdrawal symptoms after abrupt withdrawal of opioids. Opioid withdrawal symptoms develop within seconds after IV administration of naloxone. Conversely it is usually possible to abort the withdrawal syndrome by reinstituting administration of the abused opioid or by substituting methadone (2.5 mg of methadone is equivalent to 10 mg of morphine). Clonidine may also attenuate opioid withdrawal symptoms, presumably by replacing opioid-mediated inhibition with α_2-agonist–mediated inhibition of the sympathetic nervous system in the brain.

Opioid withdrawal symptoms include manifestations of excess sympathetic activity such as diaphoresis, mydriasis, hypertension, and tachycardia. Craving for the drug and anxiety are followed by yawning, lacrimation, rhinorrhea, piloerection (origin of the term *cold turkey*), tremors, skeletal muscle and bone discomfort, and anorexia. Insomnia, abdominal cramps, diarrhea, and hyperthermia may also develop. Skeletal muscle spasms and jerking of the legs (origin of the term *kicking the habit*) follow, and cardiovascular collapse is possible. Seizures are rare; their occurrence should raise suspicion of other causes of seizures, such as unrecognized withdrawal of other substances or underlying epilepsy.

Rapid opioid detoxification using high doses of an opioid antagonist administered during general anesthesia followed by naltrexone maintenance has been proposed as a cost-effective alternative to conventional detoxification approaches. There is evidence that opioid withdrawal, primarily involving the locus ceruleus, peaks and then recovers to near baseline within 4–6 hours after administration of high doses of opioid antagonists. Subsequent administration of naloxone to patients who have undergone rapid detoxification under general anesthesia should produce no evidence of opioid withdrawal, which confirms that rapid opioid detoxification has been achieved.

Unlike conventional detoxification accomplished by gradual tapering of opioid doses, the unpleasant aspects of opioid withdrawal are compressed into a few hours, during which time the patient is anesthetized. This is thought to contribute to an increased success rate. However, subsequent data indicate that the detoxification from opioids achieved with this method is *not* associated with better long-term abstinence from opioids and is associated with adverse events, some of which can be life-threatening. Indeed, a number of deaths have been reported in this regard. It is no longer a preferred treatment for opioid detoxification.

Buprenorphine is a semisynthetic alkaloid derived from brain tissue. It is a long-acting, lipid-soluble, mixed μ agonist-antagonist opioid. The half-life of buprenorphine is about 37 hours owing to its slow dissociation from receptors. Its onset is rapid, approximately 30–60 minutes with sublingual preparations and about 5–15 minutes with an IV preparation. Continued interest in buprenorphine has been attributed to its unique pharmacologic effects. It is a partial μ opioid agonist having moderate intrinsic activity, with high affinity to and slow dissociation from μ opioid receptors. Buprenorphine has a very low abuse potential and has become a widely used therapeutic agent in patients with opioid dependence.

Pharmacotherapy for opioid dependence has included μ opioid agonists, such as methadone and levomethadyl, and partial agonists. Levomethadyl is a congener of methadone that is biotransformed to active metabolites with long durations of action. The advantage of levomethadyl over methadone is the option for every-other-day dosing. Buprenorphine has pharmacodynamic effects very similar to those of typical opioid agonists such as morphine and heroin. Buprenorphine is an effective intervention for use in maintenance treatment of heroin dependence. However, if used as the sole drug, it appears to offer no advantages over methadone. Buprenorphine-carbamazepine, however, may be more effective than methadone-carbamazepine in detoxification strategies for patients addicted to opioids who also abuse other drugs. The FDA has approved marketing of buprenorphine in sublingual tablets or liquids containing buprenorphine alone (Subutex) or in combination with naloxone (Suboxone) for treatment of opioid dependence. Naloxone is added to the compound to prevent patients from dissolving the pills and then injecting them intravenously. If they try to do this, they will experience withdrawal symptoms. Buprenorphine may also have a ceiling effect that is useful in controlling opioid dependence. The FDA has reclassified buprenorphine from a schedule V drug to a schedule III drug. This imposed the regulatory controls and criminal sanctions of a schedule III narcotic on those persons who handle buprenorphine or buprenorphine-containing products. Schedule III substances by definition have less abuse potential than substances in schedules I and II, such as morphine or fentanyl. Methadone is a schedule II drug. Because of the pharmacology of buprenorphine, transfer from methadone to buprenorphine may precipitate withdrawal symptoms.

The unique pharmacologic properties of buprenorphine, with its high patient acceptance, favorable safety profile, and ease of administration, facilitate its use in the treatment of opioid dependence. Opiate detoxification with buprenorphine occurs with a minimum of discomfort. Detoxification occurs without the fatigue, sweats, unpleasant tactile sensations, aches, seizures, and confused thought processes common during traditional detoxification procedures. Buprenorphine 8–12 mg is roughly equivalent to 35–60 mg of oral methadone. Buprenorphine can be used to treat pregnant addicted patients. However, it is secreted in breast milk and should not be used by nursing mothers.

Management of Anesthesia

In patients addicted to opioids, the opioids or methadone should be maintained during the perioperative period. Preoperative medication may also include an opioid. The provider should assume a 20%–30% increase in acute opiate requirements. Nonopioid drugs such as IV or oral NSAIDs, clonidine, tramadol, gabapentin, or pregabapentin may be very useful in this patient population. Opioid agonist-antagonist drugs are *not* recommended for perioperative use because they can precipitate acute withdrawal reactions. There is no advantage to trying to maintain anesthesia with opioids, since dosages greatly in excess of normal are likely to be required. Furthermore, *long-term* opioid use leads to cross-tolerance to other CNS depressants. This may manifest as a decreased analgesic effect from inhaled anesthetics. Conversely, *acute* opioid administration *decreases* anesthetic requirements. There is a tendency for perioperative hypotension to occur, which may reflect inadequate intravascular fluid volume due to chronic infection, fever, malnutrition, or adrenocortical insufficiency. Chronic liver disease may also be present.

Management of anesthesia in patients rehabilitated from opioid addiction and in patients receiving agonist-antagonist therapy often includes a volatile anesthetic. Regional anesthesia may have a role in some patients, but it is important to remember the tendency for hypotension to occur, the increased incidence of positive results on serologic testing for HIV, the occasional presence of peripheral neuritis, and the rare occurrence of transverse myelitis.

Patients addicted to opioids often seem to experience exaggerated degrees of postoperative pain. For reasons that are not clear, satisfactory postoperative analgesia may often be achieved when average doses of meperidine are administered in addition to the usual daily maintenance dose of methadone or other opioid. Methadone and buprenorphine have minimal analgesic activity with respect to management of postoperative pain, so they are typically administered *in addition to* other opioids for postoperative analgesia. Alternative methods of postoperative pain relief include continuous regional anesthesia with local anesthetics, neuraxial opioid analgesia, and transcutaneous electrical nerve stimulation.

Barbiturates

Barbiturates have been in medical use since about 1900 but became popular in the 1960s and 1970s as treatments for anxiety, insomnia, and seizure disorders. Indeed, barbiturates were the most commonly used preanesthetic medications during that time. They also became drugs of abuse. With the development of benzodiazepines, medicinal barbiturate use decreased dramatically. Abuse of barbiturates also declined substantially.

The pharmacology of barbiturates is quite different from many other drugs of abuse, so overdose or withdrawal of barbiturates presents unique management problems. Long-term barbiturate abuse is not associated with major pathophysiologic changes. These drugs are most commonly abused orally to produce euphoria, counter insomnia, and antagonize the stimulant effects of other drugs. There is tolerance to most of the actions of these drugs, as well as cross-tolerance to other CNS depressants. Although the barbiturate doses needed to produce sedative or euphoric effects increase rapidly, lethal doses do not increase at the same rate or to the same magnitude. Thus the margin of error for individuals who abuse barbiturates, in contrast to that for those who abuse opioids or alcohol, *decreases* as barbiturate doses are increased to achieve the desired effect.

Overdose

CNS depression is the principal manifestation of barbiturate overdose. Barbiturate blood levels correspond to the degree of CNS depression (slurred speech, ataxia, irritability), with excessively high blood levels resulting in loss of pharyngeal and deep tendon reflexes and the onset of coma. No specific pharmacologic antagonist exists to reverse this barbiturate-induced CNS depression, and the use of nonspecific stimulants is not encouraged. Depression of ventilation may be profound. Maintenance of a patent airway, protection from aspiration, and support of ventilation using a cuffed endotracheal tube are often necessary. Barbiturate overdose may also be associated with hypotension because of central vasomotor depression, direct myocardial depression, and increased venous capacitance. This hypotension usually responds to fluid infusion, although occasionally vasopressors or inotropic drugs are required. Hypothermia is frequent. Acute renal failure resulting from hypotension and rhabdomyolysis may occur. Forced diuresis and alkalinization of urine promote elimination of phenobarbital but are of lesser value for many of the other barbiturates. Induced emesis or gastric lavage followed by administration of activated charcoal may be helpful in *awake* patients who ingested barbiturates less than 6 hours previously.

Withdrawal Syndrome

Abrupt cessation of excessive barbiturate ingestion is associated with potentially life-threatening responses. The time of onset, peak intensity, and duration of symptoms of withdrawal from barbiturates are delayed compared with those for opioids. Barbiturate withdrawal manifests initially as anxiety, skeletal muscle tremors, hyperreflexia, diaphoresis, tachycardia, and orthostatic hypotension. Cardiovascular collapse and hyperthermia may occur. The most serious problem associated with barbiturate withdrawal is the occurrence of grand mal seizures. Many of the manifestations of barbiturate withdrawal,

particularly seizures, are difficult to abort once they develop. If available, pentobarbital may be administered to treat barbiturate withdrawal. Phenobarbital and benzodiazepines are useful in suppressing evidence of barbiturate withdrawal.

Benzodiazepines

Benzodiazepine addiction requires ingestion of *large* dosages of the drug. As with barbiturates, tolerance and physical dependence occur with long-term benzodiazepine abuse. Benzodiazepines do not significantly induce microsomal enzymes. Symptoms of withdrawal generally occur later than with barbiturates and are less severe because of the prolonged elimination half-lives of most benzodiazepines and the fact that many of these drugs are metabolized to pharmacologically active metabolites that also have prolonged elimination half-lives.

Acute benzodiazepine overdose is *much less likely* to produce ventilatory depression than an overdose with barbiturates and many other drugs of abuse. It must be recognized, however, that the combination of benzodiazepines and other CNS depressants (e.g., alcohol) can be life threatening. Supportive treatment usually suffices for treatment of a benzodiazepine overdose. Flumazenil, a specific benzodiazepine antagonist, is useful for managing a severe or life-threatening overdose. Seizure activity suppressed by benzodiazepines could be unmasked by administration of flumazenil.

Amphetamines

Amphetamines stimulate release of catecholamines, which results in increased alertness, appetite suppression, and a decreased need for sleep. Approved medical uses of amphetamines include treatment of narcolepsy, attention deficit disorders, significant depression, and hyperactivity associated with minimal brain dysfunction in children. Tolerance to the appetite suppressant effects of amphetamines develops within a few weeks, making these drugs poor substitutes for proper dieting techniques. Physiologic dependence on amphetamines is profound, and dosages may be increased to several hundred times the therapeutic dosage. Long-term abuse of amphetamines results in depletion of body stores of catecholamines. Such depletion may manifest as somnolence and anxiety or a psychotic state. Other physiologic abnormalities reported with long-term amphetamine abuse include hypertension, cardiac dysrhythmias, and malnutrition. Amphetamines are most often abused orally but can also be inhaled or used intravenously.

Overdose

Amphetamine overdose causes anxiety, a psychotic state, and progressive CNS irritability manifesting as hyperactivity, hyperreflexia, and occasionally seizures. Other physiologic effects include hypertension and tachycardia, dysrhythmias, decreased gastrointestinal motility, mydriasis, diaphoresis, and hyperthermia. Metabolic imbalances such as dehydration, lactic acidosis, and ketosis may occur.

Treatment of oral amphetamine overdose includes induced emesis or gastric lavage followed by administration of activated charcoal and a cathartic. Phenothiazines may antagonize many of the acute CNS effects of amphetamines. Similarly, diazepam may be useful for controlling amphetamine-induced seizures. Acidification of urine promotes elimination of amphetamines.

Withdrawal Syndrome

Abrupt cessation of amphetamine use is accompanied by extreme lethargy, depression that may be suicidal, increased appetite, and weight gain. Benzodiazepines are useful in the management of withdrawal if sedation is needed, and β-blockers may be administered to control sympathetic nervous system hyperactivity. Postamphetamine depression may last for months and require treatment with antidepressant medications.

Management of Anesthesia

Pharmacologic doses of amphetamines that have been administered long term for medically indicated uses (narcolepsy, attention deficit disorder) need not be discontinued before elective surgery. Patients who require emergency surgery and who are *acutely intoxicated* from ingestion of amphetamines may exhibit hypertension, tachycardia, hyperthermia, and *increased* anesthetic requirements. Intraoperative intracranial hypertension and cardiac arrest have been attributed to amphetamine abuse. In animals, *acute* IV administration of dextroamphetamine produces dose-related increases in body temperature and anesthetic requirements. Thus it is prudent to monitor body temperature during the perioperative period. *Long-term* amphetamine abuse may be associated with markedly *decreased* anesthetic requirements, presumably as a result of catecholamine depletion in the CNS. Refractory hypotension can reflect depletion of catecholamine stores. Direct-acting vasopressors, including phenylephrine and epinephrine, should be available to treat hypotension, because the response to indirect-acting vasopressors such as ephedrine is attenuated by catecholamine depletion. Intraoperative monitoring of blood pressure using an intraarterial catheter should be considered. Postoperatively there is the potential for orthostatic hypotension once the patient begins to ambulate.

Designer/Club Drugs

MMDA (3-methoxy-4,5-methylenedioxyamphetamine, also known as *Ecstasy*), ketamine, rohypnol, phencyclidine (Angel Dust), gamma hydroxybutyrate (GHB), methamphetamine, and synthetic cathinones ("bath salts" not because they are bath salts but because they look like bath salts) are some examples of "club drugs" because they tend to be used by teenagers and young adults at nightclubs, bars, and concerts. They are also called "designer drugs" because they are manmade (rather than naturally occurring) substances, and some can be made with only a minimal knowledge of chemistry. They are becoming ever more popular, and because they are related to cocaine, amphetamines, and other hallucinogens they have the potential to cause serious, even life-threatening adverse effects. There are insufficient data in the medical literature at this time to offer recommendations regarding anesthetic management

of persons intoxicated by these substances. However, spontaneous pneumothorax and/or pneumomediastinum has been reported in several patients who had taken Ecstasy.

Forced diuresis and acidification of urine promotes elimination of phencyclidine but also introduces the risk of fluid overload and electrolyte abnormalities, especially hypokalemia.

Hallucinogens

More "traditional" hallucinogens, as represented by lysergic acid diethylamide (LSD), are usually ingested orally. Although there is a high degree of *psychological dependence,* there is no evidence of *physical dependence* or withdrawal symptoms when LSD is abruptly discontinued. The effects of these drugs develop within 1–2 hours and last 8–12 hours. They consist of visual, auditory, and tactile hallucinations and distortions of the environment and body image. The ability of the brain to suppress relatively unimportant stimuli is impaired by LSD. Evidence of sympathetic nervous system stimulation includes mydriasis, increased body temperature, hypertension, and tachycardia. Tolerance to the behavioral effects of LSD occurs rapidly, whereas tolerance to the cardiovascular effects is less pronounced.

Overdose

Overdoses of LSD have not been associated with death, although patients may experience unrecognized injuries, which reflects the intrinsic analgesic effects of this drug. On rare occasions, LSD produces seizures and apnea. It can lead to an acute panic reaction characterized by hyperactivity, mood lability, and in extreme cases, overt psychosis. Patients should be placed in a calm, quiet environment with minimal external stimuli. No specific antidote exists, although benzodiazepines may be useful for controlling agitation and anxiety reactions. Supportive care in the form of airway management, mechanical ventilation, treatment of seizures, and control of the manifestations of sympathetic nervous system hyperactivity may be needed.

Management of Anesthesia

Anesthesia and surgery have been reported to precipitate panic attacks in these patients. If such an event occurs, midazolam or diazepam is likely to be a useful treatment. Exaggerated responses to sympathomimetic drugs are likely. The analgesia and ventilatory depression of opioids are prolonged by LSD.

Marijuana

Marijuana is usually abused via smoking, which causes higher bioavailability of the primary psychoactive component, tetrahydrocannabinol (THC), than oral ingestion. Inhalation of marijuana smoke produces euphoria, with signs of increased sympathetic nervous system activity and decreased parasympathetic nervous system activity. The most consistent cardiac change is an increased resting heart rate. Orthostatic hypotension may occur. Long-term marijuana abuse leads to increased tar deposits in the lungs, impaired pulmonary defense mechanisms, and decreased pulmonary function, effects similar to cigarette smoking. There is an increased incidence of sinusitis and bronchitis. In some persons, marijuana may evoke seizures. Conjunctival reddening is evidence of vasodilation. Drowsiness is a common side effect. Tolerance to most of the psychoactive effects of THC has been observed. Although physical dependence on marijuana is not believed to occur, abrupt cessation after long-term use is characterized by mild withdrawal symptoms such as irritability, insomnia, diaphoresis, nausea, vomiting, and diarrhea. The single medical use for marijuana is as an antiemetic in patients receiving cancer chemotherapy.

The pharmacologic effects of inhaled THC occur within minutes but rarely persist longer than 2–3 hours, which decreases the likelihood that acutely intoxicated patients will be seen in the operating room. Management of anesthesia includes consideration of the known effects of THC on the heart, lungs, and CNS. Animal studies have demonstrated drug-induced drowsiness and decreased dose requirements for volatile anesthetics following *IV* administration of THC. Barbiturate and ketamine sleep times are prolonged in THC-treated animals, and opioid-induced respiratory depression may be potentiated.

Substance Abuse as an Occupational Hazard in Anesthesiology

Anesthesiologists represent 5.5% of all physicians in the United States. However, they are overrepresented in addiction treatment programs, enrolling at a rate approximately three times higher than that of any other physician group. In addition, anesthesiologists are at highest risk of relapse after drug addiction treatment. At the present time, 12%–15% of all physicians in treatment are anesthesiologists. The encouraging news is that a survey performed in 1997 revealed that the apparent incidence of substance abuse among anesthesiology residents was 1.6%, with a faculty incidence of 1.0%. Both rates represented a decline in incidence since 1986.

Why Anesthesiologists?

Numerous factors have been proposed to explain the high incidence of substance abuse among anesthesiologists. These include:

- easy access to potent drugs, particularly opioids
- high addictive potential of accessible drugs, particularly fentanyl and sufentanil
- relative simplicity of diversion of these agents, since only small doses will initially provide the effect desired by the abusing physician
- curiosity about patients' experiences with these substances
- control-oriented personality

Demographic Characteristics of Anesthesiologists Who Abuse Drugs

The curriculum on drug abuse and addiction compiled by the American Society of Anesthesiologists Committee on Occupational Health is a highly recommended in-depth source of information on this important topic. This curriculum notes the following demographic characteristics of anesthesiologists who are addicted to drugs:

- Half are younger than age 35, but this may reflect the age distribution within the specialty.
- Residents are overrepresented, possibly because increased awareness of the high risk of substance abuse among anesthesiologists has led to more careful screening for signs of addiction in anesthesiology training programs. (Interestingly, a higher proportion of anesthesiology residents who are addicted are members of the Alpha Omega Alpha Honor Society.)
- Most substance abusers are male (67%–88%) and white (75%–96%).
- Opiates are the drug of choice in 76%–90%.
- One-third to one-half abuse more than one drug.
- One-third have a family history of addictive disease, most frequently alcoholism.
- Two-thirds of anesthesiologists with a documented history of addiction are associated with academic departments.

Most Frequently Abused Drugs

Traditionally, opioids are the drugs selected for abuse by anesthesiologists. Fentanyl and sufentanil are the most commonly abused drugs, followed by meperidine and morphine. This choice is particularly evident among anesthesiologists younger than age 35. Alcohol is the abused substance found in older anesthesiologists, probably because the time to produce impairment is significantly longer than that observed with opiate addiction. The data also suggest that opiates are the substance of choice for abuse early in an anesthesiologist's career, whereas alcohol abuse is more frequently detected in anesthesia practitioners who have been out of residency for longer than 5 years.

Other drugs that have been abused include cocaine, benzodiazepines (midazolam), and more recently, propofol. Over the past few years there has been a switch to "needleless" delivery of the abused drugs. This approach provides a cleaner alternative to the more traditional IV or intramuscular routes. Every possible route of administration has been tried, including unusual IV sites (hidden veins in the feet, groin, thigh, and penis), oral-nasal administration (benzodiazepines), and sublingual and rectal routes. Volatile anesthetics have entered the abuse arena as well, with sevoflurane reported as the drug of choice among inhalational anesthetics. Regardless of the drug abused initially, after 6 months there is an increasing incidence of polydrug abuse.

Methods of Obtaining Drugs for Abuse

Anesthesiologists have developed numerous and often creative methods for obtaining drugs for abuse. The most frequently employed methods are falsely recording drug administration, improperly filling out the anesthesia record, and keeping rather than wasting leftover drugs. In addition, recent reports have highlighted a new practice involving secretly accessing multidose vials and then refilling and resealing them with other substances. It is important to be wary of the faculty member or resident who is too anxious to give breaks to others or who volunteers to take late cases. One of the most frequently reported retrospective markers of addictive behavior was the desire to work overtime, particularly during periods when supervision might be reduced, such as evenings and weekends.

Signs and Symptoms of Addictive Behavior

Regardless of which drugs are abused, any unusual and persistent changes in behavior should be cause for alarm. Classically these behaviors include wide mood swings, such as periods of depression, anger, and irritability, alternating with periods of euphoria. Key points to remember about addictive behavior include:

- Denial is universal.
- Symptoms at work are the last to appear (symptoms appear first in the community and then at home).
- The pathognomonic sign is self-administration of drugs.
- Addiction is often first detected when an individual is found comatose.
- Individuals whose addiction remains untreated are often found dead.

The most frequently overlooked symptoms of addictive behavior are:

- desire to work alone
- refusal of lunch relief or breaks
- frequent offers to relieve others
- volunteering for extra cases or call
- patient pain needs in the postanesthetic care unit that are disproportionately high given the narcotics recorded as administered
- weight loss
- frequent bathroom breaks

Associated Risks of Physician Drug Addiction

Although traditionally the risks related to substance abuse were assigned to the individual physician-abuser, it is clear there are also significant risks to patients and potential risks to the hospital staff and administration when a physician becomes impaired or addicted.

Physician

The principal risks to the anesthesia provider with addictive disease are an increased risk of suicide by drug overdose and drug-related death. Unfortunately the relapse rate for anesthesiologists after drug abuse treatment is the highest among all physician groups with a history of narcotic addiction. The risk of relapse is greatest in the first 5 years and decreases as time in recovery increases. The positive news is that 89% of anesthesiologists who complete treatment and commit to aftercare remain abstinent for longer than 2 years. However, death is the primary presenting sign of relapse in opiate-addicted anesthesiologists.

Patients can be affected by addictive behavior. The data show that impaired physicians (those who are actively abusing drugs) are at an increased risk of malpractice suits. Data from California and Oklahoma revealed a dramatic decrease in both the number and dollar value of claims filed after treatment for substance abuse.

Most states have laws requiring that hospital and medical staff report any suspected addictive behavior. Failure to report may have significant consequences depending on individual state statutes.

Process for Dealing With Suspected Substance Abuse

The process for dealing with suspected substance abuse by an anesthesiologist is significantly affected by the presence or absence of a physician assistance committee. If an institution does not have such a committee, one should be formed and policies developed so that the support required by an impaired physician is in place when it is needed. The membership of this committee should include an anesthesiologist. In addition, this group should have a consulting agreement with local addiction specialists with experience in treating and referring physicians with substance abuse issues. Ideally this treatment group would also include a physician-counselor with experience and expertise in treating anesthesiologists. Finally, this committee should have a helpline telephone number and a point of contact with at least one preselected addiction treatment program.

Reporting and Intervention

Admission to an alcohol or drug addiction treatment program is not considered a reportable event by state or national agencies. It can be dealt with as a medical leave of absence. However, intervention must be initiated as soon as there is firm evidence that substances of abuse are being diverted for personal use. This evidence needs to be clear and convincing to the physician assistance committee.

The primary goal of intervention is to get the addicted individual into a multidisciplinary medical evaluation process conducted by a team of experts at an experienced residential treatment program. *One-on-one intervention must be avoided.* The expertise of the hospital physician assistance committee and county or state medical society can be called upon to help with the intervention. After an individual has been confronted and is awaiting final disposition of his or her case, it is important not to leave the individual alone, because newly identified addicted physicians are at increased risk of suicide following this initial confrontation.

Treatment

The specifics of substance abuse treatment for physicians are beyond the scope of this chapter. However, it is important that a member of the faculty, group, or impairment committee keep in contact with the addicted physician and his or her treatment team. There is no cure for addiction, and recovery is a lifelong process. The most effective treatment programs are multidisciplinary and able to provide long-term follow-up for the impaired physician.

DRUG OVERDOSE

Acetaminophen Overdose

Acetaminophen overdose is the most common medicinal overdose reported to poison control centers in the United States. Patients typically have nausea and/or vomiting and abdominal pain at presentation. Acetaminophen toxicity is due to centrilobular hepatic necrosis caused by N-acetyl-p-benzoquinoneimine (NAPQI), which reacts with and destroys hepatocytes. Normally this metabolite constitutes only 5% of acetaminophen metabolic products and is inactivated by conjugation with endogenous glutathione. In overdose, the supply of glutathione becomes depleted and NAPQI is not detoxified.

Treatment of acetaminophen overdose begins with determination of the time of drug ingestion and with administration of activated charcoal to impede drug absorption. At 4 hours after drug ingestion, plasma acetaminophen concentration should be measured and plotted on the Rumack-Matthew nomogram, which stratifies patients into those who are not at risk of hepatotoxicity, those who are possibly at risk, and those who are probably at risk (Fig. 29.4). All patients who are possibly or probably at risk of hepatotoxicity and anyone for whom the time of ingestion is not known are treated with N-acetylcysteine, which repletes glutathione, combines directly with NAPQI, and enhances sulfate conjugation of acetaminophen. Administration of N-acetylcysteine is virtually 100% effective in preventing hepatotoxicity when administered within 8 hours of drug ingestion.

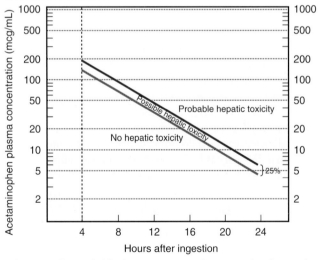

U.S. values: mcg/mL

FIG. 29.4 Rumack-Matthew nomogram for acetaminophen toxicity. The plasma concentration of acetaminophen is measured and plotted according to the time the blood sample was drawn relative to the time of overdose ingestion. Position on the nomogram indicates whether hepatotoxicity is probable, possible, or unlikely. Concentrations are expressed as mcg/mL. (Adapted from Rumack BH, Matthew H. Acetaminophen poisoning and toxicity. *Pediatrics.* 1975;55:871-876.)

POISONING

Organophosphate Poisoning

Organophosphate pesticides, carbamate pesticides, and organophosphorus compounds (nerve agents developed for chemical warfare and used in terrorist attacks) all inhibit acetylcholinesterase, which results in cholinergic overstimulation. These chemicals are absorbed by inhalation, by ingestion, and through the skin. There are several important differences between the nerve agents and insecticides. The insecticides are oily, less volatile liquids with a longer time to onset of toxicity but longer-lasting effects. Nerve agents are typically watery and volatile, acting rapidly and severely but for a shorter period of time. They are highly toxic, stable, and easily dispersed. Carbamate insecticides have more limited penetration of the CNS, bind acetylcholinesterase reversibly, and result in a shorter, milder course of toxicity than organophosphates. All can be aerosolized and vaporized. The manifestations of pesticide and nerve agent poisoning are influenced by the route of absorption, with the most severe effects occurring after inhalation. However, poisoning can also take place by absorption of the substance through the skin or eyes and by eating or drinking contaminated food or water (Table 29.13). Muscarinic signs and symptoms of organophosphate exposure include profuse exocrine secretions (tearing, rhinorrhea, bronchorrhea, salivation), gastrointestinal signs, and ophthalmic signs such as miosis. Exposure to larger doses results in stimulation of nicotinic receptors, which produces skeletal muscle weakness, fasciculations, and paralysis. Cardiovascular findings may include tachycardia or bradycardia, hypertension or hypotension. CNS effects include cognitive impairment, convulsions, and coma. Acute respiratory failure is the primary cause of

TABLE 29.13	Signs of Organophosphate Poisoning

MUSCARINIC EFFECTS
Copious secretions
  Salivation
  Tearing
  Diaphoresis
  Bronchorrhea
  Rhinorrhea
Bronchospasm
Miosis
Hyperperistalsis
Bradycardia

NICOTINIC EFFECTS
Skeletal muscle fasciculations
Skeletal muscle weakness
Skeletal muscle paralysis

CENTRAL NERVOUS SYSTEM EFFECTS
Seizures
Coma
Central apnea

death and is mediated by bronchorrhea, bronchospasm, respiratory muscle and diaphragmatic weakness or paralysis, and inhibition of the medullary respiratory center.

Treatment of organophosphate overdose involves administration of three types of drugs: an *anticholinergic drug* to counteract the acute cholinergic crisis, an *oxime drug* to reactivate inhibited acetylcholinesterase, and an *anticonvulsant drug* to prevent or treat seizures (Table 29.14). Atropine in 2-mg doses repeated every 5–10 minutes as needed is the main antidote for this poisoning. The clinical end point of atropine therapy is ease of breathing without significant airway secretions. Pralidoxime is an oxime that complexes with the organophosphate, which results in removal of the organophosphate from the acetylcholinesterase enzyme and splitting of the organophosphate into rapidly metabolizable fragments. Removal of the organophosphate from acetylcholinesterase reactivates the enzyme, and its normal functions can be resumed. Benzodiazepines are the only effective anticonvulsants for treating patients with organophosphate exposure. All patients with severe intoxication by these compounds should be given diazepam or midazolam. Respiratory muscle weakness may require mechanical ventilation.

Carbon Monoxide Poisoning

Carbon monoxide (CO) poisoning is a common cause of morbidity and the leading cause of poisoning mortality in the United States. Exposure may be accidental (inhalation of fire-related smoke, motor vehicle exhaust, fumes from a poorly functioning heating system, tobacco smoke) or intentional.

Pathophysiology
CO is a colorless, odorless, nonirritating gas that is easily absorbed through the lungs. The amount of CO absorbed depends on minute ventilation, duration of exposure, and ambient CO and oxygen concentrations. CO toxicity appears to result from a combination of tissue hypoxia and direct CO-mediated cellular damage. CO competes with oxygen for binding to hemoglobin. The affinity of hemoglobin for CO is more than 200 times greater than its affinity for oxygen. The consequence of this competitive binding is a shift of the oxyhemoglobin dissociation curve to the left, which results in impaired release of oxygen to tissues (Fig. 29.5). However, the binding

of CO to hemoglobin does not account for all the pathophysiologic consequences of CO poisoning. CO also disrupts oxidative metabolism, increases nitric oxide concentrations, causes brain lipid peroxidation, generates oxygen free radicals, and produces other metabolic changes that may result in neurologic and cardiac toxicity. CO binds more tightly to fetal hemoglobin than to adult hemoglobin, so infants are particularly vulnerable to its effects. Children, because of their higher metabolic rate and oxygen consumption, are also very susceptible to CO toxicity. CO exposure has uniquely deleterious effects in pregnant women because CO readily crosses the placenta; fetal carboxyhemoglobin (HbCO) concentration may exceed maternal HbCO concentration, and fetal elimination of CO is slower than that of the mother.

Signs and Symptoms
The initial signs and symptoms of CO exposure are nonspecific. Headache, nausea, vomiting, weakness, difficulty concentrating, and confusion are common. The highly oxygen-dependent organs—the brain and heart—show the major signs of injury. Tachycardia and tachypnea reflect cellular hypoxia. Angina pectoris, cardiac dysrhythmias, and pulmonary edema may result from the increased cardiac output

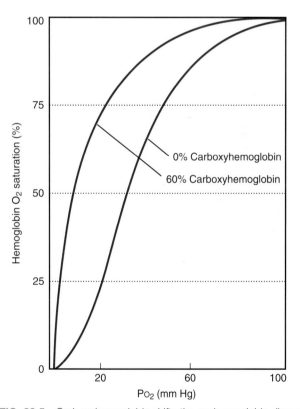

FIG. 29.5 Carboxyhemoglobin shifts the oxyhemoglobin dissociation curve to the left and changes it to a more hyperbolic shape. This results in decreased oxygen-carrying capacity and impaired release of oxygen at the tissue level. (Adapted from Ernst A, Zibrak JD. Carbon monoxide poisoning. *N Engl J Med.* 1998;339:1603-1608. Copyright 1998 Massachusetts Medical Society. All rights reserved.)

TABLE 29.14	Goals of Treatment of Organophosphate Poisoning

Reverse acute cholinergic crisis created by the poison
    Atropine 2 mg IV every 5–10 min as needed until ventilation improves
Reactivate functioning of acetylcholinesterase
    Pralidoxime 1–2 g IV
Prevent or treat seizures
    Diazepam or midazolam as needed
Provide supportive care

IV, Intravenously.

necessitated by hypoxia. Syncope and seizures may result from cerebral hypoxia and cerebral vasodilation. Of note, the degree of systemic hypotension in CO poisoning correlates with the severity of CNS structural damage. The classic finding of cherry-red lips is not commonly seen.

The effects of CO poisoning are not confined to the period immediately after exposure. Persistent or delayed neurologic effects may be seen. *Delayed neuropsychiatric syndrome,* which may include cognitive dysfunction, memory loss, seizures, personality changes, parkinsonism, dementia, mutism, blindness, and psychosis, may occur after apparent recovery from the acute phase of CO intoxication. No clinical findings or laboratory test results reliably predict which patients are at risk of delayed neuropsychiatric syndrome, but patients who are comatose at presentation, older patients, and those with prolonged exposure seem to be at greater risk.

Diagnosis

Serum HbCO concentrations should be obtained for patients suspected of CO exposure. Arterial blood sampling is not necessary, since arterial and venous HbCO levels correlate well. Measurement requires a CO-oximeter, which, by spectrophotometry, can detect and quantify all normal and abnormal hemoglobins. Routine blood gas analysis does not recognize the presence of abnormal hemoglobins, and pulse oximetry cannot distinguish HbCO from oxyhemoglobin. Oxygen saturation values measured by pulse oximetry may therefore be quite misleading.

Treatment

Treatment consists of removal of the individual from the source of CO production, immediate administration of supplemental oxygen, and aggressive supportive care (airway management, blood pressure support, cardiovascular stabilization). Oxygen therapy shortens the elimination half-time of CO by competing at the binding sites on hemoglobin and improves tissue oxygenation. Oxygen administration is continued until HbCO concentrations have returned to normal. The half-life of HbCO is 4–6 hours when patients are breathing room air, 40–80 minutes when they are breathing 100% oxygen, and approximately 15–30 minutes when they are breathing hyperbaric oxygen. Hyperbaric oxygen therapy consists of delivery of 100% oxygen within a pressurized chamber, which results in a huge increase in the amount of oxygen dissolved in blood. Hyperbaric oxygen therapy accelerates elimination of CO and may decrease the frequency of the neurologic sequelae that can result from severe CO exposure. Hyperbaric oxygen therapy is controversial, is not universally available, and has some risks. However, it may be indicated in selected patients: those who are comatose or have neurologic abnormalities at presentation, those who have HbCO concentrations in excess of 40%, and those who are pregnant and have HbCO concentrations above 15%.

KEY POINTS

- Serotonin syndrome is a potentially life-threatening adverse drug reaction that results from overstimulation of central serotonin receptors. It can be caused by an excess of

precursors, increased release, reduced reuptake, or reduced metabolism of serotonin. Many drugs are serotoninergic (i.e., involved in these serotonin processes), including selective serotonin reuptake inhibitors (SSRIs), selective serotonin-norepinephrine reuptake inhibitors (SNRIs), atypical antidepressants, MAOIs, lithium, drugs of abuse, and narcotic analgesics.

- In addition to the seizure and its neuropsychiatric effects, ECT produces significant cardiovascular effects. The typical cardiovascular response to the electrically induced seizure consists of 10–15 seconds of parasympathetic stimulation producing bradycardia and a reduction in blood pressure. This is followed by sympathetic nervous system activation resulting in tachycardia and hypertension lasting several minutes.

- *Substance abuse* may be defined as self-administration of drugs that deviates from accepted medical or social use and if sustained, can lead to physical and psychological dependence. Physical *dependence* has developed when the presence of a drug in the body is necessary for normal physiologic function and prevention of withdrawal symptoms. *Tolerance* is the state in which tissues become accustomed to the presence of a drug so that increased dosages of that drug become necessary to produce effects similar to those observed initially with smaller dosages.

- Although alcohol appears to produce widespread nonspecific effects on cell membranes, there is evidence that many of its neurologic effects are mediated by actions at receptors for the inhibitory neurotransmitter GABA. Alcohol appears to increase GABA-mediated chloride ion conductance. A shared site of action for alcohol, benzodiazepines, and barbiturates would be consistent with the ability of these different classes of drugs to produce cross-tolerance and cross-dependence.

- Acute cocaine administration is known to cause coronary vasospasm, myocardial ischemia, myocardial infarction, and ventricular dysrhythmias, including ventricular fibrillation. Associated systemic hypertension and tachycardia further increase myocardial oxygen requirements at a time when oxygen delivery to the heart is decreased by the effects of cocaine on coronary blood flow. Cocaine use can cause myocardial ischemia and hypotension for as long as 6 weeks after discontinuance of the drug.

- Anesthesiologists comprise 5.5% of all physicians in the United States but are overrepresented in addiction treatment programs, enrolling at a rate approximately three times higher than that of any other physician group. In addition, anesthesiologists are at highest risk of relapse of all physician specialists.

- Fentanyl and sufentanil are the drugs most commonly abused by anesthesiologists. This drug choice is particularly evident among anesthesiologists younger than age 35. Alcohol abuse is seen primarily among older anesthesiologists, perhaps because the time to produce impairment is significantly longer than that observed with opiate addiction. It appears that opiates are the substances of choice for abuse early in an anesthesiologist's career.

- The primary goal of an intervention is to get an addicted physician into a multidisciplinary medical evaluation process conducted by a team of experts at an experienced residential treatment program. One-on-one intervention must be avoided. After an individual has been confronted and is awaiting final disposition of his or her case, it is important not to leave the individual alone, because newly identified addicted physicians are at increased risk of suicide following the initial confrontation.
- Acetaminophen overdose is the most common medicinal overdose reported to poison control centers in the United States. Patients typically have nausea and/or vomiting and abdominal pain. Acetaminophen hepatic toxicity is caused by a metabolite of acetaminophen that reacts with and destroys hepatocytes. Normally this metabolite constitutes only 5% of acetaminophen metabolic products and is inactivated by conjugation with endogenous glutathione. In an overdose the supply of glutathione becomes depleted and the destructive metabolite is not detoxified.
- Nerve agents are organophosphate poisons that have been used in warfare and terrorist attacks. They inactivate acetylcholinesterase and create an acute, severe cholinergic crisis. Emergency management of this poisoning consists of administration of repeated large doses of atropine.
- Routine blood gas analysis does not recognize the presence of abnormal hemoglobins, and pulse oximetry cannot distinguish carboxyhemoglobin from oxyhemoglobin. Therefore in the presence of carbon monoxide poisoning, these methods provide erroneous information.
- The effects of carbon monoxide are not confined to the period immediately following exposure. *Delayed neuropsychiatric syndrome*, which may include cognitive dysfunction, memory loss, seizures, personality changes, parkinsonism, dementia, mutism, blindness, and psychosis, may occur after apparent recovery from the acute phase of carbon monoxide intoxication. Patients who are comatose at presentation, older patients, and those with prolonged exposure seem to be at greater risk.

RESOURCES

Alapat PM, Zimmerman JL. Toxicology in the critical care unit. *Chest.* 2008;133:1006-1013.

American Society of Anesthesiologists Committee on Occupational Health. *Model curriculum on drug abuse and addiction for residents in anesthesiology.* http://www.asahq.org.

Berge KH, Seppala MD, Schipper AM. Chemical dependency and the physician. *Mayo Clin Proc.* 2009;84:625-631.

Deiner S, Frost EA. Electroconvulsive therapy and anesthesia. *Int Anesthesiol Clin.* 2009;47:81-92.

Kales SH, Christiani DC. Acute chemical emergencies. *N Engl J Med.* 2004;350:800-808.

Maxwell JC, McCance-Katz EF. Indicators of buprenorphine and methadone use and abuse: what we do know? *Am J Addict.* 2010;19:73-88.

May JA, White HC, Leonard-White A, et al. The patient recovering from alcohol and drug addiction: special issues for the anesthesiologist. *Anesth Analg.* 2001;92:1608-1610.

National Poison Control Center Hotline: 800-222-1222.

Rumack BH, Matthew H. Acetaminophen poisoning and toxicity. *Pediatrics.* 1975;55:871-876.

Sadock BJ, Sadock VA, Ruiz P. *Kaplan and Sadock's Synopsis of Psychiatry.* 11th ed. Philadelphia: Lippincott Williams & Wilkins; 2014.

Smith FA, Wittmann CW, Stern TA. Medical complications of psychiatric treatment. *Crit Care Clin.* 2008;24:635-656.

Warner DO, Berger K, Sun H, et al. Risks and outcomes of substance use disorder among anesthesiology residents: a matched cohort analysis. *Anesthesiology.* 2015;123:929-936.

Weaver LK. Carbon monoxide poisoning. *N Engl J Med.* 2009;360:1217-1225.

Pediatric Diseases

MICHELLE W. DIU, THOMAS J. MANCUSO

UNIQUE CONSIDERATIONS IN PEDIATRIC PATIENTS

When caring for the pediatric patient, there are many considerations outside of the underlying medical illness(es) that one must contemplate if an age-appropriate and comprehensive care plan is to be delivered. These include (but are not limited to) age, both chronological and developmental; developmental stage, both physical and psychological; physiologic differences; and social and familial circumstances.

Anesthesia-Induced Developmental Neurotoxicity

Concerns over anesthesia-induced developmental neurotoxicity have garnered widespread attention in recent years. Mounting evidence from animal studies over the past 2 decades have consistently shown increased and accelerated neuroapoptosis upon exposure to virtually every known anesthetic agent. It is unclear whether the observed acute neuroapoptosis leads to permanent brain cell loss and how or if the degree of immediate neuronal injury correlates with subsequent neurocognitive sequelae. While inconclusive, results from studies to date generally suggest that anesthetic exposure at a young age (<3–4 years) may be associated with subsequent behavioral and learning difficulties. Single exposure of short duration appears to have little consequence. Prospective and randomized-based evidence, however, is yet lacking. As a result, at present no change in current practice is recommended for lifesaving and/or truly emergent or urgent procedures requiring anesthesia. However, nonurgent and elective surgeries should be delayed until after age 3–4 years when possible.

Anxiety

Anxiety is a normal and expected response to anticipation of surgery and anesthesia. In fact, anxiety is sometimes the only reason children or adolescents require sedation or anesthesia for nonpainful diagnostic procedures. An appreciation of circumstances that contribute to preanesthetic anxiety and recognition of factors associated with increased perianesthetic anxiety in children are important in designing an approach that minimizes apprehension and potential psychological trauma.

Age group– and developmental stage–related fears range from separation anxiety beginning around age 8–10 months, to fear of loss of control, to fear of body disfigurement and death. An understanding of the different categories of fears is essential in selecting the age-appropriate approach.

Anatomy and Physiology

Body Size and Thermoregulation

Neonates and infants are vulnerable to becoming hypothermic during the perioperative period. Body heat is lost more rapidly in this age group than in older children or adults, owing to the ratio of large body surface area to body weight/volume, the thin layer of insulating subcutaneous fat, and a decreased ability to produce heat. Shivering plays little to no role in heat production in neonates, whose primary mechanism is nonshivering thermogenesis mediated by brown fat metabolism.

It is very difficult to reestablish normothermia once hypothermia ensues in newborns and infants. As such, prevention of hypothermia is essential. Potential complications associated with intraoperative hypothermia include surgical wound infections, negative nitrogen balance, delayed wound healing, delayed postoperative anesthetic recovery, impaired coagulation, and prolonged hospitalization.

Central Nervous System

A newborn's brain comprises approximately 10% of the total body weight, compared to only 2% of total body weight of an adult's brain. Myelinization and synaptic connections are not complete until age 3–4 years. A child's brain undergoes the most rapid phase of growth in the first 2 years of life, achieving 75% of its adult size. The location of the spinal cord within the vertebrae changes with growth, with the conus medullaris reaching L3 at birth and migrating cephalad to the normal adult level of L1–L2 by the third year of life.

Airway

The airway of a term newborn differs in several ways from that of an adult. Newborns have a proportionally larger head and tongue, a larynx that is situated higher in the neck, a short and mobile epiglottis, and vocal cords whose anterior commissure is slanted inferiorly. Airway obstruction occurs more readily owing to the larger tongue size relative to the oral cavity. The cricoid cartilage (as opposed to the vocal cords in adults) is the narrowest portion of the larynx in pediatric patients. As in adults, angulation of the right mainstem bronchus favors right endobronchial intubation if the tracheal tube is inserted beyond the carina. The importance of the smaller absolute dimensions of the upper and lower airways in newborns and infants cannot be overemphasized. Transitioning from infancy to young childhood, the relative size of the head and tongue decreases, and the position of the larynx in the neck moves to the lower position as seen in adults.

Respiratory System

The functional aspects of the respiratory system (e.g., respiratory rate, tidal volume, minute ventilation) reflect a crucial physiologic difference between children and adults. Oxygen consumption (VO_2) is much greater on a per-kilogram basis in children compared to adults, owing to the difference in the ratio of surface area to volume. In addition, the high compliance of both lung parenchyma and chest wall in newborns and infants predispose to alveolar collapse, with resultant V/Q mismatching and hypoxemia.

TABLE 30.1	Holliday-Segar Formula for Caloric Expenditure		
Weight	Caloric Expenditure	Water Requirement	Fluid Maintenance[a]
0–10 kg	100 kcal/kg/day	100 mL/kg/day	4 mL/kg/h (for first 10 kg)
10–20 kg	50 kcal/kg/day	50 mL/kg/day	2 mL/kg/h (for second 10 kg)
≥20 kg	20 kcal/kg/day	20 mL/kg/day	1 mL/kg/h (for each additional kg above 20 kg)

[a]Fluid maintenance rates are additive. For example, a 25-kg child requires 4 mL/kg/h for the first 10 kg (40 mL/h) plus 2 mL/kg/h for the second 10 kg (20 mL/h) plus 1 mL/kg/h for each additional kg above 20 kg (5 mL/h), totaling 65 mL/h (40 + 20 + 5) as the hourly fluid maintenance rate.

Cardiovascular System

Pulmonary vascular resistance (PVR) gradually decreases over the first several months of life, but the vasculature remains reactive; PVR can increase dramatically under conditions of acidosis, hypoxemia, and hypercarbia. The foramen ovale and ductus arteriosus can reopen under these circumstances, with reversion to fetal circulatory patterns resulting in significantly decreased pulmonary blood flow and profound hypoxemia. Anatomic closure of the foramen ovale occurs between 3 months and 1 year of age, although 20%–30% of adults have a probe-patent foramen ovale. Functional closure of the ductus arteriosus normally occurs 10–15 hours after birth, with anatomic closure taking place in 4–6 weeks. Ductus arteriosus constriction occurs in response to increased arterial oxygenation that develops after birth. Nevertheless, the ductus arteriosus may reopen during periods of arterial hypoxemia.

Heart rate is the main determinant of cardiac output and systemic blood pressure in neonates and young infants. Contractility of the neonatal myocardium is decreased compared to that in older children and adults; this is due to a relative decrease in contractile elements. Stroke volume is also relatively fixed due to a paucity of elastic elements as well. The Frank-Starling mechanism is not operational under most circumstances. As such, increases in cardiac output in the newborn is dependent on increases in heart rate for the most part.

Fluids and Renal Physiology

Total body water content and extracellular fluid volume are increased proportionately in neonates. The extracellular fluid volume is equivalent to approximately 40% of body weight in neonates, compared with approximately 20% in adults. By 18–24 months of age, the proportion of extracellular fluid volume relative to body weight is similar to that in adults. In addition to fluid replacement, newborns and young infants may also require glucose supplementation. Maintenance glucose requirement for newborns is 6–8 mg/kg/min. Term newborns are capable of maintaining normoglycemia for up to 10 hours with no exogenous glucose administration. Perioperative fluid administration for pediatric patients can be divided into several components:

1. replacement of fluid deficits from fasting
2. maintenance fluid requirement
3. replacement of blood loss
4. replacement of evaporative losses

TABLE 30.2	Intraoperative Fluid Therapy for Pediatric Patients		
	Normal Saline or Lactated Ringer's Solution (mL/kg/h)		
Procedure	Maintenance	Replacement	Total
Minor surgery (e.g., herniorrhaphy)	4	2	6
Moderate surgery (e.g., pyloromyotomy)	4	4	8
Extensive surgery (e.g., bowel resection)	4	6	10

Fluid maintenance and replacement of deficits are based on the Holliday-Segar formula for caloric expenditure of children of different sizes. Caloric expenditure based on weight and water requirement is approximately 1 mL/kcal expended per day. This is the basis for the 4:2:1 rule (Table 30.1). Blood loss is generally replaced 3:1 for each milliliter of blood loss with isotonic crystalloid, and evaporative loss replenishments are guided by estimations based on type of procedure and associated area of surgical exposure (Table 30.2).

The glomerular filtration rate is greatly decreased in term newborns but increases nearly fourfold by 3–5 weeks. Newborns are obligate sodium losers and cannot concentrate urine as effectively as adults. Therefore adequate exogenous sodium and water must be provided during the perioperative period. Conversely, newborns excrete volume loads more slowly than adults and are more susceptible to fluid overload. Decreased renal function can also delay excretion of drugs dependent on renal clearance for elimination.

Hepatic System

At term the liver actually has significant glycogen stores that can be converted to glucose for use by the neonate. The newborn's glycogen stores, on a per-kilogram basis, are at least equal to the stores in most adults. Hepatic capacity for biotransformation and metabolism of drugs, however, is diminished until several months of postnatal life.

Hematologic System

The hematologic system undergoes significant changes after birth. In fetal life the lower p50 of fetal hemoglobin (Hb) is

TABLE 30.3	Hematologic Values in Infancy and Childhood		
Age	Hemoglobin (g/dL)	Hematocrit (%)	Leukocytes (1000/mm³)
Cord blood	14–20	45–65	9–30
Newborn	13–20	42–66	5–20
3 months	10–14	31–41	6–18
6 months to 12 years	11–15	33–42	6–15
Young adult male	14–18	42–52	5–10
Young adult female	12–16	37–47	5–10

TABLE 30.4	Estimated Blood Volumes for Neonates, Infants, and Children
Age Group	Estimated Blood Volume (mL/kg)
Premature neonate	90–100
Term neonate	80–90
Infants	75–80
Children > 1 year	70–75

TABLE 30.5	Estimation of Maximal Allowable Blood Loss[a]

A 3-kg term neonate is scheduled for intraabdominal surgery. The preoperative Hct is 50%. What is the maximum allowable blood loss (MABL) to maintain the Hct at 40%?

$MABL = EBV \times [(Hct_{high} - Hct_{low})/Hct_{average}]$

$EBV = 3\ kg \times 85\ mL/kg = 255\ mL$

$Hct_{high} - Hct_{low} = 50\% - 40\% = 10\%$

$Hct_{average} = (50\% + 40\%)/2 = 45\%$

$MABL = 255\ mL \times [(50\% - 40\%)/45\%] = 56.1\ mL$

[a]These calculations are only guidelines and do not consider the potential impact of fluid infusion therapy on the measured Hct.
EBV, Estimated blood volume; *Hct,* hematocrit.

Anesthetic Requirements

Full-term neonates require lower concentrations of volatile anesthetics than infants aged 1–6 months. Furthermore, the minimum alveolar concentration (MAC) in preterm neonates decreases with decreasing gestational age. MAC steadily increases until age 2–3 months, but after 3 months, the MAC steadily declines with age, although there are slight increases at puberty. Sevoflurane is unique among the currently used volatile anesthetics. The MAC of sevoflurane in neonates and infants remains constant.

Morphologic and functional maturation of neuromuscular junctions are not complete until approximately 2 months of age, but the implications of this initial immaturity on the pharmacodynamics of muscle relaxants are not clear. Owing to immature muscle composition, the infant's diaphragm is paralyzed at the same time as the peripheral muscles (as opposed to later in adults). This has led to the suggestion that infants may be more sensitive to the effects of nondepolarizing muscle relaxants, but the relatively large volume of distribution requires induction doses that are similar on a per-kilogram basis to those for adults. Duration of action may be prolonged because of immature hepatic and renal drug handling and excretion. Antagonism of neuromuscular blockade is generally unaffected in infants, but requirements for anticholinergics may be decreased owing to longer clearance times than in adults. Neonates and infants require more succinylcholine on a per-kilogram basis than do older children to produce similar degrees of neuromuscular blockade; this is due to the increased extracellular fluid volume and larger volume of distribution characteristic of this age group. Most practitioners limit use of succinylcholine to cases requiring rapid-sequence induction or to treatment of laryngospasm; there are risks of severe bradycardia, potential malignant hyperthermia, and other associated adverse effects in children with undiagnosed myopathies and dystrophinopathies.

Pharmacokinetics

Pharmacokinetics differ in neonates and infants compared with adults. For example, uptake of inhaled anesthetics is more rapid in infants than in older children or adults because of the

adaptive and allows the fetus to extract O_2 from maternal Hb. In the first 2 months of life, as fetal Hb is replaced by adult Hb, P_{50} increases from 19 mm Hg to 22 mm Hg and then eventually to the typical adult level of 26 mm Hg. In addition to the change in Hb type (fetal to adult), Hb concentration changes as well. Physiologic anemia occurs between 2 and 3 months of age. The nadir is typically seen between the 8th and 10th week of life. In view of the decreased cardiovascular reserve of neonates and the leftward shift of the oxyhemoglobin dissociation curve, it may be useful to maintain the neonate's hematocrit (Hct) closer to 40% than 30%, as is often accepted for older children. Typical blood cell values are delineated in Table 30.3.

The need for routine preoperative Hb determination is controversial. Routine preoperative Hb measurement in children younger than age 1 year results in detection of only a small number of patients with Hb concentrations below 10 g/dL, which rarely influences management of anesthesia or delays planned surgery. However, preoperative Hb measurement may be prudent in young infants presenting for surgery around the time of physiologic anemia. Based on estimated blood volume (Table 30.4), calculation of the maximal allowable blood loss (MABL) is useful to guide transfusion therapy (Table 30.5).

Pharmacology

Pharmacologic responses to drugs may differ in pediatric patients and adults. They manifest as differences in anesthetic requirements, responses to muscle relaxants, and pharmacokinetics.

infant's high alveolar ventilation relative to functional residual capacity. More rapid uptake may unmask negative inotropic effects of volatile anesthetics, resulting in an increased incidence of hypotension in neonates and infants upon inhalational induction of anesthesia.

An immature blood-brain barrier and decreased ability to metabolize drugs could increase the sensitivity of neonates to the effects of hypnotics. As a result, neonates might require lower doses of intravenous (IV) induction agents. On the other hand, older children and adolescents generally require a higher dose of IV induction agents compared to adults (up to 3 mg/kg of propofol in children and teenagers compared to 1.5–2 mg/kg for adults).

Decreased hepatic and renal clearance of drugs, which is characteristic of neonates, can produce prolonged drug effects. Clearance rates increase to adult levels by age 5–6 months, and during early childhood may even exceed adult rates. Protein binding of many drugs is decreased in infants, which could result in high circulating concentrations of unbound and pharmacologically active drugs.

Pediatric Cardiac Arrest During Anesthesia

The majority of children tolerate general anesthesia without incident. However, cardiac arrests do occur during anesthesia in children. Many result from either the critical health condition of the patient (especially complex congenital heart disease) or complications of the surgical procedure. The incidence of anesthesia-related cardiac arrest reported in *infants* is 15:10,000, with a range of 9.2–19:10,000. Overall, *children* experience anesthesia-related cardiac arrest at a rate of 3.3:10,000 anesthetics, with a range of 0–4.3:10,000. The incidence of anesthesia-related cardiac arrest reported for *all pediatric age groups* is 1.8:10,000.

Causes of Cardiac Arrest
More than 50% of arrests occur among infants. Patients with congenital heart disease are at significantly higher risk of perioperative cardiac arrest while undergoing noncardiac procedures. High American Society of Anesthesiologists (ASA) physical status and emergency status are also shown to be independent predictors of survival from perioperative cardiac arrest. Although no longer in use in most facilities, halothane is likely the offending agent in the majority of medication-induced perioperative cardiac arrests. Accidental IV injection of local anesthetic and/or local anesthetic toxicity due to overdose remain persistent problems.

Management
Management of a perioperative cardiac arrest depends on its cause. Initial management is guided by the same principles used for any pediatric cardiac arrest. Certification in pediatric advanced life support (PALS) is recommended for anesthesiologists regularly caring for infants and children.

TABLE 30.6   Classification of Preterm Newborns

Weight-Based Category[a]	Birth Weight (grams)	Estimated Gestational Age (weeks)
LBW	<2500	31–35
VLBW	1000 to <1500	26–30
ELBW	<1000	<26

[a]*ELBW*, Extremely low birth weight; *LBW*, low birth weight; *VLBW*, very low birth weight. VLBW and ELBW newborns are considered "micropremies."

TABLE 30.7   Age Terminology for Preterm Newborns and Infants

Term	Definition
Gestational age (GA)	First day of LMP to birth in weeks
Chronological age (CA)	Time since birth in weeks or months
Postmenstrual age	GA + CA in weeks or months
Corrected postconceptual age	CA − (40 − GA) in weeks or months

LMP, Last menstrual period.

The reader is referred to the latest PALS algorithm published by the American Heart Association (http://www.heart.org/HEARTORG/). An underlying respiratory cause of cardiac arrest should always be sought. The overall outcome for children following anesthesia-related cardiac arrest is much better than for in-hospital non–anesthesia-related arrests with respect to survival and development of new neurologic deficits.

THE PRETERM NEWBORN

Definition

As defined by the Committee on Fetus and Newborn of the American Academy of Pediatrics, preterm newborns are classified based on gestational age rather than birth weight as in the past. Preterm morbidity also correlates better with gestational age than with birth weight. A *preterm newborn* is classically defined as one born before 37 weeks' gestation. Table 30.6 illustrates the traditional classification of preterm newborns by weight and the related approximate gestational age. The term *ELGAN (extremely low-gestational-age newborn)* refers to a preterm newborn delivered at 23–27 weeks' gestation regardless of birth weight. As a group, ELGANs have immaturity of all organ systems and represent the most vulnerable of all pediatric patients, with the highest morbidity and mortality. Age terminology for preterm neonates and infants is defined in Table 30.7.

Newborns are classified as small, appropriate, or large for gestational age based on normal values established for weight at various gestational stages.

Respiratory Distress Syndrome

Lack of *surfactant* leads to development of neonatal respiratory distress syndrome (RDS). The incidence is inversely proportional to the gestational age and birth weight. Sufficient surfactant is present in most cases by 35 weeks' gestation. However, 5% of newborns diagnosed with RDS are born at term.

Signs and Symptoms

RDS usually becomes apparent within minutes of birth; it is evidenced by tachypnea, prominent grunting, intercostal and subcostal retractions, and nasal flaring. Grunting reflects the newborn's effort to mitigate alveolar collapse. Cyanosis and dyspnea progressively worsen. If untreated, apnea and irregular respirations—signs of impending respiratory failure—develop. The clinical course, chest radiograph, and blood gas analysis help establish the clinical diagnosis of RDS.

Treatment

Surfactant is administered to preterm newborns either immediately in the delivery room or later as a rescue treatment. It increases lung compliance and stabilizes the alveoli at end exhalation. Surfactant administration decreases the need for high concentrations of inspired oxygen, ventilatory support, and high ventilatory pressures. Unfortunately it has not decreased the incidence of subsequent chronic lung disease or bronchopulmonary dysplasia. In addition to the use of surfactant, newborns with RDS are being treated with delivery room nasal continuous positive airway pressure (CPAP).

Management of Anesthesia

During anesthesia the arterial oxygen saturation should be maintained near its preoperative levels. An arterial catheter (ideally in a preductal artery) is useful to monitor oxygenation, avoid hyperoxia (these preterm neonates are also at risk for developing retinal damage), and prevent respiratory and metabolic acidosis during the intraoperative and postoperative periods. Pneumothorax from barotrauma is an ever-present danger and should be considered if there is sudden cardiorespiratory decompensation. Maintaining the Hct near 40% helps optimize systemic oxygen delivery. Excessive hydration should be avoided; fluid resuscitation using smaller total volumes of colloids such as 5% albumin (10–20 mL/kg increments) should be considered over crystalloids.

Bronchopulmonary Dysplasia

Bronchopulmonary dysplasia (BPD) is a form of chronic lung disease of infancy. As already mentioned the incidence of chronic lung disease in ex–preterm newborns has not decreased despite widespread use of surfactant in the treatment of neonatal RDS.

Signs and Symptoms

BPD is a clinical diagnosis defined as oxygen dependence at 36 weeks' postconceptual age (PCA) or oxygen requirement (to maintain $PaO_2 > 50$ mm Hg) beyond 28 days of life in infants with birth weights under 1500 g. Pulmonary dysfunction in patients with BPD is most marked during the first year of life. Infants with mild BPD may eventually become asymptomatic, but airway hyperreactivity frequently persists.

Treatment

Maintenance of adequate oxygenation ($PaO_2 > 55$ mm Hg and $SpO_2 > 94\%$) is necessary to prevent or treat cor pulmonale and to promote growth of lung tissue and remodeling of the pulmonary vascular bed. Reactive airway bronchoconstriction is treated with bronchodilating agents. Diuretic administration is often needed to treat interstitial fluid retention and pulmonary edema to improve gas exchange.

Management of Anesthesia

Preoperative assessment of the child with BPD should focus on any recent respiratory decompensation and need for intervention. Ongoing drug therapy (bronchodilators, diuretics) as well as baseline oxygen saturations provide valuable clues to the severity of BPD and the child's clinical stability. The choice of drugs for anesthesia is not as important as management of the airway. In children with a history of mechanical ventilation, an endotracheal tube (ETT) one to a half size smaller than that predicted for age should be used because subglottic stenosis may be present. Tracheomalacia and bronchomalacia may also present as sequelae of previous prolonged intubation. Airway hyperreactivity is likely; thus a deep plane of anesthesia must be established prior to airway instrumentation. Indeed, children with active or prior BPD can be assumed to have reactive airway disease and should be treated similarly to those with asthma. Oftentimes, increased peak inspiratory pressures (PIPs) are required, reflecting decreased pulmonary compliance. Adequate oxygen should be delivered to maintain a PaO_2 of 50–70 mm Hg. Patients with metabolic alkalosis from furosemide therapy may exhibit a compensatory retention of CO_2. Fluid should be administered judiciously to avoid pulmonary edema.

Laryngomalacia and Bronchomalacia

Laryngomalacia is a congenital or acquired condition of excessive flaccidity of the laryngeal structures, especially the epiglottis and arytenoids. It can result from lack of normal neural control of laryngeal muscles or from pressure on the laryngeal cartilage, leading to inadequate laryngeal rigidity and thus structural collapse with normal respiratory efforts. Laryngomalacia accounts for more than 70% of persistent stridor in neonates and young infants. A congenital cause is found in 85% of cases of stridor in children who come to medical attention prior to their third birthday. Congenital vocal cord paralysis is seen in approximately 10% of infants with congenital stridor.

Bronchomalacia is seen in infants who have had a prolonged course in the neonatal intensive care unit (NICU). Risk factors include long periods of mechanical ventilation, poor nutrition, intercurrent infections, and other impediments to normal growth and development. The cartilage of the major airways is weakened; when affected infants bear down, these airways can collapse partially or completely. Infants with bronchomalacia generally also have a component of BPD. These two conditions together can lead to significant respiratory difficulties. Even a mild viral respiratory infection may worsen the situation sufficiently to require hospitalization.

Retinopathy of Prematurity

Retinopathy of prematurity (ROP) is a retinal disorder of pathologic vasculogenesis affecting preterm infants. It is a leading cause of childhood blindness and considerable visual morbidity worldwide. The risk of retinopathy is inversely related to birth weight and gestational age, occurring in up to 70% of premature infants weighing less than 1000 g at birth.

Signs and Symptoms
Disease severity is graded by 3 zones and 5 different stages according to the International Classification of ROP. The zones define the areas of the retina normally covered by physiologic vascularization. The stages, accordingly, represent (1) early ROP, (2) mild ROP, (3) intravitreal neovascularization, (4) fibrous tissue formation, and (5) retinal detachment.

Approximately 80%–90% of mild cases of ROP undergo spontaneous regression with little or no residual visual disability. However, infants with ROP have higher risks of developing visual and retinal problems later in life, including myopia, amblyopia, strabismus, glaucoma, retinal tear, and retinal detachment.

Treatment
Laser photocoagulation of the peripheral retina is the mainstay of ROP treatment. Central vision is preserved at the expense of variable peripheral visual field loss. Scleral cryotherapy and lens-sparing vitrectomy have also been used with success.

Management of Anesthesia
When dealing with an infant with ROP, challenges of limiting hyperoxemia while avoiding hypoxemia, especially during a critical period when physiologic disturbances are heightened by the stress of surgery and the effects of anesthetic drugs, must be considered. Currently there are no established guidelines for specific intraoperative goals of oxygen saturation for preterm infants presenting for surgery.

The optimal intraoperative oxygen saturation for these patients has yet to be determined, so it remains prudent to limit oxygen supplementation for preterm infants with or without ROP, especially in those less than 32 weeks' PCA. Supplemental oxygen should be used judiciously based on the patient's clinical needs. Many advocate for maintaining a stable intermediate range of oxygenation (89%–94%) and avoiding extremes (85%–89% vs. 96%–99%).

Apnea of Prematurity

Apnea of prematurity (AOP) is a result of the immaturity of the respiratory control centers in the newborn brainstem. The severity of AOP is inversely proportional to the gestational age of the newborn at birth.

Signs and Symptoms
Affected newborns exhibit both *primary (central) apnea*, in which there is simply lack of effort to breathe in the absence of any obstruction, and *obstructive apnea*. Mixed episodes of central and obstructive apnea are also seen. The CO_2 response of infants with AOP has been measured and is decreased compared to infants without AOP. Diagnosis of AOP is made on clinical grounds, and the criteria are somewhat variable. The diagnosis is made if an infant exhibits apnea longer than 15–20 seconds, apnea associated with heart rates below 80–100 beats per minute, or apnea associated with significant decreases in oxygen saturation.

Treatment
Treatment of AOP is begun once other causes of apnea (e.g., infection, CNS disorder) have been eliminated. Some cases of AOP are associated with low Hct values and resolve after sufficient packed red cell transfusion. Other nonpharmacologic treatments include nasal CPAP and (in very severe cases) mechanical ventilation. Methylxanthines are the mainstay of drug therapy for AOP. These central stimulants increase the sensitivity of the respiratory centers to CO_2. Various forms of methylxanthines are used, including aminophylline, caffeine, and caffeine citrate.

Postanesthetic Apnea

Postanesthetic apnea has many similarities with AOP. Preterm newborns who are at risk for AOP based on their corrected PCA are also at increased risk for developing postanesthetic apnea. Postanesthetic apnea is mostly seen in formerly preterm infants (birth at <37 weeks' gestation). The incidence is inversely related to PCA. Regional anesthesia without the addition of systemic sedatives and opioids appears to decrease the risk for postanesthetic apnea in at-risk infants. Regardless, it is recommended to keep infants whose PCA is less than 52–60 weeks for overnight observation after anesthesia.

Hypoglycemia

Hypoglycemia is the most common metabolic problem occurring in newborns and young infants, with many different

TABLE 30.8	Causes of Neonatal Hypoglycemia

MATERNAL FACTORS

Intrapartum administration of glucose
Drug treatment
1. β-Adrenergic antagonists (terbutaline, propranolol)
2. Oral hypoglycemic agents
3. Salicylates
Maternal diabetes/gestational diabetes

NEONATAL FACTORS

Depleted glycogen stores
1. Asphyxia
2. Perinatal stress
Increased glucose utilization (metabolic demands)
1. Sepsis
2. Polycythemia
3. Hypothermia
4. Respiratory distress syndrome
5. Congenital heart disease
Limited glycogen stores
1. Intrauterine growth retardation
2. Prematurity
Hyperinsulinism/endocrine disorders
1. Infants of diabetic mothers
2. Erythroblastosis fetalis, fetal hydrops
3. Insulinomas
4. Beckwith-Wiedemann syndrome
5. Panhypopituitarism
Decreased glycogenolysis/gluconeogenesis/utilization of alternate fuels
1. Inborn errors of metabolism
2. Adrenal insufficiency

causes (Table 30.8). Inadequate glycogen stores and immature gluconeogenesis are important risk factors. The incidence of symptomatic hypoglycemia is highest in those born small for gestational age (SGA).

Signs and Symptoms

Serum glucose levels are rarely below 35–40 mg/dL in the first 24 hours of life, or below 45 mg/dL thereafter. CNS or systemic signs of hypoglycemia such as jitteriness, seizures, apnea, lethargy, or mottling and pallor will usually be observed when serum glucose concentrations fall below 30–40 mg/dL in term infants during the first 72 hours, and less than 40 mg/dL thereafter.

Treatment

Infants with symptoms other than seizures should receive an IV bolus of 2 mL/kg (200 mg/kg) of 10% dextrose. If the infant is experiencing convulsions, an IV bolus of 4 mL/kg of 10% dextrose is indicated. Following bolus administration, a 10% dextrose infusion should be given at 8 mg/kg/min and titrated to maintain the serum glucose above 40–50 mg/dL.

Hypocalcemia

Neonates at particular risk of hypocalcemia are those born prematurely or with low birth weight, particularly infants with intrauterine growth retardation, infants of insulin-dependent diabetics, and infants with birth asphyxia associated with prolonged and difficult deliveries. Late neonatal hypocalcemia occurring 5–10 days after birth is usually due to ingestion of cow's milk, which contains high levels of phosphorous; it is not seen in breast-fed infants because human breast milk has a lower phosphate content.

Signs and Symptoms

The clinical manifestations of hypocalcemia include irritability, jitteriness, seizures, and lethargy. The classic signs of hypocalcemic tetany are very uncommon. Under anesthesia, hypocalcemia will manifest as hypotension and depressed cardiac performance. Treatment with IV calcium should be considered in newborns presenting with hypotension without an obvious cause. It is important to evaluate both total and ionized calcium.

Treatment

Management of hypocalcemia involves correction of hypocalcemia as well as hypomagnesemia and any other metabolic or acid-base abnormalities. The dose of calcium given intravenously should be based on the amount of elemental calcium administered. The starting dose is 10–20 mg/kg of elemental calcium. Calcium gluconate 10% provides 9 mg/mL of elemental calcium, and calcium chloride provides 27.2 mg/mL of elemental calcium. These doses have been shown to increase ionized calcium, blood pressure, and cardiac contractility.

Cases of bradycardia and even asystole have been seen with rapid IV administration of calcium. Thus IV calcium should be given over 5–10 minutes with electrocardiographic (ECG) monitoring. If calcium is given via an umbilical venous line, the tip should be ascertained to be in the inferior vena cava and *not too near the right atrium;* administration of calcium too close to the heart can result in dysrhythmias.

SURGICAL DISEASES OF THE NEWBORN

Congenital Diaphragmatic Hernia

Congenital diaphragmatic hernia (CDH) is a defect in the diaphragm that is associated with a variable amount of intraabdominal organ extrusion into the thoracic cavity. It has an incidence between 1:2500 and 1:3000 live births. Concomitant anomalies are seen in approximately 50% of CDH cases. Some associated congenital syndromes include Beckwith-Wiedemann, CHARGE (*c*oloboma, *h*eart defects, *a*tresia of the choanae, *r*etardation (intellectual disability), *g*enital anomalies, and *e*ar anomalies), and trisomy 21 and 18.

Signs and Symptoms

Prenatal diagnosis of CDH has increased from approximately 10% in 1985 to nearly 60% in present day. The most common findings include displacement of the heart and fluid-filled gastrointestinal segments into the thorax. Most newborns with

CDH present in the first few hours of life with respiratory distress (from mild dyspnea to cyanosis) and apparent dextrocardia in left-sided lesions. Typical physical findings include a scaphoid abdomen and a barrel-shaped chest with decreased breath sounds, distant or right-displaced heart sounds, and bowel sounds in the chest. A chest radiograph typically shows a bowel gas pattern in the chest and a mediastinal shift.

Pulmonary parenchymal and vascular hypoplasia increase pulmonary vascular resistance (PVR). This causes right-to-left shunting of blood through the ductus arteriosus, with persistence of fetal circulatory patterns. Persistent pulmonary hypertension of the newborn ensues, and if uncorrected, permanent pulmonary hypertension follows.

Treatment

Care of a newborn with a severe CDH starts immediately in the delivery room. Prompt endotracheal intubation and placement of a naso/orogastric tube for decompression of the stomach are recommended for most cases to minimize lung and even heart compression. Once considered a surgical emergency, the current approach aims at medical stabilization before surgical repair.

Specific goals of preoperative medical management include achievement of a preductal oxygen saturation of at least 90% and correction of metabolic acidosis. Crystalloid fluid and blood products are administered to maintain intravascular volume and red blood cell mass. Adequate sedation is administered in an effort to minimize increases in PVR. Mechanical ventilation should be employed with the lowest settings possible (goal, PIP < 25 cm H_2O), allowing for moderate permissive hypercarbia in an effort to minimize ventilator-induced lung injury. Surgery should be delayed until PVR has decreased and ventilation can be maintained with low PIPs and reasonable supplemental oxygen requirement. If pulmonary hypertension persists or recurs, trials of inhaled nitric oxide (iNO) and high-frequency oscillatory ventilation (HFOV) are initiated; extracorporeal membrane oxygenation (ECMO) may also be considered.

Management of Anesthesia

Endotracheal intubation should be carried out with avoidance of gastric distention. Avoiding positive-pressure mask ventilation, the patient may undergo an awake or a rapid-sequence tracheal intubation. The caveats with awake intubation include a sudden increase in PVR with agitation and ingestion of air with crying, thereby increasing risks of right-to-left shunting and lung compression, respectively. In addition to routine monitors, two pulse oximeters (preductal and postductal locations) are useful to monitor the degree of shunting. A preductal arterial cannulation (right radial) is recommended for monitoring systemic blood pressure, acid-base status, and other blood analyses. Venous access should be avoided in the lower extremities in case venous return is impaired from compression of the inferior vena cava following reduction of the hernia.

Anesthesia can be maintained with an opioid, a nondepolarizing muscle relaxant, and if tolerated, low concentrations of inhaled anesthetics. Nitrous oxide should be avoided. Vasopressors are employed based on need to maintain hemodynamic stability.

Repair of CDH via thoracoscopic approach is becoming more common, but open repair is still the preferred technique. Newborns with CDH have, almost by definition, pulmonary dysfunction that limits the patient's ability to tolerate thoracoscopy and associated CO_2 insufflation and one-lung ventilation. The primary advantages of thoracoscopic repair are smaller surgical incisions, less postoperative pain, and decreased risk of postoperative thoracic and rib deformities. However, thoracoscopic repairs tend to be longer in duration and are very challenging for the anesthesiologist, since compromise of cardiorespiratory functions may be even more significant than that seen with open repairs. The two most obvious challenges are lung compression and significant hypercarbia from CO_2 insufflation, further worsening ventilation and causing respiratory acidosis that increases PVR.

In the open surgical technique, reduction of the diaphragmatic hernia is accomplished through either a left subcostal abdominal incision or a thoracotomy incision. Depending upon the size of the defect, prosthetic material may be used to close the diaphragm. Throughout the intraoperative course, airway pressures should be monitored and maintained below 25–30 cm H_2O to minimize the risk of barotrauma and pneumothorax. After reduction of the herniated contents, an attempt to inflate the hypoplastic lung is not recommended; it is unlikely to expand, and excessive positive airway pressures may damage the contralateral lung. In addition to lung hypoplasia, these neonates are likely to have an underdeveloped abdominal cavity. Hernia reduction can cause increased intraabdominal pressure, with cephalad displacement of the diaphragm, decreased functional residual capacity, and compression of the inferior vena cava. To prevent excessively tight abdominal surgical closures in infants with large defects, it is often necessary to create a ventral hernia (which can be repaired later) and close the skin or place a Silastic pouch.

Postoperative Management

Postoperative management of neonates with CDH presents significant challenges. The long-term outcome of these patients is ultimately determined by the degree of pulmonary hypoplasia. Unfortunately there is no effective treatment for pulmonary hypoplasia.

Esophageal Atresia and Tracheoesophageal Fistula

Esophageal atresia (EA) is the most frequent congenital anomaly of the esophagus, with an approximate incidence of 1 in 4000 neonates (Fig. 30.1). More than 90% of affected individuals have an associated tracheoesophageal fistula (TEF). The most common form of EA/TEF (type C) represents 90% of all cases and presents as a blind upper esophageal pouch and a

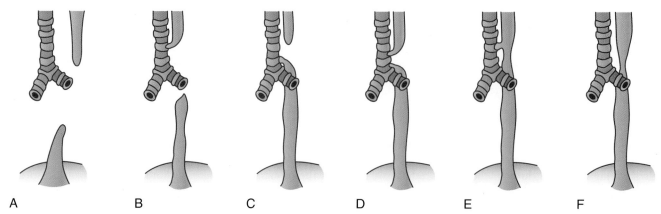

FIG. 30.1 Gross classification of congenital anomalies of the trachea and esophagus. A, Esophageal atresia (EA) without fistula. B, EA with proximal fistula. C, EA with distal fistula. D, EA with proximal and distal fistulas. E, Tracheoesophageal fistula with no EA. F, Esophageal stenosis. (With permission from Holzman RS, Mancuso TJ, Polaner DM. *A Practical Approach to Pediatric Anesthesia.* 1st ed. Philadelphia: Lippincott Williams & Wilkins; 2008:387, Fig. 18.5.)

distal esophagus that connects to the trachea via a fistula tract, typically on the posterior aspect near the carina.

More than 25% of infants with EA have other congenital anomalies, most often with the VATER (*v*ertebral defects, imperforate *a*nus, *t*racheo*e*sophageal fistula, and *r*enal dysplasia) or VACTERL (VATER with *c*ardiac and *l*imb anomalies) associations. TEF and EA are also commonly seen in some chromosomal abnormalities such as trisomy 13, 18, and 21. Approximately 20% of neonates with EA have major congenital heart defects, and 30%–40% are born preterm. Survival of neonates with EA and no associated defects approaches 100%. The mortality of infants with EA/TEF varies depending upon the birth weight and presence of a cardiac anomaly.

Signs and Symptoms

EA should be suspected if maternal polyhydramnios is present. It is usually diagnosed soon after birth when an oral catheter cannot be passed into the stomach or when the neonate exhibits cyanosis, coughing, and choking during oral feedings. Plain radiographs of the chest and abdomen will reveal coiling of a nasogastric tube in the esophageal pouch and possibly an air-filled stomach in the presence of a co-existing TEF. In contrast, pure EA may present as an airless scaphoid abdomen. Infants with an isolated TEF without EA may elude diagnosis until later in life when they may present with recurrent pneumonias and refractory bronchospasm.

Treatment

Initial therapeutic measures include maintaining a patent airway and preventing aspiration of secretions. The infant is fed nothing by mouth, given IV fluids, and placed in a head-up position to minimize regurgitation of gastric secretions through the fistula. Continuous suctioning of the proximal esophageal segment prevents aspiration of oropharyngeal secretions. Endotracheal intubation is avoided if possible because of the potential to worsen distention of the stomach,

which can lead to gastric rupture. One-lung ventilation may be necessary until the stomach can be decompressed.

Primary repair without initial gastrostomy is routine. Repair of a TEF is urgent. However, a thorough evaluation for associated anomalies, particularly congenital heart disease, should be undertaken preoperatively. If the newborn is too unstable for a complete primary repair, a staged approach with an initial gastrostomy under local anesthesia may be all the neonate can safely tolerate.

Management of Anesthesia

Awake intubation with preservation of spontaneous respiration allows for optimal positioning of the ETT while minimizing the risk of ventilatory impairment associated with gastric distention due to positive-pressure ventilation and passage of gases through the fistula. However, awake intubation may be difficult and traumatic in a vigorous infant. Induction of anesthesia can also be done via the inhalational or IV route. Regardless, spontaneous respiration should be maintained as much as possible, with any assisted positive pressure ventilatory maneuvers kept to the lowest possible inspiratory pressures. Use of muscle relaxant should be avoided if possible or at least delayed until decompressive gastrostomy is accomplished. Proper placement of the ETT is critical; it should be above the carina but below the TEF. The ETT must be above the carina because the right lung is compressed during thoracotomy. Low-dose volatile anesthetics in conjunction with air/O_2/opiate are usually well tolerated if the neonate is adequately hydrated. In addition to routine monitors, an arterial catheter may be used for blood gas monitoring. Ligation of the TEF and primary esophageal anastomosis is usually performed via a right thoracotomy. Thoracoscopic approach is also becoming more popular.

Omphalocele and Gastroschisis

Omphalocele and gastroschisis are defects of the anterior abdominal wall that permit external herniation of the

TABLE 30.9	Comparison of Omphalocele and Gastroschisis	
	Omphalocele	Gastroschisis
Gender distribution	Male > female	Male = female
Preterm birth	30%	60%
Location	Within umbilical cord	Periumbilical cord (right)
Sac	Present	Absent
Associated anomalies	>50% (cardiovascular 20%)	Rare
Surgical intervention	Not urgent	Urgent
Prognostic factors	Associated anomalies	Condition of bowel

Adapted from Christison-Lagay ER, Kelleher CM, Langer JC. Neonatal abdominal wall defects. *Semin Fetal Neonatal Med.* 2011;16:164-172, Table 1.

abdominal viscera. They are the most common congenital abdominal wall defects, with important differences between them (Table 30.9).

Signs and Symptoms
Omphalocele
Omphalocele manifests as external herniation of abdominal viscera through the base of the umbilical cord. By definition the defect is larger than 4 cm. A defect smaller than 4 cm is termed an *umbilical hernia.* The abdominal contents are contained within a sac formed by the peritoneal membrane internally and the amniotic membrane externally, without overlying skin. Most cases involve only intestinal herniation, with herniation of liver and intestine occurring half as frequently. Over 50% of cases are associated with other congenital structural (most frequently cardiac anomalies) or chromosomal anomalies. Approximately 30% of neonates with omphaloceles are born preterm. Cardiac defects and prematurity are the major causes of mortality.

Gastroschisis
Gastroschisis manifests as external herniation of abdominal viscera through a small (usually <5 cm) defect in the anterior abdominal wall. In most cases the defect occurs laterally, just to the right of the normally inserted umbilical cord. Unlike an omphalocele, a hernia sac is absent and the exposed viscera is in direct contact with amniotic fluid.

In most cases, only intestines are herniated. Gastroschisis is rarely associated with other congenital anomalies except for intestinal atresia, which occurs in 10% of cases.

Treatment
Gastroschisis requires urgent surgical intervention to limit evaporative and thermal losses. Upon delivery, the exposed viscera is at once covered in warm saline-soaked gauze, with careful positioning of the newborn to prevent kinking of the mesentery. Options for surgical management include traditional primary closure, staged closure with prefabricated silos, and more recently "sutureless" or "plastic closure" repair where the umbilical cord itself is used to cover the abdominal wall defect, which is then allowed to close with epithelialization and granulation over time. The introduction of these sutureless techniques can often avoid intubation and anesthesia in some patients (smaller, uncomplicated defects).

Decompressing the stomach with an oro/nasogastric tube decreases risks of regurgitation, aspiration pneumonia, and further bowel distention. Broad-spectrum antibiotics are started along with fluid resuscitation to replace the large evaporative losses (150–300 mL/kg/day). To address the additional considerable protein loss and third-space fluid translocation, protein-containing solutions (5% albumin) should constitute approximately 25% of the replacement fluids. A urinary catheter should be placed to monitor a goal of 1–2 mL/kg/h of urine output.

Initial medical management of omphalocele is similar to that of gastroschisis. Surgical intervention is essential but not urgent; the hernia sac of an omphalocele defect provides some protection against evaporative and thermal losses. The high incidence of associated congenital anomalies also warrants a thorough preoperative evaluation of the major organ systems, especially the heart. Although primary closure is desirable, it is not possible in most cases, owing to the large defect size and the unacceptable increase in intraabdominal pressure with one-stage reduction. Abdominal compartment syndrome can ensue with respiratory compromise, decreased venous return, poor organ perfusion, anuria, profound acidosis, and bowel necrosis. If primary closure is deemed not feasible, the viscera should be covered with a prosthetic silo and then slowly reduced over a period of several days to 1 week.

Management of Anesthesia
Important aspects of anesthetic management for omphalocele and gastroschisis closure include preservation of normothermia and fluid resuscitation. Intubation is best achieved with a rapid-sequence induction. The ETT should allow for ventilation with PIP greater than 20 cm H_2O. Primary closure may require higher PIPs, at least in the initial postoperative period. Repair of a large defect will require maximal muscle relaxation intraoperatively and during the initial postoperative period. Anesthesia is maintained with volatile anesthetics and/or opioids. Nitrous oxide is avoided because of its potential to hinder hernia reduction from potential bowel distention. These neonates have an underdeveloped abdominal cavity; tight surgical abdominal closure can result in compression of the inferior vena cava and decreased diaphragmatic excursion. Monitoring airway pressures is helpful for detecting changes in pulmonary compliance during abdominal closure. Primary closure is not recommended if inspiratory pressures are above 25–30 cm H_2O or if intravesical or intragastric pressures are above 20 cm H_2O. Any changes in ventilatory parameters and oxygen requirement must be communicated to the surgeon throughout the procedure, because this information will impact the decision to perform primary closure of the abdomen; high ventilatory pressures and excessive FIO_2 are indications for postponing immediate abdominal closure.

Evidence of unacceptably high intraabdominal pressure requires removal of fascial sutures and closure of only the skin or addition of a prosthesis such as a silo. The "silo" consists of a Silastic or Teflon mesh that is sutured to the fascia of the defect. After the silo is in place the herniated viscera is gradually returned to the peritoneal cavity over successive days and can often be done at the bedside without anesthesia. Final closure is typically done in the operating room.

Hirschsprung Disease

Hirschsprung disease, or congenital aganglionic megacolon, is the most common cause of lower intestinal obstruction in full-term neonates. The incidence is approximately 1:5000 live births, with a pronounced male predominance.

Signs and Symptoms
Hirschsprung disease may present at birth as neonatal bowel obstruction or later in childhood as chronic constipation or enterocolitis. Eighty percent of cases are diagnosed during the neonatal period, with a clinical picture of delayed passage of meconium, irritability, bilious vomiting, failure to thrive, and abdominal distention. Definitive diagnosis is obtained via a full-thickness biopsy.

Treatment
The pull-through procedure is the definitive treatment and involves removal of the aganglionic segment followed by reanastomosis of normally innervated bowels, with preservation of anal sphincter function. Laparoscopic assisted transanal pull-through procedures reportedly allow for earlier resumption of enteral feeding, better cosmetic result, less analgesic requirement, and faster time to discharge. Primary pull-through is preferable, but some patients may require an initial decompressive colostomy before definitive repair can take place. The outcome for patients with surgically treated Hirschsprung disease is reasonably good. Most patients attain fecal continence. However, patients with retained or acquired aganglionosis, complications such as severe strictures, dysfunctional bowel, and intestinal neuronal dysplasia may occur, requiring additional surgical treatment.

Management of Anesthesia
In elective cases, general anesthesia may be induced via the inhalational or IV route. Full stomach precautions should be heeded in selected cases, such as that of enterocolitis. Extra care should be taken with positioning, since these operations can be quite lengthy. A lithotomy position is required for anorectal pull-through procedures that involve both abdominal and perineal incisions. IV catheters should be placed in the upper extremities because the lower extremities may be included in the surgical field. Patients may require an initial IV bolus of 10–20 mL/kg of crystalloid to offset the volume deficit resulting from bowel preparation and fasting.

Extubation at the end of surgery is routine. In the absence of regional or neuraxial analgesia, IV opioids along with adjuncts such as acetaminophen and ketorolac are the mainstay of postoperative analgesia. Postoperative fluid requirement may be greater than maintenance in the first 24 hours.

Anorectal Anomalies

The incidence of anorectal malformations is approximately 1:5000 live births. Additional urogenital abnormalities are seen in many of these patients. Imperforate anus without fistula occurs in a small number of patients, especially in association with Down syndrome. Up to 75% of patients with anorectal malformations have other congenital anomalies such as spinal and vertebral defects and congenital cardiac lesions.

Signs and Symptoms
Anorectal malformations are apparent upon examination of the perineum. The neonate may fail to pass meconium in the first 24–48 hours of life. Male infants with imperforate anus usually require emergent surgery (diverting colostomy) to relieve the obstruction. In females the presence of a rectovaginal (rectovestibular) fistula may allow for passage of stool.

Treatment
Preliminary treatment for high lesions is a diverting colostomy followed by a posterior sagittal surgical repair. Low lesions such as perineal fistulas may be repaired during the neonatal period without an initial diverting colostomy. The majority of patients with perineal fistula and rectal atresia can attain full urinary and fecal incontinence after definitive repairs. More severe sacral malformations have significant reconstructive challenges and are associated with a lower rate of full bowel and bladder control.

Management of Anesthesia
Anesthetic management of patients presenting for decompressive colostomy or primary repair should be performed as would be for any infant with distal bowel obstruction. Rapid-sequence induction should be considered if abdominal distention is significant. Definitive anorectal reconstruction is usually performed 1–12 months later. All defects can be repaired through a posterior sagittal approach, although some patients may also require an abdominal incision to mobilize a high rectum or vagina. Extra care should be taken in positioning for these lengthy procedures. Neuromuscular blocking agents should be avoided because electrical muscle stimulation is used throughout the procedure to identify muscle structures and define the anterior and posterior limits of the new anus. Blood and third-space fluid losses are usually moderate. IV catheters should be placed in upper extremities because surgical positioning of the legs may

impede venous return and limit access to the IV catheter insertion sites.

Infantile Hypertrophic Pyloric Stenosis

Infantile hypertrophic pyloric stenosis (IHPS) is the most common cause of intestinal obstruction in infancy. It occurs in approximately 2–4 per 1000 live births and is more common in males than females (4:1), in first born males, in Caucasian infants, and in infants born prematurely compared to term infants.

Signs and Symptoms

IHPS occurs as a result of marked hypertrophy of the circular and longitudinal muscle layers of the pylorus, leading to near-complete obstruction of the gastric outlet. Affected infants typically present with nonbilious forceful or projectile vomiting occurring immediately after feeds. It most commonly occurs between the ages of 3 and 5 weeks and up to 12 weeks; although much less common, it can present earlier or later in life (up to age 6 months). The classic metabolic derangement observed is one of hypochloremic, hypokalemic, metabolic alkalosis resulting from loss of hydrogen, chloride, and potassium ions in gastric contents. The severity of dehydration can be assessed by skin turgor, mucous membranes, anterior fontanelle, urine output (number of wet diapers), and resting vital signs. Degree of serum hypochloremia correlates with severity of fluid and electrolyte loss.

On physical exam, presence of the "olive" sign is pathognomonic and is detected in 50%–90% of affected infants. It can be palpated as a firm mass at the lateral edge of the rectus abdominis muscle in the right upper quadrant. Diagnosis is confirmed by abdominal ultrasonography.

Treatment

IHPS is a medical urgency, not a surgical one. Correction of hydration status and metabolic derangement is of first priority. Severely dehydrated infants should receive an initial IV bolus (20 mL/kg) of isotonic (0.9%) normal saline. Further resuscitation is given as 5% dextrose in 0.22%–0.45% NaCl at up to 1.5–2 times the maintenance rate. Potassium chloride 10–40 mEq/L can be added based on laboratory data when adequate urine output is demonstrated. Fluid resuscitation should be guided by measurement of serum electrolyte concentrations. Once the patient is deemed medically stable, definitive surgical correction can take place.

The traditional open Ramstedt pyloromyotomy is a relatively simple procedure with minimal operative mortality (<0.5%). A longitudinal incision is made in the hypertrophic pylorus and bluntly dissected down to the level of the submucosa. More recently, minimally invasive laparoscopic pyloromyotomy has become the dominant approach in most centers.

Management of Anesthesia

All patients with pyloric stenosis should be regarded as having a full stomach and are at high risk of pulmonary aspiration of gastric contents. The stomach should be emptied as completely as possible with a large-bore orogastric catheter before induction of anesthesia and may require several passes. The airway can secured via awake or rapid-sequence intubation. Recent findings reporting safe use of inhalational induction of anesthesia in the management of pyloric stenosis must be interpreted with great caution. Maintenance of anesthesia is typically carried out with volatile agents. Muscle relaxation may be needed for surgical exposure. After tracheal intubation an orogastric tube is reinserted and left in place during surgery so that air can be insufflated into the stomach to test for mucosal perforation after pyloromyotomy.

For postoperative analgesia, IV or suppository acetaminophen should be strongly considered in additional to local anesthesia infiltration at the incision site(s) administered by the surgeon. Performance of ultrasound-guided regional analgesia, such as transversus abdominis–plane (TAP) block and rectus sheath block, has gained popularity in some centers to provide superior postoperative analgesia.

Extubation is the norm for otherwise healthy patients. However, these infants can experience increased postoperative respiratory depression. Therefore postoperatively, infants should remain in a monitored environment for several hours.

Necrotizing Enterocolitis

Necrotizing enterocolitis (NEC) is characterized by varying degrees of mucosal or transmural necrosis of the intestine, most frequently involving the terminal ileum and proximal colon. It is the most common neonatal medical and surgical emergency. The overall incidence is 1–3:1000 live births, with 90% of cases seen in preterm neonates. The incidence and case fatality rate are inversely related to gestational age and birth weight.

Signs and Symptoms

Sudden feeding intolerance with gastric distention is often the first clue. Other early signs and symptoms include recurrent apnea, lethargy, temperature instability, and glucose instability. More specific clinical manifestations of NEC are abdominal distention, high gastric residuals after feeding, evidence of malabsorption, and bloody or mucoid diarrhea. Metabolic acidosis is very common secondary to generalized peritonitis and hypovolemia. Diagnosis is based on clinical findings and confirmed with abdominal radiography. Pneumatosis intestinalis (gas bubbles in the small intestinal wall) is the hallmark of NEC. Portal venous gas and intraperitoneal free air may also be seen, the latter indicating intestinal perforation.

Treatment

Treatment is based on severity of NEC and its associated symptoms. Medical treatment consisting of empirical broad-spectrum antibiotics and supportive measures is initiated in all patients regardless of stage. Enteral feeding is held until clinical conditions improve, with parenteral nutrition and resuscitative fluid replacement tailored individually. Any existing umbilical arterial catheter should be removed to avoid compromising mesenteric blood flow. NEC carries high mortality, especially when medical management fails, in which case mortality approaches 25%. Some may require repeat bowel resections, predisposing them to short gut syndrome as well as complications from long-term parenteral nutrition.

Management of Anesthesia

As many as 50% of infants with NEC require surgical intervention, and these patients typically present with significant cardiovascular instability. Intraoperative care is often more a resuscitation effort than a general anesthetic. Aggressive fluid resuscitation should take place before induction of anesthesia. If not already intubated, induction should proceed with full stomach precautions and keeping in mind the depleted intravascular volume and possible impaired contractility. An ETT should be chosen to allow ventilation with PIPs above 20 cm H_2O because high intraabdominal pressures and decreased pulmonary compliance are likely to be encountered.

Maintenance of anesthesia is generally limited to short-acting IV opioids (fentanyl) as tolerated and muscle relaxation. There should be vigilant replacement of blood, evaporative, and third-space fluid loss. Of note, rapid fluid administration to preterm neonates may cause intracranial hemorrhage or reopening of the ductus arteriosus. Blood and platelet products should be made readily available, as should vasopressors. A peripheral artery catheter is recommended to monitor systemic blood pressure, arterial blood gases, and other laboratory data to guide fluid and blood products resuscitation. Most patients will require parenteral nutrition, and thus centrally or peripherally inserted central venous catheters should be strongly considered. Postoperative mechanical ventilation is usually required because of abdominal distention and co-existing RDS. Given the high incidence of septicemia, neuraxial analgesia is not recommended. Postoperative pain is usually managed with IV opioids, often as continuous infusions in the NICU.

Biliary Atresia

Biliary atresia is characterized by progressive and relentless obliteration of the extrahepatic bile tree, with resultant bile flow obstruction in the neonatal period. It has an overall incidence of 1:15,000 live births in Europe and North America but is much higher in east Asian countries (e.g., 1:5000 in Taiwan).

Signs and Symptoms

Biliary atresia typically presents in the early weeks after birth with persistent jaundice, dark urine, and acholic stool. Hepatomegaly and splenomegaly can both be seen, but the latter is usually a late sign. Any term infant presenting with jaundice for more than 14 days should be evaluated for underlying hepatobiliary disease. Specifically, conjugated hyperbilirubinemia is usually indicative of biliary pathologies. If left untreated, liver cirrhosis ensues, and death occurs by age 2 years. Initial diagnostic evaluation includes laboratory testing (bilirubin, transaminase, liver synthetic function tests, γ-glutamyltransferase) and ultrasonography. Endoscopic retrograde cholangiopancreatography (ERCP) and even magnetic resonance cholangiopancreatography (MRCP) are occasionally performed. Diagnosis is confirmed by liver biopsy.

Treatment

The Kasai procedure (hepatoportoenterostomy) and liver transplantation are the cornerstones of treatment for biliary atresia. The Kasai procedure involves excision of the porta hepatis to expose microscopic ductular continuity that allows for bile flow and is best performed by 8 weeks of age (Fig. 30.2). Although hepatoportoenterostomy can achieve complete resolution of jaundice and restoration of hepatic metabolic and synthetic functions, progressive inflammation of the hepatobiliary tree typically leads to recurrence of bile flow obstruction. Up to 50% of patients who have undergone the Kasai procedure will require liver transplantation by age 2.

Management of Anesthesia

Preoperative evaluation and correction of coagulopathy is important. If significant ascites is present, a rapid-sequence induction is indicated. Adequate venous access is vital, and if it cannot be obtained, a central venous catheter should be placed. A peripheral arterial catheter is strongly recommended for both hemodynamic monitoring and frequent blood sampling to guide anesthetic and fluid management.

Anesthesia can be maintained with low doses of inhaled agents along with opioids and muscle relaxants. Nitrous oxide should be avoided. Blood loss can be moderate to severe; evaporative fluid loss is invariably significant. The infant should receive postoperative care in an ICU setting. If blood and evaporative losses were small, combined with a stable hemodynamic profile, consideration can be given to early extubation after the Kasai procedure. In many cases, postoperative mechanical ventilation is appropriate.

CENTRAL NERVOUS SYSTEM DISORDERS

Cerebral Palsy

Cerebral palsy (CP) is a heterogeneous group of nonprogressive disorders with kinetic and postural abnormalities. Etiologies may differ, but the representative phenotype of motor dysfunction results from abnormalities that occurred in the *developing* brain. Being a *nonprogressive disorder* of the central nervous system (CNS), CP is also termed *static encephalopathy*. Clinical expression will vary over the course of the child's lifetime with postnatal brain development. Seizure activity and additional disturbances of sensation, perception, cognition, and behavior are common.

NORMAL

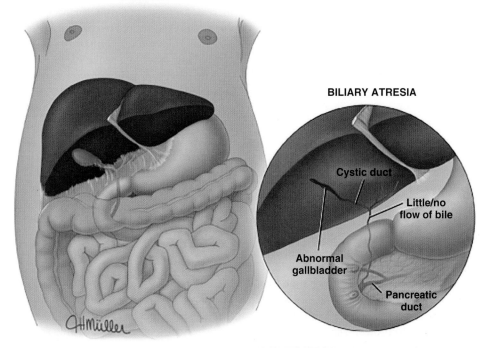

BILIARY ATRESIA

Cystic duct

Little/no
flow of bile

Abnormal
gallbladder

Pancreatic
duct

KASAI PROCEDURE

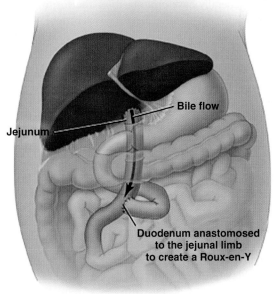

Bile flow

Jejunum

Duodenum anastomosed
to the jejunal limb
to create a Roux-en-Y

FIG. 30.2 Kasai hepatoportoenterostomy. (Reproduced with permission from Erlichman J, Loomes KM. Biliary atresia. http://www.uptodate.com/contents/biliary-atresia. Copyright © 2015 UpToDate, Inc.)

Signs and Symptoms

CP is classified based on the resting tone, extremities involved, and the presence of kinetic abnormalities. Spastic types of CP are the most common. Affected individuals manifest initial hypotonia (usually from age 6 months to 1 year) that later changes into spasticity. True hypotonic CP is rare. A history of gross motor delays is almost universal and is commonly associated with delays in reaching other milestones (fine motor, language, social interaction). Intelligence can range from normal to being severely impaired.

Truncal (postural) tone is often affected, with resultant spinal curvature deformities such as scoliosis. There is a high incidence of gastroesophageal reflux; bulbar and oromotor dysfunction can lead to recurrent aspiration events. Spasticity-induced contractures may require medical therapy (baclofen, dantrolene, botulinum toxin A injection) or surgical intervention. Dysfunctional voiding and even neurogenic bladder are seen in 30%–60% of cases. Seizure disorder is common.

Diagnosis is mostly based on a constellation of clinical findings over the course of months as symptoms surface with brain maturation. There should also be a thorough investigation of the prenatal, perinatal, postnatal, and intrapartum maternal history.

Management of Anesthesia

Patients with CP can present for a variety of surgical procedures ranging from brief dental restoration to complex posterior spinal fusion for scoliosis repair. There is no single best anesthetic plan, because each patient will have different CP-related concerns; almost any anesthetic technique can be used. CP is not associated with malignant hyperthermia. Succinylcholine is not contraindicated but should be used with discretion. In general, children with CP require a lower MAC of volatile anesthetics and have a longer emergence time than their healthy counterparts. Low pharyngeal tone and a high incidence of gastroesophageal reflux call for a low threshold for endotracheal intubation to protect against aspiration, even for brief procedures. Muscle relaxants should be used with caution because these patients generally have prolonged recovery from neuromuscular blockade. Positioning can be difficult, especially if contractures are severe. For those with seizure disorders, drug-drug interactions (e.g., cytochrome P450 induction by antiepileptics) and epileptogenic effects of some anesthetic agents (etomidate, ketamine) must be kept in mind.

Postoperative pain management can be challenging, especially for children whose verbal skills are impaired. Diazepam is an important adjunct in managing spasticity-related pain.

Supplemental regional and epidural analgesia are ideal in providing superior pain control while limiting systemic exposure to drugs with respiratory depressant effects.

Hydrocephalus

Hydrocephalus is a disorder of cerebrospinal fluid (CSF) accumulation that results in ventricular dilatation due to increased intracranial pressure (ICP). Accumulation of CSF in hydrocephalus is due to an imbalance between CSF production and absorption. Hydrocephalus has many causes and can be congenital or acquired.

Signs and Symptoms

Hydrocephalus can be acute, subacute, or chronic. The rate of CSF accumulation and the compliance of the CNS determine the clinical presentation; in general, symptoms are nonspecific. If hydrocephalus occurs before the closure of cranial sutures (between 18 and 24 months of age), the rise in ICP is generally mitigated by expansion of the intracranial space. Once cranial sutures have closed, rapid increase in ICP can occur.

In neonates and infants, hydrocephalus most often manifests as macrocephaly. The anterior fontanelle can be full or

bulging and scalp veins may be prominent secondary to increased venous pressure. Headaches along with nausea and vomiting result from stretching of the meninges and intracranial vessels. Infants are initially irritable, followed by progressive lethargy with increasing ICP.

Any newborn or infant with an enlarged head should be evaluated for hydrocephalus. Serial head circumference measurement is an easy and effective means of monitoring the progression of hydrocephalus. Most infants can be managed conservatively if head circumference increases at a slow and steady rate, unless accompanied by clinical symptoms. Any rapid increase in size usually requires surgical intervention even if the child is largely asymptomatic. Diagnosis is confirmed with neuroimaging (head ultrasonography for newborns, computed tomography [CT] and magnetic resonance imaging [MRI] for infants and older children).

Treatment

Medical therapy mainly consists of diuretic treatment (furosemide and acetazolamide decrease CSF production), although this remains controversial in children. Serial lumbar punctures have also been tried but only as a temporizing measure. The majority of children require surgical treatment either in the form of shunt placement or shuntless endoscopic third ventriculostomy (ETV). The former consists of placing a catheter into the lateral ventricle that is connected to a one-way-valve shunt system that drains into the peritoneal space, right atrium, or more rarely the pleural space. Shunt malfunction can be due to infection or mechanical failure and occurs most frequently in the first year of placement (≈40% failure rate). ETV is most successful in children older than 1 year.

Management of Anesthesia

The most important anesthetic considerations in the child with hydrocephalus relate to the presence and severity of increased ICP. Changes in position (head down, head flexion), behavior (crying), and physiology (hypercarbia) can all adversely affect ICP. As such, the child should be kept in a head-up position with as few agitating maneuvers as possible. A delicate balance must be struck between promoting calmness with pharmacologic means and minimizing the risk of hypoventilation. A careful preoperative assessment consisting of history, current clinical symptoms, and physical examination usually provides the most useful information about the severity of ICP and its impact on the child's neurologic status.

Inhalational induction may be acceptable in the child without clinical and/or radiographic evidence of severe intracranial hypertension. Volatile agents are potent cerebral vasodilators and increase ICP. This can be attenuated by preinduction hyperventilation, but this is not an easily accomplished or feasible task in most children. Children with significantly elevated ICP are usually lethargic, which permits easier awake IV catheter placement. With the exception of ketamine, virtually all IV anesthetic agents lower ICP and generally preserve cerebral perfusion pressure better than volatile agents. Ketamine is contraindicated because it can precipitate sudden increase in

ICP and rapid neurologic decompensation. The neurophysiologic effects of dexmedetomidine, an α_2-agonist, is not as well understood. Succinylcholine may be used if necessary; it can increase CBF and ICP, but the effects are transient and can be attenuated by premedication with a "defasciculating" dose of nondepolarizing muscle relaxant.

Continuation of muscle relaxation is necessary to prevent patient movement during surgical access to the intracranial ventricles. Normocapnia should be maintained for patients with normal ICP, whereas mild hypocapnia is helpful to prevent further increases in ICP; severe hypocapnia can precipitate cerebral ischemia. Invasive blood pressure monitoring is not needed in most cases of shunt surgery or ETV but may be useful to help guide anesthetic management that optimizes cerebral perfusion pressure, particularly if an ICP monitor is in place (CPP = MAP − ICP).

Finally, positional changes can have serious consequences. Extreme positioning of the head (flexion, lateral rotation) can cause further displacement of any structural abnormality (e.g., Chiari malformation) and also impair venous drainage, leading to increased ICP.

Spina Bifida

Spina bifida is the most common form of neural tube defect (Fig. 30.3), characterized by a cleft in the spinal column; this results from abnormal fusion of one or more vertebral posterior arches. This cleft can be covered by normal appearing skin, resulting in a hidden defect (*spina bifida occulta*) without involvement of the underlying neural structures. Meninges can herniate through the spinal cleft, creating a CSF-filled sac (*meningocele*) with or without skin covering. More often, both the spinal cord and meninges herniate (*myelomeningocele*) through the spinal cleft, forming a defect that lacks skin and sometimes dural covering.

Signs and Symptoms

Clinical presentation varies widely and depends on the neural elements involved and severity of the defect. *Spina bifida occulta,* as its name implies, is sometimes discovered only incidentally because normal skin hides the defect and the mild spinal cleft does not usually cause neurologic deficits. In most cases, however, the overlying skin displays an abnormal lesion

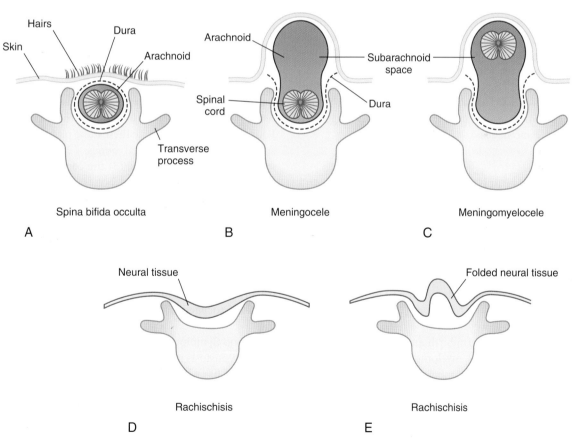

FIG. 30.3   Neural tube defects. A, Spina bifida occulta—a bony defect only, covered by skin or skin with hair. B, Meningocele—protrusion of a fluid-filled sac only (no neural tissue present). C, Meningomyelocele—protrusion of a fluid-filled sac plus neural tissue. D and E, Rachischisis—defects characterized by an open neural tube. (With permission from Holzman RS, Mancuso TJ, Polaner DM. *A Practical Approach to Pediatric Anesthesia.* 1st ed. Philadelphia: Lippincott Williams & Wilkins; 2008:203, Fig. 12.7.)

such as a dimple, hair patch, dermal sinus tract, hemangioma, or lipoma, the presence of which should alert the clinician of possible underlying spinal column and/or cord anomalies (e.g., tethered cord).

Meningoceles are normally diagnosed prenatally by fetal ultrasound or at birth by the presence of a dorsal spine mass. By definition, only the meninges are affected, without nerve tissue involvement. As such, these patients display little if any neurologic deficits and are not at noticeable risk for developing long-term neurologic sequelae. Once the meningocele is discovered, expeditious surgical repair is needed to prevent sac injury, infection, and CSF leak. Although nerves are not involved, there can be nerve root entrapment by fibrous bands in the sac. Thus nerve injury is a potential problem during surgical sac ligation.

Myelomeningocele is the most common type of spina bifida, where there is extrusion of the spinal cord into the herniated meningeal sac; oftentimes the spinal cord ends in the sac, with the spinal canal exposed in a splayed-open fashion known as the *neural placode.* Children born with a myelomeningocele have varying degrees of motor and sensory deficits as well as bowel and bladder dysfunction. Any damage to the cord and spinal nerves evident at birth is usually irreversible. Over 90% of children with a myelomeningocele also have a Chiari II malformation (also known as *Arnold-Chiari malformation*), which consists of caudal displacement of the cerebellar vermis, fourth ventricle, and the medulla down through the foramen magnum into the cervical spinal canal. Hydrocephalus and other developmental brain abnormalities are also common. Additionally, myelomeningoceles are associated with a high incidence of cardiac, esophageal, intestinal, renal, urogenital, and orthopedic anomalies.

Treatment

Meticulous care at birth is needed to prevent sac rupture and damage to the spinal cord. The defect should be covered with saline-soaked sponges, with lateral or prone positioning of the newborn to prevent compression. Nonlatex gloves should be worn to avoid latex sensitization. Surgical closure usually takes place within 24–48 hours of birth. Compared to postnatal repair, intrauterine repair of myelomeningocele has been associated with a lower rate of shunt surgery for hydrocephalus, as well as a lower rate of death at 12 months' postnatal age. Prenatal surgery, however, is only offered at a few centers and is associated with preterm birth and maternal morbidity. The majority of children with myelomeningocele have lifelong motor and sensory neurologic impairment as well as fecal and urinary incontinence.

Management of Anesthesia

Positioning is one of the first critical steps in perioperative care of the child with spina bifida defects. Maintaining the patient in the prone or lateral decubitus position is essential to avoid sac and nerve injury, particularly for myelomeningoceles. In some cases the patient may be elevated on soft rolls or a donut-shaped gel support to avoid compression of the

defect, allowing for endotracheal intubation in the supine position. Some defects may be too large to risk supine positioning, and the anesthesiologist must always be prepared for a potentially difficult intubation with lateral positioning. Surgical repair is always performed with the patient in the prone position. As such, meticulous attention must be paid to avoid compression injury to the eyes, brachial plexus, and any ventral defects such as bladder exstrophy, as well as compression of the inferior vena cava that can lead to impaired venous return.

A comprehensive preoperative assessment is necessary to identify specific anesthetic risks; myelomeningoceles are often associated with other congenital anomalies. Although an Arnold-Chiari malformation is present in almost all cases of myelomeningocele, clinically significant increases in ICP are rare, but this must always be a consideration in anesthetic management. Respiratory insufficiency and apnea (due to potential brainstem compression) are also important perioperative concerns. Intraoperative neuromonitoring is usually carried out to guide surgical repair. As such, an anesthetic plan that minimizes signal interference is important. Blood and evaporative fluid loss can be significant. This is especially true for large defects that require extensive skin undermining for closure.

Craniosynostosis

Craniosynostosis is defined as premature closure of one or more cranial sutures. At birth the cranium consists of "floating" bone plates that allow for rapid postnatal brain growth, requiring a proportionate increase in the intracranial space. Four major sutures separate these bone plates: (1) the metopic suture separates the frontal bones, (2) the sagittal suture separates the parietal bones, (3) the coronal suture separates the frontal from the parietal bones, and (4) the lambdoid suture separates the parietal bones from the occipital bone (Fig. 30.4). One or more sutures can be affected, and over 50% of cases involve the sagittal suture. The "cloverleaf" skull deformity, also known as *kleeblattschädel,* is the most severe type of craniosynostosis, where all sutures except the metopic and squamosal are fused. Single-suture craniosynostosis is usually an isolated finding, whereas multiple-suture closure is often associated with other skull base suture abnormalities.

Signs and Symptoms

Craniosynostosis is usually evident at birth or during the first 2 years of life when rapid brain growth takes place. Increase in ICP occurs when brain growth continues against a nonexpanding calvarium. As such, increased ICP is not usually seen in secondary craniosynostosis, since there is little to no brain growth. Craniosynostosis involving one or even two sutures is not generally associated with increased ICP, because the brain can still expand in at least one other direction. Premature closure of multiple sutures frequently leads to increased ICP; children may present with lethargy, nausea, vomiting, and papilledema.

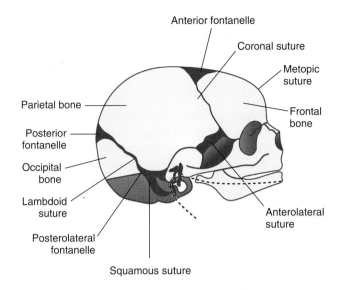

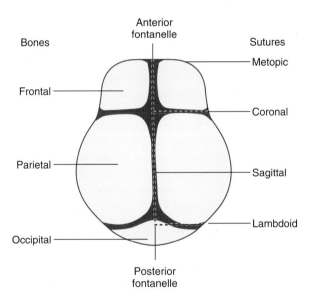

FIG. 30.4 Cranial sutures and fontanelles. (With permission from Holzman RS, Mancuso TJ, Polaner DM. *A Practical Approach to Pediatric Anesthesia*. 1st ed. Philadelphia: Lippincott Williams & Wilkins; 2008:225, Fig. 14.2.)

Most cases of nonsyndromic craniosynostosis (only one or two sutures affected) only pose cosmetic concerns with no physiologic sequelae. However, the physical deformity can adversely impact the child's psychological and social development if left untreated. Multiple-suture craniosynostosis is often associated with some degree of intellectual delay as well as hydrocephalus.

Treatment

Surgical repair can be done endoscopically (strip craniectomy) or may involve extensive calvarial reconstruction, depending on the deformity. Timing of repair is surgeon dependent and can vary between early and late infancy. Regardless, surgical correction is preferably done before the age of 1 year to take advantage of a malleable skull, optimize potential for reossification, and decrease the risk of neurologic damage, since this time period confers the greatest neural plasticity. Early intervention is also necessary to provide room for rapid brain growth during the first 2 years of life.

Management of Anesthesia

Anesthetic management must be tailored to the presence of any concomitant congenital anomalies and potential intracranial hypertension. Syndromic craniosynostosis often have other craniofacial abnormalities (midface and mandibular hypoplasia) that can make airway management extremely challenging; difficult airway equipment must be available accordingly.

Once the trachea is intubated, controlled ventilation should be set to maintain normocarbia unless hypocarbia is needed to minimize preexisting intracranial hypertension. Large-bore IV access is necessary, and insertion of an intraarterial catheter is preferred. Even with endoscopic strip craniectomy procedures, excessive blood loss can occur. Significant blood loss is usually the norm in open cranial vault reconstructive procedures (as high as one-half to one blood volume in the majority of cases). Blood products must be immediately available before skin incision. Cell salvage should be done, even for small infants, because relevant cell saver reservoir sizes (as small as 25 mL) are now available. Use of antifibrinolytics such as aminocaproic acid and tranexamic acid have shown success in reducing intraoperative blood loss and decreasing transfusion.

Other major intraoperative concerns include hypothermia, hypovolemia, and venous air embolism. Some practitioners elect to place a central venous catheter to evacuate air from the right atrium should a large venous air embolism occur. However, the small-sized catheter used in infants does not permit rapid air evacuation. Precordial Doppler has a high sensitivity for detecting venous air embolism before hemodynamic changes are evident. Nitrous oxide should be avoided.

Significant periorbital and facial edema can occur and may preclude immediate extubation. However, most infants, unless there are concomitant craniofacial anomalies, can be considered for immediate extubation if the edema is limited to the upper half of the face. In general, postoperative care in the ICU is preferred.

CRANIOFACIAL ANOMALIES

Cleft Lip and Palate

Orofacial clefts are a heterogeneous group of tissue approximation defects manifesting as cleft lip, cleft lip and palate, and cleft palate. These defects can occur in isolation or in association with a congenital syndrome.

Cleft palate results from partial or complete failure of the apposition and fusion of the palatal shelves that normally occurs between 8 and 12 weeks' gestation. *Complete cleft palate* involves cleft defects of the uvula, soft palate, and hard palate. In some cases the hard palate defect may be covered by a mucous membrane that may extend to partially cover the soft palate cleft as well; this is termed *submucous cleft palate.*

Signs and Symptoms

Newborns with orofacial clefts should have immediate evaluation and early referral to a craniofacial specialist. The child may be at risk for aspiration and airway obstruction, particularly if additional craniofacial anomalies are present. Feeding difficulty is universal because the cleft defect prevents the generation of adequate negative pressure necessary for sucking. As such, failure to thrive is a common problem in these children. Special feeding bottles and nipples are designed to help restore a more effective and energy-efficient feeding process. A multidisciplinary team consisting of physicians, dentist, nutritionist, and speech therapist is recommended to address the physical and psychological concerns that arise in different developmental stages of childhood.

Cleft palates are associated with a higher incidence of otitis media because abnormal palatal muscle insertion impairs middle ear drainage. Myringotomy with ear tube placement is generally performed at a lower threshold in these children.

Treatment

Cleft lip repair is typically performed between 6 and 12 weeks of age to restore normal feeding, whereas cleft palate repair is done later, between 9 and 14 months. Timing of cleft palate repair is aimed at preventing further speech abnormalities and at minimizing facial growth distortion (as can occur if repair is done too early).

Management of Anesthesia

Children with cleft lip or palate can undergo inhalational or IV induction of anesthesia. Concurrent cleft lip and palate defects as well as syndromic orofacial clefts may portend a difficult intubation. If a laryngeal mask airway (LMA) is considered to assist with intubation, placement of the device must be done carefully to prevent disruption of any previous cleft palate repairs.

Preformed oral right-angle endotracheal (RAE) tubes are preferred for their low profile and better fit with the retractor used during surgery. Meticulous attention must be paid to securing the ETT because frequent surgical manipulations predispose to unintentional extubation. Cleft repair may also be done in positions that increase the risk of unplanned extubation (e.g., Rose position; the patient's head is pulled over the edge of the operating table and placed in the surgeon's lap).

Significant edema of the tongue, palate, and pharyngeal tissues can occur from compression by the mouth retractor and may preclude immediate extubation. Placement of a nasopharyngeal airway by the surgeon in patients with known difficult airway or anticipated difficult extubation may be helpful in some cases.

Pain control must be balanced with the risk of respiratory depression. IV or rectal acetaminophen as well as regional anesthesia (infraorbital blocks) should be considered.

Mandibular Hypoplasia

Hypoplasia of the mandible is a common congenital anomaly. The majority occur as part of a congenital syndrome; nonsyndromic isolates are rare. Airway compromise is universal; the constricted mandibular space displaces the tongue posteriorly to cause airway obstruction. The following is a discussion of several congenital disorders that share mandibular hypoplasia as a prominent feature.

Pierre-Robin Sequence

Pierre-Robin sequence (PRS), previously termed *Pierre-Robin syndrome,* consists of the triad of micrognathia (small mandible) or retrognathia (posterior displacement of mandible), glossoptosis, and airway obstruction. Cleft palate is present in the majority of cases. PRS can be syndromic or nonsyndromic. Associated congenital disorders include Stickler syndrome, velocardiofacial syndrome, hemifacial microsomia, and fetal alcohol syndrome.

Affected newborns present with varying degrees of airway obstruction and feeding difficulties. Intervention is mostly aimed at restoring airway patency and can range from maneuvers as simple as lateral or prone positioning to surgical treatment involving tongue-lip adhesion, mandibular distraction osteogenesis, and tracheostomy. A swallowing evaluation should also be undertaken. In the absence of intrinsic skeletal growth deficiency, airway obstruction improves overtime with mandibular growth.

Hemifacial Microsomia

Hemifacial microsomia (HFM) is the one of the most common congenital facial anomalies (second only to cleft lip and palate). It is a facial asymmetry disorder affecting unilateral bone, muscle, and soft tissue structures. HFM typically affects the lower half of the face and is associated with prominent hypoplasia of the malar-maxillary-mandibular complex, with variable involvement of the ear, temporomandibular joint, and orbit, as well as the cervical spine. Goldenhar syndrome (oculoauricular-vertebral syndrome [OAV]) can be considered the most severe form of syndromic HFM, characterized by colobomas and vertebral anomalies in addition to facial asymmetry.

Treacher Collins Syndrome

Treacher Collins Syndrome (TCS), also known as *mandibulofacial dysostosis* (defective ossification or formation of bone), is a rare autosomal dominant disorder of craniofacial anomaly with variable expression. TCS facies features downward-sloping palpebral fissures, small/absent cheekbones, a normal-sized nose that may appear large with background hypoplasia, malformed pinnae, ear tags, abnormal external auditory canal, and receding chin. Occasionally, choanal atresia may be present. Intelligence is usually not affected unless hearing loss is not promptly addressed. A small percentage of patients with TCS may have concomitant congenital heart disease.

Immediate concerns revolve around establishing airway patency; tracheostomy may be indicated at birth. Swallowing difficulties lead to failure to thrive, and early gastrostomy is frequently needed for feeding. Children with TCS typically require multiple craniofacial and dental corrective surgeries throughout their childhood and adolescence.

Management of Anesthesia

Concerns central to perioperative care of patients with mandibular hypoplasia relate mainly to airway management. Concomitant congenital anomalies, especially cardiac lesions, must also be considered.

Patients with mandibular hypoplasia, especially in association with TCS and HFM, are not only difficult to intubate but may be almost impossible to mask ventilate. Therefore it is not always feasible to perform endotracheal intubation after induction of general anesthesia. When anesthesia can be safely induced, preservation of spontaneous respiration is critical before the airway is secured. Maneuvers to pull the tongue forward are helpful, since glossoptosis is a major component of airway obstruction. An LMA may serve well to assist with ventilation and as a conduit for intubation. Intubating LMA devices such as the Air-Q now exist in pediatric sizes that accommodate most neonates and infants. Direct laryngoscopy is generally difficult and unsuccessful. Alternative means for visualizing the vocal cords (e.g., fiberoscope, video laryngoscope, optical laryngoscope) must be ready for use from the outset. Some surgical treatment approaches may require nasotracheal intubation.

Drugs with respiratory depressant effects should be used sparingly. Nonopioid analgesic adjuncts and local anesthetic should be considered whenever possible. Timing of extubation is as important as initial airway management, since there may be significant postsurgical edema.

Midface Hypoplasia

Disorders with midface hypoplasia result in underdevelopment of the eye sockets, cheekbones, and upper jaw. Growth deficiency of the midface gives the characteristic concave appearance with wide set eyes (hypertelorism), proptosis, flattened nasal bridge, and a large underbite. As a result of crowding of midfacial structures, these patients often experience malocclusion and obstructive sleep apnea; proptosis increases the risk of keratoconjunctivitis.

Apert Syndrome

Apert syndrome is a rare inherited disorder (autosomal dominant) characterized by acrocephalosyndactyly. The cranium, midface, and the bones and soft tissues of the hands and feet are affected. The result is a combination of craniosynostosis, midface hypoplasia, and symmetric syndactyly of the extremities,

with cutaneous and bony fusion. Turribrachycephaly (towering skull deformity), hypertelorism, and low-set ears are also prominent features.

Most patients with Apert syndrome experience some degree of airway obstruction due to small nasopharyngeal and oropharyngeal dimensions, particularly if choanal atresia and/or tracheal stenosis are present. Obstructive sleep apnea is common and must be addressed early to avoid development of cor pulmonale. Eye complaints include proptosis with risk of corneal injury, amblyopia, strabismus, and optic nerve atrophy.

Crouzon Syndrome

Crouzon syndrome shares many clinical features with Apert syndrome, but the viscera and extremities are spared. Also known as *craniofacial dysostosis* (malformation of the face and skull bones), it is a hereditary disorder (autosomal dominant) characterized by craniosynostosis, midface hypoplasia, mandibular prognathism, and shallow eye sockets with hypertelorism and proptosis. As a result of frequent premature fusion of the coronal sutures, brachycephaly (short and broad head) is usually seen. Intellectual delay is not an intrinsic part of Crouzon syndrome but may occur secondary to increased ICP and hearing impairment. Conductive hearing loss is common and due to ear canal abnormalities (atresia or stenosis). Airway obstructive problems are similar to those seen in Apert syndrome.

Management of Anesthesia

Patients with midface hypoplasia typically present to the operating room for midface advancement procedures, adenotonsillectomy, and cranial vault reconstruction if craniosynostosis is present. Some may require tracheostomy at an early age to establish airway patency.

Both mask ventilation and tracheal intubation may be extremely difficult, especially if there are cervical spine abnormalities that limit neck extension. A plan for difficult airway management must be prepared thoughtfully.

Special attention must be paid to avoid injury to the proptotic eyes. A history of headache, vomiting, and somnolence should raise suspicion of increased ICP. Lastly, IV access may be extremely difficult in patients with Apert syndrome, depending on the severity of syndactyly.

UPPER AIRWAY DISORDERS

Acute Epiglottitis (Supraglottitis)

Historically the most common cause of epiglottitis infection was *Haemophilus influenzae* type B (HIB). This infection is now much less common in developed countries, owing to HIB immunization in children. Vaccination has shifted the median age of presentation from 3 years to between 6 and 12 years. Epiglottitis can also occur in other age groups, including adults.

Although much less common, epiglottitis may occur as a result of trauma/injury. Acute epiglottitis, also termed

TABLE 30.10   Clinical Features of Epiglottitis and Laryngotracheobronchitis

Parameter	Acute Epiglottitis	Laryngotracheobronchitis
Age group affected	2–6 yr[a]	<2 yr
Incidence	Accounts for 5% of children with stridor	Accounts for ≈ 80% of children with stridor
Etiologic agent	Bacterial	Viral
Onset	Rapid over 24 h	Gradual over 24–72 h
Signs and symptoms	4 Ds (dysphagia, dysphonia, dyspnea, drooling) High fever, tripod position	Inspiratory stridor, "barking" cough, rhinorrhea, mild fever (rarely >39°C)
Cell counts	Neutrophilia	Lymphocytosis
Lateral neck radiograph	Swollen epiglottis ("thumb sign")	Subglottic narrowing ("steeple sign")
Treatment	O_2, urgent tracheal intubation or tracheostomy during general anesthesia, fluids, antibiotics, corticosteroids (?)	O_2, aerosolized racemic epinephrine, humidity, fluids, corticosteroids, tracheal intubation for severe airway obstruction

[a]Median age of presentation is 6–12 years in postvaccination era.

supraglottitis, is a life-threatening infection of the epiglottis and adjacent supraglottic structures. Specifically it is a cellulitis of the stratified squamous epithelium of these structures, including the lingular surface of the epiglottis, the aryepiglottic folds, and the arytenoids. Occasionally the uvula is also affected. Subglottic structures are generally spared.

Signs and Symptoms

The classic presentation is a toxic-appearing, agitated child with a high fever and the "4 Ds" (dysphagia, dysphonia, dyspnea, and drooling), history of severe sore throat, and muffled voice. Typical upper respiratory infection (URI) symptoms such as rhinorrhea and cough are usually absent. A croupy cough may rarely be present and may confuse the clinical picture with laryngotracheobronchitis (Table 30.10). The child often assumes a characteristic "tripod" posture with the trunk leaning forward supported by the arms and a hyperextended neck with the chin thrust forward in an effort to maximize airflow. Inspiratory stridor is a late feature and is evidence of impending complete upper airway obstruction. The course of acute epiglottitis, particularly in small children, can deteriorate rapidly and may be fatal within 6–12 hours of presentation. Diagnosis is based principally on the clinical picture. When a lateral neck radiograph is done, it typically shows the "thumb sign," representing the shadow created by a swollen epiglottis obstructing the airway. Airway obstruction is the primary concern. Other complications of epiglottitis include epiglottic abscess, secondary infections (e.g., pneumonia, cervical adenitis, meningitis, bacteremia), and necrotizing epiglottitis.

Historically, placement of an artificial airway was universally employed. Since the median age of presentation has increased, with a concomitant increase in baseline airway caliber, selected cases may be monitored without intubation. Humidified oxygen should be administered as needed. Empirical antibiotic therapy should be initiated in all cases. Use of glucocorticoids has remained controversial.

Management of Anesthesia

Airway management is the principal goal, and care should involve both an anesthesiologist and an otolaryngologist. The child should be kept in the tripod posture. Unnecessary physical examination and IV access should be deferred until definitive airway protection is established. Expeditious transfer of the patient to the operating room by personnel with expert airway management skills is essential. Equipment for standard intubation, difficult airway, and possible emergent tracheostomy/needle cricothyrotomy must be immediately available. Styletted ETTs in 1–2 sizes smaller than that predicted for the child's age must be prepared because the airway caliber will invariably be reduced.

Anesthesia is induced via inhalation with the child in a sitting position. A calm induction with preservation of spontaneous respiration is critical. Application of moderate CPAP (10–15 cm H_2O) can help minimize further reduction in airway caliber from collapse of the pharyngeal soft tissues with anesthesia induction. Once the child is adequately anesthetized, IV access can be established, followed by direct laryngoscopy and orotracheal intubation. An air leak around the ETT (<25 cm H_2O) must be demonstrated to prevent additional tracheal damage.

Postoperative ICU care is mandatory. Timing of extubation depends on resolution of clinical signs and symptoms (resolution of fever, neutrophilia, and increasing air leak around the ETT) confirmed by repeat examination of the supraglottic structures with direct vision or flexible fiberoscopy. In most cases the child can be extubated in 24–48 hours after initiation of appropriate therapy.

Croup (Laryngotracheitis/Laryngotracheobronchitis)

Croup is a common infectious disease of the subglottic airway structures, including but not limited to the larynx and trachea. Croup is primarily a *viral* infection of the *subglottic* structures. The term "croup" has been used in the general literature to describe a variety of upper airway disorders including laryngitis, laryngotracheitis, laryngotracheobronchitis, bacterial tracheitis, and spasmodic croup. For the purpose of this discussion, *croup* refers to laryngotracheitis and laryngotracheobronchitis (involvement of the bronchi in addition to the larynx and trachea); the two are often clinically indistinguishable.

Signs and Symptoms

Croup most frequently occurs between 6 months and 3 years of age, with a peak incidence around the second year of life. In contrast to epiglottitis, croup has a more gradual onset. The child usually presents with a history of rhinorrhea, cough, sore throat, and low-grade fever that progresses to the distinctive barky or seal-like cough along with hoarse voice and inspiratory stridor. Symptoms are worse in the supine position, and thus the child with croup prefers to sit or be held upright.

Diagnosis is made clinically; radiologic and laboratory confirmatory tests are not needed. When radiographs are performed, one may see the classic *steeple sign* on an anteroposterior projection, which represents a long area of narrowing in the subglottic region. However, radiographic findings are not pathognomonic and do not correlate well with clinical severity. Inspiratory stridor is the key element in determining disease severity.

Treatment

For much of the 20th century, mist therapy (humidified air) was the cornerstone of the management of croup. This has been replaced by corticosteroid and nebulized epinephrine treatment. Steroids have proven to be effective in all cases of croup; they have emerged as the single most important outpatient treatment of croup and have significantly reduced the overall need for hospitalization. Experts recommend routine administration of corticosteroids in the treatment of croup; the most cited regimens are (1) single-dose dexamethasone (0.6 mg/kg orally or intramuscularly) and (2) nebulized budesonide (2 mg in 4 mL of water). There is still some debate over the benefit of single versus multiple doses of corticosteroids, as well as the exact dose of dexamethasone required (0.15 mg/kg vs. 0.6 mg/kg). Children with severe croup should also receive one or more nebulized epinephrine treatments (0.5 mL of 2.25% racemic epinephrine in 4.5 mL of normal saline or L-epinephrine diluted in 5 mL of normal saline at a ratio of 1:1000). Even if planned for potential discharge, children should be observed for at least 2–4 hours after the last nebulized epinephrine treatment for possible return of obstructive symptoms.

Croup is generally a self-limited infection that lasts approximately 72 hours. However, life-threatening airway obstruction can rarely occur (<1%), requiring endotracheal intubation. As in the case of acute epiglottitis, children with croup should be intubated with a smaller ETT than that predicted for their age, given the expected subglottic narrowing. Timing of extubation will depend on resolution of croup symptoms as well as treatment of any associated complications such as bacterial superinfection of the lower airways. Of note, children with recurrent croup should be evaluated for occult conditions such as subglottic stenosis, laryngeal clefts, and laryngomalacia.

TABLE 30.11	Factors Associated With Postintubation Laryngeal Edema

Age < 4 years
Tight-fitting ETT, no audible leak at or below 25 cm H_2O
Traumatic or repeated intubation
Prolonged intubation
Overinflated ETT cuff
Inadequate anesthesia during intubation
Repeated head repositioning while intubated
History of infectious or postintubation croup
Neck/airway surgery
Upper respiratory infection
Trisomy 21

ETT, Endotracheal tube.

Management of Anesthesia

Endotracheal intubation in a child with croup, as with any child with airway disorders, should be carried out in a controlled setting such as the operating room, with all necessary drugs and equipment available. Induction of anesthesia is carried out in a similar fashion to what was described for a child with acute epiglottitis.

Postintubation Laryngeal Edema

Postintubation laryngeal edema, also termed *postintubation croup* (not to be confused with infectious croup), is a potential complication of all tracheal intubations regardless of the age group. It is most commonly discussed in the context of pediatric patients because infants and children have smaller absolute tracheal diameters and thus have the highest incidence of developing clinically significant postintubation laryngeal edema. Although there may be predisposing factors (Table 30.11), this is an iatrogenic disorder as a direct result of endotracheal intubation.

Signs and Symptoms

Postintubation croup typically manifests within 30–60 minutes of extubation and is characterized by a barking or croupy cough, hoarseness, and stridor. With increasing airflow obstruction, the patient may exhibit nasal flaring, respiratory retractions, hypoxemia, cyanosis, and depressed consciousness. Treatment is aimed at reducing airway edema. Keeping the child calm is also important; crying will further exacerbate symptoms. For mild cases, mist therapy with cool humidified air may be helpful. In general, several nebulized epinephrine treatments are needed to effect sufficient mucosal vasoconstriction to help shrink the swollen mucosa. The patient must be observed for up to 4 hours after the last nebulized epinephrine treatment in case of rebound obstructive symptoms. In severe cases, heliox treatment (helium and oxygen mixtures) can also be considered. Resolution of symptoms usually occurs within 24 hours. Use of dexamethasone in both treatment and prevention of postintubation laryngeal edema is widespread, but one must recognize the slower onset of action (4–6 hours to achieve maximum effect).

Management of Anesthesia

Prevention of postintubation laryngeal edema should be a main goal in the airway management of pediatric patients. Whether one chooses to use cuffed or uncuffed ETTs, the goal should be to minimize trauma to the laryngeal and subglottic structures. Gentle laryngoscopy and ETT placement are important, as is selection of an appropriately sized ETT; confirmation of an ETT air leak at less than 25 cm H_2O should be routine.

Subglottic Stenosis

Subglottic stenosis (SGS) is a congenital or acquired narrowing of the subglottic airway. It is the most common type of laryngeal stenosis. Specifically, SGS refers to narrowing at the level of the cricoid ring. Most cases are acquired as a result of trauma.

Signs and Symptoms

Clinical presentation can range from mild respiratory symptoms to stridor and even complete airway obstruction. Mild cases of congenital SGS may not be clinically evident and are only diagnosed after the child presents with recurrent croup. SGS should always be considered in neonates and infants who have failed multiple extubation attempts.

Diagnosis of SGS is made by endoscopic examination. SGS is graded on a severity scale from I to IV, with grade I indicating less than 50% luminal obstruction; grade II, 50%–70% obstruction; grade III, 71%–91% obstruction; and grade IV with no discernible lumen. Congenital SGS is a diagnosis of exclusion made only in the absence of trauma and other identifiable postnatal causes.

Treatment

Grades I and II SGS may be amenable to medical therapy alone using antiinflammatory and vasoconstrictive agents such as corticosteroid and nebulized epinephrine. Grades III and IV SGS require surgical intervention.

Clinical symptoms ultimately dictate the need for surgical treatment regardless of grade. Less severe SGS may be treated endoscopically with steroid injection, serial dilation, and CO_2 laser ablation with or without topical mitomycin C. More severe SGS may require aggressive surgical interventions; these include anterior cricoid split, laryngotracheoplasty with cartilage graft (laryngotracheal reconstruction), and tracheotomy.

Management of Anesthesia

Since most acquired cases of SGS result from intubation-related trauma, extreme vigilance and caution must be observed in the airway management of every pediatric patient, particularly for infants and young children. There should be routine confirmation of an ETT air leak at less than 25 cm H_2O.

For patients presenting for SGS corrective procedures, standard anesthetic concerns pertaining to airway surgery should be observed. In particular, there is high risk of airway fire in the setting of laser use and electrocauterization.

In cases of open reconstruction, postoperative management is as important as the actual surgery. An ETT (often larger than that predicted for age) is left in place to act as a stent after the stenotic area has been repaired and the lumen enlarged with cartilage graft. Adequate sedation and frequently muscle relaxation are required to prevent patient movement; suture line disruption or accidental extubation can lead to disastrous airway obliteration.

Foreign Body Aspiration

Foreign body (FB) aspiration occurs when an object or substance nonnative to the laryngotracheobronchial pathway is inhaled and embedded anywhere from the level of the larynx down to the distal bronchus and beyond.

Commonly aspirated objects in the pediatric population include peanuts (up to 55% in Western societies), seeds, popcorn, other food particles, small toy parts, and metal objects. The size and shape of the aspirated object usually determine the level of entrapment. Entrapment at proximal locations can cause complete airway obstruction, asphyxiation, and death. Smaller and streamlined objects may travel down to the distal airways and present with a more subtle clinical picture. Secondary chemical or inflammatory reaction to the FB and postobstruction infection may also occur. Over half of all aspirated FBs are located in the right main bronchus, followed by the right lobar bronchi, left bronchi, trachea/carina, larynx, and bilateral locations.

Signs and Symptoms

Children between the ages of 1 and 3 years represent the overwhelming majority of victims of FB aspiration. Symptoms of bronchial aspiration include coughing, wheezing, dyspnea, and decreased air entry into the affected side. Laryngeal and tracheal FB aspiration present with frank or impending respiratory failure. Overall the classic triad of cough, wheezing, and decreased breath sounds is present in fewer than 60% of all children with FB aspiration. A reported history of choking is highly suggestive of FB aspiration, but it may be missed because choking typically lasts only seconds to minutes immediately after the aspiration event. Chronically retained airway FBs have a much more insidious presentation and are often misdiagnosed as asthma, infections of the upper or lower airways, and undefined airway abnormalities.

The diagnosis of FB aspiration can be easily established with plain radiographs if the object is radiopaque. Most aspirated objects (food items, nuts) are radiolucent, however. Diagnosis can be made based on radiographic evidence suggestive of aspiration (e.g., postobstructive atelectasis, infiltrate/consolidation, air trapping) in conjunction with the history and clinical findings.

Treatment

Rigid bronchoscopy is the procedure of choice in both diagnosis and treatment of FB aspiration. Dislodgment or fragmentation of the FB into the contralateral bronchus is a potentially lethal complication causing bilateral bronchial obstruction. When the FB cannot be removed, it is sometimes necessary to push it to a more distal location to restore ventilation to as large a portion of the lungs as possible. Rarely, FB aspiration may require thoracotomy for object retrieval.

Management of Anesthesia

There is no "gold-standard" anesthetic approach, and controversy still exists between whether to maintain spontaneous respiration or to initiate controlled ventilation. An individualized approach should be planned using information from the history, physical examination, and diagnostic images. Nitrous oxide is contraindicated if there is evidence of air trapping. Urgent/emergent need for bronchoscopic examination takes precedence over nothing-by-mouth status.

Inhalational induction of anesthesia with preservation of spontaneous respiration is generally preferred because positive pressure ventilation may move the FB into potentially more precarious positions. Total IV anesthesia should be established as early as possible after induction to provide uninterrupted anesthesia during rigid bronchoscopy. Topical anesthesia of the larynx and trachea with up to 3 mg/kg of lidocaine (2%–4%) is extremely useful in preventing laryngospasm and reaction to surgical manipulation. Anticholinergics such as atropine (10–20 μg/kg IV) or glycopyrrolate (3–5 μg/kg IV) should be readily available in case of pronounced vagal stimulation during bronchoscopy. Once the bronchoscope passes the glottis, the anesthesia circuit should be immediately connected to the side port to provide supplemental oxygen and assist spontaneous respiration, or to initiate controlled ventilation as needed. Use of a precordial stethoscope can be invaluable in assessing respiratory effort and quality in these cases.

Preservation of spontaneous respiration is ideal, but muscle relaxation is sometimes required to prevent movement during FB retrieval. At completion of the bronchoscopy, the patient may be intubated to establish definitive airway control and allow tracheal and esophageal suctioning. In general the child can be promptly extubated once appropriate criteria are met. Although rare, pneumothorax can be a complication and should always be considered in case of rapid deterioration.

Dexamethasone (0.4–1 mg/kg, maximum of 20 mg) is given prophylactically to reduce subglottic edema. Nebulized epinephrine treatment may be needed to treat postoperative croup.

Laryngeal Papillomatosis

Laryngeal papillomatosis is a common cause of hoarseness and airway obstruction in children. Also known as *recurrent respiratory papillomatosis* (warts), it is a benign neoplasm of the larynx and trachea caused by human papillomavirus (HPV). The larynx is most commonly affected, but distal involvement of the trachea and lungs can also occur.

Signs and Symptoms

Children can present between the ages of 6 months and 10 years. Dysphonia or change in voice quality (or altered cry in infants) is often the first and most prominent symptom. If left untreated, lesion growth will lead to stridor, dyspnea, and airway obstruction. Although histologically and pathologically similar in children and adults, the clinical course is quite different between the two patient populations. The main difference is the highly recurrent nature of the wart lesions in children, often necessitating numerous surgical excisions over the course of childhood. Adults usually only require a few surgical treatments for complete eradication. Lesions that begin in childhood mostly become quiescent in adolescence.

Treatment

Surgical debulking is the current standard of care in the treatment of laryngeal papillomatosis. The primary means include laser ablation (CO_2), microdébridement, and cryotherapy. Adjuvant antiviral medical therapy (cidofovir) has been used with success in moderate to severe cases. Rarely, large lesions may require tracheotomy to restore airflow. However, tracheotomy is strongly discouraged owing to the risk of inducing distal spread of disease.

Management of Anesthesia

Airway surgeries in suspension microlaryngoscopy are some of the most challenging cases in pediatric anesthesia and require close cooperation between the otolaryngologist and anesthesiologist. Patients are typically turned 90 degrees away from the anesthesia station and are suspended in a hands-free laryngoscope setup that allows for microscopic binocular operative intervention. Traditionally, intubation with a smaller ETT during surgery has been the standard approach. However, the presence of an ETT poses several problems. The most obvious is risk of airway fire because the ETT material can serve as fuel for combustion during laser surgery; alternatives such as metal, rubber, or silicone-coated ETTs wrapped in reflective foil should be used whenever possible. The physical presence of the ETT may also compromise visualization and excision of the lesion. Tubeless techniques with or without spontaneous respiration have gained popularity.

Children generally undergo inhalational induction of anesthesia with the aim to establish IV access and a steady level of total IV anesthesia as early as possible. Topical anesthesia of the larynx and trachea should be done to further decrease reaction to surgical stimuli. Muscle relaxation for cord paralysis is sometimes required for precise surgical excision of cord lesions. Most children are intubated at the completion of the surgery, even in tubeless techniques, and then allowed to awaken for extubation.

Adenotonsillar Hypertrophy/Sleep-Disordered Breathing

Adenotonsillar hypertrophy is the most common cause of snoring in children. Snoring may or may not be associated with actual obstructive hypopnea and apnea. Sleep-disordered breathing represents a spectrum of nocturnal airflow restrictive problems that may present with physiologically inconsequential snoring at one end and complete obstructive sleep apnea (OSA) at the other.

Signs and Symptoms

Children and adolescents with adenotonsillar hypertrophy present with a range of symptoms from mild snoring to obstructive sleep hypopnea and apnea. Children with OSA frequently have nonspecific behavioral difficulties such as hyperactivity and learning disability; daytime sleepiness is less common. The child will typically display audible mouth breathing, dry lips, hyponasal speech, and the so-called adenoid face (an oblong face with the mouth open and an expression of being lost or apathetic).

Tonsillar hypertrophy is graded from 0–4 depending on the percentage of the lateral oropharyngeal space occupied by the tonsillar tissues. Flexible endoscopy and lateral radiography are helpful in diagnosing adenoid hypertrophy; most cases are diagnosed clinically with examination at the time of surgery. Adenoids are located midline in the nasopharynx in close proximity to the opening of the eustachian tubes. As such, adenoid hypertrophy is frequently associated with chronic middle ear effusion, otitis media, and sinusitis.

History and physical examination alone are poor at differentiating simple snoring from OSA. As a symptom, snoring alone has relatively low positive and negative predictive values in the evaluation of children with sleep-disordered breathing. Polysomnography remains the gold standard for diagnosing OSA.

Treatment

Recognizing and treating sleep-disordered breathing is important because untreated OSA has neurocognitive, inflammatory, and cardiovascular sequelae. Adenotonsillectomy is the treatment of choice and is sometimes performed even in the absence of significant adenotonsillar hypertrophy if symptoms are progressive.

Management of Anesthesia

Preoperative anxiolytic medication is not contraindicated but should be given with discretion and used sparingly. Induction of general anesthesia is usually accomplished with inhalation of sevoflurane and oxygen, with or without nitrous oxide. Rapid airway obstruction can be expected, and oral airways of several sizes should always be readily available. Moderate CPAP is often needed to counteract the effects of relaxed upper airway muscle tone. Cuffed ETTs may be preferable to uncuffed tubes to minimize the chance of aspiration of blood. Opioids should be dosed accordingly to minimize the risk of prolonged emergence and postoperative upper airway obstruction. Nonsteroidal antiinflammatory drug (NSAID) use remains controversial and varies widely from center to center. IV acetaminophen is an excellent analgesic adjunct because it is devoid of coagulopathic and respiratory depressant effects. High-dose dexamethasone (up to 1 mg/kg IV,

maximum of 20 mg) has been shown to reduce postoperative swelling and nausea/vomiting.

Upper Respiratory Tract Infection

URI deserves a special mention because no other illness is encountered more frequently in the pediatric population presenting for surgery. As a group, URIs represent the most prevalent acute illness in the general population, with the highest overall incidence in children. Most cases of URI are mild and self-limited. However, URIs are associated with increased risk of perioperative respiratory complications such as laryngospasm, bronchospasm, and hypoxemia. Specific risk factors for respiratory complications in association with active or recent URI (within 2–4 weeks of surgery) include former prematurity, age younger than 2 years, underlying reactive airway disease, asthma, copious secretions, secondhand exposure to tobacco smoke, and prior airway surgery.

Management of Anesthesia

The traditional approach—which is to postpone elective surgery for 1–2 weeks for mild or recent URIs and for 4–6 weeks for active and more severe URIs—may be too conservative and oftentimes unrealistic. The urgency and type of surgery must be considered. Emergent procedures must proceed regardless of the severity of the URI. Type of surgery is also an important consideration; some procedures such as myringotomy and adenotonsillectomy may help relieve chronic URI-like symptoms. A detailed parental interview usually provides a helpful comparison of the child's current health status to baseline condition. In general, elective surgeries should be postponed if the child has high fever, croupy cough, general malaise, and evidence of lower respiratory tract infection.

When feasible, airway management with mask or LMA is preferable to endotracheal intubation and has been shown to have a lower incidence of perioperative respiratory complications. If intubation is required, the trachea should only be instrumented under a deep plane of anesthesia. A smaller-than-expected ETT should be considered because children with active or recent URI have a higher incidence of postintubation laryngeal edema; prophylactic dexamethasone treatment should be considered.

GENITOURINARY DISORDERS

Vesicoureteral Reflux

Vesicoureteral reflux (VUR) is abnormal reflux of urine from the bladder into the upper urinary tract, including the ureters and kidneys, and can be unilateral or bilateral. It is the most common urologic disorder in children.

Signs and Symptoms

Most children present with a febrile urinary tract infection (UTI). Some cases are discovered when confirmatory testing is prompted by prenatal urologic abnormalities or a significant family history. Evaluation for VUR should be done in children with recurrent UTIs, any male child with a first UTI, any child younger than 5 years with a febrile UTI, and children with significant renal anomalies. A voiding cystourethrogram (VCUG) is most commonly used to diagnose VUR and can be done with relative ease in most children. However, some children may require sedation or anesthesia for the urethral catheterization part of the test.

Treatment

Treatment is aimed at preventing UTI with antibiotic prophylaxis and restoring ureterovesical junction (UVJ) competence or relieving downstream bladder obstruction. Untreated reflux increases the risks of pyelonephritis and renal scarring, with subsequent reflux nephropathy. The most common surgical procedure for VUR is ureteral reimplantation or ureteroneocystostomy. The affected ureter is repositioned and retunneled into the bladder wall to create a new UVJ with the proper length-to-diameter ratio.

Management of Anesthesia

Most children with VUR are otherwise healthy and undergo general anesthesia without issues. For those with severe VUR and/or co-existing renal anomaly, baseline renal function should be evaluated. Caudal or lumbar epidural analgesia is recommended for reimplantation procedures to relieve pain and bladder spasm.

Cryptorchidism

Cryptorchidism (hidden or obscure testis) is congenital absence of one or both testes in the scrotum because of incomplete testicular descent. Undescended testes have an increased risk of malignant transformation compared to normally descended testes. Risks of infertility and testicular torsion are also increased. Additionally, there is usually a concurrent hernia with attendant risks of bowel incarceration and strangulation.

Signs and Symptoms

Cryptorchidism is diagnosed by nonpalpable testis or palpable but malpositioned testis (e.g., inguinal canal location). Physical examination must be performed in a warm environment to prevent cold-induced testicular retraction that may confound the clinical picture. Nonpalpable testes account for only one-fifth of all cases of cryptorchidism; 40% have an intraabdominal location, 40% have a high inguinal location, and the rest represent atrophy or congenital absence. Most palpable undescended testes will spontaneously descend during infancy but rarely so after 9 months of age.

Treatment

Orchiopexy is the treatment for all cases of cryptorchidism and involves identification, mobilization, and fixation of the malpositioned testis to the scrotum. Orchiopexy can be done via an inguinal, suprainguinal, or laparoscopic approach. Cases with a high intraabdominal position and short spermatic

vessels may require a two-stage procedure to allow time for collateral vessel formation after initial vessel clipping, followed by mobilization and scrotal fixation of the testis. Successful orchiopexy reduces but does not eliminate the increased risk of testicular cancer and infertility.

Management of Anesthesia

Unless the child has comorbid conditions, there are few special anesthetic considerations. An intense vagal response can be seen with surgical traction and manipulation of the spermatic cord and testicle. A high incidence of postoperative nausea and vomiting is observed; prophylactic antiemetic treatment should be routinely given. Caudal analgesia is highly recommended for the appropriate patient.

Hypospadias

Hypospadias is congenital malpositioning of the urethral meatus on the ventral aspect of the penis. The abnormal opening can occur anywhere starting from the glans penis to the penile shaft and even down to the scrotum and perineum. Hypospadias involving the glans penis, also known as *coronal hypospadias,* is the most common (50%). *Chordee,* an abnormal ventral curvature of the penis, is commonly seen with hypospadias.

Distal hypospadias imposes mostly cosmetic problems; more proximal lesions can affect urination and fertility. Treatment for hypospadias is surgical repair, and the majority can be accomplished in a single stage. Multiple corrective surgeries are needed for proximal meatal locations (scrotum and perineum) and often require preputial skin grafting. Surgery is most commonly performed between the ages of 4 and 18 months.

Hypospadias is generally an isolated finding, and most children do not present with additional health problems that pose specific anesthetic concerns. General anesthesia supplemented with caudal analgesia is the preferred technique.

ORTHOPEDIC/MUSCULOSKELETAL DISORDERS

Clubfoot (Talipes Equinovarus)

Clubfoot is a common congenital foot deformity due to malalignment of the calcaneotalar-navicular complex, resulting in a combination of (1) excessive plantar flexion, (2) a medially deviated forefoot, and (3) an inward-facing sole. Bilateral involvement is seen in 30%–50% of cases.

Signs and Symptoms

Clubfoot is evident at birth and can be diagnosed prenatally in some cases. All patients exhibit some degree of calf atrophy. Shortening of the tibia and fibula can also occur. Nonoperative treatment includes taping and serial casting for positional clubfoot; some maintain normal alignment, but there is a high rate of recurrence. Surgical Achilles tenotomy (clipping or release of the Achilles tendon) is often needed. The Ponseti method is the most popular treatment scheme for clubfoot and involves initial weekly stretching and casting (5–10 sessions), followed by percutaneous Achilles tenotomy, long leg casting with the foot in abduction and dorsiflexion, and finally a bracing program for 3–5 years.

Management of Anesthesia

Unless there are concomitant congenital problems, anesthetic management of children undergoing clubfoot corrective procedures is usually straightforward. Some procedures are done in the prone position, and some require neuromuscular blockade for adequate stretching and casting. Continuous epidural analgesia (in some cases with combined regional anesthesia) is highly recommended for more invasive procedures, because there is often significant postoperative pain.

Slipped Capital Femoral Epiphysis

Slipped capital femoral epiphysis (SCFE) literally means a slippage of the femoral end cap (*epi*, "over"; *physis*, "growth plate") over the femoral neck secondary to a fracture in the growth plate. SCFE occurs in adolescence, a period of rapid bone growth predisposing to increased growth plate instability.

Signs and Symptoms

SCFE typically presents between the ages of 10 and 16 years and affects boys more than girls. Obesity is a risk factor, and obese children tend to present at an earlier age. Other disorders associated with a higher risk of SCFE and an earlier age of onset include Down syndrome, endocrinopathies (hypothyroidism, precocious puberty, pituitary tumors), and renal osteodystrophy.

Patients present with groin, thigh, and knee pain and often hold the affected hip in an externally rotated position. Gait pattern and weightbearing ability may be affected. Twenty percent of cases have bilateral involvement even if there are only unilateral symptoms. Diagnosis is made with physical exam and plain radiography. Treatment involves surgical pinning of the growth plate to prevent further displacement.

Management of Anesthesia

Surgical treatment for SCFE is mostly done on an urgent basis to prevent further displacement with attendant risk of vascular compromise. Full stomach precautions must be observed when indicated, particularly for obese patients. There are few special anesthetic considerations unless comorbid conditions are present.

CHILDHOOD MALIGNANCIES

Wilms Tumor

Wilms tumor, or *nephroblastoma,* is the most common type of pediatric renal cancer; it is also the most common pediatric abdominal malignancy. It represents the fourth most prevalent childhood cancer. Unilateral disease is present in the overwhelming majority, with only 6% having bilateral renal involvement.

Signs and Symptoms

The peak incidence is between ages 1 and 3 years, and over 95% of cases are diagnosed before the 10th birthday. An abdominal mass, painful or painless, is the most common finding. Fever, anemia, hypertension, and hematuria may be observed. Associated congenital syndromes include WAGR syndrome (*W*ilms tumor, *a*niridia or agenesis of the iris and macular hypoplasia, *g*enitourinary anomalies, and *r*etardation/intellectual disabilities), Beckwith-Wiedemann syndrome, and Denys-Drash syndrome (triad of progressive renal disease, male pseudohermaphroditism, and Wilms tumor). Wilms tumor is typically surrounded by a pseudocapsule; it can rupture with aggressive palpation, manifesting as a rapidly enlarging abdominal mass. Metastasis to the lungs is most common, although respiratory complaints are rare. Up to 40% of cases have tumor extension into the renal vein and much less commonly into the inferior vena cava and right atrium. Coincidental acquired von Willebrand disease is seen in 8% of patients. Prognosis is dependent on tumor staging (I–V) and histology. With current therapy, children with favorable histology have an overall 80%–90% chance of survival at 5 years and 80%–90% chance of cure. Aggressive histology carries an average lifetime survival rate of 50%.

Based on the National Wilms Tumor Study Group protocol, patients with suspected Wilms tumor should undergo immediate surgical staging and concurrent radical nephrectomy when possible. Adjuvant chemotherapy and radiotherapy are guided by staging and histology.

Management of Anesthesia

Full stomach precautions should be observed if significant abdominal distention is present. Patients with known lung and vascular, particularly caval, involvement must be carefully assessed for potential cardiorespiratory compromise. Vascular invasion poses significant risk of sudden massive hemorrhage during dissection. At least one supradiaphragmatic large-bore IV should be placed in case of inferior caval clamping. Doxorubicin is a standard component of Wilms tumor chemotherapy protocol (except for a minority of cases); therefore, cardiac function by echocardiography should be assessed when applicable. Even with bilateral disease, severe renal dysfunction is rare. Nonetheless, standard laboratory tests to evaluate renal function, electrolyte balance, and cell counts should be performed. Surgical approach (laparoscopic vs. open) depends on disease burden. Continuous epidural analgesia is strongly recommended for open nephrectomy.

Hepatoblastoma

Hepatoblastoma is the most common pediatric hepatic malignancy, although liver cancer is an uncommon childhood cancer in general.

Signs and Symptoms

The median age at presentation is 1 year, and the overwhelming majority occur in children younger than age 3. There is a slight male predominance, and white children are affected five times more frequently than African American children. The most common clinical presentation is an asymptomatic abdominal mass. Anorexia may occur in advanced disease. Approximately 10% of hepatoblastomas have metastatic disease at presentation; lungs are the most common sites. The most important laboratory marker for hepatoblastoma is α-fetoprotein (AFP), although it is not specific to this disease. Regular monitoring of AFP is important in assessing disease progression and response to treatment. Diagnosis relies on tissue biopsy.

Prognosis is dependent on histology (anaplasia is unfavorable) and surgical resectability. Chemotherapy has greatly added to the success of hepatoblastoma treatment. Combined with chemotherapy, tumors that can be completely resected at diagnosis achieve a near 100% survival rate.

Management of Anesthesia

Patients with hepatoblastomas can present in relatively robust health or can be acutely ill. Other than the usual preoperative assessment, specific investigations about hepatic synthetic and metabolic functions should be made, with particular attention to coagulation status. Preoperative cardiac function should be assessed in patients receiving anthracycline chemotherapeutic agents.

Extreme hemodynamic perturbations and significant blood loss can be seen in hepatic surgeries. Large-bore IV access (preferably in the upper extremities) and invasive continuous arterial blood pressure monitoring should be established. Central venous catheter placement should also be considered, especially if peripheral venous access is inadequate. Maintaining normothermia can be challenging, given the large area of surgical exposure as well as the typical large-volume fluid resuscitation. Unless preoperative coagulation abnormalities exist, continuous epidural analgesia should be considered.

Neuroblastoma

Neuroblastoma (NB) is a group of malignant neoplasms of the sympathetic nervous system. It is the most common extracranial solid tumor in childhood and the most common neoplasm of infancy. Overall it represents the third most common pediatric cancer after leukemia and intracranial tumors. It is a disease of extreme heterogeneity in both presentation and clinical course.

Signs and Symptoms

A hallmark of NB is the broad spectrum of tumor location and clinical behavior. NB can occur anywhere throughout the sympathetic nervous system. The most common site is the adrenal gland (40%), followed by abdominal, thoracic, cervical, and pelvic sympathetic ganglia. Clinical behavior varies greatly; some can undergo spontaneous regression while others are aggressively malignant. Common sites of metastases include bone marrow, cortical bone, lymph nodes, orbits, dura, and liver; metastasis to the lungs is uncommon. Fifty percent have metastatic disease at presentation.

Two-thirds of NBs have intraabdominal primaries, and most commonly present with abdominal mass, pain, and fullness. Bone pain is another common complaint if cortical bone and bone marrow metastases are present. Orbital involvement manifests as periorbital ecchymosis and proptosis and may be the first detectable clinical sign in young infants. Tumors arising from the paraspinal ganglion may impinge on nerve roots and cause spinal cord compression.

Diagnostic evaluation begins with imaging, which may show calcified masses that help distinguish NB from the noncalcifying lesions of Wilms tumor. Tissue diagnosis is mandatory before initiating treatment. Risk stratification based on stage, histology, and age at presentation (younger age is better) helps individualize the treatment plan, consisting of surgical resection, chemotherapy, and occasionally radiotherapy. Neuroblastoma cells actively synthesize catecholamines, the metabolites of which are accumulated and secreted; urinary secretions of these substances (homovanillic acid and vanillylmandelic acid) can be measured to monitor disease activity.

Management of Anesthesia

Patients may present for a variety of procedures ranging from bone marrow biopsy to craniotomy, each with its own anesthetic considerations. Location, size, and metabolic activity of the tumor will dictate the specifics, such as need for invasive arterial pressure monitoring. Despite potential catecholamine release with tumor manipulation, intraoperative hypertension is infrequent.

Ewing Sarcoma

Ewing sarcoma is the second most common primary bone malignancy in children and adolescents after osteosarcoma. It is part of the Ewing sarcoma family of tumors that share a common neuroectodermal origin.

Signs and Symptoms

Ewing sarcoma is primarily a disease of adolescence. It can, however, occur in children younger than age 10 (30%) and also in the third decade of life (10%). It preferentially affects Caucasians and is uncommon in African Americans and Asians. Ewing sarcomas typically arise in flat and long bones of the extremities (mostly femur, then tibia, fibula, humerus) and the pelvis; soft tissues can also be involved. Localized pain, often in association with a palpable mass, is the most common presenting symptom. Pathologic fractures are seen in 15% of cases. Systemic symptoms such as fever and anorexia are uncommon (in contrast to osteosarcoma), but when present, metastatic disease is likely. Between 20% and 25% of patients have clinically detectable metastatic disease at presentation. The most common sites are lungs, bone, and bone marrow.

Definitive diagnosis is based on tissue biopsy. Plain radiography, CT, MRI, and positron emission tomography (PET) scanning are all useful diagnostic modalities.

Treatment

Neoadjuvant chemotherapy has significantly increased overall survival. Radiotherapy is also used, especially in unresectable disease and in cases with positive surgical margins. Autologous stem cell transplantation in conjunction with high-dose chemotherapy has been used with some success in selected cases of metastatic and relapsed Ewing sarcoma. Metastasis is the most important prognostic factor. The 5-year survival rate for those with localized disease is approximately 70%, compared to 30% for those with clinically detectable metastases.

Management of Anesthesia

The most important anesthetic consideration for patients with Ewing sarcoma is pain control. Significant preoperative disease-related pain is common, and risk of development of chronic pain is high. Regional and neuraxial analgesia should be heavily considered, along with a comprehensive regimen of analgesic adjuncts.

Tumors of the Central Nervous System

Primary malignancies of the CNS collectively represent the second most common cancer of childhood and adolescence (after leukemia). CNS malignancies have the highest morbidity of all childhood cancers, and the overall mortality approaches 50% despite advances in treatment options. The incidence is highest among infants and young children.

There are over 100 histologic subtypes of primary brain tumors, but the majority consists of only a few types: astrocytomas, medulloblastomas (primitive neuroectodermal tumor), ependymomas, and craniopharyngiomas. Tumor can occur anywhere within the CNS; location is primarily determined by type and age of onset. Infants most often present with supratentorial tumors, a trend also seen with adolescents. Infratentorial lesions predominate in children aged 1–10 years.

Signs and Symptoms

The clinical presentation depends primarily on tumor location. Tumors that obstruct CSF flow can cause hydrocephalus and potential intracranial hypertension. Depending on the age of the child, clinical manifestations may include macrocephaly, behavioral or personality changes, irritability, headache, and nausea and vomiting. Midline infratentorial tumors are classic examples; these lesions can also cause visual disturbances such as nystagmus, diplopia, and blurry vision. Supratentorial tumors generally cause widespread sensorimotor deficits as well as speech disturbance (aphasia) and seizures. Tumors in the suprasellar and third ventricular regions often lead to neuroendocrine abnormalities due anterior and posterior pituitary dysfunctions. Brainstem tumors are associated with cranial nerve palsies and occasionally upper motor neuron deficits (hyperreflexia). Finally, tumors in the spinal cord, either as primary lesions or as metastatic seedings from leptomeningeal spread, can cause back pain, motor and/or sensory deficits, and possible bowel and bladder dysfunction.

Diagnosis must be made expeditiously, given the high morbidity and mortality. Neuroimaging is important in both the diagnosis and planning of surgical treatment. MRI remains the gold standard. Neuroendocrine function is often perturbed in midline and suprasellar lesions.

Astrocytomas

Astrocytomas account for approximately 40% of CNS tumors and can occur throughout the CNS. As a group, astrocytomas are generally of low histologic grade and have an indolent clinical course. Juvenile pilocytic astrocytoma is the most common subtype and typically affects the cerebellum. Overall survival is 80%–100% if complete surgical resection can be achieved. Aggressive subtypes such as anaplastic astrocytoma and glioblastoma multiforme are rare in children and are mostly seen in adults.

Medulloblastomas

Medulloblastomas belong to the family of primitive neuroectodermal tumors (PNET), not to be confused with peripheral primitive neuroectodermal tumor (PPNET), which is part of the Ewing family of tumors. PNET accounts for 25% of CNS tumors, with the majority being medulloblastomas. All PNETs have a high histologic grade and demonstrate high metastatic activity within the neuraxis. These are cerebellar tumors that affect boys more than girls, with peak incidence between 5 and 7 years of age.

Ependymomas

Ependymomas arise from the ependymal lining of the ventricular system. They account for 10% of CNS tumors in children, and most are located in the posterior fossa. Surgery is the primary treatment, but it is rarely curative without adjuvant radiotherapy and chemotherapy. Overall survival is approximately 40%. Local recurrence is not uncommon.

Craniopharyngiomas

Craniopharyngiomas are the most common intracranial tumors of nonglial origin. Craniopharyngiomas can be considered benign neoplasms, although malignant transformations have been reported. Significant morbidities still exist owing to tumor proximity to major structures. Even with curative surgical resection, children are often left with serious neuroendocrine and visual complications. The modern era of treatment for craniopharyngiomas consists of surgery, radiotherapy, brachytherapy, and chemotherapy. Tumor recurrence is common.

DOWN SYNDROME (TRISOMY 21)

Down syndrome (DS), or trisomy 21, is the most common chromosomal abnormality, occurring in 1:700–1:800 live births. Advanced maternal age is a significant risk factor. Patients have characteristic dysmorphic features and experience a higher incidence of multiple diseases compared to their healthy counterparts. Although the overall life expectancy of patients with DS has dramatically improved over the years, DS still confers a shorter lifespan than would be expected for healthy individuals.

Signs and Symptoms

DS is usually apparent at birth. A constellation of characteristic dysmorphic features includes upslanting palpebral fissures, epicanthal folds, a flattened nasal bridge, flattened occiput and brachycephalic head shape, short broad hands with a distinctive transverse palmar crease, and hypotonia (Table 30.12). Diagnosis is confirmed with karyotype analysis.

Congenital anomalies of almost all organ systems are associated with DS, and it is the most common cause of intellectual disability. Almost all affected children have some degree of cognitive limitation; most cases are only mild to moderate, but severe intellectual disability can occur. Individuals with DS are also prone to developing early-onset dementia and Alzheimer's disease. Epilepsy occurs at a higher frequency than in the general population. Ocular disorders such as congenital and early-onset cataracts, strabismus, nystagmus, and refractive errors are common.

Children with DS are at increased risk of developing OSA due to soft tissue (low tone and redundancy) and skeletal (midface hypoplasia, high-arched palate) abnormalities. Poor tone and macroglossia further predispose to upper airway obstruction; a protruding tongue is commonly observed. Subglottic airway diameter is generally decreased; small insults can lead to clinically overt subglottic stenosis.

Fifty percent of patients with DS have single or multiple congenital heart defects. Endocardial cushion defects (atrioventricular septal defects [ASDs]) are the most common (40%–50%), followed by ventricular septal defects, secundum ASD, persistent patent ductus arteriosus, tetralogy of Fallot, and others.

Gastrointestinal anomalies are also common, including gastroesophageal reflux, intestinal atresia, anorectal malformations, and Hirschsprung disease. From a musculoskeletal standpoint, patients with DS have hypotonia and joint laxity. Dysplastic pelvis is also common. Atlantoaxial instability (AAI) has potentially the gravest impact on neurologic function. Subluxation of the atlas (C1) and axis (C2) joint can cause spinal cord compression with resultant sensorimotor deficits as well as loss of bowel and bladder control. AAI may be asymptomatic or can present with cord compressive symptoms including neck pain, torticollis, and gait abnormalities. Bowel and bladder dysfunction as well as paresis require immediate surgical stabilization.

Management of Anesthesia

Several clinical manifestations and associated congenital anomalies are of particular concern in the anesthetic management of children with DS. A thorough preoperative assessment must be done, with specific focus on the cardiac, respiratory,

TABLE 30.12	Clinical Findings Associated With Down Syndrome

GENERAL
Low birth weight
Short stature

CENTRAL NERVOUS SYSTEM
Intellectual disability
Seizure
Strabismus
Hypotonia

AIRWAY/RESPIRATORY SYSTEM
High-arched narrow palate
Macroglossia
Micrognathia
Subglottic stenosis
Upper airway obstruction
Increased susceptibility to postintubation croup and respiratory infections
Obstructive sleep apnea

CARDIOVASCULAR SYSTEM
Congenital heart disease
Increased susceptibility to pulmonary hypertension
Atropine sensitivity
Bradycardia with sevoflurane induction

GASTROINTESTINAL SYSTEM
Duodenal obstruction
Gastroesophageal reflux
Hirschsprung disease

MUSCULOSKELETAL SYSTEM
Atlantoaxial instability
Hyperextensibility/flexibility of joints
Dysplastic pelvis

IMMUNE/HEMATOLOGIC FUNCTIONS
Immune deficiency
Leukemia (ALL, AML)
Neonatal polycythemia

ENDOCRINE SYSTEM
Thyroid dysfunction
Low circulating levels of catecholamine

ALL, Acute lymphoblastic leukemia; *AML,* acute myeloid leukemia.
Adapted from Maxwell LG, Goodwin SR, Mancuso TJ, et al. Systemic disorders. In: Davis PJ, Cladis FP, Motoyama EK, eds. *Smith's Anesthesia for Infants and Children.* 8th ed. Philadelphia: Elsevier; 2011:1173.

and neurologic status. The presence of AAI may not be apparent because most patients are asymptomatic. A history of neck pain, head tilt, and abnormal gait suggests AAI. Older infants and toddlers can be observed for head control, passive neck range of motion, and upper motor neuron symptomatology (spasticity, hyperreflexia, clonus). Even in the absence of overt AAI, neck manipulation should be kept to a minimum at all times.

Macroglossia compounded by potential micrognathia and midface hypoplasia predispose these children to rapid airway obstruction and hypoxemia with induction of anesthesia.

Children with DS are also at higher risk for developing postintubation croup, because they have a smaller subglottic caliber. ETT sizes smaller than that predicted for age should be used. As in all children, an air leak at less than 25 cm H_2O must be demonstrated.

Significant bradycardia with inhaled sevoflurane induction occurs in up to 50% of children with DS regardless of presence or absence of co-existing congenital heart disease. It is speculated that these children have ultrastructural myocardial defects that predispose them to conduction abnormalities. Increased sensitivity to atropine is occasionally seen, manifesting as mydriasis and profound tachycardia.

The nature of any co-existing congenital heart lesions must be investigated. In general, children with DS undergoing cardiac surgery have a higher perioperative mortality than their non–trisomy 21 counterparts.

Patients must be closely observed for obstructive symptoms and hypoventilation in the postoperative period, given the high incidence of obstructive sleep apnea and obesity.

MALIGNANT HYPERTHERMIA

Malignant hyperthermia (MH) is a potentially lethal genetic disorder of muscle hypermetabolism triggered by exposure to volatile anesthetic agents and succinylcholine. It has multiple inheritance patterns, including autosomal dominant, autosomal recessive, and unclassified; penetrance and expression are extremely variable. Overall incidence is estimated to be 1:10,000 in children, much higher than that reported for adults. However, MH in children only accounts for 17%–20% of all MH cases.

Pathogenesis

The *RYR1* gene, located on chromosome 19q13.1, has been found to be the genetic culprit in the majority of cases. In 1% of cases, a mutation of the *CACNA1S* gene (chromosome 1q32) has been identified. There are numerous causative mutations in the *RYR1* gene linked to MH; 31 causative mutations have been documented to date. More will undoubtedly be discovered.

Normal muscle contraction depends on an increase in intracellular calcium (Ca^{++}). Upon membrane depolarization, Ca^{++} is released from the sarcoplasmic reticulum into the sarcoplasm via the dihydropyridine and ryanodine receptors, both of which are voltage-gated ion channels. Calcium interacts with troponin to allow cross-bridging between actin and myosin for muscle contraction to occur. MH-related mutations in the *RYR1* gene decrease receptor threshold for Ca^{++} release. Additionally, affected RYR1 receptors are resistant to negative feedback (increased Ca^{++} and magnesium levels) that normally decrease Ca^{++} conductance. Exposure to triggers causes an exaggerated Ca^{++} release at smaller degrees of membrane depolarization. Adenosine triphosphate (ATP) is consumed in all steps of intracellular Ca^{++} handling. The result is an intensely hypermetabolic process that leads to metabolic

TABLE 30.13	Differential Diagnosis of Malignant Hyperthermia
Diagnosis	Distinguishing Traits
Hyperthyroidism	Characteristic symptoms and physical findings often present; blood gas abnormalities increase gradually
Sepsis	Hypercarbia usually not seen; severe lactic acidosis may be present
Pheochromocytoma	Similar to MH except marked blood pressure swings
Metastatic carcinoid	Same as pheochromocytoma
Cocaine intoxication	Fever, rigidity, rhabdomyolysis similar to MNS
Heat stroke	Similar to MH except patient is outside the operating room
MMR	May progress to MH, ± total body spasm
MNS	Similar to MH, usually associated with use of antidepressants
Serotonergic syndrome	Similar to MH and MNS, associated with use of mood-elevating drugs

MH, Malignant hyperthermia; *MMR,* masseter muscle rigidity; *MNS,* malignant neuroleptic syndrome.
Adapted from Bissonnette B, Ryan JF. Temperature regulation: normal and abnormal [malignant hyperthermia]. In: Cote CJ, Todres ID, Goudsouzian NG, Ryan JF, eds. *A Practice of Anesthesia for Infants and Children.* 3rd ed. Philadelphia: Saunders; 2001:621.

and respiratory acidosis, hyperkalemia, rhabdomyolysis, and hyperthermia.

Signs and Symptoms

MH in humans is a vastly heterogeneous disorder. Some individuals tolerate multiple triggering anesthetics without apparent problems, whereas others demonstrate fulminant MH to only traces of volatile agents. Onset of symptoms is also variable, from immediate to hours after exposure to triggers. Early clinical signs and symptoms of MH are nonspecific and reflect a hypermetabolic state. Other disorders of hypermetabolism should be considered in the differential diagnosis (Table 30.13).

Early clinical signs include sinus tachycardia, tachypnea (if breathing is spontaneous), hypercarbia, and masseter muscle spasm (Table 30.14). Rapid exhaustion of the CO_2 absorber is usually evident, along with obvious warming of the canister. Cardiac dysrhythmias and peaked T waves may be seen owing to progressive hyperkalemia. Core temperature can rise within 15 minutes of exposure to triggering agents. However, overt hyperthermia is usually a late sign.

Laboratory analysis typically reveals mixed respiratory and metabolic acidosis (lactic acidosis), arterial hypoxemia, and hyperkalemia. Masseter muscle spasm can progress to whole body muscle rigidity with rhabdomyolysis. At this fulminant stage of MH, the patient will typically have cola-colored urine along with myoglobinuria and markedly increased serum creatinine kinase (CK; typically >20,000 U/L). Ultimately the

TABLE 30.14	Clinical Features of Malignant Hyperthermia		
Timing	Clinical Signs	Changes in Monitored Variables	Biochemical Changes
Early	Masseter spasm		
	Tachypnea	Increased minute ventilation	
	Rapid exhaustion of CO_2 absorbent	Increasing $ETCO_2$	Increased $Paco_2$
	Warm CO_2 absorbent canister		
	Tachycardia		Acidosis
	Irregular heart rate	Cardiac dysrhythmias	Hyperkalemia
		Peaked T waves	
Intermediate	Patient warm to touch	Increasing core body temperature	
	Cyanosis	Decreasing oxygen saturation	
	Dark blood in surgical site		
	Irregular heart rate	Cardiac dysrhythmias	Hyperkalemia
		Peaked T waves	
Late	Generalized skeletal muscle rigidity		Increased serum creatine kinase
	Prolonged bleeding		
	Cola-colored urine		Myoglobinuria
	Irregular heart rate	Cardiac dysrhythmias	Hyperkalemia
		Peaked T waves	
		Widened QRS	
		Ventricular dysrhythmias	

Adapted from Hopkins PM. Malignant hyperthermia: advances in clinical management and diagnosis. *Br J Anaesth*. 2000:118-128.

body's capacity to support the exaggerated oxidative metabolism is exhausted and cardiovascular collapse ensues. Severe hyperthermia is also associated with development of disseminated intravascular coagulation (DIC).

Diagnosis of MH requires a high index of suspicion based on the clinical picture supported by laboratory findings. Definitive diagnosis requires muscle biopsy for the caffeine-halothane contracture test (CHCT); however, the CHCT has a specificity of approximately 80%, so a negative result does not completely rule out MH. Early recognition and treatment are paramount. The introduction of dantrolene therapy has decreased overall mortality from 70% to less than 5%.

Anesthesia-Induced Rhabdomyolysis

Dystrophinopathies (Duchenne and Becker muscular dystrophy) have long been linked with possible increased MH susceptibility. It has now become apparent that this is not true. These patients can develop anesthesia-induced rhabdomyolysis (AIR) that is frequently accompanied by the same hypermetabolic signs as those seen in MH. An acute onset of hyperkalemic cardiac arrest (without preceding hypermetabolic signs) can be the first manifestation of AIR, a presentation *not* typical of MH. The role of dantrolene in AIR is unknown, but it likely has little efficacy because it has no membrane-stabilizing property. Although only a small percentage of patients with dystrophinopathies may develop AIR, a nontriggering anesthetic technique is recommended, given the potential life-threatening consequences.

Treatment

Dantrolene sodium is the only available treatment for MH, along with supportive measures (Table 30.15). It is thought to inhibit Ca^{++} conductance through ryanodine receptor channels and block external Ca^{++} entry into the sarcoplasm that normally occurs with membrane depolarization. Altogether, dantrolene halts further escalation of intracellular Ca^{++} levels. The most common side effects of dantrolene are muscle weakness and vein irritation. Of note, use of calcium channel blockers is contraindicated because it can worsen hyperkalemia.

Preparation of dantrolene solutions is a time-consuming and cumbersome task, requiring reconstitution of each 20 mg vial of dantrolene with 60 mL of sterile water. In 2013 the US Food and Drug Administration (FDA) approved a new dantrolene formulation, Ryanodex, that allows for much easier and faster preparation. Ryanodex is available in single-use vials, each containing 250 mg of dantrolene sodium in lyophilized powder form.

Following initial management of MH, the patient must have continued care in an ICU setting. Recrudescence occurs in up to 25% of patients, with muscular body type, temperature increase, and increased latency between exposure and onset as risk factors. Recrudescence usually occurs within the first few hours after the initial episode; late presentations (up to 36 hours after the initial episode) have been reported. As such, treatment with dantrolene should continue (1 mg/kg every 6 hours) for 48–72 hours after the last observed sign of MH. Development of DIC is an ominous sign and a common finding in fatal MH.

All patients with clinical or suspected MH should undergo CHCT. A sample size of least 1 gram of deep muscle (at least 3–5 cm in length and 1–1.5 cm in diameter) must be harvested for satisfactory testing, precluding some young children from undergoing CHCT because of their small size. Immediate family members should be counseled and possibly referred

TABLE 30.15	Treatment of Malignant Hyperthermia

ETIOLOGIC TREATMENT

Stop inhaled anesthetic immediately (add activated charcoal filters if available).

Notify surgeon immediately.

Call for help immediately.

Dantrolene (2.5 mg/kg IV) as initial bolus

Repeat every 5–10 minutes until symptoms are controlled (may require cumulative dose in excess of 10 mg/kg).

Prevent recrudescence (dantrolene 1 mg/kg IV every 6 hours for 72 hours).

SYMPTOMATIC TREATMENT

Abort or conclude surgery as soon as possible (if anesthesia is necessary, use only IV hypnotics).

Hyperventilate with 100% oxygen at >10 L/min.

Initiate active cooling (iced saline 15 mL/kg IV every 10 minutes, gastric and bladder lavage with iced saline, surface cooling) if temp > 39°C or less if rising rapidly. Stop cooling when temp < 38°C.

Consider sodium bicarbonate treatment (1–2 mEq/kg) for severe acidemia.

Treat hyperkalemia (calcium chloride 5–10 mg/kg IV, calcium gluconate 30 mg/kg, or regular insulin (0.1 unit/kg) in 1 mL/kg of 50% dextrose or 0.5 mg/kg dextrose of any percent glucose formulation.

For refractory hyperkalemia, consider β-agonist (e.g., albuterol), Kayexalate, dialysis (ECMO if cardiac arrest).

Maintain urine output (hydration, mannitol[a] 0.25 g/kg IV, furosemide 0.5–1 mg/kg IV).

For persistent and rising serum CK and K+, alkalinize urine with bicarbonate infusion at 1 mEq/kg/h for presumed imminent myoglobinuria.

Treat cardiac dysrhythmias (procainamide 15 mg/kg IV, lidocaine 2 mg/kg IV, follow PALS guidelines).

Place peripheral arterial and central venous catheter.

Check blood gas every 15 minutes until abnormalities are corrected.

Monitor in an intensive care setting for at least 24 hours.

CK, Creatine kinase; *ECMO,* extracorporeal membrane oxygenation; *IV,* intravenous; *PALS,* pediatric advanced life support.

[a]Each 20 mg vial of conventional dantrolene contains 3 g of mannitol, and each Ryanodex vial contains 125 mg of mannitol.

Adapted from Malignant Hyperthermia Association of the United States. Managing an MH crisis: emergency treatment for an acute MH event. www.mhaus.org.

TABLE 30.16	Follow-up of Patients With Malignant Hyperthermia or Masseter Muscle Rigidity

1. Medic-Alert bracelet; patient and first-degree relatives must be assumed to have MH susceptibility.
2. Refer patient to MHAUS (www.mhaus.org). MHAUS can refer patient to an MH diagnostic center.
3. Review family history for adverse anesthetic events or suggestion of heritable myopathy.
4. Consider evaluation for temporomandibular joint disorder.
5. Consider neurologic consultation to evaluate for a potential myotonic disorder.
6. For severe rhabdomyolysis, consider evaluation for a dystrophinopathy[a] or a heritable metabolic disorder (e.g., CPT II deficiency or McArdle disease).

[a]Duchenne or Becker muscular dystrophy.

CPT, Carnitine palmitoyltransferase; *MH,* malignant hyperthermia; *MHAUS,* Malignant Hyperthermia Association of the United States.

TABLE 30.17	Nontriggering Drugs for Malignant Hyperthermia

Barbiturates

Propofol

Etomidate

Benzodiazepines

Opioids

Droperidol

Nitrous oxide

Nondepolarizing muscle relaxants

Anticholinesterases

Anticholinergics

Sympathomimetics

Local anesthetics (esters and amides)

α_2-Agonists (clonidine, dexmedetomidine)

for muscle and genetic testing as well (Table 30.16). All cases of MH and significant masseter spasm should be reported to the North American Malignant Hyperthermia Registry (888-274-7899).

Management of Anesthesia

When possible, identification of susceptible patients based on personal and family history is the most important first step. Preoperative serum CK levels are generally not predictive (some patients with elevated baseline CK levels are not MH susceptible, whereas others with a normal preoperative serum CK go on to develop MH). There are currently only three disorders that have been clearly linked with MH: central core disease, King-Denborough syndrome, and Evans myopathy. Of note, a rare subset of MH-susceptible patients can develop MH to nonanesthetic triggers such as vigorous exercise, heat,

and anxiety (similar to pigs with the porcine stress syndrome). Dantrolene prophylaxis is not indicated or recommended. In addition to muscle weakness and vein irritation, other side effects of dantrolene treatment include nausea, blurred vision, and diarrhea.

Children should be given a liberal dose of oral anxiolytic(s) preoperatively (midazolam ± oral ketamine). Topical local anesthetics (EMLA, ELA-Max, Synera) may be applied to help with awake placement of an IV catheter. Use of nitrous oxide to supplement oral sedation is also helpful.

Once MH susceptibility is identified or suspected, a nontriggering anesthetic plan (Table 30.17) must be initiated, starting with elimination of triggering agents and thorough preparation of the anesthesia machine to minimize even traces of volatile agents. If available, an MH-dedicated anesthesia machine that was never exposed to volatile anesthetics should be used. Otherwise the anesthesia station must be flushed with high-flow oxygen for the recommended length of time (from 20 minutes to >100 minutes) specific to each model. Commercially available activated charcoal filters (Vapor-Clean [Dynasthetics]) can also be added to the inspiratory and expiratory ports of the anesthesia machine to remove volatile agents. These filters are reported to be effective in keeping volatile gas concentrations below 5 ppm for up to 12 hours with fresh gas flow of at least 3 L/min. Although purging is not necessary, the anesthesia machine still requires flushing with high fresh gas flows (>10 L/min) for 90 seconds prior to adding the activated charcoal filters. Of note, activated charcoal filters do not scavenge nitrous oxide. In general, external parts such as the breathing circuit, ventilation bag, and CO_2 absorber should be changed and vaporizers removed. Dantrolene and other resuscitative drugs must be immediately available.

Maintenance of anesthesia is based mostly on IV hypnotics, with or without nitrous oxide; nondepolarizing muscle relaxants may be used if necessary. Dexmedetomidine is a useful adjunct for both sedative and analgesic effects. Local anesthetic agents can be safely used. Standard ASA monitoring (pulse oximetry, end-tidal CO_2, ECG, noninvasive blood pressure, and temperature) usually suffices.

If the patient does not show clinical signs of MH within the first hour after a nontriggering anesthetic, MH is unlikely to occur later. All patients must be monitored for at least 1 hour (preferably 4 hours) in the postoperative period. Discharge to home is acceptable if the usual discharge criteria are met.

These anesthetic considerations also apply to patients who present for muscle biopsy for CHCT.

KEY POINTS

- When caring for pediatric patients—from newborns to teenagers—consideration of the physical, developmental, psychological, and physiologic implications specific to each age group is essential. Neonates, in particular preterm newborns, are the most different in terms of anatomy and physiology.
- Anesthesia-induced developmental neurotoxicity has become a much-debated topic in pediatric anesthesia. Although numerous animal studies corroborate evidence of anesthetic-induced neurotoxicity, similar human studies are lacking.
- The pediatric airway is characterized by a relatively larger head and tongue, a more cephalad larynx, a shorter cord-to-carina distance (4 mm in a term newborn), and the cricoid cartilage being the narrowest part of the airway.
- Children have a higher resting O_2 consumption rate (2×) than adults. Their functional residual capacity is similar to that in adults on a per-kilogram basis. Pulmonary and chest wall compliance is high. Anatomic differences predispose to early upper airway obstruction. All these predispose to rapid onset of hypoxemia upon induction of general anesthesia.
- Pulmonary vascular resistance (PVR) is high at birth and decreases to adult levels over days to months, but pulmonary vasculature remains reactive for a longer period of time. The ductus arteriosus and foramen ovale are only functionally closed at birth and may reopen with high PVR, hypercarbia, and hypoxemia, with resultant reversion to fetal circulation patterns.

- The immature myocardium of neonates and infants has limited contractile and elastic reserves, resulting in a relatively fixed stroke volume. Cardiac output and systemic blood pressure are dependent on heart rate.
- Physiologic anemia occurs between 2 and 3 months of age (nadir Hct 29%–31%).
- Owing to risk of apnea of prematurity and postanesthetic apnea, preterm infants less than 52–60 weeks' postconceptual age (PCA) should be observed overnight for apnea monitoring.
- The MAC for sevoflurane varies with age: newborn to 6 months, 3.3%; 6 months–12 years, 2.5%. The MAC-awake for sevoflurane in children is 0.2–0.3 of MAC.
- Children with Down syndrome may have atlantoaxial instability; cervical manipulation should be kept to a minimum. Severe bradycardia is seen in up to 50% of these children with sevoflurane inhalation induction.
- Preservation of spontaneous respiration is usually key to successful airway management of children with airway disease and craniofacial abnormalities. Close communication between surgeon and anesthesiologist is also essential.
- Confirming an air leak at less than 25 cm H_2O after intubation should be routine to minimize risk of tracheal mucosal injury. When an appropriately sized cuffed endotracheal tube is used, cuff pressure should also be kept at less than 25 cm H_2O.
- Congenital anomalies can exist as isolated findings or as part of a syndrome. Additional congenital abnormalities such as congenital heart disease and renal defects are commonly seen. A succinct but comprehensive preoperative assessment of all organ systems is usually in order.
- Antifibrinolytics (aminocaproic acid, tranexamic acid) should be considered in children undergoing surgery with expected large blood loss, such as craniosynostosis and posterior spinal fusion.
- Many childhood malignancies are treated with a multimodal approach consisting of surgery, chemotherapy, and radiation. Adverse effects related to chemotherapeutic agents should be investigated. Preoperative cardiac function should be assessed if an anthracycline-based regimen is used.
- CNS diseases may be accompanied by increased ICP, sensorimotor deficits, endocrine disturbance, and brainstem dysfunction. Signs and symptoms in infants may be nonspecific. Intraoperative monitoring for diabetes insipidus is especially important for suprasellar lesions.
- Anterior mediastinal mass presents a formidable anesthetic challenge. Preservation of spontaneous respiration (negative intrathoracic pressure) is essential. Preparation for rescue maneuvers (rigid bronchoscopy, prone positioning) must be made.
- MH and anesthesia-induced rhabdomyolysis (AIR) are distinct clinical entities that share similar clinical manifestations. Dantrolene is effective in the treatment of MH but not AIR. New dantrolene formulations (Ryanodex) allow for expedient preparation and delivery of treatment. Only central core disease, King-Denborough syndrome, and Evans myopathy have been clearly linked with MH susceptibility.

RESOURCES

Baraldi E, Filippone M. Chronic lung disease after premature birth. *N Engl J Med.* 2007;357:1946-1955.

Dede O, Motoyama EK, Yang CI, et al. Pulmonary and radiographic outcomes of VEPTR (Vertical Expandable Prosthetic Titanium Rib) treatment in early-onset scoliosis. *J Bone Joint Surg Am.* 2014;96:1295-1302.

Engle WA. American Academy of Pediatrics Committee on Fetus and Newborn. Age terminology during the perinatal period. *Pediatrics.* 2004;114:1362-1364.

Fierson WM, et al. Policy statement: screening examination of premature infants for retinopathy of prematurity. *Pediatrics.* 2013;131:189-195.

Kraemer FW, Stricker PA, Gurnaney HG, et al. Bradycardia during induction of anesthesia with sevoflurane in children with Down syndrome. *Anesth Analg.* 2010;111; 1259–1163.

Langer CL. Hirschsprung disease. *Curr Opin Pediatr.* 2013;25:368-374.

Lau CS, Chamberlain RS. Probiotic administration can prevent necrotizing enterocolitis in preterm infants: a meta-analysis. *J Pediatr Surg.* 2015;50:1405-1412.

Lin EP, Soriano SG, Loepke AW. Anesthetic neurotoxicity. *Anesthesiology Clin.* 2014;32:133-155.

Nelson P, Litman RS. Malignant hyperthermia in children: an analysis of the North American Hyperthermia Registry. *Anesth Analg.* 2014;118:369-374.

Ramamoorthy C, Haberkem CM, Bhananker SM, et al. Anesthesia-related cardiac arrest in children with heart disease: data from the Pediatric Perioperative Cardiac Arrest (POCA) registry. *Anesth Analg.* 2010;110:1376-1382.

Seiden SC, McMullan S, Sequera-Ramos L, et al. Tablet-based interactive distraction (TBID) vs oral midazolam to minimize perioperative anxiety in pediatric patients: a noninferiority randomized trial. *Paediatr Anaesth.* 2014;24:1217-1223.

Stoll BJ, Hansen NI, Bell EF, et al. Eunice Kennedy Shriver National Institute of Child Health and Human Development Neonatal Research Network. Trends in care practices, morbidity, and mortality of extremely preterm neonates, 1993-2012. *JAMA.* 2015;314:1039-1051.

Pregnancy-Associated Diseases

ZACHARY WALTON, DENIS SNEGOVSKIKH, FERNE BRAVEMAN

PHYSIOLOGIC CHANGES ASSOCIATED WITH PREGNANCY

Cardiovascular System

Most changes in the cardiovascular system are caused by the hormonal change of pregnancy. Increased activity of progesterone results in increased production of nitric oxide and prostacyclin, which together with a decreased response to norepinephrine and angiotensin result in vasodilation. Increased concentrations of relaxin lead to renal artery dilation and, through reduction in aortic stiffness, aortodilation (≈0.5-cm increase in aortic diameter is seen at term). The decrease in systemic vascular resistance during the initial weeks after conception causes a compensatory elevation of cardiac output (initially resulting from an increase in heart rate) and an increase in renin activity. Increased renin activity results in retention of sodium and, by osmotic gradient, water. About 1000 mEq of sodium will be retained by term, which results in retention of an extra 7–10 L of water. Plasma volume begins to rise in the fourth week of pregnancy, is increased by 10%–15% at 6–12 weeks, and reaches a maximum (30%–50% increase) at 28–34 weeks. The increase in plasma volume, combined with a 20%–30% increase in total red blood cell mass, results in significantly elevated total blood volume, which reaches 100 mL/kg at term. Cardiac output rises in parallel with plasma volume, increasing by 15% at 8 weeks' gestation and reaching a maximum increase of 50% by 28–32 weeks. Plasma volume and cardiac output remain stable from approximately 32 weeks until labor begins. In labor, cardiac output rises as a result of sympathetic stimulation (pain and stress) and "autotransfusion," the displacement of blood from the contracting uterus into the circulation. Compared with prelabor output, cardiac output is increased by 20% during the first stage and 50% during the second stage of labor. Just after delivery of the placenta (the end of the third stage of labor), cardiac output is elevated 80% above prelabor levels, which corresponds to a 170% increase relative to the prepregnancy level. Cardiac output falls to the prelabor level in 24–48 hours and returns to the prepregnancy level in the next 12–24 weeks. Twin pregnancy results in a 20% greater increase in cardiac output than singleton gestation.

Such an increase in cardiac workload results in ventricular hypertrophy. According to one echocardiographic study, the left ventricle increases in size by 6% and the right ventricle increases by 15%–20% by term. Increases in the size and dilations in the cardiac chamber result in a mild degree of insufficiency of all the valves except the aortic valve; it is *not* normal to see aortic insufficiency at any stage of pregnancy. Enlargement of the heart and cephalic displacement of the diaphragm cause a horizontal shift and rotation of the heart, which results in changes in the cardiac axis on the electrocardiogram. It is *not* abnormal to see a deep S wave in lead I and a large Q wave with negative T waves in leads III and aVF. The decline in systemic vascular resistance in early pregnancy reaches a nadir of 35% decrease at 20 weeks. Systemic vascular resistance slowly rises later but remains 20% lower at term than the prepregnancy level. Central venous pressure, pulmonary artery pressure, and pulmonary capillary wedge pressure remain stable throughout pregnancy.

At term the uterus can completely compress the inferior vena cava while parturients are the supine position. Twin and singleton pregnancies cause a similar degree of obstruction. The aorta is not affected by the gravid uterus. Femoral vein pressure is elevated twofold to fivefold in the supine position. Compression of the inferior vena cava by the gravid uterus results in supine hypotension syndrome, which manifests with a short period of tachycardia followed by bradycardia and profound hypotension that is resistant to treatment with pressors. Based on a study of Japanese parturients, left body tilt beyond 30 degrees can prevent development of the syndrome.

Respiratory System

Changes in the respiratory system are also caused by the hormonal changes of pregnancy. Increased activity of relaxin results in relaxation of the ligaments of the rib cage, which allows displacement of the ribs into a more horizontal position. This leads to upward displacement of the diaphragm very early in pregnancy before the gravid uterus shifts the abdominal contents. Elevation of the diaphragm and the more horizontal position of the ribs modify the shape of the chest into a barrel-like form; this decreases the vertical dimension of the chest by about 4 cm but increases the diameter of the chest by about 5 cm, which significantly increases the volume of the lungs available for gas exchange during normal spontaneous respiration. Tidal volume increases up to 40% by term. Increased activity of progesterone, a potent respiratory stimulant, leads to an increase in tidal volume and more rapid respiratory rate, so that minute ventilation is increased by 50% at term. Chronic hyperventilation results in respiratory alkalosis with a pH of 7.44, $Paco_2$ of 28–32 mm Hg, and HCO_3 concentration of 20 mmol/L. Secondary to the decline in $Paco_2$ and a lower arteriovenous oxygen difference, Pao_2 rises slightly, in the range of 104–108 mm Hg, during pregnancy. These changes increase the gradient between mother and fetus and improve maternal-fetal gas exchange.

Decrease in the vertical size of the chest secondary to elevation of the diaphragm leads to a 25% decrease in expiratory reserve volume and a 15% decrease in residual volume, which results in a 20% decrease in functional residual capacity. A 20% increase in oxygen consumption caused by an elevated basal metabolic rate, combined with the decrease in functional residual capacity, produces more rapid desaturation during periods of apnea. In a fully preoxygenated healthy nonpregnant patient, desaturation from 100% to lower than 90% occurs in approximately 9 minutes. In a healthy patient at term, desaturation occurs in only 3–4 minutes, and in a morbidly obese pregnant patient, desaturation occurs in 98 seconds.

Edema and hyperemia of the oropharyngeal mucosa, glandular hyperactivity, and capillary engorgement secondary to elevated activity of estrogen, progesterone, and relaxin result in nasal stiffness, epistaxis, and upper airway narrowing. Therefore the rates of difficult and failed intubation in pregnant women are increased—3.3% and 0.4%, respectively—which are more than eight times higher than in nonpregnant patients. When providing general anesthesia, the anesthesiologist is thus faced with a potentially difficult airway in a patient who will undergo desaturation more rapidly than a nonpregnant patient. This is one of the factors contributing to a 17-times higher mortality rate among parturient women who undergo general anesthesia than among those who undergo regional anesthesia. To minimize the likelihood/need for airway manipulation, prophylactic placement of an epidural catheter in patients assessed to have a difficult airway may help avoid airway manipulation and minimize maternal morbidity.

Hematologic System

Normal pregnancy is associated with substantial changes in hemostasis, resulting in a relatively hypercoagulable state. The activity of the majority of the coagulation factors (I, VII, VIII, IX, X, XII) is increased, whereas the activity of physiologic anticoagulants is decreased. The latter includes a significant reduction in protein S activity and an acquired activated protein C resistance. This effect (i.e., reduction in anticoagulation activity) is doubled in IVF (in vitro fertilization) pregnancies. Deep vein thrombosis occurs in 1 per 1000 deliveries, which is 5.5–6 times higher than the rate in the general female population of childbearing age, and reaches a maximum at 4–6 weeks postpartum. Procoagulant changes during normal pregnancy are counterbalanced by significant activation of the fibrinolytic system during the postpartum period.

Gastrointestinal System

Lower esophageal sphincter tone is decreased in pregnancy as a result of two factors: displacement of the stomach upward and muscle relaxation caused by the effects of progestins. Heartburn is a frequent occurrence among pregnant women. Gastric emptying is not delayed in pregnancy, although it is slowed in labor.

Bile secretion is increased during pregnancy. Bile stasis is increased owing to the effect of progesterone, and together with changes in the composition of bile acids, this results in increased gallstone formation. Cholecystectomy is the second most frequent surgery during pregnancy (after appendectomy), with a reported incidence as high as 1 in 1600 pregnancies.

Endocrine System

Pregnancy is characterized by insulin resistance caused by increased activity of hormones such as progesterone, estrogen, cortisol (2.5-fold increase at term), and placental lactogen. This insulin resistance resolves rapidly after delivery. Fasting glucose levels are lower in pregnant than in nonpregnant patients because of the high glucose utilization by the fetus.

Estrogen increases the level of thyroxin-binding globulin, which results in an elevation of total triiodothyronine (T_3) and thyroxine (T_4) levels, but levels of free T_3 and T_4 remain stable.

Other Changes

Increased levels of progesterone and endorphins elevate the pain threshold. Studies using bispectral index monitoring do not support the previous belief that pregnant patients show increased sensitivity to the effect of inhalational anesthetics.

Cerebrospinal fluid volume is decreased during pregnancy, but intracranial pressure remains stable.

Renal blood flow is increased in pregnancy. Glomerular filtration rate increases by 50% at 12 weeks' gestation, which results in a decrease in blood urea nitrogen and creatinine concentrations. Usual blood urea nitrogen and creatinine values at term are abnormal and indicate renal dysfunction (Table 31.1).

ANESTHETIC CONSIDERATIONS

Nonobstetric Surgery

Approximately 1% of all pregnant women in the United States will undergo surgery unrelated to their pregnancy (>80,000 procedures requiring anesthesia per year). The most frequent nonobstetric procedures are appendectomy, laparoscopic cholecystectomy, breast biopsy, and surgery required because of trauma.

Generally, elective surgery should be delayed until the patient is no longer pregnant and has returned to her nonpregnant physiologic state (approximately 2–6 weeks postpartum). Procedures that can be scheduled with some flexibility but that cannot be delayed until after delivery are best performed in the middle trimester. This lessons the risk of teratogenicity (greater with first-trimester medication administration) and preterm labor (greater risk in the third trimester) (Fig. 31.1).

The objective of anesthetic management in patients undergoing nonobstetric operative procedures is maternal safety, safe care of the fetus, and prevention of premature labor related

TABLE 31.1	Physiologic Changes Accompanying Pregnancy
Parameter	Average Change From Nonpregnancy Value (%)
Intravascular fluid volume	+35
Plasma volume	+45
Erythrocyte volume	+20
Cardiac output	+40
Stroke volume	+30
Heart rate	+15
Peripheral circulation	
Systolic blood pressure	No change
Systemic vascular resistance	−15
Diastolic blood pressure	−15
Central venous pressure	No change
Femoral venous pressure	+15
Minute ventilation	+50
Tidal volume	+40
Respiratory rate	+10
Pa_{O_2}	+10 mm Hg
Pa_{CO_2}	−10 mm Hg
Arterial pH	No change
Inspiratory reserve volume	+5
Tidal volume	+45
Expiratory reserve volume	−25
Residual volume	−15
Inspiratory capacity	+15
Functional residual capacity	−20
Vital capacity	No change
Total lung capacity	−5
Airway resistance	−35
Oxygen consumption	+20
Renal blood flow and glomerular filtration rate	+50
Serum cholinesterase activity	−25

to the surgical procedure or to drugs administered during or as part of the anesthesia care. To achieve these goals the effects of the patient's altered physiology must be recognized and incorporated into the anesthetic plan. Induction of and emergence from anesthesia are more rapid than in the nonpregnant state because of increased minute ventilation and decreased functional residual capacity. Supine hypotensive syndrome can occur as early as the second trimester.

Teratogenicity may occur at any stage of gestation. However, most of the critical organogenesis occurs in the first trimester. Although many commonly used anesthetics are teratogenic at high dosages in animals, few if any studies support teratogenic effects of anesthetic or sedative medications at the dosages used for anesthesia care in humans. There is some evidence of a link between maternal high-dose diazepam treatment and intrauterine growth restriction. Midazolam is safe when used to treat perioperative anxiety.

Nitrous oxide has been suggested to be teratogenic in animals when administered for prolonged periods (1–2 days). The concern regarding its use in humans is its effect on DNA synthesis. Although teratogenesis has been seen in animals only under extreme conditions that are not likely to be reproduced

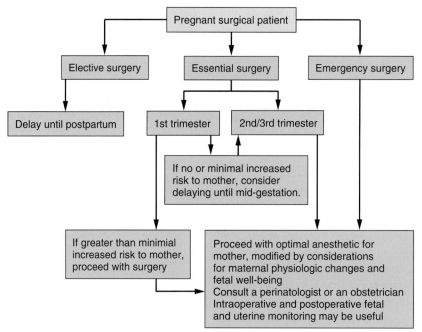

FIG. 31.1 Recommendations for management of pregnant women undergoing surgery. (Adapted from Rosen MA. Management of anesthesia for the pregnant surgical patient. *Anesthesiology.* 1999;91:1159-1163. © 1999, Lippincott Williams & Wilkins).

in clinical care, some believe that nitrous oxide use is contraindicated in the first two trimesters of pregnancy. Recent studies suggest that volatile anesthetics stimulate neuronal apoptosis in rats, but it is not obvious whether these data can be extrapolated to humans. Widespread neuronal apoptosis is associated with memory and learning deficits in laboratory animals, but again this has not been examined in humans.

Propofol and ketamine are all safe intravenous (IV) induction agents. Induction doses for these medications are unchanged in pregnancy. The choice of induction agent is usually based on provider preference and the clinical status of the patient (e.g., presence of dehydration, valvular heart disease, dysrhythmia, hypertension, or preeclampsia). None of these agents has been clearly shown to be teratogenic or have adverse effects on human brain development. Thiopental is no longer available in the United States.

Pregnant patients are more sensitive to the action of vecuronium and rocuronium but have increased clearance of both these medications. Succinylcholine dose is unchanged in pregnancy; its volume of distribution is increased, but systemic pseudocholinesterase activity is decreased, resulting in variability in duration of action.

Fetal heart rate should be monitored in the recovery room, intermittently for previable fetuses and continuously for the viable fetus. Uterine activity should also be monitored because contractions are most likely to occur proximate to the procedure and as any tocolytic effect of general anesthetics wears off. Recovery from anesthesia requires close monitoring, particularly of the airway and respiratory system, because most severe anesthetic complications occur during this period. Opioids can be used as needed to control postoperative pain.

Epidural analgesia is an option for procedures on the chest, abdomen, or lower extremities and carries less risk of opioid-induced hypoventilation when compared with IV opioids. Nonsteroidal antiinflammatory drugs (NSAIDs) should be avoided, especially after 32 weeks' gestation, because they may cause premature closure of the fetal ductus arteriosus if given for more than 48 hours.

Surgery may result in preterm labor during the intraoperative and postoperative periods. Abdominal and pelvic procedures are associated with the greatest incidence of preterm labor. The efficacy of preoperative progesterone supplementation for prevention of possible procedure-related preterm labor has not been studied.

Regional anesthesia, which includes peripheral nerve blocks as well as neuraxial anesthesia, is an option for some surgical procedures, particularly those involving the extremities. It has the advantage of avoiding the risks of general anesthesia, particularly the need to manage the airway and fetal exposure to anesthesia. Local anesthetics have an increased effect during pregnancy; thus the amount of local anesthetic administered for regional anesthesia should be reduced by 25%–30% during any state of pregnancy. Local anesthetic toxicity, especially cardiovascular toxicity, is also seen at lower plasma concentrations of those drugs.

Regional anesthesia should be considered because it minimizes fetal exposure to medications. The statement of the American College of Obstetricians and Gynecologists (ACOG) Committee on Obstetric Practice titled "Nonobstetric Surgery During Pregnancy" recommends that an obstetric consult be obtained before surgery and that use of fetal monitoring be individualized.

TABLE 31.2	Epidural Labor Analgesia		
		Infusion	
Bolus		Local Anesthetic	Opioid
Bupivacaine 0.125% with hydromorphone 10 μg/mL		Bupivacaine 0.0625%–0.125%	Hydromorphone 3 μg/mL
Bupivacaine 0.125% with fentanyl 5 μg/mL		Bupivacaine 0.0625%–0.125%	Fentanyl 2 μg/mL
Bupivacaine 0.125% with sufentanil 1 μg/mL		Bupivacaine 0.0625%–0.125%	Sufentanil 2 μg/mL
(Ropivacaine 0.075% may be used with opioid as above)		(Ropivacaine 0.075%–0.125% may be used)	(Any of the above)

Obstetric Anesthesia Care

Regional Analgesic Techniques

Use of regional techniques in parturient patients requires an understanding of the neural pathways responsible for transmission of pain during labor and delivery. The pain of labor arises primarily from receptors in the uterine and perineal structures. Afferent pain impulses from the cervix and uterus travel in nerves that accompany sympathetic nervous system fibers and enter the spinal cord at T10–L1. Pain pathways from the perineum travel to S2 and S4 via the pudendal nerves. Pain during the first stage of labor (onset of regular contractions) results from dilation of the cervix, contraction of the uterus, and traction on the round ligament. The pain is visceral and is referred to dermatomes supplied by spinal cord segments T10–L1. During the second stage of labor (complete dilation of the cervix to delivery of the fetus), pain is somatic and is produced by distention of the perineum and stretching of fascia, skin, and subcutaneous tissues.

Lumbar Epidural Analgesia

When an epidural catheter is placed for provision of analgesia during labor and delivery or anesthesia for cesarean delivery, it is important to confirm that the catheter is not in an intravascular or subarachnoid position. For this purpose it is common to administer a test dose of a solution containing the local anesthetic and epinephrine (15 μg). An epinephrine-induced increase in maternal heart rate alerts the anesthesiologist to the possibility of an intravascular catheter placement. It has been shown that patients on β-blockers may have a paradoxical bradycardia following intravascular test dose injection. For these patients an increase in systolic blood pressure of more than 15 mm Hg following a test dose may be used as evidence of *intravascular* catheter placement. Rapid onset of analgesia suggests *subarachnoid* placement. Hypotension may require administration of small doses of ephedrine (5–10 mg IV) or phenylephrine (20–100 μg IV). Use of neuraxial analgesia, specifically combined spinal-epidural analgesia, in early labor does not increase the incidence of cesarean delivery and may shorten labor compared with systemic analgesia. See Table 31.2 for analgesic choices.

Combined Spinal-Epidural Analgesia

Combined spinal-epidural analgesia has been advocated as an alternative to epidural analgesia during labor. Advantages cited for the combined technique include more rapid onset of analgesia, increased reliability, effectiveness when instituted in a rapidly progressing labor, and minimal motor block. Subarachnoid administration of low doses of opioids such as fentanyl (12.5–25 μg) or sufentanil (5–10 μg) results in rapid (5 minutes), nearly complete pain relief during the first stage of labor. Low doses of local anesthetics (e.g., 2.5 mg of bupivacaine) may also be added to the opioid solution. Disadvantages of the combined technique include the risk of fetal bradycardia, which is usually benign and very short lasting. Increased risk of postdural puncture headache has not been cited as a concern in the literature. This technique should be considered, especially when neuraxial analgesia is requested in very early labor or in a rapidly progressing multiparous labor.

Anesthesia for Cesarean Delivery

A large and growing minority (>30%) of parturient women deliver by cesarean delivery. If epidural analgesia is used for labor, this technique can easily then be converted to provide surgical anesthesia by changing the quantity and concentration of drug administered. Most elective and many urgent cesarean deliveries are performed under spinal anesthesia. Hyperbaric bupivacaine solutions provide reliable anesthesia, often with the addition of opioids for postoperative analgesia. General anesthesia is reserved for the most emergent cases in which the condition of the mother and/or fetus contraindicates regional anesthesia. For unscheduled cesarean deliveries, the consensus of ACOG and the American Society of Anesthesiologists (ASA) is that hospitals *should have the capability* to begin a cesarean delivery within 30 minutes of the decision to operate. However, not all indications for cesarean delivery require a 30-minute response time. It is noteworthy that a time interval of longer than 18 minutes, *not* 30 minutes, from the onset of severe fetal heart rate decelerations to delivery is associated with poor neonatal outcome. The anesthesiologist must consider the indication for unscheduled cesarean delivery (e.g., arrest of labor, nonreassuring fetal heart rate, maternal illness) as well as the maternal risks and benefits when choosing the anesthetic. Maternal safety and well-being are paramount in selecting an anesthetic for nonscheduled cesarean delivery.

Ideally, all patients should be assessed by the anesthesiology team on admission to labor and delivery. At a minimum the anesthesiology staff should be informed in advance and the patient evaluated when a complicated delivery is anticipated, when patient characteristics indicate increased anesthetic risk

TABLE 31.3	Factors Associated With Increased Anesthesia Risk

Obesity
Facial and neck edema
Extremely short stature
Difficulty opening mouth
Arthritis of neck, short neck, small mandible
Abnormalities of face, mouth, or teeth
Pulmonary disease
Cardiac disease

TABLE 31.4	Criteria for Diagnosis of Preeclampsia

Blood pressure > 139/89 mm Hg after 20 weeks' gestation in a woman with previously normal blood pressure
Either:
  Proteinuria (≥300 mg in a 24-hour urine specimen, or urine protein/creatinine ratio ≥ 0.3 [both measured as mg/dL])
  Or any of the following:
  Thrombocytopenia (platelet count < 100,000/μL)
  Renal insufficiency (serum creatinine > 1.1 mg/dL)
  Pulmonary edema
  Cerebral or visual symptoms

(Table 31.3), and at the first indication of a nonreassuring fetal heart rate pattern. Obviously, preanesthetic assessment must include evaluation for co-existing diseases as well as a thorough airway examination. Pulmonary aspiration and failed intubation previously accounted for three-fourths of all maternal deaths related to anesthesia care. Significant advances in anesthetic care, including the development of videolaryngoscopy, have led to a decline in the rate of aspiration and associated morbidity. In fact, according to ASA's Closed Claims Project database, between 2005 and 2013 there was only one case of aspiration associated with labor and delivery. Researchers also noted that no cases of death due to aspiration were reported in the United Kingdom between 2000 and 2005, compared to 1.5 cases per 1000 during the 1940s.

Labor is a state of high caloric demand. Most parturients do not have an appetite during active labor, but for those who do, and who do not have risk factors for aspiration (e.g., obesity, preeclampsia, treatment with opioids), at least clear liquids should be provided. The safety of a light meal (fruit, light soups, toast, light sandwiches) for healthy parturients is currently in discussion.

Urgent cesarean delivery for a nonreassuring fetal heart rate pattern does not necessarily preclude use of regional anesthesia. Rapid induction of spinal anesthesia is appropriate in many situations in which there is fetal compromise. Parturients at high risk of airway complications should undergo early induction of labor analgesia in hopes of precluding the need for general anesthesia should emergent cesarean delivery become necessary; labor analgesia can rapidly be converted to surgical anesthesia for cesarean section.

HYPERTENSIVE DISORDERS OF PREGNANCY

Hypertensive disorders of pregnancy encompass a range of disorders that include chronic hypertension, chronic hypertension with superimposed preeclampsia, gestational hypertension, preeclampsia, and eclampsia. These disorders complicate 8%–12% of all pregnancies. Hypertensive disorders result in 70 maternal deaths a year in the United States and 50,000 maternal deaths a year worldwide. The only curative treatment for hypertensive disorders that develop during pregnancy is delivery. Deteriorating maternal condition mandates urgent delivery of the fetus regardless of gestational age.

The risk of developing essential hypertension later in life is thought to be increased in women who experience gestational hypertension.

In 2013 the ACOG Task Force on Hypertension in Pregnancy updated the diagnostic and therapeutic guidelines for hypertensive disorders. The most significant update is introduction of clinical signs and symptoms that may be used in the absence of proteinuria as diagnostic criteria for preeclampsia (i.e., thrombocytopenia [platelet count < 100,000/μL], renal insufficiency [serum creatinine > 1.1 mg/dL], pulmonary edema, or cerebral or visual symptoms).

Gestational Hypertension

Gestational hypertension, or *pregnancy-induced hypertension,* is defined as an elevation of blood pressure above 139/89 mm Hg in a previously healthy woman after the first 19 weeks of pregnancy if the elevated blood pressures were recorded at least twice, with the readings taken a minimum of 4 hours apart, and no proteinuria is present. Gestational hypertension develops into preeclampsia in approximately one-fourth of these patients. It is distinguished from the onset of chronic hypertension by a postpartum return to a normotensive state.

Preeclampsia

Preeclampsia is a complex multisystem disorder of unknown etiology that is characterized by combined development of new-onset hypertension (see earlier) and new-onset proteinuria (>300 mg/24 hours) after the first 20 weeks of pregnancy. In the absence of proteinuria the following signs/symptoms are diagnostic of preeclampsia: thrombocytopenia (platelet count < 100,000/μL), renal insufficiency (serum creatinine > 1.1 mg/dL), pulmonary edema, or cerebral or visual symptoms. *Severe preeclampsia* is now defined either by blood pressure criteria (systolic blood pressure > 159 mm Hg or diastolic > 110 mm Hg) or the presence of the aforementioned nonproteinuria criteria. Tables 31.4 and 31.5 list the diagnostic criteria and clinical manifestations of preeclampsia.

Risk factors for preeclampsia include obesity, nulliparity, and advanced maternal age (Table 31.6). Of interest, smoking during pregnancy is protective against preeclampsia.

TABLE 31.5	Manifestations and Complications of Preeclampsia

Systemic hypertension
Congestive heart failure
Decreased colloid osmotic pressure
Pulmonary edema
Arterial hypoxemia
Laryngeal edema
Cerebral edema (headaches, visual disturbances, changes in levels of consciousness)
Grand mal seizures
Cerebral hemorrhage
Hypovolemia
HELLP syndrome (hemolysis, elevated liver enzymes, low platelets)
Disseminated intravascular coagulation
Proteinuria
Oliguria
Acute tubular necrosis
Epigastric pain
Decreased uterine blood flow
Intrauterine growth retardation
Premature labor and delivery
Placental abruption

TABLE 31.6	Risk Factors for Development of Preeclampsia

Factor	Relative Risk
Nulliparity	3
African American race	1.5
Age < 15 or > 35	3
Multiple gestation	4
Family history of preeclampsia	5
Chronic hypertension	10
Chronic renal disease	20
Diabetes mellitus	2
Collagen vascular disease	2–3
Angiotensinogen T235 allele	
Homozygosity	20
Heterozygosity	4

Pathophysiology

Preeclampsia is specific to human pregnancy. It is a disease of the placenta and occurs with molar pregnancies (pregnancy without the presence of fetal tissue). The hallmark of preeclampsia is an abnormal placentation-implantation. Normally, cytotrophoblasts invade the uterine wall, reaching decidual arteries and interacting with the endothelium. As a result of that interaction, cytotrophoblasts acquire an endothelial phenotype and decidual arteries become low-resistance vessels. In preeclampsia, shallow endovascular invasion precludes this cytotrophoblasts-endothelium interaction. Spiral arteries remain constricted high-resistance blood vessels that fail to provide adequate oxygen and nutrients for the growing placenta and fetus. The abnormal placenta releases vasoactive substances that cause severe endothelial dysfunction of the maternal vasculature. This injured or hyperactivated

TABLE 31.7	Diagnostic Features of Preeclampsia With Severe Features

Blood pressure > 159/110 mm Hg on 2 occasions at least 4 hours apart
Thrombocytopenia (platelet count < 100,000/μL)
Renal insufficiency (serum creatinine > 1.1 mg/dL)
Pulmonary edema
Cerebral or visual symptoms

endothelium further compromises placental blood flow. The plasma concentrations of vasodilators such as nitric oxide and prostacyclin are decreased. Severe proangiogenic and antiangiogenic imbalance has been described in patients with preeclampsia. It is unclear whether this imbalance is a cause or a consequence of abnormal implantation. Antiangiogenic proteins cause endothelial damage, especially in blood vessels with fenestrated endothelium, as is found in kidney, liver, and brain.

The sensitivity of vascular receptors to angiotensin II is significantly decreased during normal pregnancy. In preeclampsia the sensitivity increases, which contributes to vasoconstriction and placental insufficiency.

Hypoalbuminemia secondary to proteinuria and sometimes impairment of synthetic liver function results in low oncotic pressure. Endothelial injury and low oncotic pressure lead to third spacing of fluid and intravascular volume depletion.

Treatment

The definitive treatment for preeclampsia is delivery. At term a patient diagnosed with preeclampsia should be delivered. If the preeclampsia is without severe features and the patient remote from term, conservative management with bed rest and monitoring until 37 weeks' gestation or until the status of the mother or fetus deteriorates is recommended.

In women with preeclampsia with *severe* features (Table 31.7) the fetus should be delivered *immediately* in the following circumstances:
- before fetal viability
- at more than 34 weeks' gestation
- when the maternal or fetal condition is unstable, regardless of gestational age

The mode of delivery depends on fetal gestational age, the findings on cervical examination, assessment of fetal well-being, and the fetal presenting part. Only 14%–20% of women with preeclampsia with severe features are delivered vaginally.

Magnesium sulfate is administered for seizure prophylaxis (Table 31.8). It is the anticonvulsant of choice because it is 50% more effective in prevention of new and recurrent seizures than diazepam or phenytoin. The precise mechanism of action is not known. Possible explanations for its anticonvulsant effect include competitive blockade of N-methyl-D-aspartate receptors, prevention of calcium ion entry into ischemic cells, protection of endothelial cells from free radical injury, and selective dilation of cerebral blood vessels. Other benefits include an antiinflammatory effect, a decrease in maternal systemic vascular resistance, an increase in cardiac index, and fetal neuroprotection.

TABLE 31.8	Seizure Prophylaxis

Magnesium 4–6 g IV followed by 1–2 g/h IV as a continuous infusion (goal is to maintain serum concentrations of 2.0–3.5 mEq/L)
Toxicity
    7–10 mEq/L associated with loss of deep tendon reflexes
    10–13 mEq/L associated with respiratory paralysis
    ≥15 mEq/L associated with altered cardiac conduction
    >25 mEq/L associated with cardiac arrest

IV, Intravenous.

TABLE 31.9	Treatment of Systemic Hypertension Associated With Preeclampsia

Maintain diastolic blood pressure < 110 mm Hg
Hydralazine 5–10 mg IV every 20–30 min
Labetalol 5–10 mg IV or 10–20 mg PO
Nitroglycerin 0.5 μg/kg/min IV, titrated to response

IV, Intravenous; *PO,* by mouth.

There is no need to treat hypertension in women with preeclampsia *without* severe features. Indications for antihypertensive treatment during pregnancy are chronic hypertension, severe hypertension during labor and delivery, and expectant management of preeclampsia with severe features. There are only two benefits from such a treatment: prevention of placental abruption and prevention of cerebrovascular accident (which accounts for 15%–20% of maternal deaths). The goal of therapy is to maintain blood pressure below 160/110 mm Hg.

Hydralazine, labetalol, and nifedipine are all effective antihypertensives in these patients. Refractory hypertension may necessitate continuous infusion of an antihypertensive. Nitroglycerin, sodium nitroprusside, and fenoldopam are all useful as short-term therapy (Table 31.9).

Invasive hemodynamic monitoring may be useful, especially during cesarean delivery. Catheterization of the internal jugular vein during the peripartum period is associated with a higher overall risk of complications, especially infectious complications, in parturient patients compared with nonpregnant medical or surgical patients (25% vs. 15%–20%, respectively). The internal jugular vein overlies the carotid artery to a greater extent in pregnant than in nonpregnant patients, so the standard landmark approach is associated with a higher risk of carotid puncture (19% in pregnant patients vs. 10% in nonpregnant patients with the landmark approach; 6% vs. 3%, respectively, with the palpatory technique). Real-time ultrasound guidance for central line placement offers particular advantages in the pregnant population, given the ease of choosing an approach angle that reduces the risk of carotid puncture.

Management of Anesthesia

Fluid management in the patient with preeclampsia is complicated by the conflict between the need to give fluids to an intravascularly depleted patient (the degree of depletion may be reflected by a rising hematocrit [Hct]) and the obligation to avoid administration of fluids to a patient with "leaky" vasculature. As mentioned earlier, endothelial damage and low oncotic pressure make preeclamptic patients prone to third spacing of fluids and thus may lead to pulmonary edema. Invasive hemodynamic monitoring may help guide fluid therapy in patients with preeclampsia. It should be remembered, however, that catheterization of the internal jugular vein during the peripartum period carries higher risk of complications than in nonpregnant medical or surgical patients.

Labor Analgesia

In addition to providing the common benefits of epidural labor analgesia, use of neuraxial techniques in preeclamptic patients can facilitate blood pressure control during labor. Epidural analgesia will also increase intervillous blood flow in preeclampsia, which will improve uteroplacental performance and as a result fetal well-being.

Because these patients are at high risk of requiring cesarean delivery, early placement of an epidural catheter can be considered to facilitate the use of epidural anesthesia for cesarean delivery and thus avoid the risks of general anesthesia.

Spinal Anesthesia. Spinal anesthesia is the anesthetic of choice for patients with preeclampsia, unless it is contraindicated because of hypocoagulation. Neuraxial blockade causes sympathectomy and may lead to hypotension in healthy patients. In preeclamptic patients, hypertension and vasoconstriction are the result of hyperactivity of the angiotensin II receptors. Spinal anesthesia does not influence the angiotensin system and thus may result in a lesser degree of hypotension in preeclamptic patients than in healthy patients.

General Anesthesia. Not only are patients with preeclampsia subject to the common risks of general anesthesia during pregnancy, but these patients also have a higher risk of difficult intubation resulting from severe upper airway edema and a higher risk of aspiration because of the increased likelihood of difficulty in airway management. They also have an exaggerated response to sympathomimetics and methylergonovine. They have greater sensitivity to the action of nondepolarizing muscle relaxants secondary to magnesium therapy. Finally, these patients have a higher risk of uterine atony and peripartum hemorrhage resulting from the smooth muscle–relaxant effects of magnesium therapy.

HELLP Syndrome

Signs and Symptoms

*H*emolysis, *e*levated *l*iver transaminase levels, and *l*ow *p*latelet counts are the characteristic features of HELLP syndrome, a severe form of preeclampsia. Some 26% of patients with preeclampsia demonstrate 1 sign, 12% have 2 signs, and 10% show all 3 signs of the syndrome. Approximately 30% of cases present postpartum. The most frequent clinical symptoms are right upper quadrant pain (80% of patients) and edema (50%–60% of patients). Hemolysis is diagnosed by abnormalities on peripheral blood smear (presence of schistocytes), elevated bilirubin concentration (>1.2 mg/dL), decreased haptoglobin level

(<25 mg/dL), and elevated lactate dehydrogenase level (>600 units/L). Plasma concentrations of transaminases are more than twice normal levels. The platelet count is often lower than 100,000/mm³. Maternal and perinatal morbidity and mortality is increased. Formation of a subcapsular hematoma of the liver may complicate HELLP syndrome, and hepatic rupture with a very high incidence of mortality can occur.

Treatment

The definitive treatment of HELLP syndrome is delivery of the fetus. ACOG recommends that women with HELLP syndrome be delivered regardless of fetal gestational age. Patients must receive seizure prophylaxis with magnesium sulfate and correction of coagulopathy. Dexamethasone increases platelet count to a greater degree than does betamethasone.

Management of Anesthesia

Coagulopathy, risk of disseminated intravascular coagulation (DIC), and risk of severe intraabdominal bleeding resulting from rupture of a subcapsular hematoma of the liver are specific concerns in patients with HELLP syndrome. These are in addition to the general problems of anesthetic management in parturient patients with preeclampsia with severe features.

Eclampsia

Signs and Symptoms

Eclampsia is seizures or coma in the setting of preeclampsia in the absence of any other pathologic brain condition. It is by definition considered *preeclampsia with severe features* and has an incidence of 1 in 2000 pregnancies. The majority of patients are diagnosed with preeclampsia before development of seizures; however, eclampsia is the first manifestation of preeclampsia in 20%–38% of cases. The magnitude of hypertension does not correlate with the risk of eclampsia. Approximately half of patients with preeclampsia who develop seizures report prodromal symptoms such as headache or visual changes. Between 38% and 50% of eclamptic seizures occur before term; 16% of seizures occurring at term take place during labor or within 48 hours of delivery.

Typical eclamptic seizures last less than 10 minutes and are neither recurrent nor associated with focal neurologic signs. Mortality related to eclampsia is about 2%.

About one-third of eclamptic patients develop respiratory failure (with 23% of cases requiring mechanical ventilation), kidney failure, coagulopathy, cerebrovascular accident, or cardiac arrest. Fetal perinatal mortality is approximately 7% and is primarily related to issues associated with prematurity.

Management of Anesthesia

Eclampsia is not an indication for cesarean delivery.

Management of the patient with eclampsia is directed at prevention of aspiration, maintenance of airway patency, control of seizures and prevention of their recurrence, control of hypertension, and evaluation for delivery. Eclamptic seizures are self-limiting.

Magnesium sulfate is the anticonvulsant of choice because it is more effective and has a better safety profile than benzodiazepines, phenytoin, or lytic cocktails. The standard IV regimen is a loading of magnesium sulfate of 2 g every 15 minutes to a maximum of 6 g. If a patient develops seizures while receiving a magnesium infusion for seizure prophylaxis, administration of a 1- to 2-g bolus is recommended, after which a plasma magnesium level should be measured.

If the patient and fetus are in stable condition following an eclamptic seizure, management of the patient will proceed as it would for a patient with preeclampsia, and immediate delivery is not indicated unless that had been the plan before the seizure.

OBSTETRIC CONDITIONS AND COMPLICATIONS

Conditions that complicate delivery include hemorrhagic complications, amniotic fluid embolism, uterine rupture, trial of labor after cesarean delivery, vaginal birth after cesarean delivery, abnormal presentations, and multiple births.

Obstetric Hemorrhage

Obstetric hemorrhage is a leading cause of maternal morbidity and intensive care unit (ICU) admission in the United States. Although bleeding can occur at any time during pregnancy, third-trimester hemorrhage is the most threatening to maternal and fetal well-being (Table 31.10). Placenta previa and placental abruption are the major causes of bleeding during the third trimester. Uterine rupture can be responsible for uncontrolled hemorrhage that manifests during active labor. Postpartum hemorrhage occurs after 3%–5% of all vaginal deliveries. Uterine atony and placenta accreta are two leading causes of peripartum hemorrhage. Placenta accreta is the most common indication for a cesarean hysterectomy. Retained products of conception and cervical or vaginal lacerations may also lead to postpartum hemorrhage.

Because of the increased blood volume and relative good health of the average pregnant patient, parturient women tolerate mild to moderate hemorrhage with few clinical signs or symptoms. Clinical signs may be absent until 15% of total blood volume is lost. This can lead to underestimation of blood loss.

Placenta Previa

Signs and Symptoms

The cardinal symptom of placenta previa is *painless* vaginal bleeding. The first episode usually stops spontaneously. Bleeding typically manifests at approximately week 32 of gestation, when the lower uterine segment begins to form. When this diagnosis is suspected, the position of the placenta needs to be confirmed via ultrasonography or radioisotope scan.

TABLE 31.10	Differential Diagnosis of Third-Trimester Bleeding	
	Signs and Symptoms	Predisposing Conditions
Placenta previa	Painless vaginal bleeding	Advanced age Multiple parity
Placental abruption	Abdominal pain Bleeding partially or wholly concealed Uterine irritability Shock Coagulopathy Acute renal failure Fetal distress	High parity Advanced age Cigarette smoking Cocaine abuse Trauma Uterine abnormalities Compression of the inferior vena cava Chronic systemic hypertension
Uterine rupture	Abdominal pain Vaginal pain Recession of presenting part Disappearance of fetal heart tones, fetal bradycardia Hemodynamic instability	Previous uterine incision Rapid spontaneous delivery Excessive uterine stimulation Cephalopelvic disproportion Multiple parity Polyhydramnios

Diagnosis

Placenta previa occurs in up to 1% of full-term pregnancies. It is not known, although there may be an association with advanced maternal age and high parity. The greatest risk factor is previous cesarean section. Placenta previa is classified as *complete* when the entire cervical os is covered by placental tissue, *partial* when the internal os is covered by placental tissue when closed but not when fully dilated, and *marginal* when placental tissue encroaches on or extends to the margin of the internal cervical os. Approximately 50% of parturient women with placenta previa have marginal implantations. Availability of more sophisticated obstetric ultrasonography has eliminated the need for a classic/traditional "double setup" cervical examination to diagnose placenta previa. Magnetic resonance imaging (MRI) and color flow mapping during an ultrasonographic examination may identify, or at least raise suspicion for, placenta accreta.

Treatment

Once the diagnosis is made, the obstetrician will determine timing and mode of delivery. Expectant management will be chosen if the bleeding stops and the fetus is immature. When fetal lung maturity is achieved, or at 37 weeks, delivery should proceed. Obviously, delivery will occur at any time the mother exhibits cardiovascular instability. Except for patients with a marginal previa who might elect vaginal delivery, patients will be delivered by cesarean section.

Prognosis

Maternal mortality is rare. Infant perinatal mortality is 12 per 1000 births. The risk that cesarean hysterectomy will be required increases with the number of previous cesarean deliveries.

Management of Anesthesia

Anesthetic management depends on the obstetric plan and the condition of the parturient patient.

Preoperative. Mild to moderate blood loss is well tolerated by the patient and thus may result in underestimation of bleeding by the anesthesiologist. Adequate volume resuscitation is thus paramount to the patient's care. Typing and cross-matching should be performed for all patients to ensure continuous availability of packed red blood cells (PRBCs) and component products.

Intraoperative. Parturient patients with complete or partial placenta previa will be delivered by cesarean section. Anesthetic management will depend on maternal and fetal status and the urgency of the surgery. If the patient has not had recent bleeding and is scheduled for an elective procedure, regional anesthesia is preferred, as it is for all patients undergoing cesarean delivery. Large-bore IV access should be established because the patient is at greater risk of intraoperative bleeding. Cross-matched blood should be immediately available, and if the patient is in unstable condition, component products should also be available.

If hemorrhage necessitates emergency delivery, general anesthesia is the anesthetic of choice. Ketamine and etomidate are the preferred induction agents in the hypovolemic patient. Drug selection for maintenance of anesthesia will be determined by the mother's hemodynamic status.

Placenta Accreta

Placenta accreta refers to a placenta that is abnormally adherent to the myometrium but has *not* invaded the myometrium. In *placenta increta,* the placenta *has* invaded the myometrium. *Placenta percreta* is invasion through the serosa. Massive hemorrhage may occur when removal of the placenta is attempted after delivery.

Signs and Symptoms

The majority of patients with placenta accreta have no symptoms, so recognizing known risk factors is essential to early diagnosis. Retained placenta and postpartum hemorrhage occur in patients with placenta accreta.

Diagnosis

Risk factors include placenta previa and/or previous cesarean delivery, with the risk increasing for placenta previa in patients with multiple cesarean deliveries. Placenta implantation anteriorly in patients with previous cesarean deliveries also increases the risk. Additional risk factors include a short interval from cesarean delivery to conception (<18 months), advanced maternal age, and female gender of the fetus. MRI and ultrasonography with Doppler flow mapping have identified placenta accreta antenatally. However, because the predictive value of these tests is not perfect, this diagnosis is often made at the time of surgery.

Treatment

Management of placenta accreta requires close coordination among the anesthesiologist, obstetrician, interventional radiologist, gynecologic oncologist, blood bank, and specialized surgical teams. Thorough planning decreases blood loss, requirement for blood products, and perioperative morbidity and mortality. Elective cesarean delivery at 34–35 weeks' gestation to avoid emergent delivery is recommended.

A small focal placenta accreta can sometimes be excised and oversutured, allowing uterine sparing; however, in the majority of cases, cesarean hysterectomy is warranted. The magnitude of hemorrhage may be significantly reduced if attempts to separate of the placenta are avoided.

With advances in endovascular procedures, uterine-sparing management can be offered to selected patients. In this approach the placenta is left in place after delivery of the fetus, without further surgical intervention, and inflation of angioballoons or repeated selective uterine artery embolization is performed. Resorption of the poorly perfused placenta may be augmented by concurrent treatment with methotrexate. In the absence of data from large randomized controlled trials, controversy still exists about the safety and efficacy of endovascular interventions. ACOG (2012) describes both the use and efficacy of endovascular interventions as "unclear." Further, although complications are uncommon, they can be severe.

Prognosis

Maternal prognosis is good if the patient does not experience significant hemorrhage. As noted earlier, there has been some success with uterine preservation in selected cases; however, the majority of women still undergo cesarean hysterectomy. If an attempt is made to extract the placenta manually, profound hemorrhage may occur.

Management of Anesthesia

Preoperative. Significant hemorrhage should be anticipated, and thus at least two large-bore IV catheters should be placed. Insertion of an arterial catheter should be considered. PRBCs and component products should be immediately available. As soon as it is known that a patient with suspected placenta accreta will be undergoing surgical delivery, the anesthesiologist should communicate directly with the blood bank, request blood products, and provide information about the possibility for massive transfusion. The amount and type of requested products depends on the chosen transfusion strategy (goal-directed versus damage control), predicted severity of bleeding (i.e., accreta vs. percreta), baseline patient laboratory evaluation (hemoglobin, Hct, platelets, electrolytes, and coagulation), and expected limitations in supply (e.g., rare blood group or difficult match because of the presence of antibodies).

Intraoperative. A cesarean hysterectomy can be performed successfully under neuraxial anesthesia. If any of the parties involved (i.e., patient, surgeon, anesthesiologist) have particular concerns regarding neuraxial anesthesia, it is reasonable to proceed with general anesthesia.

Management of blood loss is the major issue in patients with placenta accreta. Uterine artery flow increases more than threefold during pregnancy, reaching almost 700 mL/min at term. In facilities where fast intraoperative monitoring of Hct and hemostasis (specifically fibrinogen) is available, goal-directed transfusion is the preferred strategy. In this setting, transfusion of PRBCs should be provided to prevent decrease in Hct below 21%. Transfusion of a fibrinogen-containing product (either cryoprecipitate or fibrinogen concentrate; the efficacy of these has been shown to be equivalent) should be provided to prevent decrease in fibrinogen below 2 g/dL. With this goal-directed strategy, transfusion of other blood products is usually not necessary. There is strong evidence that fibrinogen plays a central role in the pathophysiology of peripartum hemorrhage. In a study of 128 patients with postpartum hemorrhage, a fibrinogen concentration below 200 mg/dL at the time hemorrhage was diagnosed had a 100% positive predictive value for severe hemorrhage (defined as decrease of hemoglobin > 4 g/dL). The value of tranexamic acid in postpartum hemorrhage is currently under investigation in the multicenter WOMAN Trial (World Maternal Antifibrinolytic Trial).

A report from the Canadian National Advisory Committee on Blood and Blood Products found no evidence to support the use of 1:1:1 blood component ratios, and instead recommends that the ratio of blood components should be adjusted by results from either traditional coagulation tests or thromboelastography or both. In facilities where fast intraoperative monitoring of Hct and hemostasis (especially fibrinogen) is not possible, obstetrical massive transfusion protocol based on damage control resuscitation should be used.

Autologous RBC salvage can decrease the transfusion of allogeneic blood. Use of the intraoperative blood salvage machine ("cell saver") began in the 1970s in nonobstetric cases. Concerns regarding the use of cell salvage in obstetrics include the risk of amniotic fluid embolism and maternal alloimmunization. Although we do not have controlled trials to support the safety of cell salvage in obstetrics, we do have retrospective studies on over 650 cases of its use in obstetric cases without adverse sequelae. Cell salvage also offers the potential for reducing complications associated with allogeneic blood transfusion, including transfusion-related infections, mismatches related to clerical errors, and cost. ACOG and ASA have published recommendations supporting the use of intraoperative cell salvage in obstetrics.

Plasma electrolyte levels should be measured at baseline and every hour after initiation of massive transfusion, with specific assessment for hyperkalemia, hypomagnesemia, hypocalcemia, and hyperchloremia.

Placenta Abruption
Signs and Symptoms
Signs and symptoms of placental abruption depend on the site and extent of the placental separation, but abdominal pain is *always* present. When the separation involves only the placental margins, the escaping blood can appear as vaginal bleeding. On the other hand, large volumes of extravasated blood can remain concealed within the uterus. Severe blood loss from placental abruption presents as maternal hypotension, uterine irritability and hypertonus, and fetal distress or demise. Clotting abnormalities can occur. The classic hemorrhage picture includes thrombocytopenia, depletion of fibrinogen, and prolonged plasma thromboplastin times. DIC can occur and may be accompanied by acute renal failure occurring as a result of fibrin deposition in renal arterioles. Fetal distress reflects the loss of functional placenta and decreased uteroplacental perfusion because of maternal hypotension.

Diagnosis
Placental abruption is defined as premature separation of a normally implanted placenta after 20 weeks' gestation. The precise causes are unknown, but the incidence is increased with high parity, uterine abnormalities, compression of the inferior vena cava, gestational hypertension, and cocaine abuse. Placental abruption accounts for approximately one-third of third-trimester hemorrhages and occurs in 0.5%–1% of all pregnancies. Diagnosis is made before delivery using ultrasonography and at delivery by examination of the placenta.

Treatment
Definitive treatment of placental abruption is delivery of the fetus and placenta. Delivery may be vaginal if the abruption is not jeopardizing maternal or fetal well-being. Otherwise, delivery is by cesarean section.

Prognosis
Maternal complications associated with placental abruption include DIC, acute renal failure, and uterine atony, which may lead to postpartum hemorrhage. DIC occurs in approximately 10% of patients with placental abruption.

Neonatal complications are significant. Perinatal mortality is 25-fold higher if a term pregnancy is complicated by abruption. Fetal distress is also common owing to the disruption of placental blood flow.

Management of Anesthesia
If maternal hypotension is absent, clotting study results are acceptable, and there is no evidence of fetal distress due to uteroplacental insufficiency, epidural analgesia is useful to provide analgesia for labor and vaginal delivery. When the magnitude of placental separation and resulting hemorrhage are severe, emergency cesarean delivery is necessary. Most often, general anesthesia is used because regional anesthesia may be unwise in a patient with hemodynamic instability. Anesthetic management is similar to that in patients with placenta previa. Blood and blood products should be readily available because of the risk of bleeding and DIC.

It is not uncommon for blood to dissect between layers of the myometrium after premature separation of the placenta. As a result the uterus is unable to contract adequately after delivery, and postpartum hemorrhage occurs. Uncontrolled hemorrhage may require an emergency hysterectomy. Bleeding may be exaggerated by coagulopathy, in which case infusion of fresh frozen plasma and platelets may be indicated to replace deficient clotting factors. Clotting parameters usually revert to normal within a few hours after delivery of the fetus.

Postpartum Hemorrhage
Uterine Atony
Uterine atony after vaginal delivery is a common cause of postpartum bleeding and a potential cause of maternal mortality. Conditions associated with uterine atony include multiple parity, multiple births, polyhydramnios, a large fetus, and a retained placenta. Uterine atony may occur immediately after delivery or may manifest several hours later. Treatment is with IV oxytocin, which results in contraction of the uterus. Methylergonovine, administered intravenously or intramuscularly, or intramuscular or intrauterine carboprost tromethamine (or misoprostol) may also be used to control hemorrhage. In rare instances it may be necessary to perform an emergency hysterectomy.

Retained Placenta
Retained placenta occurs in approximately 1% of all vaginal deliveries and usually necessitates manual exploration of the uterus. If epidural analgesia has been used for vaginal delivery, manual removal of the retained placenta may be attempted under epidural anesthesia. Spinal anesthesia (saddle block) or low-dose IV ketamine may provide adequate analgesia if an epidural catheter is not in place. In rare cases a general anesthetic may be needed. Low doses of IV nitroglycerin (40-μg boluses) are used to relax the uterus for placental removal when indicated.

Uterine Rupture

Uterine rupture occurs in up to 0.1% of full-term pregnancies and may be associated with rapid spontaneous delivery, excessive oxytocin stimulation, multiple parity with cephalopelvic disproportion, or unrecognized transverse presentation. The risk of uterine rupture is significantly higher among patients with a history of classical uterine incision (up to 5%) compared to low transverse incision (<1%). Uterine rupture and dehiscence represent a spectrum ranging from incomplete rupture or gradual dehiscence of surgical scars to explosive rupture with intraperitoneal extrusion of uterine contents.

Signs and Symptoms
Uterine rupture may present with severe abdominal pain (often referred to the shoulder because of subdiaphragmatic irritation by intraabdominal blood) as well as maternal hypotension and disappearance of fetal heart tones.

Diagnosis
An ultrasonographic examination is useful in making the diagnosis of uterine rupture. Visual examination of the uterus at cesarean delivery will detect rupture or dehiscence. Manual examination with vaginal delivery will also detect dehiscence.

Treatment
Uterine rupture with maternal and/or fetal distress mandates immediate laparotomy, delivery, and surgical repair or hysterectomy.

Prognosis
Maternal mortality is rare. Fetal mortality is approximately 35%.

Management of Anesthesia
Anesthetic management is similar to that for patients with placenta previa who are in unstable condition.

Trial of Labor After Cesarean Delivery

Women with a history of one or two low transverse cesarean deliveries may attempt a vaginal birth (trial of labor after cesarean delivery [TOLAC]), with the goal of achieving vaginal birth after cesarean delivery (VBAC). TOLAC decreases the rate of cesarean deliveries, reduces maternal morbidity and mortality (from 13 per 100,000 to 4 per 100,000 live births), and diminishes risk of complications in future pregnancies. Some 74% of appropriately chosen candidates for TOLAC will successfully accomplish vaginal delivery. Unfortunately, many medical and nonmedical factors may increase the risk of failure when TOLAC/VBAC is used and may lead to increased maternal and perinatal morbidity.

Factors associated with a lower rate of successful VBAC include socioeconomic, ethnic, and medical factors. African American or Hispanic ethnicity, advanced maternal age, single motherhood, and fewer than 12 years of maternal education are associated with lower success. In addition, delivery at low-volume hospitals and maternal comorbid conditions (hypertension, diabetes, asthma, seizure disorders, renal disease, heart disease, obesity) also decrease the rate of a successful VBAC. Induction of labor, fetal gestational age of more than 40 weeks, fetal weight over 4000 g, and poor cervical dilation may also be predictive of failure.

The most feared obstetric emergency related to TOLAC is uterine rupture (see earlier). Factors that may increase the risk of uterine rupture among parturient women with a history of previous cesarean delivery include a classic uterine scar, induction of labor (especially after 40 weeks), two or more cesarean deliveries, maternal obesity, fetal weight over 4000 g, and delivery at a low-volume facility. In a retrospective analysis of 1787 cases of TOLAC, only two risk factors for uterine rupture were found: interdelivery interval of less than 18 months (which increased the risk threefold) and use of a single-layer closure during a prior cesarean delivery. Careful selection of candidates for TOLAC with consideration of all risk factors is necessary.

The ACOG practice bulletin for VBAC recommends that the potential complications of VBAC be thoroughly discussed with the patient and be documented before the patient is offered the option for VBAC. Both ACOG and ASA recommend that personnel—including the obstetrician, anesthesiologist, and operating room staff—be immediately available at all times to perform an emergency cesarean delivery when VBAC is being attempted. Despite the concern for uterine rupture in this patient population, the risk of uterine rupture in patients undergoing VBAC following one cesarean delivery is approximately 2%. Women who undergo VBAC rather than elective repeat cesarean delivery have reduced morbidity associated with their delivery. However, there may be a higher incidence of perinatal death in patients undergoing VBAC.

Management of Anesthesia
Neuraxial labor analgesia provides all the same benefits for parturient women attempting TOLAC as for women without a history of cesarean delivery.

The suggestion that neuraxial analgesia will mask the signs and symptoms of uterine rupture is unfounded. The pain of uterine rupture is constant (does not resolve between contractions), is much more intense, and has a different quality than the pain of contractions. Worsening of the fetal heart rate tracing will alert the obstetric and anesthesiology teams to abnormality as well. The opioid-based epidural solutions used for labor provide only analgesia and *cannot* mask the pain of uterine rupture, because these solutions *do not* provide anesthesia.

Amniotic Fluid Embolism

Amniotic fluid embolism is a rare catastrophic and life-threatening complication of pregnancy that occurs when there is disruption in the barrier between the amniotic fluid and the maternal circulation. The three most common sites for entry of amniotic fluid into the maternal circulation are the endocervical veins, the placenta, and a uterine trauma site. Multiparous parturient women experiencing tumultuous labors are at increased risk of amniotic fluid embolism.

Signs and Symptoms
The onset of the signs and symptoms of amniotic fluid embolism are dramatic and abrupt, classically manifesting as dyspnea, arterial hypoxemia, cyanosis, seizures, loss of consciousness, and hypotension that is disproportionate to blood loss. Fetal distress is present at the same time. More than

80% of these parturient women experience cardiopulmonary arrest. Coagulopathy resembling DIC with associated bleeding is common and may be the only presenting symptom.

Pathophysiology

The principal defect created by amniotic fluid embolism is a mechanical blockage of a part of the pulmonary circulation accompanied by vasoconstriction of the remaining vessels resulting from release of undefined chemicals such as prostaglandins, leukotrienes, serotonin, and histamine. As a result, pulmonary artery pressures increase, arterial hypoxemia develops owing to ventilation/perfusion mismatching, and hypotension occurs, reflecting decreased cardiac output and congestive heart failure caused by right ventricular outflow obstruction and acute right heart failure.

Diagnosis

The diagnosis of amniotic fluid embolism is based largely on clinical signs and symptoms. These include increased pulmonary artery pressures and decreased cardiac output as determined by measurements from invasive or noninvasive cardiac output monitors. Ultimately the presence of amniotic fluid material is confirmed in the parturient patient's blood aspirated from a central venous or pulmonary artery catheter. Findings of fetal squamous cells, fat, and mucin in samples of the patient's blood are indicative of amniotic fluid embolism.

Conditions that can mimic amniotic fluid embolism include inhalation of gastric contents, pulmonary embolism, venous air embolism, and local anesthetic toxicity. Pulmonary aspiration is more likely when bronchoconstriction accompanies the clinical signs and symptoms. Indeed, bronchospasm is rare in parturient women who experience amniotic fluid embolism. Pulmonary embolism is usually accompanied by chest pain.

Treatment

Treatment of amniotic fluid embolism includes tracheal intubation and mechanical ventilation of the lungs with 100% oxygen, inotropic support as guided by central venous or pulmonary artery catheter monitoring, and correction of coagulopathy. Use of positive end-expiratory pressure is often helpful for improving oxygenation. Dopamine, dobutamine, and norepinephrine have been recommended as inotropic agents to treat acute left ventricular dysfunction and associated hypotension. Fluid therapy is guided by central venous pressure monitoring, but it must be kept in mind that these patients are vulnerable to developing pulmonary edema. Treatment of DIC may include administration of fresh frozen plasma, cryoprecipitate, and platelets. Even with immediate and aggressive treatment, mortality resulting from amniotic fluid embolism remains higher than 80%.

Abnormal Presentations and Multiple Births

The presentation of the fetus is determined by the presenting part and the anatomic portion of the fetus felt through the cervix by manual examination. Description of fetal position is based on the relationship of the fetal occiput, chin, or sacrum to the left or right side of the parturient patient. Approximately 90% of deliveries are cephalic presentations in either the *occiput transverse* or *occiput anterior* position. *All* other presentations and positions are considered abnormal.

Breech Presentation
Diagnosis

Breech rather than cephalic presentations account for approximately 3.5% of all pregnancies. The cause of breech presentation is unknown, but factors that seem to predispose to this presentation include prematurity, placenta previa, multiple gestations, and uterine anomalies. Fetal abnormalities, including hydrocephalus and polyhydramnios, are also associated with breech presentations.

Treatment

Fetuses in breech presentations are delivered by elective cesarean section. Vaginal breech delivery is rare and necessitates immediate availability of anesthetic care because serious complications can occur.

Prognosis

Breech vaginal deliveries result in increased maternal morbidity. Compared with cephalic presentations, there is a greater likelihood of cervical lacerations, perineal injury, retained placenta, and shock resulting from hemorrhage. Morbidity and mortality of the neonate are also increased. These infants are more likely to experience arterial hypoxemia and acidosis during delivery because of umbilical cord compression. Prolapse of the umbilical cord occurs with increased frequency in breech presentations and is presumed to reflect failure of the presenting part to fill the lower uterine segment.

Management of Anesthesia

In parturient patients undergoing elective cesarean delivery for breech presentation, spinal anesthesia is generally used, as is routine for elective cesarean delivery.

In the case of breech presentation, vaginal delivery may be complicated by umbilical cord prolapse or fetal head entrapment, which necessitates emergency anesthesia for cesarean or instrumented vaginal delivery. Dense perineal anesthesia is needed for vaginal instrumentation and must be administered rapidly, either by using 3% 2-chloroprocaine if an epidural catheter is in place, or by inducing general anesthesia.

Multiple Gestations

The increasing use of assisted reproductive technologies has resulted in a markedly greater frequency of multiple gestations. Twin pregnancies comprise approximately 3% of all pregnancies. Triplet and higher-order gestations increased by more than 400% in the 1980s and 1990s but fell 29% from 1998–2010.

Treatment

In all triplet and higher-order gestations, delivery is by cesarean section. For twin gestations the presentation of the twins is considered when determining the mode of delivery. If both are in vertex position, vaginal delivery is appropriate. If twin A is in breech position, cesarean delivery is recommended. The route of delivery for vertex-non-vertex twins is controversial, but often cesarean delivery is recommended.

Prognosis

Maternal morbidity and mortality are increased with multiple gestations, because many obstetric complications are more common in this setting. Fetal perinatal mortality and morbidity are also increased, with preterm delivery the most common cause.

Management of Anesthesia

Preoperative. The physiologic changes associated with pregnancy may be exaggerated with multiple gestations. The larger size of the uterus causes a greater decrease in functional residual capacity. Maternal cardiac output is 20% greater in twin pregnancies.

Intraoperative. Epidural analgesia is preferred for labor analgesia because it will facilitate instrumented vaginal delivery or allow rapid induction of surgical anesthesia if needed. The risk of intrapartum and postpartum hemorrhage is increased; thus large-bore IV access should be established, and current blood type and screen results should be available. The anesthesiologist must be prepared for vaginal (forceps) or abdominal operative delivery of twin B if that twin has a nonvertex presentation.

For planned cesarean delivery, maternal and fetal status will dictate anesthetic choice.

CO-EXISTING MEDICAL CONDITIONS

Co-existing medical diseases may accompany pregnancy and thus assume importance out of proportion to the implications of the disease in the absence of pregnancy.

Heart Disease

Because of the cardiovascular changes of pregnancy, women with congenital heart disease have increased risk of peripartum cardiac complications ("cardiac events").

Cardiac pathologies are the leading cause of indirect obstetric mortality in the United States. According to the Cardiac Disease in Pregnancy (CARPREG) study in Canada, which reviewed data for 562 patients with heart disease who had 599 pregnancies and were treated in 13 Canadian hospitals, such cardiac events include pulmonary edema (documented by findings on chest radiograph or the auscultation of crackles over more than one-third of the posterior lung fields), sustained symptomatic tachydysrhythmia or bradydysrhythmia requiring treatment, stroke, cardiac arrest, and death.

The likelihood of occurrence of a cardiac event can be estimated using a scale based on the presence of certain risk factors: history of previous cardiac event; a baseline New York Heart Association (NYHA) class greater than II rating or cyanosis; left heart obstruction (mitral valve area ≤ 2 cm^2, aortic valve area < 1.5 cm^2, or peak left ventricular outflow tract gradient > 30 mm Hg by echocardiography); and reduced systemic ventricular systolic function (ejection fraction $< 40\%$). One point is assigned for each risk factor. The risk of an event is estimated to be 5% with no points, 27% with 1 point, and 75% with 2 or more points.

Pulmonary hypertension is a significant risk factor for poor maternal and neonatal outcome. Patients with pulmonary hypertension are usually advised against pregnancy. Pulmonary insufficiency has been shown to increase the risk of peripartum complications.

The ZAHARA study investigated the outcome of 1802 parturients with a history of congenital heart disease and identified similar risk factors: a history of dysrhythmia, use of cardiac medication before pregnancy, NYHA class higher than II, aortic stenosis, moderate or severe mitral and/or tricuspid regurgitation, presence of a mechanical valve, and cyanotic heart disease. A new risk score calculation for cardiac complications was offered. Among all the cardiac events observed during pregnancy, the most frequent were dysrhythmia and congestive heart failure (Table 31.11).

Cardiomyopathy of Pregnancy
Diagnosis

Left ventricular failure late in the course of pregnancy or during the first 6 weeks postpartum has been termed *cardiomyopathy of pregnancy*. The precise etiology remains unknown. Suggested causes include myocarditis or an autoimmune response. Patients have signs and symptoms of left ventricular heart failure, frequently after delivery or in the postpartum period.

Treatment

Medical treatment of peripartum cardiomyopathy is similar to treatment of other dilated cardiomyopathies. This includes preload optimization, afterload reduction, and improvement of myocardial contractility. In addition, these patients may require anticoagulant therapy because of the increased risk of thromboembolism. It is important to remember that angiotensin-converting enzyme (ACE) inhibitors, which are routinely used for afterload reduction in nonpregnant patients, are *contraindicated* during pregnancy. However, nitroglycerin or nitroprusside can be used for afterload reduction in pregnant patients.

Collaboration among the obstetrician, cardiologist, and anesthesiologist is essential to optimize care of these patients. Induction of labor is usually recommended if the patient's cardiac status can be stabilized with medical therapy. However, if acute cardiac decompensation occurs, cesarean delivery may be required because of the inability of the mother to tolerate the stresses of labor.

TABLE 31.11	Multivariable Model for Composite End Points of Cardiac and Neonatal Complications Corrected for Maternal Age and Parity	
	Odds Ratio	P value
CARDIAC COMPLICATIONS		
History of dysrhythmia	4.3	0.0011
Cardiac medication use before pregnancy	4.2	<0.0001
NYHA functional class > II	2.2	0.0298
Left-sided heart obstruction (peak gradient > 50 mm Hg, aortic valve < 1.0 cm²	12.9	<0.0001
Moderate to severe AI	2.0	0.0427
Moderate to severe PI	2.3	0.0287
Mechanical prosthetic valve	74.7	0.0014
Cyanotic heart disease (corrected or not)	3.0	<0.0001
NEONATAL COMPLICATIONS		
Twin or multiple gestation	5.4	0.0014
Smoking during pregnancy	1.7	0.007
Cyanotic heart disease (corrected or not)	2.0	0.003
Mechanical prosthetic valve	13.9	0.0331
Cardiac medication use before pregnancy	2.2	0.0009

AI, Aortic insufficiency; *NYHA,* New York Heart Association; *PI,* pulmonary insufficiency.
Adapted from ZAHARA investigators. Predictors of pregnancy complications in women with congenital heart disease. *Eur Heart J.* 2010;31:2124-2132. Epub Jun 28, 2010.

Prognosis

In approximately half of these parturient patients, heart failure is transient, resolving within 6 months of delivery. In the remaining patients, idiopathic congestive cardiomyopathy persists, and in these patients the mortality rate is as high as 25%–50%.

Management of Anesthesia

Parturient patients with peripartum cardiomyopathy will likely require invasive monitoring, including intraarterial catheterization and pulmonary artery catheterization and/or echocardiography to assess the patient's hemodynamic status and guide intrapartum management. Acute cardiac decompensation during labor may require administration of IV nitroglycerin or nitroprusside for preload and afterload reduction and dopamine or dobutamine for inotropic support. Early initiation of epidural labor analgesia is essential to minimize the cardiac stress associated with the pain of labor. Invasive monitoring will guide fluid management, titration of vasoactive drugs, and induction of epidural analgesia.

If cesarean delivery is required, epidural or spinal anesthesia may be used. In these cases, fluid management should be guided by use of invasive monitors. If spinal anesthesia is selected, a continuous technique should be implemented because use of a single-shot technique, which produces rapid hemodynamic changes, may not be well tolerated. Continuous spinal anesthesia is most often elected when an unanticipated dural puncture occurs when placing an epidural needle. It may also be selected if there is concern about obtaining a good-quality anesthetic with epidural anesthesia. In that instance the total dose of spinal drug is unchanged but is slowly titrated to allow time to correct hemodynamic perturbations should they occur.

Diabetes Mellitus

Diabetes mellitus is one of the most common co-existing medical conditions in pregnancy, occurring in approximately 2% of parturient women. The incidence is increasing because of the epidemic of obesity and the greater number of women becoming pregnant at an advanced age. Ninety percent of diabetic pregnant patients have gestational diabetes, whereas the other 10% have preexisting diabetes. Pregnancy is a state of progressive insulin resistance, as discussed earlier in the chapter. Women who cannot produce enough insulin to compensate for this resistance develop gestational diabetes. Patients who had diabetes before pregnancy have increased insulin requirements during pregnancy. Patients with type 1 diabetes are at greater risk of diabetic ketoacidosis because pregnancy is associated with enhanced lipolysis and ketogenesis and diminished ability to buffer overproduced acids. This decreased buffering ability is secondary to the lower HCO_3 concentration that results from compensation for chronic respiratory alkalosis.

Glucose can freely cross the placenta and be metabolized by the fetus. For this reason the degree of hyperglycemia seen during diabetic ketoacidosis may be lower than levels observed in nonpregnant patients (130–150 mg/dL according to some reports). In such cases, insulin therapy should be directed to normalization ("closure") of the anion gap. Administration of β-adrenergic drugs and glucocorticoids may precipitate diabetic ketoacidosis.

Diagnosis

Gestational diabetes is diagnosed in the context of a 75-g oral glucose tolerance test following a fast of at least 8 hours if any of the following conditions are met: fasting glucose 92 mg/dL or above, 1-hour glucose 180 mg/dL or above, or 2-hour glucose 153 mg/dL or above. For evaluation of risk, patients are classified by the type and duration of diabetes and the presence of comorbid conditions (Table 31.12).

Treatment

Glycemic control is the major focus of the care of pregnant women with diabetes. A blood glucose level of 60–120 mg/dL is desirable, which requires frequent changes in insulin dosage during pregnancy. In patients with gestational diabetes, dietary control is used initially. If glycemic control cannot be achieved through diet, insulin therapy is initiated.

Prognosis

Patients with gestational diabetes are at increased risk of type 2 diabetes later in life. In addition, the incidence of preeclampsia is increased, as is the incidence of polyhydramnios.

TABLE 31.12	White Classification of Diabetes Mellitus During Pregnancy
Class	**Definition**
A_1	Diet-controlled gestational diabetes
A_2	Gestational diabetes requiring insulin
B	Preexisting diabetes, without complications (duration < 10 yr or onset at age > 20 yr)
C	Preexisting diabetes, without complications (duration 10–19 yr or onset at age 10–19 yr)
D	Preexisting diabetes (duration > 20 yr or onset at age < 10 yr)
F	Preexisting diabetes with nephropathy
R	Preexisting diabetes with retinopathy
T	Preexisting diabetes with prior renal transplantation
H	Preexisting diabetes with heart disease

Fetal effects of diabetes include a greater risk of anomalies in fetuses of women with preexisting diabetes mellitus. Intrauterine fetal death, including late-trimester stillbirth, occurs more frequently in diabetic mothers, probably secondary to poor uteroplacental blood flow. Macrosomia leads to a higher incidence of cesarean delivery, shoulder dystocia, and birth trauma. Neonates are at risk for hypoglycemia and may be at greater risk of respiratory distress.

Management of Anesthesia
Preoperative
Patients with pregestational diabetes should be assessed for diabetes-related complications. Appropriate evaluation for gastroparesis, autonomic dysfunction, and cardiac, vascular, and renal involvement should be made.

Intraoperative
Epidural labor analgesia decreases pain, which results in decreased maternal plasma catecholamine levels and thus improved uteroplacental blood flow. Patients with autonomic dysfunction are especially prone to hypotension with epidural analgesia, and hypervigilance and rapid treatment are indicated.

Diabetic parturient patients are at increased risk of requiring emergent cesarean delivery. Therefore epidural analgesia may be preferred to spinal-epidural analgesia in these patients. With a functioning epidural the need for general anesthesia can be minimized in the event a cesarean section is needed.

The choice of anesthetic for cesarean delivery, as in other parturient patients, depends on the status of the mother and fetus. As for all diabetic patients undergoing surgery, blood glucose level should be checked intraoperatively.

Myasthenia Gravis

Myasthenia gravis (MG) is a disorder characterized by skeletal muscle fatigability and weakness caused by destruction or blockade of postsynaptic nicotinic acetylcholine receptors (nAChRs) by various types of autoantibodies. Muscle weakness may involve eye, limb, axial, bulbar or respiratory muscles. Pregnancy is associated with exacerbation of MG in 40% of patients, remission in 30%, and no change in the remaining 30% of patients. Exacerbations of MG most frequently happen during the first trimester of pregnancy and the early postpartum period. It has little effect on the course of the first stage of labor; however, it can impair the second stage because skeletal muscles are heavily involved. An effectively working labor epidural placed early can provide excellent pain control, alleviate the stress of labor, and thus diminish fatigue and prevent such exacerbations. Vaginal delivery requiring the use of instrumentation is easier to perform in the presence of working neuraxial analgesia. A properly placed epidural catheter can also help avoid general anesthesia in the case of unplanned cesarean delivery.

It is recommended that muscle relaxation should be achieved through inhalational agents, because nondepolarizing muscle relaxants will have prolonged effect and their reversal may precipitate a cholinergic crisis. Similarly, larger doses of succinylcholine will be necessary. Medications that cause exacerbations of MG should be avoided (refer to the website https://pharmacy.uic.edu/departments/pharmacy-practice/centers-and-sections/drug-information-group/2014 for a list of offending medications). Preeclamptic patients may develop myasthenia crisis when receiving magnesium sulfate therapy.

Neonatal myasthenia gravis occurs transiently in 20%–30% of infants born to mothers with this disorder. Manifestations usually occur within 24 hours of birth and are characterized by generalized skeletal muscle weakness and expressionless facies. When breathing efforts are inadequate, tracheal intubation and mechanical ventilation of the infant's lungs should be initiated. Anticholinesterase therapy in neonates is usually necessary for approximately 21 days after birth.

Maternal Obesity

Obesity in the United States has become a national epidemic and is a major contributor to maternal morbidity. Nearly half of US women of childbearing age are overweight or obese. The pathophysiologic features associated with obesity result in a greater incidence of pregnancy-related complications for both mother and infant than for nonobese patients and has lifelong health implications for offspring.

Prognosis
The presence of obesity during pregnancy has significant consequences for both mother and fetus. Hypertensive disorders including chronic hypertension and preeclampsia are increased in these patients. Obese patients are more likely to develop gestational diabetes and are at increased risk of thromboembolic disease. Obese patients are more likely to have an abnormal labor, and failed induction is more likely to occur. These patients are also at greater risk of postpartum hemorrhage, regardless of the route of delivery. The overall cesarean delivery rate and emergency cesarean delivery rate are increased in obese patients. Factors that lead to these increased rates included preeclampsia and diabetes, as well as an increased incidence of fetal macrosomia. Soft tissue

dystocia may also be a contributing factor. Duration of surgery can be expected to be prolonged in these patients.

Obesity has been found to increase the risk of maternal death, related to the increased incidence of preeclampsia, diabetes, pulmonary embolism, and infection. Anesthesia-related maternal mortality is also increased in the obese parturient, with airway difficulties being a major cause.

Perinatal outcome is adversely affected by obesity. The increased incidence of fetal macrosomia leads to a greater risk of birth trauma and shoulder dystocia. Meconium aspiration occurs more frequently in infants of obese women, and these infants are at greater risk of neural tube defects and other congenital abnormalities. In addition, fetal exposure to hyperglycemia in utero may result in an increased risk of developing diabetes, hypertension, and premature coronary artery disease.

Management of Anesthesia
Preanesthetic
The high incidence of medical disease associated with obesity, as well as the difficulties encountered because of the patient's body habitus, present a significant challenge in the management of obese parturient patients. Preanesthetic evaluation and preparation should include a thorough airway examination and assessment of the patient's pulmonary and cardiac status. Arterial blood gas analysis to assess for carbon dioxide retention, electrocardiography, and echocardiography may be indicated. An appropriately sized blood pressure cuff designed to fit the patient's arm must be available for management.

Local Analgesia
Epidural analgesia is a reasonable choice for labor analgesia. It provides excellent pain relief, reduces oxygen consumption, and may attenuate the cardiac responses to labor and delivery. Because obese women have a higher likelihood of requiring cesarean delivery, and the risk of general anesthesia is substantial in this patient population, early epidural analgesia offers another advantage—the ability to extend the block for surgical anesthesia.

The technical challenge of performing epidural analgesia in the obese parturient may be alleviated by the use of ultrasound. Longer needles may be required to reach the epidural space and should be readily available in the labor and delivery unit. Placement of the patient in the sitting rather than the lateral position should facilitate successful identification of the epidural space.

The high failure rate of epidural analgesia among obese patients may be reduced by proper taping technique. After placing the catheter (but before taping), repositioning to the straightened-back lateral position allows the skin to move over the catheter without pulling it out of the epidural space. After this inward movement of the catheter occurs, the catheter can taped to the skin.

Continuous spinal analgesia is an option for labor analgesia and may provide advantages over epidural analgesia in morbidly obese patients. Correct placement of the catheter is confirmed by aspiration of cerebrospinal fluid, and thus initial failure rates will be lower than with epidural analgesia. A dislodged catheter will also be more readily identified than with epidural analgesia. Continuous spinal anesthesia is associated with small but significant risk of postdural puncture headache, which may require treatment in the postpartum period.

Cesarean Delivery
The incidence of cesarean delivery is higher in obese women than in nonobese women. The continuous neuraxial technique may be preferred owing to the ability to maintain anesthesia for what may be an extended period of surgery.

If general anesthesia is unavoidable, emergency airway equipment (including appropriately sized laryngeal mask airways [LMAs]) must be immediately available. If difficult intubation is anticipated, awake intubation (most often with fiberoptic scope but also via other videolaryngoscopic devices) should be elected.

Advanced Maternal Age

In 2002, approximately 14% of all births in the United States were to women 35 years or older. In Canada in 2002, 30% of all births were to women aged 30–34, and 14% were to women aged 35–39. In 2008, births to women older than 40 years made up 3% of births in the United States, triple the rate of 2 decades earlier. Patients and healthcare professionals believe that advanced maternal age results in poor outcomes. The rationale for this view is the higher incidence of chronic medical conditions in older patients. Indeed, advanced maternal age is independently associated with maternal morbidities such as gestational diabetes, preeclampsia, placental abruption, and cesarean delivery. In addition, older parturient women are more likely to weigh more than 70 kg and have preexisting hypertension or diabetes. Multiple gestations are more common in older pregnant women, as are miscarriage, preterm delivery, and fetal complications such as congenital anomalies, low birth weight, and intrauterine and neonatal death.

Cesarean delivery is performed more frequently in women of advanced maternal age. In some, the need for cesarean delivery is related to confounding problems. However, advanced maternal age is also independently associated with an increased likelihood of cesarean delivery, and rates of patient-requested cesarean delivery are much higher in women older than age 34 than in women aged 25 or younger.

Management of Anesthesia
As with obstetric management, anesthetic care of the parturient patient of advanced maternal age is related to the patient's comorbid conditions, the most frequent of which have been discussed in other sections of this chapter.

Substance Abuse

Diagnosis
Diagnosis of substance abuse is often by history. Many commonly abused substances are mind altering or affect the

cardiovascular system when the patient is in an acutely intoxicated state. Diagnosis of substance abuse in a patient who is not under the influence of a substance at admission may be made when that patient or her infant develops withdrawal symptoms, or the newborn is diagnosed with a syndrome related to in utero exposure.

Substances abused in pregnancy parallel those abused in society at large: alcohol, tobacco, opioids, and cocaine are frequently abused.

Alcohol Abuse
Signs and Symptoms
Approximately 4% of pregnant women are heavy alcohol users. Maternal signs and symptoms may include abnormal results on liver function tests, but often the diagnosis is not made until delivery, when fetal alcohol syndrome is diagnosed in the neonate. Fetal alcohol syndrome occurs in approximately one-third of infants born to mothers who drink more than 3 oz of alcohol per day during pregnancy. However, studies have reported neurobehavioral deficit, intrauterine growth restriction, and other congenital abnormalities in infants of moderate alcohol consumers. Current recommendations reflect the view that there is *no safe level* of alcohol consumption during pregnancy.

Management of Anesthesia
Management of anesthesia in pregnant patients who abuse alcohol entails the same considerations as anesthetic care of nonpregnant alcohol abusers.

Tobacco Abuse
Signs and Symptoms
Cigarettes are the most commonly abused drug during pregnancy. Because pregnant smokers are relatively young, often there are minimal signs and symptoms associated with tobacco abuse in this population. A strong association is found between cigarette smoking and low infant birth rate, placental abruption, and impaired respiratory function in newborns. In those who smoke more than 20 cigarettes per day, the incidence of premature delivery doubles. Sudden infant death syndrome occurs much more frequently in infants of mothers who smoke. Paradoxically, smoking has a protective effect against the development of preeclampsia.

Management of Anesthesia
As with alcohol abuse, anesthetic considerations for care of tobacco-using parturients are similar to those for care of nonpregnant patients who smoke.

Opioid Abuse
There are numerous medical complications of injected drug use. These include infectious complications such as human immunodeficiency virus infection and hepatitis. Patients may develop local abscesses or, more significantly, may have endocarditis or thrombophlebitis. A pregnant patient admitted while receiving long-term opioid therapy should be maintained on that therapy during her pregnancy and into the postpartum period. It is not recommended that these patients undergo detoxification during pregnancy. In fact, withdrawal from opioids during the third trimester can result in perinatal asphyxia or death of the neonate. Withdrawal of the neonate from opioids can present as respiratory distress, seizures, hyperthermia, and sudden infant death syndrome. Neonates should be observed and treated for withdrawal symptoms as necessary.

Management of Anesthesia
Labor and delivery analgesia and postpartum pain management in the opioid-dependent parturient presents a particular set of concerns. Many of these concerns also apply to chronic pain patients, who may be on chronic opioid therapy. Opioid agonist-antagonist drugs (nalbuphine, butorphanol, pentazocine, and others), and even tramadol should be avoided in patients receiving maintenance opioid therapy (except buprenorphine), because these substances may provoke acute withdrawal. For the same reason, buprenorphine should not be given to a parturient who takes methadone. Patients receiving maintenance opioid therapy have been shown to have higher opioid requirements following cesarean section. Fentanyl patient-controlled analgesia (PCA) may be a preferable option in management of postoperative pain in a parturient taking buprenorphine, because of the higher fentanyl affinity to μ receptors than buprenorphine. Ultrasound-guided transversus abdominis–plane (TAP) block may be beneficial for postcesarean pain control among opioid-dependent patients. There is a need for close monitoring of these patients for respiratory depression. During the postoperative period, moderate sedation was observed significantly more frequently (50% vs. 19%) among opioid-dependent patients than opioid naïve patients. At the same time, postoperative pain score was also higher in the opioid-dependent group.

Methadone and buprenorphine maintenance therapy prevents development of maternal withdrawal. The MOTHER (Maternal Opioid Treatment: Human Experimental Research) study prospectively compared safety and effectiveness of buprenorphine versus methadone maintenance therapy during pregnancy. It demonstrated some advantage of buprenorphine treatment for neonatal outcome (less severe neonatal abstinence syndrome, better neurobehavioral function) but more frequent self-discontinuation of therapy (33% vs. 18%) when compared to mothers treated with methadone. It is recommended that parturients receive satisfactory analgesia during the peripartum period, because inadequate pain control could promote drug-seeking behavior and potential addiction recurrence.

Cocaine Abuse
Signs and Symptoms
Cocaine abuse among parturient women affects multiple organs, including the cardiovascular, respiratory, neurologic, and hematologic systems. Cocaine is associated with maternal cardiovascular complications such as systemic

TABLE 31.13	Obstetric Complications Associated With Cocaine Abuse During Pregnancy

Spontaneous abortion
Preterm labor
Premature rupture of membranes
Placental abruption
Precipitous delivery
Intrauterine fetal demise
Maternal hypertension
Meconium aspiration
Low Apgar score at birth

hypertension, myocardial ischemia and infarction, cardiac dysrhythmias, and sudden death. Sudden increases in systemic blood pressure may be the primary cause of cerebral hemorrhage. Alternatively, cerebrovascular spasm can produce local ischemia and infarction. Subarachnoid hemorrhage, intracerebral bleeding, aneurysmal rupture, and seizures have been associated with cocaine use during pregnancy. Thrombocytopenia may occur following cocaine use and result in prolonged bleeding times. Maternal use of cocaine may lead to metabolic and endocrine changes in both the fetus and mother, which presumably reflects cocaine-induced release of catecholamines. Pulmonary complications (asthma, chronic cough, dyspnea, pulmonary edema) occur most often in parturient women who smoke freebase cocaine.

An increased incidence of significant obstetric complications is seen in parturient women who abuse cocaine during pregnancy (Table 31.13). The incidence of placental abruption, intrauterine fetal demise, and preterm labor is increased. High spontaneous abortion rates may be related to cocaine-induced vasoconstriction, enhanced uterine contraction, and abrupt changes in systemic blood pressure.

Diagnosis
Identification of parturient women abusing cocaine is difficult because urine checks detect metabolites of cocaine for only 14–60 hours after use. One of most important predictors of cocaine abuse is the absence of prenatal care.

Management of Anesthesia
Preoperative. Evaluation of parturient patients suspected of cocaine abuse includes electrocardiography and possibly echocardiography to check for the presence of valvular heart disease. In parturient patients who have severe cocaine-induced cardiovascular toxicity, hemodynamic stabilization must be established before induction of anesthesia.

Intraoperative. Cocaine-induced thrombocytopenia must be excluded if regional anesthesia is planned. Epidural anesthesia is instituted gradually, with attention to hydration and left uterine displacement to prevent hypotension. Ester-based local anesthetics, which undergo metabolism by plasma cholinesterase, may compete with cocaine, so metabolism may be decreased for both drugs. Body temperature increases, and

sympathomimetic effects associated with cocaine may mimic malignant hyperthermia.

FETAL ASSESSMENT AND NEONATAL PROBLEMS

Electronic Fetal Monitoring
Electronic fetal monitoring permits evaluation of fetal welfare by following changes in fetal heart rate as recorded using an external (Doppler) monitor or fetal scalp electrode. The basic principle of fetal monitoring is to correlate changes in fetal heart rate with fetal well-being and uterine contractions. In 2010, ACOG published a revised practice bulletin updating the nomenclature for intrapartum fetal monitoring. A three-tier interpretation system was established that combines the assessment of baseline rate, beat-to-beat variability, accelerations, and periodic decelerations.

Baseline Heart Rate
Normal fetal heart rate is 110–160 beats per minute (bpm).
Bradycardia is less than 110 bpm for longer than 10 minutes.
Tachycardia is more than 160 bpm for longer than 10 minutes.

Beat-to-Beat Variability
The fetal heart rate varies by 5–20 bpm in a manner that is irregular in amplitude and frequency. This normal heart rate variability is thought to reflect the integrity of neural pathways from the fetal cerebral cortex through the medulla, vagus nerve, and cardiac conduction system. Fetal well-being is confirmed when beat-to-beat variability is present. Conversely, fetal distress resulting from arterial hypoxemia, acidosis, or central nervous system damage is associated with minimal to absent beat-to-beat variability.

Drugs administered to parturient patients may blunt or eliminate fetal heart rate variability even in the absence of fetal distress. Drugs most frequently associated with loss of beat-to-beat variability are benzodiazepines, opioids, barbiturates, anticholinergics, and local anesthetics, as used for continuous lumbar epidural analgesia. These drug-induced effects do not appear to be deleterious but may cause difficulty in interpreting the results of fetal heart rate monitoring. In addition, lack of heart rate variability may be present normally in the premature fetus and during fetal sleep cycles.

Terms used to describe fetal heart rate variability are defined as follows:
absent: variability undetectable
minimal: 5 bpm or less
moderate: 6–25 bpm
marked: more than 25 bpm

Accelerations
An acceleration is a visually apparent abrupt increase in fetal heart rate. A prolonged acceleration lasts longer than 2 minutes but less than 10 minutes. If an acceleration lasts 10 minutes or longer, it is a change in baseline.

Decelerations

Early Decelerations

Early decelerations are characterized by a slowing of the fetal heart rate that *begins with the onset of uterine contractions.* Slowing is maximum at the peak of the contraction, with a return to near baseline at its termination. Decreases in heart rate are usually not more than 20 bpm or below an absolute rate of 100 bpm. This deceleration pattern is thought to be caused by vagal stimulation secondary to compression of the fetal head. Early decelerations are *not* prevented by increasing fetal oxygenation but are blunted by administration of atropine. Traditionally this fetal heart rate pattern is *not* associated with fetal distress.

Late Decelerations

Late decelerations are characterized by a slowing of fetal heart rate that *begins 10–30 seconds after the onset of uterine contractions.* Maximum slowing occurs after the peak intensity of the contraction. A *mild late deceleration* is defined as a decrease in heart rate of less than 20 bpm; *profound slowing* is present when the decrease is more than 40 bpm. Late decelerations may be associated with fetal distress and most likely reflect myocardial hypoxia secondary to uteroplacental insufficiency. Primary factors contributing to the appearance of late decelerations include maternal hypotension, uterine hyperactivity, and chronic uteroplacental insufficiency, such as may be seen with maternal diabetes mellitus or hypertension. When this pattern persists, there is a predictable correlation with development of fetal acidosis. Late decelerations can be corrected by *improving fetal oxygenation.* When beat-to-beat variability persists despite late deceleration, the fetus is still likely to be born vigorous.

Variable Decelerations

Variable decelerations are the most common pattern of fetal heart changes observed during the intrapartum period. As the term indicates, these decelerations are variable in magnitude, duration, and time of onset relative to uterine contractions. For example, this pattern may begin before, with, or after the onset of uterine contractions. Characteristically, deceleration patterns are abrupt in onset and cessation. The fetal heart rate almost invariably decreases to less than 100 bpm. Variable decelerations are thought to be caused by *umbilical cord compression.* Atropine diminishes the severity of variable decelerations, but administration of oxygen to the mother is *without* effect. If deceleration patterns are not severe and repetitive, there are usually only minimal alterations in the fetal acid-base status. Severe variable deceleration patterns that persist for 15–30 minutes are associated with fetal acidosis.

Prolonged Decelerations

A prolonged deceleration is a decrease in the fetal heart rate from baseline of more than 15 bpm that lasts longer than 2 minutes and less than 10 minutes. If the deceleration lasts longer than 10 minutes, it represents a baseline change.

TABLE 31.14	Three-Tiered System for Interpretation of Electronic Fetal Heart Rate (FHR) Monitoring
Category	Characteristics
Category I *(Must include all characteristics)*	**Rate:** 110–160 beats/min **Variability:** moderate **Late or variable decelerations:** absent **Early decelerations:** present or absent **Accelerations:** present or absent
Category II	*All FHR tracings not classified as category I or III*
Category III *(Includes either of the characteristics listed)*	**Absence of baseline FHR variability** and **any of the following:** • Recurrent late decelerations • Recurrent variable decelerations • Bradycardia **Sinusoidal pattern**

Sinusoidal Pattern

Sinusoidal heart rate variability is a visually smooth, undulating sine wave–like pattern with a cyclical frequency of 3–5 minutes persisting for 20 minutes or longer.

Three-Tiered Classification of Fetal Heart Rate Tracings

Table 31.14 presents a three-tiered system for categorizing the tracings obtained in fetal heart rate monitoring based on baseline rate, degree of variability, and pattern of decelerations and/or accelerations.

Category I tracings are normal. These tracings are strongly predictive of normal acid-base status. No specific action is required.

Category II tracings are indeterminate. Although they are not predictive of abnormal acid-base status, there is not enough evidence to classify them as normal or abnormal. Ancillary testing or intrauterine resuscitation may be indicated.

Category III tracings are abnormal and are associated with abnormal fetal acid-base status. Evaluation of the fetus and measures to resolve the abnormal pattern are required. If the tracing does not improve with intervention, delivery should be expedited.

Fetal Scalp Sampling

Fetal scalp sampling may be indicated to evaluate a fetus with an abnormal fetal heart rate pattern. Based on the results, suspected fetal hypoxia may be confirmed, which establishes a need for urgent delivery. Good neonatal outcomes are associated with a pH of 7.20 or greater, whereas a pH of 7.20 or lower suggests fetal compromise necessitating immediate delivery.

Fetal Pulse Oximetry

Fetal pulse oximetry is a newer technique evaluating intrapartum fetal oxygenation. It is currently employed as an adjunct to electronic fetal heart rate monitoring and may be used when heart rate monitoring produces a nonreassuring tracing. The fetal pulse oximeter provides continuous fetal arterial

TABLE 31.15	Determination of Apgar Score for Evaluating Neonates		
	Points		
Parameter	0	1	2
Heart rate (beats/min)	Absent	<100	>100
Respiratory effort	Absent	Slow Irregular	Crying
Reflex irritability	No response	Grimace	Crying
Muscle tone	Limp	Flexion of extremities	Active
Color	Pale Cyanotic	Body pink Extremities cyanotic	Pink

oxygen saturation readings when placed through the cervix to lie alongside the fetal cheek or temple. Normal fetal oxygen saturations range between 30% and 70%. Saturations less than 30% are suggestive of fetal acidemia.

Ultrasonography

Ultrasonographic examination of the fetus when the mother is in labor may be useful to determine the fetal presenting part. Also, if fetal heart tones are undetectable using Doppler scanning, ultrasonography may confirm intrauterine fetal health or demise. Ultrasonography may also be used to determine the quantity of amniotic fluid present in the uterus and to diagnose placental abruption and placenta previa.

Evaluation of the Neonate

Assessment of the infant immediately after birth is important so that neonates in distress who require active resuscitation can be identified promptly. As a guide to identifying and treating neonates with depressed function, the Apgar score has not been surpassed.

The Apgar score assigns a numerical value to five signs measured or observed in neonates 1 minute and 5 minutes after delivery (Table 31.15). Of the five factors, heart rate and quality of respiratory effort are the most important; color is the least informative in identifying neonates in distress. A heart rate of less than 100 bpm generally signifies arterial hypoxemia. Disappearance of cyanosis is often rapid when ventilation and circulation are normal. Nevertheless, many healthy neonates still have cyanosis at 1 minute owing to peripheral vasoconstriction in response to cold ambient temperatures in the delivery room. Acidosis and pulmonary vasoconstriction are the most likely causes of persistent cyanosis.

Apgar scores correlate well with acid-base measurements performed immediately after birth. When scores are higher than 7, neonates have either normal blood gas concentrations or mild respiratory acidosis. Infants with scores of 4–6 have moderately depressed function; those with scores of 3 or below have combined metabolic and respiratory acidosis. Infants with mild to moderately depressed function (Apgar scores of

3–7) frequently improve in response to oxygen administration by face mask, with or without positive pressure ventilation of the lungs. Tracheal intubation and external cardiac massage are indicated according to the Neonatal Resuscitation Program (NRP) algorithm. The NRP is a standardized training and certification program administered by the American Academy of Pediatrics (AAP).

Period Immediately After Birth

Major changes in the neonatal cardiovascular system and respiratory system occur immediately following delivery. For example, with clamping of the umbilical cord at birth, systemic vascular resistance increases, left atrial pressure increases, and flow through the foramen ovale ceases. Expansion of the lungs decreases pulmonary vascular resistance, and the entire right ventricular output is diverted to the lungs. In normal newborns the increase in Pao_2 to more than 60 mm Hg causes vasoconstriction and functional closure of the ductus arteriosus. When adequate oxygenation and ventilation are not established after delivery, a fetal circulatory pattern persists that is characterized by increased pulmonary vascular resistance and decreased pulmonary blood flow. Furthermore, the ductus arteriosus and foramen ovale remain open, which results in large right-to-left intracardiac shunts with associated arterial hypoxemia and acidosis.

A high index of suspicion must be maintained for serious abnormalities that can be present at birth or manifest shortly after delivery. These include meconium aspiration, choanal stenosis and atresia, diaphragmatic hernia, hypovolemia, hypoglycemia, tracheoesophageal fistula, and laryngeal anomalies.

Hypovolemia

Newborns with mean arterial pressures of less than 50 mm Hg at birth are likely to be hypovolemic. Poor capillary refill, tachycardia, and tachypnea will be present. Hypovolemia frequently follows intrauterine fetal distress, during which larger-than-normal proportions of fetal blood are shunted to the placenta and remain there after delivery and clamping of the umbilical cord. Umbilical cord compression is also frequently associated with hypovolemia.

Hypoglycemia

Hypoglycemia can manifest as hypotension, tremors, and seizures. Infants with intrauterine growth restriction and those born to diabetic mothers or after severe intrauterine fetal distress are vulnerable to hypoglycemia.

Meconium Aspiration

Meconium is the breakdown product of swallowed amniotic fluid, gastrointestinal cells, and secretions. It is seldom present before 34 weeks' gestation. After approximately 34 weeks, intrauterine arterial hypoxemia can result in increased gut motility and defecation. Gasping associated with arterial hypoxemia causes the fetus to inhale amniotic fluid and debris into the lungs. If delivery is delayed, meconium is broken down and excreted from the lungs. If birth occurs within 24 hours of aspiration, the meconium is still present in the major airways and is distributed to the lung periphery with the onset of spontaneous breathing. Obstruction of small airways causes ventilation/perfusion mismatching. The breathing rate may be more than 100 breaths per minute, and lung compliance decreases to levels seen in infants with respiratory distress syndrome. In severe cases, pulmonary hypertension and right-to-left shunting through the patent foramen ovale and ductus arteriosus (persistent fetal circulation) lead to severe arterial hypoxemia. Pneumothorax is also a common problem in the presence of meconium aspiration.

In the past, treatment of meconium aspiration consisted of placing a tracheal tube immediately after delivery and attempting to suction meconium from the newborn's airways. Currently a more conservative approach is recommended because routine tracheal intubation of all infants with meconium staining ($\approx$10% of all newborns) may cause unnecessary airway complications. In 2010, NRP guidelines were updated such that they do *not* recommend routine intrapartum oropharyngeal and nasopharyngeal suctioning for infants born with either clear or meconium-stained amniotic fluid. Endotracheal suctioning *is* indicated for nonvigorous meconium-stained newborns.

Choanal Stenosis and Atresia

Nasal obstruction should be suspected in neonates who have good breathing efforts but in whom air entry is absent. Cyanosis develops if these infants are forced to breathe with their mouths closed. Unilateral or bilateral choanal stenosis is diagnosed based on the inability to pass a small catheter through each naris. Such failure may reflect congenital (anatomic) obstruction or, more commonly, function atresia resulting from obstruction by blood, mucus, or meconium. The congenital form of choanal atresia must be treated surgically during the neonatal period. Use of an oral airway may be necessary until surgical correction can be accomplished. Functional choanal atresia is treated by nasal suctioning. Opioids often cause congestion of the nasal mucosa and obstruction. Such congestion can be treated with phenylephrine nose drops.

Diaphragmatic Hernia

Severe respiratory distress at birth in association with cyanosis and a scaphoid abdomen suggests a diaphragmatic hernia. Chest radiographs demonstrate abdominal contents in the thorax. Initial treatment in the delivery room includes tracheal intubation and ventilation of the lungs with oxygen. A pneumothorax on the side opposite the hernia is likely if attempts are made to expand the ipsilateral lung.

Tracheoesophageal Fistula

A tracheoesophageal fistula should be suspected when polyhydramnios is present. An initial diagnosis in the delivery room is suggested when a catheter inserted into the esophagus cannot be passed into the stomach. Copious amounts of oropharyngeal secretions are usually present. Chest radiographs taken with the catheter in place confirm the diagnosis.

Laryngeal Anomalies

Stridor is present at birth as a manifestation of laryngeal anomalies and subglottic stenosis. Insertion of a tube into the trachea beyond the obstruction alleviates the symptoms. *Vascular rings* are anomalies of the aorta that may compress the trachea, producing both inspiratory and expiratory obstruction. It may be difficult to advance a tracheal tube beyond the obstruction produced by vascular rings.

KEY POINTS

- Physiologic changes of pregnancy affect all organ systems. They influence maternal compensation for comorbid conditions and maternal response to anesthesia.
- There is less fetal drug exposure with regional anesthesia. Any well-managed anesthetic is safe.
- Blood pressure, oxygenation, and normocarbia should be maintained during delivery.
- Delivery is the definitive treatment for pregnancy-induced hypertension. Delivery should be delayed only if the risk of neonatal immaturity outweighs maternal risk.
- Co-existing medical diseases may result in maternal (and fetal) decompensation related to the physiologic changes of pregnancy.
- Fetal assessment permits evaluation of fetal well-being and guides neonatal management.

RESOURCES

American College of Obstetricians and Gynecologists. ACOG practice bulletin no. 116: management of intrapartum fetal heart rate tracings. *Obstet Gynecol.* 2010;116:1232.

American College of Obstetricians and Gynecologists. ACOG practice bulletin no. 115: vaginal birth after previous cesarean delivery. *Obstet Gynecol.* 2010;116(Pt 1):450.

American College of Obstetricians and Gynecologists. Postpartum hemorrhage. ACOG practice bulletin no. 76. *Obstet Gynecol.* 2006;108:1039-1047 (Reaffirmed 2011.)

American College of Obstetricians and Gynecologists. ACOG practice bulletin no. 474: nonobstetric surgery during pregnancy. *Obstet Gynecol.* 2011;117:420-421 (Reaffirmed 2015.)

American College of Obstetricians and Gynecologists. Hypertension in pregnancy. Report of the American College of Obstetricians and Gynecologists Task Force on Hypertension in Pregnancy. *Obstet Gynecol.* 2013;122:1122.

Brearton C, Bhalla A, Mallaiah S, Barclay P. The economic benefits of cell salvage in obstetric haemorrhage. *Int J Obstet Anesth.* 2012;21:329-333.

Cheek TG, Baird E. Anesthesia for nonobstetric surgery: maternal and fetal considerations. *Clin Obstet Gynecol.* 2009;52:535-545.

Cunningham FG, Bangdiwala S, Brown SS, et al. National Institutes of Health consensus development conference statement: vaginal birth after caesarean: new insights. *Obstet Gynecol.* 2010;115:1279-1290.

Drenthen W, Biersma E, Balci A, et al. Predictors of pregnancy complications in women with congenital heart disease. *Eur Heart J.* 2010;31:2124-2132.

Dzik WH, Blajchman MA, Fergusson D, et al. Clinical review: canadian National Advisory Committee on Blood and Blood Products—massive transfusion consensus conference 2011: report of the panel. *Crit Care.* 2011;15:242.

Hull AD, Resnick R. Placenta accreta and postpartum hemorrhage. *Clin Obstet Gynecol.* 2010;53:228-236.

Ko JY, Leffert LR. Clinical implications of neuraxial anesthesia in the parturient with scoliosis. *Anesth Analg.* 2009;109:1930-1934.

Lee SW, Khaw KS, Ngan Kee WD, et al. Haemodynamic effects from aortocaval compression at different angles of lateral tilt in non-labouring term pregnant women. *Br J Anaesth.* 2012;109:950-956.

Leffert LR, Schwamm LH. Neuraxial anesthesia in parturients with intracranial pathology: a comprehensive review and reassessment of risk. *Anesthesiology.* 2013;119:703-718.

Liumbruno GM, Meschini A, Liumbruno C, Rafanelli D. The introduction of intra-operative cell salvage in obstetric clinical practice: a review of the available evidence. *Eur J Obstet Gynecol Reprod Biol.* 2011;159:19-25.

Martin JA, Hamilton BE, Ventura SJ, et al. Births: final data for 2010. *Natl Vital Stat Rep.* 2012;61:1-72.

McDonnell NJ, Paech MJ, Clavisi OM, Scott KL, ANZCA Trials Group. Difficult and failed intubation in obstetric anaesthesia: an observational study of airway management and complications associated with general anaesthesia for caesarean section. *Int J Obstet Anesth.* 2008;17:292-297.

Ouyang DW, Khairy P, Fernandes SM, et al. Obstetric outcomes in pregnant women with congenital heart disease. *Int J Cardiol.* 2010;144:195-199.

Perlman JM, Wyllie J, Kattwinkel J, et al. Part 11: neonatal resuscitation: 2010 international consensus on cardiopulmonary resuscitation and emergency cardiovascular care science with treatment recommendations. *Circulation.* 2010;122:S516-S538.

Pereira L. Surgery in the obese pregnant patient. *Clin Obstet Gynecol.* 2009;52:546-556.

Ralph CJ, Sullivan I, Faulds J. Intraoperative cell salvaged blood as part of a blood conservation strategy in caesarean section: is fetal red cell contamination important? *Br J Anaesth.* 2011;107:404-408.

Siu SC, Sermer M, Colman JM, et al. Prospective multicenter study of pregnancy outcomes in women with heart disease. *Circulation.* 2001;104:515-521.

Index

Page numbers followed by "*b*" indicate boxes; "*f*" figures; "*t*" tables